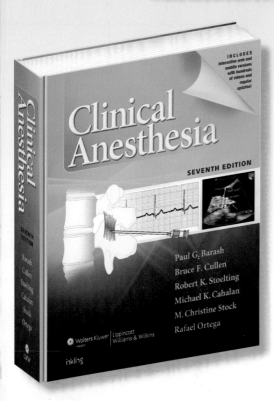
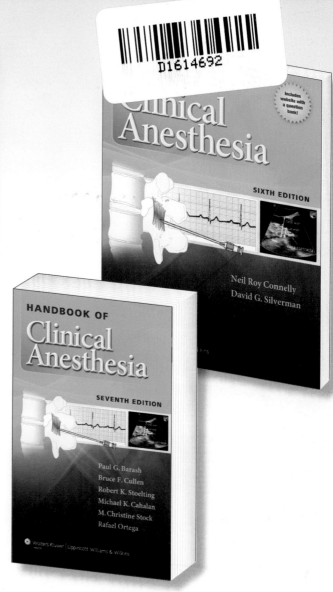
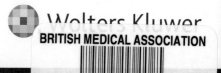

Clinical Anesthesia Fundamentals

Clinical Anesthesia Fundamentals

EDITED BY

Paul G. Barash, MD
Professor
Department of Anesthesiology
Yale University School of Medicine
Attending Anesthesiologist
Yale-New Haven Hospital
New Haven, Connecticut

Bruce F. Cullen, MD
Emeritus Professor
Department of Anesthesiology
University of Washington School of Medicine
Seattle, Washington

Robert K. Stoelting, MD
Emeritus Professor and Past Chair
Department of Anesthesia
Indiana University School of Medicine
Indianapolis, Indiana

Michael K. Cahalan, MD
Professor and Chair
Department of Anesthesiology
The University of Utah School of Medicine
Salt Lake City, Utah

M. Christine Stock, MD
Professor and Chair
Department of Anesthesiology
Northwestern University Feinberg School
of Medicine
Chicago, Illinois

Rafael Ortega, MD
Professor
Vice-Chairman of Academic Affairs
Department of Anesthesiology
Boston University School of Medicine
Boston, Massachusetts

Sam R. Sharar, MD
Professor
Department of Anesthesiology and Pain
Medicine
University of Washington School of Medicine
Seattle, Washington

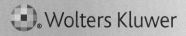

Philadelphia • Baltimore • New York • London
Buenos Aires • Hong Kong • Sydney • Tokyo

Acquisitions Editor: Brian Brown
Product Development Editor: Nicole Dernoski
Editorial Assistant: Lindsay Burgess
Production Project Manager: Priscilla Crater
Design Coordinator: Doug Smock
Illustration Coordinator: Jennifer Clements
Manufacturing Coordinator: Beth Welsh
Marketing Manager: Daniel Dressler
Prepress Vendor: Aptara, Inc.

9 8 7 6 5 4 3 2 1

Printed in China

Library of Congress Cataloging-in-Publication Data
Clinical Anesthesia Fundamentals / edited by Paul G. Barash, Bruce F. Cullen, Robert K. Stoelting, Michael K. Cahalan, M. Christine Stock, Rafael Ortega, Sam R. Sharar.
    p. ; cm.
    Includes bibliographical references and index.
    ISBN 978-1-4511-9437-1 (alk. paper)
    I. Barash, Paul G., editor.
    [DNLM: 1. Anesthesia. 2. Anesthesiology. 3. Anesthetics. WO 200]
    RD81
    617.9′6—dc23
                                                                                2014047607

LWW.com

For all students of anesthesiology

Contributors

Ron O. Abrons, MD
Assistant Professor
Department of Anesthesiology
The University of Iowa Carver College of Medicine
Director, Airway Management Training and
  Research
The University of Iowa Hospitals and Clinics
Iowa City, Iowa

Ashley N. Agerson, MD
Assistant Professor
Department of Anesthesiology
Northwestern University Feinberg School
  of Medicine
Attending Physician
Northwestern Memorial Hospital
Chicago, Illinois

Shireen Ahmad, MD
Professor and Associate Chair Faculty
  Development
Department of Anesthesiology
Northwestern University Feinberg School
  of Medicine
Chicago, Illinois

Shamsuddin Akhtar, MD
Associate Professor
Department of Anesthesiology
Yale University School of Medicine
New Haven, Connecticut

Aymen A. Alian, MD, MB, BCh
Associate Professor
Department of Anesthesia
Yale University School of Medicine
Associate Director of Ambulatory Surgery
Yale New Haven Hospital
New Haven, Connecticut

Abbas Al-Qamari, MD
Assistant Professor
Department of Anesthesiology
Northwestern University Feinberg School
  of Medicine
Chicago, Illinois

Yogen G. Asher, MD
Assistant Professor of Anesthesiology
Northwestern University Feinberg School
  of Medicine
Chicago, Illinois

Gina C. Badescu, MD
Bridgeport Anesthesia Associates
Bridgeport, Connecticut

Paul G. Barash, MD
Professor
Department of Anesthesiology
Yale University School of Medicine
Attending Anesthesiologist
Yale-New Haven Hospital
New Haven, Connecticut

John F. Bebawy, MD
Assistant Professor
Departments of Anesthesiology and Neurological
  Surgery
Northwestern University Feinberg School
  of Medicine
Chicago, Illinois

Honorio T. Benzon, MD
Professor
Department of Anesthesiology
Northwestern University Feinberg School
  of Medicine
Attending Anesthesiologist
Northwestern Memorial Hospital
Chicago, Illinois

Wendy K. Bernstein, MD, MBA
Associate Professor
Department of Anesthesiology
University of Maryland School
  of Medicine
Director, Simulation Program
University of Maryland Hospital
Baltimore, Maryland

Sanjay M. Bhananker, MD, FRCA
Associate Professor
Department of Anesthesiology and Pain
  Medicine
University of Washington School
  of Medicine
Harborview Medical Center
Seattle Children's Hospital
Seattle, Washington

Jessica Black, MD
Resident in Anesthesiology
Department of Anesthesiology
Boston University School of Medicine
Boston Medical Center
Boston, Massachusetts

Sorin J. Brull, MD, FCARCSI (Hon)
Professor
Department of Anesthesiology
Mayo Clinic College of Medicine
Jacksonville, Florida

Louanne M. Carabini, MD
Assistant Professor
Department of Anesthesiology
Northwestern University Feinberg School
  of Medicine
Attending Anesthesiologist
Northwestern Memorial Hospital
Chicago, Illinois

Niels Chapman, MD
Professor
Department of Anesthesiology
University of New Mexico School
  of Medicine
Albuquerque, New Mexico

Casper Claudius, MD, PhD
Staff Specialist
Department of Intensive Care
Copenhagen University Hospital
Copenhagen, Denmark

Christopher W. Connor, MD, PhD
Assistant Professor
Departments of Anesthesiology and Biomedical
  Engineering
Boston University School
  of Medicine
Director of Research
Boston Medical Center
Boston, Massachusetts

Armagan Dagal, MD, FRCA
Associate Professor
Department of Anesthesiology and Pain
  Medicine
University of Washington School of Medicine
Harborview Medical Center
Seattle, Washington

Alexander M. DeLeon, MD
Assistant Professor
Department of Anesthesiology
Northwestern University Feinberg School
  of Medicine
Associate Chair, Education
Northwestern Memorial Hospital
Chicago, Illinois

Talmage D. Egan, MD
Professor
Department of Anesthesiology
University of Utah School of Medicine
Salt Lake City, Utah

Ryan J. Fink, MD
Assistant Professor of Anesthesiology
Anesthesiology and Perioperative Medicine
Oregon Health and Science University
Portland, Oregon

Jorge A. Gálvez, MD
Associate Professor
Department of Anesthesiology and Critical Care
University of Pennsylvania Perelman School
  of Medicine
Pediatric Anesthesiologist
The Children's Hospital of Philadelphia
Philadelphia, Pennsylvania

Susan Garwood, MB, ChB
Associate Professor
Department of Anesthesiology
Yale University School of Medicine
Attending Physician
Yale New Haven Hospital
New Haven, Connecticut

R. Mauricio Gonzalez, MD
Clinical Assistant Professor
Department of Anesthesiology
Boston University School of Medicine
Vice Chair of Clinical Affairs, Quality and
  Patient Safety
Boston Medical Center
Boston, Massachusetts

Andreas Grabinsky, MD
Assistant Professor
Department of Anesthesiology and Pain
  Medicine
University of Washington School of Medicine
Harborview Medical Center
Seattle, Washington

Loreta Grecu, MD
Assistant Professor
Department of Anesthesiology
Yale University School of Medicine
Attending Anesthesiologist
Yale New Haven Hospital
New Haven, Connecticut

Dhanesh K. Gupta, MD
Associate Professor
Departments of Anesthesiology and Neurological
  Surgery
Northwestern University Feinberg School of
  Medicine
Director of Neuroanesthesia Research
Northwestern Memorial Hospital
Chicago, Illinois

Matthew R. Hallman, MD, MS
Assistant Professor
Department of Anesthesiology and Pain
  Medicine
University of Washington School of Medicine
Director, Critical Care Medicine Fellowship
Harborview Medical Center
Seattle, Washington

Elizabeth E. Hankinson, MD
Chief Resident
Department of Anesthesiology
University of Washington
Harborview Medical Center
Seattle, Washington

Christopher J. Hansen, DO
Resident in Anesthesiology
Department of Anesthesiology
Boston School of Medicine
Boston, Massachusetts

Thomas K. Henthorn, MD
Professor and Chair
Department of Anesthesiology
University of Colorado School of
  Medicine
University Hospital
Aurora, Colorado

Natalie F. Holt, MD, MPH
Assistant Professor
Department of Anesthesiology
Yale University School of Medicine
Medical Director
Ambulatory Procedures Unit
Veterans Affairs CT Healthcare System
West Haven, Connecticut

Robert S. Holzman, MD, MA (Hon.), FAAP
Professor
Department of Anesthesia
Harvard Medical School
Senior Associate in Perioperative Anesthesia
Boston Children's Hospital
Boston, Massachusetts

Yulia Ivashkov, MD
Assistant Professor
Department of Anesthesiology and Pain Medicine
University of Washington School of Medicine
Harborview Medical Center
Seattle, Washington

Aaron M. Joffe, DO
Associate Professor
Department of Anesthesiology and Pain Medicine
University of Washington School of Medicine
Harborview Medical Center
Seattle, Washington

Kyle E. Johnson, MD
Cardiothoracic Anesthesiologist
Department of Anesthesiology
Medical Anesthesia Consultants
McLeod Regional Medical Center
Florence, South Carolina

Antoun Koht, MD
Professor of Anesthesiology, Neurological Surgery,
  and Neurology
Department of Anesthesiology
Northwestern University Feinberg School
  of Medicine
Chicago, Illinois

Tom C. Krejcie, MD
Professor and Associate Chair of Medical
  Technology
Department of Anesthesiology
Northwestern University Feinberg School
  of Medicine
Associate Chief Medical Officer
Northwestern Memorial Hospital
Chicago, Illinois

Sundar Krishnan, MBBS
Clinical Assistant Professor
Divisions of Cardiothoracic Anesthesia
    and Critical Care
University of Iowa Carver College
    of Medicine
University of Iowa Hospitals and
    Clinics
Iowa City, Iowa

Kelly A. Linn, MD
Assistant Professor
Department of Anesthesiology
Medical College of Wisconsin
Staff Physician
Clement J. Zablocki Veterans Affairs Medical
    Center
Milwaukee, Wisconsin

Joseph Louca, MD
Assistant Professor of Anesthesiology
Department of Anesthesiology
Boston University School of Medicine
Boston, Massachusetts

Sofia Maldonado-Villalba, MD
Resident in Anesthesiology
Department of Anesthesiology
Boston University School of Medicine
Boston, Massachusetts

Jonathan B. Mark, MD
Professor
Department of Anesthesiology
Duke University Medical Center
Chief, Anesthesiology Service
Veterans Affairs Medical Center
Durham, North Carolina

Katherine Marseu, MD
Lecturer
Department of Anesthesia and Pain
    Medicine
University of Toronto
Staff Anesthesiologist
University Health Network-Toronto General
    Hospital
Toronto, Ontario, Canada

Roger S. Mecca, MD
Clinical Professor of Anesthesiology
Department of Anesthesiology and Perioperative
    Care
University of California at Irvine
Orange, California

Candice R. Montzingo, MD, FASE
Associate Professor
Department of Anesthesiology
University of Utah
Salt Lake City, Utah

Wissam Mustafa, MD
Resident in Anesthesiology
Department of Anesthesiology
Boston Medical Center
Boston University
Boston, Massachusetts

Naveen Nathan, MD
Assistant Professor
Department of Anesthesiology
Northwestern University Feinberg School
    of Medicine
Northwestern Memorial Hospital
Chicago, Illinois

R. Dean Nava, Jr., MD
Assistant Professor
Department of Anesthesiology
Northwestern University Feinberg School
    of Medicine
Chicago, Illinois

Isuta Nishio, MD
Assistant Professor
Department of Anesthesiology and Pain Medicine
University of Washington School of Medicine
Attending Anesthesiologist
VA Puget Sound Health Care System
Seattle, Washington

Mark C. Norris, MD
Director of Obstetric Anesthesia
Department of Anesthesiology
Boston Medical Center
Boston, Massachusetts

Adriana Dana Oprea, MD
Assistant Professor
Department of Anesthesiology
Yale University School of Medicine
Associate Director, Preadmission Testing Clinic
Yale New Haven Hospital
New Haven, Connecticut

Rafael Ortega, MD
Professor
Vice-Chairman of Academic Affairs
Department of Anesthesiology
Boston University School of Medicine
Boston, Massachusetts

Paul S. Pagel, MD, PhD
Staff Physician
Department of Anesthesiology
Clement J. Zablocki Veterans Affairs
   Medical Center
Milwaukee, Wisconsin

Melissa L. Pant, MD
Attending Anesthesiologist
Department of Anesthesiology
Northwestern Lake Forest Hospital
Lake Forest, Illinois

Ramesh Ramaiah, MD, FCARCSI, FRCA
Assistant Professor
Department of Anesthesiology and Pain Medicine
University of Washington School of Medicine
Attending Anesthesiologist
Harborview Medical Center
Seattle, Washington

Glenn Ramsey, MD
Professor
Department of Pathology
Northwestern University Feinberg School
   of Medicine
Medical Director, Blood Bank
Northwestern Memorial Hospital
Chicago, Illinois

Meghan E. Rodes, MD
Assistant Professor
Department of Anesthesiology
Northwestern University Feinberg School
   of Medicine
Attending Physician
Northwestern Memorial Hospital
Chicago, Illinois

Gerardo Rodriguez, MD
Assistant Professor
Department of Anesthesiology
Boston University School of Medicine
Director, East Newton Surgical Intensive Care Unit
Boston Medical Center
Boston, Massachusetts

William H. Rosenblatt, MD
Professor of Anesthesiology
Department of Anesthesiology
Yale University School of Medicine
Attending Physician
Yale New Haven Hospital
New Haven, Connecticut

Babak Sadighi, MD
Resident
Department of Anesthesiology
Boston University School
   of Medicine
Boston Medical Center
Boston, Massachusetts

Roya Saffary, MD
Resident
Department of Anesthesiology
Boston Medical Center
Boston, Massachusetts

Francis V. Salinas, MD
Clinical Assistant Professor
Department of Anesthesiology and Pain
   Medicine
University of Washington School
   of Medicine
Staff Anesthesiologist
Virginia Mason Medical Center
Seattle, Washington

Barbara M. Scavone, MD
Professor
Department of Anesthesia and Critical Care;
   Obstetrics and Gynecology
University of Chicago
Chief, Division of Obstetric Anesthesia
University of Chicago Medicine
Chicago, Illinois

Alan Jay Schwartz, MD, MSEd
Professor
Department of Anesthesiology and Critical Care
University of Pennsylvania Perelman School
   of Medicine
Director of Education
Children's Hospital of Philadelphia
Philadelphia, Pennsylvania

Sam R. Sharar, MD
Professor
Department of Anesthesiology and Pain
   Medicine
University of Washington School of Medicine
Harborview Medical Center
Seattle, Washington

Benjamin M. Sherman, MD
TeamHealth Anesthesia
Legacy Good Samaritan Hospital
Portland, Oregon

Sasha Shillcutt, MD, FASE
Associate Professor
Department of Anesthesiology
University of Nebraska Medical Center
Director of Perioperative Echocardiography
The Nebraska Medical Center
Omaha, Nebraska

Peter Slinger, MD, FRCPC
Professor
Department of Anesthesia
University of Toronto
Staff Anesthesiologist
Toronto General Hospital
Toronto, Ontario, Canada

Karen J. Souter, MB, BS, FRCA
Professor
Department of Anesthesiology and Pain Medicine
University of Washington School of Medicine
Vice Chair for Education
University of Washington Medical Center
Seattle, Washington

Paul A. Stricker, MD
Assistant Professor
Department of Anesthesiology and Critical Care
    Medicine
University of Pennsylvania Perelman School
    of Medicine
Attending Anesthesiologist
The Children's Hospital of Philadelphia
Philadelphia, Pennsylvania

James E. Szalados, MD, MBA, Esq., FCCP, FCCM, FCLM
Director, Surgical Critical Care and SICU
Director Critical Care Telemedicine Services
Rochester Regional Health System
Rochester General Hospital
Rochester, New York
Professor of Anesthesiology and Medicine
University of Rochester School of Medicine
Chief, Surgical Critical Care and Critical Care
    Telemedicine
Medical Director, Surgical and Neurocritical
    Care Units
Rochester General Hospital
Rochester, New York

Elizabeth M. Thackeray, MD, MPH
Associate Professor
Department of Anesthesiology
University of Utah School of Medicine
Salt Lake City, Utah

Joshua M. Tobin, MD
Director, Trauma Anesthesiology
Department of Anesthesiology
University of Southern California Keck School
    of Medicine
Los Angeles County Hospital
Los Angeles, California

Amy E. Vinson, MD, FAAP
Instructor in Anesthesia
Department of Anesthesiology, Perioperative, and
    Pain Medicine
Harvard Medical School
Assistant in Perioperative Anesthesia
Boston Children's Hospital
Boston, Massachusetts

Peter von Homeyer, MD, FASE
Assistant Professor
Department of Anesthesiology and Pain Medicine
University of Washington School of Medicine
Attending Physician
University of Washington Medical Center
Seattle, Washington

Mary E. Warner, MD
Department of Anesthesiology
Mayo Clinic
Rochester, Minnesota

James R. Zaidan, MD, MBA
Professor and Past Chair
Department of Anesthesiology
Emory University Hospital
Atlanta, Georgia

Preface

In the current era of health care reform, we are surrounded by changes in every aspect of clinical patient care, from incorporation of electronic health records to the emergence of novel health care delivery models. Concurrent with these new paradigms in health care delivery is an equally exciting evolution in medical education, as teachers at all levels—from basic science instructors to clinical care mentors—face three critical challenges: (1) exposing trainees to the rapidly expanding volumes of biomedical and biopsychosocial discovery, (2) translating such advances into cost-effective and patient-centered clinical applications, and (3) using novel teaching methods that target the cognitive needs and learning tools demanded by "digital native" learners of the millennial generation.

Clinical Anesthesia Fundamentals is our response to these challenges, specifically designed to fill the void in anesthesia and perioperative care education exemplified by the early trainee's question "Where can I go to most efficiently learn the fundamentals of anesthesia care?" *Clinical Anesthesia Fundamentals* is a complete, yet succinct introduction to the essential clinical principles and practices for early learners of anesthesia – students and residents. In contrast to *Clinical Anesthesia, 7th Edition* and other compendium textbooks of anesthesia that typically comprise 1,500 to 3,000 pages in print form and are comprehensive references for both the veteran practitioner and the seasoned trainee, *Clinical Anesthesia Fundamentals* is a fraction this size in its print form, and its liberal use of graphic and tabular presentations emphasize elemental concepts that facilitate trainees to thoughtfully apply their basic science knowledge to the clinical setting.

More importantly, *Clinical Anesthesia Fundamentals* capitalizes on novel and emerging digital teaching tools designed both to appeal to millennial learners and to reinforce content acquisition through complementary methods of content delivery. First, the book was designed from the "ground up" as a fully interactive digital resource that includes enhanced and innovative displays of text content, figures, and tables, over 130 videos and animated graphics, and quick links to Web-based reference citation sources. Second, content delivery and eventual mastery are reinforced by several novel tools including "Did You Know" statements of key clinical pearls, multiple-choice questions and explanatory answers in both written and video formats, and interactive video exercises that review key content. All electronic components of the book are viewable through any browser and as a download to one's smartphone or tablet, thus providing immediate and ubiquitous access for the reader.

The 44 concise chapters are organized into three sections targeting the early learner of anesthesia—an Introduction to the History and Future of Anesthesiology; the Scientific and Technical Foundations of Anesthesia (including relevant organ anatomy and physiology, pharmacology, and basic clinical technology); and the Clinical Practice of Anesthesia (including basic and specialty aspects of perioperative care both within and outside the operating room, pain management, critical care, and provider wellness).

Consistent with the unique purpose of the book, 57 of the 74 contributing authors are new to the *Clinical Anesthesia* series, including many whose specific academic interests in medical education bring new perspective and energy to the presentation of fundamental clinical content. The book concludes with a series of Appendices, carefully selected for their reference value and clinical relevance to early anesthesia trainees, including essential physiologic formulas/definitions, an electrocardiography atlas, pacemaker/defibrillator protocols, common herbal medications, and key standards/algorithms from the American Society of Anesthesiologists, American Heart Association, Anesthesia Patient Safety Foundation, and Malignant Hyperthermia Association of the United States.

In summary, *Clinical Anesthesia Fundamentals* provides early anesthesia learners with effortless print and digital access to essential anesthesia principles, procedures, and protocols in a succinct and user-friendly format that leverages complementary learning tools to reinforce content delivery. By avoiding the comprehensive (and potentially overwhelming) detail of compendium textbooks that is no doubt indispensable for advanced trainees and veteran practitioners, we hope that *Clinical Anesthesia Fundamentals* will provide early anesthesia learners with a solid foundation to begin their careers, and prepare them for both more advanced and lifelong learning in our specialty.

We wish to express our appreciation to all our knowledgeable and dedicated contributors who exceeded our challenge to present fundamental content in a novel, yet highly concise format. We also are indebted to the anesthesia trainees who provided invaluable advice and feedback on the scope and content of the book in its various development phases. Lastly, we would like to thank our editors at Wolters Kluwer, Brian Brown and Keith Donnellan, for their commitment to excellence. Finally, we owe a debt of gratitude to Nicole Dernoski, Product Development Editor at Wolters Kluwer; Chris Miller, Production Manager at Aptara; and Dan Dressler, Marketing Manager at Wolters Kluwer whose day-to-day management of this endeavor resulted in a publication that exceeded the Editors' expectations.

Paul G. Barash, MD
Bruce F. Cullen, MD
Robert K. Stoelting, MD
Michael K. Cahalan, MD
M. Christine Stock, MD
Rafael Ortega, MD
Sam R. Sharar, MD

Contents

SECTION III: Clinical Practice of Anesthesia

SECTION IV: Appendices

Contents

Introduction

1

History and Future

Rafael Ortega
Christopher J. Hansen

Most medical textbooks begin by discussing the history of the subject. Why? Succinctly stated, we only learn from the past. Although modern anesthesiology is practiced in today's future-driven environment, there is much to learn by analyzing the historical evolution of the specialty.

The field of anesthesiology is at a turning point that will define the future course of the profession. Today, anesthesiologists face new challenges, from expanding their roles in perioperative medicine and critical care to confronting professional competition and health care reform.

Understanding how and why anesthetics came into use, how they have evolved, and how the profession has grown is essential for a true understanding of the specialty and anticipating new forays into the future.

I. Pain and Antiquity

From early Mesopotamian and Egyptian cultures to Asian and Central American cultures, practices for the relief of pain have existed for centuries. For instance, the Greek physician Dioscorides reported on the analgesic properties of the mandrake plant, 2,000 years ago. With the advent of surgical medicine, various combinations of substances, including opium, alcohol, and marijuana, were inhaled by diverse cultures for their mind-altering and analgesic effects. The "soporific sponge," which was popular between the 9th and 13th centuries, became the primary mode of delivering pain relief to patients during surgical operations. The sponges were saturated with a solution derived from the combination of poppies, mandrake leaves, and various herbs. Before the surgical procedure, the sponge was moistened with hot water to reconstitute the ingredients and then placed over the mouth and nose so the patient could inhale the anesthetic vapors. *Laudanum*, an opium derivative prepared as a tincture, was produced in the 16th century by Paracelsus (1493–1541). Laudanum was used as an analgesic. However, like other medications of the time, it was also prescribed for a variety of diseases such as meningitis, cardiac disease, and tuberculosis. In Indian culture, avatars such as Dhanwantari used

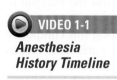

VIDEO 1-1

Anesthesia History Timeline

3

anesthetics for surgical pain and severed nerves for relief of neuralgia. Chinese physicians have used acupuncture and various herbal substances to ease surgical pain for centuries. In 1804, *Seishu Hanaoka* (1760–1835), a surgeon from Japan, induced general anesthesia with a herbal combination containing anticholinergic alkaloids capable of inducing unconsciousness. Hanaoka developed an enteral formulation called *Tsusensan*. His patients would ingest this concoction before Hanaoka would begin the surgical procedure (1).

II. Inhaled Anesthetics

A. Nitrous Oxide

Joseph Priestley (1733–1804), an English chemist and clergyman known for his isolation of oxygen in its gaseous form, was also the first to isolate *nitrous oxide*. Although he did not report on nitrous oxide's possible medical applications, it was his discovery and isolation of this and various other gases that would allow for modern methods of inhaled anesthesia. Sir Humphry Davy (1778–1829) described nitrous oxide's effect on breathing and the central nervous system. In 1800, he stated, "As nitrous oxide in its extensive operation appears capable of destroying physical pain, it may probably be used with advantage during surgical operations in which no great effusion of blood takes place." Despite his insight, Davy did not employ nitrous oxide as an anesthetic, and his lasting legacy to history was coining of the phrase *"laughing gas,"* which describes nitrous oxide's ability to trigger uncontrollable laughter.

Horace Wells (1815–1848) was the first individual to attempt a public demonstration of general anesthesia using nitrous oxide. Wells, a well-known dentist from Hartford, Connecticut, had used nitrous oxide for dental extractions. In 1845, he attempted to publicly perform the painless extraction of a tooth using nitrous oxide. However, possibly due to inadequate administration time, the patient was not fully insensible to pain and was said to have moved and groaned. Because of this, Wells was discredited and became deeply disappointed at his failed demonstration. Wells spent the better part of his remaining life in self-experimentation and unsuccessfully pursuing recognition for the discovery of inhaled anesthesia (2).

B. Diethyl Ether

Although the origin of diethyl ether's discovery is debated, it may first have been synthesized by eighth-century Arabian philosopher Jabir ibn Hayyan or 13th-century European alchemist Raymundus Lully.

By the 16th century, Paracelsus and others were preparing this compound and noting its effects on consciousness. Paracelsus documented that diethyl ether could produce drowsiness in chickens, causing them to become unresponsive and then wake up without any adverse effects. In the 17th and 18th centuries, ether was sold as a pain reliever, and numerous famous scientists of the time examined its properties. Because of its effects on consciousness, it also became a popular recreational drug in Britain and Ireland as well as in America, where festive group events with ether were called "ether frolics."

Although many were aware of the effects of inhaled ether, it was a physician from Georgia who first administered ether with the deliberate purpose of producing surgical anesthesia. *Crawford Williamson Long* (1815–1878) administered ether as a surgical anesthetic on March 30, 1842, to James M. Venable for the removal of a neck tumor. However, his results were not published until 1849, three years after William T. G. Morton's famous public demonstration.

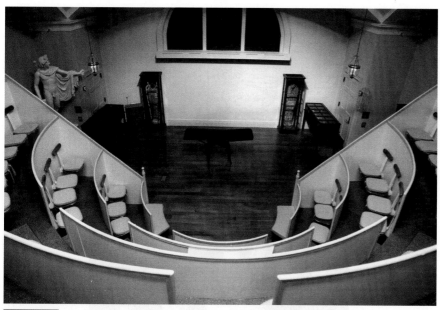

Figure 1-1 The surgical amphitheater at the Massachusetts General Hospital, today known as the Ether Dome, where Morton's demonstration took place on October 16, 1846.

This was not from a lack of insight, but rather a lack of desire for recognition. When he finally did publish his experiments with ether, he stated he did so at the bequest of his friends who felt he would be remiss not to state his involvement in the history of inhalation anesthesia.

On October 16, 1846, William T. G. Morton induced general anesthesia with ether, which allowed surgeon John Collins Warren (1778–1856) to remove a vascular tumor from Edward Gilbert Abbott (Fig. 1-1). The anesthetic was delivered through an inhaler consisting of a glass bulb containing an ether-soaked sponge and a spout at the other end through which the patient could breathe. The glass bulb was open to room air, allowing the patient to breathe in fresh air that mixed with the ether inside the bulb before passing through the spout and into the patient's lungs. The event occurred in a surgical amphitheater at the Massachusetts General Hospital, known today as the *Ether Dome*. News of the demonstration spread quickly, and, within a matter of months, the possibility of painless surgery was known around the world.

C. The Ether Controversy
In all, Morton completed three trials at the Massachusetts General Hospital before the hospital deemed it safe for use. Although today Morton is usually credited with this discovery, at the time, those involved were aware that Charles T. Jackson was the intellectual discoverer of this process and Morton was simply its executor. Charles Jackson, a notable Boston physician, chemist, and Morton's preceptor, stated that he counseled Morton on the use of inhaled ether for insensibility to pain (3).

Shortly after Morton's demonstration, Henry Jacob Bigelow (1818–1890), professor emeritus in the Department of Surgery at Harvard Medical School, described his famous account of the events that transpired at Massachusetts General Hospital, proclaiming that Morton and Jackson had discovered how to render patients insensible to pain. The article, published in the *Boston*

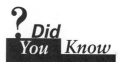

The ether controversy refers to the acrimonious arguments that ensued among the various individuals who believed they deserved the credit for having introduced inhalation anesthesia.

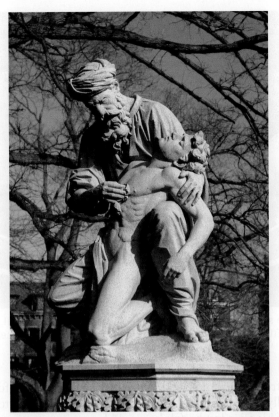

Figure 1-2 The sculpture atop the Ether Monument in the Public Garden in Boston symbolizing the relief of human suffering.

Medical and Surgical Journal (the predecessor to the *New England Journal of Medicine*), was widely distributed (4). The news reached Horace Wells, who contended that he had discovered inhaled anesthetics through his use of nitrous oxide. It was these assertions that would lead to what is now called the *"ether controversy."* The debate was made worse by what was most likely an attempt for monetary reward, with Morton's subsequent denial of Jackson's share in the discovery, leading to all three being pitted against one another (5).

The controversy would destroy both the reputations and lives of those involved, and to this day it lives on through various monuments throughout New England and other areas of the nation avowing credit to those depicted. It should be noted that, although not usually cited as being involved in the ether controversy, Crawford Long did publish his accounts of his use of ether. As such, there are various monuments asserting his place in the history of anesthesia (Fig. 1-2).

D. Spread of Ether

After Morton's famous demonstration, Henry Jacob Bigelow and his father Jacob Bigelow wrote letters to English physicians Francis Boott and Robert Liston, respectively. Boott, a general practitioner, and Liston, a surgeon, conducted Europe's first successful administration of surgical anesthesia with ether in December 1846, leading to Liston's famous words, "Well gentlemen, this Yankee Dodge sure beats *mesmerism* hollow." News traveled fast, and use of ether anesthesia swiftly found its way throughout the European continent.

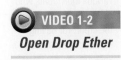

VIDEO 1-2

Open Drop Ether

E. Chloroform

Although *chloroform* had been discovered nearly two decades earlier, it was not used as a surgical anesthetic until a year after Morton's demonstration in 1847. James Young Simpson, a Scottish obstetrician, had learned of ether's effects after Liston's successful operation and had employed it with some of his patients. Although it did relieve some of the suffering associated with childbirth, Simpson was not satisfied and began to search for a better solution. Through the advice of a chemist, he became aware of chloroform and its anesthetizing effects. On November 4, 1847, he and two friends imbibed the contents of a bottle containing chloroform. Needless to say, they were satisfied by their self-experimentation and Simpson began using chloroform to relieve the pain of childbirth.

F. Critics of Anesthesia

The anesthetic use of chloroform and ether was not without its skeptics, and arguments against its use were made on moral, religious, and physiologic grounds. However, unlike ether, in Europe, chloroform use was more easily legitimized through the scientific logic of *John Snow*, who proclaimed its safety over ether and would eventually administer it to Queen Victoria during the birth of Prince Leopold. Perhaps because of the widespread use of chloroform and the effect a monarch can have on its citizens, the use and study of surgical anesthesia prospered in 19th-century Europe, while in the United States it remained comparatively stagnant.

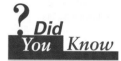

The scientific study of surgical anesthesia prospered in 19th-century Europe, while in the United States it remained comparatively stagnant for decades.

G. The Birth of Modern Surgical Anesthesia

London physician John Snow, best known for his epidemiologic work on cholera and the introduction of hygienic medicine, could also be called the first true anesthetist. As was his manner, he delved deeply into the study and understanding of volatile anesthetics. Unlike Morton, Wells, and Jackson, Snow was not worried about his role and potential legacy in medicine, but rather with the safe and proper administration of anesthesia. His calm and attentive attitude in the operating theater and focus on the patient's well-being, rather than his self-pride, is a model to be emulated.

H. Modern Inhaled Anesthetics

Perhaps Snow's intense study of the mechanism of action and possible side effects of inhaled anesthetics inspired the quest for an ideal inhalation anesthetic. Throughout the 20th century, various drugs such as ethyl chloride, ethylene, and cyclopropane were used for surgical anesthesia. But these were eventually abandoned due to a variety of drawbacks such as their pungent nature, weak potency, and flammability. The discovery that *fluorination* contributed to making anesthetics more stable, less toxic, and less combustible led to the introduction of halothane in the 1950s. The 1960s and 1970s would bring about various fluorinated anesthetics such as methoxyflurane and enflurane. These were eventually discontinued due to untoward side effects. Although initially more difficult to synthesize and purify, isoflurane, an isomer of enflurane, had fewer side effects than previous agents. It has been used since the late 1970s and is still a popular inhalation anesthetic today. There were no further advances in inhaled anesthetics until the introduction of desflurane in 1992 and sevoflurane in 1994. Both of these agents, along with isoflurane and nitrous oxide, are the most widely used inhaled agents used today.

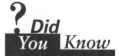

Inhaled anesthetics such as cyclopropane and ether were abandoned among other reasons due to their high flammability.

III. Intravenous Anesthetics and Regional Anesthesia

In 1853, Alexander Wood administered intravenous morphine for the relief of neuralgia through a hollow needle of his invention. This extraordinary accomplishment allowed for the administration of intravenous agents for both anesthesia and analgesia.

A. Intravenous Anesthesia

Phenobarbital was the first drug to be used as an intravenous induction agent. This barbiturate, synthesized in 1903 by Emil Fischer and Joseph von Mering, caused prolonged periods of unconsciousness followed by slow emergence and as such was not an ideal anesthetic. However, its success in producing anesthesia and the promotion and study of intravenous anesthetics by men such as John Lundy opened new possibilities in anesthesia. In 1934, Ralph Waters (1883–1979) from the University of Wisconsin and John Lundy (1894–1973) from the Mayo Clinic administered thiopental (a potent barbiturate) as a successful intravenous induction anesthetic agent. Lundy emphasized the approach, referred to as *"balanced anesthesia,"* that consisted of a combination of several anesthetic agents and strategies to produce unconsciousness, neuromuscular block, and analgesia. Through use of this approach, Lundy allowed for a safer and more complete administration of anesthesia. Thiopental's popularity led to the introduction of several other types of intravenous hypnotics including ketamine (1962), etomidate (1964), and propofol (1977). Since that time, other intravenous agents such as benzodiazepines and new opioids have been added to the specialty's armamentarium and further research continues.

B. Regional Anesthesia

Cocaine, originally described by Carl Koller in 1884 as a local anesthetic, became a mainstay for regional anesthesia through the early 1900s. During this time period, various nerve and plexus blocks were described, as was the technique of spinal anesthesia, all using cocaine as a local anesthetic. However, early cases of regional anesthesia were not without incident. Adverse effects, including postdural puncture headache, vomiting, and cocaine's addictive quality, necessitated the development of local anesthetics such as procaine in 1905 and lidocaine in 1943, which were much safer.

Throughout the 1940s, advances continued in the field of regional anesthesia with the advent of continuous spinal anesthesia by William T. Lemmon in 1940 and Edward Tuohy's eponymous needle in 1944. Tuohy's modification of the spinal needle allowed a catheter to pass into the epidural space and administer doses of local anesthetics. From that point to the present, subarachnoid and epidural administration methods of local anesthetics and opioids are commonly employed for analgesia during labor and delivery as well as for managing postoperative pain. Innovations such as ultrasound imaging and nerve stimulators are now used to facilitate locating and identifying nerves, thus improving the quality of the block.

IV. Neuromuscular Blocking Agents

Curare has been used for centuries by Amerindians of South America. Applied to arrows and darts, its paralyzing effects were originally employed for hunting and warfare. Through accounts from Spanish exploration of the area, news of curare and its effects reached Europe. Initially, medical applications for curare were limited; however, with the introduction of endotracheal intubation and mechanical ventilation, curare could be used to prevent laryngospasm during laryngoscopy and relax abdominal muscles during surgical procedures. In 1942, Griffith and Johnson introduced the first drug form of curare called Intocostrin. Intocostrin facilitated both tracheal intubation and abdominal muscle relaxation, allowing for a more optimized surgical patient. Although other muscle relaxants were studied, they were subsequently discarded due to undesirable autonomic nervous system effects. The next great step in neuromuscular blocking agents came in 1949 with the synthesis of the depolarizing neuromuscular blocking agent *succinylcholine* by Nobel Laureate Daniel Bovet (1907–1992). Nondepolarizing neuromuscular-blocking agents such as vecuronium and rocuronium, as well as atracurium and cis-atracurium, were introduced into clinical practice in the late 20th century.

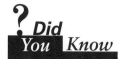

? Did You Know

The first drug form of curare was first introduced in 1942, marking the beginning of the use of neuromuscular blocking agents during surgical procedures.

V. Anesthesiology as a Medical Specialty

Anesthesiology as a medical specialty developed gradually in the United States during the 20th century. For decades after Morton's demonstration, there was no formal instruction in anesthesia. In the first part of the 20th century, Ralph Waters advocated for dedicated anesthesia departments and training programs. Later, anesthesiologists such as Thomas D. Buchanan and John Lundy established formal anesthesia departments in the New York Medical College and the Mayo Clinic, respectively, and Waters at the University of Wisconsin–Madison established the first anesthesiology postgraduate training program in 1927.

VI. Modern Anesthesiology Practice

Although advances such as Sir Robert Macintosh's and Sir Ivan Magill's contributions to airway management were made in the early 1900s, anesthesiology further evolved in the second half of the 20th century with a strong emphasis on safety. In 1985, the *Anesthesia Patient Safety Foundation* was established with a mission "to ensure that no patient is harmed by anesthesia." Additional monitoring tools such as pulse oximetry and capnometry notably decreased mortality rates during anesthetic procedures. Furthermore, the refinements in anesthesia delivery systems have been remarkable.

Presently, the *American Society of Anesthesiologists* provides the *guidelines* for anesthesiology. The stated goals of this professional organization are to establish "an educational, research and scientific association of physicians organized to raise and maintain the standards of anesthesiology and to improve the care of patients."

The history of nurses administering anesthesia in the United States is intertwined with the rapid development of the country after the 1840s and the relative scarcity of physicians. It is known that nurses provided anesthesia as early as the Civil War, but it was not until 1956 that the term *certified registered nurse anesthetist (CRNA)* was introduced. In 2013, the Emery Rovenstine Memorial Lecture, considered by many the main event during the American Society of Anesthesiologists' annual meeting, addressed the competition between anesthesiologists and nurse anesthetists to provide anesthesia care. The American Society of Anesthesiologists supports a physician-led model for anesthesia care known as the *anesthesia care team*. On the other hand, the *American Association of Nurse Anesthetists*, the organization representing nurse anesthetists, promotes independent practice and is aggressively lobbying in legislative and regulatory arenas to achieve their goal. In 2001, Medicare allowed states to opt out of a regulation that required CRNAs to administer anesthetics under the supervision of a physician, and today there are more than a dozen states allowing CRNAs to practice independently. The controversy over who can administer anesthesia independently, which may have financial and quality of care implications, continues to be debated.

The current economic environment will test anesthesiology as a service to patients and as an area of specialization for physicians. The diversity in the composition of the anesthesia care team varies across the country and will continue to change as economic pressures evolve. Although some may view the current challenges as a menace for this medical specialty, many find opportunities for improvement.

Three different approaches to the delivery of anesthesia care in the United States are currently used. Most anesthetics are delivered by a team typically comprising an anesthesiologist and a CRNA and an anesthesiologist assistant or a resident. However, there are anesthesiologists delivering anesthesia care themselves in a "physician-only" model, and in some areas of the country, there are CRNAs working alone. In recent years, individual practices have merged into large groups, and anesthesia practice management has become more demanding and complex.

Today anesthesiologists act as perioperative physicians capable of coordinating pre-, intra-, and postoperative care. Students interested in pursuing a career in anesthesiology must be passionate about the specialty, excel academically, and have a unique predisposition blending a calm and poised attitude with the ability to make swift decisions and take immediate action. Considering the aging population and the ever increasing need for health care, including surgical procedures, anesthesiology as a profession has a bright future.

References

1. Ortega RA, Mai C. History of anesthesia. In: Vacanti CA, Sikka PK, Urman RD, et al., eds. *Essential Clinical Anesthesia.* Cambridge: Cambridge University Press; 2011:1–6.
2. Haridas RP. Horace Wells' demonstration of nitrous oxide in Boston. *Anesthesiology.* 2013;119(5):1014–1022.
3. Zeitlin GL. Charles Thomas Jackson, "The Head Behind the Hands." Applying science to implement discovery in early nineteenth century America. *Anesthesiology.* 2009;110(3):687–688.
4. Bigelow HJ. Insensibility during surgical operations produced by inhalation. *Boston Med Surg J.* 1846;16:309–317.
5. Ortega RA, Lewis KP, Hansen CJ. Other monuments to inhalation anesthesia. *Anesthesiology.* 2008;109(4):578–587.

Questions

1. The first successful public demonstration of the use of ether anesthesia during a surgical procedure is generally credited to whom?
   A. Joseph Priestley
   B. William Morton
   C. Charles Jackson
   D. Henry Bigelow

2. Advantages of fluorinating anesthetic agents include all of the following EXCEPT:
   A. Greater potency
   B. Greater stability
   C. Greater toxicity
   D. Less combustibility

3. Which of the following neuromuscular blocking agents (NMBA) was first used in clinical practice?
   A. Vecuronium
   B. Succinylcholine
   C. Pancuronium
   D. Curare

4. The term balanced anesthesia was introduced to refer to:
   A. A combination of anesthetic agents to produce unconsciousness, neuromuscular block, and analgesia
   B. The combined use of spinal anesthesia and sedation
   C. General anesthesia with a barbiturate and morphine
   D. Total intravenous anesthesia

5. The correct historical order of introduction of the following local anesthetics is:
   A. Lidocaine, procaine, bupivacaine
   B. Procaine, cocaine, lidocaine
   C. Cocaine, procaine, lidocaine
   D. Cocaine, bupivacaine, procaine

Scientific and Technical Foundations of Anesthesia

PART A

Core Organ Functions: Anatomy & Physiology

2 The Respiratory System

Abbas Al-Qamari
R. Dean Nava, Jr.

I. Introduction

It is of paramount importance for any anesthesia provider to understand the basic concepts of the respiratory system and the mechanics of ventilation and gas exchange. The principles described in this chapter are put to use every day in operating rooms and intensive care units around the world. Understanding these principles can help guide clinical decision making as well as having informed discussions with other consulting services in the perioperative care of patients.

II. Muscles of Ventilation

A. Diaphragm

The diaphragm is the main muscle of ventilation, and, during nonstrenuous breathing, it does the vast majority of the work. A mobile central tendon that originates from the vertebral bodies, lower ribs, and sternum anchors it. As the diaphragm contracts, negative pressure is generated in the intrapleural space, causing inflow of air into the lungs. As the diaphragm relaxes, the volume within the thoracic cavity decreases and air moves out. During nonstrenuous breathing, exhalation is mainly passive. Approximately 50% of the diaphragm's musculature is composed of fatigue-resistant, slow twitch muscle fibers (1,2).

B. Accessory Muscles

As the work of breathing increases, more skeletal muscles become involved. The external intercostal muscles assist in inhalation, and to some degree the internal intercostal muscles provide support for exhalation. The abdominal muscles (the most important expiratory accessory muscles) contract, assisting with depressing the ribs and producing forced exhalation through an increase in intra-abdominal pressure. They are also important for generating the propulsive expiratory force involved with coughing and maintaining adequate bronchial hygiene. The cervical strap muscles (the most important inspiratory

? *Did* *You Know*

During nonstrenuous breathing, the diaphragm does the vast majority of work and that exhalation is mainly passive.

15

accessory muscles) help to elevate the sternum and upper chest to increase thoracic cavity dimensions. The scalenes help prevent inward motion of the ribs and the sternocleidomastoids help to elevate the upper part of the rib cage. As the work of breathing continues to increase, the large back and paravertebral muscles become involved. All of these muscles are prone to fatigue (1,2).

III. Structures of the Lung

A. Thoracic Cavity and Pleura

The lungs are contained within the bony thoracic cage, consisting of the 12 thoracic vertebrae, 12 pairs of ribs, and the sternum. The intercostal muscles lie between each pair of ribs. The diaphragm makes up the inferior border of the thoracic cavity. The mediastinum separates the lungs medially.

Each lung weighs approximately 300 to 450 g. The right lung is slightly larger than the left and has three lobes as opposed to the left's two. *Fissures* separate the lobes. Each lung is composed of 10 segments, the anatomic divisions of which correspond to the branching of the proximal conducting airways. The lung parenchyma is invested by a layer of visceral pleura. The visceral pleura also covers the surfaces of the interlobar fissures. As this visceral layer is reflected back upon itself at the level of the hilum and pulmonary ligament, it becomes the parietal pleura. This pleura covers the entirety of the thoracic cage and diaphragm. A fluid layer 20 µm thick separates the two layers. This fluid layer allows for the smooth movement of the lung against the thoracic cavity as the respiratory cycle occurs (1–3).

B. Airways

Immediately distal to the larynx begins the trachea. A series of C-shaped cartilaginous rings support this large airway anteriorly and laterally. The posterior, or membranous, portion of the trachea lacks this rigid support structure, thereby allowing flexibility for food boluses that traverse the esophagus posteriorly.

At the distal end of the trachea lies the carina—the first branch point in the respiratory tree, beyond which lay the left and right main-stem bronchi. The right main bronchus has a significantly less acute angle of branching. This "straight shot" allows for a less circuitous path for aspirated material and is the primary reason aspiration events occur more often in the right lung.

The right lung then divides into the right upper lobe bronchus and bronchus intermedius. The bronchus intermedius divides almost immediately into the right middle and right lower lobe bronchi. The left main bronchus divides into the left upper and left lower lobe bronchi. It is at this lobar level that the cartilage rings evident proximally are replaced by plate-like islands of cartilage within the wall of the airway.

Collateral Ventilation

Each lobar branch then further divides into segmental branches. The airways continue to divide for another 5 to 25 generations depending on their position within the lung. As branching progresses, the amount of cartilage contained within the wall continues to decrease. The point at which cartilage is totally absent from the airway wall is termed the **terminal bronchiole** and is the final conducting airway before reaching the functional unit of the lung known as the *acinus.*

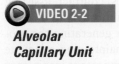

Alveolar Capillary Unit

Each acinus comprises respiratory bronchioles, alveolar ducts, alveolar sacs, and grape-like clusters of alveoli. The alveolus serves as the main point of gas exchange between lung parenchyma and the pulmonary vasculature. Approximately 300 million alveoli are present in an average adult male. In the upright position, the largest alveoli are found at the apex of the lung and the smallest at the bases. This size difference becomes less pronounced as inspiration occurs. Each alveolus is comprised mainly of type I cells, which form the majority of the epithelial surface of the alveolus, and type II cells, which produce surfactant and function as reserve precursor cells for type I cells (1–3).

C. Vasculature

Within the pulmonary system, there exist two types of vascular supply. The first is the bronchial circulation, which arises from the aorta and the intercostal arteries and is oxygenated systemic blood that provides nutrition to the tissues of the bronchi, visceral pleura, and pulmonary vasculature. It is not involved with alveolar gas exchange.

The second vascular system is the pulmonary circulation. This vascular supply takes deoxygenated systemic blood and sends it to the pulmonary capillaries for interface with the alveoli. It is here that alveolar gas exchange occurs—oxygen is absorbed and carbon dioxide is excreted. The newly oxygenated blood is then sent back into the systemic circulation for distribution to the rest of the body.

The pulmonary arterial trunk arises directly from the right ventricle. It very quickly bifurcates into the left and right main pulmonary arteries. These pulmonary arteries further divide into separate lobar arteries. It is at this level that the vessels enter the hilum of their respective lungs.

After entering the lung, the pulmonary vasculature divides along with its corresponding airway. They subdivide into arterioles, and then finally into capillaries at the level of the alveolus. As one moves past the alveolus, the vessels become venules. These eventually coalesce into lobular veins, then further on to the four pulmonary veins, two each from left and right lung. These pulmonary veins drain into the left atrium, where the oxygenated blood is then circulated systemically until it returns to the right atrium and ventricle for recirculation through the pulmonary system. It should be noted that blood in the pulmonary arteries is typically deoxygenated and the pulmonary venous blood is oxygenated. This is opposite of the systemic circulation; the nomenclature is based on which vessels arise from and return to the heart (1,2).

IV. Breathing and Lung Mechanics

The generation of a breath, which allows the inflow of atmospheric air into the lungs and outflow of carbon dioxide–rich air from the alveoli, is a function of periodic changes in partial pressure gradients. The way these pressure gradients are achieved depends on whether the breath is spontaneously or mechanically generated.

A. Spontaneous Ventilation

Except in the case of alveolar collapse, the pressure within the alveoli is greater than the intrathoracic pressure surrounding the lung parenchyma. This alveolar pressure is generally atmospheric at end expiration and end inspiration. Intrapleural pressure, which is used as a surrogate for intrathoracic pressure by convention, is approximately −5 cm water (H_2O) at end expiration. Using zero as a reference for atmospheric pressure during a no-flow state at end expiration, the end-expiratory transpulmonary pressure can be calculated:

$$P_{transpulmonary} = P_{alveolar} - P_{intrapleural}$$
$$P_{transpulmonary} = 0 \text{ cm } H_2O - (-5 \text{ cm } H_2O)$$
$$P_{transpulmonary} = 5 \text{ cm } H_2O$$

When the diaphragm and intercostal muscles contract and inspiration occurs, the intrathoracic volume increases and a new intrapleural pressure is generated, approximately −8 to −9 cm H_2O. Alveolar pressure also decreases to −3 to −4 cm H_2O, maintaining the transpulmonary pressure at 5 cm H_2O, but generating a pressure gradient between the alveoli and upper airway. This change allows for air to flow down the gradient into the alveoli and participate in gas exchange and also expands the alveoli.

When the diaphragm and intercostals relax, the intrapleural pressure returns to −5 cm H_2O. Transpulmonary pressure does not support the expanded alveoli at these intrathoracic volumes, and they begin to collapse. The air flows from the alveoli out toward the upper airway and the previous end-expiratory pressures and alveolar size are reestablished.

B. Mechanical Ventilation

Most mechanical ventilation modes involve the application of positive pressure with each breath. As positive pressure is delivered, the alveoli expand, and gas flows to the alveoli until alveolar pressure equals that in the upper airway. When the positive pressure breath is stopped, expiration occurs passively until another positive pressure breath is delivered (2,3) (see Chapter 41).

C. Movement of the Lung Parenchyma

The movement of the lung tissue itself is passive and depends on overcoming two types of resistance: (a) elastic resistance of the lung parenchyma, chest wall, and gas–liquid interface in the alveoli and (b) nonelastic resistance of the airways to gas flow. The work necessary to overcome these two resistances is the physiologic work of breathing.

D. Elastic Resistance

Both the lung parenchyma and thoracic cavity have their own elastic recoil properties. The tendency of the lungs is to collapse due to the high number of elastin fibers within the tissue as well as the surface tension at the air–fluid interface of the alveoli. The tendency of the chest wall is to move outward due to its structural makeup that resists deformation and the muscle tone of the chest wall.

E. Surface Tension

Fluid lines each alveolus. Thus, the air that enters the alveolus first makes contact with this fluid layer. This gas–fluid interface is much the same as a bubble and as such behaves much like one. Like a bubble, the surface tension of the gas–fluid interface favors collapse of the alveolus. In order for a bubble to remain inflated, the gas pressure within the bubble contained by a surface tension must be greater than the gas pressure on the outside of the bubble. Laplace's law helps to quantify the pressure within the alveolus with a given surface tension:

$$Pressure = \frac{2 \times Surface\ tension}{Radius}$$

As demonstrated by the equation, the higher the surface tension, the greater the propensity of the alveolus to collapse. To overcome this tendency to collapse, the lung produces surfactant at the gas–fluid interface. Surfactant reduces surface tension, allowing the alveolus to more readily stay expanded.

The higher the concentration of surfactant in an alveolus, the more the surface tension is reduced. Conversely, as the concentration decreases, the effect on surface tension decreases. This relationship helps to stabilize the alveoli. As the alveolus decreases in size, the concentration of surfactant increases, helping to prevent collapse. As the alveolus begins to overdistend, the surfactant concentration decreases and alveolar shrinkage is favored (2,3).

F. Compliance

A useful measure of elastic recoil is **compliance.** It is defined as a change in volume divided by the change in pressure:

$$C = \Delta V/\Delta P$$

The higher the pressure needed to produce a specific change in volume, the lower the compliance of the system and the higher is the elastic recoil of that same system.

Compliance can be calculated both for the lung and the chest wall separately. Normal lung compliance is 150 to 200 mL/cm H_2O and is defined as:

$$C_{Lung} = \frac{\text{Change in lung volume}}{\text{Change in transpulmonary pressure}}$$

Chest wall compliance is normally 100 mL/cm H_2O and is defined as:

$$C_{Chest\ wall} = \frac{\text{Change in chest volume}}{\text{Change in transthoracic pressure}}$$

where transthoracic pressure equals atmospheric pressure minus intrapleural pressure.

Total compliance is the combination of chest wall and lung compliances and is normally 100 mL/cm H_2O. It is defined mathematically as:

$$1/C_T = (1/C_{Lung}) + (1/C_{Chest\ wall})$$

$$C_T = \text{total compliance}$$

Compliance can be affected by the presence of secretions, inflammation, fibrosis, fluid overload, and a host of other factors. It is a useful measure, especially in the setting of mechanical ventilation, to demonstrate worsening or improvement of lung mechanics (2,3).

V. Resistance to Gas Flow

There are two types of gas flow: laminar and turbulent. Both of these are present simultaneously during a respiratory cycle, although the physics of both are very different.

A. Laminar Flow

At flow rates below those that produce turbulent flow, gas flows through a straight, unbranched tube in a series of concentric cylinders that slide over one another. The velocity of the gas in the cylinder abutting the tube walls is zero, and the maximal flow velocity is in the innermost cylinder. Thus, gas that flows through the center of the tube reaches the end of the conduit before

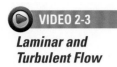

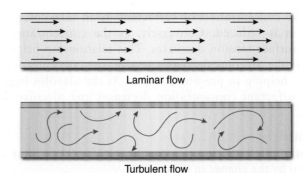

Laminar flow

Turbulent flow

Figure 2-1   Graphic representation of laminar and turbulent flow.

the rest of the tube has filled with gas. This type of flow is usually inaudible. Resistance to laminar flow is described by the following equation:

$$R = \frac{8 \times \text{length} \times \text{viscosity}}{\pi \times (\text{radius})^4 \, \text{flow}} = P_B - P_A$$

where P_B equals barometric pressure and P_A equals alveolar pressure.

Notice that airway radius influences resistance by a power of four. Note also that gas density has no effect on the resistance to laminar flow; only viscosity influences resistance. Less-dense gases such as helium (which has a similar viscosity to air) will not improve gas flow in the setting of laminar flow.

B. Turbulent Flow

Flow through branched or disordered tubes often produces a disruption of laminar flow, which produces random movement of gas through a tube, known as *turbulent flow*. Especially at high flow rates, turbulent flow can occur even in an unbranched, straight tube. In contrast to the parabolic shape of the advancing laminar flow cone, the front of the advancing turbulent flow stream is square. Hence, the flowing gas almost completely fills the tube before advancing to the end of the conduit. The mathematical computation of turbulent flow is complex and beyond the scope of this chapter, although there are some basic concepts that should be mentioned. The resistance during turbulent flow is generally proportional to the flow rate of the gas. During laminar flow, resistance is inversely proportional to the flow rate, at least until a critical flow rate is reached that changes the flow from laminar to turbulent. Although laminar flow is sensitive to changes in radius, turbulent flow is even more exquisitely sensitive; changes in radius result in a change in resistance to a power of five of the change in radius. Finally, resistance to turbulent flow is directly proportional to gas density rather than viscosity. As gas density decreases, resistance decreases as well. It is in cases of turbulent flow and increased airway resistance that less dense gases such as helium are useful (2,3) (Fig. 2-1).

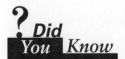

? Did You Know

Helium is useful to decrease resistance to flow only if flow is turbulent—as one might observe during asthma.

VI. Ventilation

Arguably the central function of the pulmonary system is oxygen and carbon dioxide gas exchange. *Ventilation,* movement of gas in and out of the lungs, is essential for continued exchange to occur at the level of the alveolus and pulmonary capillary membrane. Respiratory centers in the brain normally control ventilation.

As anesthetic management often alters normal ventilation, a thorough understanding of ventilatory physiology is essential to the practice of anesthesiology.

A. Respiratory Centers

Basal ventilation is controlled by respiratory centers located in the brainstem, particularly the medulla and the pons. They process an array of information to determine a ventilation rate and pattern and are able to function independent of an intact cerebrum (4).

The medulla oblongata contains the most basic ventilation control centers, the *dorsal respiratory group (DRG)* and the *ventral respiratory group (VRG)*. The DRG provides for a ventilation rate by rhythmically stimulating inspiration. The VRG, conversely, coordinates exhalation. The DRG stimulates inspiration, which is followed by a signal by the VRG to extinguish the stimulation from the DRG, halting active inspiratory effort and allowing for passive exhalation. Without the VRG, DRG activity results in an irregular breathing pattern characterized by maximum inspiratory efforts and bouts of apnea. In this manner, the DRG and VRG work in combination, resulting in rhythmic ventilation.

The pontine respiratory centers, the apneustic center and the pneumotaxic respiratory center communicate with respiratory centers in the medulla oblongata to alter the ventilation pattern and rate. The apneustic center sends signals to the DRG to prolong inspiration, whereas the pneumotaxic center functions to limit inspiration. With increased stimulation the pneumotaxic center will also increase the ventilatory rate in addition to decreasing inspiratory volume. In this fashion, the pontine respiratory centers are able to alter ventilation.

Respiratory centers in the medulla and pons are the primary centers of ventilation control. However, the midbrain and cerebral cortex may also affect the ventilatory pattern. For example, the reticular activating system in the midbrain increases rate and volume of inspiration with activation. Reflexes can also alter ventilation. Both the swallowing and vomiting reflex result in a cessation of inspiration to avoid aspiration. The cough reflex is stimulated by irritation of the trachea and requires a deep inspiration followed by a forced exhalation to be effective at clearing irritants. Smooth muscle spindles in the airways of lungs likely react to pressure changes from pulmonary edema or atelectasis, providing proprioception for the lung and resulting in ventilatory alterations. Golgi tendon organs, tendon spindles primarily located in intercostal muscles, are stimulated when stretched, inhibiting further inspiration. The Hering-Breuer reflex, although weakly present in humans, may also alter ventilation by inhibiting inspiration during lung distention. In this manner, reflexes and higher brain centers affect ventilation patterns established by respiratory centers in the brainstem.

B. Chemical Ventilatory Control

The respiratory centers regulate ventilation based on the relative chemical content of oxygen and carbon dioxide. Central and peripheral chemoreceptors provide chemical environmental data to the respiratory centers (5).

Central chemoreceptors are located in the medulla and relay information on ventilation needs based on pH. Despite not being directly sensed, carbon dioxide has a potent effect on central chemoreceptors by conversion to hydrogen ions altering the pH:

$$CO_2 + H_2O \rightarrow H_2CO_3 \rightarrow H^+ + HCO_3^-.$$

As carbon dioxide readily passes the blood–brain barrier, it is converted into hydrogen ions, stimulating the central chemoreceptors in the medulla.

The response to elevations in carbon dioxide is rapid, resulting in increases in tidal volume and ventilation rate within 1 to 2 minutes. Over several hours, the response to sustained elevations in carbon dioxide diminishes as bicarbonate ions are likely transported into the cerebrospinal fluid, neutralizing the stimulating hydrogen ions formed by elevated carbon dioxide levels. The ability of the cerebrospinal fluid to alter and neutralize its hydrogen ions over time explains the respiratory center's response to chronic versus acute elevations in carbon dioxide levels. Of note, central chemoreceptors will also decrease ventilation secondary to hypothermia, but most important, they respond to changes in hydrogen ion concentrations secondary to carbon dioxide concentrations.

Carotid body chemoreceptors deliver signals to the respiratory centers based on oxygen and carbon dioxide content from the periphery. These peripheral chemoreceptors are found at the bifurcation of the common carotid artery and communicate to the respiratory centers via the afferent glossopharyngeal nerve. Carotid body chemoreceptors also deliver signals of acidosis, both from metabolic and elevated carbon dioxide causes, although signals of increased acidosis from peripheral chemoreceptors have minimal effects on ventilation. Aortic body chemoreceptors found around the aortic arch also deliver signals regarding partial pressure of oxygen via the vagus nerve. This leads primarily to changes in circulation with minimal effects on ventilation.

Breath-holding and the ventilatory response to altitude aptly illustrate chemoreceptor signal integration by respiratory centers. Knowing that central carbon dioxide sensing chemoreceptors override peripheral oxygen sensing chemoreceptors aids in understanding the process of chemoreceptor ventilatory control. With significant altitude elevation, the arterial partial pressure of oxygen (PaO_2) decreases, thereby stimulating the peripheral carotid body chemoreceptor to acutely increase ventilation. The increased ventilation in turn lowers carbon dioxide levels, decreasing the hydrogen ion concentration, resulting in inhibition of ventilation from the central chemoreceptors. The increased signal from the peripheral chemoreceptors coupled with the decreased drive from the central chemoreceptors results in a new equilibrium. This causes increased ventilation but continued hypoxemia, likely the cause of the headache associated with altitude sickness. With time, renal compensation allows bicarbonate ions to be removed from the cerebrospinal fluid to normalize hydrogen ion concentration. The normalization removes inhibition of ventilation from the central chemoreceptors, allowing the respiratory centers to comply with the ventilatory signal transmitted by the peripheral chemoreceptors responding to hypoxemia. Mountain climbers routinely practice acclimatization to allow chemoreceptors to function with physiologically appropriate outcomes.

Breath-holding, a common childhood game, also clearly demonstrates chemoreceptor ventilatory physiology. The combination of stimulating signals from the central chemoreceptors, at arterial carbon dioxide partial pressure ($PaCO_2$) of 50 mm Hg and peripheral chemoreceptors at PaO_2 of 65 mm Hg, compels adults to ventilate. With breath-holding, the PaO_2 decreases to approximately 65 mm Hg within 1 minute, while the $PaCO_2$ increases 12 mm Hg in the first minute and then 6 mm Hg per minute thereafter (6). Most adults are able to hold their breath for a minute, reaching $PaCO_2$ levels of 65 mm Hg and PaO_2 levels of 50 mm Hg. If one inhales supplemental oxygen, minimizing ventilatory signals from the peripheral chemoreceptors, ventilation does not occur until $PaCO_2$ levels reach 60 mm Hg or in 2 to 3 minutes.

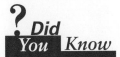

Did You Know

Signaling to the respiratory centers is initiated at arterial partial pressure of oxygen (PaO_2) <100 mm Hg, but ventilation is not altered until oxygen partial pressure falls below 65 mm Hg, at which point tidal volume and ventilation rate are increased.

Did You Know

Peripheral carotid body chemoreceptors respond primarily to lack of oxygen, while central chemoreceptors react to elevations in carbon dioxide.

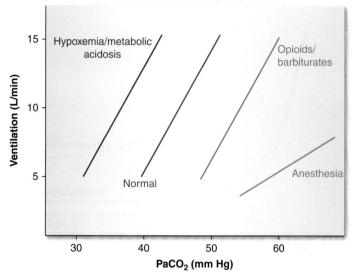

Carbon dioxide ventilatory response curve

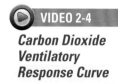

VIDEO 2-4

Carbon Dioxide Ventilatory Response Curve

Figure 2-2 Carbon dioxide ventilatory response curve. The linear ventilatory response to carbon dioxide in the normal physiologic range is illustrated by the blue curve. Ventilation response is increased with hypoxemia and metabolic acidosis and decreased with respiratory depressants as depicted by the red and green curves, respectively. Anesthesia results in a decreased rate of ventilatory response, as seen with the yellow curve.

Hyperventilation with supplemental oxygen can depress $PaCO_2$ to 20 mm Hg, allowing breath-holding to continue for approximately 5 minutes. Notably, hyperventilation without supplemental oxygen can be deleterious and result in unconsciousness as the hypoxemic ventilatory drive from peripheral oxygen-sensing chemoreceptor is outweighed by central carbon dioxide–sensing chemoreceptors. Thus, hyperventilating room air prior to a prolonged underwater swim is highly inadvisable!

Graphic representation of carbon dioxide and oxygen response curves allows for quantitative understanding of ventilation control. The $PaCO_2$ and PaO_2 ventilation response curves represent resultant ventilation at different levels of $PaCO_2$ and PaO_2, respectively. The $PaCO_2$ ventilation response curve is fairly linear in the normal range (Fig. 2-2). The change in ventilatory response increases at $PaCO_2$ >80 mm Hg, resulting in a parabolic graph and peaks at about 100 mm Hg, at which point carbon dioxide becomes a ventilatory depressant. The $PaCO_2$ response curve may be shifted left with arterial hypoxemia, the peripheral chemoreceptor response, metabolic acidosis, or a central nervous system etiology. The left shift will result in an increase in minute ventilation at constant $PaCO_2$ levels. The response to $PaCO_2$ may be decreased with opioids or barbiturates, which act as ventilatory depressants, shifting the response curve to the right. Opioids result in decreased minute ventilation with decreased respiratory rates, while barbiturates and inhaled anesthetics initially result in increased ventilatory rates with decreased tidal volumes. Continued administration of barbiturates or inhalational anesthetics will eventually depress the ventilatory response to $PaCO_2$, resulting in a flatter curve.

The PaO_2 ventilation response curve depends on the concurrent $PaCO_2$ level (7). Holding $PaCO_2$ levels constant illustrates the sole effect of PaO_2

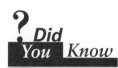

? *Did You Know*

With $PaCO_2$ levels >80 mm Hg, CO_2 acts as a ventilatory depressant and hypnotic.

Oxygen ventilatory response curve

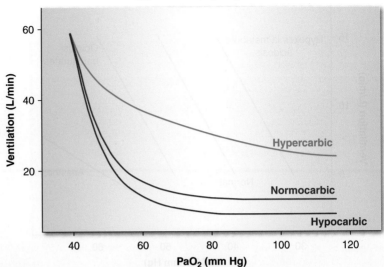

Figure 2-3 Oxygen ventilatory response curve. At normocarbic and hypocarbic levels, ventilation is stimulated at arterial carbon dioxide partial pressure (PaO_2) of 60 mm Hg, as illustrated by the blue and red curves, respectively. With hypercarbia, ventilation is stimulated at PaO_2 levels below 100 mm Hg, as seen with the green curve. Importantly note that carbon dioxide levels are constant along curves in this figure.

on ventilation (Fig. 2-3). At normocarbic levels, peripheral chemoreceptors will stimulate ventilation at levels of PaO_2 below 65 mm Hg. With hypercarbia, the signals from peripheral chemoreceptors lead to increased ventilation only when PaO_2 levels are below 100 mm Hg, the level at which peripheral chemoreceptors begin to send impulses to the respiratory centers. Normally, however, as humans increase ventilation $PaCO_2$ levels decrease. As $PaCO_2$ levels decrease, the ventilatory impulse from central chemoreceptors is decreased to the point where ventilation signals from the peripheral chemoreceptors are muffled, leading to a decrease ventilatory response. This phenomenon results in depressed oxygen-mediated ventilatory response compared to situations where $PaCO_2$ levels are normal.

Oxygen at supratherapeutic levels may be detrimental. In patients who depend on peripheral chemoreceptors for hypoxic ventilatory drive, PO_2 >65 mm Hg will likely suppress ventilation and result in hypercarbia. Supratherapeutic oxygen delivery may also lead to free radical injury, resulting in acute lung injury.

A low level of carbon dioxide leads to suppression of ventilatory drive, cerebral vasoconstriction, and lowered plasma calcium ion concentration secondary to alkalosis. Conversely, elevated carbon dioxide may result in increased sympathetic output, causing tachycardia and hypertension. Elevated carbon dioxide can also act to cause disorientation with further increases leading to unconsciousness. Thus, the respiratory centers rely on impulse generation from chemoreceptors to maintain carbon dioxide and oxygen at physiologic levels.

VII. Oxygen and Carbon Dioxide Transport

Introduction of oxygen and removal of carbon dioxide are essential to normal cellular metabolism. Movement of these gases between the environment and tissue is complex, relying on both simple diffusion and carrier molecules.

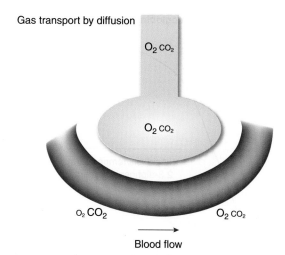

Gas transport by diffusion

O_2 CO_2

O_2 CO_2

O_2 CO_2 O_2 CO_2

Blood flow

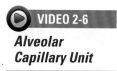

VIDEO 2-6

Alveolar Capillary Unit

Figure 2-4 The transport of oxygen and carbon dioxide in terminal airways and across the alveolar capillary membrane is dependent on diffusion. A larger font indicates a relative higher partial pressure of carbon dioxide or oxygen compared with a smaller font. Carbon dioxide and oxygen molecules move along a diffusion gradient from higher to lower partial pressures.

A. Oxygen and Carbon Dioxide Transport in Lungs

Oxygen is first inhaled from the environment and travels down the airways as a component of air by convection secondary to the force generated from the energy of inspiration. As air reaches the distal airways, diffusion becomes the predominant mode of gas transport (Fig. 2-4). Diffusion allows for movement of molecules across a distance to an area of lower concentration in an energy independent manner. The pulmonary capillaries arrive at the alveoli with blood that has a lower partial pressure of oxygen than the air entrained in the alveoli. The lower partial pressure of oxygen in blood creates a diffusion gradient, allowing oxygen to diffuse across the alveolar membrane into the pulmonary capillary bed. Relative concentrations of oxygen drive the movement of oxygen into the blood. This also allows oxygenation in the absence of ventilation, apneic oxygenation, provided a diffusion gradient is present. Similarly, pulmonary capillary blood arrives at the alveoli with a relatively rich carbon dioxide concentration, allowing carbon dioxide to diffuse from the blood into the alveoli. The pulmonary diffusion capacity or the ability of carbon dioxide to pass between the alveoli to blood is 20 times greater than oxygen, allowing for it to diffuse across the alveolar membrane with greater efficiency. After oxygen diffuses from the alveoli to the pulmonary capillary bed, oxygen from terminal airways will then diffuse into the alveoli. Concurrently, carbon dioxide newly introduced into the alveoli is transported along a diffusion gradient in a reverse pathway until it reaches the upper airways for exhalation by ventilation. The pulmonary capillary blood, which has now absorbed oxygen from and released carbon dioxide to the alveoli, propagates forward. This allows for new oxygen-poor and carbon dioxide–rich blood to interact with the alveoli. By this process, diffusion allows for oxygen and carbon dioxide to be exchanged at the alveoli–pulmonary capillary interface. Note that diffusion is a passive process. Oxygen and carbon dioxide are not actively selected. If the partial pressure of oxygen in the alveoli is decreased by significantly elevated carbon dioxide levels, diffusion hypoxia may result as the diffusion gradient for oxygen is diminished. Diffusion allows gas exchange

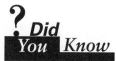

? *Did You Know*

The diffusing capacity of carbon dioxide is 20 times greater than that of oxygen.

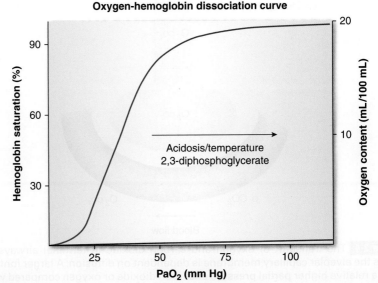

VIDEO 2-7

Oxygen
Hemoglobin
Dissociation
Curve

Oxygen-hemoglobin dissociation curve

Figure 2-5 The oxygen–hemoglobin dissociation curve demonstrates that a majority of oxygen content is bound to hemoglobin at partial pressures of 60 mm Hg. The linear portion of the curve allows for oxygen unloading at partial pressures of oxygen found in the peripheral systemic capillary beds, the site of tissue oxygenation. Furthermore, increases in acidosis, temperature, and 2,3-diphosphoglycerate decrease hemoglobin's affinity for oxygen, allowing for increased oxygen supply to areas with increased metabolic needs as evidenced by increase temperature, acidosis, and deoxygenated hemoglobin. Of note, the majority of oxygen content is found bound to hemoglobin, as seen by the small portion of oxygen content supplied by oxygen dissolved in blood (*red curve*).

to occur along a concentration gradient from the airways across the alveolar–capillary membrane to the blood.

B. **Oxygen and Carbon Dioxide Transport in Blood**

The transport of oxygen and carbon dioxide in the lungs is dependent on hemoglobin (8). Oxygen is transported in the blood both bound to hemoglobin and dissolved in blood. Oxygen dissolved in blood is a small fraction of the amount bound to hemoglobin. Hemoglobin is a complex molecule consisting of four heme subunits, with each subunit binding a molecule of oxygen. The binding of oxygen to hemoglobin is illustrated by the oxygen–hemoglobin dissociation curve (Fig. 2-5). The curve demonstrates two important concepts. First, it demonstrates that hemoglobin allows the blood to carry a large content of oxygen, even at the low partial pressure of 60 mm Hg of oxygen. Second, the linear part of the curve allows for delivery of a significant amount of oxygen with just a slight change in partial pressures of oxygen, allowing for oxygen unloading at tissues. The affinity of hemoglobin for oxygen is altered under certain conditions. Affinity for oxygen by hemoglobin is decreased by acidosis, elevation in temperature, and increased levels of 2,3-diphosphoglycerate, a by-product of red blood cell metabolism, which aids partially deoxygenated hemoglobin to release further oxygen. This decreased affinity, however, is beneficial as it allows for unloading of oxygen from hemoglobin in tissue with higher metabolic requirements. This is evidenced by increased acidosis, temperature, and deoxygenated hemoglobin. The Bohr effect specifically describes hemoglobin's decreased affinity for oxygen in environments with carbon dioxide elevation or acidosis.

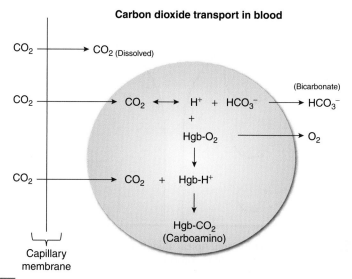

Carbon dioxide transport in blood

CO_2 ———→ CO_2 (Dissolved)

CO_2 ———→ CO_2 ⟷ H^+ + HCO_3^- ———→ HCO_3^- (Bicarbonate)

+

$Hgb-O_2$ ———→ O_2

CO_2 ———→ CO_2 + $Hgb-H^+$

$Hgb-CO_2$
(Carboamino)

Capillary
membrane

Figure 2-6 Three forms of carbon dioxide (CO_2) transport in blood are illustrated. CO_2 enters the capillary and a portion is dissolved in blood. A majority of CO_2 enters the red blood cells and is converted to bicarbonate (HCO_3^-), which is transported in the blood. The conversion of CO_2 to HCO_3^- results in hydrogen ions (H^+), which are stabilized by deoxyhemoglobin as depicted by $Hgb-H^+$. Stabilization of the H^+ favors the formation of more HCO_3^- and allows $Hgb-H^+$ to form a carboamino compound, the third form taken by carbon dioxide.

Carbon dioxide is transported in the blood in three different forms (Fig. 2-6). It is either dissolved in blood or transported as bicarbonate or as a carboamino compound. The solubility of carbon dioxide is much greater than oxygen, accounting for approximately 10% of the carbon dioxide transported in venous blood. Bicarbonate, the form in which the bulk of carbon dioxide is transported, is formed by carbonic anhydrase enzymes in the red blood cells. The formation of bicarbonate results in hydrogen ions as a by-product. As hemoglobin releases oxygen, it becomes deoxygenated and readily accepts hydrogen ions, acting as buffer and favoring the formation of further bicarbonate. Additionally, deoxygenated hemoglobin buffered with hydrogen ions is able to bind carbon dioxide, allowing transport in the form of a carboamino compound. The *Haldane effect* is the ability of deoxygenated hemoglobin to transport carbon dioxide by facilitating the formation of bicarbonate and acting as a buffer for formed hydrogen ions and as a carboamino compound. Basically the ability of blood to transport carbon dioxide is increased with lower oxygen concentrations.

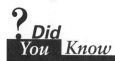

? *Did*
You Know

Ten percent of carbon dioxide in blood is dissolved, and the bulk of carbon dioxide is transported and stored as bicarbonate.

VIII. Ventilation and Perfusion

In order for gas exchange to occur, ventilated alveoli must be exposed to blood within pulmonary capillaries. Physiologically, lungs are heterogeneous. Alveoli are exposed to varying amounts of ventilation and perfusion (9). However, the matching of ventilation and perfusion is paramount to oxygen and carbon dioxide exchange.

A. Ventilation and Perfusion Distribution

Ventilation distribution within the lung depends on the compliance of alveoli and the relative distending pressure. Theoretically, the pressure within all the alveoli in the lung is constant, but the pressure outside the alveoli is

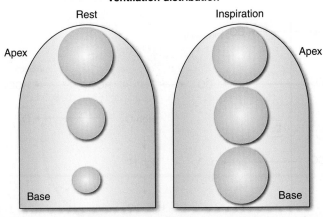

Ventilation distribution

Figure 2-7 Ventilation distribution. Apical alveoli are distended compared with basal alveoli at rest secondary to greater compressive force at the base of the lung, as depicted by the three different alveolar positions at rest. The less distended basal alveoli are therefore resting at a more compliant position than the distended apical alveoli. With inspiration, the basal alveoli are exposed to greater ventilation, while the apical alveoli see minimal ventilation, as illustrated by the change in distention between the alveoli from rest to inspiration.

heterogeneous throughout the lung, resulting in different-sized alveoli (Fig. 2-7). In the upright position, alveoli are resting at larger inflated volumes at the apex compared with the base of the lung secondary to greater compressing gravitational pressure outside the alveoli at the base. The alveoli at the base are relatively less inflated but resting at a more compliant position. As the lungs are inflated, the basal alveoli receive more ventilation because they are at a more compliant point than apical alveoli and the distending pressure is greater. Ventilation distribution is also affected by anatomy and flow rates. Central regions of the lung are preferentially ventilated, but as flow rates are increased, this ventilatory difference is minimized. Simply stated, during spontaneous ventilation, more gas is distributed to gravity-dependent areas.

Alveolar perfusion is also heterogeneous in the lung and dependent mainly upon gravity (Fig. 2-8). Gravity increases the flow of blood to dependent areas. West et al. (10) divided the lung into three zones based on relative alveolar pressure (P_A), pulmonary artery pressure (P_a) and pulmonary venous pressure (P_v). Physiologically, the pulmonary artery pressure must always exceed pulmonary venous pressure; the zones are described by the degree of alveolar pressure in relation to pulmonary artery and venous pressure. Perfusion depends on the relative resistance to the pulmonary artery pressure in each of the zones. Zone 1 is the area of the lung in which $P_A > P_a > P_v$ and is found in the least gravity-dependent area of the lung. The pulmonary artery pressure is low enough that the alveolar pressure can result in pulmonary capillary compression, limiting perfusion. Zone 2 occurs where $P_a > P_A > P_v$. Fortunately, this zone comprises the majority of the lung, allowing for matching of perfusion and ventilation. Perfusion in zone 2 is determined by the relative pressure difference between pulmonary artery and alveolar pressure. In the most gravity dependent area, zone 3, $P_a > P_v > P_A$. In zone 3, perfusion depends on the pulmonary artery and venous pressure gradient. Anatomy also affects the perfusion of the lung. Areas of the lung exposed to greater pulmonary pressures tend to be anatomically closer to the source of pulmonary

Perfusion distribution

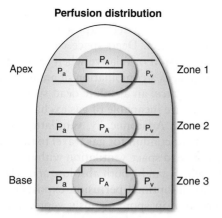

Figure 2-8 Perfusion distribution is heterogeneous throughout the lung. Font size indicates the relative alveolar pressure (P_A), pulmonary arterial pressure (P_a), and pulmonary venous pressure (P_v). At the apex, P_A is greater than P_a and P_v, limiting perfusion as illustrated by the compression of the red capillary resulting in zone 1. At the base, P_a and P_v are greater than P_A, resulting in increased perfusion as depicted by the dilated red capillary resulting in zone 3. P_A is between P_a and P_v in zone 2.

perfusion, the pulmonary artery. Again, similar to ventilation, perfusion is greater at gravity-dependent areas.

B. Ventilation and Perfusion Relationship

Matching ventilation with perfusion is vital to ensuring carbon dioxide and oxygen gas exchange. Ideally, ventilation would be perfectly matched with perfusion, optimizing the possibility for gas diffusion across the alveolar and pulmonary capillary membranes. The distribution of ventilation and perfusion, however, is heterogeneous in the lung, resulting in mismatches of ventilation and perfusion (Fig. 2-9). Mismatches in ventilation and perfusion routinely occur along a continuum.

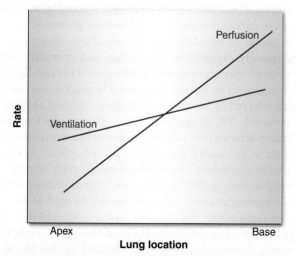

Figure 2-9 Ventilation perfusion matching. Both ventilation and perfusion of alveoli increase at the base compared with the apex, but the rate of increase is greater for perfusion than for ventilation, with progression to the base of the lung. The intersection point indicates where ventilation and perfusion are evenly matched. The area to the right of the intersection point is relative dead space, and the area to the left of the intersection point is relative shunt.

Ventilation in the excess of perfusion is termed *dead space*. Dead space is the portion of ventilation inadequately exposed to perfusion, primarily altering carbon dioxide elimination. Dead space can be absolute if the ventilation is exposed to no perfusion or relative when the ventilation is exposed to poor perfusion. Dead space is a combination of anatomical and alveolar dead space. *Anatomical dead space,* an absolute dead space, is the portion of ventilation to structures that are incapable of gas exchange, such as the pharynx, trachea, and large airways. Anatomically, ventilation must first supply anatomical dead space as it is a conduit for gas travel to the alveoli, resulting in an increased proportion of dead space ventilation with decreases in tidal volume. *Alveolar dead space,* which can be both absolute and relative, consists of ventilation to alveoli with suboptimal perfusion exposure. Approximately one-third of minute ventilation in spontaneously ventilating individuals is dead space. With positive pressure ventilation, dead space ventilation may further increase.

Increased dead space ventilation is a result of either increased ventilation in poorly perfused alveoli, decreases in perfusion locally or globally, or both. Dead space ventilation most often is increased secondary to decreased cardiac output, which results in decreased pulmonary perfusion. Pulmonary perfusion can also be decreased by embolic phenomenon in the pulmonary vasculature. A routine assessment of dead space ventilation is a comparison of end-tidal carbon dioxide and arterial carbon dioxide. If ventilation and perfusion were perfectly matched, end-tidal carbon dioxide and arterial carbon dioxide would, for clinical purposes, be equal as all the ventilated gas would equilibrate with the arterial carbon dioxide. As some of the ventilated gas is not exposed to capillaries carrying carbon dioxide, dead space gas picks up negligible carbon dioxide. This dilutes the carbon dioxide from the perfusion-exposed ventilation and results in a gradient between alveolar and end-tidal carbon dioxide. As the gradient between end-tidal carbon dioxide to arterial carbon dioxide increases, concerns for pulmonary perfusion are raised. Dead space ventilation is most often a consequence of decreased perfusion when ventilation is stable. Thus, changes in dead space ventilation should be evaluated for changes in cardiac output and pulmonary perfusion.

Perfusion in excess of ventilation is termed *shunt.* Shunt is the portion of perfusion inadequately exposed to ventilation and primarily affects oxygenation. Similar to dead space, shunt may be absolute if the capillary blood flow is exposed to no ventilation or relative if exposed to inadequate ventilation. Relative shunt is also referred to as venous admixture. Normal absolute anatomical shunt is approximately 5% of cardiac output. This results from pleural, bronchial, and thebesian arteries that supply oxygen to the structures of the lung but do not participate in gas exchange with the alveoli. Shunt, both absolute and relative, may also be secondary to pathologic states, such as atelectasis, pulmonary edema, and pneumonia. Shunt is the most common cause of poor oxygenation. Arterial oxygen saturation, however, cannot be used as an assessment for shunt. It does not incorporate the effect of mixed venous blood, the blood that leaves the right heart for gas exchange. If blood leaving the right heart has high oxygen saturation, shunt could be underestimated as this blood would need minimal oxygenation to appear normal. Shunt is better assessed by comparing arterial oxygen and mixed venous saturation levels, requiring a pulmonary artery catheter. Placement of a pulmonary artery catheter is not without consequence. Caregivers often rely on clinical acumen to determine the cause of poor oxygenation, realizing that shunt is often the causative pathophysiology.

Ventilation and perfusion matching is critical. Physiologic mechanisms help to optimize matching. Hypocapnic pulmonary bronchoconstriction is provoked by low carbon dioxide. Dead space ventilation results in low carbon dioxide levels. Bronchoconstriction of dead space airways diverts ventilation to areas with better perfusion, decreasing dead space ventilation. Hypoxic pulmonary vasoconstriction is triggered by low oxygen levels as seen with shunt. Vasoconstriction of shunt pulmonary vasculature diverts blood to better-ventilated regions, decreasing shunt. Hypocapnic pulmonary bronchoconstriction decreases dead space ventilation by decreasing ventilation in lung regions with poor perfusion. Pulmonary hypoxic vasoconstriction decreases shunt by decreasing perfusion to lung areas with poor ventilation. These processes help to improve ventilation and perfusion matching.

IX. Tissue Oxygenation Assessment

Appropriate tissue oxygenation is a central tenet of anesthetic practice. Quantitative evaluations of oxygenation allow for a better understanding of the etiology of hypoxia or poor tissue oxygenation (Appendix A). The alveolar gas equation calculates the highest possible alveolar partial pressure of oxygen. Also of importance, the equation demonstrates how increased carbon dioxide concentration will result in decreased arterial oxygenation. As described by the equation, increasing the inspired concentration of oxygen can overcome the deficiency in the oxygen gradient caused by hypoventilation. The equation also allows comparisons of alveolar and arterial oxygen partial pressures. Significant differences between alveolar and arterial partial pressure of oxygen may indicate ventilation–perfusion mismatch or alveolar–pulmonary capillary diffusion impairment. Fortunately, alveolar–pulmonary capillary diffusion impairment is rarely clinically significant and can be overcome with supplemental oxygen except for the most extreme situations.

Ventilation–perfusion mismatch in the form of shunt is the most common cause of poor oxygenation. The amount of shunt can be calculated using the shunt fraction equation or ventilation–perfusion ratio but requires a pulmonary artery to measure mixed venous saturation. If arterial oxygenation is adequate and tissue oxygenation is still poor, the ability to deliver oxygen is investigated. Assuming delivery of blood is adequate with normal cardiovascular function, the oxygen-carrying capacity of blood is analyzed with the oxygen content equation. The oxygen-content equation highlights the reliance on hemoglobin to meet tissue oxygen needs. If tissue oxygenation is poor despite adequate arterial oxygenation and hemoglobin content, abnormal hemoglobin or tissue metabolism should be considered. Tissue oxygenation requires complex physiologic processes, which may be better elucidated quantitatively when problems arise.

X. Lung Volumes

Lung volume varies by the size of the individual, and as such, normal values are generally based on height. Combinations of two or more lung volumes are known as *capacities* (Fig. 2-10).

A. Functional Residual Capacity

The functional residual capacity (FRC) is the amount of air left in the lungs at end exhalation after a normal breath. It is the combination of the residual volume and expiratory reserve volume. One of its main purposes is to serve as an oxygen

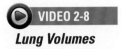

VIDEO 2-8

Lung Volumes

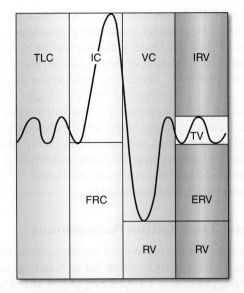

Figure 2-10 Graphic representation of lung volumes and capacities; the four volumes on the right side combine to form total lung capacity. The remainder of the boxes demonstrates the various lung capacities and their relationship to the overlying spirograph. ERV, expiratory reserve volume; FRC, functional residual capacity; IC, inspiratory capacity; IRV, inspiratory reserve volume; RV, residual volume; TLC, total lung capacity; TV, tidal volume; VC, vital capacity. (From Tamul PC, Ault ML. Respiratory function in anesthesia. In: Barash P, Cullen B, Stoelting R, et al., eds. *Clinical Anesthesia*. 7th ed. Philadelphia: Wolters Kluwer/Lippincott Williams & Wilkins, 2013:263–285, with permission.)

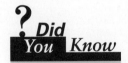

? Did You Know

Arterial hypoxemia does not occur instantaneously during apnea because the capillary blood that continues to perfuse the alveoli extracts oxygen from within the FRC.

reservoir during periods of apnea. During apnea, there is still perfusion to the lungs. It is the stored oxygen within the FRC that is obtained by the pulmonary circulation. For this reason, arterial hypoxemia does not occur instantaneously during apnea but rather over a longer period of time. Reductions in FRC can result in a much shorter period of time to arterial hypoxemia during apnea.

There are a number of reasons that FRC is reduced. Conditions that affect the lung parenchyma directly are pulmonary edema, atelectasis, pulmonary fibrosis, and acute lung injury. Mechanical or functional causes include pleural effusion, posture (simply lying down decreases FRC by 10%), pregnancy, obesity (due to a decrease in chest wall compliance), and abdominal compartment syndrome. Ventilatory muscle weakness is also a functional cause.

B. Closing Capacity

Small distal airways with little or no cartilaginous support depend on traction from the elastic recoil of surrounding tissue to remain open. Along with this, small airway patency is dependent on lung volume. The lung volume at which these small airways begin to close is known as the *closing capacity*.

In young individuals, the FRC far exceeds the closing capacity. As one ages, however, the closing capacity steadily increases until it equals or even surpasses that of the FRC. When the closing capacity is reached, alveoli in the affected portions of lung are perfused but not ventilated, which leads to intrapulmonary shunting. This intrapulmonary shunt in combination with a low oxygen reserve in the setting of a low FRC can lead to significant arterial hypoxemia.

Unlike FRC, closing capacity is unrelated to posture; because of this, the relation of the FRC (which is affected by posture) to closing capacity can change with patient position. In older individuals, the FRC can exceed the closing capacity in the upright position and fall below it in the supine position. In elderly patients, the closing capacity may be greater than the FRC, even in the upright position.

C. Vital Capacity

Vital capacity is the maximum amount of air that can be expelled from the lungs after both a maximal inspiration and maximal expiration: tidal volume plus inspiratory reserve volume plus expiratory reserve volume. This value is important for determining the patient's ability to maintain bronchial hygiene by coughing, as explained in the next section on pulmonary function testing. It is dependent upon respiratory muscle function and chest wall compliance. Normal values for vital capacity are 60 to 70 mL/kg (2,11).

XI. Pulmonary Function Testing

A. Forced Vital Capacity

The forced vital capacity (FVC) test is performed by having the patient inhale maximally and then forcefully exhaling as rapidly and thoroughly as possible into a spirometer. The overall volume should be equal to the vital capacity. The value of the FVC is that the measurement is done at maximal expiratory effort over a certain amount of time. As a result, maximal flows can be calculated at particular lung volumes. Because the flow cannot be increased above a maximum rate for a given lung volume at maximal effort, the test results are generally very reproducible with adequate patient cooperation. Normal values of this test are dependent on the patient's size, age, sex, and race.

B. Forced Expiratory Volume

The forced expiratory volume in 1 second (FEV_1) test is performed by measuring the volume of air expired at maximal effort in the first 1 second of exhalation at maximal effort after a maximal inhalation. Because it is a measurement of volume over a specific period of time, it is a measure of flow. The FEV_1 can be decreased by both obstructive conditions and restrictive conditions.

C. FEV_1/FVC Ratio

One of the more useful calculations is the ratio of the FEV_1 to the FVC. It helps to elucidate whether a patient has a restrictive or obstructive etiology of decreased FEV_1 and is expressed as a percentage. A normal patient is able to expel 75% to 85% of his or her FVC in the first second of maximal expiratory effort. In patients with a predominantly obstructive process, the FEV_1/FVC ratio is reduced. In restrictive lung processes, the FEV_1 and FVC are generally reduced proportionally to each other, so the ratio is normal to even slightly elevated due to increased elastic recoil of the lung.

D. Forced Expiratory Flow

Another common measurement is the forced expiratory flow (FEF). There are a number of different types of FEF measurements. They are differentiated by the point during exhalation of the FVC at which they are measured. One of the more common values is the $FEF_{25-50\%}$. It is an average FEF of the middle 50% of the FVC. It is thought to be more sensitive for detection of early, mild obstructive pulmonary processes. Other measures are the $FEF_{50\%}$ and $FEF_{75\%}$, which are the flows present after 50% of the FVC has been exhaled and 75% has been exhaled, respectively. All of these values are decreased in the setting of obstructive pulmonary disease.

Table 2-1   Pulmonary Function Tests in Restrictive and Obstructive Lung Disease

Value	Restrictive Disease	Obstructive Disease
Definition	Proportional decreases in all lung volumes	Small airway obstruction to expiratory flow
FVC	↓↓↓	Normal or slightly ↑
FEV$_1$	↓↓↓	Normal or slightly ↓
FEV$_1$/FVC	Normal	↓↓↓
FEF$_{25-75\%}$	Normal	↓↓↓
FRC	↓↓↓	Normal or ↑ if gas trapping
TLC	↓↓↓	Normal or ↑ if gas trapping

FEV, forced expiratory volume; FRC, functional residual capacity; FVC, forced vital capacity; TLC, total lung capacity; ↓↓↓, ↑↑↑, large decrease or increase, respectively; ↓, ↑, small/moderate decrease or increase, respectively.
From Tamul PC, Ault ML. Respiratory function in anesthesia. In: Barash P, Cullen B, Stoelting R, et al., eds. *Clinical Anesthesia.* 7th ed. Philadelphia: Wolters Kluwer/Lippincott Williams & Wilkins, 2013:263–285, with permission.

E. Maximal Voluntary Ventilation

Maximal voluntary ventilation (MVV) is a pulmonary function test that is used to evaluate a patient's exercise capacity as well as his or her ability to tolerate major surgery. The patient is asked to breathe as hard and as fast as he or she can for 10 to 15 seconds. The total volume over this time is measured and then extrapolated to 1 minute. Numerous conditions can cause a reduction in MVV. These include obstructive and restrictive lung conditions, heart disease, neuromuscular impairment, and lack of patient cooperation or understanding (Table 2-1) (2,11).

F. Flow–Volume Loops

Flow–volume loops are graphic representations of the respiratory cycle. The gas flow rate is represented on the x-axis and lung volume is on the y-axis (Fig. 2-11). Notice that expiratory flow in Figure 2-11 is above zero on the x-axis and inspiratory flow is below. These graphic representations were previously very commonly used to ascertain whether obstruction of large airways was intrathoracic or extrathoracic. With the advent of modern imaging modalities, this method has become less useful, although it is important to note the change in morphology of the curve with different types of obstruction (Fig. 2-12). As demonstrated in Figure 2-12, a variable nonfixed extrathoracic obstruction will produce a flattened curve in the inspiratory part of the cycle. A variable nonfixed intrathoracic obstruction will result in a flattened expiratory portion of the loop. A fixed obstruction produces flattened curves in both parts of the cycle regardless of its position (2,11).

G. Carbon Monoxide Diffusing Capacity

The transfer of oxygen from the alveolus to erythrocyte is done through diffusion. Three main variables affect the diffusion of oxygen into the bloodstream. They are:

1. Area of the interface between alveolus and capillary—the greater the area, the greater the capacity for diffusion.

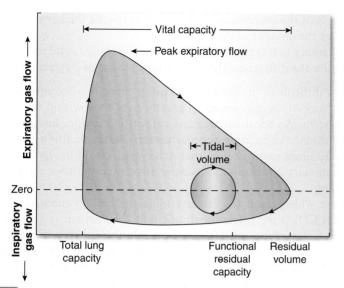

Figure 2-11 Flow–volume loop in a normal patient. (From Tamul PC, Ault ML. Respiratory function in anesthesia. In: Barash P, Cullen B, Stoelting R, et al., eds. *Clinical Anesthesia*. 7th ed. Philadelphia: Wolters Kluwer/Lippincott Williams & Wilkins, 2013:263–285, with permission.)

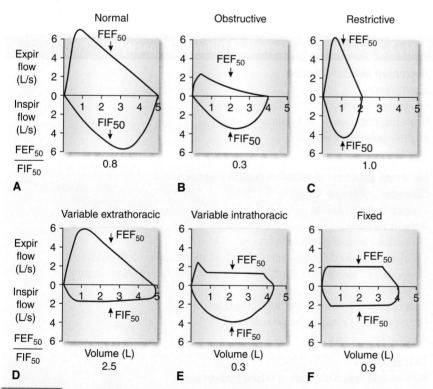

Figure 2-12 Flow–volume loops in various disease states. (From Spirometry: Dynamic lung volumes. In: Hyatt R, Scanlon P, Nakamura M, eds. *Interpretation of Pulmonary Function Tests: A Practical Guide*. 3rd ed. Philadelphia: Lippincott Williams & Wilkins, 2009:5–25, with permission.)

2. Thickness of the membrane between the two—the thicker the membrane, the lower the amount of diffusion.
3. The difference in oxygen tension between alveolar gas and venous blood—the greater the difference, the greater the amount of oxygen diffused.

It is very difficult to measure the diffusing capacity of oxygen because the partial pressure of oxygen varies so greatly over time within the pulmonary vascular system. An ideal surrogate is carbon monoxide. Its normal partial pressure within the circulation approaches zero. It has an affinity for hemoglobin that is 20 times stronger than that of oxygen. Therefore, its level throughout the pulmonary circulation remains relatively constant for the purposes of measurement.

The most widely used test to determine the carbon monoxide diffusing capacity (DLCO) is the single breath method. The patient is asked to exhale completely, followed by inhalation to total lung capacity of a gas mixture containing a low concentration of carbon monoxide and an inert gas such as helium. After reaching total lung capacity, the patient is asked to hold his or her breath for 10 seconds, then exhale completely again to residual volume. The concentration of carbon monoxide is then measured in the exhaled sample.

Decreases in the DLCO can be caused by a host of reasons. These can be divided mainly into conditions that affect the area available for diffusion or increase the thickness of the alveolar–capillary membrane (Table 2-2) (12).

Table 2-2   Causes of a Decreased Diffusing Capacity
Decreased *area* for diffusion:
Emphysema
Lung/lobe resection
Bronchial obstruction, as by tumor
Multiple pulmonary emboli
Anemia
Increased *thickness* of alveolar–capillary membrane:
Idiopathic pulmonary fibrosis
Congestive heart failure
Asbestosis
Sarcoidosis involving parenchyma
Collagen vascular disease—scleroderma, systemic lupus erythematosus
Drug-induced alveolitis or fibrosis—bleomycin, nitrofurantoin, amiodarone, methotrexate
Hypersensitivity pneumonitis, including farmer's lung
Histiocytosis X (eosinophilic granuloma)
Alveolar proteinosis
Miscellaneous
High carbon monoxide back pressure from smoking
Pregnancy
Ventilation–perfusion mismatch

From Diffusing capacity of the lungs. In: Hyatt R, Scanlon P, Nakamura M, eds. *Interpretation of Pulmonary Function Tests: A Practical Guide*. 3rd ed. Philadelphia: Lippincott Williams & Wilkins, 2009:41–49, with permission.

XII. Preoperative Pulmonary Assessment

Much of the preoperative assessment in regard to pulmonary function is aimed at identifying patients who may be at greater risk for postoperative pulmonary complications. It is also an opportunity to assess the baseline pulmonary characteristics of the patient that may guide clinical decision making intra- and postoperatively. For any patient, the most important part of the preoperative evaluation is the history and physical examination. Beyond this, ancillary tests that can be considered are:

• Chest radiography
• Arterial blood gas
• Spirometry

The decision to pursue further testing and the specific tests one orders should be tailored both to the individual patient's condition as well as the operation or procedure the patient is about to undergo. The American Society of Anesthesiologists guidelines on preoperative pulmonary evaluation state that clinicians should "balance the risks and costs of these evaluations against their benefits. Clinical characteristics to consider include type and invasiveness of the surgical procedure, interval from previous evaluation, treated or symptomatic asthma, symptomatic COPD, and scoliosis with restrictive function" (13).

Some conditions that predispose to derangements in pulmonary function are:

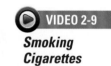

VIDEO 2-9

Smoking Cigarettes

• Chronic lung disease
• Smoking history, persistent cough, or wheezing
• Chest wall and spinal deformities
• Morbid obesity
• Requirement for single-lung ventilation or lung resection
• Severe neuromuscular disease

Again, the most important part of any evaluation in regard to pulmonary status is the history and physical examination. Any test that is ordered should be done with a specific purpose in mind, for example, knowing the baseline $PaCO_2$ or PaO_2 of a patient with severe chronic obstructive pulmonary disease in order to help guide the decision to extubate at the conclusion of the anesthetic course (2).

XIII. Anesthetic Considerations in Obstructive and Restrictive Lung Disease

A. Obstructive Lung Disease

Patients with obstructive lung disease are predisposed to having more reactive airways that could potentially lead to bronchoconstriction and significant wheezing. Because of this, one should consider administering preoperative bronchodilators and a dose of intravenous corticosteroids. The patient should also be at a relatively deep plane of anesthesia before instrumenting the airway to help lessen the chance of bronchoconstriction; opioids and lidocaine preintubation are also helpful in this regard.

During mechanical ventilation, it is advisable to avoid high respiratory rates to prevent gas trapping and to allow for a longer expiratory time. This also requires that the selected tidal volume may need to be higher. If tracheal extubation is planned at the conclusion of the procedure, care must be taken to prevent bronchoconstriction and the resultant increase in airway resistance. Extubating the patient at a deep plane of anesthesia and using mask ventilation for emergence is a useful strategy.

B. Restrictive Disease

Patients with restrictive disease have a decrease in all measured lung volumes, including the FRC. As discussed previously, the FRC acts as an oxygen reservoir during periods of apnea. With this reservoir reduced in capacity, patients with restrictive disease tolerate much shorter periods of apnea than normal patients. Rapid desaturation during apnea is common.

These patients also will require smaller tidal volumes and may have elevated peak inspiratory pressures during mechanical ventilation due to reduced lung compliance. They will likely require higher respiratory rates as well. Care must be taken during mechanical ventilation to not allow inspiratory pressures to become too elevated in an effort to prevent barotrauma.

XIV. Postoperative Pulmonary Function and Complications

A. Postoperative Pulmonary Function

The main alteration in postoperative lung mechanics is a restrictive defect. This occurs in nearly all patients, and as a result, patients tend to breath faster and shallower. With any type of operation under general anesthesia, the FRC does not return to its preoperative level for up to a week, perhaps even a few weeks for operations involving a sternotomy (2).

B. Postoperative Pulmonary Complications

Two significant postoperative complications specifically related to the respiratory system are atelectasis and pneumonia. The incidence of these two complications is related to the site of surgery. Open upper abdominal operations have a much higher rate, lower abdominal and thoracic have a slightly lower rate than upper abdominal surgery, and all other peripheral operations have the lowest risk. There are a number of strategies to consider to prevent pulmonary complications. Most of them focus on improving lung expansion. The use of incentive spirometry is widespread and very helpful when used appropriately. Many patients use the device incorrectly or not often enough, so training and monitoring by the staff caring for the patient is crucial. Early patient ambulation is vital to prevent postoperative pulmonary complications. Having adequate analgesia is also helpful so that the above strategies can effectively be used. This can be achieved through the use of parenteral or intravenous medications, neuraxial analgesics, or regional techniques. The analgesic techniques employed depend on the surgical site and individual patient characteristics (2).

References

1. Tomashefski JF, Farver CF. Anatomy and histology of the lung. In: Tomashefski JF, Cagle PT, Farver CF, et al., eds. *Dail and Hammar's Pulmonary Pathology*, Vol. II. 3rd ed. New York: Springer; 2008:20–48.
2. Tamul PC, Ault ML. Respiratory function in anesthesia. In: Barash P, Cullen B, Stoelting R, et al., eds. *Clinical Anesthesia*. 7th ed. Philadelphia: Wolters Kluwer/Lippincott Williams & Wilkins, 2013:263–285.
3. Butterworth JF, IV, Mackey DC, Wasnick JD. Respiratory physiology & anesthesia. *Morgan & Mikhail's Clinical Anesthesiology*. 5th ed. New York: McGraw-Hill; 2013.

4. Guz A. Regulation of respiration in man. *Annu Rev Physiol.* 1975;37:303–323.
5. Berger AJ, Mitchell RA, Severinghaus JW, et al. Regulation of respiration. *N Engl J Med.* 1977;297(2,3,4):92–97, 138–143, 194–201.
6. Stock MD, Downs JB, McDonald JS, et al. The carbon dioxide rate of rise in awake apneic humans. *J Clin Anesth.* 1988;1:96.
7. Weil JV, Byrne-Quinn E, Sodal IE, et al. Hypoxic ventilatory drive in normal man. *J Clin Invest.* 1970;49:1061–1072.
8. Tyuma I. The Bohr effect and the Haldane effect in human hemoglobin. *Jpn J Physiol.* 1984;34(2):205–216.
9. Galvin I, Drummond GB, Nirmalan M. Distribution of blood flow and ventilation in the lung: Gravity is not the only factor. *Br J Anaesth.* 2007;98(4):420–428.
10. West JB, Dollery CT, Naimark A. Distribution of blood-flow and pressure-flow relations of the whole lung. *J Appl Physiol.* 1965;20:175–183.
11. Hyatt R, Scanlon P, Nakamura M. Spirometry: Dynamic lung volumes. *Interpretation of Pulmonary Function Tests: A Practical Guide.* 3rd ed. Philadelphia: Lippincott Williams & Wilkins, 2009:5–25.
12. Hyatt R, Scanlon P, Nakamura M. Diffusing capacity of the lungs. *Interpretation of Pulmonary Function Tests: A Practical Guide.* 3rd ed. Philadelphia: Lippincott Williams & Wilkins, 2009:41–49.
13. American Society of Anesthesiologists Task Force on Preanesthesia Evaluation. Practice advisory for preanesthesia evaluation: An updated report by the American Society of Anesthesiologists task force on preanesthesia evaluation. *Anesthesiology.* 2012;116: 522–539.

Questions

1. At what arterial partial pressure of oxygen (PaO_2) would you expect a patient who breathes from hypoxic respiratory drive to begin to increase minute ventilation in response to a low PaO_2?
   A. 120 mm Hg
   B. 100 mm Hg
   C. 65 mm Hg
   D. 45 mm Hg

2. During spontaneous ventilation, what is true of ventilation and perfusion in the gravity-dependent lung relative to other areas of the lung?
   A. Ventilation is greater; perfusion is greater
   B. Ventilation is greater; perfusion is less
   C. Ventilation is less; perfusion is greater
   D. Ventilation is less; perfusion is less

3. Why do humans not become instantaneously hypoxemic when we become apneic?
   A. The work of breathing becomes zero during apnea, so there is no oxygen consumption
   B. Because total lung capacity is not affected by apnea
   C. Because lung perfusion decreases during apnea
   D. Because there is still oxygen available in the alveoli at end-expiration

4. During normal, resting breathing, which combination is true?
   A. Inspiration is active; exhalation is active
   B. Inspiration is active; exhalation is passive
   C. Inspiration is passive; exhalation is active
   D. Inspiration is passive; exhalation is passive

5. Which combination is true with respect to the peripheral carotid body and central chemoreceptors?
   A. Both peripheral chemoreceptors and central chemoreceptors respond to lack of oxygen.
   B. Peripheral chemoreceptors respond to lack of oxygen; central chemoreceptors respond to elevation in carbon dioxide.
   C. Peripheral chemoreceptors respond to elevation in carbon dioxide; central chemoreceptors respond to lack of oxygen.
   D. Both peripheral chemoreceptors and central chemoreceptors respond to elevation in carbon dioxide.

3 Cardiovascular Anatomy and Physiology

Sam R. Sharar
Peter von Homeyer

I. Cardiac Anatomy

The normal heart is about the size of an adult fist, weighs approximately 300 g, and has a trapezoid shape with its apex oriented leftward and anterior in the chest (Fig. 3-1) (1). The anterior thoracic surface projections of the heart and great vessels, relative to the bony ribs, sternum, and xiphoid process, are shown in Figure 3-2. As the central blood pump of the human body, it contracts about 100,000 times per day and propels blood into the pulmonary and systemic circulations. The right and the left chambers are anatomically separated by septa. Only in the fetal circulation or in the setting of certain pathologies (e.g., atrial septal defect) is there direct communication of blood flow between the right and left sides. On each side, blood first flows from veins into a thin-walled atrium. It then flows through an *atrioventricular* (AV) *valve* into a muscular ventricle, and finally through a *semilunar valve* into the great arteries—the aorta on the left and the *pulmonary artery* (PA) on the right (Fig. 3-3).

The *heart wall* has three layers: the thin, inner, endocardium; the thick, middle myocardium; and the outer epicardium (i.e., the visceral pericardium). The myocardium is anchored to the cardiac *fibrous skeleton*, a system of dense collagen forming two rings and connective trigones that separate the atria and ventricles to prevent uncontrolled conduction of electrical impulses and also serve as anchors for the AV valves.

The *right atrium* (RA), *superior vena cava* (SVC), and *inferior vena cava* (IVC) form the right lateral border of the heart. Venous return from the heart itself enters the RA through the *coronary sinus* (CS), which collects blood from the major cardiac veins. The internal wall of the RA includes the right-sided wall of the *interatrial septum* (IAS). The center of the IAS features the oval fossa, a small groove that is a remnant of the foramen ovale. It allows oxygenated blood to cross from right to left in the fetal circulation. It usually closes after birth, but remains patent in 25% to 30% of the population.

The *right ventricle* (RV) forms most of the anterior surface of the heart, some of its inferior surface, and has about a sixth of the muscle mass of the

(text continues on page 44)

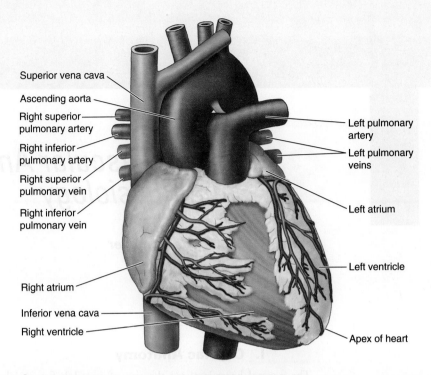

Superior vena cava

Ascending aorta

Right superior pulmonary artery

Right inferior pulmonary artery

Right superior pulmonary vein

Right inferior pulmonary vein

Left pulmonary artery

Left pulmonary veins

Left atrium

Left ventricle

Right atrium

Inferior vena cava

Right ventricle

Apex of heart

A   Anterior view

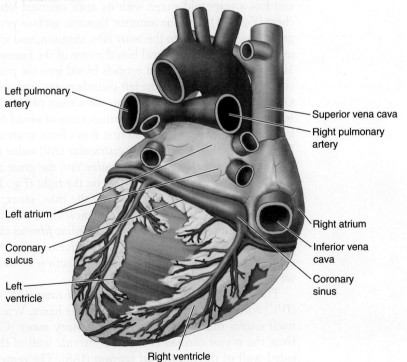

Left pulmonary artery

Superior vena cava

Right pulmonary artery

Left atrium

Coronary sulcus

Left ventricle

Right atrium

Inferior vena cava

Coronary sinus

Right ventricle

B   Postero-inferior view

Figure 3-1 Key anatomic features of heart from the anterior view (**A**) and posterior-inferior view (**B**). (From Moore KL, Agur AMR, Dalley II AF. Thorax. In: Moore KL, Agur AMR, Dalley II AF. *Clinically Oriented Anatomy*, 7th ed. Philadelphia: Lippincott Williams & Wilkins, 2013:131–149, with permission.)

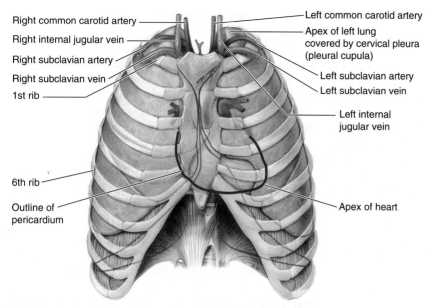

Right common carotid artery

Right internal jugular vein

Right subclavian artery

Right subclavian vein

1st rib

6th rib

Outline of pericardium

Left common carotid artery

Apex of left lung covered by cervical pleura (pleural cupula)

Left subclavian artery

Left subclavian vein

Left internal jugular vein

Apex of heart

Figure 3-2 Anterior surface projections of the heart and great vessels relative to the lungs and ribs. Note the close relation of the lung apices to the internal jugular and subclavian veins (relevant to placement of central venous catheters) and the bare area of the pericardium that can be accessed for pericardiocentesis with needle placement under and to the left of the xiphoid process of the sternum. (From Moore KL, Agur AMR, Dalley II AF. Thorax. In: Moore KL, Agur AMR, Dalley II AF. *Clinically Oriented Anatomy,* 7th ed. Philadelphia: Lippincott Williams & Wilkins, 2013:131–149, with permission.)

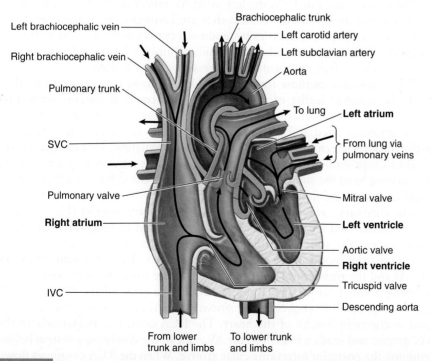

Left brachiocephalic vein

Right brachiocephalic vein

Pulmonary trunk

SVC

Pulmonary valve

Right atrium

IVC

Brachiocephalic trunk

Left carotid artery

Left subclavian artery

Aorta

To lung

Left atrium

From lung via pulmonary veins

Mitral valve

Left ventricle

Aortic valve

Right ventricle

Tricuspid valve

Descending aorta

From lower trunk and limbs

To lower trunk and limbs

Figure 3-3 The course of normal blood flow from the great venous vessels through the right and left heart chambers to the systemic aorta. (From Moore KL, Agur AMR, Dalley II AF. Thorax. In: Moore KL, Agur AMR, Dalley II AF. *Clinically Oriented Anatomy,* 7th ed. Philadelphia: Lippincott Williams & Wilkins, 2013:131–149, with permission.)

left ventricle (LV). The muscular *interventricular septum* (IVS) functions as a contractile wall for both the RV and the LV.

The *tricuspid valve* (TV) has three distinct leaflets (anterior, septal, and posterior) that are attached to tendinous cords. It connects to papillary muscles that tighten to draw the valve cusp edges together in ventricular systole and prevent regurgitant flow through this AV valve. The RV wall is heavily trabeculated, with one prominent trabecula (moderator band) connecting the IVS with the anterior RV wall. It houses the right branch of the AV conduction bundle (see below).

The *pulmonic valve* (PV) is a semilunar valve with three defined cusps (anterior, left, right) that are pushed toward the wall of the *right ventricular outflow tract* (RVOT) with ventricular contraction in systole. After relaxation in diastole, the cusps close like an umbrella to prevent regurgitation. The main PA quickly bifurcates into right and left branches that lead deoxygenated blood to the pulmonary circulation for subsequent gas exchange.

Oxygenated blood returning from the lungs enters the *left atrium* (LA) through four pulmonary veins, normally two originating from each lung. The LA forms the majority of the base of the heart, with the small LA appendage as part of its anterolateral wall. The IAS has a small semilunar indentation representing the left-sided aspect of the oval fossa.

The LV forms the apex of the heart, as well as most of its left (lateral) and diaphragmatic (inferior) surfaces, and its normal maximal wall thickness is 10 mm (compared with 3 mm in the RV). The IVS is concave to the highly trabeculated LV wall, resulting in an almost circular LV chamber on anatomic cross-section.

Unlike the right-sided TV, the left-sided AV *mitral valve* (MV) is bicuspid, with anterior and posterior leaflets that are connected to anterolateral and posteromedial papillary muscles by tendinous cords similar to those of the TV. Both MV leaflets receive cords from papillary muscles that keep this valve shut in the setting of high intraventricular pressure during systole.

The inflow and outflow tracts of the LV lie almost parallel to each other, with the anterior leaflet of the mitral valve forming a natural separation between these two structures. The *left ventricular outflow tract* (LVOT) is more smooth walled and of round or oval shape, and it contains the *aortic valve* through which blood enters the systemic circulation. This valve has three distinct cusps named after the presence or absence of coronary artery ostia originating from the sinuses of Valsalva just above the valve: the left coronary, right coronary, and noncoronary cusps (Fig. 3-4).

The coronary vasculature consists of the *coronary arteries* (Fig. 3-5) and the CS (described earlier). The arteries carry blood to most of the myocardium except the subendocardial layers, which receive oxygen directly via diffusion from blood inside the cardiac chambers. The *left coronary artery* (LCA) and the *right coronary artery* (RCA) arise from the respective sinuses in the proximal aorta. The RCA travels to the right of the PA in the AV groove and sends branches to the *sinoatrial* (SA) *node* (inside the RA wall) and to the right border of the heart. The RCA continues posteriorly in the AV groove and sends a branch to the AV node of the conducting system before entering the posterior interventricular groove. When the RCA continues down that groove to form the posterior interventricular branch, this is termed *right dominant* circulation (~70% of individuals). The LCA travels between the PA and the LA appendage and splits early in its course into the *left anterior descending* (LAD) artery and the circumflex branch. The LAD continues

? Did You Know

Coronary artery anatomy is termed either right dominant or left dominant depending on which main coronary artery feeds the posterior descending branch (in the interventricular groove) to the posterior-inferior surface of the heart. Right dominant circulation is most common, found in 70% of the population.

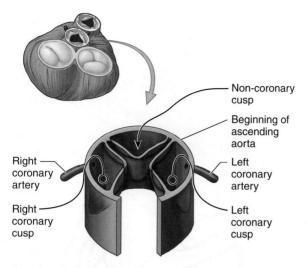

- Non-coronary cusp
- Beginning of ascending aorta
- Right coronary artery
- Left coronary artery
- Right coronary cusp
- Left coronary cusp

Anterior view of aortic valve

Figure 3-4 Relation between the aortic valve cusps and the coronary arteries. Like the pulmonary valve, the aortic valve has three semilunar cusps: right, posterior, and left. During systole, ejected blood forces the cusps apart. During diastole, the cusps close and coronary artery flow occurs. (From Moore KL, Agur AMR, Dalley II AF. Thorax. In: Moore KL, Agur AMR, Dalley II AF. *Clinically Oriented Anatomy,* 7th ed. Philadelphia: Lippincott Williams & Wilkins, 2013:131–149, with permission.)

in the anterior interventricular groove all the way to the LV apex and around the inferior aspect of the heart where it often forms anastomoses with the branches of the posterior interventricular branch. The LAD also sends many septal branches to the IVS throughout its course, as well as prominent diagonal branch to the lateral wall. When the circumflex branch gives rise to the posterior interventricular branch, this is termed *left dominant* circulation (~30% of individuals). Such variable coronary artery anatomy is important when trying to understand the relation between coronary artery disease and regional dysfunction of ischemic myocardium.

Normal *electrical conduction* is initiated by an electrical impulse generated in the SA node, a locus of specialized cardiac cells in the RA wall that have no contractile function. As the pacemaker center of the heart, the SA node autonomically generates an impulse at about 60 to 80 beats per minute. From the SA node, bundles of cells lead to the AV node located above the right fibrous trigone of the heart at the AV border. From the AV node, the impulse is conducted in the AV bundle that pierces the fibrous skeleton of the heart and splits just above the muscular IVS into right and left bundles. The right bundle continues toward the apex of the heart and then splits into smaller subendocardial RV branches. The left bundle splits close to its origin into a left anterior and a left posterior branch, which then further split into subendocardial LV branches near the apex of the heart (Fig. 3-6).

The *pericardium* is a double-layered sac around the heart. The visceral serous layer (epicardium) covers most of the heart's surface. It extends to and reflects at the proximal portion of the great vessels and turns into the parietal pericardial sac. Between the two layers, a small amount of fluid is considered physiologic. The pericardium protects and restrains the heart, reduces friction associated with its constant movement within the mediastinum, and separates the heart and origin of the great vessels from other structures inside the

VIDEO 3-1

Pericardium

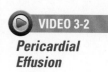

VIDEO 3-2

Pericardial Effusion

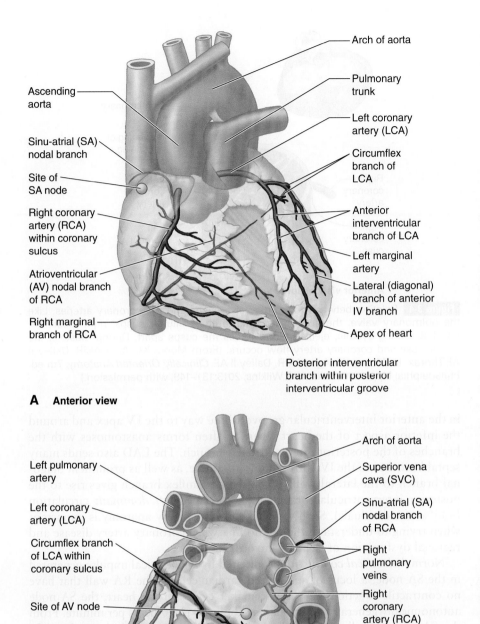

A   Anterior view

B   Postero-inferior view

Figure 3-5 Coronary artery anatomy for the typical right dominant pattern (see text for details) is shown from the anterior view (**A**) and the posterior view (**B**). (From Moore KL, Agur AMR, Dalley II AF. Thorax. In: Moore KL, Agur AMR, Dalley II AF. *Clinically Oriented Anatomy,* 7th ed. Philadelphia: Lippincott Williams & Wilkins, 2013:131–149, with permission.)

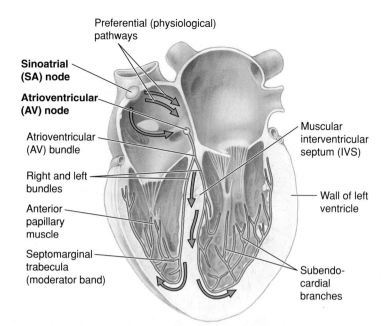

Preferential (physiological) pathways

Sinoatrial (SA) node

Atrioventricular (AV) node

Atrioventricular (AV) bundle

Right and left bundles

Anterior papillary muscle

Septomarginal trabecula (moderator band)

Muscular interventricular septum (IVS)

Wall of left ventricle

Subendo-cardial branches

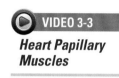

VIDEO 3-3

Heart Papillary Muscles

Figure 3-6 Impulses initiated at the sinoatrial (SA) node are propagated through the atrial musculature to the atrioventricular (AV) node, followed by conduction through the AV bundle and its right and left branches in the intraventricular septum (IVS) to the myocardium. (From Moore KL, Agur AMR, Dalley II AF. Thorax. In: Moore KL, Agur AMR, Dalley II AF. *Clinically Oriented Anatomy,* 7th ed. Philadelphia: Lippincott Williams & Wilkins, 2013:131–149, with permission.)

mediastinum. Abnormal pericardial fluid collections (e.g., pericardial tamponade) can be accessed and withdrawn as described in Figure 3-2.

II. The Cardiac Cycle

The *cardiac cycle* consists of an orchestrated sequence of spontaneous electrical and contractile events occurring simultaneously in both the right and left sides of the heart. When combined with the flow-directing influence of the four unidirectional heart valves, a sequential rise and fall of fluid pressures within each of the four heart chambers results in a predictable pattern of chamber volumes and pressures that produces forward cardiac output and accompanying heart sounds associated with valve closure (2). These synchronized electrical and mechanical events are depicted under normal anatomic and physiologic conditions in Figure 3-7. Anatomic or physiologic abnormalities in any of these components can alter events of the cardiac cycle and ultimately impact cardiac performance.

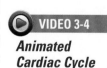

VIDEO 3-4

Animated Cardiac Cycle

Focusing on the left heart, depolarization of the LV associated with the QRS complex of the electrocardiogram (ECG) initiates LV contraction and begins the period of *systole* with closure of the mitral valve contributing to the first heart sound (S_1). During early systole, both the mitral and aortic valves are closed; the mitral valve due to the positive LV → LA pressure gradient and papillary muscle contraction, and the aortic valve due to the positive aortic root → LV pressure gradient. Because LV volume is fixed during early systole, LV contraction results in a brief, yet rapid isovolumic elevation in LV pressure. The maximum rate of rise in LV pressure (+dP/dt) occurs during this

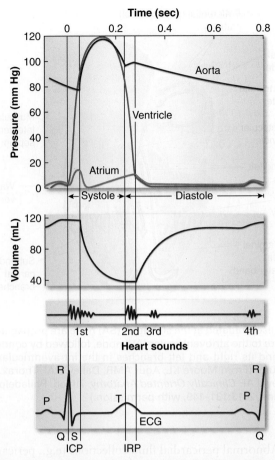

Figure 3-7 Mechanical and electrical events of the cardiac cycle also showing the left ventricular (LV) volume curve and the heart sounds. Note the LV isovolumic contraction period (ICP) and the relaxation period (IRP) during which there is no change in LV volume because the aortic and mitral valves are closed. The LV decreases in volume as it ejects its contents into the aorta. During the first third of systolic ejection (the rapid ejection period), the curve of emptying is steep. ECG, electrocardiogram. (From Pagel PS, Kampine JP, Stowe DF. Cardiac anatomy and physiology. In: Barash PG, Cullen BF, Stoelting RK, et al. *Handbook of Clinical Anesthesia*, 7th ed. Philadelphia: Lippincott Williams & Wilkins, 2013:239–262, with permission.)

brief *isovolumic contraction period* and is commonly used as the index of LV contractility (as discussed later).

Once the rapidly rising LV pressure exceeds aortic root pressure, the aortic valve passively opens and pulsatile aortic flow begins. Both the LV and aortic pressures continue to rise, then quickly peak and fall during the remainder of systole as ventricular contraction ceases and the LV repolarizes. The stroke volume ejected during systole is approximately two-thirds of the end-diastolic LV volume.

Systole ends when the slowly declining aortic root pressure exceeds the more rapidly falling LV pressure, resulting in passive closure of the aortic valve and its contribution to the second heart sound (S_2). As *diastole* begins, both the mitral and aortic valves are briefly closed. During this short-lived, *isovolumic relaxation period*, LV pressure rapidly falls, while LA pressure slowly rises due to pulmonary inflow. When LA pressure exceeds LV pressure, the MV passively opens and diastolic filling of the LV begins. Diastole consists of four phases—isovolumic relaxation, early diastolic filling, diastasis, and atrial systole (LA contraction)—until the cardiac cycle is repeated with LV depolarization and contraction.

Similar parallel events occur in the right heart during the cardiac cycle with corresponding chamber volumes (i.e., right and left ventricular stroke volumes are equal under normal anatomic conditions) and tricuspid/pulmonic valve movements mirroring the mitral/aortic movements. As a result of peristaltic inflow, lesser cardiac muscle mass, and lesser contractile strength of the RV, there is no isovolumic contraction period in the RV. The RV and PA pressures are significantly lower than corresponding left-sided pressures. Right-sided systolic ejection time may exceed the left-sided time, resulting in later closure of the pulmonic valve (compared with the aortic valve) and a split S_2. During spontaneous inspiration, ***venous return*** is increased to the right ventricle and decreased to the left ventricle, resulting in prolongation of the splitting of S_2, referred to as *physiologic splitting*.

III. Control of Heart Rate

Heart rate is determined by the constantly and often instantaneously changing balance between multiple intrinsic and extrinsic factors. Key intrinsic factors include autonomic efferent innervation (both ***sympathetic nervous system*** [SNS] and ***parasympathetic nervous system*** [PNS]) (see Chapter 4), neural reflex mechanisms, humoral influences, and cardiac rhythm. Extrinsic factors include direct- and indirect-acting pharmaceutical and recreational drugs, fear, hyperthermia, and others that affect heart rate through modulation of intrinsic factors.

Efferent autonomic tone to the heart is initiated in the anterior (PNS) and posterior (SNS) hypothalamus and is modulated by the cardiac acceleration and cardiac slowing centers in the medulla prior to peripheral distribution. Sympathetic preganglionic fibers arising from T1 to T4 spinal levels enter the nearby paravertebral sympathetic chain, inferior cervical (stellate) ganglion, and middle cervical ganglion. They synapse with postganglionic SNS neurons that directly innervate the SA node, AV node, and myocardium via β_1-adrenergic norepinephrine receptors. PNS preganglionic fibers to the heart arise from the brainstem and are carried in the vagus nerve. Both the right and left vagus nerves exit the jugular foramena, traverse the neck within the carotid sheaths posterior to the carotid arteries. They course directly to the heart where they synapse with short postganglionic PNS neurons that moderate the SA and AV nodes via muscarinic acetylcholine receptors. The opposing effects of the SNS (tachycardia) and PNS (bradycardia) on the SA node normally favor vagal inhibition. As a result of this vagal predominance, load-induced increases in heart rate are first achieved by release of PNS tone and thereafter by SNS activation. Several neural reflex mechanisms can also affect heart rate, including the ***baroreceptor response, atrial distention response (Bainbridge reflex), carotid chemoreceptor reflex, Cushing reflex***, and ***oculocardiac reflex*** (Table 3-1).

Humoral factors (e.g., circulating catecholamines) also influence heart rate independent of the SNS and PNS. For example, the denervated heart following heart transplantation responds to exercise load with tachycardia owing to increased circulating catecholamine levels. Myocardial β_1-adrenergic receptors can also be activated and heart rate is increased by direct pharmacologic agonists (isoproterenol, epinephrine), agents that indirectly cause release of endogenous catecholamines (ephedrine), or drugs that impair catecholamine metabolism or reuptake (cocaine).

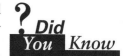

? ***Did You Know***

With spontaneous inspiration, venous return to the right ventricle is increased, resulting in prolonged ejection time compared with the left ventricle. This causes the pulmonic valve to close later than the aortic valve, producing respiration-induced variation in splitting of S_2 (physiologic splitting).

Table 3-1 Cardiac Reflexes that Affect Heart Rate

Reflex	Afferent Sensor	Efferent Response
Baroreceptor	Baroreceptors sense blood pressure in carotid sinus (CN IX) and aortic arch (CN X)	*Low blood pressure* → increased SNS tone → increased heart rate, inotropy, and vasoconstriction *High blood pressure* → increased PNS tone (CN X) → reduced heart rate and inotropy
Atrial Receptor (Bainbridge)	Stretch receptors in the right atrium sense CVP (CN X)	*High CVP* → increased SNS tone and decreased PNS tone (CN X) → increased heart rate
Chemoreceptor	PaO2 and pH sensors in carotid bodies (CN IX) and aortic bodies (CN X)	*Low PaO2 and pH* → increased ventilation and PNS tone → decreased heart rate and inotropy
Oculocardiac	Stretch receptors in extra-ocular muscles sense pressure on globe (ciliary nerves and CN V)	*High globe pressure* → increased PNS tone (CN X) → decreased heart rate
Cushing	Increased ICP	*High ICP* → increased SNS tone → increased inotropy and vasoconstriction → low heart rate (baroreceptor reflex)

CN, cranial nerve; SNS, sympathetic nervous system; PNS, parasympathetic nervous system; CVP, central venous pressure; PaO2, arterial partial pressure of oxygen; ICP, intracranial pressure.

IV. Coronary Physiology

Resting *coronary blood flow* is approximately 250 mL/min (~5% of total cardiac output) and can be increased up to fivefold during strenuous physical exercise. Coronary blood flow is influenced by physical, neural, and metabolic factors. The primary physical factor is *coronary perfusion pressure*—the difference between aortic pressure and either LV pressure (left coronary artery) or RV pressure (right coronary artery). Extravascular coronary artery compression (due to contracting myocardium), heart rate (altering the duration of diastole), vessel length, and blood viscosity also impact coronary perfusion. The primary neural factor is SNS tone to the heart, which increases coronary blood flow when increased aortic pressure outweighs reduced coronary flow associated with stronger myocardial contraction and shortened diastolic filling time (tachycardia). Active vasodilation of coronary arteries is limited because vagal stimulation has no apparent effect on vessel caliber and, unlike skeletal muscle vasculature, sympathetic cholinergic innervation is not present in coronary arteries. However, β_2-adrenergic receptor–mediated vasodilation can occur in small coronary arterioles and accounts for ~25% of coronary vasodilation observed during exercise-induced hyperemia. Lastly, increased myocardial metabolism is associated with the bulk of coronary vasodilation through the action of yet-to-be-defined local metabolic factors.

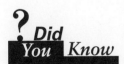

? Did You Know

Because the subendocardium is exposed to higher pressures during systole than the subepicardial layer, the former is more susceptible to ischemia, particularly in settings of coronary stenosis, ventricular hypertrophy, or tachycardia.

Coronary blood flow varies with the cardiac cycle, and is determined by the difference between aortic pressure and tissue (wall) pressure. LCA flow is highly variable—it peaks during early diastole when perfusion pressure is highest and approaches zero in early systole when LV contraction (and coronary compression) is greatest. In contrast, RCA flow is more constant throughout the cardiac cycle and peaks during systole due to the lesser muscle mass and contraction of the RV. Because the subendocardium is exposed to higher pressures during systole than the subepicardial layer, the former is more susceptible to ischemia, particularly in settings of coronary stenosis, ventricular hypertrophy, or tachycardia. However, *subendocardial ischemia* is partially offset by enhanced capillary anastomoses and local metabolic vasodilation in this layer.

VIDEO 3-5
Coronary Perfusion

The heart has the highest *oxygen extraction ratio* of any organ (~70%); as a result, under normal conditions the venous oxygen saturation of blood in the coronary sinus (~30%) is lower than that in the right atrium (~70%). *Myocardial oxygen consumption* is determined by heart rate, myocardial contractility, and ventricular wall stress (including preload and afterload), with the major determinants being the heart rate and the magnitude of LV pressure developed during the isovolumic contraction period. Because of this high extraction ratio, increased myocardial oxygen demand can only be met through increased coronary blood flow. Thus, the dominant controller of coronary blood flow is myocardial oxygen consumption. The coronary circulation is ideally constructed for this purpose, as its myocardial capillary density is approximately eight times greater than that of skeletal muscle (approximately one capillary for each cardiac muscle fiber). When myocardial oxygen supply is unable to meet increases in myocardial oxygen demand (e.g., coronary artery stenosis), *myocardial ischemia* occurs. Ischemia is first clinically manifested by increased LV end-diastolic volume and decreased LV compliance and can progress to wall motion abnormalities, decreased ejection fraction, ECG abnormalities (ST-segment changes), *congestive heart failure* (CHF), and ultimately *cardiogenic shock*.

VIDEO 3-6
Myocardial Oxygen Supply-Demand

V. The Pressure-Volume Diagram

The mechanical events in the LV cardiac cycle depicted in Figure 3-7 can also be presented graphically as the LV *pressure-volume* (P-V) *diagram*, shown in Figure 3-8. With pressure plotted on the vertical axis and volume on the horizontal axis, a near-rectangular "loop" is formed in a counterclockwise path beginning in the lower right at end diastole (low LV pressure and high LV volume). It consists of four phases of the cardiac cycle: isovolumic contraction period (vertical right line), systole (horizontal top line), isovolumic relaxation period (vertical left line), and diastole (horizontal bottom line). The line drawn from the origin to the end-systolic "corner" of the P-V loop defines the *end-systolic pressure-volume relation* (ESPVR), with the slope of this line being an index of myocardial contractility. Similarly, the line drawn from the origin to the end-diastolic corner of the P-V loop defines the *end-diastolic pressure-volume relation* (EDPVR), the slope that can be used to quantify LV compliance.

VIDEO 3-7
Pressure-Volume Loop

The size and shape of the P-V diagram, as well as the slopes of the ESPVR and EDPVR lines, allow recognition of various cardiac events without ECG correlation and will change predictably across a range of pathologic states such as ventricular dysfunction or valvular heart disease (2,3). For example, the area of the P-V diagram defines LV *stroke work* for the cardiac cycle,

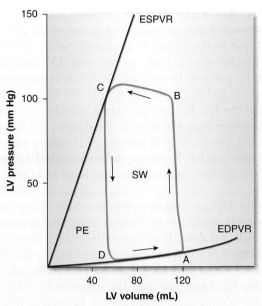

Figure 3-8 A steady-state left ventricular (LV) pressure volume diagram. The cardiac cycle proceeds in a time-dependent counterclockwise direction (*arrows*). Points A, B, C, and D correspond to LV end diastole (closure of the mitral valve), opening of the aortic valve, LV end systole (closure of the aortic valve), and opening of the mitral valve, respectively. Segments AB, BC, CD, and DA represent isovolumic contraction, ejection, isovolumic relaxation, and filling, respectively. The LV is constrained to operate within the boundaries of the end-systolic and end-diastolic pressure-volume relations (ESPVR and EDPVR, respectively). The area inscribed by the LV pressure-volume diagram is stroke work (SW) performed during the cardiac cycle. The area to the left of the LV pressure-volume diagram between ESPVR and EDPVR is the remaining potential energy (PE) of the system. (From Pagel PS, Kampine JP, Stowe DF. Cardiac anatomy and physiology. In: Barash PG, Cullen BF, Stoelting RK, et al. *Handbook of Clinical Anesthesia*, 7th ed. Philadelphia: Lippincott Williams & Wilkins, 2013:239–262, with permission.)

whereas a right shift in the vertical right portion of the diagram indicates an increase in LV preload. Examples of P-V diagrams indicating impaired LV contractility and diastolic dysfunction associated with decreased LV compliance are shown in Figure 3-9.

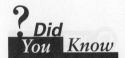

? Did You Know

In isolated cardiac muscle, contractile tension increases with stimulation frequency and is maximal at 150 to 180 contractions per second (Bowditch effect). However, such high heart rates reduce diastolic filling time in the intact heart and are only seen in special settings (dysrhythmias, strenuous exercise).

VI. Factors that Determine Systolic Function

A. Left Ventricular Pump

Each ventricle essentially operates as a hydraulic pump whose performance is defined by its ability to collect blood (diastolic function) and eject blood (systolic function), which is determined by the factors summarized in Figure 3-10. The key determinants of systolic function are the blood volume ejected (*stroke volume*), the volume efficiency of blood ejection (*ejection fraction*), the pumping frequency (*heart rate*), the volume of blood filling the pump (*preload*), the downstream resistance the ejected blood must overcome (*afterload*), and the contractile ability of the ventricle (*myocardial contractility*).

B. Cardiac Output and Ejection Fraction

Pump performance of the LV is practically measured as the *cardiac output*, defined as the stroke volume (SV) times the heart rate. The SV is the difference between the *end-diastolic volume* (EDV) and *end-systolic volume* (ESV). As shown in

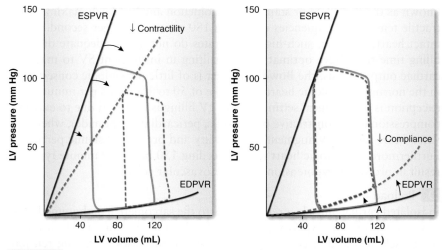

Figure 3-9 These schematic illustrations demonstrate alterations in the steady state left ventricular (LV) pressure-volume diagram produced by a reduction in myocardial contractility as indicated by a decrease in the slope of the end-systolic pressure-volume relation (end-systolic pressure-volume relations [ESPVR]; *left*) and a decrease in LV compliance as indicated by an increase in the position of the end-diastolic pressure-volume relation (end-diastolic pressure-volume relations [EDPVR]; *right*). These diagrams emphasize that heart failure may result from LV systolic or diastolic dysfunction independently. (From Pagel PS, Kampine JP, Stowe DF. Cardiac anatomy and physiology. In: Barash PG, Cullen BF, Stoelting RK, et al. *Clinical Anesthesia*, 7th ed. Philadelphia: Lippincott Williams & Wilkins, 2013:239–262, with permission.)

Figure 3-8, a normal EDV of ~120 mL and ESV of ~40 mL would yield a SV of ~80 mL. The normal LV ejection fraction (SV/EDV) is therefore 67%. Thus, pump efficiency is impaired (i.e., low ejection fraction) in settings such as a dilated LV with elevated EDV and normal SV (e.g., dilated cardiomyopathy) or a normal-sized LV with poor contractility and low SV (e.g., myocardial infarction).

C. Heart Rate

In isolated heart muscle, contractile tension increases with stimulation frequency due to an increase in intracellular calcium content. This effect is

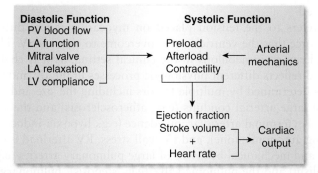

Figure 3-10 The major factors that determine left ventricular (LV) diastolic (*left*) and systolic (*right*) function. Note that pulmonary venous (PV) blood flow, left atrial (LA) function, mitral valve integrity, LA relaxation, and LV compliance combine to determine LV preload. (From Pagel PS, Kampine JP, Stowe DF. Cardiac anatomy and physiology. In: Barash PG, Cullen BF, Stoelting RK, et al. *Handbook of Clinical Anesthesia*, 7th ed. Philadelphia: Lippincott Williams & Wilkins, 2013:239–262, with permission.)

known as the Bowditch or staircase phenomenon and results in maximal contractile tension at frequencies of 150 to 180 contractions per second. In the intact heart, however, such high heart rates do not allow adequate diastolic filling time to achieve optimal EDV, resulting in insufficient SV to maintain cardiac output. Thus, the Bowditch effect is of little physiologic consequence in the normal physiologic heart rate range of 50 to 150 beats per minute. The exception is with clinical settings where LV filling is impaired due to extrinsic compression (e.g., constrictive pericarditis, pericardial tamponade), where elevated heart rates may augment contractility and preserve systemic perfusion. Furthermore, pathologic heart rates exceeding 150 beats per minute typically result in profound hypotension and cardiovascular collapse.

D. Preload

In isolated cardiac muscle, preload refers to the sarcomere length immediately prior to contraction. Applying force (preload) to the resting muscle stretches the muscle to the desired length and results in increases in resting tension, initial velocity of contraction, and peak contractile tension. This relation between preload (resting myocardial length) and contractile performance is termed the *Frank-Starling relationship*. In the intact ventricle, this relation is between preload (EDV) and systolic ventricular pressure and SV, both of which influence cardiac output (SV times heart rate) and ventricular stroke work (SV times mean arterial pressure).

Because EDV influences both systolic pressure and SV, preload is an important determinant of cardiac output and is moderated by circulating blood volume, venous tone, and posture. Furthermore, when afterload is held constant, the effects of preload on SV and cardiac output are strongly influenced by ventricular performance. For example, the failing LV is less preload sensitive than the normal LV; as a result, increases in EDV produce a lesser response in SV, resulting in pulmonary congestion. Conversely, when contractility is enhanced by circulating or endogenous catecholamines, the LV is more preload sensitive, with increases in EDV leading to an amplified SV response. Preload is most reliably assessed by echocardiographic measurement of EDV (4). In clinical practice, however, a variety of surrogates for EDV may also be considered indicators of preload, each of which can potentially be affected by specific anatomic and physiologic conditions that can introduce inaccuracies in preload assessment (Fig. 3-11).

VIDEO 3-8
The Starling Curve

E. Afterload

Afterload refers to the tension placed on myocardial fibers during systole and is the force that the ventricle must overcome to eject its SV. The concept of afterload can seem nebulous in the clinical setting, as it is challenging to measure and reflects different physiologic processes in the LV and the RV. LV afterload is determined by multiple factors including the size and mechanical behavior of large arterial conduits (e.g., atherosclerosis) and the aortic valve (e.g., stenosis), terminal arteriolar impedance (e.g., hypoxia-induced vasodilation, varying autonomic tone), and LV wall stress. RV afterload is determined by the size and mechanical behavior of large pulmonary arteries (e.g., pulmonary embolism) and the pulmonic valve (e.g., stenosis), pulmonary arteriolar impedance (hypoxia- and hypercarbia-induced vasoconstriction), and RV wall stress.

The important relation between ventricular volume, wall stress, and myocardial work is based on the balance of opposing forces that help maintain a spherical shell at a certain size, which is described by *Laplace's law*

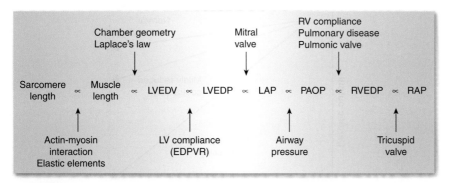

Figure 3-11 This schematic diagram depicts factors that influence experimental and clinical estimates of sarcomere length as a pure index of the preload of the contracting left ventricular (LV) myocyte. LVEDV, LV end-diastolic volume; LVEDP, LV end-diastolic pressure; EDPVR, end-diastolic pressure-volume relation; LAP, left atrial pressure; PAOP, pulmonary artery occlusion pressure; RV, right ventricle; RVEDP, RV end-diastolic pressure; RAP, right atrial pressure. (From Pagel PS, Kampine JP, Stowe DF. Cardiac anatomy and physiology. In: Barash PG, Cullen BF, Stoelting RK, et al. *Clinical Anesthesia*, 7th ed. Philadelphia: Lippincott Williams & Wilkins, 2013:239–262, with permission.)

(Fig. 3-12). As an idealized spherical shell, the LV maintains any given size due to the balance between ventricular pressure (acting to enlarge the LV) and wall stress (acting to resist LV enlargement). Laplace's law relates LV pressure (p) and wall stress (σ) in the equation $[p = (2 * \sigma * h)/r]$, where r is the sphere's radius and h is the LV wall thickness. Thus, increases in either LV pressure (e.g., essential hypertension) or LV size (e.g., chronic mitral insufficiency) result in increased wall stress and increased afterload. In order for myocardial cells to generate greater tension and wall stress in these settings, greater energy expenditure is required, thereby increasing both myocardial oxygen consumption and the risk of myocardial ischemia.

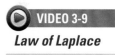

VIDEO 3-9

Law of Laplace

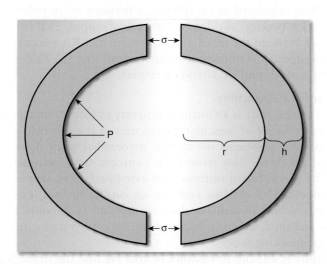

Figure 3-12 This schematic diagram depicts the opposing forces within a theoretical left ventricular (LV) sphere that determines Laplace's law. LV pressure (P) pushes the sphere apart, whereas wall stress (σ) holds the sphere together. r, LV radius; h, LV thickness. (From Pagel PS, Kampine JP, Stowe DF. Cardiac anatomy and physiology. In: Barash PG, Cullen BF, Stoelting RK, et al. *Clinical Anesthesia*, 7th ed. Philadelphia: Lippincott Williams & Wilkins, 2013:239–262, with permission.)

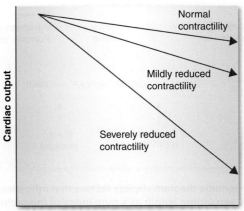

Figure 3-13 The effects of increasing afterload (systemic vascular resistance) on ventricular performance (cardiac output) are shown for three different states of contractility. Under normal conditions, increases in afterload reduce left ventricle (LV) performance. However, the failing LV is more afterload sensitive than the healthy LV; thus, a greater decrease in cardiac output occurs as myocardial contractility is progressively impaired.

As with preload, changes in afterload can significantly influence SV and cardiac output, particularly when ventricular performance is abnormal. For example, the failing LV with reduced contractility is more afterload sensitive than the healthy LV and will demonstrate a proportionately greater decrease in cardiac output when afterload is increased (Fig. 3-13).

As with preload, direct measurement of afterload in the clinical setting is challenging. The most common surrogate assessment of afterload is the calculation of vascular resistance using measurements of cardiac output and pressure changes across either the pulmonary vasculature (*pulmonary vascular resistance* [PVR]) or the systemic vasculature (*systemic vascular resistance* [SVR]). PVR is calculated as the difference between mean pulmonary artery pressure and LA pressure divided by the cardiac output. SVR is calculated as the difference between the mean aortic pressure and RA pressure divided by the cardiac output. It is important to understand that the PVR and SVR are only estimates of RV and LV afterload, respectively.

F. Myocardial Contractility

Myocardial contractility is an intrinsic property of cardiac muscle. It refers to the force and velocity of muscular contraction of the ventricle under conditions of load and represents the systolic myocardial work done for a given preload and afterload. Also termed the inotropic state, contractility can be influenced by a number of intrinsic and extrinsic factors that increase inotropy (autonomic SNS activity, endogenous catecholamines, exogenous catecholamines, calcium, digitalis) or decrease inotropy (autonomic PNS activity, myocardial ischemia, hypoxia, hypercarbia, cardiomyopathy, hypocalcemia, β_1-adrenergic blocking drugs).

Contractility is difficult to measure in vivo because the strength of cardiac contraction is also determined by preload and afterload. As noted earlier, the maximum rate of rise in LV pressure (+dP/dt) that occurs during the brief isovolumic contraction period is one useful indirect index of LV contractility, in part because it is largely afterload independent. In contrast, the Frank-Starling relationship dictates that +dP/dt is highly dependent on preload. LV pressure

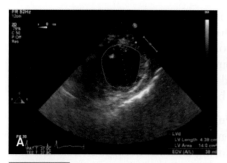 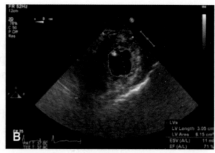

Figure 3-14 Calculation of fractional area change from left ventricle (LV) midpapillary short axis images obtained at end diastole (**A**) and end systole (**B**). The LV endocardial border surrounding the black LV chamber is manually traced (excluding the papillary muscles), and the inscribed area is calculated by integrating software. The LV ejection fraction is determined as the difference between the end-diastolic area and the end-systolic area, divided by the end-diastolic area. (From Pagel PS, Kampine JP, Stowe DF. Cardiac anatomy and physiology. In: Barash PG, Cullen BF, Stoelting RK, et al. *Clinical Anesthesia,* 7th ed. Philadelphia: Lippincott Williams & Wilkins, 2013:239–262, with permission.)

(and hence +dP/dt) can only be directly measured invasively during cardiac catheterization but can be estimated by transesophageal echocardiography (TEE). The two most practical surrogate assessments of contractility by TEE are the ejection fraction (Fig. 3-14) and P-V diagram analysis of the ESPVR (Figs. 3-8 and 3-9).

VII. Factors that Determine Diastolic Function

A. Heart Chambers

In addition to its ability to eject blood during ventricular systole, pump performance of the heart is also dependent on its diastolic function—the ability to fully and efficiently collect blood prior to ventricular contraction. The atria contribute to this process as thin-walled, low-pressure chambers that function more as large reservoir conduits, in contrast to their respective thick-walled, high-pressure ventricles that function as forward propelling blood pumps.

B. Left Ventricular Response to Load

Diastolic loading of the ventricle generally occurs by adding volume (preload) to the chamber or by increasing resistance (afterload) to outflow. The ventricle responds to load by lengthening its myocardial fibers, increasing wall stress, or both, thereby modulating ventricular relaxation, filling, and compliance. Because such changes in load are dynamic and occur frequently both in daily activities (e.g., exercise) and in the perioperative setting (e.g., blood loss, fluid resuscitation, volatile anesthetics), the ability of the ventricle to rapidly adjust to such changes and ultimately maintain cardiac output (termed *homometric autoregulation*) defines diastolic function.

For the LV, *diastolic dysfunction* occurs when the ventricle cannot rapidly adjust to increases in load, resulting in persistently elevated LV volumes or pressures that precipitate LV failure. Diastolic dysfunction occurs when LV relaxation or filling is impaired or when the LV becomes less compliant. This can occur as an isolated abnormality (with intact systolic function) or in association with systolic dysfunction (5). Diastolic dysfunction is more common in the elderly and often associated with conditions that increase ventricular wall stiffness or afterload (e.g., LV hypertrophy). Because prior knowledge of patients' diastolic function can affect clinical management, an understanding of its assessment strategies is vital. Unfortunately, no single index of diastolic function completely characterizes this portion of the cardiac cycle or accurately predicts those at greatest risk of developing heart failure in response to changing load conditions. Thus, both invasive and noninvasive assessments of ventricular relaxation, filling, and compliance may be needed.

C. Invasive Assessment of Diastolic Function

Complete and rapid *LV relaxation* is necessary to facilitate efficient passive ventricular filling and maximize EDV during diastole. Because LV relaxation is an active, energy-dependent process involving dissociation of contractile proteins in myocardial cells, myocardial ischemia is a frequent cause of impaired LV relaxation. Thus, ischemia can impair cardiac output and precipitate CHF through both diastolic and systolic mechanisms. Invasive assessment of LV relaxation is performed during cardiac catheterization by directly measuring the time course of LV pressure decline (–dP/dt) during the isovolumic relaxation period. The two most commonly calculated indices of LV relaxation from this method are the maximal rate of LV pressure reduction (smaller values of –dP/dt indicate impaired LV relaxation) and the time constant of LV relaxation (prolonged time constants indicate impaired LV relaxation). Although these indices have prognostic value, noninvasive techniques have largely supplanted them.

D. Noninvasive Assessment of Diastolic Function

As noted earlier, P-V diagram analysis of the EDPVR by echocardiography is one common method for assessing LV compliance (Figs. 3-8 and 3-9). Also, because the isovolumic relaxation period for the LV is defined as the portion of the cardiac cycle between when the aortic valve closes and the mitral valve opens (Fig. 3-7), the length of this period is related to LV relaxation. Impaired LV relaxation results in a prolonged *isovolumic relaxation time* (IVRT). The IVRT can be measured by observing aortic and mitral valve closure by echocardiography and, in the absence of aortic or mitral valve disease, is inversely proportional to LV relaxation.

A second method of assessing LV relaxation uses Doppler echocardiographic measurement of blood flow velocities across the mitral valve. During diastole, two distinct flow patterns occur at this location: an early E peak associated with early LV filling and a later A peak corresponding to LA contraction. When LV relaxation is prolonged, the E wave deceleration time is prolonged, the A wave velocity is increased, and the ratio of these two flow velocities decreases (E/A < 1). As diastolic function worsens and LA pressures increase, the E wave velocities increase, first to an E/A ratio in the normal range (E/A > 1), then to higher ratios (E/A > 2) (6).

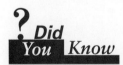

In the elderly, age-related autonomic nervous system dysfunction interferes with the baroreceptor reflex arc, such that hypotension-induced compensatory increases in blood pressure and heart rate are less pronounced than in young adults.

VIII. Blood Pressure

A. Systemic, Pulmonary, and Venous

Cardiac output enters the systemic and pulmonary circulations from the LV and RV, respectively, each of which contain serial arterial, microcirculatory, and venous components. Systemic blood pressures exceed pulmonary blood pressures due to differing anatomic structures and pump capabilities of the RV and LV, significantly lower vascular impedance of the pulmonary circulation compared with the systemic circulation, and nearly identical cardiac outputs in both circulations, the fluid mechanics analog of *Ohm's law* (pressure = flow × resistance).

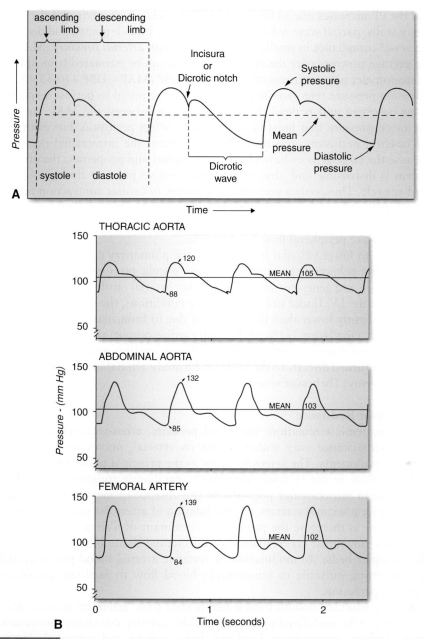

Figure 3-15 The typical aortic pulse pressure waveform is shown (**A**), with each pulse consisting of a brief, sharp ascending limb, followed by a more prolonged descending limb. Each pulse is easily separated into systole and diastole by the dicrotic notch, with the peak pressure corresponding the systolic pressure and the lowest pressure being the diastolic pressure. Mean arterial pressure is the average pressure over the entire pulse period (**B**). The pulse pressure waveform changes as one moves distally in the systemic arterial tree due to arterial branching and changes in vessel elasticity.

The typical aortic *pressure waveform* is shown in Figure 3-15. The peak of the wave is the *systolic blood pressure* (SBP) and the nadir is the *diastolic blood pressure* (DBP), with the difference between the two termed the *pulse pressure* (PP). As the pressure wave moves distally in the arterial tree, the sharp dicrotic notch becomes more scooped, the SBP increases, the DBP decreases, and the PP increases due to the combination of elastic properties of the large artery walls, partial wave reflection at large artery branch points, and decreasing vessel compliance in smaller arteries. The *mean arterial pressure* (MAP) is the average pressure over the entire period and can be estimated from sphygmomanometer measurements of the SBP and DBP (MAP = DBP + [0.33 × PP]). Perfusion pressure refers to the driving pressure required to perfuse a specific tissue or organ and is defined as the difference between the MAP and the resistance pressure that must be overcome to affect perfusion. For example, the cerebral perfusion pressure is the MAP minus the intracranial pressure. Because the large arteries have elastic components and properties, the arterial system is distensible and able to maintain positive pressure throughout the cardiac cycle. Thus, only a portion of the energy of cardiac contraction results in forward capillary flow, with the remainder stored as potential energy in the elastic recoil of the arteries, a property known as the *Windkessel effect*, which serves to make peripheral flow less pulsatile.

Because of lower vascular impedance in the pulmonary circulation, the RV accomplishes pulmonary perfusion with lower systolic pressures and less oxygen consumption and generates significantly lower arterial outflow pressures compared with the LV. Under normal anatomic conditions, the cardiac output of the RV is slightly lower than that of the LV due to bronchial blood flow from the systemic circulation (~1% of the total cardiac output) that returns deoxygenated blood directly to the left atrium. A very small portion of the cardiac output is returned directly to the LV from coronary arterial luminal shunts and coronary veins (Thebesian veins).

B. Vascular Resistance

For the systemic circulation, the blood pressure, cross-sectional area, and volume capacitance vary widely across its arterial, microcirculatory, and venous components. The arterioles serve as the principal points of resistance to blood flow in the systemic circulation, producing roughly 95% reduction in mean intravascular pressure. In the absence of mechanical obstruction in more proximal arteries, the modulation of arteriolar vascular smooth muscle tone is therefore the principal determinant of SVR and serves three important functions: (a) regulation of differential tissue blood flow to specific vascular beds; (b) modulation of systemic arterial blood pressure; and (c) converting pulsatile to nonpulsatile blood flow to facilitate consistent capillary perfusion.

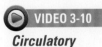

VIDEO 3-10

Circulatory System Blood Flow and Pressures

Resting vascular smooth muscle exerts mild tonic arteriolar vasoconstriction that can be modulated by autonomic SNS activity, circulating hormones, drugs, ambient temperature, local metabolic activity, and autoregulation to achieve further vasoconstriction or vasodilation. For example, autonomic SNS stimulation results in norepinephrine release that activates a β-adrenergic receptors in vascular smooth muscle to augment resting vasoconstriction. In vascular beds containing both α- and β$_2$-adrenergic receptors (e.g., skeletal muscle), exogenous epinephrine at low doses will selectively activate β$_2$-adrenergic receptors and cause vasodilation. Whereas high doses will result in predominate activation of α-adrenergic receptors and lead to enhanced vasoconstriction. Local metabolic activity plays an important role in regional control of vascular resistance because arterioles lie within the organ itself and are exposed to the local environment. When blood flow to tissue is inadequate to meet metabolic needs, local factors (e.g., high carbon dioxide [CO$_2$], low pH) result in vasodilation and increased blood flow to meet metabolic demand.

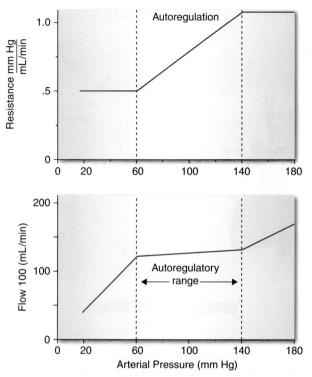

Figure 3-16 Autoregulation occurs when blood flow (*lower panel*) is maintained relatively constant over a wide range of mean arterial pressures (in this case 60 to 140 mm Hg). This process is accomplished by changes in vascular resistance (*upper panel*) that are independent of neural and hormonal influence.

Autoregulation refers to the intrinsic tendency of a specific organ or tissue bed to maintain constant blood flow despite changes in arterial pressure, independent of hormonal or neural mechanisms. Autoregulation is typically active within a specific range of arterial pressures, within which constant flow is achieved by changes in vascular resistance (Fig. 3-16). Outside this range, blood flow varies proportionately to arterial pressure, with clinical consequences of ischemia (low pressure) or hyperemia (high pressure). The human organs with the most clinically relevant autoregulation features are those whose perfusion is physiologically critical—the brain, kidney, and heart (7).

C. Baroreceptor Function

In addition to the immediate regulation of blood flow by autoregulation at the tissue level, more widespread and short-term adjustments in systemic arterial pressure are also regulated by the baroreceptor reflex (Table 3-1, Fig. 3-17). This inverse relation between arterial blood pressure and heart rate was first described by Etienne Marey in 1859 and serves to preserve cardiac output and arterial pressure under varying conditions such as postural changes, exercise, and hypovolemia. The afferent limb of the reflex is initiated by pressure-sensitive stretch receptors in the carotid sinus and the aortic arch that relay sensory information to the medullary vasomotor center via the glossopharyngeal and vagus nerves. The efferent limb of the reflex includes two possible responses: (a) elevated arterial pressure results in increased vagal PNS tone and decreased SNS tone, which modifies heart rate downward at the SA and AV nodes and reduces both myocardial contractility and arteriolar

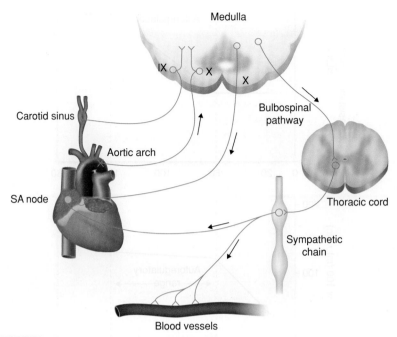

Figure 3-17 The afferent limb of the baroreceptor reflex is initiated by baroreceptors in the carotid sinus (glossopharyngeal nerve) and aortic arch (vagus nerve) with transmission to the medulla. Elevated blood pressure results in efferent vagal nerve traffic to the heart that slows heart rate and reduces contractility (to reduce blood pressure). In contrast, low blood pressure results in efferent sympathetic tone via the spinal cord and sympathetic chain that increases both heart rate and contractility, and also results in peripheral vasoconstriction. SA, sinoatrial.

vasoconstriction to diminish both cardiac output and arterial pressure; (b) low arterial pressure results in increased SNS traffic at various levels of the sympathetic chain to modify heart rate upward at the SA node and augment ventricular contractility to enhance cardiac output, as well as increase arteriolar vasoconstriction to rapidly increase arterial pressure.

One clinical application of the baroreceptor reflex is the performance of external carotid massage in patients with supraventricular tachycardia. This will stimulate afferent glossopharyngeal nerve traffic and enhance reflex PNS vagal tone to slow pathologic tachycardias. The baroreceptor reflex also underlies the typical observation of compensatory tachycardia in patients with hypovolemic hypotension. Conversely, abnormal baroreceptor reflex responses can occur in patients with neurologic impairments at any point along the reflex arc. For example, age-related autonomic dysfunction in the elderly is often manifest by postural syncope due to reductions in cerebral perfusion pressure and flow.

IX. Venous Return

A. Vascular Compliance, Capacitance, and Control

As blood exits the capillary bed, it passes first through venules and then a steadily decreasing number of veins of increasing size. The vascular system cross-sectional area in the small and large veins is similar to that in the small and large arteries. Compared with their corresponding arterial structures, however, venous structures are generally slightly larger in diameter, have thinner walls containing less vascular smooth muscle, and possess far greater capacitance (lower vascular resistance). This 10 to 20 times higher compliance means that veins can accommodate large changes in blood volume with only a small change in pressure. Venous smooth muscle receives SNS innervation, which when activated decreases venous compliance and promotes venous return to the RA.

B. Muscle Action, Intrathoracic Pressure, and Body Position

Venous return to the RA contributes to ventricular preload and is primarily determined by extravascular factors. These include skeletal muscle contraction in the limbs (*muscle pump*), intrathoracic pressure changes associated with respiratory activity (*thoraco-abdominal pump*), external vena cava compression, and forces of gravity associated with postural changes (8,9). Skeletal muscle contractions in the arms and legs, in combination with pressure-passive one-way venous valves in peripheral veins, augment venous return, particularly during exercise. Muscle contraction compresses veins within large muscle groups and forces venous blood centrally, whereas skeletal muscle relaxation decompresses veins and draws in blood from the distal limb and adjacent veins. Repeated compression–decompression cycles rapidly propel venous blood centrally and enhance venous return. Patients with incompetent venous valves are unable to augment their venous return with exercise or postural changes and may experience syncope under these conditions.

Spontaneous respiration changes the transmural pressure in veins passing through the intrathoracic cavity and modifies venous return. During inspiration, diaphragmatic descent and thoracic cage expansion create negative intrathoracic pressure, while at the same time elevating intra-abdominal pressure. These combined forces increase the pressure gradient favoring blood return from the subdiaphragmatic vena cava to the RA. Negative intrathoracic pressure also reduces thoracic vena cava and RA pressures and further enhances venous return from the head, neck, and upper extremities. Conversely, spontaneous expiration increases intrathoracic pressure and impairs venous return. The overall effect of spontaneous ventilation is to enhance venous return compared with apneic conditions because mean intrathoracic pressures are slightly negative over the entire respiratory cycle. In contrast, positive pressure ventilation increases mean intrathoracic pressures, impairs venous return, and can negatively impact cardiac output.

C. Blood Volume and Distribution

Total body water constitutes ~60% of body weight (42 L in a 70-kg person), with ~40% (28 L) in the intracellular space and ~20% (14 L) in the extracellular space. Plasma volume accounts for one-fifth (3 L) of the extracellular volume, and erythrocyte volume (2 L) is part of the intracellular volume; therefore, blood volume is ~5 L in a 70-kg person. Blood volume is nonuniformly distributed throughout the circulatory tree, with approximately 65% in the systemic venous system, 15% in the systemic arterial system, 10% in the pulmonary circulation, and the remainder in the heart and systemic microcirculation.

X. Microcirculation

A. Capillary Diffusion, Oncotic Pressure, and Starling's Law

The ultimate purpose of the cardiovascular system is to deliver oxygen and nutrients to tissues, and to remove CO_2 and metabolic waste products from the cellular level. This process occurs in the rich network of capillaries that are only 5 to 10 μm in diameter, yet so overwhelming in number that the overall surface area of the network is 20 times greater than that of all the small and larger arteries. Capillary density is greatest in metabolically active tissues (e.g., myocardium, skeletal muscle) and lowest in less active tissues (e.g., fat, cartilage).

Water and solutes diffuse in both directions across the capillary wall, with water and water-soluble molecules (e.g., sodium chloride, glucose) traversing the wall through clefts between adjacent endothelial cells, lipophilic molecules (oxygen, CO_2) moving directly across the endothelial cells, and large molecules traversing through large clefts or by pinocytosis within endoplasmic vesicles. Thus, the capillary wall acts as a semipermeable membrane across which water, gases, and small substrates move primarily by diffusion according to concentration gradients (10). In addition, when there is a difference between hydrostatic forces and osmotic forces across the capillary wall, water movement also occurs by filtration. In the microvasculature, osmotic pressure is largely determined by protein concentration (particularly albumin) and is termed *oncotic pressure*. According to the *Starling hypothesis*, fluid filtration across the porous capillary wall is determined by the balance between the hydrostatic and oncotic pressure gradients across the wall, as well as by the size and number of intercellular clefts. The hydrostatic pressure gradient favors water movement out of the capillary and is slightly greater than the oncotic pressure gradient that favors water movement into the capillary. The relation between these factors is governed by the *Starling equation*:

$$F = Kf * ([Pc - Pt] - \sigma [\pi c - \pi i]),$$

where F is the fluid movement across the capillary wall, Kf is the filtration constant of the capillary membrane (reflecting its permeability), Pc is the capillary hydrostatic pressure (higher on the arteriolar side of the capillary than on the venular side of the capillary), Pt is the tissue hydrostatic pressure (typically near zero), σ is the reflection coefficient (a correction factor for protein permeability of the capillary wall), πc is the plasma oncotic pressure, and πi is the interstitial oncotic pressure.

A high Kf indicates a highly water permeable capillary, such as in the presence of histamine, whereas a low Kf indicates low capillary permeability. The factors in the Starling equation including typical pressure values are illustrated in Figure 3-18.

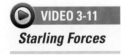
VIDEO 3-11
Starling Forces

The bulk flow of water and proteins across the capillary membrane is generally in the direction from the intravascular to the interstitial space. Highly permeable lymphatic capillaries collect this bulk flow in tissues and return the fluid and proteins (predominately albumin) through lymphatic vessels of progressively increasing size, facilitated by intermittent skeletal muscle activity, smooth muscle in the lymphatic walls, and one-way valves. The volume of fluid returned to the circulation (largely through the thoracic duct) in 24 hours is approximately equal to the total plasma volume.

B. Precapillary and Postcapillary Sphincter Control

Capillary blood flow in any given tissue bed is highly variable and is controlled by the precapillary and postcapillary sphincters. Transmural pressure (intravascular minus extravascular pressure) and contraction/relaxation of the precapillary and postcapillary sphincters are the primary determinants of capillary flow, with the latter mediated by both neural and local humoral factors. Unlike vasoconstriction in more proximal arteriolar beds that adjust but do not abolish tissue blood flow, precapillary sphincter can fully occlude

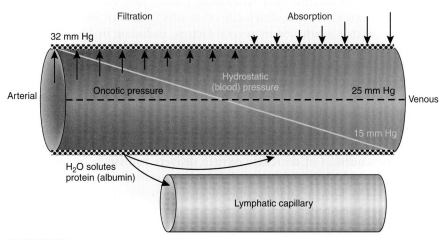

Filtration

Absorption

32 mm Hg

Hydrostatic
(blood) pressure

Arterial

Oncotic pressure

25 mm Hg

Venous

15 mm Hg

H_2O solutes
protein (albumin)

Lymphatic capillary

Figure 3-18 Fluid movement across the capillary membrane is determined by the permeability of the membrane to water, solutes, and protein; the hydrostatic pressure difference across the membrane; and the oncotic pressure difference across the membrane, and is summarized by the Starling equation (see text). The hydrostatic pressure gradient varies across the length of the capillary, favoring fluid movement out of the capillary to a greater degree on the arterial end. The oncotic pressure gradient is uniform and favors fluid movement into the capillary. Net fluid movement is toward the interstitium, with lymphatic capillaries collecting the excess filtrate and returning it to the circulation.

the vessel lumen, directing flow away from capillary beds into nearby arteriovenous shunts. For example, in cold environments precapillary sphincter tone is increased to shunt blood away from cutaneous beds to retain heat. Abnormal perioperative thermoregulation occurs when this tone is impaired by various anesthetic agents. In addition, by reducing capillary flow, precapillary sphincter contraction also reduces fluid filtration due to a reduction in Pc. Postcapillary sphincter contraction also reduces capillary flow, but increases fluid filtration due to an increase in Pc.

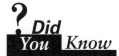

? Did You Know

Unlike vasoconstriction in systemic arteriolar beds that adjust but do not abolish tissue blood flow, precapillary sphincters can completely occlude the vessel lumen and direct flow away from selected capillary beds (e.g., shunting of blood away from the cutaneous circulation in cold environments).

C. Viscosity and Rheology

The flow of any fluid in any tube is always dependent on the pressure difference between ends of the tube; in the absence of a gradient, no flow will occur. As noted earlier, the simplest description of this phenomenon is the fluid mechanics analog of Ohm's law (flow = Δ pressure/resistance). However, both tube size and physical characteristics of the fluid, particularly its viscosity (a measure of its resistance to deformation by shear forces), require a more detailed relation between flow and pressure that applies to the vascular system. Through a series of experiment in glass tubes, Poiseuille described such a relation—the *Poiseuille equation*:

$$F = (\Delta \text{ pressure} * \pi * r^4)/(8 * L * \eta),$$

where r is the tube radius, L is the tube length, and η is the *fluid viscosity* (a measure of a fluid's resistance to deformation by shear or tensile stress). Thus, although the tube radius is the most powerful determinant of flow, fluid viscosity also impacts flow.

Fluids with a constant viscosity (*Newtonian fluids*) include those with low η (water) or high η (maple syrup), and for flow within any given tube geometry, their flow is linearly related to pressure difference. However, for fluids whose viscosity is variable (***non-Newtonian fluids***), flow varies not only with pressure difference, but also with factors that affect viscosity. Blood has a variable viscosity that is affected by several factors, including by blood constituents and blood shear rate—the velocity gradient of blood as one moves from vessel wall (low velocity) to the vessel lumen (high velocity). Because blood is rheologically a suspension of erythrocytes in plasma, increasing the concentration of erythrocytes (hematocrit) causes the blood viscosity to increase. For example, increasing the hematocrit from 45% to 70% (polycythemia) doubles the blood viscosity, with a proportionate reduction in blood flow for any given tube diameter and pressure difference (by Poiseuille's equation), with potential clinical consequences of decreased oxygen delivery to tissues. In addition, in the ventricle, high shear rates occurring during systole decrease blood viscosity and facilitate flow, in contrast to low shear rates occurring during diastole increase blood viscosity.

References

1. Moore KL, Agur AMR, Dalley II AF. Thorax. In: Moore KL, Agur AMR, Dalley II AF, eds. *Clinically Oriented Anatomy,* 7th ed. Philadelphia: Lippincott Williams & Wilkins, 2013:131–349.
2. Pagel PS, Kampine JP, Stowe DF. Cardiac anatomy and physiology. In: Barash PG, Cullen BF, Stoelting RK, et al. *Clinical Anesthesia,* 7th ed. Philadelphia: Lippincott Williams & Wilkins, 2013:239–262.
3. Grossman W. Diastolic dysfunction and congestive heart failure. *Circulation.* 1990; 81(2 Suppl):III1–III7.
4. Schober P, Loer SA, Schwarte LA. Perioperative hemodynamic monitoring with transesophageal Doppler technology. *Anesth Analg.* 2009;109(2):340–353.
5. Borlaug BA, Kass DA. Invasive hemodynamic assessment in heart failure. *Heart Fail Clin.* 2009;5(2):217–228.
6. Cohen GI, Pietrolungo JF, Thomas JD, et al. A practical guide to assessment of ventricular diastolic function using Doppler echocardiography. *J Am Coll Cardiol.* 1996; 27:1753–1760.
7. Dagal A, Lam AM. Cerebral autoregulation and anesthesia. *Curr Opin Anaesthesiol.* 2009;22(5):547–552.
8. Funk DJ, Jacobsohn E, Kumar A. Role of the venous return in critical illness and shock: Part I—physiology. *Crit Care Med.* 2013;41(1):255–262.
9. Funk DJ, Jacobsohn E, Kumar A. Role of the venous return in critical illness and shock: Part II—shock and mechanical ventilation. *Crit Care Med.* 2013;41(2):573–579.
10. Parker JC, Guyton AC, Taylor AE. Pulmonary transcapillary exchange and pulmonary edema. *Int Rev Physiol.* 1979;18:261–315.

Questions

1. Which one of the following statements is TRUE?
   A. In the presence of coronary stenosis, sub-endocardial tissues are more susceptible to ischemia than subepicardial tissues.
   B. As blood traverses the coronary circulation, oxygen content normally decreases from 20 to 15 mL O_2/100 mL blood.
   C. Resting coronary blood flow in an adult is normally about 10 percent of total cardiac output.
   D. Blood supply to the left ventricle ·is directly dependent on the difference between mean aortic pressure and left ventricular end-systolic pressure.

2. Cardiac output is determined by all of the following EXCEPT:
   A. Myocardial contractility
   B. End-diastolic left ventricular volume
   C. End-diastolic left atrial pressure
   D. Systemic vascular resistance

3. Factors contributing to left ventricular diastolic dysfunction include all of the following EXCEPT:
   A. A heart rate of 150 bpm
   B. Mitral valve stenosis
   C. A large thymoma
   D. A mixed venous $pO_2 = 45$ mm Hg

4. A sample of blood is withdrawn from the distal port of a pulmonary artery catheter that has been placed in an adult without cardiovascular or pulmonary disease. The blood sample has a $pO_2 = 23$ mm Hg. This is consistent with which of the following?
   A. The catheter is properly positioned in the pulmonary artery
   B. The catheter tip is near effluent flow from the coronary sinus
   C. Moderate anemia
   D. An elevated cardiac output

5. The S_2 heart sound is normally split because:
   A. Systemic arterial pressure is higher than pulmonary artery pressure
   B. Left ventricular compliance is lower than right ventricular compliance
   C. The aortic valve closes slightly before the pulmonic valve
   D. Left ventricular wall thickness exceeds right ventricular wall thickness

6. The sign of myocardial ischemia most likely to appear first is:
   A. ST segment change
   B. Decreased left ventricular ejection fraction
   C. Regional ventricular wall motion abnormalities
   D. Increased left ventricular end-diastolic volume

7. The area within the left ventricular pressure-volume loop corresponds to:
   A. Cardiac output
   B. Stroke volume
   C. Left ventricular stroke work
   D. Myocardial oxygen consumption

8. Which of the following is NOT required to construct a Starling ventricular function curve?
   A. Cardiac output
   B. Systemic vascular resistance
   C. Pulmonary artery wedge pressure
   D. Left ventricular stroke work

9. A 30-year-old male is undergoing retinal eye surgery under general endotracheal anesthesia, including positive pressure ventilation and pharmacologic paralysis. All of the following statements regarding venous return are true EXCEPT:
   A. Venous return is impaired by skeletal muscle paralysis
   B. Trendelenburg (head down) position will enhance venous return
   C. Venous return is enhanced by positive pressure ventilation
   D. Valves in extremity veins remain competent during general anesthesia

10. A 30-year-old female has severe hypoalbuminemia due to chronic alcoholic liver disease. Which one of the following statements is TRUE regarding her systemic microcirculation?
    A. Capillary hydrostatic pressure is increased and will increase extravascular fluid movement.
    B. Capillary membrane permeability is increased and will increase extravascular fluid movement.
    C. Plasma oncotic pressure is decreased and will decrease extravascular fluid movement.
    D. Plasma oncotic pressure is decreased and will increase extravascular fluid movement.

4 Central and Autonomic Nervous Systems

Loreta Grecu

I. Anatomy and Physiology

A. The Central Nervous System

The central nervous system (CNS) is comprised of the brain and the spinal cord (Fig. 4-1). The brain is subdivided into four areas: triencephalon, diencephalon, cerebellum, and brainstem.

The Triencephalon (Cerebrum)

The human intellect is considered to be at the level of the cerebrum. It is organized into two cerebral hemispheres and includes the basal ganglia and cerebral cortex. *Basal ganglia* are a group of nuclei that include the caudate nucleus, putamen, and globus pallidus and, together with the thalamus and cerebral cortex, coordinate motor function. The cerebral cortex is the main terminal for independent thought, consciousness, language, memory, and learning. The function of the cerebral cortex is divided into sensory, motor, and associative areas. The basic sensory and motor functions are responsible for receiving and processing information. The associative function is responsible for the highest level of mental activity, which includes abstract thinking, speech, musical and mathematical skills, as well as intercommunication.

The Diencephalon

The diencephalon contains two structures: thalamus and hypothalamus. The thalamus is involved in motor control as well as with sleep–wake cycles and, if injured, can develop profound coma. The *hypothalamus* is a major autonomic control center with essential survival functions such as food intake, thirst, water balance, and control of body temperature, blood pressure, and rage. It is the gatekeeper that connects with both the autonomic nerve centers in the brain as well as with the endocrine system. It synthesizes and releases two hormones—oxytocin and antidiuretic hormone—and indirectly controls the release of the pituitary gland hormones.

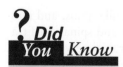

? Did You Know

The olfactory nerve is the only cranial nerve whose input reaches the cerebral cortex *without* going through the thalamus.

VIDEO 4-1

Pituitary Gland Hormones

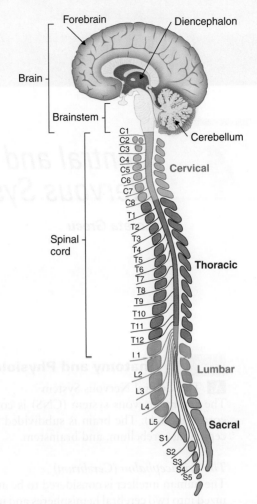

Forebrain

Diencephalon

Brain

Brainstem

Cerebellum

C1
C2
C3
C4
C5   Cervical
C6
C7
C8
T1
T2
T3
T4
T5
T6   Thoracic
T7
T8
T9
T10
T11
T12

Spinal
cord

l 1
L2
L3   Lumbar
L4
L5
S1   Sacral
S2
S3
S4
S5

Figure 4-1 Components of central nervous system. (From Preston RR, Wilson TE. Sensory and motor systems. In: Harvey RA, ed. *Physiology*. Baltimore: Lippincott Williams & Wilkins; 2013:53–90, with permission.)

The Brainstem

The brainstem has several components, namely, the medulla, pons, and midbrain. All the information that passes between the brain and spinal cord traverses the midbrain. Most of the cranial nerves, except cranial nerves I and II, have their origin in the midbrain as well. The cranial nerves provide sensory and motor innervation to the head and neck as well as ensure the primordial senses such as vision, hearing, smell, and taste.

The Cerebellum

The cerebellum is relatively small, but it contains more neurons than the remainder of the brain. This is because it is responsible for coordination of movements such as posture, balance, coordination and speech, overall motor function, as well as learning motor behaviors.

B. The Spinal Cord

The spinal cord is located in the spinal canal and is divided into several regions: cervical, thoracic (dorsal), lumbar, sacral, and coccygeal (Fig. 4-1). The spinal cord is divided into 31 segments that correspond to 31 pairs of spinal nerves,

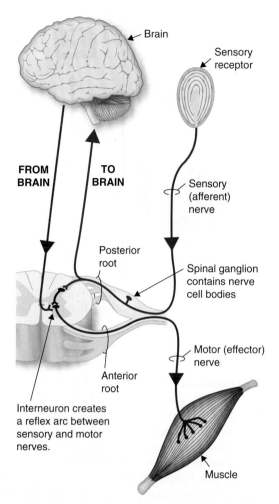

Brain

Sensory
receptor

**FROM
BRAIN**

**TO
BRAIN**

Sensory
(afferent)
nerve

Posterior
root

Spinal ganglion
contains nerve
cell bodies

Motor (effector)
nerve

Anterior
root

Interneuron creates
a reflex arc between
sensory and motor
nerves.

Muscle

Figure 4-2 Typical sensory and motor pathways. (From Preston RR, Wilson TE. Sensory and motor systems. In: Harvey RA, ed. *Physiology.* Baltimore: Lippincott Williams & Wilkins; 2013:53–90, with permission.)

one on each side of the body. Although the spinal cord terminates at L2 vertebral body, the spinal nerves continue caudally until they reach the appropriate dermatome level (cauda equina). The filum terminale marks the tract of regression of the spinal cord. Sensory and motor fibers cross the midline, so in reality the left side of the brain controls the right side of the body and vice versa.

The spinal nerves have components of both sensory afferent and motor efferent fibers and emerge from C2 to S2-3 to control all body functions as well as movement. The sensory component travels toward the spinal cord via a posterior root and enters the spinal canal via the intervertebral foramen (Fig. 4-2). The cell body is located in a spinal ganglion, and the fibers travel upward to synapse with nuclei to the brain or synapse directly with a motor neuron, allowing the cord-mediated reflexes to *reflex arc.*

The motor component travels caudally from the brain and synapses with peripheral motor neurons within the spinal cord, exits the spinal column via the anterior root, and travels toward the periphery along the sensory fibers of the spinal nerves.

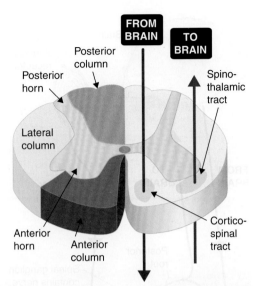

Figure 4-3 Organization of the spinal cord. (From Preston RR, Wilson TE. Sensory and motor systems. In: Harvey RA, ed. *Physiology.* Baltimore: Lippincott Williams & Wilkins; 2013:53–90, with permission.)

The spinal cord is organized like a butterfly (Fig. 4-3) with gray matter that contains neuronal cell bodies, dendrites, and unmyelinated axons in the center and white matter that contains myelinated axons surrounding it. The white matter contains bundles of nerve fibers organized into *tracts*, ascending and descending, which transfer information between the brain and peripheral nervous system. The tracts are named based on their origin and destination (e.g., spinothalamic tract, corticospinal tract, etc.) (see Figs. 37.1 and 37.2). The gray matter is organized into anterior and posterior horns that allow the traveling neurons to synapse. It has commissures that allow information to travel between the two sides.

Cerebrospinal Fluid

The protection of the CNS is ensured by bone, both at the level of the spinal cord as well as at the level of the brain, three membranes called meninges, as well as a layer of cerebrospinal fluid (CSF). The meninges are comprised of three layers: pia mater (the thinnest), the arachnoid mater (a fibrous membrane), and the thick membrane is dura mater.

The CSF is a sterile colorless fluid produced in the choroid plexus that surrounds the CNS and has a significant function in absorption of shock, providing buoyancy (floatability), allowing some volume changes, and providing homeostasis to ensure a perfect functionality of the CNS.

? Did You Know

The total volume of cerebral spinal fluid is 150 mL, of which 50 mL is in the subarachnoid space of the spinal cord.

II. The Autonomic Nervous System

The autonomic nervous system (ANS) is the core of the human organism. It regulates the functions of the visceral organs, including the heart, lungs, gastrointestinal system, hormonal release, as well as body temperature, all of which are not under conscious control.

The ANS is separated into two divisions: sympathetic (adrenergic, SNS), and parasympathetic (cholinergic, PNS) nervous system. These two divisions fine tune organ function and have opposing effects (Table 4-1 and Fig. 4-4) (2,3).

Table 4-1   Functions of the Autonomic Nervous System

Organ, Tract, or System		Effect of Sympathetic Stimulation[a]	Effect of Parasympathetic Stimulation[b]
Eyes	Pupil Ciliary body	Dilates pupil (admits more light for increased acuity at a distance)	Constricts pupil (protects pupil from excessively bright light) Contracts ciliary muscle, allowing lens to thicken for near vision (accommodation)
Skin	Arrector muscles of hair	Causes hairs to stand on end ("goose-flesh" or "goose bumps")	No effect (does not reach)[c]
	Peripheral blood vessels	Vasoconstricts (blanching of skin, lips, and turning fingertips blue)	No effect (does not reach)[c]
	Sweat glands	Promotes sweating[d]	No effect (does not reach)[c]
Other glands	Lacrimal glands	Slightly decreases secretion[e]	Promotes secretion
	Salivary glands	Secretion decreases, becomes thicker, more viscous[e]	Promotes abundant, watery secretion
Heart		Increases the rate and strength of contraction; inhibits the effect of parasympathetic system on coronary vessels, allowing them to dilate[e]	Decreases the rate and strength of contraction (conserving energy); constricts coronary vessels in relation to reduced demand
Lungs		Inhibits effect of parasympathetic system, resulting in bronchodilation and reduced secretion, allowing for maximum air exchange	Constricts bronchi (conserving energy) and promotes bronchial secretion
Digestive tract		Inhibits peristalsis, and constricts blood vessels to digestive tract so that blood is available to skeletal muscle; contracts internal anal sphincter to aid fecal continence	Stimulates peristalsis and secretion of digestive juices Contracts rectum, inhibits internal anal sphincter to cause defecation
Liver and gall-bladder		Promotes breakdown of glycogen to glucose (for increased energy)	Promotes building/conservation of glycogen; increases secretion of bile
Urinary tract		Vasoconstriction of renal vessels slows urine formation; internal sphincter of bladder contracted to maintain urinary continence	Inhibits contraction of internal sphincter of bladder, contracts detrusor muscle of the bladder wall causing urination
Genital system		Causes ejaculation and vasoconstriction resulting in remission of erection	Produces engorgement (erection) of erectile tissues of the external genitals
Suprarenal medulla		Release of adrenaline into blood	No effect (does not innervate)

[a]In general, the effects of sympathetic stimulation are catabolic, preparing body for the fight-or-flight response.
[b]In general, the effects of parasympathetic stimulation are anabolic, promoting normal function and conserving energy.
[c]The parasympathetic system is restricted in its distribution to the head, neck, and body cavities (except for erectile tissues of genitalia); otherwise, parasympathetic fibers are never found in the body wall and limbs. Sympathetic fibers, by comparison, are distributed to all vascularized portions of the body.
[d]With the exception of the sweat glands, glandular secretion is parasympathetically stimulated.
[e]With the exception of the coronary arteries, vasoconstriction is sympathetically stimulated; the effects of sympathetic stimulation on glands (other than sweat glands) are the indirect effects of vasoconstriction.
Reused from Moore KL, Dalley AF II, Agur AMR. *Moore Clinically Oriented Anatomy.* 7th ed. Baltimore: Lippincott Williams & Wilkins/WK Health; 2013:65, with permission.

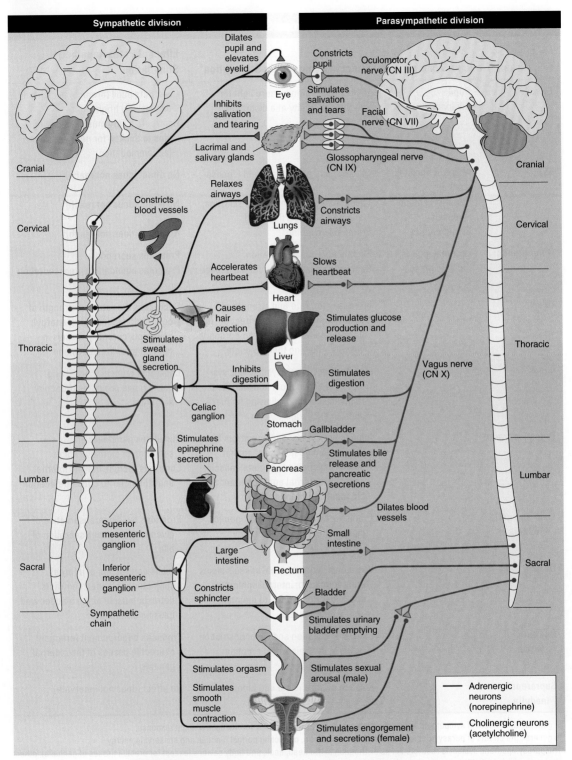

Figure 4-4 Organization of the autonomic nervous system. (From Preston RR, Wilson TE. Sensory and motor systems. In: Harvey RA, ed. *Physiology*. Baltimore: Lippincott Williams & Wilkins; 2013:53–90, with permission.)

The SNS aids the body with fight-or-flight responses and is catabolic (energy expending) system. The role of PNS is quite the opposite; it contributes mainly to body conservation and restoration and is considered a homeostatic or anabolic (energy-conserving) system. The central components of the ANS include the cerebral cortex, hypothalamus, amygdala, stria terminalis, brainstem, and intermediate reticular zone of the medulla.

Both SNS and PNS have afferent and efferent fibers that close a loop between the spinal cord and visceral organs and determine reflexes that aim toward an equilibrium state of the body.

The afferent pathways have receptors in the visceral organs that are sensitive to mechanical and chemical stimuli as well as temperature variations. The impulses are transmitted along the somatic or autonomic nerves through the dorsal roots toward the spinal cord or the cranial nerves toward the brainstem.

The afferent fibers play an important role in both conducting visceral pain impulses and regulating visceral function. The difference between the ANS and somatic innervation is that the transmission of the impulses from the CNS toward the effector organs is conducted by connecting two multipolar neurons for both divisions of the ANS. Although the somatic motor innervation contains only one neuron (Fig. 4-5). The ANS contains efferent fibers and ganglia that are clustered into two separate groups, the **thoracolumbar** (for SNS) from T1-L2 and **craniosacral** for PNS (Fig. 4-4). The preganglionic axons are

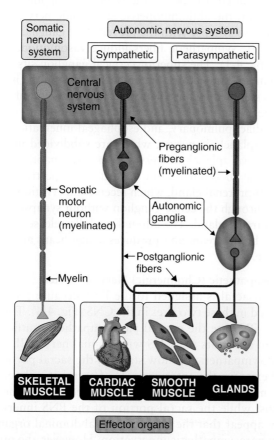

Figure 4-5 Efferent pathways of somatic and autonomic nervous systems. (From Preston RR, Wilson TE. Sensory and motor systems. In: Harvey RA, ed. *Physiology.* Baltimore: Lippincott Williams & Wilkins; 2013:53–90, with permission.)

short, myelinated, and cholinergic and exit the spinal cord and enter the white rami communicans that connect with prevertebral or paravertebral ganglia. The postganglionic axons continue through the gray rami communicans and continue together with blood vessels and nerves toward the end organs. These axons are long, unmyelinated, and primarily adrenergic with the exception of sweat glands, which are cholinergic. The PNS exits the CNS via the cranial nerves III, VII, IX, and X as well as through the sacral roots. The preganglionic fibers are myelinated, cholinergic, and fairly long, because the ganglia are located close to the end organ. The postganglionic fibers are short and cholinergic.

A. The Sympathetic (Adrenergic) Nervous System

The cell bodies of the SNS are found in the intermediolateral cell columns of the thoracic and upper lumbar T1-L1, L2, L3 region of the spinal cord and are organized somatotopically (Fig. 4-4). The next connection is with the paravertebral or prevertebral ganglia. The paravertebral ganglia are organized into right and left sympathetic chains that parallel the length of the thoracolumbar column. The prevertebral ganglia are located in plexuses that surround the main branches of the abdominal aorta, with the best example being the celiac ganglia that are around the celiac artery's branch takeoff.

The presynaptic sympathetic fibers that exit the spinal cord follow several possible courses; most connect to the paravertebral ganglia in the immediate vicinity of the spinal cord either at the same level or immediately adjacent. The fibers that form the abdominopelvic splanchnic nerve pass through the sympathetic trunk to synapse with the prevertebral ganglia.

The postsynaptic sympathetic fibers induce vasomotion, pilomotion, and sudomotion (Table 4-1). The superior cervical ganglion sits at the top of the sympathetic chain and innervates the organ function in the head. Innervation for the viscera is supplied by the splanchnic nerves, commonly distributed into two subcategories (Fig. 4-4). First are the cardiopulmonary splanchnic nerves that provide cardiac, pulmonary, and esophageal innervation. Second are the abdominopelvic splanchnic nerves, which are subdivided into greater, lesser, thoracic, and lumbar splanchnic nerves with postsynaptic fibers that follow the branches of the abdominal aorta toward the respective organs. The only exception is the suprarenal gland, which receives innervation from presynaptic fibers that pass through the celiac ganglion without synapsing and end on the cells of the suprarenal gland. The adrenal medulla releases neurotransmitters directly into the bloodstream and produces a significant and impressive sympathetic response.

B. The Parasympathetic (Cholinergic) Nervous System

The name craniosacral is assigned to the PNS because the presynaptic cell bodies are located in these two sites in the CNS (Fig. 4-4). Thus, the two subdivisions of the PNS are the cranial parasympathetic outflow, which starts in the brainstem and exits the CNS with cranial nerves III, VII, IX, and X. The sacral parasympathetic outflow starts in the sacral portion of the spinal cord S2-4 and exits via the anterior roots of sacral spinal nerve and the pelvic splanchnic nerves. The innervation is directed toward the head from the cranial portions, while the sacral portion of the PNS innervates the pelvic organs. It may appear that the thoracic and abdominal organs are less well represented by parasympathetic innervation. However, the outflow from the cranial portion of PNS via the vagus nerve (X) controls all thoracic and abdominal organs and most of the gastrointestinal tract from the esophagus

Table 4-2 Classification and Conduction Velocities of Nerve Fibers			
Description of Nerve Fibers	**Group**	**Diameter (µm)**	**Conduction Velocity (m/s)**
Myelinated somatic	A { Alpha α	20	120
	Beta β		
	Gamma γ		5–40 (pain fibers)
	Delta δ	3–4	5–40 (pain fibers)
	Epsilon ε	2	5
Myelinated visceral (Preganglionic autonomic)	B	<3	3–15
Unmyelinated somatic	C	<2	0.5–2 (pain fibers)

From Grecu L. Autonomic nervous system: Physiology and Pharmacology. In: Barash PG, Cullen BF, Stoelting RK, et al., eds. *Clinical Anesthesia.* 7th ed. Philadelphia: Lippincott Williams & Wilkins; 2013: 362–407, with permission.

to the left colic flexure. The rest of the colon is innervated by the sacral outflow.

As opposed to the SNS, the PNS has a more limited distribution. Also, different from the SNS, the presynaptic fibers of the PNS are long, while the postsynaptic fibers are short.

C. Autonomic Nervous System Transmission

Nerve conduction is initiated with an action potential (Fig. 4-6A). The speed of conduction is dependent on a number of factors: the number of synapses, nerve fiber diameter, neural insulation, and salutatory conduction (Fig. 4-6B–D and Table 4-2). Transmission of excitation across the synaptic clefts is accomplished by releasing specific chemical substances, which in turn connect with a receptor on an organ and is ultimately followed by a biologic response. The ANS can again be divided based on the specific transmitter that is released at the synaptic level. The preganglionic transmission of both SNS and PNS involves secretions of *acetylcholine (ACh)*. At the effector level though, the SNS releases predominantly *norepinephrine (NE)*, with few exceptions at the vascular sympathetic nerve terminals. At the effector level the PNS releases ACh.

D. Parasympathetic Nervous System Transmission

ACh, as opposed to the other mediators, cannot be recycled. Therefore, it needs to be constantly manufactured in the presynaptic terminal. This chemical process is catalyzed by choline acetyl transferase and includes acetylation of choline by acetyl coenzyme A. The release of ACh is dependent on the release of calcium (Ca^{2+}) from the interstitial space. The rapid recovery to baseline state is essential for an adequate regulation of function of an effector organ. Thus, ACh needs to be quickly removed from the synaptic cleft by hydrolysis (acetylcholinesterase and pseudocholinesterase [plasma cholinesterases]), which are found at the level of neurons at the neuromuscular junction. These enzymes hydrolyze ACh and other drugs such as ester-type local anesthetics, succinylcholine, among others.

E. Sympathetic Nervous System Transmission

The main mediators for the SNS are NE and *epinephrine (EPI)*, with a significant predominance of NE. ACh is the transmitter for the preganglionic

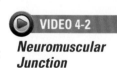
VIDEO 4-2

Neuromuscular Junction

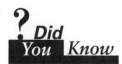
Did You Know

Neurotransmitters norepinephrine and epinephrine released into the circulation from the adrenal medulla are called hormones.

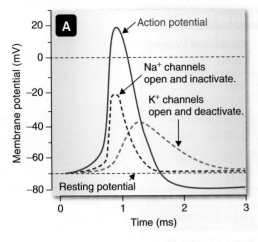

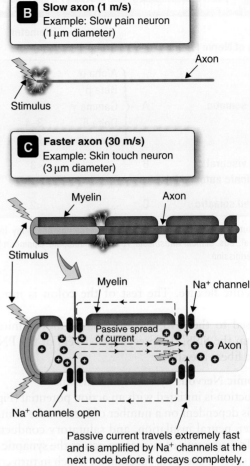

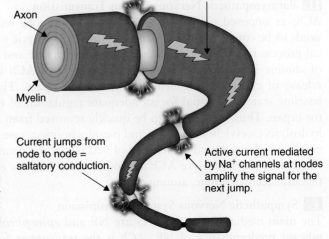

Figure 4-6 **A:** Time sequence of channel events during an action potential. **B–D:** Axonal conduction velocity related to myelin sheath and diameter neuronal fiber diameter. (From Preston RR, Wilson TE. Sensory and motor systems. In: Harvey RA, ed. *Physiology.* Baltimore: Lippincott Williams & Wilkins; 2013:53–90, with permission.)

fibers for the SNS. At the level of the adrenal gland (medulla), there is a significant release of both EPI and NE in circulation by the chromaffin cells, with EPI being preponderant. When these mediators are released into the circulation, they are considered hormones, because they are synthesized, stored, and released by the adrenal gland (4).

There are three possible mechanisms for NE inactivation. NE is removed from the synaptic cleft by: (a) reuptake into the presynaptic terminals (the predominant mechanism), (b) extraneuronal uptake by effector cells, and (c) diffusion. The NE and EPI, cleared by extraneuronal uptake, are metabolized by monoamine oxidase (MAO) and the catechol-O-methyltransferase (COMT) to a final product, vanillylmandelic acid, which is eliminated in the urine. Thus, the endogenous catecholamines are mainly inactivated by reuptake into the synapse. The liver and kidneys mainly metabolize the exogenous catecholamines, and this mechanism confers a longer duration of action.

F. Receptors
Cholinergic Receptors
Ach is the common mediator for a variety of substrates, including the PNS, the presynaptic transmission of the SNS, and the neuroeffector junction of striated muscle (Fig. 4-7). Cholinergic receptors are further divided into two

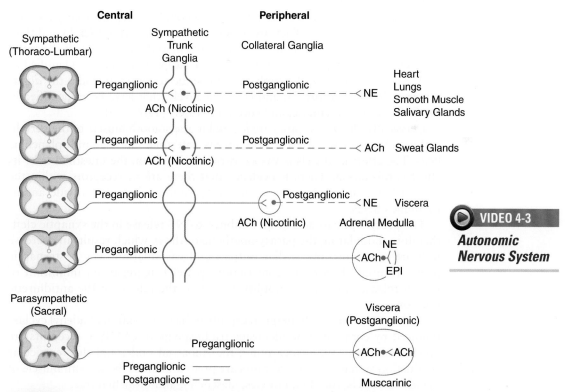

VIDEO 4-3

Autonomic Nervous System

Figure 4-7 Schematic diagram of the efferent autonomic nervous system. Afferent impulses are integrated centrally and sent reflexively to the adrenergic and cholinergic receptors. Sympathetic fibers ending in the adrenal medulla are preganglionic, and acetylcholine (ACh) is the neurotransmitter. Stimulation of the chromaffin cells, acting as postganglionic neurons, releases epinephrine (EPI) and norepinephrine (NE). (From Grecu L. Autonomic nervous system: Physiology and pharmacology. In: Barash PG, Cullen BF, Stoelting RK, et al., eds. *Clinical Anesthesia.* 7th ed. Philadelphia: Lippincott Williams & Wilkins; 2013:362–407, with permission.)

subcategories—nicotinic and muscarinic—based on their stimulation predominantly by nicotine or muscarine, respectively, although both types respond to ACh. Muscarinic receptors are located at the postganglionic PNS terminals within the cardiac and smooth muscle. Its stimulation induces bradycardia, bronchoconstriction, miosis, salivation, and increased gastrointestinal motility. These effects can be inhibited by blocking the receptors with atropine. These receptors are subclassified into five subgroups so that M_1, M_4, and M_5 are mainly located in the CNS and are involved in complex processes such as memory arousal, attention, and analgesia. M_1 receptors are found in the autonomic ganglia and in the gastric parietal cells; M_2 receptors are mainly located at the heart; and M_3 receptors are located at the smooth muscle level. M_4 is found in CNS and inhibits cyclic adenosine 3′,5′-monophosphate (cAMP). M_5 regulates intracellular Ca^{2+} as a signaling pathway.

Nicotinic receptors are localized at the synaptic junction of both SNS and PNS ganglia, with low doses of nicotine being stimulating and elevated doses being inhibitory. SNS stimulation is followed by tachycardia and hypertension due to release of EPI and NE from the adrenal medulla. If the nicotine dose is increased further, the symptoms become those of hypotension and neuromuscular weakness, as it becomes an inhibitor instead.

Adrenergic Receptors

Adrenergic receptors are a class of G protein–coupled receptors that are stimulated by catecholamines. They are divided into two types *α and β*. In addition, each category is subdivided into α_1 and α_2 and β_1 and β_2, respectively. Recently another category, a β_3 receptor present in the adipose tissue, was identified as well. Another category of peripheral adrenergic receptors includes the *dopaminergic (DA) receptors*, D_1 and D_2, respectively, that have been identified in the CNS, renal, mesenteric, and coronary vessels (Table 4-3).

Classically, the α_1 receptors are located in the smooth muscle of the peripheral vessels, coronary arteries, skin, uterus, intestinal mucosa, and splanchnic beds. The effect in vessels is vasoconstriction, while on the intestinal tract its effect is relaxation. There is evidence that there are α_1 receptors within the myocardium, such that using α_1-adrenergic antagonists can provide antiarrhythmic effects.

The presynaptic α_2 acts as an inhibitor to NE release in the synaptic cleft, therefore modulating the parasympathetic outflow, which results in decrease in heart rate, inotropy, cardiac output, and vasodilation. The postsynaptic α_2 are responsible for vasoconstriction, platelet aggregation, inhibition of insulin release, and bowel motility as well as the release of the antidiuretic hormone.

Activation of the β-adrenergic receptors induces activation of adenyl cyclase followed by conversion of adenosine triphosphate to cAMP. β_1 receptors are present mainly in the myocardium, the sinoatrial node, and the ventricular conduction system. The β_2 receptors are predominant in the smooth muscle of the blood vessels, the skin, muscles, mesentery, and bronchial tree.

The dopaminergic receptors are found in the CNS, blood vessels, and postganglionic sympathetic nerves. They are divided into several subcategories, with the clinically important ones being DA_1 and DA_2. DA_1 is postsynaptic only, and its effect is mainly vasodilation; DA_2 is both pre- and postsynaptic. The presynaptic DA_2 is similar to the presynaptic α_2 and thus inhibits the

Table 4-3   Adrenergic Receptors

Receptor	Synaptic Site	Anatomic Site	Action	LV Function and Stroke Volume
α_1	Postsynaptic	Peripheral vascular smooth muscle	Constriction	Decreased
		Renal vascular smooth muscle	Constriction	
		Coronary arteries, epicardial	Constriction	
		Myocardium 30–40% of resting tone	Positive inotropism	Improved
		Renal tubules	Antidiuresis	
α_2	Presynaptic	Peripheral vascular smooth muscle release	Inhibit NE	
		Coronaries	Secondary vasodilation ?	Improved
		CNS	Inhibition of CNS activity Sedation Decrease MAC	
	Postsynaptic	Coronaries, endocardial	Constriction	Decreased
		CNS	Inhibition of insulin release Decreased bowel motility Inhibition of antidiuretic hormone Analgesia	
		Renal tubule	Promotes Na^{2+} and H_2O excretion	
β_1	Postsynaptic NE sensitive	Myocardium	Positive inotropism and chronotropism	Improved
		Sinoatrial (SA) node Ventricular conduction Kidney Coronaries	Renin release Relaxation	
β_2	Presynaptic NE sensitive	Myocardium	Accelerates NE release	Improved
		SA node ventricular conduction vessels	Opposite action to presynaptic α_2 agonism Constriction	
	Postsynaptic (extrasynaptic) (EPI sensitive)	Myocardium	Positive inotropism and chronotropism	Improved
		Vascular smooth muscle	Relaxation	Improved
		Bronchial smooth muscle	Relaxation	Improved
β_3		Adipose tissue	Enhancement of lipolysis	
		Renal vessels	Relaxation	

(continued)

Table 4-3   Adrenergic Receptors (*Continued*)

Receptor	Synaptic Site	Anatomic Site	Action	LV Function and Stroke Volume
DA$_1$	Postsynaptic	Blood vessels (renal, mesentery, coronary)	Vasodilation	Improved
		Renal tubules	Natriuresis Diuresis	
		Juxtaglomerular cells	Renin release (modulates diuresis)	
		Sympathetic ganglia	Minor inhibition	
DA$_2$	Presynaptic	Postganglionic sympathetic nerves	Inhibit NE release	Improved
			Secondary vasodilation	
	Postsynaptic	Renal and mesenteric vasculature	? Vasoconstriction	

Na^{2+}, sodium ion; MAC, monitored anesthesia care; CNS, central nervous system; SA, sinoatrial; NE, norepinephrine; EPI, epinephrine; DA, dopamine; LV, left ventricular; NE, norepinephrine; EPI, epinephrine; DA, dopamine.
From Grecu L. Autonomic nervous system: Physiology and pharmacology. In: Barash PG, Cullen BF, Stoelting RK, et al., eds. *Clinical Anesthesia*. 7th ed. Philadelphia: Lippincott Williams & Wilkins; 2013:362–407, with permission.

release of NE and induces vasodilation, while the postsynaptic DA$_2$ is similar to the postsynaptic α$_2$ and induces vasoconstriction.

Other receptors include adenosine receptors that have the role to reduce NE release, which decreases blood pressure, especially in circumstances that involve hypoxic conditions (reduce oxygen demand). *Serotonin* decreases the release of NE at the synaptic level by reducing the available calcium ions. Prostaglandins E$_2$, histamine, and some opioids seem to act by decreasing the release of NE at certain levels. Their direct antagonists do not act by increasing the release of NE at the synaptic level.

The number of receptors fluctuates depending on physiologic, genetic, and developmental factors. Receptors are produced by the sarcoplasmic reticulum and are externalized to the synaptic membrane. At times the same receptors may be internalized in order to be recycled. Catecholamines induce a direct effect on the number or the concentration of the receptors, which is termed upregulation or downregulation, and these can be altered by changing or discontinuing the administration of adrenergic drugs.

G. Autonomic Nervous System Reflexes

When the autonomic pathways are disrupted due to a variety of pathologic conditions, loss of normal function is expected. One example is Horner syndrome, which is associated with ptosis, myosis, and anhydrosis (eyelid droop, inability to increase the diameter of the pupil, and inability to sweat, respectively), which is determined by disruption of the respective sympathetic pathways (e.g., nerve blocks such the interscalene nerve block). Tests that are used to determine *autonomic dysfunction* include monitoring of cardiac parameters during changes in posture (tilt table test), cold pressor test (hand immersion in ice-cold water), Valsalva maneuver, and even nerve conduction studies monitoring sweating and thermal changes. The most common feature of autonomic dysfunction is orthostatic hypotension with a decrease of at least 20 mm Hg in systolic blood pressure or a decrease of 10 mm Hg

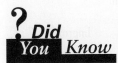
? Did You Know

In general, the number of adrenergic receptors is inversely proportional to the concentration of circulating catecholamines.

? Did You Know

Orthostatic hypotension is a harbinger of an increase in perioperative morbidity and mortality and should be considered an additional risk factor for a given patient.

in the diastolic blood pressure upon standing upright for 3 minutes. Valsalva maneuver requires forced expiration against resistance, which has the purpose of decreasing the venous blood return into the thorax, with a subsequent decrease in the blood pressure. A normal response is sensed by the baroreceptors and a reflex increase in the heart rate that is sympathetically mediated should be expected. On the other hand, patients with dysautonomia will not have the expected increase in the heart rate.

References

1. Preston RR, Wilson TE. Sensory and motor systems. In: Harvey RA, ed. *Physiology*. Baltimore: Lippincott Williams & Wilkins; 2013:53–90.
2. Moore KL, Dalley AF II, Agur AMR. *Moore Clinically Oriented Anatomy*. 7th ed. Baltimore: Lippincott Williams & Wilkins; 2013.
3. McGrane S, Atria NP, Barwise JA. Perioperative implications of the patient with autonomic dysfunction. *Curr Opin Anaesthesiol*. 2014;27:365–370.
4. Grecu L. Autonomic nervous system: Physiology and pharmacology. In: Barash PG, Cullen BF, Stoelting RK, et al., eds. *Clinical Anesthesia*. 7th ed. Philadelphia: Lippincott Williams & Wilkins; 2013:362–407.

Questions

1. An 80-year-old female received midazolam 2 mg for premedication for an uneventful 30-minute gynecologic procedure (propofol infusion and fentanyl). Ten minutes after arrival in the PACU, the patient exhibits new onset delirium. You elect to treat with:
   A. Physostigmine or pyridostigmine, since they both cross the blood brain barrier.
   B. Physostigmine or pyridostigmine, since neither crosses the blood brain barrier.
   C. Physostigmine since it crosses the blood brain barrier.
   D. Pyridostigmine since it crosses the blood brain barrier.

2. On a postoperative visit, 8 hours after operation on the upper arm under interscalene block, the patient complains of diplopia and hoarseness. You note the following on physical examination. This complication is the result of:

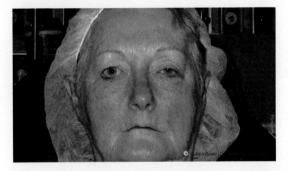

   A. Anesthetic block of the stellate ganglion and recurrent laryngeal nerve
   B. Myasthenia gravis
   C. Intracerebral hemorrhage
   D. Migraine headache

3. A 45-year-old female underwent open abdominal hysterectomy 24 hours previously under spinal anesthesia. On the postoperative visit, she complains of throbbing headache, and diplopia in the sitting or standing position, which is relieved when she lies flat. Your assessment of the patient includes

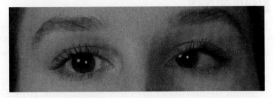

   A. Immediate neurosurgical consult
   B. Treat with an epidural blood patch immediately
   C. Observe, bed rest, and fluids for 24 hours because this represents a stretch of cranial nerve III
   D. Observe, bed rest, and fluids for 24 hours because this represents a stretch of cranial nerve VI

4. The only hormones synthesized in the hypothalamus are:
   A. Growth hormone somatostatin
   B. Oxytocin and vasopressin
   C. Antidiuretic hormone and oxytocin
   D. Epinephrine and norepinephrine

5. The difference between a somatic efferent nerve and the typical autonomic nerve efferent pathway is:
   A. Sympathetic ganglia located at distance from spinal cord
   B. Parasympathetic ganglia are located near the target organ
   C. Somatic efferent nerve cell bodies traverse the posterior root of the spinal cord
   D. Somatic efferent nerve interneuron is in the spinal ganglion

6. **The nerve fiber with the fastest transmission speed is:**
   A. Pain fiber
   B. Touch axon
   C. Motor neuron
   D. Unmyelinated fibers

7. **In the preoperative assessment clinic you suspect a patient has autonomic dysfunction. You test your diagnosis with a Valsalva maneuver. Which of the following supports your theory?**
   A. Increase of mean arterial pressure by 20% from resting state
   B. Decrease in heart rate by 15%
   C. Reduction of systolic arterial pressure by 30 mm Hg from resting state
   D. Tachycardia and increase cardiac output

6. The nerve fiber with the fastest transmission speed is:

A. Pain fiber

B. Touch axon

C. Motor neuron

D. Unmyelinated fibers

7. In the preoperative assessment clinic you suspect a patient has autonomic dysfunction. You test your diagnosis with a Valsalva maneuver. Which of the following supports your theory?

A. Increase of mean arterial pressure by 20% from resting state.

B. Decrease in heart rate by 15%

C. Reduction of systolic arterial pressure by 50 mm Hg from resting state

D. Tachycardia and increase cardiac output

The Renal System

Susan Garwood

I. Renal Anatomy and Physiology

A. Anatomy

The kidneys are paired retroperitoneal organs that lie obliquely in the upper part of the paravertebral gutters (Fig. 5-1). The kidneys are supplied by the renal arteries, and the right renal artery passes posterior to the inferior vena cava. The renal artery enters the hilum and usually divides to form the anterior and posterior branches. The renal veins drain the kidneys and also receive venous drainage from the suprarenal gland, gonads, diaphragm, and body wall. Lymph drains to lumbar nodes via locally situated nodes. The sympathetic innervation arises from the celiac and intermesenteric plexuses and travels with the renal arteries. The parasympathetic innervation is derived from the splanchnic nerves which include pain fibers.

The renal parenchyma is enclosed by a tough but thin fibrous membrane (except for the hilus) and is divided into two distinct regions: the cortex and the medulla (Fig. 5-1). The *cortex* is the outer portion of the kidney and contains alternating bands of cortical labyrinth (glomeruli and convoluted tubules) and parallel arrays of straight tubules (medullary rays). The *medulla* is the deeper part of the parenchyma and is divided into an outer region, which contains the thick ascending limb of the loop of Henle, and the inner region, which is marked by the absence of loops of Henle. The outer region of the medulla is itself divided into an outer and inner stripe, which are defined by the presence (outer) or absence (inner) of proximal tubules (Fig. 5-1). Tubules in the medulla are arranged into pyramids, which are oriented with the base toward the cortex and the tip (papilla) toward a minor calyx to where urine drains.

B. Physiology: Correlation of Structure and Function

The Nephron

The *nephron* is the structural and functional unit of the kidney and is responsible for urine formation. It plays a dominant role in water and electrolyte homeostasis, acid base balance, and blood pressure control. The nephron comprises a glomerulus and a tubule (Fig. 5-2). The glomerulus

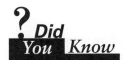

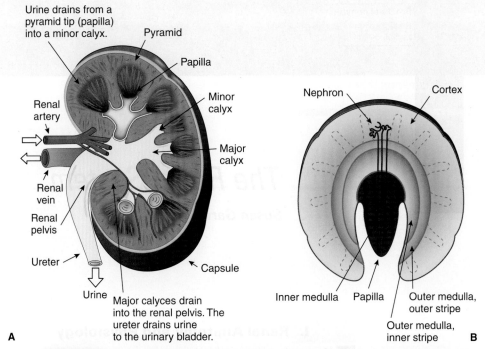

Urine drains from a pyramid tip (papilla) into a minor calyx.

Pyramid

Papilla

Renal artery

Minor calyx

Nephron

Cortex

Major calyx

Renal vein

Renal pelvis

Ureter

Capsule

Urine

Major calyces drain into the renal pelvis. The ureter drains urine to the urinary bladder.

Inner medulla   Papilla   Outer medulla, outer stripe

Outer medulla, inner stripe

A

B

Figure 5-1 **A:** Gross anatomy of the kidney. **B:** Medullary inner and outer stripes. (From Preston RR, Wilson TE. Filtration and micturition. In: Harvey RA, ed. *Physiology.* Philadelphia: Lippincott Williams & Wilkins, 2013, with permission.)

is a capillary tuft encased in a fibrous structure called Bowman's capsule, together known as the *renal corpuscle.* This is where filtration of blood occurs. Absorption and secretion occur in the renal tubule (proximal convoluted tubule, loop of Henle, and distal convoluted tubule). Filtrate from each nephron drains into the collecting duct system and pass toward the renal calyces.

The Glomerulus

The *glomeruli* are supplied by an afferent arteriole and drained by an efferent arteriole. They can be divided into *superficial glomeruli* (80% to 85% of glomeruli; located near the renal capsule and associated with short loops of Henle) and *juxtamedullary glomeruli* (15% to 20% of glomeruli, which have long loops of Henle extending deep into the medulla) (Fig. 5-3). The capillaries have three layers (fenestrated endothelium on the blood side, visceral epithelium on the filtrate side, and a basement membrane in between), which create a filtration barrier and provide selective filtration of the blood.

The Juxtaglomerular Apparatus

The juxtaglomerular apparatus comprises the afferent and efferent arterioles, extraglomerular mesangial cells, and the macula densa (Fig. 5-4). The macula densa is a region of the specialized, distal, thick ascending limb of the *loop of Henle* of the parent nephron. It is formed from low columnar cells that have their apical membranes exposed to the tubular fluid and the basilar aspect in contact with cells of the mesangium and the afferent arteriole. Gap junctions exist between the mesangial cells, serving as a functional link between the macula densa, glomerular arterioles, and mesangium.

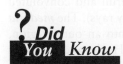

? *Did You Know*

The macula densa cells are positioned to sense changes in the tubular fluids and interact with the effector cells of the juxtaglomerular apparatus, creating changes in blood flow and glomerular filtration rate (tubuloglomerular feedback).

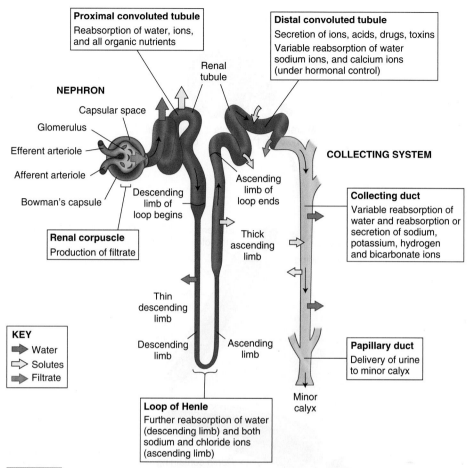

Proximal convoluted tubule
Reabsorption of water, ions, and all organic nutrients

Distal convoluted tubule
Secretion of ions, acids, drugs, toxins
Variable reabsorption of water sodium ions, and calcium ions (under hormonal control)

Renal tubule

NEPHRON

Capsular space

Glomerulus

Efferent arteriole

Afferent arteriole

Bowman's capsule

Descending limb of loop begins

COLLECTING SYSTEM

Renal corpuscle
Production of filtrate

Ascending limb of loop ends

Thick ascending limb

Collecting duct
Variable reabsorption of water and reabsorption or secretion of sodium, potassium, hydrogen and bicarbonate ions

Thin descending limb

Descending limb

Ascending limb

KEY
→ Water
⇨ Solutes
→ Filtrate

Papillary duct
Delivery of urine to minor calyx

Minor calyx

Loop of Henle
Further reabsorption of water (descending limb) and both sodium and chloride ions (ascending limb)

Figure 5-2 The nephron: Structure and function.

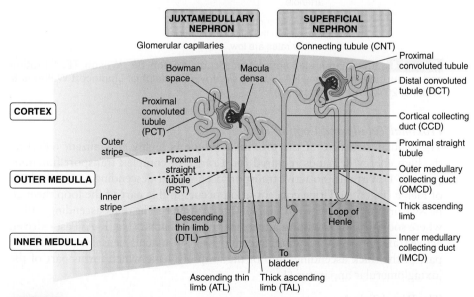

JUXTAMEDULLARY NEPHRON

SUPERFICIAL NEPHRON

Glomerular capillaries

Connecting tubule (CNT)

Proximal convoluted tubule

Bowman space

Macula densa

Distal convoluted tubule (DCT)

CORTEX

Proximal convoluted tubule (PCT)

Cortical collecting duct (CCD)

Outer stripe

Proximal straight tubule

Proximal straight tubule (PST)

Outer medullary collecting duct (OMCD)

OUTER MEDULLA

Inner stripe

Thick ascending limb

Descending thin limb (DTL)

Loop of Henle

Inner medullary collecting duct (IMCD)

INNER MEDULLA

To bladder

Ascending thin limb (ATL)

Thick ascending limb (TAL)

Figure 5-3 Nephron types and the collecting duct system. (From Preston RR, Wilson TE: Filtration and micturition. In: Harvey RA, ed. *Physiology*. Philadelphia: Lippincott Williams & Wilkins, 2013, with permission.)

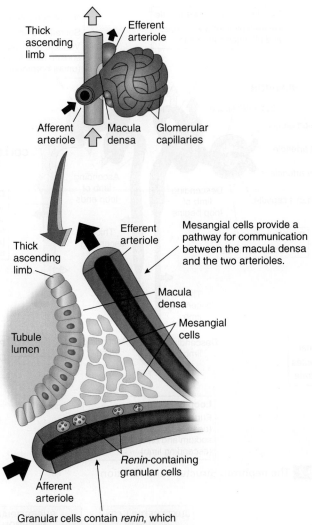

Thick ascending limb

Efferent arteriole

Afferent arteriole   Macula densa   Glomerular capillaries

Efferent arteriole

Thick ascending limb

Mesangial cells provide a pathway for communication between the macula densa and the two arterioles.

Macula densa

Tubule lumen

Mesangial cells

Renin-containing granular cells

Afferent arteriole

Granular cells contain *renin*, which is released into the circulation when tubule flow rates are low.

Figure 5-4 Juxtaglomerular apparatus. (From Preston RR, Wilson TE. Filtration and micturition. In: Harvey RA, ed. *Physiology*. Philadelphia: Lippincott Williams & Wilkins, 2013, with permission.)

Proximal Tubule and Loop of Henle

The cellular structure of the *proximal tubule* is highly specialized, reflecting the high energy demands required for a range of complex transport functions (Table 5-1). Virtually no active transport occurs in the descending part of the loop of Henle (Fig. 5-4). Urine concentration occurs in this part of the loop through passive urea transporters and simple water channels. The thick ascending limb is where sodium and potassium adenosine triphosphatase (Na, K-ATPase)–driven active transport resorbs sodium and chloride. The macula densa, is the modified part of the thick ascending limb of the loop of Henle which forms part of the juxtaglomerular apparatus (1).

The Distal Tubule

The *distal tubule* is composed of the distal convoluted tubule, the connecting segment, and the initial collecting tubule (Fig. 5-3). The cells of the distal

Table 5-1	Relations of Cellular Structure and Function in the Proximal Tubule		
Segment	**Location**	**Structure**	**Function**
Proximal convoluted tubule (S1)	Cortical labyrinth	Tall cuboidal cells, long brush border and villi, long mitochondria situated at deep infoldings of the basolateral membrane, apical vesicles, abundant lysosomes and peroxisomes	Bulk reabsoption of water, electrolytes, glucose, and other solutes, driven by transporters and channels in apical and basolateral membranes. Reabsorption of LMW proteins and peptides by receptor-mediated endocytosis
Straight tubule S2	Medullary rays of the cortex and outer stripe of the outer medulla	Cuboidal cells less tall than S1, shorter brush border and fewer villi, fewer mitochondria, vesicles and lysosomes, less basolateral infoldings, fewer peroxisomes	Secretion of organic acids, lipid biosynthesis, catalase-mediated destruction of hydrogen peroxide
Straight tubule S3	Predominantly outer medulla	Cuboidal cells with long brush border, less complex basolateral border than S1 and S2, few mitochondria, vesicles and lysosomes	

Na, K-ATPase, sodium and potassium adenosine triphosphatase; LMW, low molecular weight; S, segment.

convoluted tubule actively transport sodium and have calcium ATPase, which is important in the reabsorption of divalent cations. The connecting segments lie within the cortical labyrinth, where several join together to form the collecting duct. Cells of the connecting segment are similarly involved in sodium and cation transport but, unlike the distal convoluted tubule cells, they have water channels.

C. Glomerular Filtration Rate

The glomerular filtration rate is the volume of filtrate formed by both kidneys per minute. This is approximately 125 mL/min in an average patient with normal renal function. Fluid and solutes are forced under pressure from the glomerulus (afferent arteriole) into the capsular space (enclosed by *Bowman's capsule*) of the renal corpuscle. A filtration membrane allows the passage of fluid and small solutes into the capsular space based on their physical size and charge. Filtration occurs by bulk flow driven by the hydrostatic pressure of the blood; small molecules pass rapidly through the filtration membrane while larger molecules are retained within the arteriole. The relatively large diameter of the afferent arterioles and small diameter of the efferent arterioles result in a high capillary pressure (~60 mm Hg). This driving pressure is opposed by the back pressure of the capsular hydrostatic pressure (~15 mm Hg). Although the concentration of the small solutes is the same across the filtration membrane, large proteins are retained and the osmotic pressure of the blood increases as the fluid moves out of the glomerulus. This results in an overall net filtration pressure of approximately 17 mm Hg. There is a direct relation between the net filtration pressure and the glomerular filtration rate.

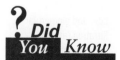
? Did You Know

Glomerular filtration is the primary determinant of urine composition.

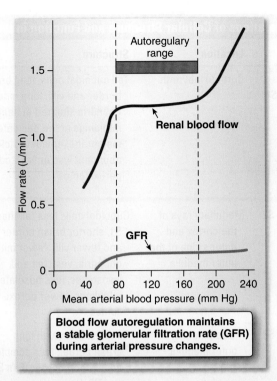

Figure 5-5   Autoregulation of renal blood flow. (From Preston RR, Wilson TE. Filtration and micturition. In: Harvey RA, ed. *Physiology*. Philadelphia: Lippincott Williams & Wilkins, 2013, with permission.)

If either the hydrostatic or osmotic pressure of the glomerular capillaries or the hydrostatic pressure of the capsular space changes, the glomerular filtration rate will also change.

D. Autoregulation of Renal Blood Flow and Glomerular Filtration

Autoregulation of renal blood flow and glomerular filtration rate are intimately related. In normal humans, renal blood flow is maintained nearly constant over the range of 70 to 120 mm Hg mean systemic arterial pressure (Fig. 5-5). There are three main mechanisms whereby renal blood flow and thus glomerular filtration rate are regulated: myogenic response, tubuloglomerular feedback, and sympathetic nervous system stimulation.

Myogenic Response

The myogenic response is the intrinsic property of vascular smooth muscle, whereby arterioles constrict in response to increased transmural pressure and allow a relatively constant blood flow and glomerular filtration rate (2).

The Tubuloglomerular Feedback

The tubuloglomerular feedback mechanism occurs via the macula densa. By virtue of its proximity to the afferent arteriole (Fig. 5-4), it is perfectly positioned to create a feedback loop controlling blood flow through the glomerulus. If the myogenic response does not fully regulate blood flow through the glomerulus, the increased capillary pressure increases the glomerular filtration rate, inhibiting sodium reabsorption in the proximal tubule. The increased delivery of sodium chloride in the tubular fluid reaching the macula densa in the distal tubule results in vasoconstriction of the afferent arteriole (tubuloglomerular feedback). Increased sodium transport in the distal tubule is not the only mechanism triggering tubuloglomerular feedback. Tubular fluid flow, independent of sodium concentration, is sensed by primary cilia located on the apical (luminal) aspect of the macula densa cells.

Sympathetic Nervous System

During periods of stress, such as hypotension or hemorrhage, sympathetic stimulation overrides autoregulation. Increased sympathetic discharge causes intense constriction of all of the renal vessels, reducing the glomerular filtration rate and subsequent fluid and electrolyte losses. Increased renal sympathetic activity decreases sodium and water excretion by 1) increasing tubular water and sodium reabsorption throughout the nephron, 2) decreasing renal blood flow and glomerular filtration rate by vasoconstriction of the arterioles, and 3) increasing activity of the renin angiotensin system by releasing renin from the juxtaglomerular granular cells (3).

E. Tubular Reabsorption of Sodium and Water

Sodium moves freely from the glomerulus across the filtration membrane into Bowman's capsule and has the same concentration in the tubular fluid as it has in the plasma. Approximately two-thirds of the filtrate reaching the proximal tubule is reabsorbed and is regulated both acutely and chronically by blood pressure, extracellular fluid volume, renin angiotensin system, sympathetic nervous system, and an intrarenal dopamine natriuretic system (4). The bulk of sodium chloride, bicarbonate, phosphate, glucose, water, and other substrates is reabsorbed into the tubular cells as they move *passively* down their concentration gradients (Fig. 5-6). Sodium potassium ATPase in the basolateral membrane then *actively* pumps sodium out of the cell into the interstitial fluid, maintaining a low intracellular concentration. This maintains the driving force for sodium entry from the tubular fluid at the luminal side. The *colloid oncotic pressure* in the capillaries accompanying the proximal tubules is high because large molecules are retained by the filtration membrane of Bowman's capsule. Sodium and water are reabsorbed from the interstitial fluid into the capillaries by bulk flow mediated by both hydrostatic and osmotic forces. The fraction of sodium reabsorbed in the proximal tubule varies according to prevailing conditions (Table 5-2). Water reabsorption occurs passively in the proximal tubule by osmosis and is coupled with sodium transport through the cells. Water also passes through the tight junctions between cells, which allows for diffusion of water and small ions.

The loop of Henle has three distinct regions: the thin descending segment, the thin ascending segment, and the thick ascending segment. The thin segments have thin membranes with no brush borders and few mitochondria

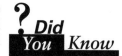

? Did You Know

The renal sympathetic nerves innervate the arterioles, the tubules, and the juxtaglomerular apparatus. This regulates blood flow, glomerular filtration, sodium and water reabsorption, and activity of the renin angiotensin system.

Table 5-2 Factors Affecting Sodium Reabsorption by the Renal Tubule	
Factors Decreasing Sodium Reabsorption	**Factors Increasing Sodium Reabsorption**
Increased blood pressure	Reduced blood pressure, hemorrhage
High salt intake	Low salt diet
Increased extracellular volume	Sympathetic stimulation
Inhibition of angiotensin II	Angiotensin II

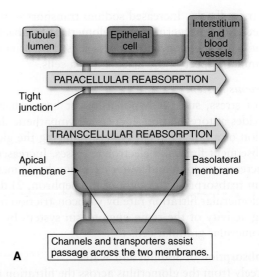

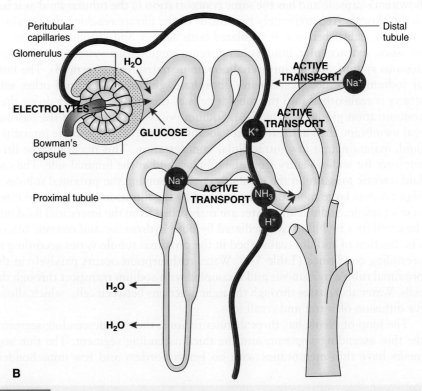

Figure 5-6 **A:** Reabsorption from tubular lumen. (From Preston RR, Wilson TE. Filtration and micturition. In: Harvey RA, ed. *Physiology*. Philadelphia: Lippincott Williams & Wilkins, 2013, with permission.) **B:** Transport of substances across glomerulus. (From *Straight A's in Anatomy and Physiology*. Ambler, PA: Lippincott Williams & Wilkins; 2007:313, with permission.)

(Fig. 5-3) because of low metabolic requirements. There is *little active* reabsorption of water or solutes within these segments. However, the thin descending segment is highly permeable to water, but not to solutes. Therefore, as water diffuses passively out of the cells, the osmolarity of the tubular fluid increases to a maximum at the very tip of the loop of Henle. In contrast, both the thin and thick part of the ascending limb are impermeable to water (Fig. 5-6). Sodium moves into the cell along its gradient which is maintained by basolateral sodium potassium ATPase. At the same time, sodium cotransports potassium into the cell against its gradient.

The remainder of the *distal nephron* includes the connecting segment (or connecting tubule) and collecting duct (Figs. 5-2 and 5-3). Only a small percentage of the original filtrate reaches these segments, but the reabsorption of water and solutes is highly regulated here and accounts for the fine tuning of fluid and electrolyte homeostasis by the kidney. There are distinct cell populations in the distal nephron. The connecting segment consists of connecting cells and intercalated cells, while the collecting duct consists of principal cells and intercalated cells. Sodium reabsorption in the connecting segment and collecting duct is mediated by the connecting cells and principal cells via hormone-sensitive (aldosterone) apical epithelial sodium channels. The *intercalated cells* are of two types: type A, which secretes protons and reabsorbs potassium, and type B, which secretes bicarbonate and reabsorbs chloride. Water reabsorption, which occurs to a much greater extent in the collecting duct than the connecting segment, is under the influence of antidiuretic hormone (arginine vasopressin). The collecting duct is normally relatively impermeable to water. However, it becomes highly permeable in the presence of antidiuretic hormone.

F. The Renin-Angiotensin-Aldosterone System

The renin-angiotensin-aldosterone system (RAAS) traditionally considers that *angiotensinogen (AGT)* is generated by the liver, cleaved by renin, and released from the juxtaglomerular cells of the kidneys to form *angiotensin I (Ang I)*. This is in turn further cleaved by *angiotensin-converting enzyme (ACE)* produced by the lungs to form the active hormone *angiotensin II (Ang II)* (Fig. 5-7).

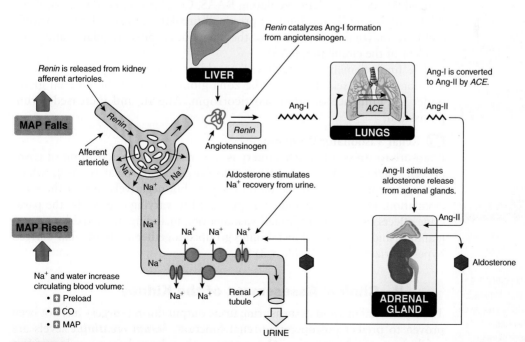

Figure 5-7 The renin angiotensin aldosterone system. (From Preston RR, Wilson TE. Filtration and micturition. In: Harvey RA, ed. *Physiology*. Philadelphia: Lippincott Williams & Wilkins, 2013, with permission.)

Table 5-3   Renal Vasodilators

Factor	Site of Action	Mainly Counteracts	Time Course	Contribution to Vasodilation
Nitric oxide	Medulla +++ Cortex ++	Renal sympathetic nerve stimulation	Later prolonged effect	50–70%
Prostaglandins	Medulla +++ Cortex +/–	Angiotensin II Vasopressin	Later prolonged effect	20–40%
EDHF	Medulla +++ Cortex 0	RAS	Initial response, short lived	<20%

EDHF, endothelial-derived hyperpolarizing factor; RAS, renin angiotensin system.

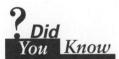

? Did You Know

The net result of aldosterone action is reabsorption of sodium and water in the collecting duct, resulting in an increase in intravascular volume and systemic blood pressure.

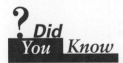

? Did You Know

Serum creatinine level does not rise until at least half of the kidney's nephrons are destroyed or damaged. Consequently, creatinine levels are often preferred to monitor renal function on a more long-term basis.

Ang II then binds to specific receptors in the adrenal cortex, releasing aldosterone. The combined effect of RAAS produces vasoconstriction, increased blood pressure, and aldosterone-mediated sodium retention in the collecting duct. The main effector peptide is Ang II, which binds to two distinct receptors: angiotensin type-1 receptor (AT_1R) and angiotensin type-2 receptor (AT_2R). AT_1Rs are more numerous than AT_2Rs throughout the body, and they mediate vasoconstriction, tubular sodium reabsorption sympathetic stimulation and secretion of aldosterone, vasopressin, and endothelin.

Actually, RAAS is a much more complex scheme, involving ACE-independent pathways and, more importantly, local (paracrine) and even intracellular (intracrine) RAAS within the kidneys (5). In the normal physiological state, sodium and water balance is thought to be predominantly under the control of local RAAS rather than circulating RAAS. Cellular studies have colocalized AGT, Ang I, Ang II, and renin in proximal tubular and juxtaglomerular cells and have shown that the release of these peptides is finely regulated and independent of the circulating RAAS.

The final element of the RAAS is aldosterone, the mineralocorticoid hormone that is secreted from the zona glomerulosa of the adrenal gland under the influence of adrenocorticotropin, Ang II, and increased serum potassium.

G. Renal Vasodilator Response

Exposure to stress, of which surgery is one, results in the activation of *vasopressor factors* (RAAS, sympathetic discharge, vasopressin release), which maintain or increase systemic blood pressure but negatively impact the renal circulation. However, the kidney is protected to varying degrees by the paracrine effects of several intrarenal vasodilators, including nitric oxide, prostaglandins, and a number of metabolites grouped together as endothelial-derived hyperpolarizing factor (Table 5-3) (6).

II. Clinical Assessment of the Kidney

The traditional method of measuring urine output during surgery has not been proven to predict postoperative renal function. *Serum creatinine* levels are similarly nonpredictive of renal outcome as they depend on a number of factors, some of which may change dramatically during the perioperative period (Table 5-4). Changes in serum creatinine during the perioperative period have

Table 5-4	Factors Affecting Serum Creatinine Levels
Physiologic Factors Affecting Serum Creatinine	**Drugs Affecting Serum Creatinine**
Age, gender, ethnicity	Cimetidine, trimethoprim, sulfamethoxalate, fibric acid derivative—decrease tubular secretion
Muscle mass, muscle diseases	Some cephalosporins—interfere with assay
Protein intake	Corticosteroids, vitamin D metabolites—affect production and release

been found to be more predictive of renal outcome. The now established *RIFLE* (Risk, Injury, Failure, Loss, End stage) and *AKIN* (Acute Kidney Injury Network) classifications (Fig. 5-8) of renal risk based on increases in serum creatinine or glomerular filtration rate are accepted as the standard for predicting and reporting renal outcomes (7,8). In a study of patients undergoing infrarenal abdominal aortic aneurysm surgery, AKIN was more robust in predicting mortality (9). Other renal function tests, which may be helpful, are based on the filtration ability of the kidney. Glomerular filtration rate is estimated from the ***Cockcroft-Gault equation*** or the ***Modification of Diet in Renal Disease (MDRD)*** formula both, of which are available online (10,11). The kidney's ability to filter and reabsorb electrolytes can be estimated from a spot sample of blood and urine as the fractional excretion of sodium (FE_{Na}) and can be used to differentiate between hypovolemia and renal injury in oliguria. A urinary sodium <20 mmol/L and a FE_{Na} <1% are suggestive of prerenal failure; while a urinary sodium >40 mmol/L and a FE_{Na} >1% are suggestive of intrinsic renal failure (Table 5-5).

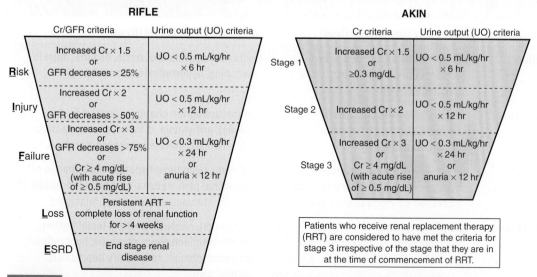

Figure 5-8 The RIFLE (Risk, Injury, Failure, Loss, End stage renal disease) and AKIN (Acute Kidney Injury Network) classifications of acute kidney injury. (From Cruz DN, Ricci Z, Ronco C. Clinical review: RIFLE AKIN—Time for reappraisal. *Crit Care.* 2009;13(3):211–219, with permission.)

Table 5-5   Laboratory Indices in Renal Failure

	Prerenal	Renal	Postrenal
Creatinine (mg/dL)	↑	↑	↑
BUN (mg/dL)	↑↑	↑	↑
Spot urine Na$^+$ (mEq/L)	<20	>40	>20
Urine osmolality (mOsm/L)	>500	<400	<350
FE$_{NA}$ (%)	<1	>2	>2

BUN, blood urea nitrogen; Na, sodium; FE$_{NA}$, fraction sodium excreted in urine.

III. Perioperative Nephrology

A. Pathophysiology

Traditionally, *perioperative renal dysfunction* has been divided into prerenal (hypovolemia, shock, hemorrhage), intrarenal (intrinsic, renal parenchyma damage), and postrenal (obstructive) causes of oliguria (Table 5-5). As noted previously oliguria is not a good marker for either renal function or renal outcome in the perioperative period. Efforts are now being concentrated on developing earlier detection of kidney injury. A number of biomarkers that have been investigated in translational research protocols are now recommended as part of the clinical approach to diagnose renal dysfunction in critical care settings (8).

B. Electrolyte Disorders

The most common electrolyte disorders encountered in the perioperative period and critical care setting are those involving sodium, potassium, calcium, magnesium, and phosphorus, with significant effects predominantly on the cardiac, neuromuscular, and central nervous systems (Table 5-6). Of these,

Table 5-6   Signs and Symptoms of Electrolyte Disorders

Electrolyte	Abnormally Low Levels (Hypo)	Abnormally High Levels (Hyper)
Sodium	Anorexia, nausea, lethargy, cerebral edema, convulsions, coma, arrhythmia, death	Confusion, convulsions, coma, oliguria, muscle twitching, hyperreflexia, spacticity
Potassium	Electrocardiogram changes (flat T waves, U waves), arrhythmia, muscle weakness	Electrocardiogram changes (peaked T waves), arrhythmia, malaise, gastrointestinal disturbances, muscle weakness, paralysis
Calcium	Paresthesia, irritability, seizures, hypotension, myocardial depression, increased QT interval, laryngospasm	Confusion, hypotonia, hyporeflexia, lethargy, abdominal pain, nausea, vomiting, decreased ST and QT intervals, polyuria, nephrolithiasis
Magnesium	Arrhythmias, weakness, muscle twitching, tetany, apathy, seizures	Hypotension, nausea, vomiting, facial flushing, urinary retention, ileus, paralysis, hyporeflexia, bradyarrhythmias, respiratory depression, cardiac arrest
Phosphate	Muscle weakness, respiratory failure, hemolysis	Calcium precipitation, decreased intestinal calcium absorption

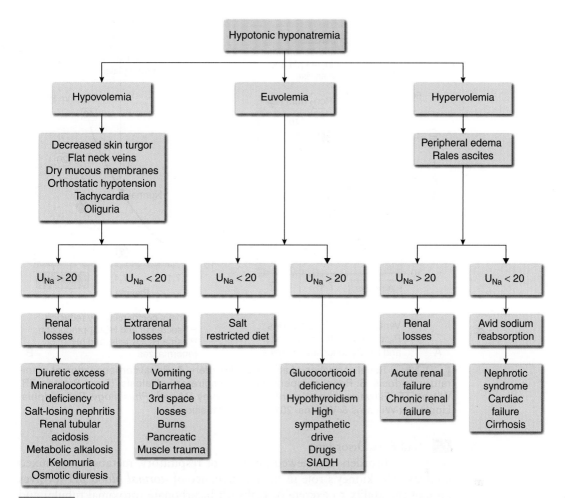

Figure 5-9 Diagnostic algorithm for hypotonic hyponatremia. SIADH, syndrome of inappropriate secretion of antidiuretic syndrome; U_{NA}, urinary sodium concentration (mEq/L) in a spot urine sample. (From Schrier RW. *Manual of Nephrology*. 6th ed. Philadelphia: Lippincott Williams & Wilkins, 2006, with permission.)

hyponatremia is the most common abnormality (up to 15% of hospitalized patients), which can occur in the context of a normal, expanded, or contracted extracellular volume (Fig. 5-9). Assessment of the volume status of the patient along with a measure of urinary sodium excretion is the first step in diagnosing the cause. *Hypernatremia* is usually the result of water loss (diabetes insipidus, osmotic diuretic, burns) rather than sodium gain.

Potassium balance is normally tightly controlled via gastrointestinal and renal excretion and reabsorption. In the kidney, 70% of potassium reabsorption occurs in the proximal tubule, 15% to 20% in the loop of Henle, and the remainder of the reabsorbed potassium is under the influence of aldosterone in the collecting duct. Ninety-eight percent of total body potassium is intracellular, and imbalances often occur because of shifts across cellular membranes (insulin therapy, beta-agonism, and acid base disturbances). Frank losses are due to vomiting and diarrhea or drug and hormone effects. Hyperkalemia may be caused by renal failure, potassium-sparing diuretics, intravenous therapy, and acidosis.

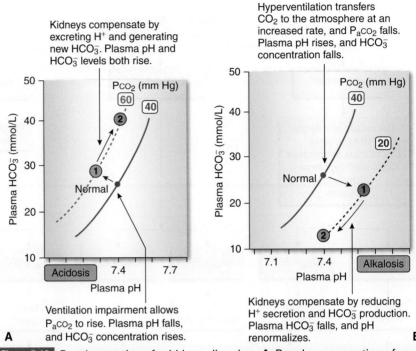

Figure 5-10 Renal correction of acid-base disorders. **A:** Renal compensation of respiratory acidosis. **B:** Renal compensation of respiratory alkalosis. (From Preston RR, Wilson TE. Filtration and micturition. In: Harvey RA, ed. *Physiology*. Philadelphia: Lippincott Williams & Wilkins, 2013, with permission.)

C. Acid Base Disorders

Acid base disorders are viewed as being of respiratory, metabolic, or mixed etiology. The kidney's role in the maintenance of *normal blood pH* revolves around the ability to excrete or reabsorb bicarbonate (proximal tubule) and hydrogen ions (distal tubule and collecting duct) (Fig. 5-10). Hydrogen ion excretion in the urine regenerates the bicarbonate originally consumed by buffering a hydrogen ion in the extracellular fluid. The excreted hydrogen ions are themselves buffered by titratable renal buffers (predominantly ammonia) and lost in the urine.

D. Acute Kidney Injury

Patients who develop acute kidney injury (AKI) in the perioperative period have a worse clinical outcome and an increased risk of death. One-third of patients surviving with AKI will go on to develop significant chronic kidney disease, while only one-half of the remainder will return to baseline renal function. The pathogenesis of AKI is complex. It involves both the vascular endothelium and tubular epithelium and the release of inflammatory and immune mediators and other cascades (12). Factors precipitating the events that culminate in AKI are typically ischemic (hypoperfusion, vasoconstriction) or toxic (e.g., contrast media, aminoglycosides, myoglobin) (7). Several clinical renal risk indices exist that may be helpful in planning surgery and anesthesia. No specific pharmacologic agent has been shown to consistently benfit AKI in the perioperative setting. Management of patients at risk for, or with AKI, is predicated on the use of adequate hemodynamic monitoring to aid goal-oriented therapy and provide appropriate intravascular volume repletion, mean arterial pressure, cardiac output, and oxygen-carrying capacity. All

Table 5-7 Effects of Chronic Kidney Disease on Other Organ Systems		
System	**Derangement**	**Causes**
Cardiac	Hypertension Myocardial dysfunction Pericarditis Tamponade Congestive heart failure	Hypervolemia, activation of RAAS Activation of SNS Uremia, dialysis
Respiratory	Pulmonary edema Restrictive lung disease	Reduced oncotic pressure Uremic pleuritis

Metabolic	Metabolic acidosis
	Hyperkalemia
	Hypoglycemia
		Inability to conserve bicarbonate
		  and excrete titratable acids
		Reduced clearance of insulin/other
		  hypoglycemic drugs; reduced
		  renal gluconeogenesis

Hematologic	Anemia
	Platelet dysfunction
		Loss of erythropoietin
		Action of uremic toxins, abnormal
		  nitric oxide production, von
		  Willebrand factor abnormalities
		  and drugs

Immunologic	Cell-mediated defects Humoral immunity defects	Reduced clearance of cytokines
Gastrointestinal	Nausea and vomiting Delayed gastric emptying Anorexia	Uremia, drug therapy, dialysis

Neuromuscular	Encephalopathy
	Seizures, tremors, and
	  myoclonus
	Autonomic dysfunction
	Polyneuropathy
		Electrolyte, cation, and fluid
		  abnormalities

RAAS, renin angiotensin aldosterone system; SNS, sympathetic nervous system.

nonessential and potentially nephrotoxic agents must be avoided or at least minimized. Careful consideration should be given to the level of postoperative care and surveillance required as AKI typically does not manifest until several days later.

E. Chronic Kidney Disease

Chronic kidney disease (CKD) is defined by the International Society of Nephrology and Kidney Disease Improving Global Outcomes as abnormalities of kidney structure or function, present for more than 3 months, with implications for health (Table 5-7). CKD is classified based on cause, glomerular filtration rate (GFR), and albuminuria (13). Grades of CKD have been established according to GFR and albuminuria, and risk can be apportioned according to these grades (Fig. 5-11). Because hypertension and diabetes are the leading causes of CKD, accounting for >70% of cases, there is significant comorbidity associated with the cause of CKD and by CKD itself (Table 5-7).

Prognosis of CKD by GFR and albuminuria categories

Prognosis of CKD by GFR and albuminuria categories: KDIGO 2012			Persistent albuminuria categories Description and range		
			A1	**A2**	**A3**
			Normal to mildly increased	Moderately increased	Severely increased
			<30 mg/g <3 mg/mmol	30–300 mg/g >30 mg/mmol	>300 mg/g >30 mg/mmol
GFR categories (mL/min/1.73 m²) Description and range	G1	Normal or high	≥90		
	G2	Mildly decreased	60–89		
	G3a	Mildly to moderately decreased	45–59		
	G3b	Moderately to Severely decreased	30–44		
	G4	Severely decreased	15–29		
	G5	Kidney failure	<15		

Green: Low risk (if no other markers of kidney disease, no CKD); Yellow: Moderately increased risk; Orange: High risk; Red: Very high risk; CKD: Chronic Kidney Disease; GFR: Glomerular filtration rate; KDIGO: Kidney Disease Improvement for Global Outcome.

Figure 5-11 Prognosis of chronic kidney disease by glomerular filtration rate and albuminuria categories. (From KDIGO 2012 Clinical Practice Guideline for the Evaluation and Management of Chronic Kidney Disease. Kidney International Supplements. 2013;3(1):x. www.kdigo.org/clinical_practice_guidelines/pdf/CKD/ KDIGO_2012_CKD_GL.pdf.)

The National Kidney Foundation's Kidney Disease Outcomes Quality Initiative provides evidence-based clinical practice guidelines for all stages of CKD and their related complications, including the management of hyperglycemia, hyperlipidemia, and anemia. Although a large proportion of CKD patients have diabetes, they are prone to hypoglycemia (Table 5-7). The current NKF guidelines for anemia is a hemoglobin >13 mg/dL.

Patients with *end-stage renal disease (ESRD)* require dialysis for survival. These patients have added physiologic derangements because of the dialysis therapy itself and the means of delivering that dialysis (Tables 5-8 and 5-9). Patients undergoing chronic dialysis are at risk for the development of infection, protein calorie deficiency malnutrition, amyloidosis, and psychological deterioration.

F. Drug Prescribing in Renal Failure

Drug prescribing in renal failure is based on altered *drug kinetics*, which occur in kidney disease. Limitations are placed on both drugs and dosing because of reduced renal clearance, increased volume of distribution, decreased plasma

Table 5-8	Complications of Dialysis or Hemofiltration Access
Access Route	**Complications**
Temporary venous access (usually internal jugular vein, subclavian vein)	Bleeding, hypotension, hematoma (increased BUN, pigmenturia), thrombosis, stricture (SVC syndrome), pneumothorax, chylothorax, nerve injury
Peritoneal (becoming rare mode of access)	Ileus, increased abdominal pressure, increased risk of aspiration, raised diaphragm, reduced lung volumes, restrictive respiratory pattern
Upper limb arteriovenous fistula	Restricted limb access, thrombosis, interference with blood sampling and pulse oximetry, shunting, reduced vascular resistance

BUN, blood urea nitrogen; SVC, superior vena cava.

protein binding, acidemia, coexisting liver disease, and changes in gastrointestinal uptake. Knowledge of a drug's pharmacokinetics will assist in modifying dose and interval timing and may help predict and prevent unwanted side effects (14,15) (see also Chapter 7).

G. Anesthetic Agents in Renal Failure

The pharmacokinetics of volatile anesthetics are not dependent on renal function, protein binding, or volume of distribution. However, the *fluoride ion* released during the metabolism of methoxyflurane and possibly enflurane have been attributed to nephrotoxicity in patients who have had long exposure to these agents. Drugs eliminated unchanged by the kidneys (some nondepolarizing muscle relaxants, cholinesterase inhibitors, many antibiotics) have increased elimination half-times, which are inversely related to GFR in CKD patients. Many anesthetic drugs are protein bound to varying degrees, and consequently, the free (active) fraction is increased in CKD. Of the induction agents, thiopental is most extensively protein bound and

Table 5-9	Acute Complications of Dialysis
Hypotension	Ultrafiltration-induced volume depletion; osmolar shifts across the dialysis membrane; myocardial ischemia; arrhythmias, pericardial effusion
Arrhythmia	Acute potassium flux; rapid pH changes
Hypersensitivity reaction	Exposure to polyacrylonitrile surfaces of dialysis membrane, residual ethylene oxide from sterilization of equipment
Dialysis disequilibrium	Characterized by nausea, vomiting, seizures, and even coma due to rapid changes in pH and solutes across CNS membranes

CNS, central nervous system.

therefore most affected in ESRD, with ketamine and etomidate being less affected. Propofol is not affected by ESRD because it is rapidly biotransformed by the liver into inactive metabolites, which are then excreted by the kidneys. In general, benzodiazepines are highly protein bound, and the increased availability in ESRD is further enhanced by reduced renal excretion of active metabolites (e.g., midazolam, lorazepam, and alprazolam).

Single doses of narcotics are generally not greatly affected by ESRD, although protein-bound narcotics require a smaller dose. The ultrashort-acting narcotics are preferable in ESRD, and fentanyl and remifentanil appear to be safe. Sufentanil, however, has been reported to cause prolonged narcosis. Short-acting muscle relaxants are preferable in patients with renal disease, and the two agents atracurium and cis-atracurium, which are metabolized by spontaneous nonenzymatic degradation, are the drugs of choice. Nevertheless, these two drugs have a toxic metabolite, laudanosine, which may accumulate during infusion of the parent drug.

IV. Diuretic Drugs: Effects and Mechanisms

A. The Physiologic Basis of Diuretic Action

Diuretics are typically classified according to their site of action in the nephron. In general terms, diuretic drugs act on the mechanism that moves sodium ions from the tubular lumen into the cell where they can then be pumped across the basolateral surface by Na-K ATPase and reabsorbed (Table 5-10).

B. Dopaminergic Agents

In the kidney, dopamine is synthesized in the proximal tubule from circulating L-dopa, via the enzyme L-amino acid decarboxylase. Circulating and locally formed dopamine activates a number of *dopamine receptors* via adenylyl cyclase, phospholipase C, and phospholipase A_2 on arterioles and tubules affecting both sodium excretion and renal hemodynamics (Table 5-11). Sodium reabsorption is reduced in the proximal tubule, producing a diuresis and natriuresis. Although dopamine is an effective diuretic, it has other effects on the cardiovascular system, which may include tachycardia and increased blood pressure even at so-called renal doses (1 to 3 µg/kg/min).

Table 5-10	Site and Mechanism of Action of Diuretics	
Site of Action	**Mechanism of Action**	**Common Drug Names**
Proximal tubule	Carbonic anhydrase inhibition	Acetazolamide
	Osmotic diuresis	Mannitol
Thick ascending limb of the loop of Henle	NKCC2 inhibition	Furosemide, ethacrynic acid, bumetanide, torsemide
Distal convoluted tubule	Sodium chloride cotransporter inhibition	Hydrochlorothiazide, metolazone
Collecting duct	Epithelial sodium channel inhibition	Amiloride, triamterene
	Aldosterone inhibition	Spironolactone

NKCC2, sodium-potassium-dichloride cotransporter.

Table 5-11	Effects of Dopamine on Renal Blood Flow and Tubular Function	
Effects on Renal Blood Flow	**Tubular Effects**
Renal vasodilation by increasing prostaglandin production	Reduces activity of Na-H exchanger in luminal membrane of proximal tubule
Increased renal blood flow which causes increased GFR	Inhibits Na-K-ATPase pump on basolateral membrane of proximal tubule Inhibits renal renin expression and release in macula densa by inhibiting COX-2

Na-H, sodium hydrogen ion; Na-K-ATPase, sodium potassium adenosine triphosphatase; GFR, glomerular filtration rate; COX-2, cylooxygenase-2.

Dopamine has not been shown to protect against or ameliorate either AKI or CKD and is no longer recommended for these roles. The selective dopamine 1 agonist fenoldopam is also an efficient diuretic, and there are some data suggesting that it may be effective in preventing cardiac surgery–associated AKI. It is, however, not in widespread use as a renoprotective agent and is only U.S. Food and Drug Administration approved as an antihypertensive in hypertensive crises due to systemic vasodilation and diuresis.

References

1. Sipos A, Vargas A, Peti-Peterdi J. Direct demonstration of tubular fluid flow sensing by macula densa cells. *Am J Physiol Renal Physiol.* 2010;299:F1087–F1093.
2. Burke M, Pabbidi MR, Farley J, et al. Molecular mechanisms of renal blood flow autoregulation. *Curr Vasc Pharmacol.* 2014;12:1–14.
3. DiBona GF. Nervous kidney: Interaction between renal sympathetic nerves and the renin-angiotensin system in the control of renal function. *Hypertension.* 2000;36:1083–1088.
4. McDonough AA. Mechanisms of proximal tubule sodium transport regulation that link extracellular fluid volume and blood pressure. *Am J Physiol Regul Integr Comp Physiol.* 2010;298:R851–R861.
5. Carey RM. The intrarenal renin-angiotensin and dopaminergic systems: Control of renal sodium excretion and blood pressure. *Hypertension.* 2013;61:673–680.
6. Sadowski J, Badzynska B. Intrarenal vasodilator systems: NO, prostaglandins and bradykinin: An integrative approach. *J Physiol Pharmacol.* 2008;59(Suppl 9):105–119.
7. Bagshaw SM, Bellomo R, Devarajan P, et al. Review article: Acute kidney injury in critical illness. *Can J Anesth.* 2010;57:985–998.
8. McCullough PA, Shaw AD, Haase M, et al. Diagnosis of acute kidney injury using functional and injury biomarkers: Workgroup statements from the Tenth Acute Dialysis Quality Initiative Consensus Conference. *Contrib Nephrol.* 2013;182:13–29.
9. Bang J-Y, Lee JB, Yoon Y, et al. Acute kidney injury after infrarenal abdominal aortic aneurysm: A comparison of AKIN and RIFLE criteria for risk prediction. *BJA.* 2014;113:9093–1000.
10. U.S. Department of Health and Human Services. National Kidney Disease and Education Program. Estimating GFR. Available at: http://nkdep.nih.gov/lab-evaluation/gfr/estimating.shtml.
11. MD+CALC. Creatine clearance (Cockcroft-Gault equation). Available at: http://www.mdcalc.com/creatinine-clearance-cockcroft-gault-equation/.
12. Sharfuddin AA, Molitoris BA. Pathophysiology of ischemic acute kidney injury. *Nat Rev Nephrol.* 2011;7:189–200.

13. KDIGO 2012 Clinical Practice Guideline for the Evaluation and Management of Chronic Kidney Disease. Kidney International Supplements. 2013;3(1):x. Available at: www.kdigo.org/clinical_practice_guidelines/pdf/CKD/KDIGO_2012_CKD_GL.pdf.
14. Griffiths RS, Olyaei AJ. Drug dosing in patients with chronic disease. In: *Nephrology Secrets*. 3rd ed. Philadelphia: Wolters Kluwer; 2012:197–206.
15. Gabardi S, Abramson S. Drug dosing in chronic kidney disease. *Med Clin North Am.* 2005;89(3):649–687.

Questions

1. Which compound is actively transported in the thin descending loop of Henle?
   A. Water
   B. Sodium
   C. Glucose
   D. None

2. Autoregulation of renal blood flow in the normal adult:
   A. Occurs between mean arterial pressure 70 to 120 mm Hg
   B. Maintains renal blood flow at 1.25 L/min
   C. Maintains glomerular filtration rate at 125 mL/min
   D. All of the above

3. Autoregulation of renal blood flow occurs with all of the following EXCEPT:
   A. Myogenic response
   B. Tubuloglomeric response
   C. Arterial oxygen saturation
   D. Sympathetic nervous system response

4. The intrinsic renal vasodilator with the greatest contribution to vasodilation is:
   A. Prostaglandin
   B. Nitric oxide
   C. Endothelial derived hyperpolarizing factor
   D. Aldosterone

5. This graph depicts the relationship between:

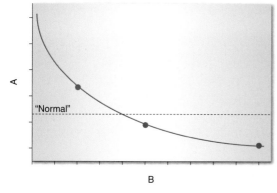

   A. Axis A = serum creatinine; Axis B = glomerular filtration rate
   B. Axis A = serum creatinine; Axis B = renal blood flow
   C. Axis A = mean arterial pressure; Axis B = glomerular filtration rate
   D. Axis A = serum creatinine; Axis B = blood urea nitrogen (BUN)

6. The major difference between the RIFLE (Risk, Injury, Failure, Loss, End stage) and AKIN (Acute Kidney Injury Network) classification of renal injury is:
   A. Use of glomerular filtration rate (GFR)
   B. Use of urine output
   C. Use of creatinine
   D. Use of blood urea nitrogen (BUN)

7. An 80-year-old male intensive care unit patient with a history of chronic obstructive pulmonary disease has the following: arterial blood gas (40% oxygen by facemask) pH 7.30, arterial carbon dioxide partial pressure ($PaCO_2$) 60 mm Hg, and arterial partial pressure of oxygen (PaO_2) 60 mm Hg. The renal compensation for this blood gas profile is:
   A. Excrete H^+
   B. Decrease HCO_3^- production
   C. Reabsorb HCO_3^- in distal tubule
   D. Reabsorb K^+ in collecting duct

8. In a patient with renal failure, dopamine administration:
   A. Increases Na^+ in proximal tubule
   B. Is protective against acute and chronic kidney injury
   C. Causes renal effects due to cardiac actions alone
   D. Is inferior to fenoldopam for renal protection

9. An 80-year-old male is seen preoperatively with a clinically significant gastrointestinal bleed. His blood pressure is 70/40, pulse 110, respiration 24, oxygen saturation as measure by pulse oximetry (SpO_2) 94%. What part of his kidney is likely to sustain the most damage?
   A. Tubule
   B. Loop of Henle
   C. Glomerulus
   D. Basement membrane

10. One week following discharge after left knee replacement, a 65-year-old female is prescribed ibuprofen for postoperative analgesia. Following ibuprofen treatment, her creatinine will likely:
    A. Increase
    B. Not increase, but her BUN will increase
    C. Not change
    D. Decrease

6 Liver Anatomy and Physiology

Niels Chapman

I. Gross Anatomy

The human liver is the largest solid organ, comprising 2% of total body mass and weighing approximately 1,500 g. Anatomically, the liver has *four lobes (right, left, caudate, and quadrate)* and can be further subdivided into eight segments, according to Couinaud's classification. Residing behind the rib cage in the right upper quadrant of the abdomen, the liver is covered in a thin connective tissue layer *(Glisson's capsule)* and is attached to the anterior abdominal wall by the falciform ligament and round ligament of the liver (umbilical cord remnant) and to the diaphragm by the coronary ligament (Fig. 6-1).

Key related structures of the hepatobiliary system include the *gallbladder* and its *cystic duct* outflow tract, which combines with the common hepatic duct to form the *common bile duct*. More distally, the common bile duct joins the pancreatic duct to form the *hepatopancreatic ampulla (ampulla of Vater)*, which then drains bile and pancreatic secretions into the second portion of the duodenum through the *sphincter of Oddi* (Figs. 6-1 and 6-2).

II. Microscopic Anatomy

Hepatocytes are arranged within *hepatic sinusoids* surrounding a central hepatic vein and are bordered by interlobular *portal triads* consisting of a biliary duct, hepatic artery, and portal vein (Figs. 6-3 and 6-4). This functional anatomy results from a complicated embryologic ballet in which the growing organ forms around portal veins, with bile ducts originating out of precursor ductal plates situated on the portal veins. Hepatic sinuses run from the peripheral portal triads to the centrolobar hepatic veins and are lined with fenestrated endothelial cells, featuring intracytoplasmic pores and loose intercellular junctions. In addition to the endothelial cells, other resident cell populations of the sinusoidal wall include *Kupffer cells* (macrophages),

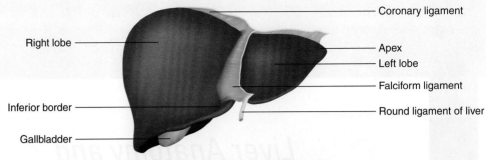

(A) Anterior view, diaphragmatic surface

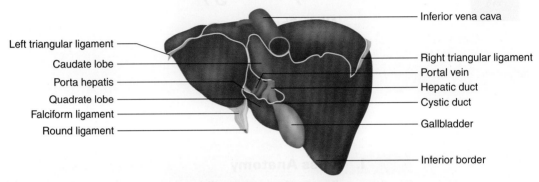

(B) Posterior-inferior view, visceral surface

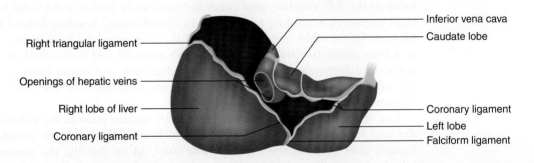

(C) Superior view

Figure 6-1 Gross anatomy of the liver. (From Moore KL, Agur AMR, Dalley AF. *Clinically Oriented Anatomy.* 7th ed. Philadelphia: Wolters Kluwer; 2013, with permission.)

stellate cells (responsible for extracellular matrix production and capable of contractile function to regulate sinusoidal blood flow), and *pit cells* (lymphocytes). The space separating the sinusoids from hepatocyte bars is known as the *perisinusoidal space of Disse,* and it contains extracellular matrix generated by stellate cells, Kupffer cells, and dendritic cells. These latter two cell types are involved in microbial and antigen host defense and contribute to the significant immune function of the liver as well as to the fibrosis observed with hepatic cirrhosis.

Bile is produced by hepatocytes and secreted into biliary canaliculi via *canals of Hering,* which are trough-like structures bordered by both hepatocytes and cholangiocytes that then drain into bile ducts.

Gallbladder, bile and pancreatic ducts (anterior view)

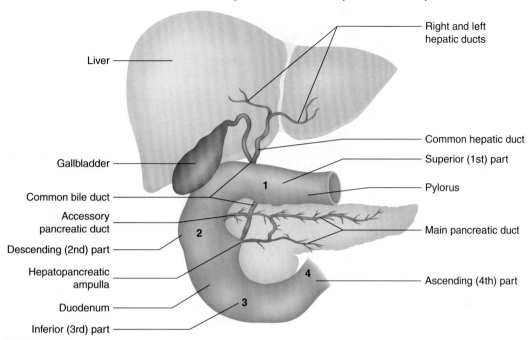

Figure 6-2 Gallbladder, bile, and pancreatic ducts. (From Moore KL, Agur AMR, Dalley AF. *Clinically Oriented Anatomy*. 7th ed. Philadelphia: Wolters Kluwer; 2013, with permission.)

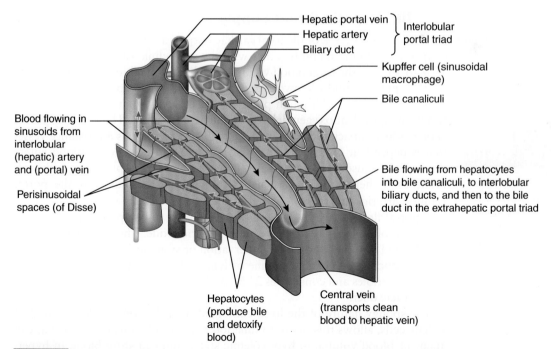

Figure 6-3 Section of hepatic lobule with functional diagram of bile and blood flow. (From Moore KL, Agur AMR, Dalley AF. *Clinically Oriented Anatomy*. 7th ed. Philadelphia: Wolters Kluwer; 2013, with permission.)

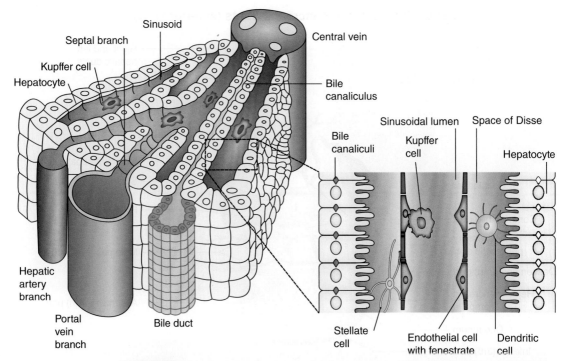

Figure 6-4 Portion of hepatic lobule: Microanatomy. (From Adams DH, Eksteen B. Aberrant homing of mucosal T cells and extra-intestinal manifestations of inflammatory bowel disease. *Nature Rev Immunol.* 2006;6:244–251, with permission.)

III. Hepatic Blood Supply

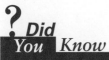

VIDEO 6-1

Liver Blood Volume

? Did You Know

Due to its high blood flow (25% of cardiac output) and immense blood filtration capacity, the liver produces up to 50% of all lymph volume flowing in the thoracic duct.

The liver receives 25% of the total cardiac output, accounts for 20% of resting oxygen consumption, and together with the splanchnic vascular bed contains 10% to 15% of the total blood volume. The liver's dual blood supply consists of 75% portal blood (deoxygenated blood) and 25% hepatic arterial blood (oxygenated blood). Although portal blood is deoxygenated, its higher flow results in equivalent oxygen delivery to the hepatic artery. The valveless *portal vein* acts as a capacitance vessel, while the *hepatic artery* is a resistance vessel that is dependent on systemic arterial pressure and flow. Most blood enters the hepatic sinusoids from portal venules through inlet sphincters, although branches of hepatic arterioles also terminate in sinusoids near the portal venules (arteriosinus twigs).

If portal flow decreases, arterial blood supply can be upregulated by vasodilatory molecules such as adenosine and nitric oxide. These mechanisms are not affected by either autonomic innervation or systemic humoral factors. The liver produces a significant volume of lymph through direct exudation from hepatic arterioles and constitutes 25% to 50% of the total lymph flow through the thoracic duct.

The spongy nature of the liver, combined with the contractile potential of stellate cells, allows this organ to function as an autologous reservoir that can augment blood volume in hypovolemic states and can store blood in hypervolemic states. This latter phenomenon can be observed in conditions of right heart failure (congestive hepatopathy), hypervolemia (renal failure), and iatrogenic overresuscitation.

IV. Hepatic Metabolic, Synthetic, and Excretory Functions

The liver performs a remarkable spectrum of metabolic and excretory functions, ranging from nutritional substance uptake from the portal and systemic circulations, to synthesis of various proteins and bile components, to regulation of circulating nutrients and toxins, to immune host defense (1). Examples of these functions include:

- *Bile synthesis and regulation: **Bile** is composed of various hepatic metabolic products, including cholesterol, phospholipids, bilirubin, and bile salts. Its secretion into the intestinal tract facilitates lipid emulsification, lipid absorption, and excretion of toxins and lipophilic drugs. Impaired bilirubin metabolism or bile secretion (e.g., gallstones) can lead to jaundice and malabsorption of dietary fats (steatorrhea).
- *Protein synthesis:* Most blood proteins (except antibodies) are synthesized in and secreted by the liver, including albumin, the ***vitamin K–dependent coagulation factors (II, VII, IX, and X),*** and the ***vitamin K–independent factors (V, XI, XII, and XIII and fibrinogen).*** These can be assessed clinically as indirect indicators of hepatic synthetic function. Amino acid synthesis and breakdown also occur in the liver, the latter by transamination and oxidative deamination, with formation of keto acids, ammonia, and glutamine. Disruption of these synthetic functions can be observed in extreme starvation or liver failure, leading to hypoproteinemia, ascites formation, and bleeding disorders.
- *Production of cholesterol and lipoproteins:* The liver transforms ingested **cholesterol** and synthesizes various lipoprotein species that act as blood-borne, transportable, emulsified packages that allow transport of essential cell metabolism elements around the body.
- *Nutrient storage:* The liver converts excess glucose into **glycogen** for storage and blood glucose regulation and also stores **fat-soluble vitamins (A, D, E, and K)** and minerals. As a result, liver failure is often accompanied by profound hypoglycemia.
- *Hemoglobin metabolism:* The liver processes iron-containing heme (in the form of unconjugated **bilirubin** generated by erythrocyte destruction and hemoglobin release in the spleen) so that its iron content can by recycled for various uses. The liver conjugates bilirubin with glucuronic acid to form water-soluble bilirubin that is excreted in bile.
- *Detoxification of drugs and other poisonous substances:* On an evolutionary basis, the position of the liver as the first organ to encounter products of intestinal absorption allowed survival in an environment in which plants produced toxins aimed at prohibiting consumption by animals. As the biochemical arms race evolved, the cytochrome apparatus in the liver has become capable of processing an extremely wide array of natural and synthetic substances to less- or nontoxic compounds. Nonetheless, some ingested toxins and drugs are capable of causing liver damage, if not liver failure (e.g., acetaminophen). Similarly, the endogenous toxin **ammonia** (absorbed across the intestine or created during hepatic protein metabolism) is converted in the liver to water-soluble urea for subsequent renal excretion. Impaired liver function results in ammonia accumulation and can lead to hepatic encephalopathy.
- *Immune host defense:* The ***mononuclear phagocyte system*** (formerly known as the reticuloendothelial system) comprises multiple cell types distributed

across various organs in a coordinated function of host defense, which includes the Kupffer and dendritic cells noted above. Impaired liver function can result in more frequent or severe systemic infections (e.g., spontaneous bacterial peritonitis). Kupffer cells also lyse erythrocytes into heme and globin components, thereby augmenting splenic release of unconjugated bilirubin into the circulation, where it combines with circulating albumin, eventually returning to the liver for hemoglobin metabolism, as described above.

V. Assessment of Hepatic Function

Due to the multiple "functions" of the liver and its sizable metabolic capacity, there is no single liver function test that is specific or accurate in identifying impaired hepatic function. Rather, assessment of hepatic function is more typically a triangulation process that incorporates clinical findings (history, physical examination), hepatobiliary imaging studies (ultrasound, computed tomography, magnetic resonance imaging, contrast radiography), and various laboratory tests (2,3). Laboratory tests are categorized as static and dynamic (Fig. 6-5). *Static tests* generally measure blood levels of individual hepatic enzymes (typically elevated when liver injury is present) or

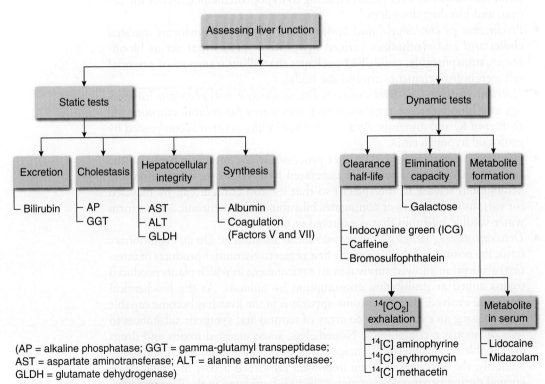

(AP = alkaline phosphatase; GGT = gamma-glutamyl transpeptidase;
AST = aspartate aminotransferase; ALT = alanine aminotransferasee;
GLDH = glutamate dehydrogenase)

Figure 6-5 Laboratory tests of hepatic function. Laboratory tests of hepatic function generally fall into two categories: the commonly used static tests of circulating blood compounds, proteins, and coagulation factors, and the infrequently used dynamic tests of liver metabolism, elimination, and clearance functions. (From Beck C, Schawrtges I, Picker O. Perioperative liver protection. *Curr Opin Crit Care.* 2010;16:142–147, with permission.)

hepatic synthesis products (typically reduced when liver injury is present) and are widely available. *Dynamic tests* measure functional pathways of substrate clearance and elimination or metabolite formation, but they are infrequently available and expensive. Routine laboratory testing of liver function is not advised because commonly used static liver function tests do not accurately reflect organ function, but instead indicate varying degrees of liver inflammation or damage. Instead, testing should be performed if the medical history, current disease process, or physical examination arouses suspicion of acute or chronic hepatic disease or if surgery involving the liver is planned.

Standard laboratory assays can potentially indicate organ injury (transaminases, bilirubin), impaired synthetic function (serum albumin, prothrombin time, fibrinogen), or systemic effects of advanced organ dysfunction (platelet count). Specific static laboratory tests include the hepatic transaminases aspartate aminotransferase (AST), alanine aminotransferase (ALT), alkaline phosphatase (AP), and γ-glutamyl transpeptidase (GGT). The AST enzyme is also found in muscle and other nonhepatic tissues, and AP is also found in bone, placenta, and intestine. In contrast, ALT and GGT are almost exclusively found in the liver; therefore, ALT and GGT are felt to be more specific indicators of liver pathology. Both AST and ALT can be elevated in settings of acute liver damage when the enzymes leak out of injured hepatocytes into the blood. In chronic liver disease, elevations in AST and ALT may not be present; however, the AST/ALT ratio is typically elevated in patients with alcoholic hepatitis or cirrhosis. An AST/ALT ratio >2 is present in ~70% of these patients compared with 26% of patients with postnecrotic cirrhosis, 8% with chronic hepatitis, 4% with viral hepatitis, and none with obstructive jaundice. If AP or GGT levels are elevated, a problem with bile flow is most likely present. Bile flow problems can be due to a bile duct pathology within the liver, the gallbladder, or the extrahepatic ducts.

As noted previously, unconjugated bilirubin is a breakdown product of heme from erythrocytes and is then conjugated with glucuronic acid in the liver for excretion in the bile. Elevated blood levels of "indirect bilirubin" (unconjugated bilirubin) indicate excessive hemoglobin breakdown (e.g., hemolysis) or impaired hepatic conjugation function. Elevated blood levels of "direct bilirubin" (conjugated bilirubin) occur when hepatic function is normal but bilirubin excretion is impaired (e.g., common bile duct obstruction). Bilirubin elevation is associated with abnormal physical examination findings of scleral icterus and cutaneous jaundice.

Albumin is a major protein formed by the liver; thus, chronic liver disease can impair albumin production and result in reduced blood albumin levels. Hypoalbuminemia has significant systemic effects on both protein binding of drugs (e.g., hypoalbuminemia results in larger fractions of unbound drug [see Chapter 7]) and oncotic pressure (e.g., hypoalbuminemia results in lower plasma oncotic pressure, favoring water movement to extravascular tissues in the form of edema and ascites [see Chapter 3]).

Because many protein coagulation factors are synthesized in the liver, liver injury can result in abnormal blood clotting or reductions in circulating coagulation factors. Indirect assessment of liver function by coagulation testing is most commonly done by measuring the prothrombin time and calculating its associated international normalized ratio (INR). Blood fibrinogen is the most frequently tested individual coagulation factor.

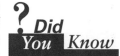

? Did You Know

Much like the combination of cardiac imaging and cardiac enzyme measurements is used to assess heart function and cardiac injury, the combination of hepatic imaging (computed tomography, ultrasound) and hepatic enzyme measurements (transaminases) is used to assess liver function and hepatic injury.

VI. Metabolism and Drug Disposition

The majority of all pharmaceuticals used in medical practice, including those used routinely in the perioperative period and the critical care setting, undergo *biotransformation* or *elimination* in the liver. Liver metabolism of such drugs, as well as other natural and synthetic substances (collectively known as xenobiotics), occurs by drug metabolizing enzymes that are genetically determined, yet can be environmentally modulated by both *enzyme induction* and *enzyme inhibition* (4,5). The general goal of such drug metabolism is to render the compounds more hydrophilic so that renal elimination of the modified drug or its metabolites can occur.

Hepatic drug metabolism occurs through two enzyme systems, either alone or in combination. *Phase 1 enzymes* generally alter existing functional groups to make the molecule more polar, thereby increasing its water solubility. Phase 1 enzymes consist of the *cytochrome P450* (CYP superfamily) class of enzymes that hydrolyze, oxidize, or reduce the parent compound (see Chapter 7). *Phase 2 enzymes* act primarily to conjugate polar compounds, thereby further increasing their hydrophilicity. Both phase 1 and phase 2 enzymes are inducible but can also be inhibited (usually by other drugs).

A more functional description of hepatic drug disposition of pharmaceuticals draws a distinction between substances cleared rapidly (essentially on the first pass through the liver from the portal or systemic venous circulations) and those that require considerable time for metabolism. Substances that undergo significant *first-pass elimination* are said to have a *high extraction ratio*. Elimination of these drugs is largely determined by hepatic blood flow. Drugs that require a prolonged time for biotransformation are said to have a *low extraction ratio*. Such drugs are often protein bound in the circulation and therefore are not readily available to drug metabolizing enzymes in the liver. Intermediate between these two extremes are substances that do not clearly fall into either category are said to have an intermediate extraction ratio. Elimination of these drugs is equally dependent on blood flow and metabolic activity. Examples of drugs commonly used in the practice of anesthesiology and pain medicine are listed for each of these three categories in Table 6-1.

Table 6-1	Examples of Hepatic Clearance Patterns of Common Pharmaceuticals	
High Clearance (high extraction ratio that is blood flow dependent)	**Intermediate Clearance**	**Low Clearance (low extraction ratio that is blood flow independent)**
Morphine	Aspirin	Warfarin
Lidocaine	Quinine	Phenytoin
Propofol	Codeine	Rocuronium
Propranolol	Nortriptyline	Methadone
Fentanyl	Vecuronium	Diazepam
Sufentanil	Alfentanil	Lorazepam

References

1. Steadman RH, Braunfeld MY. The liver: surgery and anesthesia. In: Barash PG, Cullen BF, Stoelting RK, et al. *Clinical Anesthesia*. 7th ed. Philadelphia: Lippincott Williams & Wilkins; 2013:1294–1325.
2. Beck C, Schawrtges I, Picker O. Perioperative liver protection. *Curr Opin Crit Care*. 2010;16:142–147.
3. Hoetzel A, Ryan H, Schmidt R. Anesthetic considerations for the patient with liver disease. *Curr Opin Anesthesiol*. 2012;25:340–347.
4. Sweeney BP, Bromilow J. Liver enzyme induction and inhibition: Implications for anaesthesia. *Anaesthesia*. 2006;61:159–177.
5. Gupta DK, Henthorn TK. Basic principles of clinical pharmacology. In: Barash PG, Cullen BF, Stoelting RK, et al. *Clinical Anesthesia*. 7th ed. Philadelphia: Lippincott Williams & Wilkins; 2013:156–188.

Questions

1. The dual blood supply to the liver can best be described by which of the following statements?
   A. Liver blood supply is 75% from the hepatic artery and 25% from the portal vein.
   B. Liver blood supply is 50% from the hepatic artery and 50% from the portal vein.
   C. Liver blood supply is 25% from the hepatic artery and 75% from the portal vein.
   D. Liver blood supply is 10% from the hepatic artery and 90% from the portal vein.

2. A 55-year-old man with end-stage liver disease from alcoholic cirrhosis would be expected to demonstrate all of the following abnormalities EXCEPT:
   A. Increased susceptibility to bacterial infection
   B. Ascites
   C. Hyperglycemia
   D. Increased susceptibility to bruising

3. Dynamic laboratory tests are more accurate measures of liver function than static laboratory tests, and both are easily obtained in most medical settings. TRUE or FALSE?
   A. True
   B. False

4. A 47-year-old woman with acute right upper quadrant pain and scleral icterus undergoes a series of static laboratory blood tests, demonstrating elevated levels of AST and ALT, with an AST/ALT ratio of 2.9. Which of the following clinical or diagnostic findings is also likely to be present?
   A. Ultrasound examination showing a 7-mm common bile duct stone with proximal bile duct dilation
   B. Elevated blood alcohol content
   C. Computed tomography scan showing a 7-cm mass in the head of the pancreas
   D. Serology indicating acute hepatitis A

5. Drug X has a high extraction ratio and is given by mouth to two different, yet otherwise healthy, adult patients: one with a normal cardiac output (Patient NL) and one in hypovolemic shock (Patient HS). Which of the following statements is most likely to be TRUE?
   A. Drug X will be rapidly cleared by both patients.
   B. Drug X will be slowly cleared by both patients.
   C. Drug X will be cleared more rapidly by Patient NL.
   D. Drug X will be cleared more rapidly by Patient HS.

PART B *Pharmacology*

7
Principles of Pharmacokinetics and Pharmacodynamics

Dhanesh K. Gupta
Thomas K. Henthorn

This chapter will review the fundamentals of clinical pharmacology to enable the anesthesia practitioner to use the information in subsequent chapters to develop anesthetic and postoperative analgesic plans that minimize exposure of patients to supratherapeutic and subtherapeutic concentrations and decrease patient morbidity. Opioids are used as a prototype drug class to explain these pharmacokinetic and pharmacodynamic principles.

I. Pharmacokinetics

In order to produce a drug effect, it is necessary to deliver the drug to the site of action. Most drugs used outside the perioperative or intensive care environment are administered in a manner in which their effects are achieved over days, weeks, or even years. In contrast, in the acute care environment, the clinician often needs to achieve onset of drug effect in a matter of minutes. Mathematical models that describe the drug plasma concentration versus time profile are readily available and easily implemented on model-based infusion pumps, personal computers, and even mobile devices. This initial section will qualitatively describe pharmacokinetic concepts that are necessary in order to rationally choose dosing regimens for opioids, hypnotics, and neuromuscular junction blocking agents.

A. Routes of Drug Administration

In order to produce a drug effect, it is necessary to deliver the drug to the site of action. Although the most familiar routes of drug administration are the oral and intravenous (IV) routes, there are a wide range of other sites for administering drugs into the body (Table 7-1). Blood flow is the usual means by which drug is delivered to the site of action. Thus, IV drug administration is considered the gold standard to which all other methods of drug administration are compared (i.e., *bioavailability* is defined as the ratio of drug exposure of a dose delivered by another route vs. IV administration). The IV route is preferred for several fundamental reasons. First, the IV route of drug administration provides almost immediate changes in drug concentrations

Table 7-1　Routes of Drug Administration Using Opioids as a Prototype

Formulation	Bioavailability	Time to Maximum Plasma Concentration	Comments
Intravenous	100%	<1 minute	• Gold standard
Oral (gastrointestinal)	0–50%	1–3 hours	• Hepatic first-pass metabolism reduces bioavailability in high hepatic extraction ratio drugs • Intestinal metabolism contributes to decreased bioavailability
Oral transmucosal	65–75%	15–30 minutes	• Bypasses hepatic first pass metabolism • Requires high lipophilicity, otherwise passes to gastrointestinal tract
Sublingual	75%	30–45 minutes	• Bypasses hepatic first-pass metabolism • Requires high lipophilicity, otherwise passes to gastrointestinal tract
Intranasal	90%	10–20 minutes	• Bypasses hepatic first pass metabolism • Limited for low lipophilicity
Rectal transmucosal	20–70%	0.75–2 hours	• Partially bypasses hepatic first-pass metabolism
Subcutaneous	>75%	15–30 minutes	• Not limited by lipophilicity compared to transmucosal, transdermal, or intranasal routes
Transdermal	>90%	10–20 hours	• Limited by permeability through skin • Constant concentration from 10–48 hours
Intramuscular	100%	5–30 minutes	• Not limited by lipophilicity compared to transmucosal, transdermal, or intranasal routes
Inhalational	>90%	5–30 minutes	• Ventilation-perfusion mismatch results in some delayed uptake and bioavailability <100%
Intrathecal	Not reported	0.5–4 hours	• Spinal and supraspinal sites of action
Epidural	100%	15–45 minutes	• Bolus opioids act at spinal sites, despite plasma absorption

in blood because the drug does not need to be absorbed into the systemic circulation. Furthermore, the vascular system is able to immediately deliver drugs to the site of drug action by intravascular mass transport to tissue capillary beds. Once drug reaches the capillary, it can enter tissue by diffusion or active transport. If extensive alveolar endothelial, epithelial drug uptake, or metabolism is present for inhalation anesthetics and vaporized drugs, bioavailability will be limited. Finally, the intravascular space is the easiest and most relevant biologic fluid to sample for drug concentration measurements.

When multiple blood samples are obtained, the resultant drug concentration versus time data can be mathematically modeled to describe and interpret the pharmacokinetic properties of the drug. When injected or rapidly infused, IV drug administration results in rapid increases in drug–blood concentration, rapid transfer to tissues of the effect site, and rapid onset of drug effect. In general, the maximum drug effect is proportional to the maximum plasma concentration achieved.

Routes of drug administration such as oral, intramuscular, and subcutaneous usually result in a slower onset of drug effect and a lower peak drug effect (Table 7-1). The rate and extent of drug absorption into the systemic circulation are important determinants of the time course of drug effect. The rate of drug absorption is dependent on a complex interplay of the physiochemical properties of the drug, the physiochemical properties of the delivery vehicle, and the perfusion of the tissue where the drug is administered.

A few generalizations can be made regarding *drug absorption*. First, lipophilic drugs are absorbed faster than hydrophilic drugs because diffusion across lipid cellular barriers is faster. Furthermore, drug delivery vehicles or devices can be designed that slow the rate of drug absorption by such mechanisms as physically binding a drug molecule to decrease its lipophilicity (e.g., sustained-release drug formulations of pills) or adding additional diffusion barriers (e.g., transdermal patch layers). Finally, the perfusion of the tissue where the drug is administered can significantly alter its absorption profile. For example, inhaled fentanyl via a microvaporization device has a plasma concentration profile that is similar to that of IV drug administration. This is because nearly all the drug reaches the alveoli, where there is a minimal diffusion barrier and perfusion by the entire cardiac output. In contrast, oral administration of drugs produces a peak plasma concentration that is substantially lower than IV administration. There is a delayed time to peak concentration because of the limited perfusion of the gastrointestinal mucosa and the metabolism of drug in the liver before entering the systemic circulation, thus limiting both the rate and extent of absorption, respectively. This *first-pass metabolism* by the liver is the major determinant of the limited bioavailability of many drugs administered via the gastrointestinal tract. For neuraxial routes, the physiochemical properties of the drug and the physiochemical delivery of the vehicle determine the rate by which drug diffuses locally into adjacent neural tissue. Uniquely, systemic absorption and the plasma drug concentration profile are not related to the drug effect profile by these routes.

The slower rate of systemic absorption and the lower peak plasma concentration of the non-IV methods of drug administration may lead clinicians to believe that the only benefit of this route of drug administration is convenience in avoiding IV access. However, a commonly overlooked benefit of the non-IV methods of drug administration is that the same impediments to rapid systemic absorption can provide a prolonged drug effect. As long as the plasma concentration is maintained at a level above the therapeutic threshold concentration, the drug will produce an effect (Fig. 7-1) (1).

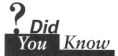

Did You Know

Blood is rarely the site at which a drug produces its desired and undesired actions.

Did You Know

For anesthetic gases and inhaled vaporized drugs, the bioavailability is close to 100%. Thus, the inhaled route mimics IV administration.

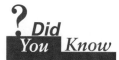

Did You Know

There are two non-IV routes for which tissue perfusion does not affect drug onset of effect because the drug is delivered adjacent to the site of action—the intrathecal space and the epidural space.

B. Drug Distribution and Drug Elimination
Drug Distribution
Once drug is in the central circulation, it travels by intravascular blood flow to the tissue capillary beds where it is free to leave and re-enter the intravascular space by diffusion or active transport at the blood–tissue interface. Drug transport, either into or from the tissue, is usually not saturable, so drug uptake by

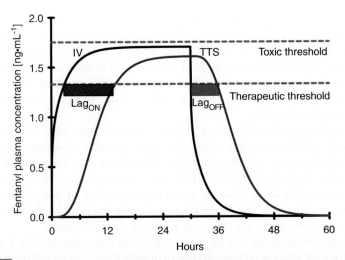

Figure 7-1 The plasma concentration profile achieved with 75 μg/hr of transdermal therapeutic systems fentanyl (*blue line,* TTS-fentanyl) or intravenous fentanyl (*black line,* IV-fentanyl). The TTS-fentanyl "simulation" is based on a compartmental model developed to mimic the output of published observations, whereas the IV-fentanyl simulation was generated from the most robust three-compartment fentanyl pharmacokinetic-pharmacodynamic (PK-PD) model available. Although there is a brief delay until the IV-fentanyl achieves a plasma concentration above the *therapeutic threshold* (*lower dashed green line*), the delay until the TTS-fentanyl produces a plasma concentration above the therapeutic threshold is much longer (*black crosshatched bar,* Lag$_{ON}$). This delay results from a combination of the time that it takes the TTS-fentanyl system to establish and equilibrate with a subcutaneous depot of fentanyl and the continuous tissue distribution and systemic elimination of intravenously absorbed fentanyl. Similarly, when fentanyl administration is discontinued 30 hours after initiation of therapy, there is a rapid decrease in the plasma concentration in the IV-fentanyl profile, whereas the continued uptake of fentanyl from the subcutaneous depot maintains the plasma concentration above the therapeutic threshold for several hours in the TTS-fentanyl profile and then slows the rate at which the plasma concentration decreases. This delay (*blue crosshatched bar,* Lag$_{OFF}$) is not due to an alteration in the plasma distribution or the systemic elimination of fentanyl, but rather to the continued absorption from the subcutaneous depot.

the tissue is mostly limited by the blood flow to the tissue (flow-limited drug uptake). The distribution of cardiac output to the different tissue beds and the cellular mass of the tissue determine the rate of drug equilibration with the plasma in each tissue bed. For example, the brain and the kidneys equilibrate over a matter of minutes due to their high blood flow and relatively low tissue volume (2). In contrast, the well-perfused muscle and splanchnic tissues take hours to approach equilibrium due to their large tissue volumes relative to blood flow (Fig. 7-2). Despite having the highest blood to tissue solubility ratio, the body's adipose tissue is relatively poorly perfused and therefore does not approach equilibrium with the plasma for days.

Unless the tissue metabolizes or excretes the drug, drug transport between the blood and the tissue is a bidirectional process that is governed by the law of mass action. When the concentration of drug in the tissue becomes higher than the plasma concentration, the overall movement of drug is from the tissue to the plasma (Fig. 7-2). This *redistribution* of an opioid or hypnotic from the highly perfused but low tissue volume brain back into the plasma will eventually decrease the concentration of drug at its site of action below the therapeutic threshold and thereby halt its effect. It is important to note that the brain

Figure 7-2 **A:** The concentration profiles produced by an intravenous bolus of fentanyl for the concentration in the plasma (*solid black line*), fast equilibrating tissue (*solid blue line*), and slow equilibrating tissue (*solid red line*). Note that the plasma concentration of fentanyl decreases rapidly after administration while it increases rapidly in the fast equilibrating tissue. From the point when the concentration in the fast equilibrating tissue exceeds that in the plasma (*green arrow*), there will be continued transfer of drug from the fast equilibrating tissue to the plasma (redistribution). Throughout this time there is continuous, slow uptake of drug by the slow equilibrating tissue and there is no redistribution of drug from this tissue to the plasma. **B:** The concentration profiles produced by repeated intravenous boluses of fentanyl every 5 minutes for the concentration in the plasma (*solid black line*), fast equilibrating tissue (*solid blue line*), and slow equilibrating tissue (*solid red line*). Note that the plasma concentration of fentanyl rapidly decreases after each bolus, while it rapidly increases throughout the entire 30-minute period in fast equilibrating tissue. For each bolus from the second bolus onward, there is redistribution of drug from the fast equilibrating tissue to the plasma at any of the times when the plasma concentration is lower than the fast equilibrating tissue concentration (initial time of redistribution is at the *green arrow, R*). With each subsequent bolus, the duration of redistribution is longer and longer. There is still no redistribution between the slow equilibrating tissue and the plasma. **C:** The concentration profiles produced by a 12-hour continuous infusion of fentanyl for the concentration in the plasma (*solid black line*) and slow equilibrating tissue (*solid red line*). Note that the fast equilibrating tissue is not shown because *on this time scale it essentially overlaps that of the plasma,* although, in reality there is a small difference that results in transfer of drug from the plasma to the fast equilibrating tissue until the infusion is stopped, at which time there is redistribution of drug from the fast equilibrating tissue to the plasma. Note that once the infusion is stopped, there is redistribution of drug from the slow equilibrating tissue to the plasma (*green arrow*). In addition, the elimination half-life is related to the slope of the washout curve (after the infusion is terminated).

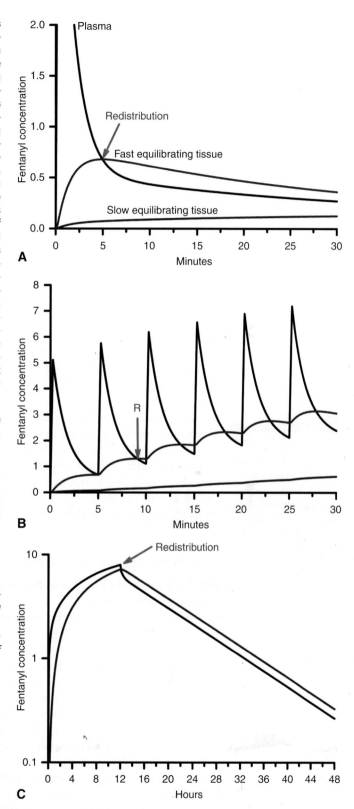

may redistribute drug minutes after a bolus of drug has been administered. But tissue beds such as the muscle, which are slower to equilibrate because of the large capacity for drug uptake, will continue to take up drug until the plasma concentration decreases below the tissue concentration as drug is metabolized, excreted, and drug distributed throughout the body. With repeated injections or an infusion of drug, tissue uptake of drug will continue as long as the blood–drug concentration remains above that of tissue–drug concentration. Thus, when drug administration is stopped or the rate is decreased, these tissues begin to act like depots, causing net transfer of drug to blood and slowing the rate of further decrease of the plasma concentrations (Fig. 7-2). When the rate of net tissue transfer of drug to blood is equal to the elimination rate of drug from the body, then the blood–drug concentration versus time profile enters into the terminal elimination phase where the rate of change (or half-life) remains constant (3).

Drug Elimination
The only way to decrease the total amount of drug in the body is to eliminate it from the body. Some drugs are sufficiently hydrophilic to be excreted via passive filtration or active transport unchanged by the kidneys. But the majority of opioids and hypnotics are sufficiently lipophilic (they must cross the blood–brain barrier) that they must be metabolized to a more hydrophilic form that can be excreted. Biotransformation of drugs into more hydrophilic compounds is usually achieved by enzymatic reactions that are oxidative or, rarely, reductive. Together these are referred to as phase I reactions that occur in the endoplasmic reticulum of liver cells, but also in some cases the kidney, intestinal mucosa, and lung. The cytochrome P450 (CYP P450) superfamily of enzymes, which are found in the endoplasmic reticulum of hepatocytes and some other cells, is primarily responsible for phase I reactions. These new molecularly altered drugs can then be conjugated to such molecules as glucuronide by enzymes, in this case, glucuronidase. Some drugs, such as propofol and morphine can be directly conjugated to glucuronide without phase I reactions. Regardless of whether there was a phase I step, conjugations are referred to as phase II reactions and occur in the cytosol of hepatocytes (and other cells). Glucuronides and other conjugates can then be eliminated into the urine or gastrointestinal tract via the bile.

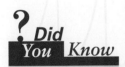

? Did You Know

Genetic polymorphisms of the enzymes involved in drug metabolism are the most common cause of interindividual variability in the rate of drug elimination from the body.

C. Mathematical Concepts in Pharmacokinetics
Volume of Distribution
In a purely physical sense, the amount (mass) of solute divided by a known physical volume of fluid will equal the concentration of the solute in the fluid. In a patient, this is strictly true as well, but one would have to homogenize the patient in order to measure the correct concentration in the resultant fluid volume. In pharmacokinetics, the sample fluid is typically plasma and the amount of solute (or drug) put into the body can also be measured. So the *plasma-apparent volume* of distribution becomes the drug (or solute) dose divided by the plasma drug concentration. If one could homogenize the patient, the volume of fluid in the patient would always be the volume of distribution of the solute (or drug). Almost always, what is reported in pharmacokinetic tables is the plasma-apparent volume of distribution. It rarely corresponds to any known true physical fluid volume and, instead, is what the volume appears to be based on the plasma–drug concentration (2,3).

Volumes of distribution of drugs can range from a practical low of the body's extracellular fluid volume (for drugs that are excluded from entering cells) to volumes that are many times larger than the weight of a patient (for drugs that partition into tissues because of active transport, binding, or physicochemical preference for the lipid constituents of cells over the watery environment of plasma).

Elimination Clearance

As drug is delivered to excretory organs such as the liver or kidneys, the drug is subject to permanent removal or biotransformation to another chemical entity (i.e., it ceases to exist as the drug administered). If an organ perfectly removed all drug from the blood as it flowed through, the clearance would equal the blood flow to that organ. If only a fraction of the drug present in the blood to the organ can be removed in the time of passage dictated by blood flow, then clearance is the fraction removed on one pass multiplied by the organ's blood flow. Thus, clearance is stated in terms of flow (e.g., liters per minute), and *elimination clearance* represents the total of all the clearances of all the eliminating organs for a particular drug.

Usually, drugs that have clearances near that of liver blood flow are very efficiently biotransformed by phase I reactions (e.g., fentanyl) or phase II reactions (e.g., propofol) in the liver and, in the case of propofol, also in the kidneys. With such drugs, the elimination clearance is considered to be *flow limited,* meaning the clearance will only decrease if blood flow to the organ decreases (e.g., with low cardiac output). For other drugs that are less efficiently biotransformed (e.g., midazolam), the clearance is more (or even solely) influenced by the enzymatic rate.

Many factors can influence the performance of the enzymatic process, such as the presence of other drugs (inhibition), disease (hepatitis), tight plasma protein binding, and genetic modification of the enzyme protein, and can limit the fraction of drug eliminated from the blood flowing to the organ. In these cases, blood flow is less of a factor in determining elimination clearance, and these drugs' clearance are referred to as *capacity limited.*

Clearance is typically calculated by dividing the dose of drug administered (D) by the total area under the plasma drug concentration versus time curve (AUC). Often, elimination clearance follows the rules of physiology for organs such as the liver (as in the examples in the previous paragraph) or the kidney (e.g., pancuronium, gentamicin). However, elimination clearance can also be estimated by D/AUC for drugs eliminated in other ways, such as tissue cholinesterases (e.g., remifentanil) or even spontaneous autodegradation by Hofmann elimination (e.g., cis-atracurium).

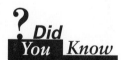

Half-life

Most drugs are eliminated as a fixed fraction per unit of time. This circumstance is known as *first-order kinetics* and the fraction eliminated is the *rate constant* (units of time^{-1}), and drug concentration decreases exponentially. Exponential functions are made to appear linear by plotting them as the natural log of concentration versus time. This relation is easy to conceptualize by converting the rate constant to a half-life using the natural log of ½ (−0.693), making half-life equal to 0.693 divided by the rate constant. Half-life is also useful in estimating the rise toward steady state during constant dosing using the same relation (e.g., concentrations increase to 50%, 75%, and 90% of steady state in 1, 2, and 3.3 half-lives, respectively).

Half-life (t$_{1/2}$) combines the concepts of volume of distribution (Vd) and elimination clearance Cl$_E$ in the following relation: $t_{1/2} = 0.693 \times Vd/Cl_E$.

? Did You Know

The rate of decline of drug concentrations in plasma and the effect site can be easily estimated using the half-life concept (e.g., concentrations decrease by 50%, 75%, and 90% in 1, 2, and 3.3 half-lives, respectively).

VIDEO 7-1

*Two-Compartment
Kinetics*

Compartmental Models

Several conditions arise in the practice of administering anesthesia to make the simple rules regarding half-life of limited value. First, these rules require the assumption of the body as a single compartment. A pharmacokinetic compartment is a mathematical construct in which the overall shape or behavior of the drug concentration versus the time curve can be described by a particular and definable exponential set of rules. Following oral dosing, for instance, the kinetics of absorption tends to mask the early drug distribution to tissues, and a single compartment is sufficient to well describe the pharmacokinetic events of a single or multiple doses. Thus, monoexponential kinetics applies in these cases and permits full use of the half-life rules presented above. However, when rapid IV drug doses or drug infusions, in which the duration is measured in minutes or hours (as opposed to days), are used, the drug concentration versus time relation is dramatically multiexponential and requires multiple rate constants to describe the varying steepness of the curve (2,3).

A *pharmacokinetic compartment* is a mathematical construct that assumes instantaneous and continuously uniform mixing of drug (or solute) within it. Clearance is calculated as the volume of distribution times the exiting transfer rate constant. A monoexponential drug concentration versus time curve is equivalently described by a one-compartment model. Likewise, a multiexponential concentration versus time curve (usually with two or three exponential terms) is equivalently described by a multicompartment model with two or three compartments. It is conceptually easier to envision a central compartment connected by transfer rate constants to rapid and slow equilibrating compartments (in the case of a three-compartment model) than a multiexponential equation. Additionally, computing power has removed the use of the multiexponential equation, which can be solved with a simple hand-held calculator. Now, applications running on phones can easily solve the differential equations of multicompartmental models, merging both conceptual and computational ease.

Context-sensitive Decrement Times

To one extent or another, all tissues in the body act as drug depots. The rates that they accumulate drug as tissues equilibrate their drug concentrations with blood–drug concentrations varies with the blood flow to the tissue in relation to the tissue mass and its propensity to sequester the drug (i.e., the blood–tissue partition coefficient or the concentration ratio at complete blood–drug equilibrium). These depots continue to accumulate drug until a steady state is reached. For large depots with relatively low blood flow, a day or more is required to reach steady state. Thus, for drug administration times that are less than those required to bring all tissues to steady-state blood–tissue drug concentration ratios, the degree to which each tissue depot is "full" will vary as will the rates at which the various tissues will release drug back into the blood as the net transfer reverses after administration ceases.

Clinicians need to predict when drug concentrations in blood (or effect site) will fall (or decrement) from that needed to maintain the desired anesthetic drug effect to a drug concentration associated with another state, say, wakefulness. Duration of action after a single IV bolus dose is usually readily available or known. However, when there has been continuous or repeated drug administration, the duration of action depends on the length of drug administration (or context sensitivity).

Using pharmacokinetic-pharmacodynamic models, the time needed to decrement from a predicted therapeutic concentration during administration to a

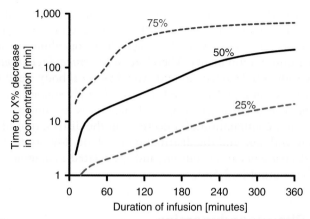

Figure 7-3 The context-sensitive 25%, 50%, and 75% decrement times after fentanyl infusions of 1 to 360 minutes in duration. Note that the y-axis is plotted as a logarithmic scale. While a 25% decrease in the plasma concentration after a 360 minute infusion takes less than 20 minutes (*green dashed line*), it takes over 240 minutes for a 50% decrease in plasma concentration after the same 360-minute infusion (*solid black line*). In addition, a 75% decrease in plasma concentration takes approximately 500 minutes for infusions of 180 minutes or longer (*red dashed line*).

drug concentration that will be nontherapeutic following termination of infusions of variable lengths can be simulated (4). These are plotted as time for a percentage drug concentration decrement, say, 50% (or half-time), on the y-axis versus the length of time the drug was continuously infused on the x-axis (Fig. 7-3). Typically, the length of decrement time will rise as the infusion duration increases, but the shape of the curve is unique to each drug.

D. Covariates that Effect Pharmacokinetics

There are several physiologic factors that can alter the pharmacokinetics of a drug. Most of the focus in the clinical pharmacology literature is on the effects of hepatic or renal disease on pharmacokinetic parameters. Any good estimate of glomerular filtration rate will correlate well with the elimination clearance of a drug that is filtered by the kidneys. But the elimination clearance of a drug that is excreted by active transport into the tubules is not as strongly correlated with glomerular filtration rate. Unfortunately, clinical liver function tests (e.g., transaminases and liver synthetic function) are not good estimates of the remaining metabolic capacity of the liver for drug elimination. Therefore, it is difficult to quantitatively or even qualitatively estimate how to adjust dosing of drugs with liver disease. Fortunately, recovery from a single bolus, repeated boluses, and even short infusions depends as much, if not more, on drug distribution to and redistribution from tissue than elimination clearance. Therefore, unless severe end-organ disease is present, a small decrease in the frequency or repeated boluses or the infusion rate can be made and adjusted based on clinically observed drug effect.

Increasing weight alters pharmacokinetic parameters because increasing tissue volumes and blood volume increase the tissue available for drug uptake. Increases in the blood flow to these tissues increase the volume of distribution for each of the tissues and the total body. Although most hypnotics and opioids are relatively lipophilic, dosing these drugs to the actual body weight overshoots the target concentration. Yet dosing these drugs to the ideal body weight undershoots the target concentration. This is because the relative poor perfusion of the fat results in very little contribution of this compartment

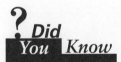

to the increased volume of distribution and distributional clearances during the first several hours of drug infusion. However, the increased muscle mass required to carry the increased body weight does contribute substantially to the increased dose requirements. Therefore, a *pharmacologic body weight*—ideal body weight + 0.33 × (actual body weight – ideal body weight)—is often employed when dosing propofol and opioids. The physiologic bases for age-related changes in drug distribution and clearances are unclear. They most likely represent a combination of a decrease in the distribution of lean tissue versus muscle with age and the distribution of blood flow to these tissues, an age-related decrease in cardiac output, and age-related changes in the distribution of cardiac output (1,2,5,6).

II. Pharmacodynamics

A. Dose–Response and Concentration–Effect Relations

Anyone who has ever taken an analgesic understands that as the dose of a drug is increased, the analgesic response is also increased. In addition, the probability that he or she has a satisfactory analgesic response is increased with a higher dose. Furthermore, more painful injuries require higher doses of drug to achieve a satisfactory response. However, as the dose is increased above a certain point, there is minimal improvement in the analgesic response, in that the maximum drug effect is achieved. The interindividual variability in the relation of the dose needed to produce a given pharmacologic effect varies considerably, even in normal patients. The interindividual variability in the dose–response relation is caused by interindividual variability in the relation between the drug concentration and pharmacologic effect (pharmacodynamic variability) superimposed on interindividual variability in the concentration of drug produced by a given dose of drug (pharmacokinetic variability). This highlights the major disadvantage of the dose–response relation versus the concentration–response relation. The dose–response relation is unable to correctly identify whether the interindividual variability is caused by differences in pharmacokinetics, pharmacodynamics, or both.

Most drugs produce their physiologic effects (both therapeutic and toxic effects) by binding to a ***drug-specific receptor*** on the cell membrane, in the cytoplasm, or in nucleoplasm of the cell. This produces a change in cellular function. Drug binding to the receptor is a reversible process that follows the law of mass action—higher concentrations of drug result in higher numbers of drug-receptor complexes and a larger drug effect. The relation between drug concentration and the intensity of the response is most often characterized by a curvilinear relation (Fig. 7-4). For most drugs, there is a minimum concentration that needs to be achieved before an effect can be observed (therapeutic threshold). Once a pharmacologic effect is produced, small increases in drug concentration usually produce relatively large increases in drug effect. As the drug effect reaches near maximum, increases in concentration produce minimal changes in effect.

B. Therapeutic Thresholds and Therapeutic Windows

The previous discussion alluded to the fact that in a given individual, there may not only be interindividual variability but also significant intraindividual variability in the concentration that produces the desired clinical effect without side effects. This intraindividual variability depends on several physiologic factors.

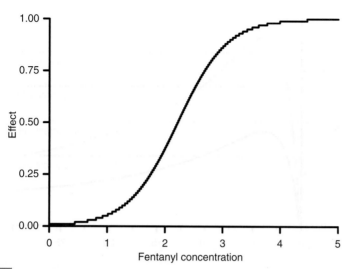

Figure 7-4 The concentration versus effect curve for fentanyl. Note the sigmoidal-shaped curve. Between a 25% to 75% effect, the curve is approximately linear, and small changes in the concentration of fentanyl result in a large change in effect. In contrast, below 25% and above 75% effect, the curve is relatively flat, and large changes in fentanyl concentration are required to produce a small change in clinical effect.

First, the *minimum effective concentration* that produces a clinically significant effect (therapeutic threshold) can vary depending on the magnitude of the stimulation requiring treatment (Fig. 7-5). For example, as shown in Figure 7-5, the patient who is recovering from an excision of a melanoma requires a lower opioid concentration for adequate analgesia than the patient recovering from a lumbar spine fusion. Therefore, the dose of fentanyl that produces analgesia in the melanoma patient may not produce discernable analgesia in the spine fusion patient (i.e., below the therapeutic threshold). In contrast, the dose of fentanyl that produces analgesia in the spine fusion patient will produce analgesia in the melanoma patient, and it will have a faster onset of analgesia because it reaches the therapeutic threshold quicker. In addition, because the magnitude of the painful stimulus is lower in the melanoma patient than the spine fusion patient, it is likely that the concentration at which the patient will have significant ventilatory depression will also be lower. Although the therapeutic window (toxic threshold – therapeutic threshold) may be the same magnitude, the spine fusion patient will have the entire window "shifted higher." Therefore, a dose of fentanyl that may have been therapeutic and safe for the spine fusion patient will possibly cause major ventilatory depression for the melanoma patient for the time that the concentration is above the toxic threshold for the melanoma patient (toxic threshold M). Furthermore, the duration of adequate analgesia (time above the therapeutic threshold M) will be longer for the melanoma patient if given the larger dose of fentanyl.

C. The Effect Site

Ideally drug should be delivered to the site of drug action, and the concentration in that tissue should be measured to determine the drug's concentration–effect relation. However, for most drugs, it is difficult, if not impossible, to safely and repeatedly access and measure the site of drug action. Therefore, most pharmacokinetic-pharmacodynamic studies involve repeated measurement of blood concentrations of drugs and repeated measurements of a drug

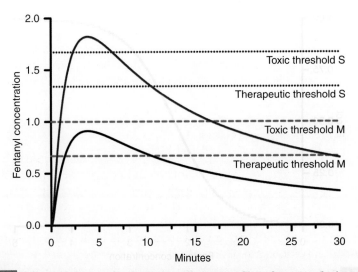

Figure 7-5 The effect site concentration versus time profiles after a 1 μg/kg intravenous bolus (*solid black line*) and a 2.5 μg/kg intravenous bolus (*solid blue line*) of fentanyl. The linearity of doses is demonstrated by the fact that the 2.5 μg/kg bolus results in a similar profile to that of the 1 μg/kg bolus but with a peak concentration 2.5 times higher. Representative therapeutic thresholds (the minimum concentration required to produce analgesia) and toxic threshold (the concentration above which ventilatory depression occurs) are demonstrated for a patient after superficial melanoma surgery (*green dashed lines,* M) and for a patient after lumbar spine fusion surgery (*dotted red lines,* S). A given bolus of fentanyl only produces analgesia from the time it produces an effect site concentration above the therapeutic threshold concentration for a patient until the time when the effect site concentration decreases below the therapeutic threshold concentration. If the effect site concentration does not exceed the toxic threshold for a patient, then it does not produce excessive ventilatory depression. In contrast, if the bolus does produce an effect site concentration above the toxic threshold concentration, it will produce severe ventilatory depression until the effect site concentration decreases below the toxic threshold concentration. For example, in a patient after superficial melanoma resection, a 1 μg/kg bolus of fentanyl (*solid black line*) will initially produce detectable analgesia approximately 2 minutes after administration (when it crosses the therapeutic threshold M, *lower dashed green line*), which will last approximately 10 minutes after administration (when the concentration decreases below the therapeutic threshold, *lower green dashed line*). Because dose does not produce a concentration above the toxic threshold (*upper dashed green line*), there will be no ventilatory depression after this single bolus. In contrast, in the same melanoma patient, a 2.5 μg/kg bolus of fentanyl (*solid blue line*) will initially produce detectable analgesia <1 minute after administration (when it crosses the therapeutic threshold M, *dashed green line*), which will last until approximately 30 minutes after administration (when the concentration decreases below the therapeutic threshold, *lower green dashed line*). Because the dose produces an effect site concentration above the toxic threshold for the melanoma resection patient (*upper dashed green line*), it will produce significant ventilatory depression from approximately 2 minutes until the effect site concentration decreases below the same toxic threshold at approximately 18 minutes. So, although the larger bolus produces a quicker onset of analgesia and a longer duration of action, it produces toxicity for a portion of this time. For the spine surgery patient (*dotted red lines* for therapeutic threshold and toxic threshold, S), a 1 μg/kg bolus will be subtherapeutic and ineffective (*black solid line*) because it does not produce a concentration above the therapeutic threshold (*lower dotted red line*). In contrast, a 2.5 μg/kg bolus produces analgesia from approximately 2 through 10 minutes after administration (time that *blue line* is above lower *red dotted line*), however, there is a period of time where this dose will produce severe ventilatory depression (from 2.5 through 8 minutes after administration, when the *solid blue line* is above the *upper dotted red line*). Therefore, a smaller dose of 2 μg/kg may be preferable to prevent an effect site concentration outside the therapeutic window (the area above the therapeutic threshold but below the toxic threshold).

effect. Because drug effect actually does not occur in the blood, pharmacokinetic models incorporate a *"virtual" effect site* that acts as a mathematical link between observed drug concentration changes in the blood and the measured drug effect. This effect site describes the time lags observed between the onset and offset of drug effect relative to the change in blood–drug concentration (Fig. 7-4) (7).

III. Drug Interactions

The perioperative period is characterized by the administration of varying doses of multiple drugs to induce, maintain, and antagonize anesthetics along with antibiotics, antiepileptics, and each patient's preoperative medications. Therefore, it should not be surprising that there is the potential for multiple drug interactions, some of which are part of the anesthetic plan (i.e., coadministration of an opioid with a volatile anesthetic to decrease the minimum alveolar concentration, and others which are inadvertent consequences of the polypharmacy of the perioperative period). An unintended consequence of many drugs is alterations in the physiologic mechanisms of drug absorption, distribution, and elimination. These pharmacokinetic alterations result in subtherapeutic or supratherapeutic concentrations with unintentional drug toxicity. In order to anticipate which drug–drug interactions may occur, it is useful to understand the mechanism of most drug interactions.

A. Absorption

With the increasing use of preoperative oral medications to attenuate cardiovascular risk (e.g., β-receptor antagonists) or decrease opioid requirements after surgery (e.g., cyclooxygenase inhibitors, gabapentinoids, sustained release opioids, etc.), anesthesiologists can no longer ignore drugs that alter absorption. In addition, foods, such as grapefruit juice, can alter *jejunal cytochrome P450 enzyme* activity and expression and intestinal P-glycoprotein expression. Increased intestinal metabolism and increased intestinal drug efflux can both decrease drug bioavailability. Fortuitously, the most common perioperative adjuvant drugs—metoprolol, the cyclooxygenase-2 inhibitors, the gabapentinoids, and the sustained release opioids—are minimally affected by these mechanisms. However, as more oral medications are routinely added to the perioperative period, it is important to consider whether their bioavailability will be altered from these mechanisms.

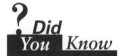

? *Did You Know*

Drugs that alter the gastric pH (e.g., ranitidine) or alter gastric emptying and intestinal transit time (e.g., metoclopramide) can alter drug dissolution and drug absorption.

B. Distribution

Although often forgotten in the pharmacology literature, drug alterations of distribution are the most common pharmacokinetic drug–drug interactions observed during anesthesia. The clinical pharmacology literature dedicates extensive effort to drug displacement from protein binding sites by competing drugs. This form of *drug–drug interaction* increases the unbound concentration of a drug and potentially produces exposure to supratherapeutic concentrations and potential toxicity. However, this mechanism of drug–drug interaction is not clinically important for anesthetic drugs because (a) there is a tremendous excess of unoccupied binding sites for most anesthetic drugs and (b) the hepatic metabolism of most anesthetic drugs is flow limited. Therefore, the liver will normalize the free concentration to predisplacement concentrations. The more common but less commonly discussed method by which drug–drug interactions affect the distribution of anesthetic drugs is by changing cardiac output and the distribution of cardiac output (2). These alterations in the tissue distribution of a drug (intercompartmental clearances) will change the exposure of the effect site to the drug. Although it is obvious that vasoactive agents can alter regional blood flow even if the cardiac output is constant, it is often forgotten that volatile anesthetics and propofol can alter the distribution of regional blood flow and therefore alter the plasma drug concentration profile.

C. Metabolism

The most commonly discussed mechanism of pharmacokinetic drug–drug interactions in the clinical pharmacology literature is the induction or *inhibition of drug metabolism*. There are many commonly used drugs that induce (or inhibit) cytochrome P450 isozymes, which increase (or decrease) hepatic drug metabolism and decrease (or increase) drug exposure. Increased drug metabolism by induction of cytochrome P450 3A4 by the antiepileptics is one of the most common examples in the perioperative literature. Fortunately, with the anesthetic drugs that have CYP P450 3A4 metabolism, it is relatively easy to increase the dose or dosing frequency to titrate to the desired effect of the neuromuscular junction blocking agent, opioid, or intravenous hypnotic. It may be more difficult to avoid drug overdose when there is a decrease in drug metabolism by this mechanism. For example, with the concomitant administration of protease inhibitors that inhibit opioid metabolism, it is necessary to start with lower doses and then slowly increase the dose or dosing frequency to avoid prolonged exposure to supratherapeutic concentrations and toxicity, such as prolonged ventilatory depression. An additional therapeutic challenge is when the conversion of a prodrug to its active drug is inhibited by another drug. Because of the variability of the amount of CYP 2D6 inhibition by selective serotonin reuptake inhibitors, it may be easier to avoid opioids that require CYP 2D6 conversion (i.e., codeine, oxycodone, and hydrocodone) rather than attempt to predict adequate analgesia in patients taking these drugs, especially with the acetaminophen in its commonly available formulations (8).

D. Direct and Indirect Antagonists

The easiest pharmacodynamic drug–drug interactions to understand are the methods anesthesiologists use to antagonize the clinical effects of opioids and nondepolarizing neuromuscular blocking agents. The opioid antagonist naloxone is an example of a pharmacodynamic drug–drug interaction in which a *direct antagonist* of the μ-opioid receptor is administered that displaces the opioid from the μ-opioid receptor and reverses opioid-induced ventilatory depression and decreases the pain threshold. In contrast, the cholinesterase inhibitors (e.g., neostigmine) increase the amount of acetylcholine available at the neuromuscular junction. Therefore, they are *indirect antagonists* of the nondepolarizing neuromuscular junction blocking agents.

E. Unintended Toxicity

Over the past two decades, the age of surgical patients has expanded, as has the overall use of chronic medications. The majority of outpatient medications have very little pharmacodynamic interaction with the perioperative medications. Excessive central nervous system (CNS) serotonin levels from antidepressants that inhibit the CNS monoamine oxidase degradation of serotonin or decrease the reuptake of serotonin can result in toxic serotonin concentrations if combined with other monoamine oxidase inhibitors (e.g., methylene blue) or serotonin reuptake inhibitors (e.g., opioids, such as methadone, meperidine, and tramadol). Unfortunately, washout of these antidepressants can take over 4 weeks and are not without side effects, such as worsening pain or depression. When methylene blue administration is required, it is recommended that the antidepressant not be restarted for at least 24 hours after the previous dose of it. In addition, if signs or symptoms of serotonin toxicity develop, a serotonin receptor antagonist (e.g., oral cyproheptadine or IV chlorpromazine) should be administered as well as required supportive care (9).

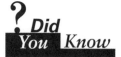

F. Opioid-Hypnotic Synergy

Although it is possible to produce the clinical state of general anesthesia solely with the administration of high-effect site concentrations of a volatile anesthetic or an IV anesthetic, the unintended consequences of these included a prolonged time for washout (emergence) and undesired hemodynamic side effects (arterial dilation and venodilation). The combination of an opioid and a hypnotic is synergistic (i.e., supra-additive) and not only produces a clinical anesthetic state that is indistinguishable from that produced by a hypnotic alone, but often allows for faster washout (emergence). Analysis of the combinations of an opioid and a hypnotic that produce the same clinical anesthetic state generates a three-dimensional surface that, when projected onto the concentration–effect plane, produces a family of *concentration–response curves*. These models allow the conceptualization of this complex drug–drug interaction that can not only be used to compute via simulation the optimal opioid-hypnotic combinations that minimize the time to emergence with adequate analgesia but can also be used qualitatively to describe the difference in adequate opioid-hypnotic combinations for education of anesthesia providers (Fig. 7-6) (10).

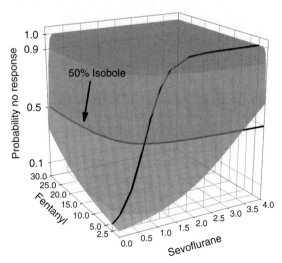

Figure 7-6 A response surface model characterizing the fentanyl–sevoflurane interaction for analgesia to electrical tetanic stimulation. The projection of the response surface onto the horizontal plane (sevoflurane vs. fentanyl plane) results a collection of effect isoboles, while the projection of the response surface onto the vertical plane (sevoflurane vs. effect vertical plane) results in a collection of sevoflurane concentration–response curves for a variety of remifentanil concentrations. (Adapted from Manyam SC, Gupta DK, Johnson KB, et al. Opioid-volatile anesthetic synergy: A response surface model with remifentanil and sevoflurane as prototypes. *Anesthesiology*. 2006;105:267–278.)

References

1. Gupta DK, Avram MJ. Rational opioid dosing in the elderly: Dose and dosing interval when initiating opioid therapy. *Clin Pharmacol Ther.* 2012;91:339–343.
2. Henthorn TK, Krejcie TC, Avram MJ. Early drug distribution: A generally neglected aspect of pharmacokinetics of particular relevance to intravenously administered anesthetic agents. *Clin Pharmacol Ther.* 2008;84:18–22.
3. Shafer SL, Stanski DR. Improving the clinical utility of anesthetic drug pharmacokinetics. *Anesthesiology.* 1992;76:327–330.
4. Shafer SL, Varvel JR. Pharmacokinetics, pharmacodynamics, and rational opioid selection. *Anesthesiology.* 1991;74:53–63.
5. Minto CF, Schnider TW, Egan TD, et al. Influence of age and gender on the pharmacokinetics and pharmacodynamics of remifentanil. I. Model development. *Anesthesiology.* 1997;86:10–23.
6. Schnider TW, Minto CF, Gambus PL, et al. The influence of method of administration and covariates on the pharmacokinetics of propofol in adult volunteers. *Anesthesiology.* 1998;88:1170–1182.
7. Kern SE, Stanski DR. Pharmacokinetics and pharmacodynamics of intravenously administered anesthetic drugs: Concepts and lessons for drug development. *Clin Pharmacol Ther.* 2008;84:153–157.
8. Crews KR, Gaedigk A, Dunnenberger HM, et al. Clinical pharmacogenetics implementation consortium guidelines for cytochrome p450 2d6 genotype and codeine therapy: 2014 update. *Clin Pharmacol Ther.* 2014;95:376–382.
9. Boyer EW, Shannon M. The serotonin syndrome. *N Engl J Med.* 2005;352:1112–1120.
10. Manyam SC, Gupta DK, Johnson KB, et al. Opioid-volatile anesthetic synergy: A response surface model with remifentanil and sevoflurane as prototypes. *Anesthesiology.* 2006;105:267–278.

Questions

1. Which route of drug administration results in the least bioavailability?
   A. Intravenous
   B. Subcutaneous
   C. Epidural
   D. Oral

2. As compared to intravenous administration, oral administration produces:
   A. Similar peak plasma concentration
   B. Similar time to peak plasma concentration
   C. Affected by first pass metabolism
   D. Plasma concentrations are not affected by perfusion of the gastro-intestinal mucosa

3. The rate of drug equilibration between the tissue and the plasma is determined by:
   A. Flow limited drug uptake
   B. Plasma colloid oncotic pressure
   C. Tissue drug saturation
   D. Blood-to-tissue solubility ratio

4. To undergo biotransformation, fentanyl:
   A. Must be converted to a lipophilic compound
   B. Must undergo phase I reaction in the brain
   C. Must be conjugated by the enzyme glucuronidase
   D. Glucuronide is eliminated only by the kidney

5. Clearance of fentanyl and propofol is:
   A. Biotransformed only by phase I reactions
   B. Flow limited
   C. Similar to midazolam
   D. Limited by intrinsic clearance

6. During constant dosing, the half-life ($t_{1/2}$) useful in estimating the rise to steady state concentration (50%, 75%, 90% steady state) is:
   A. 1, 3, 5 half-lives
   B. 1, 2, 3.3 half-lives
   C. 6.6
   D. 9.9

7. A 115-kg, 30-year-old female (body mass index [BMI] 40) is scheduled for bariatric surgery. The appropriate dose of propofol for this patient is:
   A. 2.0 mg/kg ideal body weight
   B. 2.0 mg/kg of actual weight
   C. 2.0 mg/kg pharmacologic body weight
   D. 2.5 mg/BMI unit

8. Interpatient variability in the dose required to produce a given pharmacologic effect is based on all of the following EXCEPT:
   A. Pharmacodynamics
   B. Pharmacokinetics
   C. Dose–response relation
   D. Concentration–response relation

9. A clinical example of a drug-drug interactions is:
   A. Isoproterenol alters the distribution of cardiac output and increases the plasma concentration of propofol
   B. Selective serotonin reuptake inhibitors (SSRI's) inhibit CYP 2D6 activity and increase clinical effectiveness of codeine as an analgesic
   C. Remifentanil effects (synergistic) the end tidal concentration of sevoflurane that is required to provide immobility and attenuate the hemodynamic responses to noxious stimulation
   D. Methylene blue administration to patients who have been taking selective serotonin reuptake inhibitors (SSRI's) is associated with malignant hyperthermia syndrome

10. In the following figure, identify the context sensitive half-time ($CSt_{1/2}$) for remifentanil (**R**).

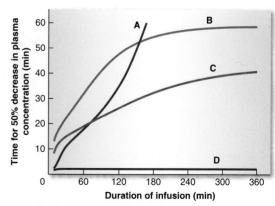

    A. A
    B. B
    C. C
    D. D

8 Inhalational Anesthetic Agents

Ramesh Ramaiah
Sanjay M. Bhananker

The value of inhaled gases as effective pain relievers was discovered in the 1840s. Nitrous oxide was effective for analgesia and sedation, whereas diethyl ether could produce general anesthesia. Since then, several pure gases and volatile anesthetics (liquids that have been vaporized to be inhaled) have been synthesized, studied, and used in clinical practice.

I. Pharmacologic Principles

A. Terminology

The behavior of administered drugs is best described in terms of *pharmacodynamics* (what the drug does to the body) and *pharmacokinetics* (what the body does to the drug). Pharmacodynamics describes the effects of drugs on organ systems, tissues, and specific receptors. Pharmacokinetics describes the way in which drugs are absorbed upon their administration, their distribution within various body compartments, their metabolism, and their elimination or excretion.

B. Classification of Inhaled Anesthetics

Some inhaled anesthetics are in a gaseous state at room temperature and are stored in tanks. Examples of such anesthetic gases include nitrous oxide, xenon, and an explosive gas, cyclopropane, which is no longer in use. Most inhaled anesthetics in current use are termed volatile anesthetics because they are liquids at room temperature. These are stored in bottles and converted to a gas phase using special agent-specific vaporizers that can deliver a precise concentration of the drug into the anesthetic circuit. Outdated examples of volatile anesthetics include diethyl ether, halothane, and enflurane. Current volatile anesthetics include sevoflurane and isoflurane. Desflurane is an inhaled anesthetic that has characteristics of both a pure gas and a volatile anesthetic. That is, because its boiling point is 24 °C, it changes from a liquid to a gas at a temperature very near normal room temperature. Vaporization of desflurane requires a vaporizer that is more complex than necessary for the other volatile anesthetics.

Table 8-1	Physical Properties of Commonly Used Inhalational Anesthetic Agents				
Property	Sevoflurane	Desflurane	Isoflurane	Nitrous Oxide	Xenon
Boiling point (°C)	59	24	49	−88	−108
Vapor pressure at 20°C (mm Hg)	157	669	238	38,770	—
Blood:gas partition coefficient	0.65	0.42	1.46	0.46	0.115
Oil:gas partition coefficient	47	19	91	1.4	1.9
Minimum alveolar concentration (MAC)	1.8	6.6	1.17	104	63 to 71
Metabolized in the body (%)	2–5	0.02	0.2	0	0

C. Physical Characteristics of Inhaled Anesthetics

Table 8-1 describes some of the properties of inhaled anesthetic agents currently in use. A *partition coefficient* (e.g., blood:gas or brain:blood) is expressed in various media as the solubility of these anesthetics. If a container with equal volumes of blood and air was exposed to enough isoflurane to produce a 1% concentration of isoflurane in the gas phase (1 mL isoflurane/100 mL of air) and allowed to come to equilibrium (total pressure equal in both air and blood), then 1.46 mL of isoflurane would be dissolved in each 100 mL of blood. The isoflurane would be "partitioned" between the blood and air in a ratio of 1.46:1, so the partition coefficient would be 1.46.

The *blood:gas* partition coefficient determines the speed of anesthetic induction, recovery, and change of anesthetic depth. An agent with a relatively high blood:gas partition coefficient (e.g., isoflurane = 1.46) will require a longer time for induction (and recovery) compared with an anesthetic with a lower blood:gas partition coefficient (e.g., sevoflurane = 0.65). Anesthesia results when the anesthetic is fully dissolved in the blood and an effective partial pressure of the anesthetic is attained in the blood (and brain). It takes longer for induction of anesthesia with an anesthetic with a high blood:gas partition coefficient because more anesthetic is dissolved in blood. And it takes longer for the blood to become "saturated" and the partial pressure exerted by the anesthetic to be high enough to produce a surgical level of anesthesia.

The *oil:gas* partition coefficient is a measure of lipid solubility of an inhaled anesthetic. The higher the oil:gas partition coefficient, the more potent the anesthetic and the lower the partial pressure (i.e., concentration) required to achieve a surgical plane of anesthesia (see below for a discussion of the minimum alveolar concentration).

II. Uptake and Distribution of Inhaled Anesthetic Agents

It is common to discuss the pharmacokinetic behavior of inhaled anesthetics in terms of their uptake and distribution because they are delivered to the patient by inhalation, absorbed or taken up by the blood, and then distributed to organs throughout the body (including the brain!). Furthermore, because it is difficult to measure blood concentrations of inhaled anesthetics, but relatively easy to measure the concentration, or fraction, inspired (F_I), expired (F_E), and in the alveolae (F_A) (which is nearly equivalent to that in the blood and brain), the pharmacokinetcs of inhaled anesthetics are typically described in terms of these readily measured values.

A. Alveolar/Inspired Anesthetic Concentration

The speed with which the alveolar anesthetic concentration rises and approaches the inspired concentration determines the speed of onset of action of the anesthetic and correlates with the rapidity of induction of anesthesia. The rise in F_A/F_I is faster with agents that have a low blood:gas partition coefficient (e.g., nitrous oxide, sevoflurane, desflurane). If the minute ventilation is high, as with overzealous manual or mechanical ventilation, an increased amount of anesthetic is brought to the alveoli. If cardiac output is low, as from hypovolemia, less anesthetic is carried away from the lungs and the blood becomes "saturated" with anesthetic more rapidly. As a result, the rise in F_A/F_I is faster, induction of anesthesia is more rapid, and unwanted side effects of anesthetics (such as hypotension) can be more profound under these conditions (Fig. 8-1).

B. Concentration Effect and Overpressurization

Concentration effect and overpressurization refer to two similar but distinct methods used to speed up the time needed for induction of anesthesia with

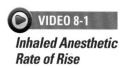

VIDEO 8-1

Inhaled Anesthetic Rate of Rise

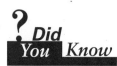

?Did You Know

Sevoflurane (alone or in conjunction with nitrous oxide) is the most common agent used for inhalational induction in children.

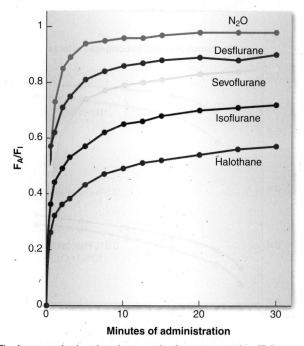

Figure 8-1 The increase in the alveolar anesthetic concentration (F_A) toward the inspired anesthetic concentration (F_I) is most rapid with the least-soluble anesthetics (nitrous oxide, desflurane, and sevoflurane) and intermediate with the more soluble anesthetics (isoflurane and halothane). After 10 to 15 minutes of administration (about three time constants), the slope of the curve decreases, reflecting saturation of vessel-rich group tissues and subsequent decreased uptake of the inhaled anesthetic. (From Inhaled anesthetics. In: Barash PB, Cullen BF, Stoelting RK, et al. *Handbook of Clinical Anesthesia*. 7th ed. Philadelphia: Lippincott Williams & Wilkins, 2013:227–251, with permission.)

an inhaled anesthetic (or an increase in depth of anesthesia during an anesthetic). The *concentration effect* refers to the fact that the higher the F_I of an inhaled anesthetic agent, the faster the rise in the F_A/F_I ratio. Uptake of a large volume of anesthetic by the blood causes an increase in alveolar ventilation, which in turn promotes a rapid rise of the F_A/F_I ratio. Although theoretically this applies to all inhaled anesthetics, practically it only has clinical relevance to nitrous oxide and xenon because they are delivered at relatively high concentrations. *Overpressurization* refers to the use of a higher F_I than the desired F_A for the patient to achieve a faster rise in the F_A/F_I ratio. Thus, one might use 8% inspired sevoflurane during induction of anesthesia in order to rapidly achieve the 2% alveolar sevoflurane concentration required for surgical anesthesia.

C. Second Gas Effect

The *second gas effect* is more of a theoretic than practical phenomenon. It occurs when an anesthetic in high concentration, the "second" gas (e.g. nitrous oxide), is acutely added to an already inhaled low concentration "first" gas (e.g., sevoflurane). The initial, rapid uptake of a high volume of nitrous oxide (into the blood) concentrates the sevoflurane in the alveoli and results in a faster rise of the F_A/F_I ratio of sevoflurane. In addition, due to an uptake of large volumes of the nitrous oxide, the resulting replacement of that gas increases inspired ventilation, which also augments the concentration of sevoflurane present in the alveoli. In theory, but probably not clinically obvious, this speeds the induction of anesthesia or more rapidly deepens the level of existing anesthesia (Fig. 8-2).

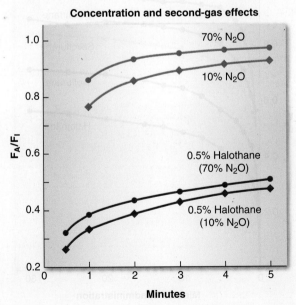

Figure 8-2 The concentration effect is demonstrated in the top half of the graph in which 70% nitrous oxide (N_2O) produces a more rapid increase in the alveolar anesthetic concentration (F_A)/inspired anesthetic concentration (F_I) ratio of N_2O than does administration of 10% N_2O. The second-gas effect is demonstrated in the lower lines in which the F_A/F_I ratio for halothane increases more rapidly when administered with 70% N_2O than with 10% N_2O. (From Inhaled anesthetics. In: Barash PB, Cullen BF, Stoelting RK, et al. *Handbook of Clinical Anesthesia.* 7th ed. Philadelphia: Lippincott Williams & Wilkins, 2013:227–251, with permission.)

Table 8-2	Tissue Groups and Their Perfusion		
Group	Body Mass (%)	Cardiac Output (%)	Perfusion (mL/100 g/min)
Vessel rich	10	75	75
Muscle	50	19	3
Fat	20	6	3

D. Distribution

Inhaled anesthetics delivered to the alveoli diffuse into the blood and are distributed to various organs in accordance with the amount of blood flow to those organs (Table 8-2). The organs that will be exposed to the most anesthetic early will be in the vessel-rich group, such as the heart, lung, brain, and liver. These organs receive about 75% of the normal cardiac output. The second group of perfused tissues are in the muscle group (including skin) and take longer to become saturated with anesthetic. The least perfused tissues (such as fat) take the longest amount of time to become saturated with anesthetic. But they also take the longest amount of time to be rid of anesthetic when the surgical procedure is terminated. Theoretically, the anesthetic in fat could serve as a depot of anesthetic, which is slowly released back into the circulation and could prolong awakening. In reality, this is not a significant problem with modern anesthetics with low solubility in blood. The dose, duration of anesthetic, and solubility of the agent in various tissues are the primary determinants of the magnitude of this depot or reservoir.

E. Metabolism

Only a small proportion of modern inhaled anesthetics undergo metabolism. Most of the anesthetic is exhaled in an unchanged state (Table 8-1). The pharmacokinetic and pharmacodynamic properties of these anesthetics are not significantly affected by their metabolism. Metabolism of halogenated hydrocarbons anesthetics, such as sevoflurane or desflurane, in the liver may be a factor in rare cases of postanesthetic hepatotoxicity.

III. Neuropharmacology of Inhaled Anesthetics

As with other drugs, the clinical effects of inhaled anesthetics are dependent on the administered dose. However, because the concentration of gas in the blood is difficult to measure, the depth of inhaled anesthesia is generally expressed in terms of the more readily measured end-exhalation, or alveolar, concentration. Thus, a 1% alveolar concentration of sevoflurane is equivalent at one atmosphere (760 mm Hg) to a partial pressure of 76 mm Hg in the blood (and brain).

The concept of *minimum alveolar concentration (MAC)* is commonly used to compare the pharmacologic effects of one inhaled anesthetic to another. One MAC is the concentration of an inhaled anesthetic at which 50% of patients do not move in response to a standard surgical stimulation (such as a skin incision). Consequently, if only an inhaled anesthetic is used for a surgical procedure, then more than 1 MAC must be administered to ensure all patients are unresponsive. MAC values are additive. For example, 0.5 MAC of sevoflurane and 0.5 MAC of nitrous oxide is equivalent to 1 MAC. Similarly, concomitant administration of opioids and sedatives reduces MAC. Some of the many factors that may increase or decrease MAC are listed in Table 8-3.

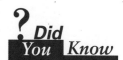

MAC values are more useful to compare potency of different inhaled anesthetic agents. Administering at least 0.7 MAC end-tidal concentration of inhaled anesthetics is needed for prevention of recall and intraoperative awareness.

Table 8-3 Factors that Influence Minimum Alveolar Concentration (MAC) of Inhaled Anesthetics

MAC increases with:
Chronic ethanol use
Hyperthermia
Hypernatremia
Monoamine oxidase inhibitors
Acute dextroamphetamine administration
Cocaine
Ephedrine
Levodopa

MAC decreases with:
Increasing age
Barbiturates
Benzodiazepines
Opioids
Ketamine/verapamil/lithium
Acute ethanol intoxication
Clonidine and dexmedetomidine
Hypothermia/hyponatremia
Pregnancy

All the newer inhaled anesthetics depress cerebral metabolic rate in a similar fashion, resulting in an isoelectric electroencephalogram. They usually produce a loss of consciousness and amnesia at relatively lower inspired concentrations (25% to 35% of MAC), although there is considerable variation in sensitivity among individuals. There is controversy whether sevoflurane has any pro-convulsant effects, and its use in patients with epilepsy is questioned. All the potent agents cause a dose-dependent increase in cerebral blood flow (Fig. 8-3). Changes in intracranial pressure parallel the increase in cerebral

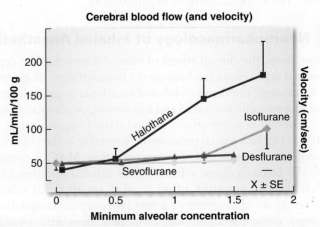

Figure 8-3 Cerebral blood flow (CBF) measured in the presence of normocapnia and in the absence of surgical stimulation in volunteers. At light levels of anesthesia, halothane (but not isoflurane, sevoflurane, or desflurane) increases CBF. Isoflurane increases CBF at 1.6 minimum alveolar concentration. (From Inhaled anesthetics. In: Barash PB, Cullen BF, Stoelting RK, et al. *Handbook of Clinical Anesthesia*. 7th ed. Philadelphia: Lippincott Williams & Wilkins, 2013:227–251, with permission.)

blood flow at a dose of 1 MAC or above. Inhalation anesthetics offer some degree of cerebral protection from ischemic or hypoxic insults. However, conclusive evidence in humans for sevoflurane and desflurane is lacking. The effects of nitrous oxide on cerebral physiology are not very clear as its effects vary among different species. Nitrous oxide may even have antineuroprotective properties. All the inhaled anesthetics can produce a dose-dependent depression of sensory and motor-evoked potentials. Visual-evoked potentials are the most sensitive to the effects of volatile agents. There is increasing evidence that the inhalation anesthetics may be one of the main contributing factors for the development of short-term cognitive impairment following surgery, particularly in elderly adults.

IV. Cardiovascular Effects

Inhalation anesthetics produce dose-dependent myocardial depression and a decrease in systemic arterial blood pressure. The decrease in blood pressure is mainly due to a reduction of systemic vascular resistance. Heart rate is relatively unchanged by the inhaled anesthetics, although desflurane and to some extent isoflurane can cause sympathetic stimulation, leading to tachycardia and hypertension during induction or when the inspired concentration is abruptly increased (Fig. 8-4). Nitrous oxide also causes some increased

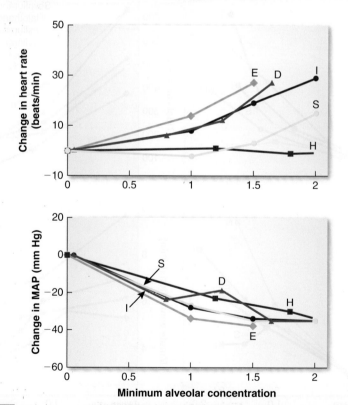

Figure 8-4   Heart rate and systemic blood pressure changes (from awake baseline) in volunteers receiving general anesthesia with a volatile anesthetic. Halothane and sevoflurane produced little change in heart rate at <1.5 minimum alveolar concentration. All anesthetics caused similar decreases in blood pressure. MAP, mean arterial pressure; S, sevoflurane; I, isoflurane; D, desflurane; E, enflurane; H, halothane. (From Inhaled anesthetics. In: Barash PB, Cullen BF, Stoelting RK, et al. *Handbook of Clinical Anesthesia*. 7th ed. Philadelphia: Lippincott Williams & Wilkins, 2013:227–251, with permission.)

sympathetic activity. Its direct cardiac depressive effects are neutralized by this increased sympathetic activity in healthy individuals. Unlike the outdated anesthetic halothane, the newer inhaled anesthetics (isoflurane, sevoflurane, desflurane) do not sensitize the myocardium to circulating catecholamines or predispose patients to dysrhythmias. Inhaled anesthetics are capable of providing myocardial protection against some ischemic and reperfusion injuries that last beyond the elimination of the anesthetic gases. Recent evidence suggests that some inhaled anesthetics, including xenon, also may offer protection against ischemic injury in the kidneys, liver, and brain.

V. Respiratory Effects

Inhaled anesthetics produce dose-dependent respiratory depression with a decrease in both tidal volume and respiratory rate. The increase in arterial carbon dioxide partial pressure as a result of respiratory depression is somewhat offset by the stimulation of the attendant surgical procedure. All of the inhaled anesthetics produce a dose-dependent depression of the ventilatory response to hypercarbia and the chemoreceptor response to hypoxia, even at subanesthetic concentrations (as low as 0.1 MAC).

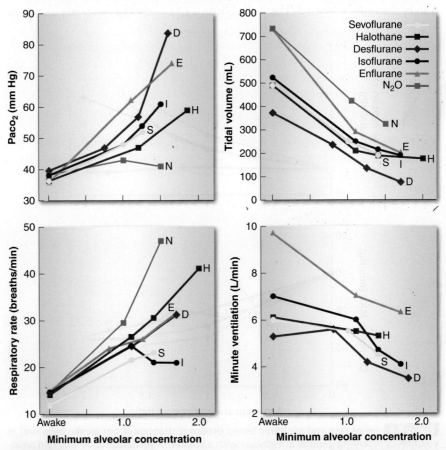

Figure 8-5 Comparison of mean changes in resting arterial carbon dioxide partial pressure (PaCO$_2$), tidal volume, respiratory rate, and minute ventilation in patients receiving an inhaled anesthetic. N$_2$O, nitrous oxide. (From Inhaled anesthetics. In: Barash PB, Cullen BF, Stoelting RK, et al. *Handbook of Clinical Anesthesia*. 7th ed. Philadelphia: Lippincott Williams & Wilkins, 2013:227–251, with permission.)

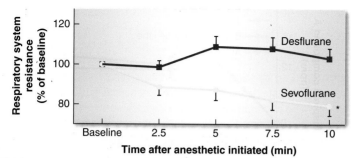

Figure 8-6 Changes in airway resistance before (baseline) and after tracheal intubation were significantly different in the presence of sevoflurane compared with desflurane. (From Inhaled anesthetics. In: Barash PB, Cullen BF, Stoelting RK, et al. *Handbook of Clinical Anesthesia*. 7th ed. Philadelphia: Lippincott Williams & Wilkins, 2013:227–251, with permission.)

Inhalation of the volatile anesthetics (especially isoflurane and desflurane) during induction of anesthesia can produce airway irritation and may precipitate coughing, laryngospasm, or bronchospasm. This is more likely in patients who smoke or have asthma. At surgical levels of anesthesia, equipotent doses of inhaled anesthetics produce some bronchodilation, with the exception of desflurane, which causes mild bronchoconstriction. Desflurane has higher pungency than other anesthetics and is not suitable for induction of anesthesia by inhalation of gas alone. Sevoflurane is the ideal agent for an inhaled induction both in children and adults. All of the inhaled anesthetics inhibit hypoxic pulmonary vasoconstriction in animals, producing an intrapulmonary shunt, but their effects in humans during one lung ventilation may be less severe (Figs. 8-5 and 8-6).

Following anesthesia with nitrous oxide, if the nitrous oxide is abruptly discontinued and the patient is allowed to breathe room air, there is a risk of transient *diffusion hypoxia*. A large volume of nitrous oxide diffuses from mixed venous blood into the alveoli. But simultaneously, the large volume of nitrogen being inhaled is not absorbed as quickly into the blood because it is so much less soluble than nitrous oxide. Consequently, the concentration of oxygen in the lung is reduced. This effect is short lived (2 to 3 minutes), and hypoxia can easily be avoided by having the patient breathe 100% oxygen when discontinuing nitrous oxide.

VI. Effects on Other Organ Systems

Inhaled anesthetics other than nitrous oxide directly relax skeletal muscles; this effect depends on the dose administered. They also potentiate the actions of nondepolarizing neuromuscular blocking drugs. All inhaled anesthetics other than nitrous oxide and xenon can precipitate malignant hyperthermia in susceptible patients.

All volatile inhaled anesthetics directly depress uterine muscle tone in a dose-dependent fashion similar to vascular smooth muscle. This can contribute to excessive uterine bleeding for women undergoing cesarean delivery or a therapeutic abortion, when the concentration of anesthetic exceeds 1 MAC. The anesthetic will also affect the newborn infant in terms of wakefulness, but the effect is short lived. It is common practice to administer lower concentrations of inhaled anesthetics (0.5 to 0.75 MAC) along with nitrous oxide when general anesthesia is necessary for cesarean delivery. In contrast, the

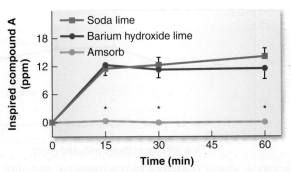

Figure 8-7 Compound A levels produced from three carbon dioxide absorbents during 1 minimum alveolar concentration sevoflurane anesthesia delivered at a fresh gas flow of 1 L/min (mean $\neq$ SE). *Asterisk* indicates $P <.05$ versus soda lime and barium hydroxide lime. (From Inhaled anesthetics. In: Barash PB, Cullen BF, Stoelting RK, et al. *Handbook of Clinical Anesthesia.* 7th ed. Philadelphia: Lippincott Williams & Wilkins, 2013:227–251, with permission.)

uterine relaxant effects of volatile anesthetics may be desirable in patients with a retained placenta.

Some older inhaled anesthetics are known to decrease liver blood flow. However, the new ether-based anesthetics (isoflurane, desflurane, sevoflurane) maintain or increase hepatic artery blood flow while decreasing or not changing portal vein blood flow. Rarely, patients may develop hepatitis secondary to exposure of an inhaled anesthetic, most notably from halothane (halothane hepatitis), which is an immune-mediated reaction to oxidatively derived metabolites of the anesthetic. Inhaled anesthetics may cause a decrease in renal blood flow as a result of decreased cardiac output and blood pressure or an increase in renal vascular resistance.

VII. Potential Toxicity of Inhaled Anesthetics

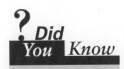

Inhaled anesthetics and nitrous oxide are greenhouse gases. Nitrous oxide is also destructive to the ozone layer. The global warming potential (GWP) of desflurane is the highest, followed by isoflurane. Sevoflurane has the least GWP. Xenon has none.

Sevoflurane can be degraded to vinyl ether, also called *Compound A,* by the carbon dioxide (CO_2) absorbent in the anesthesia breathing circuit. The production of Compound A is enhanced when a low total flow of oxygen or nitrous oxide is used, during use of a closed-circuit breathing system, and when the CO_2 absorbent is warm or very dry. Compound A is toxic to the renal system of animals; however, there has been no evidence of renal toxicity with sevoflurane usage in humans. Figure 8-7 shows the extent to which Compound A is produced with various CO_2 absorbents.

Desflurane can be degraded to carbon monoxide by CO_2 absorbents. This is most likely when the absorbent is new or dry (water content <5%) and when the absorbent contains barium.

All the modern volatile anesthetics contain fluoride. This was a problem for older anesthetics, such as methoxyflurane, because metabolism of the drug to a free fluoride ion caused renal toxicity. However, the newer anesthetics undergo limited metabolism, and fluoride-induced renal toxicity has not been demonstrated.

VIII. The Nonvolatile Anesthetics

A. Nitrous Oxide

For many reasons, the clinical use of nitrous oxide is on the decline. First, because it is relatively weak (the MAC is 105%), it cannot be used as the sole anesthetic agent. Second, it can readily diffuse into closed air spaces such as the middle ear, bowel, cranial air sinuses, a pneumoperitoneum (e.g., during laparoscopic procedures), a pneumothorax, and gas bubbles inserted during ocular surgery. This can result in either an increase in volume of the space (e.g., distension of bowel) or an increase in pressure (e.g., in the eye or middle ear). Third, it is associated with a high incidence of postoperative nausea and vomiting when it is used for longer than 1 hour. Fourth, due to its interference with folate metabolism, it has the potential for toxic effects on the developing embryo. Nitrous oxide oxidizes the cobalt atom on vitamin B_{12}, thereby irreversibly inhibiting the B_{12}-dependent enzyme *methionine synthetase* and resulting in elevated levels of homocystine. This end product leads to endothelial dysfunction, oxidative stress, and destabilizes arterial plaque. Prolonged administration of nitrous oxide, as for sedation in the intensive care unit, is associated with severe anemia. Finally, nitrous oxide, like CO_2, causes ozone depletion in the upper atmosphere. Despite the declining use of nitrous oxide intraoperatively, the administration of a 50:50 mixture of oxygen and nitrous oxide (Entonox) remains useful for brief analgesia in pediatric dentistry, labor analgesia, burn dressing changes, and related procedures.

B. Xenon

Xenon is a rare noble gas occurring naturally in air at 0.05 parts per million. Recently, there has been renewed interest in the use of xenon as an anesthetic gas. Xenon has several advantages when compared with not only nitrous oxide but also to the potent volatile anesthetics. Xenon has rapid onset and offset of action due to its extremely low blood:gas partition coefficient (Table 8-1). Its effects on cardiovascular, neuronal, and respiratory systems are minimal, and it is not a trigger for malignant hyperthermia. Xenon also can be used in low concentrations for analgesia. This action is mediated through inhibition of N-methyl-D-aspartate receptors in the central nervous system. The only limitation to routine use of xenon is its cost. The gas exists at very low concentrations in our atmosphere, and there is a high cost associated with its extraction and recycling. New anesthetic systems are being developed that will allow use of xenon in small volumes and will recycle the gas after it is exhaled.

IX. Clinical Use of Inhaled Anesthetics

Due to a lack of pungency and a low blood:gas partition coefficient, sevoflurane is the agent of choice for an inhaled induction of anesthesia in both children and adults, such as when intravenous access is not possible or desirable. Inhaled anesthetics remain the most popular drugs for maintenance of anesthesia during surgery as they are easy to administer and the dose can be easily titrated in response to highly variable surgical stimuli. Despite their popularity, inhaled anesthetics have some significant drawbacks. These can include profound respiratory depression, hypotension, lack of analgesia at low concentrations, postoperative nausea and vomiting, the potential for triggering malignant hyperthermia in susceptible individuals, and rare toxicity such as hepatitis. The volatile anesthetics also interfere with monitoring of sensory-evoked potentials when administered in doses of more than 0.5 MAC. Nevertheless, despite these drawbacks, when inhaled anesthetics are administered for surgical procedures by appropriately trained specialists, the morbidity and mortality from general anesthesia are remarkably low.

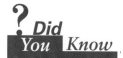

All volatile anesthetic agents increase the incidence of postoperative nausea and vomiting (PONV) and the risk increases with the duration of exposure to the anesthetic. They should be avoided in patients at high risk of PONV.

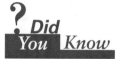

Shutting off the fresh gas flows (rather than shutting off the vaporizer) during intubation or airway instrumentation is the best approach to prevent operating room pollution with anesthetic gases and reduce wastage.

Suggested Readings

Becker DE, Rosenberg M. Nitrous oxide and the inhalation anesthetics. *Anesth Prog.* 2008; 55(4):124–132.

Derwall M, Coburn M, Rex S, et al. Xenon: Recent developments and future perspectives. *Minerva Anestesiol.* 2009;75(1–2):37–45.

de Vasconcellos K, Sneyd JR. Nitrous oxide: are we still in equipoise? A qualitative review of current controversies. *Br J Anaesth.* 2013;111(6):877–885.

Eger EI 2nd. The pharmacology of isoflurane. *Br J Anaesth.* 1984;56(Suppl 1):71s–99s.

Eger EI 2nd. New inhalational agents—desflurane and sevoflurane. *Can J Anaesth.* 1993; 40(5 Pt 2):R3–R8.

Eger EI 2nd. Age, minimum alveolar anesthetic concentration, and minimum alveolar anesthetic concentration-awake. *Anesth Analg.* 2001;93(4):947–953.

Harris PD, Barnes R. The uses of helium and xenon in current clinical practice. *Anaesthesia.* 2008;63(3):284–293.

Hirota K. Special cases: ketamine, nitrous oxide and xenon. *Best Pract Res Clin Anaesthesiol.* 2006;20(1):69–79.

Jones RM. Desflurane and sevoflurane: inhalation anaesthetics for this decade? *Br J Anaesth.* 1990;65(4):527–536.

Kharasch ED. Biotransformation of sevoflurane. *Anesth Analg.* 1995;81(6 Suppl):S27–S38.

Leighton KM, Koth B. Some aspects of the clinical pharmacology of nitrous oxide. *Can Anaesth Soc J.* 1973;20(1):94–103.

Sanders RD, Franks NP, Maze M. Xenon: no stranger to anaesthesia. *Br J Anaesth.* 2003; 91(5):709–717.

Smith I. Nitrous oxide in ambulatory anaesthesia: does it have a place in day surgical anaesthesia or is it just a threat for personnel and the global environment? *Curr Opin Anaesthesiol.* 2006;19(6):592–596.

Smith WD. Pharmacology of nitrous oxide. *Int Anesthesiol Clin.* 1971;9(3):91–123.

Questions

1. All of the following inhaled anesthetics must be administered using an agent-specific calibrated vaporizer EXCEPT:
   A. Xenon
   B. Isoflurane
   C. Sevoflurane
   D. Desflurane

2. Which of the following properties of inhaled anesthetics is the primary determinant of the rapidity with which it can induce anesthesia?
   A. The vapor pressure at room temperature
   B. The oil:gas partition coefficient
   C. The blood:gas partition coefficient
   D. The minimum alveolar concentration (MAC)

3. The rate at which the alveolar concentration (F_A) of an inhaled anesthetic approaches that being inspired (F_I) is most rapid under which of the following conditions:
   A. Increased blood pressure
   B. Increased cardiac output
   C. Increased ventilation
   D. Increased body fat

4. Which of the following organs or tissue groups has the LEAST effect in determining the rapidity of induction with an inhaled anesthetic?
   A. Skeletal muscle
   B. Skin
   C. Liver and kidney
   D. Fat

5. The minimum alveolar concentration (MAC) of an inhaled anesthetic is the concentration necessary to:
   A. Produce adequate anesthesia for minor surgical procedures (e.g., tonsillectomy)
   B. Produce adequate anesthesia for all surgical procedures
   C. Produce analgesia without a loss of consciousness
   D. Prevent movement in response to a skin incision in 50% of patients

6. All of the following are decreased during general anesthesia with sevoflurane EXCEPT:
   A. Myocardial contractility
   B. Systemic vascular resistance
   C. Cerebral blood flow
   D. Minute ventilation

7. A patient with a long history of smoking and asthma requires an inhaled induction of anesthesia. The preferred anesthetic is:
   A. Nitrous oxide
   B. Sevoflurane
   C. Desflurane
   D. Isoflurane

8. A spontaneously breathing anesthetized patient becomes accidently disconnected from the anesthetic circuit and breathes room air. A fall in oxygen saturation measured with a pulse oximeter is most likely to occur most rapidly when the anesthetic is:
   A. 8.0% desflurane
   B. 1.2% isoflurane
   C. 2.5% sevoflurane
   D. 75% nitrous oxide

9. Anesthesia with isoflurane, as opposed to a combination of nitrous oxide and opioids, is most likely to contribute to excessive bleeding during which of the following procedures:
   A. Cesarean delivery
   B. Resection of an intracranial meningioma
   C. Transurethral prostatectomy
   D. Repair of a femoral artery laceration

10. What is the primary reason why xenon is NOT routinely used for general anesthesia?
    A. It cannot be used as the sole anesthetic (MAC is too high)
    B. It has a high blood:gas partition coefficient
    C. It has a metabolite that is potentially nephrotoxic
    D. High cost

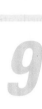

9 Intravenous Anesthetics and Sedatives

Christopher W. Connor
Babak Sadighi
Jessica Black

Before examining any anesthetic medication in detail, it is important to consider what occurs when an intravenous sedative is administered. Unlike inhaled agents, the mechanisms of action for intravenous sedatives and anesthetics are well characterized.

Initially, the medication will be transported and diluted within the patient's cardiovascular system. There will be no change in the patient's level of consciousness. Some of the medication will be transported across the blood–brain barrier where it will become redistributed to its effect site and bind to the receptors for which it has affinity.

As the medication binds to its *target receptors*, the onset of sedation can be observed. There will be a progressive diminution in the patient's level of consciousness, continuing until chemical equilibrium is reached at the effect site. Depending on the medication and the quantity administered, this decreased level of consciousness may range from light sedation with preserved spontaneous ventilation to general anesthesia with apnea.

The medication that is circulating in the cardiovascular system is eventually eliminated from the body, metabolized into an inactive or degraded form, or redistributed and sequestered into other peripheral tissues in which it produces no effect. The concentration of the medication within the cerebral circulation will start to fall, and the concentration gradient will draw the medication away from its effect site. Binding at the target receptors within the brain then decreases, and recovery toward consciousness begins.

If it is desired to prolong the patient's sedation, additional medication can be administered. In response to these further doses, the concentration of medication will instead approach a new equilibrium concentration with a corresponding level of clinical sedation. Eventually, the patient can be allowed to recover by discontinuing the infusion. The additional medication administered must then be eliminated, metabolized, or redistributed. The medication will return into circulation from the peripheral tissues into which it had been sequestered. The quantity of medication present may also temporarily exceed the metabolic capacity of the pathways by which it is degraded. Consequently, the clinical return to consciousness will now be slower than before and will depend on the quantity and duration of the medication's administration. Finally, it must be considered that an individual may not respond as expected or may have an unanticipated adverse reaction to the medication instead.

In this vignette, there are four pharmacologic themes, illustrating the clinical use of an intravenous anesthetic or sedative:

1. Mechanism of action: molecular interaction of a medication with a receptor
2. Pharmacokinetic profile: the trafficking, *redistribution*, and elimination of the medication within the body
3. Pharmacodynamic profile: the behavior of a concentration of this medication at the population of receptors within the brain
4. Adverse reactions: the extent to which the medication may produce allergic or *hypersensitivity reactions*.

I. General Pharmacology of Intravenous Anesthetics

A. Mechanism of Action

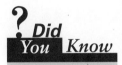

The most commonly used intravenous anesthetic agents—the barbiturates, propofol, the benzodiazepines, and etomidate—all act at the site of the γ-aminobutyric acid A (GABA$_A$) receptor, as shown schematically in Figure 9-1. GABA is the main inhibitory neurotransmitter within the central nervous system, and its action at the GABA$_A$ receptor causes increased transport of chloride (Cl$^-$) ions across the membrane and into the *postsynaptic neuron*. The postsynaptic neuron becomes hyperpolarized, which functionally inhibits further propagation of nerve signals. The GABA$_A$ receptor is therefore a ligand-activated ion channel composed of five subunits. Intravenous anesthetics that bind to the GABA$_A$ receptor do not bind at the same location as GABA itself (the orthosteric binding site), instead they bind at other locations (allosteric sites) and change the effect of GABA upon the receptor. These intravenous anesthetics are therefore

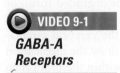

VIDEO 9-1

GABA-A Receptors

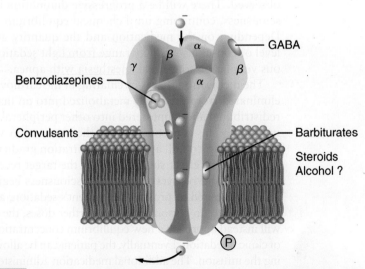

Figure 9-1 Schematic model of the γ-aminobutyric acid A (GABA$_A$) receptor complex, illustrating recognition sites for many of the substances that bind to the receptor. (From White PF, Eng MR. Intravenous anesthetics. In: Barash PG, Cullen BF, Stoelting RK, et al. *Clinical Anesthesia*. 7th ed. Philadelphia: Wolters Kluwer Health/LWW, 2013:480, with permission.)

positive allosteric modulators of the $GABA_A$ receptor and cause receptor conformational changes such that the action of GABA itself is potentiated and sedation occurs. The subunit composition of $GABA_A$ receptors can vary: there are 19 different possible subunits arising from eight different subunit classes (α_{1-6}, β_{1-3}, γ_{1-3}, δ, ε, θ, π, and ρ). Intravenous anesthetic agents may only be active at receptors expressing certain combinations: the benzodiazepine allosteric binding site occurs only at the interface of α and γ_2 subunits, and etomidate is active primarily at $GABA_A$ receptors that contain β_2 or β_3 subunits.

B. Pharmacokinetics and Metabolism

The redistribution and elimination of intravenous anesthetics within the body can be approximated with a simplified *three-compartment model* of the body. In this model, medications are administered into a first well-mixed central compartment. Diffusion occurs back and forth between this first compartment and the additional second and third peripheral compartments. The diffusion constants (shown as *k* in Fig. 9-2) are such that one peripheral compartment equilibrates quickly with the central compartment and one equilibrates more slowly. The drug is not pharmacologically active in these peripheral compartments. Instead, they act as reservoirs into which medications are redistributed and sequestered. These peripheral compartments model how the action of the medication may be terminated by redistribution. They also model the way in which accumulation of medication within these peripheral compartments can lead to progressively increasing context-sensitive half-times as medication diffuses back into the central compartment. An effect site compartment models the receptor population at which the medication has its mechanism of action. Diffusion also occurs between the central and the effect site compartments. But because the quantity of drug bound to the receptors at any given moment

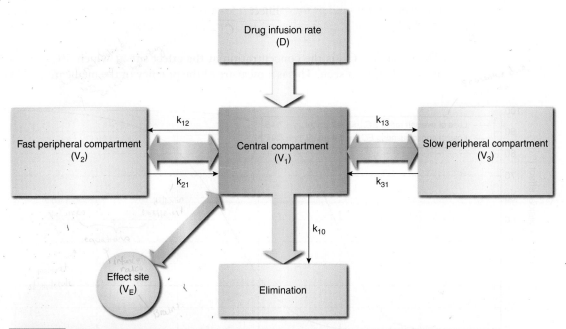

Figure 9-2 Three-compartment model for the pharmacokinetic modeling of intravenous medication administration, redistribution, and elimination. Additionally, an effect site compartment is present. The volume of this compartment is assumed to be sufficiently small that the effect on the quantity of medication in the central compartment is negligible.

is minor compared with the total quantity of medication in the body, the effect site compartment is assumed to be sufficiently small that its effect on the mass of medication within the central compartment is negligible.

The structure of these compartments, with their associated volumes and diffusion coefficients, allows a series of differential equations to be produced that model the trafficking of medication in response to changes in infusion rates. A computer can be used to determine an ideal sequence of infusion rate changes so that the concentration of drug at the effect site is brought to the desired concentration within the optimum time (1). This practice is known as *target-controlled infusion*.

C. Pharmacodynamic Effects

Many combinations of GABA$_A$ *receptor subunits* are possible. However, in practice, these variations are not directly accounted for between individual receptors when predicting the clinical effect of a dosage of a medication. Instead, the effect site in the pharmacokinetic model represents the combined population of all the receptors, and the likely clinical effect is determined by a statistical model relating this concentration to a particular clinical outcome. These pharmacodynamic models are created for different clinical outcomes with different medications. Figure 9-3 shows two separate pharmacodynamic models: the leftmost model relates the concentration of propofol at the effect site to the loss of the eyelash reflex, and the rightmost model relates the concentration of propofol to loss of consciousness (2). The most notable characteristic is the strong nonlinearity of these relationships. It is possible, with only a small increase in concentration of propofol, to transition rapidly from consciousness to unconsciousness. These nonlinear models have a standard form, known as the sigmoid-E_{max} model or the Hill equation (3):

$$\frac{\text{Effect}}{E_{max}} = \frac{C^{\gamma}}{C^{\gamma} + EC_{50}^{\gamma}}$$

The variable EC_{50} is the concentration at the effect site at which 50% of the maximal effect is seen. This is a measure of the potency of the medication. The

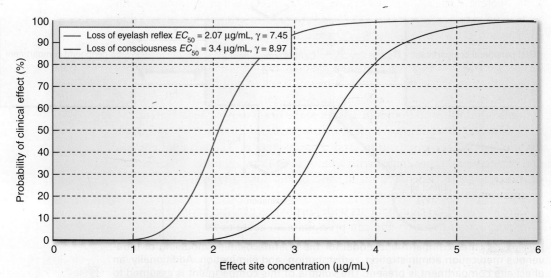

Figure 9-3 Pharmacodynamic models for the probability of loss of eyelash reflex and for the probability of loss of consciousness based on propofol effect site concentration.

γ variable is the sigmoid coefficient, and greater values of γ yield more abrupt transitions. A small change in propofol effect site concentration can cause a large, even unexpected, clinical effect.

D. Hypersensitivity (Allergic) Reactions

The most common causes of hypotension following induction with intravenous anesthetic agents are unrecognized hypovolemia and unexpected drug interactions. True hypersensitivity reactions are rare, although case reports of histamine release with all intravenous anesthetic agents, with the exception of etomidate, have been alleged. Propofol does not normally cause histamine release but *anaphylactoid reactions* have been reported in patients with multiple drug allergies. Barbiturates can precipitate acute intermittent porphyria in susceptible patients.

II. Comparative Physiochemical and Clinical Pharmacologic Properties

A. Barbiturates

The most commonly used barbiturates are the thiobarbiturates: thiopental (Pentothal, 5-ethyl-5-[1-methylbutyl]-2-thiobarbituric acid), thiamylal (Surital, 5-allyl-5-[1-methylbutyl]-2-thiobarbituric acid), and the oxybarbiturate methohexital (Brevital, 1-methyl-5-allyl-5-[1-methyl-2-pentanyl] barbituric acid).

Barbiturates depress the reticular activating system in the brainstem and are believed to potentiate the action of $GABA_A$ receptors, increasing the duration of an associated chloride ion channel opening. Barbiturates decrease cerebral metabolic rate of oxygen ($CMRO_2$), cerebral blood flow (CBF), and intracranial pressure (ICP). Barbiturates can induce an isoelectric electroencephalogram (EEG), maximally decreasing $CMRO_2$.

Barbiturates are formulated as sodium salts and are reconstituted in water or isotonic sodium chloride (0.9%) to prepare 2.5% thiopental, 1% to 2% methohexital, and 2% thiamylal. These preparations are highly alkaline (pH 9 to 10). When they are added to lactated ringers or other acidic drug preparations, crystalline precipitation will occur and may irreversibly occlude intravenous tubing and catheters. Barbiturates rarely cause pain on injection but will cause significant tissue irritation if extravasated. Inadvertent intra-arterial injection of thiobarbiturates causes serious complications, including intense vasoconstriction, thrombosis, and tissue necrosis. Immediate treatment may require intra-arterial papaverine and lidocaine or procaine, regional anesthesia-induced sympathectomy (stellate ganglion block, brachial plexus block), and heparinization.

The anesthetic action of the barbiturates is primarily terminated by redistribution from the central lipophilic tissues of the brain to peripheral lean muscle compartments. Barbiturates undergo slow *terminal elimination* via hepatic metabolism, biliary conjugation, and renal excretion. The terminal elimination of thiopental is prolonged with a half-life of 10 to 12 hours. Methohexital clearance is more dependent on hepatic blood flow, allowing for a shorter elimination half-life of 4 hours.

Care should be taken in patients with porphyrias because barbiturates stimulate porphyrin formation and can precipitate an acute crisis.

B. Propofol

Propofol (Diprivan) is an alkylphenol compound prepared in an egg lecithin emulsion consisting of soybean oil, glycerol, egg phosphatide, and ethylenediaminetetraacetic acid or metabisulphite as an antimicrobial.

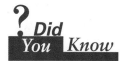

? Did You Know

Commonly used intravenous anesthetic agents such as the barbiturates, propofol, the benzodiazepines, and etomidate act at the site of the $GABA_A$ receptor.

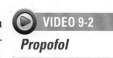

VIDEO 9-2

Propofol

Propofol increases the binding affinity of GABA with the GABA$_A$ receptor. Coupled to a chloride channel, the activation leads to the *hyperpolarization* of the nerve membrane and is similar to the mechanism of action of the barbiturates. Propofol causes a decrease in arterial blood pressure due to a simultaneous decrease in systemic vascular resistance, a decrease in preload (caused by inhibition of sympathetic tone and direct vascular smooth muscle effect), and direct myocardial depression. These effects are dose and concentration dependent. Propofol decreases CMRO$_2$, CBF, and ICP. However, in patients with increased cranial pressure, the depressant effect of propofol on systemic arterial pressure will dramatically decrease cerebral perfusion pressure (CPP). Propofol does not affect cerebrovascular regulation or cerebral reactivity to carbon dioxide tension. Its neuroprotective qualities include EEG burst suppression similar to thiopental, anticonvulsive properties, and the decrease of intraocular pressure. Propofol also has antipruritic and antiemetic properties.

Propofol emulsion often causes pain upon injection into small hand veins. This pain can be minimized by injection into larger veins and by mixing lidocaine with the propofol prior to injection.

The anesthetic action of propofol is primarily terminated by redistribution from the central lipophilic tissues of the brain to peripheral compartments. Whether used as a single-bolus, an induction agent, or as a continuous infusion, the *redistribution half-life* is very short (2 to 8 minutes) and the context-sensitive half-life for infusions up to 8 hours is less than 40 minutes. Metabolism is primarily hepatic and inactive water-soluble metabolites are eliminated renally. However, the presence of even clinically significant hepatic and renal disease does not markedly change propofol pharmacokinetics (4).

An egg allergy is not necessarily a contraindication to the utilization of propofol. Most egg allergies involve egg albumin found in egg whites. The egg lecithin in the propofol emulsion is an egg yolk extract. Propofol must be handled with sterile technique as the emulsion can support bacterial growth. Unused propofol should be discarded 6 hours after opening. The use of long-term, high-dose infusion in critically ill children and adults may cause *propofol infusion syndrome (PRIS)* characterized by cardiac failure, rhabdomyolysis, metabolic acidosis, renal failure, hyperkalemia, hypertriglyceridemia, and hepatomegaly. PRIS is rare, and its pathophysiology is uncertain, but it is often fatal. If suspected, propofol must be immediately discontinued and an alternative sedative employed.

C. Benzodiazepines

Benzodiazepine compounds consist of a benzene ring and a diazepine ring. Side-chain variations from this molecular backbone have produced dozens of medications with various potencies and clearance rates. The most commonly used benzodiazepines in anesthesia are midazolam (Versed), lorazepam (Ativan), and diazepam (Valium). Midazolam is water soluble at low pH values. Lorazepam and diazepam are insoluble and are formulated with propylene glycol. Venoirritation is sometimes seen on administration.

Benzodiazepines bind to the same GABA$_A$ receptors as barbiturates but at a different site on the receptor. The frequency of the associated chloride ion channel opening is increased with binding of GABA to the receptor, causing sedation along the same downstream pathway as propofol and the barbiturates. Benzodiazepines similarly decrease CMRO$_2$, CBF, and ICP. Although benzodiazepines are unable to completely suppress EEG bursts, they are effective in suppressing and controlling grand mal seizures.

Unlike propofol and the barbiturates, sedation with benzodiazepines can be pharmacologically reversed. *Flumazenil* is a specific competitive antagonist for benzodiazepines with a high affinity for the benzodiazepine receptor site. The dosage of flumazenil is 0.5 to 1 mg intravenously. It is cleared more rapidly than the benzodiazepines, so patients must be monitored as resedation may occur and repeated doses of flumazenil may be required.

Benzodiazepines are hepatically metabolized and are susceptible to hepatic dysfunction and the coadministration of other medications. Being highly protein bound, the free drug fraction is increased in severe liver disease and chronic kidney disease (CKD), with the elimination half-life being either prolonged or shortened, respectively. Hepatic clearance is enhanced if hepatic function is unaffected in the CKD patient. Primary diazepam metabolites, desmethyldiazepam and 3-hydroxydiazepam, are pharmacologically active and prolong the sedative effects. These metabolites are further conjugated to form inactive water-soluble glucuronidated products. A conjugated midazolam metabolite, α-hydromidazolam, may also accumulate in CKD patients receiving large doses of midazolam.

Although benzodiazepines are not known to be significant teratogens, there is concern that they may increase the incidence of cleft palette in susceptible patients. Newborns may exhibit withdrawal syndrome from benzodiazepines administered to the mother. Consequently, benzodiazepines are usually avoided during pregnancy (5).

D. Etomidate

Structurally, etomidate (Amidate) is unrelated to other anesthetic agents. It has an imidazole ring that, under physiologic pH, makes it lipid soluble. Etomidate is a *stereoisomer*. Only the R^+ isomer possesses clinical anesthetic activity. To allow for an injectable solution, the drug is dissolved in propylene glycol. This solution may cause pain on injection, which may be reduced by preadministration of intravenous lidocaine.

Etomidate also acts through binding to $GABA_A$ receptors, increasing the affinity of the receptors for GABA, although etomidate appears to operate preferentially at $GABA_A$ receptors that express only a subset of the possible β subunits (6). Etomidate is thought to cause subcortical disinhibition, explaining the involuntary myoclonic movements and trismus commonly encountered during induction with this medication. Etomidate decreases $CMRO_2$, CBF, and ICP, while maintaining good CPP secondary to hemodynamic stability. Etomidate is capable of producing convulsion-like EEG potentials in epileptic patients without creating actual convulsions, helping to localize seizure foci during intraoperative mapping. Although etomidate may create these potentials, it has anticonvulsant properties and may be used against status epilepticus. Etomidate also increases the amplitude of somatosensory-evoked potentials (SSEP), helping in situations where interpretation is needed and SSEP signal quality is poor. Postoperative nausea and vomiting is more common with etomidate than with propofol or thiopental and it lacks any analgesic properties. Etomidate transiently inhibits *11-β-hydroxlase*, an enzyme involved in the production of steroids, which causes adrenocortical suppression. Even after a single induction dose, suppression can be seen for 5 to 8 hours. In its favor, however, etomidate does not cause histamine release and causes minimal hemodynamic depression and bronchoconstriction, even in the presence of cardiovascular and pulmonary disease. It is this hemodynamic stability that underlies the continued use of etomidate in clinical practice.

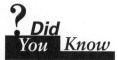

? Did You Know

Unlike propofol and the barbiturates, sedation with benzodiazepines can be pharmacologically reversed with flumazenil, a specific competitive antagonist for benzodiazepines.

? Did You Know

Etomidate transiently inhibits 11-β-hydroxlase, an enzyme involved in the production of steroids, even after a single induction dose.

Awakening from etomidate occurs primarily by redistribution to peripheral tissues. Terminal elimination occurs by hepatic biotransformation to inactive metabolites that are then renally excreted.

E. Ketamine

Ketamine (Ketalar) is a highly lipid-soluble *phencyclidine* derivative. In the United States, ketamine is sold as a racemic mixture. Of the two forms, S^+ ketamine is more potent than the R^- stereoisomer and exhibits a greater rate of clearance and a faster recovery from anesthesia (7). Ketamine has unique properties to distinguish it from other intravenous anesthetics: it stimulates the sympathetic nervous system, has minimal respiratory depression, and it causes potent bronchodilation. Ketamine has several routes of administration, making it an excellent choice for uncooperative patients and pediatrics. Its major effects are mediated through its potent antagonism of the *N-methyl-D-aspartate (NMDA) receptor*, rather than action at the $GABA_A$ receptor.

Ketamine is a cerebral vasodilator, causing increased CBF and increased ICP. It also increases $CMRO_2$. Ketamine is relatively contraindicated in patients with space occupying lesions within the central nervous system (CNS), especially those with elevated ICP. Research has shown that normocapnia will blunt the undesirable effects of ketamine on increased CBF. But other induction agents are more appropriate and almost always available. Additionally, although ketamine causes myoclonus and increased EEG activity, it is still considered an anticonvulsant and may be used as a last-line agent in *status epilepticus*.

The NMDA receptor is an excitatory receptor found throughout the CNS, including areas in the spinal cord, thalamolimbic system, and nucleus tractus solitarius (NTS). Glutamate, the most prominent excitatory neurotransmitter within the CNS, binds to the receptor and (among many other functions) transduces signals for pain, associates sensory signals between the thalamus and cortex, and causes global excitation. Ketamine causes analgesia not only by blocking the pain signal at the spinal cord but also by "disassociating" the communication of pain between the thalamus and limbic system. This state of *dissociative amnesia* causes the patient to appear conscious (eyes open, staring) but remain unresponsive to sensory input (pain, verbal stimulus).

The mechanism of action of ketamine is complex. It is theorized that ketamine blockades the NMDA receptors within the NTS and prevents these neurons from inhibiting the vasomotor center, resulting in a positive release of catecholamines. In isolation, ketamine is a direct myocardial depressant, but secondary to this indirect release of catecholamines, it acts as a cardiac stimulant, causing increased blood pressure, heart rate, and cardiac output. Some caution is required in patients with pre-existing sympathetic blockade, such as those with spinal cord lesions or those with exhaustion of their catecholamine stores (e.g. shock trauma patients), because they will not produce these indirect cardiac stimulatory effects. Ketamine also blocks sodium channels, which contributes to its analgesic effects.

Termination of the clinical effect of ketamine is primarily due to redistribution from the brain to the peripheral tissues. Ketamine is hepatically metabolized by the cytochrome P450 system into several metabolites, of which one, norketamine, retains some anesthetic properties. The metabolites are renally excreted. Although lipid soluble, ketamine is the least protein-bound molecule of all intravenous anesthetics.

Respiratory drive and upper airway reflexes remain minimally affected. However, patients who are at risk for aspiration should be intubated during general anesthesia with ketamine. Ketamine causes increased lacrimation and salivation that may lead to laryngospasm. Pretreatment with an anticholinergic agent such as glycopyrrolate can attenuate this response. Unfortunately, ketamine tends to produce unpleasant emergence reactions such as hallucinations, out of body experiences, and fear, which have limited its widespread use as a primary anesthetic medication. These emergence reactions are better tolerated in the pediatric population and should be of major consideration in psychiatric patients. Nevertheless, the unique properties of ketamine and its multiple documented routes of administration (intravenous, intramuscular, oral, rectal, and even epidural and intrathecal) give it many adjunct clinical uses.

F. Dexmedetomidine

Dexmedetomidine (Precedex) is the S-enantiomer of medetomidine and is a centrally-acting, highly-selective α_2 agonist. It produces sedation and analgesia without substantial respiratory depression.

The α_2 receptors are located presynaptically and in the locus ceruleus, an area of brain responsible for arousal and sympathetic activity. The α_2 receptors are inhibitory receptors and, when activated, decrease the amount of downstream neurotransmitter released. For sympathetic nerves, this results in less catecholamine release, which causes decreased blood pressure and heart rate. The α_2 receptors are also located on axons in the spinal cord involved in pain transmission. When these receptors are activated, nociceptive transmission is decreased and the perception of pain is attenuated. Activating α_2 receptors in the *locus ceruleus* causes sedation and decreased sympathetic activity. Because dexmedetomidine acts only on α_2 receptors, which are not involved with respiration, minimal respiratory depression is observed.

The liver rapidly metabolizes dexmedetomidine through mechanisms involving uridine 5'-diphosphoglucuronosyl transferase. The drug is rapidly cleared, and metabolites are excreted via bile and urine. Renal or hepatic insufficiency may delay excretion of the metabolites.

As dexmedetomidine provides sedation and analgesia without causing respiratory depression, it has clinical uses in both the operating room and intensive care unit setting. In the operating room, dexmedetomidine has been used primarily as an adjunct to general anesthesia for patients who require alternative mechanisms of analgesia. It is used either in the setting of preexisting opioid tolerance in patients with chronic pain or to reduce opioid administration in those patients at risk of opioid-related postoperative respiratory depression, such as for the morbidly obese or patients with obstructive sleep apnea.

When used as the sole, systemic medication, dexmedetomidine is a good choice of anesthetic for awake fiberoptic intubation or in combination with regional anesthesia. In the intensive care unit, dexmedetomidine can be helpful for weaning intubated patients from the ventilator as it provides sedation with minimal respiratory depression. Compared with benzodiazepines in the intensive care unit, dexmedetomidine is associated with a reduced incidence of delirium and a more physiologic sleep state (8). Dexmedetomidine, however, should not be infused continuously for more than 24 hours, as there is concern for rebound hypertension, rebound excitability, and arrhythmia.

III. Clinical Use of Intravenous Anesthetics

A. Use of Intravenous Anesthetics as Induction Agents

Barbiturates

The induction dose of thiopental is 3 to 5 mg/kg in adults, 5 to 6 mg/kg in children, and 6 to 8 mg/kg in infants. Induction doses are reduced in the geriatric population by 30% to 40%, in obstetric patients in early term (7 to 13 weeks' gestation), in patients with advanced American Society of Anesthesiologists physical status (3 or 4), and when used in conjunction with other medications. The induction of anesthesia occurs in less than 30 seconds, and spontaneous awakening from an induction dose occurs within 20 minutes.

The induction dose of methohexital is 1 to 1.5 mg/kg in adults. At lower doses, methohexital can paradoxically increase or activate cortical EEG seizure discharges in patients with temporal lobe epilepsy. However, this property makes a bolus dose of methohexital the intravenous anesthetic of choice for electroconvulsive therapy.

Propofol

The induction dose of propofol in adults is 1.5 to 2.5 mg/kg; lean body weight should be used in the morbidly obese. Decreased induction doses should be considered for the elderly due to decreased volume of distribution and slowed clearance. Propofol causes decreased systemic arterial pressure on induction, due partially to direct action on vascular smooth muscle. Because this effect is related to plasma concentration rather than effect site concentration, it may be possible to blunt the effect by administering the bolus more gradually or in divided doses.

Benzodiazepines

The induction dose of midazolam is 0.1 to 0.2 mg/kg intravenously. However, the prolonged recovery from induction with even short-acting benzodiazepines limits their usefulness as induction agents in routine clinical use (9).

Etomidate

Etomidate has a very favorable hemodynamic profile on induction, with minimal depression in blood pressure. It is often used for anesthetizing patients who have significant cardiovascular disease or for emergent situations, such as *shock trauma*, in which the need to preserve hemodynamic stability takes precedence over etomidate's drawbacks. Etomidate is only administered intravenously, and the induction dose for adults is 0.2 to 0.3 mg/kg. The onset is extremely rapid, at approximately one arm-to-brain circulation time. The myoclonus and trismus that may follow induction with etomidate can make initial attempts at ventilation and intubation difficult unless the induction is promptly accompanied with a neuromuscular blocker. Etomidate does not inhibit the sympathetic response to laryngoscopy and intubation unless combined with an analgesic.

Ketamine

The induction dose of ketamine in adults is 1 to 2 mg/kg when administered intravenously. However, induction with ketamine via intramuscular administration is frequently used when the patient is unable to tolerate placement of an intravenous line, such as pediatric patients, uncooperative patients, or patients with cognitive impairments. An intramuscular injection of 4 to 6 mg/kg provides induction of an anesthetic state with maintained spontaneous ventilation, allowing for an intravenous line to be placed and the further management of the patient to proceed.

B. Use of Intravenous Drugs for Maintenance of Anesthesia
Barbiturates
Barbiturates are used to improve brain relaxation during neurosurgery and may protect brain tissue from transient episodes of focal ischemia by decreasing $CMRO_2$ (10). However, the dosing required to maintain EEG suppression is associated with prolonged emergence and delayed extubation. In general, the use of barbiturate infusions to maintain anesthesia is not recommended because the capacity of the body to redistribute barbiturates is relatively limited. Continuous administration of barbiturates rapidly causes the concentration of medication in the peripheral compartments to approach the concentration within the central compartment. Termination of the anesthetic effect then depends solely on terminal elimination, leading to a very prolonged context-sensitive half-life.

Propofol
Propofol is commonly used to maintain a state of general anesthesia without the use of inhaled anesthetic agents. In this practice, known as *total intravenous anesthesia*, an infusion of propofol provides the hypnotic component of the general anesthetic. Infusion rates with propofol range between 100 to 200 µg/kg/min for hypnosis. However, propofol alone provides no analgesia, so concurrent infusion of an opioid such as fentanyl or remifentanil is usually necessary.

Benzodiazepines
Infusion rates for midazolam for maintaining hypnosis and amnesia are 0.25 to 1.0 µg/kg/min when also combined with an inhalational agent or opioid analgesic. Midazolam is the preferred benzodiazepine for continuous infusion due to the long context-sensitive half-lives of diazepam and lorazepam. However, infusions of benzodiazepines for anesthesia are associated with prolonged emergence and are typically used only in patients who are expected to remain intubated.

Etomidate
When etomidate was introduced, its hemodynamic stability appeared to make it an appropriate choice for prolonged sedation. However, it is now known to be unsafe for this indication. Etomidate potently inhibits *steroid synthesis* at the 11-β-hydroxylase enzyme, and its use results in a significant increase in mortality in sedated intensive care unit patients. Maintenance infusions of etomidate are contraindicated.

Ketamine
Ketamine infusions are sometimes used during general anesthesia as an adjunct medication. A subanalgesic infusion (3 to 5 µg/kg/min) during general anesthesia can be used in patients with opioid-resistant chronic pain in whom postoperative pain management is likely to be difficult. In the developed world, general anesthesia is not maintained by ketamine infusion. However, the technique is recognized by the International Committee of the Red Cross (ICRC) and is stipulated as the anesthetic of choice for major war surgery in conditions of limited resources. The ICRC protocol calls for dilution of 500 mg of ketamine in 1 L of normal saline to produce a concentration of 0.5 mg/mL. The infusion is titrated against the patient's response, both for induction and

maintenance of anesthesia. A usual maintenance dose of ketamine is around 4 mg/kg/hr, which corresponds to an infusion of approximately 500 mL/hr of this dilution in a 60- to 70-kg patient.

C. Use of Intravenous Anesthetics for Sedation

Barbiturates

Propofol and modern benzodiazepines have largely supplanted the use of barbiturates for sedation. Nevertheless, a small 25- to 50-mg dose of thiopental can be very efficacious if it is necessary to premedicate a patient who is agitated or hostile. There is usually no pain on administration, unlike propofol, and there is usually no sense of the onset of sedation or of *disinhibition*, unlike midazolam.

Propofol

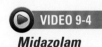

Propofol Infusion Dosing

Propofol infusions, or intermittent bolus doses of comparable quantities of medication, are commonly used for moderate procedural sedation. Maintenance infusion rates for satisfactory sedation usually range between 25 to 75 µg/kg/min, although higher initial infusion rates may be required to establish a suitable concentration at the effect site. Children require higher dosages due to a larger volume of distribution and an accelerated clearance rate. Propofol exhibits respiratory depression in a dose-dependent fashion. A decrease in tidal volumes and an increased respiratory rate are seen with infusion. Inhibition of the hypoxic ventilatory drive and hypercarbic response is observed even at sedating doses of propofol. However, bronchodilation is also observed in patients with asthma or chronic obstructive pulmonary disease.

Benzodiazepines

The multiple administration routes of benzodiazepines allow this class to be a key component in sedation. In addition to the intravenous route of administration, midazolam is routinely given orally to children, although this indication has never been U.S. Food and Drug Administration approved. Intramuscular, intranasal, transbuccal, and sublingual routes are also possible. Intramuscular diazepam should be avoided due to unreliable absorption and pain. When primarily used as premedications and adjuvants, benzodiazepines are dose-dependent anxiolytics, sedatives, anterograde amnestics, anticonvulsants, and muscle relaxants. Midazolam dosing for anesthesia premedication is 0.02 to 0.04 mg/kg intravenously or intramuscularly in adults, 0.4 to 0.8 mg/kg orally in children. Benzodiazepines display minimal cardiorespiratory depression except when large doses are administered or when synergistically administered with opioids. Used alone, they slightly decrease arterial blood pressure, cardiac output, and peripheral vascular resistance. Midazolam can cause *vagolysis*, resulting in changes in heart rate. Midazolam can be used for procedural sedation with minimal risk of respiratory depression, although in practice a carefully titrated propofol infusion will produce both superior amnesia and a faster recovery. However, the availability of flumazenil to acutely reverse sedation with benzodiazepines can provide a margin of safety that is unavailable when using propofol. Consequently, midazolam may be preferred for sedation in the setting of a jeopardized airway, such as for an awake tracheostomy, because it can be pharmacologically reversed.

Dexmedetomidine

Dexmedetomidine is an intravenous formulation that can also be administered orally, nasally, intramuscularly, or rectally. The oral dose is 2.6 to 4 µg/kg and takes about 30 to 60 minutes before sedation is appreciated. The intranasal dose of 1 to 2 μg/kg has a quicker onset of action. Dexmedetomidine sedation is most commonly administered intravenously as an infusion, ranging from 0.3 to 0.7 μg/kg/hr. This rate is titrated based on sedation level and hemodynamic stability. An initial loading dose of 1 μg/kg may be given, infused over 10 minutes. Some centers forgo the loading dose as it increases the risk of hemodynamic instability.

References

1. Shafer SL, Gregg KM. Algorithms to rapidly achieve and maintain stable drug concentrations at the site of drug effect with a computer-controlled infusion pump. *J Pharmacokinet Biopharm.* 1992;20:147–169.
2. Vuyk J, Engbers FH, Lemmens HJ, et al. Pharmacodynamics of propofol in female patients. *Anesthesiology.* 1992;77:3–9.
3. Felmlee MA, Morris ME, Mager DE. Mechanism-based pharmacodynamic modeling. *Methods Mol Biol.* 2012;929:583–600.
4. Servin F, Cockshott ID, Farinotti R, et al. Pharmacokinetics of propofol infusions in patients with cirrhosis. *Br J Anaesth.* 1990;65:177–183.
5. ACOP Bulletins—Obstetrics. ACOG Practice Bulletin: Clinical management guidelines for obstetrician-gynecologists number 92, April 2008 (replaces practice bulletin number 87, November 2007). Use of psychiatric medications during pregnancy and lactation. *Obstet Gynecol.* 2008;111:1001–1020.
6. Vanlersberghe C, Camu F. Etomidate and other non-barbiturates. *Handb Exp Pharmacol.* 2008;182:267–282.
7. Kharasch ED, Labroo R. Metabolism of ketamine stereoisomers by human liver microsomes. *Anesthesiology.* 1992;77:1201–1207.
8. Riker RR, Shehabi Y, Bokesch PM, et al. Dexmedetomidine vs midazolam for sedation of critically ill patients: A randomized trial. *JAMA.* 2009;301:489–499.
9. Reves JG, Fragen RJ, Vinik HR, et al. Midazolam: Pharmacology and uses. *Anesthesiology.* 1985;62:310–324.
10. Shapiro HM. Barbiturates in brain ischaemia. *Br J Anaesth.* 1985;57:82–95.

Questions

1. Which of the following is correct regarding barbiturates?
   A. They stimulate the reticular activating system in the brainstem.
   B. They potentiate the action of $GABA_A$ receptors.
   C. They increase cerebral metabolic rate of oxygen.
   D. They decrease the duration of chloride ion channel opening.

2. Which of the following drugs can have its effects reversed with a pharmacologic antagonist?
   A. Sodium thiopental
   B. Propofol
   C. Etomidate
   D. Diazepam

3. Which of the following is correct regarding etomidate?
   A. Unlike propofol, it does not cause pain upon injection.
   B. Etomidate is capable of producing convulsion-like EEG potentials in epileptic patients.
   C. Etomidate transiently inhibits methionine synthetase.
   D. It produces hypotension.

4. Which of the following drugs acts by antagonizing the NMDA receptor?
   A. Ketamine
   B. Dexmedetomidine
   C. Propofol
   D. Etomidate

5. Which of the following is correct regarding dexmedetomidine?
   A. It produces significant respiratory depression.
   B. It is metabolized in the kidney.
   C. It produces analgesia.
   D. Compared to benzodiazepines in the intensive care unit, dexmedetomidine is associated with a greater incidence of delirium.

10 Analgesics

Elizabeth M. Thackeray
Talmage D. Egan

I. Brief History and Overview

Analgesics are an essential resource for the provision of anesthesia and treatment of postoperative pain. Both opioid and nonopioid analgesics will be reviewed in this chapter. Opioid analgesics predate modern medicine while nonsteroidal anti-inflammatory drugs (NSAIDs), with their anti-inflammatory, antipyretic, and analgesic qualities, have become integral parts of perioperative medicine in the past 30 years.

The first NSAIDs to be isolated were salicylic acid derivatives. Traditional NSAIDs inhibit prostanoid synthesis through nonspecific inhibition of the cyclooxygenase (COX) enzymes. Prostanoids are produced in response to tissue injury and inflammation, both peripherally and centrally. This contributes to peripheral pain sensitization, general pain perception, and the sickness syndrome consisting of fever, anorexia, and changes in mood and sleep patterns (1). Prostanoids are also involved in homeostatic functions in the kidneys, gastric mucosa, platelets, and central nervous system (CNS). They are derived from arachidonic acid, which is released from cell membranes during tissue injury and inflammation, and consist of prostaglandins, including prostacyclin, and thromboxane A2. Multiple enzymes are involved in the transformation of arachidonic acid into prostaglandins and thromboxane A2, including isoforms of the COX enzymes (Fig. 10-1). The characterization of the COX-2 isoform as "inducible" (by neurotransmitters, growth factors, and proinflammatory cytokines) and the COX-1 isoform as "constitutive" is based on the predominant function of each isoform. But this is an oversimplification and both isoforms have some constitutive and some inducible functions. The COX-3 isoform remains poorly understood. Although aspirin irreversibly inhibits cyclooxygenase and thus platelet aggregation (see discussion below), the other NSAIDs reversibly inhibit cyclooxygenase so that enzymatic function is restored as the drug is cleared from the circulation, leading to a dose-dependent and drug-dependent effect on platelet aggregation.

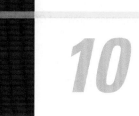

? Did You Know

Aspirin irreversibly inhibits platelet aggregation for the life of the platelet, while other non-COX-2 specific, nonsteroidal anti-inflammatories reversibly inhibit aggregation in a dose-dependent manner until the drug is cleared from the circulation.

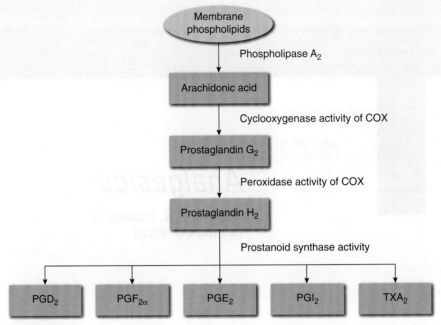

Figure 10-1 Schematic view of prostanoid synthesis. COX, cyclooxygenase enzymes; PG, prostaglandin; TX, thromboxane; PGD_2, prostaglandin D_2; $PGF_{2\alpha}$, prostaglandin $F_{2\alpha}$; PGE_2, prostaglandin E_2; PGI_2, prostaglandin I_2; TXA_2, thromboxane A_2.

II. Nonopioid Analgesics

A. Acetaminophen

Indications, Contraindications, and Dose

Acetaminophen (also known as paracetamol, APAP, para-acetylaminophenol, N-acetyl-para-aminophenol) is widely used as an analgesic and antipyretic for both children and adults. Although it has been reported to suppress inflammation in animals and in dental tissue, the anti-inflammatory effect is considered low to nonexistent (2). *Centrilobular hepatotoxicity* occurs with acute overdose and may occur at smaller doses in chronic alcoholics, although the relation between acetaminophen use and alcohol ingestion is not straightforward. Use of acetaminophen in patients with chronic liver disease who do not regularly consume alcohol is not contraindicated, although the maximum safe dose has not been determined (3). It is available in oral, rectal, and intravenous preparations. The dose is 10 to 15 mg/kg every 4 to 6 hours in children (every 6 to 8 hours in neonates) and 325 to 650 mg every 4 to 6 hours in adults. The maximum dose in children is 75 mg/kg/day and, historically, no more than 4 g/day in adults. However, due to the availability of combination products (over-the-counter cough and cold preparations and hydrocodone- and oxycodone-acetaminophen combinations) and cases of liver failure in patients taking <4 g/day, the U.S. Food and Drug Administration (FDA) requested in 2011 that manufacturers limit combination products to 325 mg. Soon after, the manufacturer changed the maximum daily dose to 3 g/day, and in 2014 the FDA asked prescribers and pharmacies to discontinue prescribing or dispensing products with more than 325 mg of acetaminophen.

Mechanism of Action

The mechanism of action of acetaminophen is unknown, although there is strong evidence for a central site of action. Multiple sites of action have been

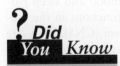

? Did You Know

In 2011 the U.S. Food and Drug Administration requested that manufacturers of acetaminophen-containing products limit those products to a maximum of 325 mg of acetaminophen per dose to decrease the chance of hepatic toxicity.

postulated, including COX-1, -2, and -3 inhibition, and modulation of the opioidergic, serotonergic, and endocannabinoid systems (2).

Pharmacokinetics and Pharmacodynamics
Acetaminophen is highly bioavailable after oral administration, and it crosses the blood–brain barrier. Time to peak effect is approximately 20 minutes (2).

Metabolism and Excretion
The major metabolic pathway of acetaminophen is *glucuronidation* and *sulfation* in the liver. The nontoxic conjugates that are formed are largely excreted in the urine and bile. Between 5% and 9% of acetaminophen is oxidized by the cytochrome P450 (CYP) system, resulting in N-acetyl-p-benzoquinone-imine (NAPQI), the toxic metabolite that can cause hepatocellular injury if the hepatic detoxification process is overwhelmed by a large dose of acet-aminophen. NAPQI is highly reactive and is rapidly metabolized by conjuga-tion with glutathione transferase to a nontoxic compound that is eventually excreted as mercapturic acid and cysteine conjugates. Approximately 2% of ingested acetaminophen is excreted unchanged by the kidneys (3).

Drug Interactions and Adverse Effects
Acetaminophen is a dose-related hepatotoxin due to the small amount of NAPQI produced. Depleted glutathione stores due to overdose, malnutrition, or alcohol ingestion may increase the risk of hepatotoxicity. Drugs that induce the CYPs, such as anticonvulsants (phenytoin, carbamazepine, phenobarbital), and isoniazid may increase the risk of acetaminophen toxicity, although the evidence for clinically significant drug–acetaminophen interactions is incom-plete. Acetaminophen poisoning was the leading cause of acute liver failure between 1995 and 2003 in the United States, with 48% of acetaminophen-related cases due to *unintentional overdose* (3). Fifty-one percent of patients had used a *single* over-the-counter acetaminophen product.

B. Acetylsalicylic Acid
Indications, Contraindications, and Dose
Acetylsalicylic acid (also called aspirin or ASA) can be used for relief from mild to moderate pain. It has both anti-inflammatory and antipyretic effects. Today it is prescribed most commonly for its antiplatelet effects and has indications including acute myocardial infarction, unstable angina, transient ischemic attacks, preven-tion of arterial and venous thrombosis, and platelet disorders. Aspirin *irreversibly* inhibits platelets aggregation by inhibiting platelet thromboxane A2 synthesis and by preventing adenosine diphosphate release from platelets. Its antiplatelet effect lasts for the life of the platelet (8 to 10 days) (4). Contraindications to aspirin use include the presence of gastric and duodenal ulcers, as aspirin may cause upper gas-trointestinal (GI) bleeding from erosive gastritis. Enteric coating, taking aspirin and other NSAIDs with meals, histamine 2 antagonists, and proton pump inhibitors are helpful in minimizing mucosal damage. Aspirin is contraindicated in children due to the association with *Reye syndrome*, a life-threatening acute liver failure seen after certain viral infections. The antithrombotic effects of aspirin do not seem to be dose dependent, while the GI side effects and risk of bleeding increase with increasing doses. Therefore, a daily dose of 81 to 325 mg is prescribed for most indications (4).

Mechanism of Action
Aspirin is a nonselective, irreversible COX inhibitor. It also affects the kal-likrein system, decreasing granulocyte attachment to injured vessels, among other effects (4).

Pharmacokinetics and Pharmacodynamics
Aspirin can be administered orally or per rectum, with a 40% to 50% bio-availability. Aspirin has a short (15 minutes) plasma half-life, while the plasma half-life of its primary metabolite, salicylic acid, is much longer and dose dependent, between 2 and 12 hours. Of note is the difference between aspirin's short pharmacokinetic half-life and its *prolonged pharmacodynamic effects* due to the irreversible platelet inhibition.

Metabolism and Excretion
Aspirin undergoes extensive first-pass metabolism and is metabolized to salicylic acid, which has less pharmacologic activity in the liver, plasma, and red blood cells. Aspirin is highly bound to albumin. Only a small amount of aspirin is excreted unchanged in the urine; the rest is excreted as salicylic acid or glycine.

Drug Interactions and Adverse Effects
Aspirin can *erode gastric mucosa,* cause *acute tubular necrosis* secondary to decreased renal blood flow, and *precipitate bronchospasm* in patients with asthma or aspirin sensitivity. Because aspirin blocks the cyclooxygenase enzymes, substrate is shifted into the alternative pathway, thus increasing the generation of leukotrienes. Aspirin overdose may present with acid-base abnormalities, renal failure, dehydration, abnormal blood glucose, seizures, or coma. These patients require management in the intensive care unit with alkaline diuresis to promote salicylate excretion and may require hemodialysis. Activated charcoal may prevent absorption of aspirin after overdose.

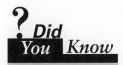

C. Other Nonsteroidal Anti-inflammatories: Ibuprofen, Ketorolac, and Celecoxib
Nonselective NSAIDs (nsNSAIDs) carry a side-effect profile that includes dose-related inhibition of platelet aggregation, GI bleeding, renal dysfunction, altered bone healing, hypertension, and bronchospasm. The COX-2 inhibitors were developed in an attempt to eliminate some of these adverse effects, particularly the GI side effects and interference with platelet aggregation. In 2004, the manufacturer voluntarily withdrew rofecoxib from the market after an interim analysis of a long-term study in patients with colon polyps demonstrated an increased risk for cardiovascular events, including myocardial infarction and stroke. For similar reasons, the FDA asked the manufacturer to voluntarily withdraw valdecoxib from the market in 2005. Celecoxib, with its intermediate levels of COX-2 selectivity compared with rofecoxib and valdecoxib, remains the only COX-2 inhibitor available in the United States. The FDA groups all NSAIDs, whether COX-2 selective NSAIDs or nsNSAIDs, *together* with regard to skin, cardiovascular, renal, and GI side effects.

Indications, Contraindications, and Dose
Ibuprofen, ketorolac, and celecoxib are indicated for pain, inflammation, and fever. When used in the perioperative period, nsNSAIDs demonstrate an *opioid-sparing effect.* Thus, they decrease the common opioid side effects such as postoperative nausea and vomiting, constipation or ileus, and cardiorespiratory depression (5). Because celecoxib has no effect on platelet function, it is especially useful in the perioperative period. Ketorolac is generally considered to be contraindicated in tonsillectomy, adenoidectomy, total joint replacements, and major plastic surgery because of the increased risk of bleeding on the "raw" surface areas. Note, however, that in the studies demonstrating increased blood loss, ketorolac had been administered pre-emptively, either before surgical incision or before achieving primary hemostasis. No controlled studies in the peer-reviewed

? Did You Know

The rate of upper gastrointestinal complications is highest with ketorolac compared with other nonsteroidal anti-inflammatories and therefore it should not be used for more than 5 consecutive days.

literature demonstrate an increase in blood loss when ketorolac was administered near the end of surgery or postoperatively (5). A 2013 meta-analysis published by the Cochrane Collaboration found both an increased and decreased risk of bleeding after pediatric tonsillectomy. It concluded that although there is insufficient evidence to exclude an increased risk of bleeding when NSAIDs are administered during pediatric tonsillectomy, the use of NSAIDs did confer the benefit of a decrease in postoperative vomiting (6). Concerns about bone healing from animal models and human experiments have long limited the use of NSAIDs in orthopedic surgery. However, a meta-analysis revealed no increased risk of nonunion associated with NSAIDs and spinal fusion surgery when only high-quality studies were included (5). Other studies show poor fracture healing when nsNSAIDs as well as COX-2 inhibitors are used. Some experts advocate avoiding NSAID use in patients or procedures with a high risk of nonunion.

The risk of GI complications is present for all NSAIDs, including COX-2 inhibitors. A recent meta-analysis concluded that the relative risk for upper GI complications of celecoxib and ibuprofen are among the lowest of the NSAIDs studied, while ketorolac had one of the *highest* relative risks for upper GI complications (7). Proton pump inhibitors offer effective protection against peptic ulcers when administered with nsNSAIDs, but COX-2 selective NSAIDs may be more protective of the small intestine.

Ibuprofen and ketorolac are contraindicated in patients with *renal insufficiency,* as even short courses (<5 days) can produce transient reductions in renal function. This transient reduction is clinically unimportant in patients with normal preoperative renal function, and there are no reports of renal failure when ketorolac was administered for ≤5 days (5). Celecoxib appears to have the same rate of renal dysfunction as the nsNSAIDs. Celecoxib is contraindicated after coronary artery bypass surgery because it is associated with a greater overall risk of adverse events compared with placebo. Celecoxib is also contraindicated in patients with active gastrointestinal bleeding, history of allergy to sulfonamides (due to the presence of a sulfa moiety), and history of asthma or allergic-type reactions to NSAIDs. However, celecoxib has *no effect* on platelet function or bleeding time.

Ibuprofen is available over the counter with a recommended oral dose of 200 to 400 mg every 6 hours. Inflammatory conditions may require 400 to 800 mg orally every 6 to 8 hours. Children should receive 5 to 10 mg/kg every 6 to 8 hours. In 2009, an intravenous preparation was approved by the FDA. Ketorolac is dosed at 15 to 30 mg intramuscularly or intravenously every 6 hours for no more than 5 days. A single dose of 60 mg may be used. The pediatric dose is 0.5 mg/kg. Celecoxib is available in 50 mg, 100 mg, 200 mg, and 400 mg capsules. Acute pain in adults is dosed at 400 mg orally, then 200 mg orally twice a day. It is approved for use in children older than 2 years old. For children weighing 10 to 25 kg, the dose is 50 mg twice a day; patients weighing >25 kg may receive 100 mg twice a day.

Mechanism of Action
Ibuprofen and ketorolac are nsNSAIDs that inhibit the cyclooxygenase enzymes (see above). Celecoxib is a COX-2 inhibitor, predominantly inhibiting the COX-2 isoform of the cyclooxygenase enzyme.

Pharmacokinetics and Pharmacodynamics
Ibuprofen has close to 100% oral bioavailability and a time to peak effect of 1 to 2 hours. Seventy percent to 90% of the dose is excreted within 24 hours. It is *highly protein bound,* as are the other conventional NSAIDs. Protein binding may be an important determinant in its distribution into the synovial fluid, thus,

its efficacy in rheumatoid arthritis. Ibuprofen distributes into the cerebrospinal fluid and has a longer half-life in the cerebrospinal fluid than in the plasma.

Ketorolac has a rapid onset when administered intravenously, with a time to peak plasma concentrations of 5 minutes. The half-life of ketorolac is approximately 5 hours, and more than 90% is excreted within 2 days (8). Celecoxib reaches peak plasma concentrations in 2 to 4 hours after oral administration and is extensively protein bound.

Metabolism and Excretion

Elimination and metabolism of NSAIDs occur largely through **hepatic biotransformation** and **renal excretion**. Patients with hepatic and renal disease may have higher and more prolonged plasma concentrations. Ibuprofen is oxidized by the CYP enzymes, as well as conjugated with glucuronic acid in the liver. The drug and its metabolites are rapidly excreted in both urine and feces. Excretion in breast milk is minimal, and the American Academy of Pediatrics considers ibuprofen to be compatible with breastfeeding. Ketorolac is metabolized by glucuronidation, and more than 90% is excreted in the urine within 2 days. Celecoxib undergoes biotransformation to carbolic acid and glucuronide metabolites, which are excreted in urine and feces. It is metabolized by the CYP enzymes and has an elimination half-life of about 11 hours.

Drug Interactions and Adverse Effects

The nsNSAIDs carry a side-effect profile that includes dose-related inhibition of platelet aggregation, GI bleeding, renal dysfunction, bone healing, hypertension, and bronchospasm. Short-term (<5 days) use of ketorolac does not increase the risk of perioperative complications, except the risk of bleeding in high-risk surgeries with raw surface areas (tonsillectomy or adenoidectomy, major plastic surgery, total joint replacement). Ketorolac demonstrates a high rate of GI ulceration, which limits its use to <5 days.

The cardiovascular risk of COX-2 inhibitors has been a subject of much concern since two studies investigating colon polyp prevention with COX-2 inhibitors were stopped early because of significantly increased risk for the composite of **cardiovascular death, myocardial infarction, stroke,** or **heart failure**. Two COX-2 inhibitors (rofecoxib and valdecoxib) were taken off the market in response.

The cardiovascular outcomes are probably due to the elevations in blood pressure that occur with all NSAIDs rather than to any particular risk associated with COX-2 inhibitors. Cardiovascular outcomes of nsNSAIDs had not yet been studied prospectively with sufficient power to document an increased risk of NSAIDs compared with placebo. It should be noted that after the withdrawal of rofecoxib and valdecoxib, studies have shown that older adults prescribed opioids are more likely to die than patients receiving NSAIDs; even cardiovascular complications are higher in patients taking opioids when compared with NSAIDs (9).

GI prophylaxis is often recommended to patients who are prescribed NSAIDs, and concurrent treatment with protective medications (ranitidine, cimetidine, misoprostol, aluminum and magnesium hydroxide suspension) had no significant effects on ibuprofen pharmacokinetics.

D. N-Methyl-D-Aspartate Receptor Blocker: Ketamine
Indications, Contraindications, and Dose

Ketamine can be used as a general anesthetic, but at subanesthetic doses, it is effective in treating neuropathic, ischemic, and acute pain, as well as regional pain syndromes. Because of its minimal effect on the respiratory system and unique mechanism of action, it is appealing for use in a variety of patients. *N-methyl-D-aspartate (NMDA)* overactivity is one mechanism for decreased opioid responsiveness. Therefore, ketamine may be especially useful in patients taking opioids chronically. After intraoperative ketamine administration, patients report lower postoperative pain intensity for up to 48 hours and have lower morphine requirements for 24 hours. In anesthetic doses (>1 mg/kg), ketamine causes tachycardia, hypertension, and increased systemic and pulmonary vascular resistance (SVR and PVR, respectively). Its use may be contraindicated in patients in whom tachycardia and hypertension may lead to morbidity, such as those with ischemic heart disease, heart failure, and stroke. Because ketamine has a negative inotropic effect, the combination of negative inotropy and increased SVR and PVR can lead to hemodynamic decompensation in patients with severe heart failure. At subanesthetic doses, ketamine does not generally increase blood pressure. Ketamine has long been considered contraindicated in patients with elevated intracranial pressure (ICP). However, recent meta-analyses concluded that ketamine does not increase ICP in sedated and ventilated patients, and in fact, may decrease ICP in some cases (10). Induction doses of ketamine are 1 to 4 mg/kg intravenously or 2 to 4 mg/kg intramuscularly. Intraoperative bolus dosing is 0.1 to 0.5 mg/kg, and infusions are generally administered between 0.1 to 0.2 mg/kg/hr. In addition to intravenous and intramuscular administration, ketamine has been given by the subcutaneous, oral, rectal, and intranasal routes.

Mechanism of Action
Ketamine is an NMDA receptor antagonist. The NMDA receptor is found throughout the CNS and in the same locations as opioid receptors. The NMDA receptor is a transmembrane protein that affects neuronal hyperexcitability, which is seen clinically as hyperalgesia, allodynia, spontaneous generation of painful impulses, and radiation of pain.

Pharmacokinetics and Pharmacodynamics
The onset of action after intravenous administration is rapid (within seconds) and the half-life is 2 to 3 hours. Intramuscular administration is 93% bioavailable. Bioavailability is much lower for intranasal and oral administration, although intranasal administration is associated with a rapid onset of action.

Metabolism and Excretion
Ketamine undergoes extensive hepatic metabolism by the cytochrome 3A4 to the active metabolite norketamine. Substantial first-pass metabolism results in greater norketamine production after oral administration. Small amounts of unmetabolized drug are excreted in the urine.

Drug Interactions and Adverse Effects
No significant drug interactions are reported with ketamine. Adverse events after ketamine administration are dose related and more likely at anesthetic doses (>1 mg/kg) than at analgesic doses. The most common adverse events associated with ketamine are *psychomimetic,* including hallucinations, emergence phenomena, vivid dreams, and blunted affect. Ketamine is twice as likely as placebo to cause hallucinations, although this effect may be attenuated by premedication with a benzodiazepine. Patients are also twice as likely to report pleasant dreams after ketamine administration when compared with placebo. Ketamine can have significant cardiovascular effects, including tachycardia, hypertension, and increased systemic and pulmonary vascular

resistance. Because ketamine also has a negative inotropic effect, the combination of negative inotropy and increased SVR and PVR can lead to hemodynamic decompensation in patients with severe heart failure. Ketamine is a sialogogue and may cause other GI effects such as nausea, vomiting, and anorexia. Ulcerative cystitis is seen with ketamine abuse.

E. Alpha$_2$ Adrenergic Agonists: Clonidine and Dexmedetomidine

Indications and Dose

The α_2 adrenergic receptor agonists clonidine and dexmedetomidine are indicated for sedation and analgesia (11). Because of the reduction in sympathetic activity and agitation, dexmedetomidine causes a state reminiscent of non–rapid eye movement physiologic sleep without impaired cognitive function. These agents also do not inhibit *respiratory drive* any more than natural sleep. This combination makes them appealing for use in the intensive care setting to facilitate early extubation. There is also evidence of postoperative morphine-sparing effect and decreased emergence delirium in children.

Clonidine is available as a tablet, as an injectable solution, and as a transdermal patch. When used in the perioperative period for anxiolysis, sedation, and analgesia, typical oral doses are between 0.2 and 0.3 mg. Intravenous dosing is between 1 and 5 µg/kg over 30 to 60 minutes, sometimes followed by an infusion of 0.3 µg/kg/hr (11). Dexmedetomidine is administered as an intravenous infusion at a rate of 0.2 to 1 µg/kg/hr. A bolus dose is generally administered over several minutes to promote the achievement of steady state. However, significant hemodynamic derangements can occur with the oft-recommended bolus dose of 1 µg/kg over 10 minutes, so caution is warranted.

Mechanism of Action

Dexmedetomidine and clonidine are agonists of the α_2 receptors, which are found throughout the brain and are important in the regulation of dopamine and norepinephrine as well as involved in multiple physiologic processes. The posterior horn of the spinal cord is the most significant site of analgesic activity, although pain transmission in the sensory nerves may also be affected. Dexmedetomidine is more specific to the α_2A receptors than clonidine; α_2A receptors mediate sedation, analgesia, and hypotension in the locus ceruleus.

Pharmacokinetics and Pharmacodynamics

Clonidine has close to 100% oral bioavailability, with peak plasma concentrations occurring at 1 to 3 hours; half of the initial dose is recovered unchanged in the urine. Clonidine is considered a long-acting drug, while dexmedetomidine is somewhat shorter acting. Clonidine and dexmedetomidine undergo hepatic and renal metabolism and elimination.

Drug Interactions and Adverse Effects

Bradycardia, hypotension, and hypertension may occur with both dexmedetomidine and clonidine. Despite causing sedation, the α_2 agonists do not seem to prolong postoperative recovery time (11).

III. Opioids

A. Endogenous Opioids

Endogenous opioids and opioid receptors are located throughout the peripheral and central nervous systems. Endogenous opioids include the enkephalins, dynorphins, and β-endorphins, which are produced from large protein precursors by proteolytic cleavage. The opioid system has a central role in nociception and analgesia and also affects multiple physiologic processes, including the stress response, endocrine and immune functions, GI transit, ventilation, and mood and well-being. β-endorphins and enkephalins have the greatest affinity for μ and δ receptors, while dynorphins preferentially bind to the κ receptors.

B. Opioid Receptors

The opioid receptors are G-protein coupled receptors, with seven transmembrane portions, intracellular and extracellular loops, and significant homology among the opioid receptor subtypes. Binding of opioid agonists leads to G-protein activation and primarily inhibitory effects that decrease neuronal excitability (decreased cyclic adenosine monophosphate production and calcium ion influx, increased potassium ion efflux), although it should be noted that opioid binding *increases* production of prostaglandins and leukotrienes. Four opioid receptors, μ, κ, δ, and nociception or orphanin opioid receptor, have been identified (MOP, KOP, DOP, and NOP, respectively). Each is antagonized by naloxone and provides spinal and supraspinal analgesia. The μ and δ agonists are involved in positive reinforcement, whereas κ agonists produce aversion, hallucinations, and malaise. The μ and δ antagonists thus overcome the euphoric effects of opiate drugs, while κ antagonists produce positive effects. Opioid receptors are found throughout the CNS, including the substantia gelatinosa of the spinal cord, the periaqueductal gray region, the limbic system, the area postrema, thalamus, and cerebral cortex. Opioid receptors are also found outside the CNS in peripheral neurons, neuroendocrine tissue, immune cells, GI, biliary, and other tissues (Fig. 10-2).

C. Mechanism of Opioid Analgesia

In the spinal cord, opioids inhibit the release of *substance P* from primary sensory neurons in the dorsal horn, attenuating the transmission of painful stimuli from peripheral nerves to the cerebral cortex. In the brainstem, opioids act at descending inhibitory pathways to attenuate painful stimuli. There is also activity of opioid agonists in the forebrain and the reward structures of the brain.

D. Opioid-induced Hyperalgesia, Tolerance, and Dependence

Opioid *tolerance* is a well-described phenomenon in which chronic opioid use leads to a requirement for increasing doses of opioids to reach a similar analgesic effect. Chronic opioid exposure leads to an increase in substance P activity and an NMDA-mediated increase in the synthesis and release of prostaglandins, collectively contributing to opioid tolerance. Acute opioid tolerance, or increasing opioid requirements after only brief exposure to opioids, has also been suggested, but its existence is controversial. Analgesic tolerance increases more than tolerance to the respiratory depressant effects, thus narrowing the therapeutic window of these agents (12). Opioid-induced *hyperalgesia* is less well understood, and, in contrast to opioid tolerance, refers to an increased response to normally painful stimuli. Three mechanisms have been proposed: NMDA receptor activation as part of activation of the central glutaminergic system, increased release of excitatory spinal neuropeptides, and descending spinal facilitation. Although both opioid tolerance and opioid-induced hyperalgesia may manifest as increasing opioid requirements to reach the desired analgesic effect, distinguishing between the two is important because opioids worsen the problem of opioid-induced hyperalgesia. In both cases, use of multimodal analgesia and NMDA antagonists may be helpful in achieving analgesic goals. Opioid dependence is characterized by an unpleasant and complex

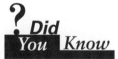
? Did You Know

With continued use, the tolerance to the analgesic effects of opioids increases more than tolerance to the respiratory depressant effects, thus narrowing the therapeutic window.

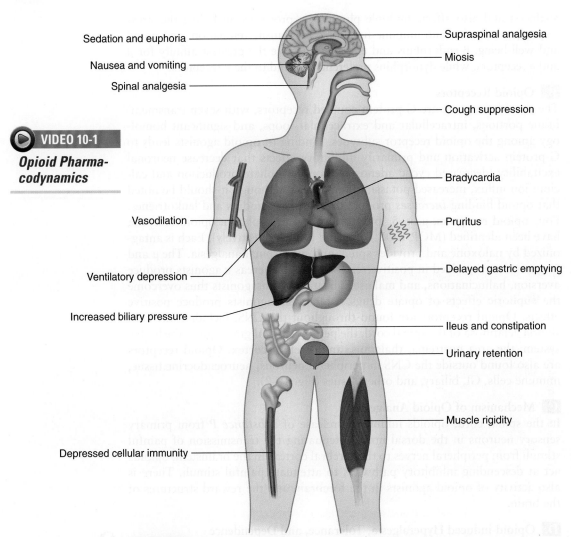

VIDEO 10-1

Opioid Pharma-codynamics

Sedation and euphoria

Nausea and vomiting

Spinal analgesia

Vasodilation

Ventilatory depression

Increased biliary pressure

Depressed cellular immunity

Supraspinal analgesia

Miosis

Cough suppression

Bradycardia

Pruritus

Delayed gastric emptying

Ileus and constipation

Urinary retention

Muscle rigidity

Figure 10-2 Opioid pharmacodynamics. A summary chart of the selected effects of the fentanyl congeners.

withdrawal syndrome that includes physical signs and a disagreeable emotional state.

E. Routes of Administration

Opioids are available in oral and intravenous preparations. Several are available only as intravenous agents and may be administered as a bolus dose or as an infusion. Fentanyl is also available in transdermal and transmucosal forms and has been given by the intranasal and transpulmonary routes. Fentanyl, morphine, and sufentanil (in preservative-free formulations) are routinely used in the intrathecal space, and fentanyl is commonly used in the epidural space.

F. Pharmacokinetics and Pharmacodynamics

Rational opioid selection requires consideration of concepts such as *time to peak effect after bolus injection, time to steady state after beginning an infusion, and the context-sensitive half-time,* or time to 50% decrease in effect-site concentrations after an infusion is stopped. These concepts are probably best understood when presented as computer simulations of drug effect. Figure 10-3A

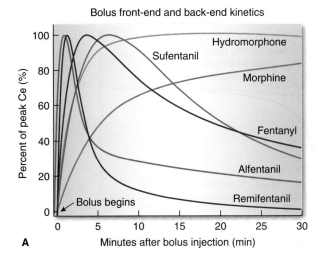

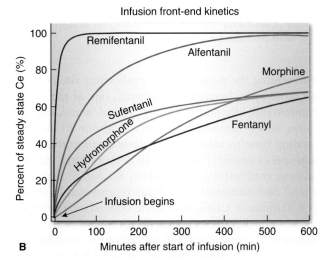

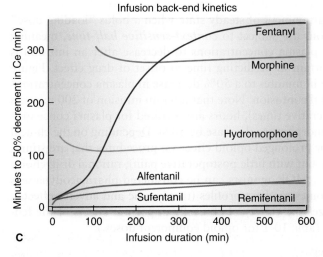

Figure 10-3 Opioid pharmacokinetics. Simulations illustrating front-end and back-end pharmacokinetic behavior after administration by bolus injection or continuous infusions for morphine, hydromorphone, fentanyl, alfentanil, sufentanil, and remifentanil using pharmacokinetic parameters from the literature. **A:** Percent of peak effect-site concentrations after bolus dosing. **B:** Percent of steady-state effect-site concentrations after beginning an infusion. **C:** Context-sensitive half-time, or time in minutes to a 50% decrease in effect-site concentrations after an infusion is stopped. (From Hemmings HC, Egan TD. *Pharmacology and Physiology for Anesthesia: Foundations and Clinical Application.* Philadelphia: Elsevier; 2013, with permission.)

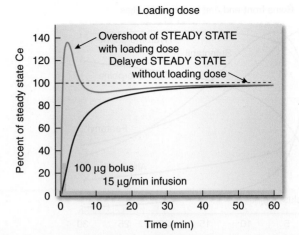

Figure 10-4 Simulation demonstrating plasma concentrations after administration of a bolus dose of remifentanil followed by an infusion, showing the rapid attainment of steady state when a bolus is used. (From Hemmings HC, Egan TD. *Pharmacology and Physiology for Anesthesia: Foundations and Clinical Application.* Philadelphia: Elsevier; 2013, with permission.)

presents a simulation representing the percentage of peak effect site concentrations over time. When rapid opioid analgesia is desired, one of the rapid-onset opioids, such as remifentanil, alfentanil, fentanyl, or sufentanil, may be more useful than morphine, which reaches peak effect at about 90 minutes after injection. Understanding time to *steady-state plasma concentration* is critical when using an infusion of opioid. Figure 10-3B demonstrates the percentage of steady-state plasma concentrations over time. Recognize that with two exceptions (remifentanil and alfentanil), the drugs represented have not reached steady state after 600 minutes. Clinicians should understand the implications of this simulation; namely, that plasma concentrations will continue to rise for hours after an infusion is begun (with the exception of remifentanil) even though the infusion rate may not have changed. Figure 10-4 represents the administration of a bolus dose of remifentanil followed by an infusion and shows the rapid attainment of steady state when a bolus "loading dose" is used. Lastly, infusions are subject to *context-sensitive half-time,* meaning the time required for plasma concentrations to decrease after an infusion is stopped. This is important in predicting time to offset of drug effect. Figure 10-3C shows the time in minutes to a 50% decrease in plasma concentrations versus the duration of the infusion. Note that after an infusion of 200 minutes (well within many operative times), hours are required for plasma concentrations of fentanyl and morphine to decrease by 50%. Depending on the clinical requirements (need for prolonged opioid effect vs. procedures that are stimulating intraoperatively but with little postoperative pain), rational drug choice can be informed. Most MOP agonists can be considered pharmacodynamics equivalents when it comes to effect profiles (therapeutic and adverse effects). Figure 10-2 summarizes the variety of clinically important effects of the fentanyl congeners. (See Table 10-1 for opioid equipotent doses.)

G. Therapeutic Effects

The primary effect of opioids is analgesia. Opioids act on peripheral nerves and in the spinal cord to attenuate noxious stimuli and act centrally by altering the affective response. The µ agonists are more effective at treating sensations

Table 10-1 Opioid Equipotent Doses	
Opioid	**Dose**
Morphine	1 mg
Meperidine	10 mg
Methadone	1 mg
Hydromorphone	0.2 mg
Fentanyl	50 μg
Alfentanil	150 μg
Sufentanil	5 μg
Remifentanil	50 μg

carried by the slow, *unmyelinated C fibers* and less effective at treating neuropathic pain and stimuli transmitted by fast, myelinated A-δ fibers. Opioids produce sedation and δ-wave activity on the electroencephalogram that resemble natural sleep. Although increasing doses of opioid reliably produce sedation, they do not reliably produce unresponsiveness and amnesia. Opioids suppress the cough reflex in the medulla. Conversely, a bolus dose of an opioid can produce an increase in coughing; this is often noted during induction of anesthesia that includes an opioid.

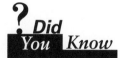

H. Adverse Effects

The μ agonists suppress ventilatory drive in the medulla and alter the ventilatory response to carbon dioxide and hypoxia. Normally, minute ventilation increases as arterial carbon dioxide partial pressure ($PaCO_2$) increases, with a sharp increase in minute ventilation as $PaCO_2$ increases above 40 mm Hg. Under the influence of opioids, minute ventilation still increases with increasing $PaCO_2$ but at a lower rate, so that the ventilatory response to carbon dioxide is decreased. A gradual increase in opioid levels, for example, after morphine administration, will cause progressive respiratory depression and hypercapnia, thus helping to maintain ventilation. In contrast, a rapid rise in opioid levels, as with an intravenous bolus of remifentanil or alfentanil, may cause apnea until the $PaCO_2$ levels rise above the *apneic threshold*. The apneic threshold is the $PaCO_2$ level below which a patient will not breathe while under the influence of opioid agonists. Both respiratory rate and tidal volume are decreased, with respiratory rate decreases occurring at lower doses of opioids and tidal volume decreases occurring at higher doses. Factors that increase the risk of opioid-induced ventilatory depression include high dose, natural sleep, old age, other CNS depressants, and decreased clearance due to hepatic or renal insufficiency.

The fentanyl congeners directly increase *vagal tone* in the brainstem, sometimes causing bradycardia. This can be treated with an antimuscarinic agent if necessary. Opioids cause arterial and venous dilation without affecting myocardial contractility by decreasing vasomotor activity in the brainstem and by direct action on vessels. In most patients, this is clinically insignificant, but it may cause hypotension in patients with chronic hypertension or congestive heart failure. Rapidly administered high bolus doses of the fentanyl congeners

? Did You Know

The factors that increase the risk of opioid ventilatory depression include high dose, natural sleep, old age, other CNS depressants and decrease clearance due to hepatic or renal insufficiency.

can result in muscle rigidity, which can be severe enough to prevent effective bag-mask ventilation. The rigidity tends to coincide with unresponsiveness and can be prevented with neuromuscular blockers. The mechanism of rigidity is unknown. This phenomenon leads some practitioners to preoxygenate patients receiving a remifentanil bolus as part of monitored anesthesia care (MAC).

I. Metabolism and Active Metabolites
Opioids are generally lipid-soluble, highly protein-bound, weak bases that are ionized at physiologic pH. Although there are unique characteristics of individual opioids, opioids are typically metabolized by the hepatic CYP system. Hepatic conjugation followed by excretion by the kidneys can also be significant. Remifentanil is the major exception to this rule (see subsequent discussion).

J. Drug Interactions
Sedative-hypnotic agents and opioids are *synergistic,* with greater analgesia and sedation resulting from combinations than from either alone. Figure 10-5 illustrates this concept in which a small dose of fentanyl and midazolam results in a higher probability of sedation and analgesia in combination than either would alone, while the probability of ventilatory depression is minimal. A similar effect is seen when propofol and opioids are combined (Fig. 10-6). Opioids decrease the MAC of volatile anesthetics significantly (>75%) at moderate doses of opioid.

K. Pharmacogenetics and Special Populations
Although codeine has a limited role in the intraoperative period, its unique pharmacogenomics are clinically significant. Codeine is a *pro-drug,* with 5% to 10% metabolized to morphine by an isoform of the cytochrome P450 system, CYP2D6. In the approximately 10% of the white population who lack this enzyme, or in patients whose CYP2D6 enzyme is inhibited by another drug like fluoxetine, paroxetine, bupropion, or quinidine, there will be a limited response to codeine, although the response to morphine is maintained (13). The opioids tramadol, hydrocodone, and oxycodone are also metabolized, at least in part, by CYP2D6. There seems to be a decreased analgesic response to tramadol in codeine "poor metabolizers," but the data are less clear with regard to hydrocodone and oxycodone. Another subset (~1% to 2%) of the population is known as codeine *"ultra-rapid metabolizers"* and carry duplicated, functional CYP2D6 genes. These patients convert a greater percentage of codeine to morphine. The increased clinical effect of codeine has been implicated in pediatric deaths following tonsillectomy with or without adenoidectomy, and in 2013 the FDA issued a black box warning against the use of codeine in children undergoing tonsillectomy.

With the exception of the anhepatic phase of orthotopic liver transplantation, the degree of liver failure encountered in most surgical patients is not usually significant enough to dramatically alter opioid metabolism. However, patients with hepatic encephalopathy may be particularly sensitive to the sedative effects of opioids. Remifentanil's unique metabolism makes its disposition unaffected even during the anhepatic phase. Renal failure causes clinically significant accumulation of metabolites of morphine and meperidine. Disposition of the fentanyl congeners is less affected by renal failure, and as with hepatic failure, remifentanil's pharmacology is unaltered by renal failure.

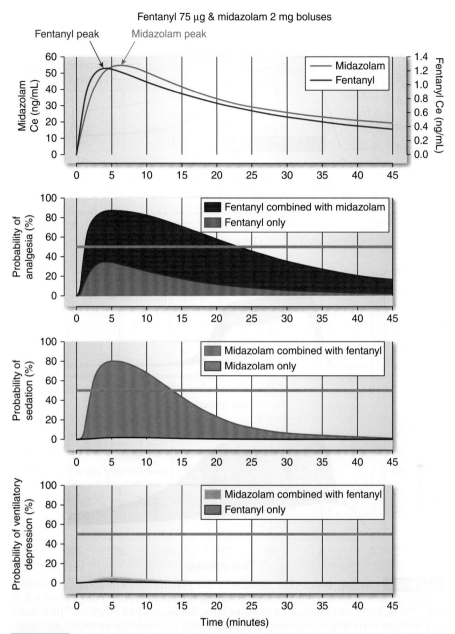

Figure 10-5 Simulation of 75 µg fentanyl and 2 mg midazolam administered by intravenous bolus at the same time. The top simulation illustrates the time to peak plasma concentration of each drug. The middle simulations demonstrate the synergistic effect of combining fentanyl and midazolam for the clinical effects of analgesia and sedation. The bottom simulation illustrates the low probability of ventilatory depression with this combination, in contrast to the high probability of analgesia and sedation. (From Safe Sedation Training. https://www.safesedationtraining.com/, accessed October 6, 2014, with permission.)

Morphine undergoes conjugation in the liver and kidney to morphine-3-glucuronide and morphine-6-glucuronide, both of which accumulate in renal failure. Morphine-6-glucuronide is an active metabolite with similar potency to morphine, and severe respiratory depression can result from its accumulation. Normeperidine is the active metabolite of meperidine, which

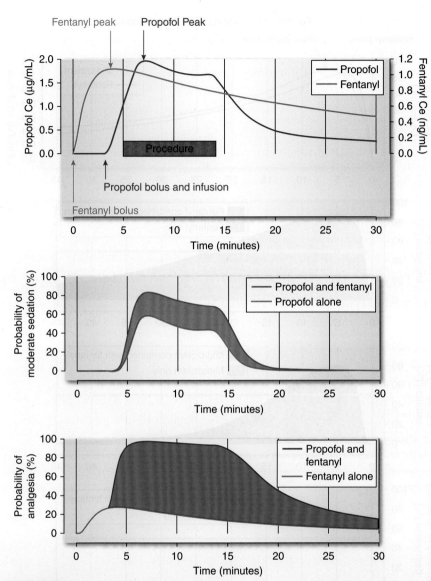

Figure 10-6 The top simulation represents the plasma concentrations of fentanyl and propofol. The fentanyl is administered as a bolus intravenous dose at time 0. A propofol bolus is administered 4 minutes later, followed by an infusion. The middle and bottom simulations represent the probability of moderate sedation and analgesia, respectively, and illustrate the principle of synergism between opioids and propofol. (From Safe Sedation Training. https://www.safesedationtraining.com/, accessed October 6, 2014, with permission.)

is normally excreted by the kidneys and thus accumulates during renal failure. It causes CNS excitation, including anxiety, tremulousness, myoclonus, and seizures; therefore, meperidine is contraindicated in patients with renal failure.

Studies examining sex differences in responses to opioids have produced mixed results. Authors of three small studies observed a greater respiratory depressant effect of opioids in women than in men. Processed electroencephalogram (used as a surrogate measure of opioid effect) demonstrates that the potency of the fentanyl congeners is directly related to increasing age. In patients over age 65, the dose of remifentanil (and presumably other opioids as well) should be reduced by as much as 50%.

With the exception of remifentanil, limited work has characterized the behavior of opioids in obese patients. The key to administering opioids to obese patients is the choice of a *dosing scalar:* dosing an obese patient based on total body weight will reliably result in excessive plasma concentrations, while dosing based on lean body mass or fat free mass may be inadequate. Dosing remifentanil to fat free mass in obese patients most closely mimics total body weight dosing in lean patients. One approach is to estimate opioid needs based on modified fat free mass (MFFM = fat free mass + 0.4 [total body weight – fat free mass]) and titrate to the clinical effect.

L. Indications, Doses, and Special Considerations

Morphine

Morphine is the prototypic opioid and a very effective analgesic. It has a slow onset time because it is almost completely ionized at physiologic pH and is *poorly lipid soluble;* thus it enters the CNS slowly and peaks about 90 minutes after intravenous injection. Although this prolonged onset time allows partial pressure of carbon dioxide levels to climb gradually, reducing the risk of acute respiratory depression, it may also result in clinicians inappropriately redosing morphine before the peak effect is achieved. Histamine release causing hypotension may be observed after large bolus doses. Morphine undergoes extensive *first-pass metabolism* after oral administration, resulting in high morphine-6-glucuronide levels. This high hepatic extraction ratio means that orally administered morphine has lower bioavailability than parenteral morphine (13). (See Table 10-2 for typical bolus doses of opioids.)

Hydromorphone

Hydromorphone is a potent synthetic opioid with an onset time that is similar to morphine but reaches peak effect more quickly, within about 15 minutes. It has a prolonged clinical effect (~2 hours) and is suitable for use in patient-controlled analgesia.

Meperidine

Due to the accumulation of meperidine's active metabolite, normeperidine, in renal failure and potential CNS sequelae (see earlier discussion), meperidine

Table 10-2	Typical Opioid Bolus Doses
Opioid	**Typical Bolus Dose**
Morphine	1–5 mg IV
Hydromorphone	0.2–0.4 mg IV
Meperidine	12.5–50 mg IV
Fentanyl	50–150 μg IV
Sufentanil	5–15 μg IV
Alfentanil	150–300 μg IV
Remifentanil	25–100 μg IV Common infusion dose: 0.05–0.15 μg/kg/min

IV, intravenous.

is seldom used as an analgesic today. It is indicated for anesthetic-related rigors.

Fentanyl

Fentanyl can be administered intravenously as well as by the transdermal, transmucosal, intranasal, and transpulmonary routes. Fentanyl has a peak onset 3 to 5 minutes after intravenous administration, and its analgesic effect lasts 30 to 45 minutes. Peak respiratory depression occurs between 3 and 5 minutes after an intravenous dose. These pharmacokinetic features, combined with fentanyl's mild hemodynamic effects, make it a useful drug for sedation during minor procedures as well as during the induction and maintenance phases of anesthesia. Fentanyl's prolonged context-sensitive half-time (Fig. 10-3C) makes infusions of limited use unless carefully dosed with an understanding of the pharmacokinetics.

Sufentanil

Sufentanil is the most *potent* opioid commercially available for human use; 5 µg of intravenous sufentanil is the analgesic equivalent to 50 µg of fentanyl.

Alfentanil

Alfentanil reaches peak effect rapidly, ~90 seconds after bolus intravenous dose, and plasma concentrations fall rapidly, similar to remifentanil (Fig. 10-1). In contrast to remifentanil, however, termination of the effect of alfentanil after an infusion (context-sensitive half-time) is comparable to that of sufentanil. The combination of rapid onset of effect after bolus dosing and relatively prolonged termination of effect after an infusion may make alfentanil an attractive anesthetic adjunct during a stimulating surgery in which significant postoperative pain is anticipated. Hepatic metabolism of alfentanil is less predictable than fentanyl and sufentanil due to significant interindividual variability of hepatic CYP3A4, the enzyme primarily responsible for biotransformation of alfentanil.

Remifentanil

Remifentanil is a potent fentanyl congener characterized by rapid onset (within 90 seconds), short duration (~3 minutes), and short context-sensitive half-time (~5 minutes). It is metabolized by *ester hydrolysis* in the blood and tissues and is thus unaffected by hepatic or renal failure. Because it does not accumulate and its termination of effect is so reliable, it is suitable to use as a bolus dose for short, painful procedures performed under sedation, as an infusion for longer sedation procedures, and as an infusion during general anesthesia. It is an eminently titratable drug and allows the anesthesiologist to respond effectively to changing levels of surgical stimulation. Its very short context-sensitive half-time will terminate the analgesic effect shortly after the infusion is stopped. Therefore, if postoperative analgesia is required, a longer-acting analgesic should be administered instead.

Methadone

Methadone is available in oral and intravenous forms and is most commonly used in the treatment of opioid addiction because its prolonged pharmacokinetics makes acute withdrawal symptoms unlikely. The dextrorotatory isomer of methadone also has **NMDA antagonism** activity, which may attenuate the effects of opioid tolerance. Methadone prolongs the QT interval.

M. Reversal Agents and Associated Effects

Naloxone is an opioid receptor competitive antagonist with the greatest affinity for the µ receptor. In the absence of opioid, naloxone administration has no effect. In the presence of opioid, naloxone can reverse all clinical effects of opioids when dosed appropriately and is most often used to reverse opioid-induced ventilatory depression. Naloxone is rapidly metabolized in the liver and has a high clearance; thus, its *duration of action* is usually shorter than the opioid whose effects it is intended to reverse. Patients should be carefully monitored after administration of naloxone for a recurrence of ventilatory depression. Naloxone can cause tachycardia and, rarely, pulmonary edema and even sudden death in previously healthy individuals (14). The mixed opioid agonist-antagonists include nalbuphine, pentazocine, and butorphanol. These agents are partial κ agonists and complete, competitive μ antagonists. The analgesic and respiratory effects of these agents reach a ceiling effect and do not decrease MAC as profoundly as morphine or fentanyl. These *"partial agonists"* have less abuse potential than opioid agonists but are also less effective at treating pain. They are most commonly used to attenuate side effects of opioids (ventilatory depression, pruritus) while maintaining some analgesia (the partial κ agonism). The μ antagonism will precipitate withdrawal in opioid dependent patients. Buprenorphine is a similar drug but is a κ antagonist and a partial μ agonist.

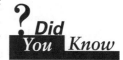

? Did You Know

Naloxone duration of action is usually substantially shorter than the opioids whose effects it is intended to reverse.

References

1. Chen L, Yang G, Grosser T. Prostanoids and inflammatory pain. *Prostaglandins Other Lipid Mediat.* 2013;104–105:58–66.
2. Toussaint K, Yang XC, Zielinski MA, et al. What do we (not) know about how paracetamol (acetaminophen) works? *J Clin Pharm Therapeut.* 2010;35(6):617–638.
3. Bunchorntavakul C, Reddy KR. Acetaminophen-related hepatotoxicity. *Clin Liver Dis.* 2013;17(4):587–607.
4. Gaglia MA Jr, Clavijo L. Cardiovascular pharmacology core reviews: Aspirin. *J Cardiovasc Pharmacol Therapeut.* 2013;18(6):505–513.
5. White PF, Raeder J, Kehlet H. Ketorolac: Its role as part of a multimodal analgesic regimen. *Anesth Analg.* 2012;114(2):250–254.
6. Lewis SR, Nicholson A, Cardwell ME, et al. Nonsteroidal anti-inflammatory drugs and perioperative bleeding in paediatric tonsillectomy. *Cochrane Database Syst Rev.* 2013;7:003591.
7. Castellsague J, Riera-Guardia N, Calingaert B, et al. Individual NSAIDs and upper gastrointestinal complications: A systematic review and meta-analysis of observational studies (the SOS project). *Drug Saf.* 2012;35(12):1127–1146.
8. Evers AM, ed. *Anesthetic Pharmacology: Physiologic Principles and Clinical Practice.* Philadelphia: Churchill Livingstone; 2004.
9. Katz JA. COX-2 inhibition: What we learned—a controversial update on safety data. *Pain Med.* 2013;14(Suppl 1):S29–S34.
10. Zeiler FA, Teitelbaum J, West M, et al. The ketamine effect on ICP in traumatic brain injury. *Neurocrit Care.* 2014;21(1):163–173.
11. Blaudszun G, Lysakowski C, Elia N, et al. Effect of perioperative systemic alpha2 agonists on postoperative morphine consumption and pain intensity: Systematic review and meta-analysis of randomized controlled trials. *Anesthesiology.* 2012;116(6): 1312–1322.
12. Pasternak GW, Pan YX. Mu opioids and their receptors: evolution of a concept. *Pharmacol Rev.* 2013;65(4):1257–1317.
13. Crews KR, Gaedigk A, Dunnenberger HM, et al. Clinical Pharmacogenetics Implementation Consortium guidelines for cytochrome P450 2D6 genotype and codeine therapy: 2014 update. *Clin Pharmacol Therapeut.* 2014;95(4):376–382.
14. Olofsen E, van Dorp E, Teppema L, et al. Naloxone reversal of morphine- and morphine-6-glucuronide-induced respiratory depression in healthy volunteers: A mechanism-based pharmacokinetic-pharmacodynamic modeling study. *Anesthesiology.* 2010; 112(6):1417–1427.

Questions

1. Nonsteroidal anti-inflammatory drugs (NSAIDs) relieve pain by what mechanism?
   A. Inhibition of prostanoid synthesis
   B. Inhibition of thromboxane A2 effects
   C. Inhibition of prostacycline effects
   D. Inhibition of arachidonic acid synthesis
   E. None of the above

2. Which currently available nonsteroidal anti-inflammatory drug (NSAID) does not inhibit platelet aggregation?
   A. Rofecoxib
   B. Valdecoxib
   C. Celecoxib
   D. Ketorolac
   E. None of the above

3. Clonidine and dexmedetomidine relieve pain by what mechanism?
   A. Augmentation of endogenous opioid binding
   B. Cyclooxygenase inhibition
   C. μ receptor downregulation
   D. α_2 receptor stimulation
   E. None of the above

4. What is the context-sensitive half-time of a drug?
   A. The time it takes for the plasma concentration of a drug to decrease by 50% after the infusion of the drug is stopped.
   B. The time it takes for the plasma concentration of a drug to reach 50% of its steady-state concentration during a constant infusion.
   C. The time it takes to increase the plasma concentration of a drug by 50% when the drug infusion rate is doubled.
   D. The time it takes to decrease the plasma concentration of a drug by 50% when the drug infusion rate is halved.
   E. None of the above.

5. Which opioid is the most potent?
   A. Fentanyl
   B. Sufentanil
   C. Hydromorphone
   D. Methadone
   E. None of the above

6. In a patient weighing 140 kg with a fat free mass (lean body mass) of 70 kg, what would be the modified fat free mass to use for the initial calculation of the infusion rate of remifentanil?
   A. 120 kg
   B. 100 kg
   C. 90 kg
   D. 80 kg
   E. None of the above

11 Neuromuscular Blocking Agents

Sorin J. Brull
Casper Claudius

I. Physiology and Pharmacology

A. Morphology of the Neuromuscular Junction

The *neuromuscular junction (NMJ)* consists of the presynaptic motor neuron, the postsynaptic muscle fiber, and the intervening 50 to 70 nm gap (synaptic cleft) between the two, which contains the enzyme acetylcholinesterase (AChAse) (Fig. 11-1). The NMJ has a highly ordered mechanism that converts the electrical signal of the motor nerve into a chemical signal (release of *acetylcholine [ACh]*), which in turn is converted into an electrical event (muscle membrane depolarization), leading to a mechanical response (muscle contraction). The *motor unit* consists of the motor neuron and the muscle fiber it innervates. *Nicotinic muscle type acetylcholine receptors* (muscle type nAChRs) are located in folds of the postsynaptic muscle membrane in very high concentrations (10,000 receptors per squared micrometer) and are not normally found extrasynaptically. More than 90% of all nAChRs in a muscle fiber are located at the synapse, an area that represents <0.1% of the total muscle membrane surface area (1).

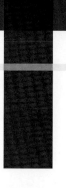
Nerve Stimulation

ACh mediates transmission of an impulse from nerve to muscle. When depolarization of the motor nerve reaches the nerve terminal, voltage-gated calcium ion (Ca^{2+}) channels open, and the vesicles (quanta) that contain ACh are released by exocytosis from the nerve terminal into the cleft. This release of ACh quanta (each containing 5,000 to 10,000 ACh molecules) is antagonized by hypocalcemia and hypermagnesemia. The potassium ion (K^+) channels in the nerve terminal area limit the extent of Ca^{+2} entry into the terminal and limit the transmitter quantal release, initiating nerve membrane repolarization.

B. Presynaptic Events: Mobilization and Release of Acetylcholine

ACh is synthesized in the presynaptic nerve terminal from acetate and choline and is divided into two functional pools. The "immediately available pool"

185

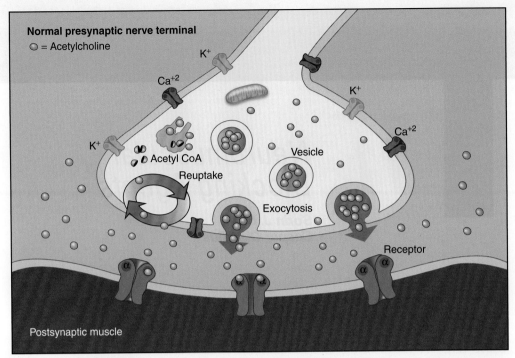

Figure 11-1 Normal neuromuscular transmission across the myoneural junction.

consists of a small fraction of all ACh available in the nerve terminal. Most of the ACh is contained in the "reserve pool," which must first be transported (mobilized) to the area adjacent to the membrane (the active zone) and become part of the immediately available pool before it can be released into the cleft. Once nerve depolarization occurs and the intracellular Ca^{+2} concentration increases, ACh quanta are released into the synaptic cleft. Released ACh can then bind to the postsynaptic nAChRs to initiate muscle contraction followed by rapid hydrolysis by AChAse into choline and acetic acid. Choline is then reuptaken into the presynaptic nerve terminal. ACh can also bind to presynaptic neuronal nAChRs to facilitate ACh mobilization.

C. Postsynaptic Events

Small quantities of ACh are released spontaneously into the cleft, resulting in small depolarizations (5 mV) of the muscle membrane. These miniature end-plate potentials may represent the membrane effects of a single ACh quantum. When sufficient ACh quanta are released (200 to 400), the postjunctional muscle membrane depolarization reaches an end-plate potential and the excitation-contraction sequence is activated. ACh binds to both recognition sites of the α subunits of the nAChRs, inducing a conformational change of the receptor that results in the formation of a central channel (pore). The central channel allows sodium ion (Na^+) influx and K^+ efflux, resulting in muscle cell membrane depolarization. Voltage-gated Na^+ channels on the muscle membrane propagate the action potential across the membrane, leading to development of muscle tension (the excitation–contraction coupling).

D. Receptor Up- and Downregulation

When the frequency of stimulation at the NMJ decreases over days (or longer), resulting from severe burns, immobilization, infection or sepsis, prolonged use of neuromuscular blocking agents (NMBAs) in the intensive care unit, or cerebrovascular accidents, the number of immature (fetal) nAChRs increases (upregulation). The immature nAChRs have increased sensitivity to agonists (ACh and succinylcholine [SCh]) and decreased sensitivity to nondepolarizing NMBAs. The channel opening time of the immature nAChRs is up to tenfold longer and may allow systemic release of lethal doses of intracellular K^+ in response to administration of SCh. Downregulation of mature nAChRs occurs during periods of sustained agonist stimulation, for instance, chronic neostigmine use (in patients with myasthenia gravis), or organophosphorus poisoning, which leads to resistance to SCh but extreme sensitivity to nondepolarizing NMBAs.

II. Neuromuscular Blocking Agents

A. Pharmacologic Characteristics of Neuromuscular Blocking Agents

Potency of a drug is determined by the dose required to produce a certain effect and is expressed as a dose versus response sigmoidal curve. For NMBAs, the effect is depression of normal muscle contraction. Thus, a dose that depresses the maximal muscle contraction by 50% is termed 50% effective dose or ED_{50}. Most NMBA potencies are expressed as the dose required for 95% depression of the single twitch (ST) during nerve stimulation, or ED_{95}. Onset of action (onset time) for all NMBAs is defined as the time from its administration (usually intravenous) until maximal neuromuscular block (disappearance of ST). Onset time is inversely related to dose and can be affected by rate of delivery to action site (blood flow, speed of injection, etc.), receptor affinity, mechanism of action (depolarizing vs. competitive), and plasma clearance (metabolism, redistribution). Duration of action until recovery to 25% (DUR 25%) is defined as the time from drug administration until recovery of ST to 25% of baseline (normal) strength. The total duration of action is defined as the time from drug administration until recovery of train-of-four (TOF) ratio to 0.90 (DUR 0.90). Duration of action is directly related to the dose of NMBA administered. Recovery index is defined as the time of spontaneous recovery of ST from 25% to 75% of control (RI_{25-75}), a period during which the spontaneous recovery is relatively linear and is not affected significantly by the NMBA dose.

NMBAs can be classified based on their mode of action: *depolarizing* NMBAs (e.g., SCh) produce muscle relaxation by directly depolarizing the nAChRs (Fig. 11-2). This occurs because SCh (made up of two ACh molecules joined end to end) acts as a "false transmitter," mimicking ACh (Fig. 11-3). *Nondepolarizing* NMBAs compete with ACh for the two α subunit recognition sites, preventing normal nAChR function. Nondepolarizing agents can be classified according to their chemical structure (benzylisoquinolinium or steroidal) or to their duration of action (short, intermediate, or long duration).

III. Depolarizing Neuromuscular Blocking Drugs: Succinylcholine

A. Neuromuscular Effects

Succinylcholine is the only depolarizing NMBA available clinically (Table 11-1, Fig. 11-3). Because of its molecular similarity to ACh, SCh depolarizes both postsynaptic and extrajunctional receptors, but because it is not

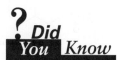

? Did You Know

Succinylcholine has the fastest onset, the shortest duration, and greatest reliability (i.e., narrowest onset variability around the mean) of any NMBA.

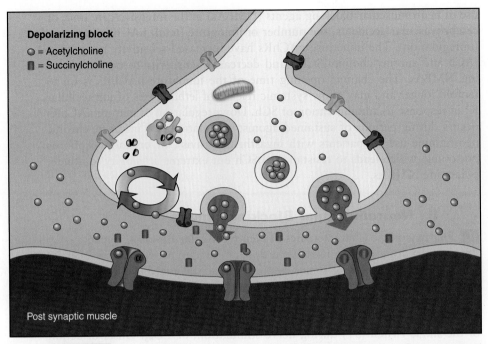

Figure 11-2 The effects of a depolarizing neuromuscular block at the myoneural junction.

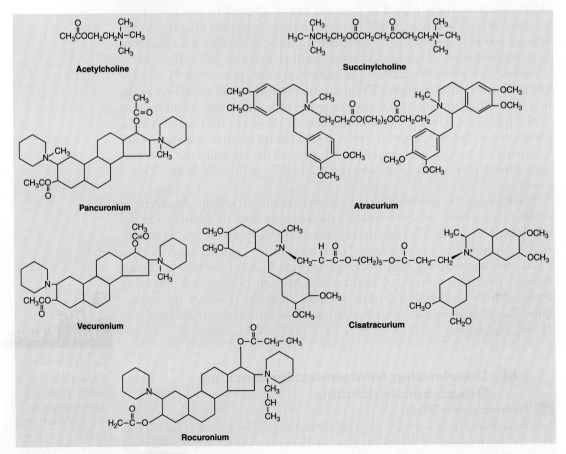

Figure 11-3 Chemical structures of acetylcholine and the clinically available neuromuscular blocking agents.

Table 11-1	Dosing Regimens and Characteristics of Depolarizing and Nondepolarizing Aminosteroid Neuromuscular Blocking Agents			
Agent[a]	SCh	Panc	Vec	Roc
Type (structure)	Depolarizing	Nondepolarizing	Nondepolarizing	Nondepolarizing
Type (duration)	Ultrashort	Long	Intermediate	Intermediate
Potency: ED95 (mg/kg)	0.3	0.07	0.05	0.3
Intubation dose (mg/kg)	1.0	0.1	0.1	0.6
Onset time (min)	1.0	2–4	3–4	1.5–3
Clinical duration (min)	7–10	60–120	25–50	30–40
Recovery index (R25–75) (min)	2–4	30–45	10–15	8–12
Maintenance dose (mg/kg)	N/A	0.02	0.01	0.1
Infusion dose (µg/kg/min)	Titrate to single twitch (ST) muscle response	20–40 (not recommended)	1–2	5–10
Elimination route	Plasma cholinesterase	Renal 40–70%; hepatic 20%	Renal 10–50%; hepatic 30–50%	Renal 30%; hepatic 70%
Active metabolites	No active metabolites	3-OH, 17-OH pancuronium	3-OH vecuronium (desacetyl)	No active metabolites
Side effects	Myalgias; bradycardia/asystole in children or with repeated dosing; dual block	Vagal block (tachycardia), catecholamine release	Vagal blockade at large doses	Minimal
Contraindications (other than specific allergy)	High K^+; MH; muscular dystrophy, children, receptor upregulation, pseudocholinesterase deficiency	Short surgical procedures (<60 min); not recommended for continuous infusion	None	None
Comments	Fastest onset, most reliable for rapid tracheal intubation	Significant accumulation, prone to residual block (3-OH metabolite)	Not for prolonged intensive care administration (myopathy); reversible by sugammadex (except in the U.S.)	Pain on injection; easily reversible by sugammadex (except in the U.S.)

ED_{50}, effective dose 50%; SCh, succinylcholine; Panc, pancuronium; Vec, vecuronium; Roc, rocuronium; K^+, potassium; MH, malignant hyperthermia.
[a]Agents in current clinical use in the United States. The data are averages obtained from published literature, assume there is no potentiation from other coadministered drugs (such as volatile inhalational anesthetics), and the effects are measured at the adductor pollicis muscle. Other factors, such as muscle temperature, mode of evoked response monitoring, type or site of muscle monitoring, will affect the data.

VIDEO 11-1

Fasciculations After Succinylcholine

degraded by AChAses, it depolarizes the muscle membrane for a longer period of time, leading to desensitization. This desensitization then leads to flaccid paralysis after the initial receptor activation (manifested clinically as muscle "fasciculations").

B. Characteristics of Depolarizing Blockade
As with all NMBAs, increasing the dose of SCh leads to a progressive decrease in force of muscle contraction (ST). However, the response to repetitive stimulation (TOF and tetanus patterns, see below) is maintained (no fade) because SCh has no affinity for the presynaptic (neuronal) nAChRs, despite progressive but equivalent decrease in the force of contractions. Additionally, after a brief period of high-frequency stimulation (tetanus), there is no increase or amplification in the force of subsequent muscle contractions (no posttetanic potentiation). Large doses (>10 times ED_{95}) or prolonged (>30 minutes) exposure to SCh or presence of abnormal (atypical) plasma cholinesterases (pseudocholinesterase/butyrylcholinesterase deficiency) may lead to dual (or phase II, or nondepolarizing) block. This is characterized by fade of responses to repetitive stimulation and amplification of muscle responses after high-frequency stimulation (posttetanic potentiation), similar to nondepolarizing block.

C. Pharmacology of Succinylcholine
The onset of SCh at peripheral muscles (such as adductor pollicis muscle [APM]) is the fastest of any NMBA (1 to 2 minutes). Its ED_{95} is approximately 0.30 mg/kg, and at doses of 1 to 1.5 mg/kg (3 to 5 × ED_{95}), the DUR 25% of SCh is 10 to 12 minutes, but is prolonged beyond 15 minutes with larger doses. Despite paralysis at APM, the diaphragm (and other central muscles) starts to contract and spontaneous breathing may resume 5 minutes after 1 mg/kg SCh administration. SCh is most commonly administered intravenously (IV), but intraosseous, intralingual, and intramuscular routes have been reported if an IV cannot be established. Onset is delayed, particularly with intramuscular administration. Hydrolysis of SCh by pseudocholinesterase (also known as butyrylcholinesterase or plasma cholinesterase) occurs in the plasma.

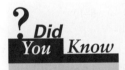

? Did You Know

Almost 90% of the intravenous dose of SCh is hydrolyzed in the plasma before reaching the myoneural junction.

D. Side Effects
SCh can induce significant bradycardia and asystole, particularly in children, and after redosing. Premature ventricular escape beats are also common. Cardiac effects can be attenuated by pretreatment with anticholinergics. Disorganized muscle contractions (*fasciculations*) after SCh administration are very common (80% to 90% of patients). *Myalgias* are also very common 1 to 2 days postoperatively (in 50% to 60% of patients). Fasciculations have been considered a possible etiology for myalgia, but systematic reviews have not established a clear relationship. A "defasciculating" pretreatment with a small dose of nondepolarizing NMBA (10% ED_{95}) is sometimes used to decrease the incidence of fasciculations and myalgia. However, this technique may render some patients at risk of *regurgitation* and *pulmonary aspiration* because of partial paralysis of pharyngeal muscles. Furthermore, because of the large individual variability, pretreatment may be ineffective in other patients. If pretreatment is used, the dose requirement for SCh is increased (up to 2 mg/kg). The most effective prophylaxis for myalgia without using nondepolarizing NMBAs is pretreatment with nonsteroidal anti-inflammatory drugs (e.g., aspirin or diclofenac), with a number-needed-to-treat of 2.5.

Although SCh may *increase intragastric pressure,* the lower esophageal sphincter tone is also increased, such that the intragastric–esophageal pressure gradient remains the same. Thus, there is no increase in the risk of aspiration from the use of SCh. *Intraocular pressure (IOP)* also increases with SCh (up to a 15 mm Hg increase), and pretreatment does not attenuate this increase. However, despite fears that this SCh-induced increase in IOP may induce extrusion of ocular contents in patients with an "open-globe" injury, clinical practice in thousands of patients has not reported this complication. *Elevation in intracranial pressure* from SCh may occur, and this increase is attenuated by defasciculation. Inadequate levels of anesthesia during laryngoscopy and tracheal intubation, however, are much more likely to increase intracranial pressure. Although SCh administration induces an elevation in the plasma level of potassium of 0.5 mEq/L, severe *hyperkalemia* with attendant cardiac arrest has only been reported in cases in which there is a proliferation of immature nAChRs (see "Receptor Up- and Downregulation"). Particularly important is the association between pediatric myotonia and muscle dystrophies with SCh administration, leading to fatal hyperkalemia and rhabdomyolysis. For this reason, the U.S. Food and Drug Administration has a black box warning on the use of SCh, and clinicians should reserve its use in children for emergency tracheal intubation. SCh may also trigger lethal malignant hyperthermia (MH), especially in patients anesthetized with volatile anesthetics (see Appendix G). Some patients (both adults and children) may exhibit masseter muscle spasm after SCh administration, making intubating conditions difficult. In some cases, particularly in pediatrics, masseter spasm is associated with MH. SCh can produce *allergic reactions (anaphylaxis)* in about 1 of 10,000 administrations, more commonly than any other anesthetic drug.

E. Clinical Uses

SCh is indicated for rapid attainment of optimal intubating conditions and prevention of regurgitation and pulmonary aspiration of gastric contents in patients at risk (those unfasted, with gastroparesis or gastrointestinal obstruction) in the rapid sequence induction and intubation (RSII) scenario. In this setting, SCh is the drug closest to the "ideal" NMBA: it has the shortest clinical duration (5 to 10 min at 1 mg/kg dose), so most patients will resume some diaphragmatic function before significant apnea-induced hypoxia occurs. It has the shortest onset time (1 minute at 1.5 mg/kg); and it has the highest reliability, with the fewest outliers (patients whose intubating conditions are poor at the time of intubation). In obese individuals who need RSII, the dose of SCh should be calculated on the basis of actual body weight, rather than ideal body weight. Children are more resistant than adults to the actions of SCh, and the usual dose (see "Side Effects") is 1.5 to 2.0 mg/kg (up to 3 mg/kg in infants).

F. Contraindications to Use of Succinylcholine

Use of SCh is contraindicated in patients (and their relatives) with a history of MH. The relative risk of MH with SCh administration (vs. without SCh) is 20 times higher when combined with volatile anesthetics (2). Other settings in which SCh is contraindicated include states of receptor upregulation due to the potential for *lethal hyperkalemia*, critical care patients or those immobilized for prolonged periods (e.g., weeks), and patients with *pseudocholinesterase deficiency*. Approximately 1 in 25 patients may be heterozygous and 1 in 2,500 individuals may be homozygous for the "atypical" deficiency gene and may require prolonged (hours) postoperative mechanical ventilation. In patients with renal failure, SCh may be administered if the plasma K^+ is not elevated. Lethal hyperkalemia following administration of SCh has been reported in severely acidotic and hypovolemic patients.

IV. Nondepolarizing Neuromuscular Blocking Agents

A. Characteristics of Nondepolarizing Blockade

Nondepolarizing NMBAs compete with ACh for binding to one or both of the α subunits of the nAChRs. With repetitive stimulation at frequencies between 0.1 and 2 Hz during partial block, muscle contraction fatigue (fade) develops. The degree of fade can be determined by a sequence of four stimuli delivered at a 2 Hz frequency by calculating the ratio of the amplitude of the fourth response (T4) to the amplitude of the first response (T1). This ratio is the TOF ratio, or T4/T1. Another characteristic of nondepolarizing block is the transient amplification of responses that follows a 5-second period of tetanic stimulation (posttetanic potentiation [PTP] or facilitation) that lasts about 2 to 3 minutes following tetanic stimulation. Unlike depolarizing blockade, which is potentiated by the administration of anticholinesterases, the nondepolarizing block can be antagonized by these agents as long as the depth of block at the time of reversal is not excessive.

B. Pharmacology of Nondepolarizing Neuromuscular Blocking Drugs

Nondepolarizing NMBAs can be classified as long, intermediate, and short acting, and their duration of action depends on metabolism, redistribution, and elimination (Tables 11-1 and 11-2; Figs. 11-3 and 11-4). They also can be classified based on their chemical structure as benzylisoquinolinium (atracurium, cisatracurium, mivacurium) or aminosteroid (pancuronium, rocuronium, vecuronium) compounds. Nondepolarizing NMBAs are almost always administered intravenously. Intramuscular delivery leads to very slow and variable onset of action. Since they are positively charged, nondepolarizing NMBAs are distributed mostly in the extracellular fluid (ECF). Thus, in

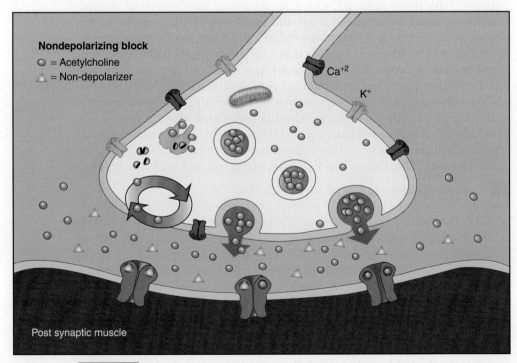

Nondepolarizing block

◯ = Acetylcholine
△ = Non-depolarizer

Ca^{+2}

K^+

Post synaptic muscle

Figure 11-4 The effects of a nondepolarizing (competitive) block at the myoneural junction.

Table 11-2   Dosing Regimens and Characteristics of Benzylisoquinolinium Nondepolarizing Neuromuscular Blocking Agents

Agent[a]	Atrac	Cisatrac
Type (duration)	Intermediate	Intermediate
Potency: ED95 (mg/kg)	0.25	0.05
Intubation dose (mg/kg)	0.5	0.15
Onset time (min)	3–4	5–7
Clinical duration (min)	30–45	35–50
Recovery index (R25–75) (min)	10–15	12–15
Maintenance dose (mg/kg)	0.1	0.01
Infusion dose (μg/kg/min)	10–20	1–3
Elimination route	Renal 10%; Hofmann 30%; ester hydrolysis 60%	Hofmann 30%; ester hydrolysis 60%
Active metabolites	No active metabolites	No active metabolites
Side effects	Histamine release; laudanosine and acrylates production	None; histamine release at high doses
Contraindications (other than specific allergy)	Hemodynamically unstable patients	None
Comments	Organ-independent elimination	Trivial histamine, laudanosine and acrylate levels

ED_{95}, effective dose 95%; Atrac, atracurium; Cisatrac, cisatracurium.
[a]Agents in current clinical use in the United States. The data are averages obtained from published literature, assume there is no potentiation from other coadministered drugs (such as volatile inhalational anesthetics), and the effects are measured at the adductor pollicis muscle. Other factors, such as muscle temperature, mode of evoked response monitoring, type or site of muscle monitoring, will affect the data.

patients with renal or hepatic failure (who have increased ECF), larger initial doses may be required.

C.   Onset and Duration of Action

Onset of nondepolarizing NMBAs generally depends on potency; less potent agents such as rocuronium (ED_{95} of 0.300 mg/kg) have more molecules per equivalent dose than a potent NMBA such as vecuronium (ED_{95} of 0.05 mg/kg). Thus, an ED_{95} dose of rocuronium will have six times more molecules than an equipotent dose of vecuronium, and the plasma concentration of rocuronium will be greater than that of vecuronium. This greater concentration difference between plasma and the biophase partly explains the more rapid onset of rocuronium. A similar plasma or biophase concentration gradient might be achieved by administering, for example, six times the ED_{95} of vecuronium. Although this will speed up the onset, the much larger dose will also markedly prolong the total duration of action. Typically, a dose of 2 to 3 × ED_{95} of a nondepolarizing NMBA is used to facilitate tracheal intubation.

D.   Nondepolarizing Agents

Pancuronium is one of the oldest nondepolarizing NMBAs. DUR 25% is often more than 1 to 2 hours, but it can be prolonged further in renal or hepatic failure or with repeated administrations (Table 11-1; Fig. 11-3). Pancuronium has vagolytic effects, as well as direct sympathomimetic effects; it blocks norepinephrine presynaptic reuptake. Because of its high potency, it is slow in onset of neuromuscular block, so doses $>2 \times ED_{95}$ are usually needed for intubation in <5 minutes. It has traditionally been used in cardiac surgery because its vagolytic effects counteract the bradycardic effects associated with high-dose opioid techniques. Today, many clinicians find use of pancuronium obsolete because of the risk of significant postoperative residual neuromuscular weakness.

Vecuronium is an intermediate-duration NMBA that is devoid of cardiovascular effects; because it is more potent than rocuronium, its onset of action is slower (Table 11-1; Fig. 11-3). Vecuronium precipitates in the IV tubing if administered immediately after thiopental but does not precipitate after propofol administration. Since the introduction of rocuronium, vecuronium is no longer recommended for RSII.

Rocuronium is structurally similar to pancuronium and vecuronium (Table 11-1; Fig. 11-3). Because of its low potency, the high plasma concentration achieved after bolus administration decreases rapidly, so that its duration of action in patients with normal renal and hepatic function is determined mostly by its redistribution, not its elimination. Unlike vecuronium, rocuronium metabolites are minimal, with very low neuromuscular blocking activity (17-OH rocuronium), so the risk of accumulation is minimal. In the vast majority of cases, it has replaced the use of SCh in the RSII clinical setting. At doses of 3.5 to $4 \times ED_{95}$ (1.0 to 1.2 mg/kg), the onset rivals that of SCh, with similar intubation conditions (3). The DUR 25%, however, at these doses is 50 to 70 minutes. Similar to vecuronium, rocuronium is hemodynamically stable, releases no histamine, and rare allergic reactions (similar to all aminosteroid NMBAs) have been documented. Reports from Europe suggest that the incidence of anaphylaxis following rocuronium may be higher than with other NMBAs. This propensity has been ascribed to sensitization to an antitussive medication, pholcodine, which was previously available in some European countries. Potency appears to be greater in women than in men and in North American than in European patients. In the pediatric population, onset and duration of action are shorter, and dose requirements are slightly increased.

Because of its rapid onset, rocuronium can be used in high doses (1.2 mg/kg) in the RSII setting, particularly in those patients in whom the use of SCh is contraindicated. It must be noted, however, that although the mean onset time at this dose approaches that of SCh (60 seconds), the variability of onset is greater with rocuronium, so it is more likely that some rare outliers may have poor intubating conditions at the time of attempted laryngoscopy. It also must be kept in mind that after large doses, the DUR 25% is significantly prolonged (>60 minutes), and spontaneous (diaphragmatic) ventilation cannot be relied upon for maintenance of oxygenation in the "cannot-intubate, cannot-ventilate" scenario. In such emergencies, the administration of a large dose (16 mg/kg) of sugammadex (see below) may be life-saving, as long as spontaneous ventilatory drive has not been blocked by the administration of opioids or anesthetics.

Atracurium is a bis-benzylisoquinolinium compound of the curare family and is made up of a mixture of 10 optical isomers (Table 11-2; Fig. 11-3). It shares, with most of the isoquinolinium compounds, a unique, dual metabolic pathway: a nonenzymatic degradation that is directly proportional with temperature and pH (Hofmann reaction) and a secondary pathway that involves hydrolysis by nonspecific plasma esterases. At the usual dose for tracheal intubation ($2 \times ED_{95}$), atracurium has a relatively long onset (3 to 5 minutes). Onset can be shortened by increasing the dose, but above this level (0.5 mg/kg), atracurium induces histamine release, resulting in skin flushing, tachycardia, and hypotension. DUR 25% is intermediate (30 to 45 minutes) and similar to the other intermediate-duration agents, but it is slightly more predictable, likely because of the dual metabolic pathway. Unlike aminosteroid NMBAs, atracurium potency is similar for both men and women and is not affected appreciably by age or organ failure. Allergic reactions have been reported with the same frequency as the other benzylisoquinolinium compounds. The breakdown products of laudanosine and acrylates have no clinical significance.

Cisatracurium has been developed in an attempt to reduce the propensity for histamine release (Table 11-2; Fig. 11-3). It is a potent cis-cis isomer of atracurium, so its onset time is longer than that of atracurium. Because five times less cisatracurium is administered than atracurium, it does not induce histamine release. Metabolism is similar to that of atracurium, and because of the dual elimination pathways that are organ function independent and its hemodynamic stability, cisatracurium is preferred for use in the intensive care setting. The incidence of anaphylactic reactions is similar to that of atracurium.

?Did You Know

Atracurium metabolism is by the same enzymes that degrade esmolol and remifentanil.

V. Drug Interactions

A. Additive and Synergistic Effects

Nondepolarizing NMBAs can have either *additive* or *synergistic effects* when combined. Usually, combining two chemically similar drugs with similar duration of action (e.g., atracurium and cisatracurium) results in an additive potency interaction with no effect on total duration. When drugs of different classes are combined (e.g., cisatracurium and rocuronium), the effects in term of total dose are synergistic, where, for instance, ED_{25} of rocuronium plus ED_{25} of cisatracurium will have an ED_{95} effect. Combining different drugs with different duration of action is a special case of interaction. When an intermediate-duration drug (vecuronium) is added at the end of a long-acting drug-based (pancuronium) block, recovery will follow the duration of the long-acting agent pancuronium. In contrast, when pancuronium is added during recovery from vecuronium, the pancuronium recovery will be shorter, similar to that of vecuronium. This apparent paradox is due to the fact that recovery will always be that of the drug that blocked the majority (70% to 90%) of the receptors (loading dose drug). The second, maintenance drug dose is in comparison very small and only blocks a small proportion (10% to 15%) of the free receptors. Thus, the predominant characteristics of recovery will be those of the loading drug.

B. Antagonism

Adding depolarizing and nondepolarizing NMBAs results in mutual antagonism. For instance, defasciculating doses of a nondepolarizing NMBA prior to administration of SCh will increase the SCh dose requirement and shorten the SCh duration of action.

C. Potentiation

Inhalational anesthetic agents potentiate neuromuscular block (desflurane > sevoflurane > isoflurane > halothane > nitrous oxide), likely by direct effects at the postjunctional receptors. Higher concentration (minimum alveolar concentration) and longer agent exposure will potentiate the neuromuscular block to a greater extent. The intravenous agent propofol has no effect on neuromuscular transmission.

Local anesthetics potentiate the effects of both depolarizing and nonde-polarizing NMBAs but are insufficient to significantly shorten the onset time; however, most NMBAs' duration of action is prolonged.

The new generation *antibiotics* have little, if any, propensity for prolonging the effects of NMBAs. Older antibiotics, such as streptomycin and neomycin, which are known to depress neuromuscular function, are rarely used today, and the aminoglycosides have limited effects. Hypercarbia, acidosis, and hypothermia, however, may further potentiate the depressant effects of antibiotics in the critically ill. In patients receiving acute administration of *anticonvulsants* (phenytoin, carbamazepine), neuromuscular block is potentiated, while chronic administration significantly decreases the duration of action of aminosteroids while having little effect on benzylisoquinolinium compounds. *Beta-receptor* and *calcium channel antagonists* have insignificant effects on NMBAs, but *ephedrine*, likely by increasing cardiac output, has been shown to hasten the onset of rocuronium.

Corticosteroids, particularly when administered in critical illness for prolonged periods in conjunction with neuromuscular blockade, will markedly increase the risk of myopathy (up to 50% of mechanically ventilated patients who receive both drugs).

VI. Altered Responses to Neuromuscular Blocking Agents

Multiple factors affect the *pharmacokinetics* of all drugs, including NMBAs. Intraoperative *hypothermia* prolongs the duration of NMBAs by decreasing the receptor sensitivity and ACh mobilization, decreasing the force of muscle contraction, and reducing renal and hepatic metabolism and the Hofmann degradation pathway (prolonging the action of benzylisoquinolinium drugs atracurium and cisatracurium).

Aging results in decreased total body water and serum albumin concentration, reducing the volume of distribution of NMBAs. The decreased cardiac function, glomerular filtration rate, and liver blood flow decrease the rate of NMBA elimination (especially the steroidal compounds pancuronium, vecuronium and rocuronium).

Acid-base and electrolyte imbalance affect the duration of action of NMBAs and their metabolism and elimination. Hypokalemia potentiates non-depolarizing block and decreases the effectiveness of anticholinesterases (neostigmine) in antagonizing nondepolarizing block. Hypermagnesemia prolongs the duration of action of NMBAs by inhibition of Ca^{+2} channels (both pre- and postsynaptically). Acidosis interferes with the effects of anticholinesterases in reversing a nondepolarizing block. *Hypercarbia* also leads to acidosis and interferes with NMBA antagonism.

Organ dysfunction (aside from changes induced by aging) affects all NMBAs. All drugs with significant hepatic and renal metabolism (aminosteroids) will be affected and their duration of action prolonged by liver and kidney dysfunction. For this reason, benzylisoquinolinium-class NMBAs are preferred in patients with organ dysfunction (such as critically ill patients in the intensive care unit), because the nonenzymatic Hofmann degradation is less dependent on normal organ function.

VII. Monitoring Neuromuscular Blockade

A. Monitoring and Risk–Benefit Ratio

The introduction of NMBAs into clinical medicine (curare in 1942 and succinylcholine in 1949) has facilitated major advances in anesthesiology. Despite the tremendous advances afforded by NMBAs, these agents have their own set of complications. *Allergic reactions* and *anaphylaxis* (with an incidence of 1 in 6,000 to 20,000 administrations depending on NMBA), although rare, are significant problems. Use of NMBAs without the ability to secure the airway may be lethal, and a substantial minority (30% to 40%) of patients who receive NMBAs have significant postoperative residual neuromuscular weakness (mistermed residual curarization because curare is no longer used). Given that there are over 230 million major surgeries performed every year worldwide, the number of patients exposed to potential complications is huge, and appropriate *monitoring* is a major patient safety issue. Aside from the cost of the monitors and related disposables (electrodes), there are no significant potential complications from monitoring neuromuscular function, so the risk–benefit ratio is heavily in favor of monitoring. Several anesthesiology organizations around the world have recently started publishing best-practice guidelines that include routine neuromuscular monitoring.

B. Characteristics of Nerve Stimulators and Neuromuscular Monitors

Monitoring involves the stimulation of a peripheral nerve and evaluating the response (contraction, or twitch) of the innervated muscle. Nerve stimulators have been in use for over 60 years. They are generally battery-operated, hand-held units that provide the stimulus via wires connected to surface (skin) electrodes. Nerve stimulators (Fig. 11-5) should not be confused with neuromuscular monitors. The monitors not only provide nerve stimulation, they also *measure* the evoked muscle response by using different technologies. Neuromuscular monitors are either battery-operated, hand-held devices or can be incorporated into the anesthesia workstations as modular units. Nerve stimulators (and the stimulation units of the neuromuscular monitors) deliver a

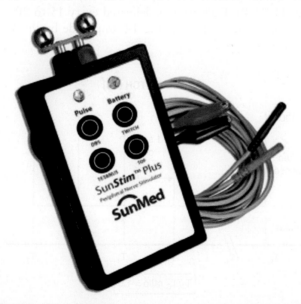

Figure 11-5 Typical nerve stimulator used in clinical practice, which has the following modes of stimulation: twitch, tetanus, double burst, and train-of-four. (http://www.medline.com/product/SunStim153-Plus-by-Sun-Medical/Machines/Z05-PF60828)

range of currents between 0 to 70 mA. The current should be constant over the duration of the impulse (which is at least 100 μsec to ensure depolarization of all nerve endings, but ≤300 μsec to avoid exceeding the nerve refractory period), and the impulse should be square-wave.

The current is delivered via surface (skin) stimulating electrodes that have a silver–silver chloride interface with the skin, reducing its resistance. Surface electrodes are preferred to the invasive, transcutaneous needle electrodes. The optimal conducting surface area is circular, with a diameter of 7 to 8 mm; this area provides sufficient current density to depolarize peripheral nerves. Skin can have very high resistance (up to 100,000 ohms), and "curing" the skin (i.e., placing the electrodes over the abraded, cleaned skin and allowing at least 15 minutes for the silver chloride gel to penetrate the dermis) will decrease skin resistance to below 5,000 ohms and ensure delivery of a constant, maximal current.

C. Monitoring Modalities

The first nerve stimulators delivered single repetitive stimuli at frequencies between 0.1 and 10 Hz. The muscle response was a ST to each stimulus (Fig. 11-6). The frequency of stimulation cannot be >0.1 Hz (1 stimulus every 10 seconds) because muscle fatigue may occur. To measure the degree of neuromuscular block, the current intensity is increased progressively (prior to NMBA administration) from 0 mA in 5 to 10 mA steps. The amplitude of the evoked muscle response is plotted over time and has a sigmoidal shape. Once the amplitude of the muscle response no longer increases as current intensity increases, the response is maximal, and the current required is called *maximal current*. Increasing the current value by 20% above maximal ensures that all fibers in the innervated muscle will depolarize, despite skin resistance changes over time. This is termed *supramaximal current*. Because a baseline control value is needed to compare the force of contraction over time, this modality (ST) is used clinically to determine onset of neuromuscular block, not recovery.

TOF stimulation was introduced clinically in 1971 and consists of four sequential ST stimuli (named T1, T2, T3, and T4) delivered at a frequency of 2 Hz (Fig. 11-7A,B). Each train is delivered every 15 to 20 seconds. The TOF ratio is calculated by dividing the T4 amplitude by the T1 amplitude.

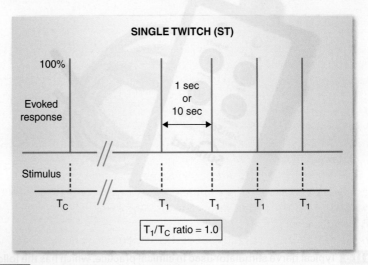

Figure 11-6 Single twitch nerve stimulation.

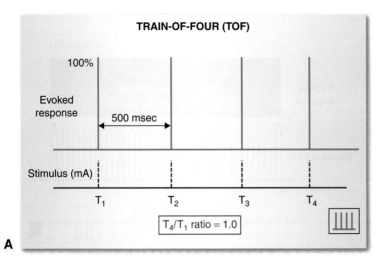

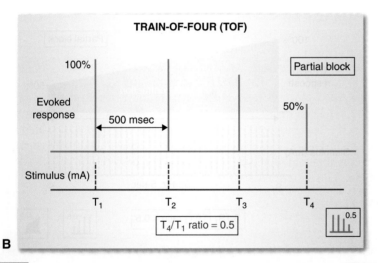

Figure 11-7 **A:** Following train-of-four (TOF) stimulation, TOF baseline ratio (T4/T1 = 1.0) is observed. **B:** Following TOF stimulation, depression of response to TOF (T4/T1 = 0.5) is noted following administration of a nondepolarizing neuromuscular blocking agent.

The control TOF ratio (before administration of NMBA) is 1.0 (100%). During a partial nondepolarizing block, the ratio decreases (fades) as the degree of block increases. TOF has multiple benefits over ST monitoring: at supramaximal stimulation, T1 and ST amplitudes are the same, so TOF does not require a baseline measurement—all subsequent responses are then measured as a fraction of T1. By eliciting four responses, the clinician sometimes is able to assess the degree of fade subjectively by visual or tactile means, or, more reliably, by counting the number of evoked responses (twitches) of TOF (TOF count). Additionally, the TOF ratio remains consistent over a range of stimulating currents, so it can be used to measure the degree of neuromuscular recovery in patients recovering from anesthesia (currents of 20 to 30 mA are not associated with the high degree of discomfort of supramaximal, 60 to 70 mA stimulation).

Tetanic stimulation (tetanus) describes repetitive stimulation at a frequency >30 Hz (Fig. 11-8A,B). Below this threshold, repetitive nerve stimulations result in individual, rapid contractions. At frequencies above 30 Hz, the

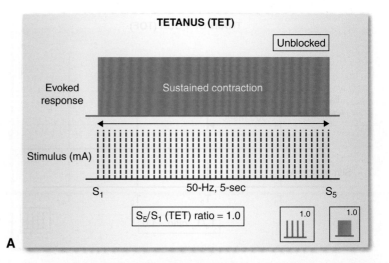

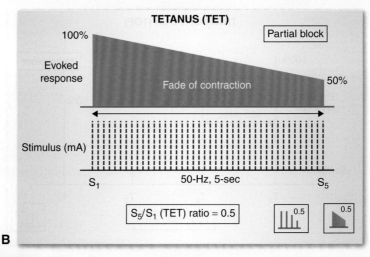

Figure 11-8 **A:** Following tetanic stimulation, at baseline, no fade is observed. **B:** Following tetanic stimulation, after administration of a neuromuscular blocking agent, fade is observed (0.5). (S_1, S_5 = the ratio of the amplitude at the end of the fifth second to the amplitude at the beginning of the first second.)

The control TOF ratio (before administration of NMBA) is 1.0 (100%). Dur-

muscle responses become fused into a sustained contraction. The maximal voluntary muscle contraction is approximately 60 Hz, so frequencies above this level are supraphysiologic and may result in muscle contraction fade, even in the absence of NMBAs. Tetanus has been studied extensively for durations of 5 seconds, so clinicians should always use 5-second durations to evaluate neuromuscular function. When tested during partial nondepolarizing block, the high frequency of tetanic stimulation will cause a temporary increase in the amount of ACh released, so that subsequent responses will be increased transiently (period of PTP). Depending on the tetanic frequency, this period of potentiated responses may last 1 to 2 minutes after a 5-second, 50 Hz tetanus, or 3 minutes after 100 Hz tetanus. The response to stimulation during the period of PTP can be used to evaluate the degree of block when there are no responses to TOF stimulation (i.e., when the TOF count is 0).

Posttetanic count (PTC), which is used during periods of profound block, consists of a 5-second, 50-Hz tetanic stimulus, followed 3 seconds later by a

? Did You Know

The fade of TOF in response to nondepolarizing NMBAs corresponds to the fade of tetanic stimulation.

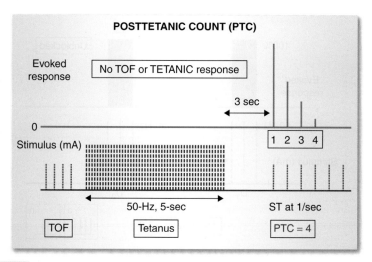

Figure 11-9   Posttetanic count (PTC). The number of posttetanic twitches is inversely related to the degree of neuromuscular block.

series of 15 to 30 ST at a frequency of 1 Hz (Fig. 11-9). The number of posttetanic twitches is inversely proportional to the depth of block: the fewer posttetanic twitches there are, the deeper the block. From a depth of block of PTC equal to 1 until recovery to a TOF count of 1, intermediate-acting NMBAs require 20 to 30 minutes (4). By delivering two (instead of four) intense stimuli (minitetanic bursts) separated by 0.75 second, the two fused responses can be evaluated as a direct comparison instead of comparing the fourth response of TOF to the first. This modality is termed *double burst stimulation* (DBS$_{3,3}$) (Fig. 11-10A,B). The numbers 3,3 signify that each burst contains three stimuli at a frequency of 50 Hz. Because the two individual bursts are tetanic in frequency, a longer recovery period between successive DBS stimulations is necessary (20 seconds). Using DBS subjectively, clinicians are able to detect fade when the TOF is <0.60, an improvement over the subjectively detected TOF fade. The relationship between TOF ratio and DBS$_{3,3}$ ratio is linear and identical between 0.0 and 1.0. In order to further increase the ability to detect small degrees of fade, another pattern of DBS only uses two minitetanic stimuli in the second burst. This is called DBS$_{3,2}$, and the baseline control DBS$_{3,2}$ ratio is 0.8 when the TOF ratio and DBS$_{3,3}$ ratio is 1.0.

D. Recording the Response
There are different modalities to assess the degree of neuromuscular block: *subjective* and *objective evaluation* (4,5). There are also different technologies for measuring the evoked response (objective evaluation). *Clinical testing* has been advocated for decades; tests such as grip strength, vital capacity, tidal volume, or leg lift are notoriously poor at detecting residual fade. In fact, none of these tests has a positive predictive value for detection of fade above 0.5. The best clinical test, the ability to resist removal of a tongue blade from the clenched teeth, cannot be used in patients whose tracheas are still intubated.

For decades, investigators have shown that regardless of the NMBA used, over 40% of patients managed intraoperatively by clinical criteria or subjective evaluation had residual paralysis (TOF <0.90) when tested objectively in the postanesthesia acute care unit (6). Given that postoperative pulmonary complications are relatively common in patients with residual neuromuscular

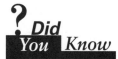

Did You Know

Both visual and tactile (subjective) evaluation of fade to TOF stimulation failed to recognize significant degrees of residual block (when TOF ratio is >0.40).

Did You Know

Even the often-used test of 5-second head lift has the same poor predictive value as other clinical tests (PPV ≤0.5). A majority of volunteers were able to maintain head lift for >5 seconds at a TOF ratio of 0.5.

Did You Know

It is estimated that postoperative mortality is increased 90-fold if patients have residual paralysis that requires unplanned tracheal reintubation and intensive care postoperatively.

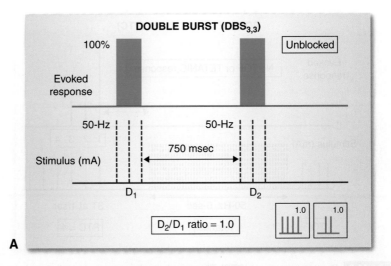

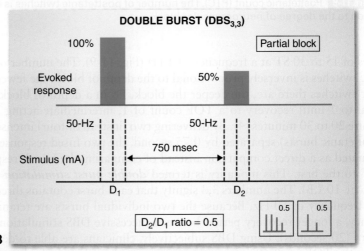

Figure 11-10 **A:** Double burst stimulation (DBS$_{3,3}$). **B:** Double burst stimulation (DBS$_{3,3}$) ratio = 0.5.

block, *objective monitoring* of adequacy of reversal prior to tracheal extubation is strongly recommended.

Electromyography (EMG) is one of the oldest methods of measuring neuromuscular transmission. For EMG monitoring, a peripheral nerve (usually the ulnar nerve) is stimulated via surface (skin) electrodes, and the action potential generated at the innervated muscle (the APM) is measured. Measurement of the evoked response involves either area under the curve of the muscle action potential, the peak-to-baseline, or the peak-to-peak amplitude of the signal.

Acceleromyography (AMG) has been the most commonly used clinical method of measuring muscle function in the past two decades (Fig. 11-11). AMG consists of an accelerometer mounted to a moving muscle (usually the thumb) that measures the acceleration in response to nerve stimulation (the ulnar nerve). Although it is the most commonly used monitor, it has several major limitations that prevent it from becoming the standard of care. The AMG setup can be simple, but is relatively time consuming, if performed properly. The thumb must be allowed to move freely throughout surgery, and arm movement may change the vector of thumb adduction, necessitating

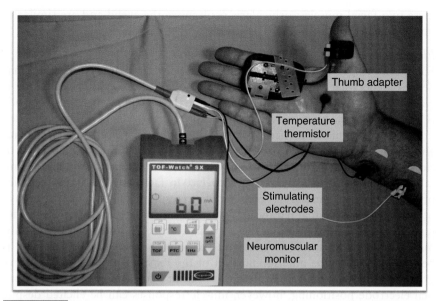

Figure 11-11 An accelerometer in position (between thumb and forefinger) to monitor the response to ulnar nerve stimulation of the thumb muscle and send information to a monitor. A thermistor is included to ensure consistency of temperature measurement during the measurement periods.

recalibration. AMG monitors cannot be used in procedures that require the patient's arms be tucked under the surgical drapes. During recovery from neuromuscular block, the TOF ratio can reach 140% of baseline, introducing a 40% error in baseline calculation. Newer models are employing two-dimensional and even triaxial vectoring to improve consistency and reliability, but most of the rest of its limitations remain.

E. Differential Muscle Sensitivity

It has long been known that NMBAs do not affect all muscles at the same time nor produce the same depth of relaxation. It is also important to note that NMBAs are administered to produce good intubating conditions, vocal cord paralysis, abdominal muscle relaxation, or diaphragmatic immobility. Yet, laryngeal muscles, abdominal muscles, and the diaphragm are not monitored. Understanding the relation between the response of the different muscles to the effects or NMBAs is therefore clinically important.

The APM is most commonly monitored (subjectively or objectively). Being a peripheral muscle, the onset time at the APM is longer than in centrally located muscles, where blood flow (and thus drug delivery) is greater. At the same time, APM is more sensitive to nondepolarizing NMBAs, so recovery is delayed in comparison to central muscles (diaphragm, laryngeal muscles). Even monitoring of similar, peripheral muscles can induce error: stimulation of the ulnar nerve produces flexion of the fifth finger as well as APM contraction. However, the recovery of the fifth finger contraction occurs more rapidly than at the APM, so making a clinical decision based on recovery of the fifth finger will overestimate the degree of recovery elsewhere.

When the patient's arms are not available for intraoperative monitoring, clinicians will monitor facial muscles: innervation of the facial nerve and evaluation of contractions of the eye muscles, either orbicularis oculi, or the corrugator supercilii. However, the time course of recovery is not the same for

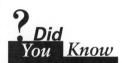

Did You Know

The eyebrow muscle, corrugator supercilii, has a similar time course of recovery to the laryngeal adductors.

these two facial muscles: orbicularis oculi move the eyelid and are similar in time course to APM.

Electrode Placement

For monitoring the APM, stimulating electrodes are placed along the ulnar nerve on the volar surface of the forearm. The distal (negative) electrode is placed 2 cm proximal to the wrist crease, and the proximal (positive) electrode is placed along the ulnar nerve, 3 to 4 cm proximal to the negative electrode.

A common clinical practice is to place the stimulating electrodes on the face and to monitor the eyelid (orbicularis oculi) muscle. Improper placement of electrodes on the temple and lower jaw leads to direct muscle stimulation and false assessment of neuromuscular recovery. In fact, current clinical practice of monitoring eye muscles has been shown to result in a fivefold increased risk of postoperative residual paralysis (7). Placement of the stimulating electrodes just lateral to the eye or along the zygomatic arch, as done most commonly, may activate other facial muscles and confound assessment. Facial nerve is best stimulated at the anterior portion of the mastoid process, as the nerve exits the skull, with the second electrode in front of the ear. Even with the optimal electrode positioning, however, muscle responses can be elicited despite complete block due to direct muscle stimulation.

Stimulation of the posterior tibial nerve along the medial malleolus produces flexion contraction of the great toe, which has a time course similar to APM.

F. Clinical Applications

Knowledge of time course for onset, duration, and recovery of neuromuscular block of NMBAs is important for optimal care. For assessing the quality of intubating conditions, monitoring of central muscles (or peripheral muscles with time course similar to central muscles) is paramount. When the dose of nondepolarizing NMBA is sufficiently large to offset the relative resistance of central muscles, onset at the laryngeal muscles will be faster than at the APM because of the greater blood flow (and drug delivery).

A special clinical challenge presents when surgery requires a deep (profound) level of intraoperative block. This can be accomplished with larger doses of nondepolarizing NMBAs but at the expense of markedly prolonging the duration of block and increasing the likelihood of residual neuromuscular block and its complications. If a level of block that prevents diaphragmatic movement is required, the depth of block can be monitored with PTC—a PTC of 1 or 2 should be sufficient for most surgeries. In contrast, spontaneous recovery of at least TOF count of 2 or 3 should have occurred before attempting pharmacologic reversal with anticholinesterases.

Patients managed with deep intraoperative block are particularly at risk for postoperative residual paralysis, which is associated with an increased risk of silent aspiration, hypoxemia, need for reintubation, and prolonged stay in the postanesthesia care unit (5). Recent studies have shown a significant reduction in forced vital capacity and peak expiratory flow in postanesthesia care unit patients who had received pharmacologic reversal with anticholinesterase agents and were deemed ready for tracheal extubation.

VIII. Reversal of Neuromuscular Blockade

A. Anticholinesterase Agents

Blocking the breakdown of ACh by AChAse results in an increase in the available pool of ACh at the synaptic cleft and better chances of competing with the nondepolarizing NMBA, resulting in normal transmission. There are three clinically available AChAse inhibitors (anticholinesterase agents): *neostigmine*, *edrophonium*, and *pyridostigmine*. Their duration of action, at equivalent doses, is similar (60 to 120 minutes), but onset of action is fastest for edrophonium, intermediate with neostigmine, and longest with pyridostigmine. Because edrophonium is even less effective at reversing deep block than neostigmine, it is used infrequently. Neostigmine is the most frequently used anticholinesterase agent today.

All cholinesterase inhibitors, including neostigmine, block AChAse at all cholinergic synapses and therefore have significant parasympathomimetic effects. For this reason, they are generally coadministered with either glycopyrrolate (preferred because of similar onset of action with neostigmine) or with atropine (which has a faster onset of tachycardia similar to edrophonium and crosses the blood–brain barrier). All cholinesterase inhibitors are quaternary compounds and do not cross the blood–brain barrier. Neostigmine, as a reversal agent, has a ceiling effect and may be limited in its ability to reverse the neuromuscular block beyond neuromuscular function equivalent to a TOF ratio of 0.6 (8).

B. Factors Affecting Neostigmine Reversal

The rate of neostigmine-aided recovery depends on several factors. When administered at a deep degree of block, such as PTC of 1 or 2, duration of neostigmine-induced reversal may be >50 to 60 minutes. In contrast, when administered at a TOF count of 4, reversal to TOF >0.90 may only take 15 to 20 minutes (although it may take as long as 60 to 90 minutes, especially in the presence of volatile anesthetics). Regardless of when administered, neostigmine-induced reversal is always faster than spontaneous recovery. Larger doses of neostigmine will also be more effective than lower doses in effecting neuromuscular block reversal, within the dose ranges in which neostigmine is effective (i.e., at doses less than the maximum 70 μg/kg). Although there is no difference in the speed of recovery induced by neostigmine among the intermediate-acting nondepolarizing NMBAs, reversal is prolonged when used with long-acting agents such as pancuronium. Age also affects neostigmine-induced speed of reversal, being faster (and likely more complete) in children than in adults and slower in the elderly. Finally, drugs and conditions that potentiate the effect of nondepolarizing NMBAs will also prolong the neostigmine-induced recovery: volatile anesthetics, aminoglycoside antibiotics, magnesium, opioids (because of hypercarbia and acidosis they induce), and hypothermia.

C. Neostigmine: Other Effects

Neostigmine (and the other anticholinesterases) induce vagal stimulation, so anticholinergic agents are usually coadministered. *Atropine* is faster in onset than *glycopyrrolate*, produces more tachycardia, and crosses the blood–brain barrier. For these reasons, glycopyrrolate is generally chosen. It is slower in onset and induces less of a tachycardic response, and for these reasons it is preferred in cardiac patients. Other side effects of neostigmine include increased salivation and bowel motility; although the anticholinergic agents are effective in preventing salivation, their effects on bowel motility are limited. Several recent meta-analyses of the effects of neostigmine on postoperative nausea and vomiting have not been able to conclusively show a connection.

D. Clinical Use

When the depth of block is deep (PTC of 1 or 2), neostigmine should not be administered. When spontaneous recovery is evident (TOF count of 2 or 3),

? Did You Know

Increasing the dose of neostigmine beyond 70 μg/kg is not recommended. This dose may induce neuromuscular dysfunction. At a time when recovery of neuromuscular function is almost complete, administration of even small doses of neostigmine (30 μg/kg) may produce upper airway collapse and decrease the activity of the genioglossus muscle, rendering the patient susceptible to aspiration.

a full dose could be contemplated, although administration of 50 µg/kg once TOF count is 4 would induce a faster and more complete recovery. When the TOF appears by subjective means to have no fade (or once the measured TOF is 0.4 and above), a small dose of neostigmine (20 µg/kg) is recommended. If the objectively measured *TOF is 0.9* or above, no neostigmine should be administered (5). Routine reversal with AChAse does not exclude significant residual weakness and it is therefore recommended to monitor the block objectively until TOF is >0.90.

E. Selective Relaxant Binding Agents: Sugammadex

Sugammadex is a γ-cyclodextrin that has been developed as a selective binding agent (9) and is currently not available for clinical use in the United States. It has a central cavity that perfectly encapsulates the steroid nucleus of steroidal intermediate-acting NMBAs (rocuronium > vecuronium >> pancuronium >> pipecuronium) but has no affinity for any of the other depolarizing or nonde-polarizing *NMBAs*. Binding to rocuronium is extremely tight, with no clini-cally relevant dissociation. Binding to vecuronium is one-third as tight, but because the equivalent vecuronium dose has one-sixth as many molecules as rocuronium, the effectiveness of reversal is similar for both drugs. The affin-ity to pancuronium (and pipecuronium) may be too low to attempt reversal with sugammadex. The sugammadex-rocuronium complexes are excreted via the kidneys, with an elimination half-life of 100 minutes. Currently, it is rec-ommended to wait 24 hours for repeated administration of rocuronium after sugammadex reversal of NMBAs. However, recent studies suggest earlier re-administration of rocuronium may be acceptable if a high dose of sugamma-dex has not been used.

Clinical Use, Side Effects, and Safety

Sugammadex is biologically inactive and does not have affinity for any known receptors; therefore, it is devoid of hemodynamic and coagulation side effects. Sugammadex has been marketed in Europe since 2009 without changes in its safety profile.

Studies have suggested that high-dose rocuronium for RSII and sugammadex-induced reversal may currently provide near-ideal neuromuscular block man-agement without significant side effects. In the morbidly obese patients, the dose of sugammadex has been calculated based on ideal body weight plus 40%. When used in the obese patient in suboptimal doses of 1 to 2 mg/kg, reparalysis has been reported. Importantly, if no neuromuscular monitor is used, there is a risk of significant residual weakness, even with administration of sugammadex 2 to 4 mg/kg. Therefore, monitoring neuromuscular function to determine the appropriate dose of sugammadex and minimize the risk of residual block is strongly recommended.

References

1. Naguib M, Flood P, McArdle JJ, et al. Advances in neurobiology of the neuromuscular junction: Implications for the anesthesiologist. *Anesthesiology.* 2002;96:202–231.
2. Dexter F, Epstein RH, Wachtel RE, et al. Estimate of the relative risk of succinylcholine for triggering malignant hyperthermia. *Anesth Analg.* 2013;116:118–122.
3. Andrews JI, Kumar N, van den Brom RH, et al. A large simple randomized trial of rocuronium versus succinylcholine in rapid-sequence induction of anaesthesia along with propofol. *Acta Anaesthesiol Scand.* 1999;43:4–8.
4. Viby-Mogensen J, Jensen NH, Engbaek J, et al. Tactile and visual evaluation of the response to train-of-four nerve stimulation. *Anesthesiology.* 1985;63:440–443.

5. Brull SJ, Murphy GS. Residual neuromuscular block: Lessons unlearned. Part II: Methods to reduce the risk of residual weakness. *Anesth Analg.* 2010;111:129–140.
6. Grosse-Sundrup M, Henneman JP, Sandberg WS, et al. Intermediate acting nondepolarizing neuromuscular blocking agents and risk of postoperative respiratory complications: Prospective propensity score matched cohort study. *BMJ.* 2012;345:e6329.
7. Thilen SR, Hansen BE, Ramaiah R, et al. Intraoperative neuromuscular monitoring site and residual paralysis. *Anesthesiology.* 2012;117:964–972.
8. Herbstreit F, Zigrahn D, Ochterbeck C, et al. Neostigmine/glycopyrrolate administered after recovery from neuromuscular block increases upper airway collapsibility by decreasing genioglossus muscle activity in response to negative pharyngeal pressure. *Anesthesiology.* 2010;113:1280–1288.
9. Schaller SJ, Fink H. Sugammadex as a reversal agent for neuromuscular block: An evidence-based review. *Core Evid.* 2013;8:57–67.

Questions

1. The release of acetylcholine "packets" are antagonized by:
   A. Hypercalcemia
   B. Hypermagnesemia
   C. Hypokalemia
   D. Hyponatremia

2. Clinically the potency of neuromuscular blocking drugs is expressed as:
   A. ED_{50}
   B. ED_{95}
   C. RI_{25-75}
   D. Duration of drug administration until recovery of TOF >0.9

3. A phase II block with succinylcholine exhibits the following characteristics EXCEPT:
   A. Fade to repetitive stimulation
   B. Posttetanic potentiation
   C. Reversed by an anticholinesterase
   D. Fade to double burst suppression 3,3

4. The most effective prophylaxis for postsuccinylcholine myalgia is:
   A. Nonsteroidal anti-inflammatory drugs
   B. Pretreatment with a nondepolarizing muscle relaxant
   C. Hydrocortisone
   D. Lidocaine

5. A 200-kg female is scheduled for exploratory laparotomy for intestinal obstruction. Your management plan calls for the use of a rapid sequence induction/intubation (RSII). The appropriate dose of succinylcholine for this patient is calculated on the basis of:
   A. Ideal body weight
   B. Actual body weight
   C. Body Mass Index
   D. ([Ideal body weight] + [Actual body weight])/2

6. The onset of action of nondepolarizing muscle relaxants is explained, in part by:
   A. Potency
   B. Higher ED_{95}
   C. The plasma/biophase concentration gradient
   D. Lower ED_{50}

7. By direct effects on the postjunctional receptors, which of the following inhalation agents potentiates the effects of rocuronium the most?
   A. Sevoflurane
   B. Desflurane
   C. Isoflurane
   D. Nitrous oxide

8. The administration of methylprednisolone (500 mg) to a 70-kg male intensive care patient with sepsis who is receiving vecuronium for ventilatory management will:
   A. Increase risk of myopathy
   B. Have no effect on incidence of myopathy
   C. Decrease risk of myopathy
   D. Not occur with rocuronium

9. An 80-kg patient has had a laparoscopic cholecystectomy with propofol/sevoflurane/rocuronium. The TOF is ≥0.90. She meets signs for extubation of the endotracheal tube. Your management includes:
   A. Neostigmine 2.5 mg plus 1.0 mg glycopyrrolate
   B. Neostigmine 5.0 mg plus 1.0 mg glycopyrrolate
   C. Edrophonium 20 mg
   D. No reversal of the rocuronium is indicated

10. You decide to administer an anticholinergic agent to a patient who has received a general anesthetic with pancuronium for muscle relaxation. Which reversal agent is most appropriate to administer with glycopyrrolate?
    A. Edrophonium
    B. Pyridostigmine
    C. Neostigmine
    D. Physostigmine

12

Local Anesthetics

Francis V. Salinas

Local anesthetics are a class of drugs that transiently and reversibly inhibit the conduction of sensory, motor, and autonomic neural impulses. Clinically, local anesthetics are primarily used to provide perioperative anesthesia or analgesia. This chapter presents the mechanism of action of local anesthetics, the physiochemical properties that determine their clinical pharmacology, clinical applications, and potential for toxicity. Relevant peripheral nerve anatomy and physiology are briefly reviewed here, with more detailed information presented in Chapter 4. Chapters 21 and 31 will present common clinical applications for local anesthetics.

I. Mechanism of Action of Local Anesthetics

A. Anatomy of Nerves

The neuron is the basic functional unit responsible for the conduction of neural impulses. It typically consists of a cell body attached to several branching processes (dendrites) and a single axon that carries neural impulses toward and away from the cell body (Fig. 12-1A). Axons are cylinders of axoplasm encased within a lipid bilayer cell membrane that is embedded with various proteins, including voltage-gated sodium (Na^+; VG_{Na}) channels. Glial cells (oligodendrocytes in the central nervous system [CNS] and Schwann cells in the peripheral nervous system) are closely associated with neurons and function to support, insulate, and nourish axons. A nerve fiber is composed of an axon, its associated glial cell, and the surrounding endoneural connective tissue.

Peripheral nerve fibers are organized within three layers of connective tissue (Fig. 12-1B). Individual nerve fibers are immediately surrounded by *endoneurium*, consisting of delicate connective tissue that consists of Schwann cells and fibroblasts along with capillaries. A dense layer of collagenous connective tissue, the *perineurium*, encloses bundles of nerve fibers into a fascicle. It functionally provides an effective barrier against penetration of the nerve fibers by foreign substances. The *epineurium* is also a dense connective tissue layer that surrounds and encases bundles of fascicles together into a cylindrical sheath

209

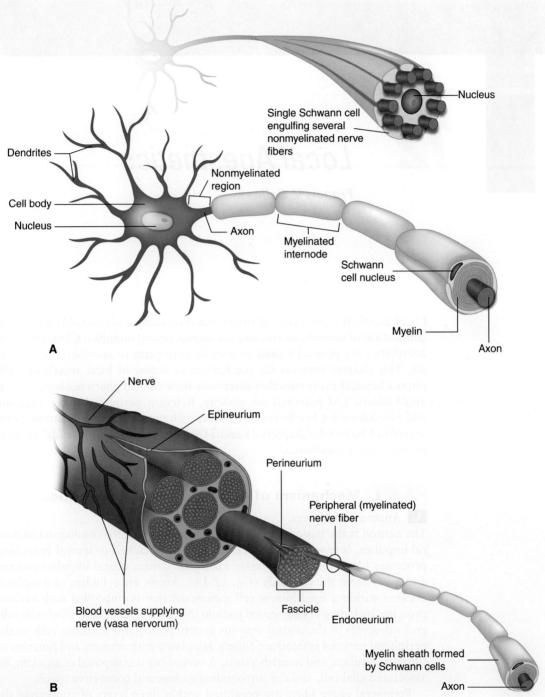

Figure 12-1 **A:** Representative neuron and myelinated and nonmyelinated axon. The neuron consists of a cell body (soma), dendrites, and an axon. Myelinated nerve fibers have a sheath composed of a continuous series of neurolemma (derived from Schwann cells) that surround the axon and form a series of myelin segments. Multiple nonmyelinated nerve fibers are individually encased within a single neurolemma that does not produce myelin. **B:** Arrangement of perineural connective tissue layers in a representative nerve. Peripheral nerves consist of bundles of nerve fibers, the layers of the connective tissues (endoneurium, perineurium, and epineurium) that serve to bind them, and associated blood vessels (vasa nervorum) that supply them. All but the smallest peripheral nerves are arranged in bundles called fascicles.

Table 12-1 Classification of Peripheral Nerve Fibers

Fiber Classification	Diameter (μm)	Myelination	Conduction Velocity (m/s)	Anatomical Location	Function	Local Anesthetic Susceptibility
Aα	6–22	Yes	30–120	Efferent to muscles	Motor	++
Aβ	6–22	Yes	30–120	Afferent from skin and joints	Touch and proprioception	++
Aγ	3–6	Yes	15–35	Efferent to muscle spindles	Muscle tone	++++
Aδ	1–4	Yes	5–25	Afferent sensory	Distinct, well-localized (fast) pain, cold temperature, touch	+++
B	<3	Yes	3–15	Preganglionic sympathetic	Autonomic	++
C	0.3–1.3	No	0.7–1.3	Afferent sensory, postganglionic sympathetic	Autonomic, warm temperature, touch, and diffuse (slow) pain	+

+ (least susceptible), ++, +++, ++++ (most susceptible) to conduction blockade.

structurally similar to a coaxial cable. An additional connective tissue layer that forms a *paraneural* sheath further encases peripheral nerves. Together, these tissue layers offer protection to peripheral nerves but also present a significant barrier to passive diffusion of local anesthetics toward the axonal cell membrane.

Peripheral nerves are mixed nerves containing both afferent and efferent nerve fibers that are either myelinated or nonmyelinated (Fig. 12-1A). The cell membrane (neurolemma) of Schwann cells envelops axons. Nonmyelinated nerve fibers consist of multiple axons that are simultaneously encased by the neurolemma of a single Schwann cell. Voltage-gated sodium channels (VG_{Na}) are uniformly distributed along the entire axon of nonmyelinated nerve fibers. In contrast, a myelinated nerve fiber is segmentally encased by a myelin sheath that is derived from a continuous series of neurolemma that concentrically wraps around a single axon. Specialized regions, known as the nodes of Ranvier, where the VG_{Na} are concentrated along the axons of myelinated nerve fibers, periodically interrupt the myelin sheath. Along myelinated axons, Na^+ conductance is restricted to the nodes of Ranvier. This allows action potential propagation to jump from one node to the next via saltatory conduction, which significantly enhances the speed of signal transmission (Table 12-1).

B. Electrophysiology of Neural Conduction and Voltage-gated Sodium Channels

Neurons maintain a resting membrane potential of approximately –60 to –70 mV. The Na^+-K^+ (potassium) pump actively cotransports three Na^+ ions out of the cell for every two K^+ ions into the cell. This creates an electro-chemical concentration gradient across the semipermeable cell membrane. The resulting ionic disequilibrium favors the movement of Na^+ ions into the cell and K^+ ions out of the cell. However, despite the concentration gradient for both ions, the resting cell membrane is relatively more permeable to K^+ ions. This facilitates a net passive efflux of K^+ ions out of the cell and leaves a relative net excess of negatively charged ions (polarized) within the axoplasm.

Neural impulses are conducted along axons as action potentials, which are transient membrane depolarizations initiated by various mechanical, chemical, or thermal stimuli. Depolarization is mediated primarily via rapid intracellular influx of Na^+ ions flowing down its electrochemical gradient through VG_{Na}. The VG_{Na} spans the axonal membrane and consists of an α-subunit and one or two varying auxiliary β-subunits. The α-subunit forms the ion-conducting pore of the VG_{Na} and it comprises four homologous domains (I to IV), each with six α-helical transmembrane segments. The loops that link the S5 and S6 segments of the α-helices of each of the four domains are located extracellular, extending inward to form the narrowest section of the channel pore. They are believed to provide its ion selectivity.

At the resting membrane potential, the channel pore is in a resting (closed) conformation. Upon an initial depolarization, movement of the S1-S4 voltage-sensing segments leads to rearrangement of the S6 segment. This results in activation (opening) of the channel pore, inducing a sudden increase in Na^+ ion permeability. The resultant rapid inward Na^+ current activates and opens additional VG_{Na}. This further accelerates depolarization until a threshold membrane potential is reached, triggering an action potential. During the depolarization phase, the inward Na^+ current flows into the axoplasm and spreads to the adjacent (inactive) cell membrane, resulting in a wave of sequential depolarization (and the action potential) propagating along the axon. Although the wave of depolarization spreads from the initial area of excitation in both directions, the just activated membrane behind the impulse is temporarily refractory to subsequent depolarization. Thus, the propagation of the impulse is unidirectional. The activated VG_{Na} is inactivated within milliseconds by an additional conformational change. This leads to binding of the cytoplasmic loop located between domains III and IV to the cytoplasmic opening of the VG_{Na} to form the rapid inactivation gate. The rapid inactivation gate functions as an intracellular blocking particle that folds into and blocks the channel pore. This rapid inactivation process is required for repetitive firing of action potentials in neural circuits and for control of excitability in neurons. Repolarization occurs due to a combination of a progressive decrease in the driving force for the inward Na^+ current and inactivation of VG_{Na}. In addition, membrane depolarization simultaneously activates voltage-gated K^+ channels. This leads to an outward positive current of K^+ ions, which in conjunction with VG_{Na} inactivation, eventually returns the axonal membrane to or just beyond (hyperpolarization) its resting membrane potential. In summary, inward positive currents, mediated by Na^+ ions, depolarize the membrane, and in contrast, outward positive currents, mediated by K^+ ions, repolarize the membrane.

C. Voltage-gated Sodium Channels and Interactions with Local Anesthetics

Local anesthetics act at the axonal membrane by binding to a specific region within the α-subunit. This prevents VG_{Na} activation, thus inhibiting the inward Na^+ current that mediates membrane depolarization. The binding site for local anesthetics is located within the channel pore and is formed from amino acid residues in the S6 segments of domains I, III, and IV. The binding site may be approached from two pathways: from the intracellular aspect of the channel pore (hydrophilic pathway) or laterally from within the lipid membrane (hydrophobic pathway). As the amount of administered local anesthetic increases, an increasing percentage of VG_{Na} bind to local anesthetics, further inhibiting the inward Na^+ current. Subsequently, the rate of depolarization (in response to stimulation) is attenuated, inhibiting the achievement of the threshold membrane potential. Consequently, achievement of an action potential becomes increasingly difficult. With a sufficient number of local anesthetic-bound VG_{Na}, an action potential can no longer be generated and impulse propagation is blocked. Local anesthetic binding to VG_{Na} does not alter the resting membrane potential nor does it alter the threshold potential.

Local anesthetics bind more avidly to VG_{Na} in the activated (open) and inactivated (channel pore is *open* but closed by movement of the inactivation gate) conformations. The difference in binding affinity is attributable to the difference in the availability of the two pathways for local anesthetic to reach the binding site. Local anesthetics produce a concentration-dependent decrease in inward Na^+ current characterized as *tonic blockade*, representing a decrease in the number of open confirmation VG_{Na} (1). With repeated depolarization, a greater number of VG_{Na} are in either the activated or inactivated conformations. Therefore, they can be bound at a given local anesthetic concentration. Additionally, the dissociation rate of local anesthetics from their binding site is slower than the rate of transition from the inactivated to the resting conformation. Thus, repeated stimulation results in accumulation of local anesthetic-bound VG_{Na} characterized as *frequency-dependent blockade*.

D. Mechanisms of Nerve Block

In order for local anesthetics to bind VG_{Na}, they must reach the neural membrane. Thus, local anesthetics must penetrate through variable amounts of perineural tissue and still maintain a sufficient concentration gradient to diffuse through the lipid bilayer. Only a small fraction (1% to 2%) of local anesthetic reaches the neural membrane even when deposited in close proximity to peripheral nerves. Peripheral nerves that have been desheathed in vitro require about a hundredfold lower local anesthetic concentration than peripheral nerves in vivo. In contrast, central neuraxial nerves are encased in three layers of meninges: the pia mater, arachnoid membrane, and dura mater. The pia mater is adherent to the nerves themselves and is separated from the arachnoid membrane by cerebrospinal fluid that fills the space between these two layers. The *subarachnoid* space, where the spinal nerves are only covered by the pia mater, is the target location for spinal anesthesia. The dura mater further encases the arachnoid membrane, forming the dural sac, a tough covering around the central neuraxis. The epidural space consists of everything located within the vertebral canal but outside the dural sac. The presence of the arachnoid membrane and dura mater result in tenfold higher local anesthetic dose requirements to produce complete epidural blockade compared with that required in the subarachnoid space.

The quality of nerve block is determined not only by the intrinsic potency of the chosen local anesthetic but also by the concentration and volume of the administered local anesthetic. The potency of a local anesthetic can be expressed as the minimum effective concentration required to establish complete nerve blockade. The volume of local anesthetic is also important, as a sufficient length of axon or successive nodes of Ranvier must be blocked in

? Did You Know

Not only do local anesthetics prevent nerve impulse propagation by adhering to binding sites on voltage-gated sodium channels in the cell membrane (tonic blockade), but they also dissociate from the binding site more slowly than the site can return to its resting conformation (frequency-dependent blockade).

order to inhibit regeneration of the neural impulse. This is due to the phenomenon of ***decremental conduction***. Membrane depolarization passively decays with distance away from the front of the action potential to the point that impulse propagation stops when depolarization falls below the threshold for VG_{Na} activation. If less than a critical length of axon is blocked, the action potential may still be regenerated in the proximal neural membrane segment or node of Ranvier when the decaying depolarization is still above the threshold potential.

Different types of nerve fibers demonstrate varying minimal blocking concentrations and local anesthetic susceptibilities (Table 12-1). Clinically, there is a predictable progression of sensory and motor function blockade, starting first with loss of temperature sensation, followed by proprioception, motor function, sharp pain, and lastly light touch. Termed ***differential block***, this progression was initially attributed to differences in axon diameter, with smaller fibers inherently more susceptible to conduction blockade compared with that of larger fibers. However, small myelinated fibers (Aγ and Aδ) are the most susceptible to conduction blockade. Next in order of block susceptibility are large myelinated fibers (Aα and Aβ), and the least susceptible are small, nonmyelinated C fibers.

Within peripheral nerves, longitudinal and radial diffusion of local anesthetic will produce varying drug concentrations along and within the nerve during the onset and recovery from clinical block. When local anesthetics are deposited around a peripheral nerve, diffusion progresses from the outer surface (mantle) toward the center (core) along a concentration gradient. Consequently, nerve fibers arranged in the mantle of mixed peripheral nerves are blocked initially. These outer nerve fibers are typically distributed to more proximal anatomic structures, whereas core fibers innervate more distal structures. This topographical arrangement explains the initial development of proximal, followed by distal anesthesia, as local anesthetic diffuses to the more centrally located core nerve fibers. In summary, the sequence of onset and recovery from peripheral nerve block depends on a combination of the topographical arrangement of the nerve fibers within a mixed peripheral nerve and their inherent susceptibility to local anesthetic blockade.

II. Local Anesthetic Pharmacodynamics

A. Physiochemical Properties and Relationship to Activity and Potency

Local anesthetics in solution are weak bases that typically carry a positive charge at the amine group at physiologic pH. The prototypical local anesthetic structure consists of a hydrophobic group (typically a lipid-soluble aromatic ring) connected to a hydrophilic group (charged amine) by either an amide or ester linkage (Fig. 12-2). The nature of the chemical bond is the basis for classification of local anesthetics as either an aminoamide or aminoester (Table 12-2). Although the nature of the linkage determines the basis for metabolism (aminoamides are metabolized in the liver, whereas aminoesters are metabolized by plasma cholinesterase), the physiochemical properties are largely determined by the nature of the alkyl substitutions on either the aromatic ring or the amine group, the charge of the amine group, or the stereochemistry of the related isomers (Table 12-2). These physiochemical properties largely determine the potency, onset and duration of action, and tendency for differential nerve block.

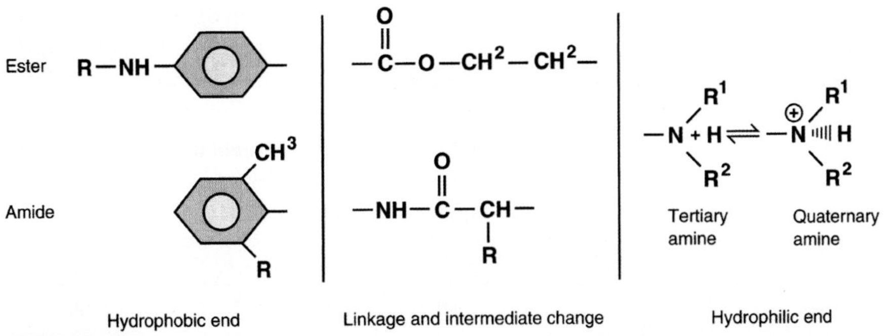

Figure 12-2 The prototypical structures of aminoester and aminoamide local anesthetics. (From Mulroy F, Bernards CM, McDonald SB, Salinas FV. A Practical Approach to Regional Anesthesia. 4th Edition. Philadelphia: Wolters Kluwer, 2009:2.)

Lipid solubility is determined by the degree of alkyl substitutions on either the aromatic ring or the amine group. Lipid solubility is typically expressed by the partition coefficient in a hydrophobic solvent (typically octanol). Compounds with increased octanol solubility are more lipid soluble (Table 12-2). Increased lipid solubility enhances the ability to penetrate the lipid membrane and deliver local anesthetic in closer proximity to the membrane bound VG_{Na}, which in turn correlates with the potency and, to a lesser extent, the duration of action. Although lipid solubility correlates with octanol solubility (and inherent potency in vitro), the minimum in vivo local anesthetic concentration that will block impulse conduction may be affected by numerous factors such as fiber size, type, and myelination, tissue pH (see below), local tissue redistribution and sequestration into lipid-rich perineural compartments, and inherent vasoactive properties of the specific local anesthetic.

At physiological pH, local anesthetics are weak bases that exist in equilibrium between either the lipid soluble base form or the water-soluble ionized form. The relative percentage of each form is determined by the dissociation constant (pKa) and surrounding tissue pH. The pKa is the pH at which the percentage of each form is equal (Table 12-2), which is defined by the Henderson-Hasselbalch equation:

$$pKa = pH + \log [BH^+]/[B]$$

where $[BH^+]$ is the concentration of the charged, lipid-insoluble form of the local anesthetic, and $[B]$ is the concentration of the uncharged lipid-soluble form of local anesthetic.

The lower the pKa for a given local anesthetic, the higher the percentage of the lipid-soluble base form that exists to more readily penetrate the lipid cell membrane, thus speeding the onset of action. After penetration through the cell membrane into the axoplasm, equilibrium between the base form and the charged form is re-established. It is the charged form within the axoplasm that more avidly binds to local anesthetic binding sites within the channel pore of the VG_{Na}.

The majority of clinically useful local anesthetics are formulated as racemic compounds. These are one-to-one mixtures of enantiomeric stereoisomers bearing identical chemical composition, but with a different three-dimensional spatial orientation around an asymmetric carbon atom. Although enantiomers of local anesthetics have identical physiochemical properties, they exhibit different clinical pharmacodynamics (potency) due to subtle differences in interaction and binding of VG_{Na}. For example, levobupivacaine (the S-enantiomer

Table 12-2   Chemical Structure and Physiochemical Properties of Clinically Useful Local Anesthetic Agents

Local Anesthetic	Chemical Structure	Partition Coefficient (Lipid Solubility)	pKa	Percentage Ionized at pH 7.4	Percentage Protein Bound
Aminoamides					
Lidocaine		366	7.9	76	65
Prilocaine		129	7.9	76	55
Mepivacaine		130	7.6	61	78
Bupivacaine		3420	8.1	83	96
Ropivacaine		775	8.1	83	94
Aminoesters					
Procaine		100	8.9	97	6
2-Chloroprocaine		810	8.7	95	N/A
Tetracaine		5822	8.5	93	76

of bupivacaine) and ropivacaine (the S-enantiomer of the bupivacaine, but with a propyl alkyl group rather than the butyl group found in bupivacaine) appear to have equipotent clinical efficacy for neuronal conduction block. However, they have a lower potential for cardiac systemic toxicity than either the R-enantiomer or the racemic mixtures.

B. Additives to Augment Local Anesthetic Activity

Local anesthetics are formulated as hydrochloride salts to increase their solubility and stability. The pH of commercially prepared local anesthetic solutions ranges from 3.9 to 6.47 and is especially acidic when prepackaged with epinephrine (see below). Given that the pKa of the most commonly used local anesthetics ranges from 7.6 to 8.9 (Table 12-2), <3% of the local anesthetic solution is in the lipid-soluble neutral form at physiologic pH. This slows penetration through the cell membrane and delays the onset of conduction block. An even lower lipid-soluble fraction may be encountered clinically when local anesthetics are injected into infected tissues that have a more acidic pH. Thus, alkalinization of local anesthetic solutions by the addition of sodium bicarbonate may potentially increase the onset and the quality of conduction block by increasing the percentage of lipid-soluble base form. Clinical experience demonstrates that the addition of sodium bicarbonate may speed the onset of intermediate-acting local anesthetics (lidocaine and mepivacaine). However, this modification has minimal effect with the longer acting, more potent amide local anesthetics (bupivacaine or ropivacaine) (2).

Epinephrine is commonly added to local anesthetic solutions to induce vasoconstriction at the site of injection. The α_1-adrenoreceptor–mediated vasoconstrictive effect of epinephrine augments local anesthetic activity by antagonizing the inherent vasodilating effect of most local anesthetics. Consequently, decreased vascular absorption facilitates and maintains intraneural local anesthetic uptake. The reported clinical benefits include enhancement of the quality of conduction block and prolongation of the duration of action. It also decreases the peak systemic local anesthetics levels, potentially limiting toxic effects (3). The extent to which epinephrine prolongs the duration of conduction block largely depends on the physiochemical properties of the local anesthetic as well as the site of injection. For example, the addition of epinephrine to lidocaine typically extends the conduction block by at least 50%, but the addition of epinephrine to bupivacaine has little or no clinically relevant effect on the duration of blockade. Additional analgesic effects due to epinephrine (and clonidine) may also occur through interaction with α_2-adrenoreceptors in the CNS, directly activating endogenous analgesic mechanisms.

Clonidine is a direct-acting α_2-agonist, but it also possesses direct inhibitory effects on neural conduction (A and C peripheral nerve fibers) (4). In contrast to epinephrine, clonidine will improve the duration of conduction block, regardless of whether lidocaine or bupivacaine is used. However, potential clonidine-associated side effects of bradycardia and orthostatic hypotension have limited its more widespread clinical use.

III. Local Anesthetic Pharmacokinetics

Local anesthetics are most commonly delivered to extravascular tissue in close proximity to the intended target site. The resulting plasma concentration is influenced by the total dose of administered local anesthetic, the extent of systemic absorption, tissue redistribution, and the rate of elimination. Patient-specific factors such as age, cardiovascular and hepatic function, and plasma protein binding also influence subsequent plasma levels. An understanding of these factors should maximize the clinical application of local anesthetics, while minimizing potential complications associated with toxic systemic drug levels.

A. Systemic Absorption

In general, decreased systemic local anesthetic absorption provides a greater margin of safety in clinical practice. The rate and extent of systemic absorption are influenced by a number of factors, including total local anesthetic dose, site of administration, physiochemical properties of individual local anesthetics, and addition of vasoconstrictors (epinephrine). For any given site of administration, the greater the total dose of local anesthetic, the greater the extent of systemic absorption and peak plasma levels (C_{max}). Furthermore, an increased rate of absorption will also decrease the time to peak plasma levels (T_{max}). Within the clinical range of commonly used doses, the dose–response relationship is nearly linear and is relatively unaffected by anesthetic concentration or speed of injection. The extent of perineural tissue perfusion significantly influences systemic absorption, so that local anesthetic administration in highly perfused perineural tissues results in higher C_{max} and shorter T_{max}. Thus, the rate of systemic absorption from highest to lower is intrapleural > intercostal > caudal > epidural > brachial plexus > sciatic/femoral > and subcutaneous tissue. The rate of systemic absorption is also influenced by the physiochemical properties of the individual local anesthetic agents. In general, the more potent, lipid-soluble local anesthetics will result in decreased systemic absorption. The greater the lipid solubility, the more likely it will be sequestered in the lipid-rich compartments of both the axonal membrane and perineural tissues. The effects of epinephrine have been previously discussed and counteract the inherent vasodilator characteristics of most local anesthetics. The reduction in C_{max} associated with epinephrine is more pronounced for the less lipid-soluble local anesthetics, while increased neural and perineural tissue binding may be a greater determinant of systemic absorption with increased lipid solubility.

B. Distribution

After systemic absorption, local anesthetics are rapidly distributed throughout all body tissues and can be described by a two-compartment model (see Chapter 7). The pattern of distribution (and relative tissue concentration) is influenced by the perfusion, partition coefficient, and mass of specific tissue compartments. The highly perfused organs (brain, lung, heart, liver, and kidneys) are responsible for the initial rapid uptake (α-phase), which is followed by a slower redistribution (β-phase) to less perfused tissues (muscle and gut). In particular, the lung extracts significant amounts of local anesthetic. Consequently, C_{max} and the threshold for systemic toxic effects require much lower doses of local anesthetics following arterial injections compared with that for venous injections.

C. Elimination

The chemical linkage determines the biotransformation and elimination of local anesthetics (see Fig. 12-2). Aminoamides are metabolized in the liver by cytochrome P-450 enzymes via N-dealkylation and hydroxylation. Aminoamide metabolism is highly dependent on hepatic perfusion, hepatic extraction, and enzyme function. Therefore, local anesthetic clearance is decreased by conditions such as cirrhosis and congestive heart failure. Excretion of the aminoamide metabolites occurs by renal excretion, with <5% of unmetabolized local anesthetic excreted by the kidney. Prilocaine is the only aminoamide local anesthetic that is hydrolyzed to o-toluidine, which can oxidize hemoglobin to methemoglobin in a dose-dependent fashion. Prilocaine doses as low as 8 mg/kg may be expected to produce sufficient methemoglobin levels to cause cyanosis (methemoglobinemia).

Aminoester local anesthetics are rapidly metabolized by plasma cholinesterase. Procaine and benzocaine are metabolized to *para-aminobenzoic acid (PABA)*, which has been associated with rare anaphylactic reactions with the use of these local anesthetics. Patients with genetically abnormal plasma cholinesterase or those who are taking cholinesterase inhibitors have decreased aminoester metabolism. They would theoretically be at increased risk for systemic toxic effects, but clinical evidence is lacking.

D. Clinical Pharmacokinetics

The metabolism of local anesthetics is of significant clinical relevance as systemic toxicity (determined principally by C_{max}) depends on the balance between systemic absorption and elimination. Local anesthetics are largely bound to tissue and plasma proteins, yet systemic toxicity is related to the free (unbound) plasma concentration. Thus, plasma protein binding of local anesthetics reduces the free concentration in the systemic circulation and also reduces the risk of systemic toxicity. The extent of plasma protein binding is primarily dependent on the level of α_1-acid glycoprotein and albumin, and it is also influenced by the pH of the plasma. Clinical conditions that decrease plasma proteins (cirrhosis, pregnancy, newborn status) decrease binding capacity. Furthermore, the percentage of protein binding decreases as the pH decreases. Thus, in the presence of acidosis (seizures, cardiac arrest, renal failure), the amount of unbound drug increases. Altered hepatic clearance may also influence the elimination of local anesthetics. For example, neonates have immature hepatic microsomal enzymes, leading to decreased elimination of aminoamide local anesthetics. Some medications such as beta-blockers, H_2 receptors, and fluvoxamine inhibit specific hepatic microsomal enzymes and may also contribute to decreased aminoamide local anesthetic metabolism. All of the previously described factors that influence systemic absorption, distribution, and patient-specific factors should be taken into account to minimize the risk for systemic toxicity. These factors form the basis for current recommendations of "maximal doses" of local anesthetics (5).

IV. Toxicity of Local Anesthetics

Clinically significant adverse effects of local anesthetics include local anesthetic systemic toxicity (LAST), local tissue toxicity, allergic reactions, and local anesthetic-specific effects. LAST results from excessive plasma concentrations of local anesthetic, either due to unintentional direct intravascular injection or from systemic absorption of larger doses of local anesthetics performed during peripheral nerve blocks, epidural anesthesia, or even large-volume infiltration (*tumescent*) anesthesia. As previously discussed, plasma concentration is determined by the balance between systemic absorption and elimination. Clinically significant symptoms of LAST manifest primarily in the CNS and cardiovascular system (CVS).

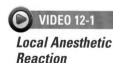

VIDEO 12-1

Local Anesthetic Reaction

A. Central Nervous System Toxicity

Local anesthetics readily cross the blood–brain barrier and produce dose-dependent signs and symptoms of CNS toxicity. Initial symptoms may include drowsiness, circumoral numbness, facial tingling, restlessness, tinnitus, or auditory hallucinations. Objective signs of progressive CNS excitation may manifest as tremors or muscle twitching and can progress to generalized tonic-clonic convulsions (6). If local anesthetic plasma levels are sufficiently elevated or the rate of rise is rapid, CNS excitation may progress to generalized CNS depression, leading to coma or respiratory or even cardiac arrest. The apparent biphasic pattern of CNS toxicity reflects neuronal depression by local anesthetics. At lower plasma concentrations, selective depression of cortical inhibitory neurons permits relatively unopposed actions of excitatory neurons, manifesting as CNS excitation. In contrast, markedly elevated plasma levels reflect the added inhibition of excitatory neurons and present clinically as profound CNS depression. The potential for CNS toxicity directly parallels the intrinsic potency of local anesthetics and can be augmented by various clinical factors. Untreated convulsions, for example, can rapidly cause both respiratory and metabolic acidosis, increasing the risk for CNS toxicity by decreasing plasma protein binding, increasing cerebral perfusion, and favoring intracellular trapping of the uncharged form of the local anesthetic.

B. Cardiovascular System Toxicity

In general, significantly larger doses of local anesthetics are required to produce CVS toxicity compared with the doses needed for CNS toxicity. Local anesthetic–induced CVS toxicity can lead to hemodynamic instability due to a combination of direct myocardial depression, direct arteriolar vasodilation, the potential to cause significant dysrhythmias, and impaired autonomic regulation of the CVS system. Similar to CNS toxicity, the more potent lipid-soluble local anesthetics appear to have greater inherent CVS toxicity compared with the less potent local anesthetics. For example, the ratio of the dose required for irreversible CVS collapse relative to that required for CNS toxicity is much lower for bupivacaine than for lidocaine. Additionally, the more potent lipid soluble agents (e.g., bupivacaine) produce a different pattern of CVS toxicity compared with the less potent agents. At progressively increasing plasma concentrations, all local anesthetics can cause hypotension, myocardial depression, and dysrhythmias. However, toxic levels of bupivacaine can result in sudden cardiovascular collapse caused by malignant ventricular dysrhythmias that are often resistant to traditional resuscitation protocols.

The more potent lipid-soluble local anesthetics display greater potential for direct electrophysiologic toxicity (prolongation of the PR and QRS intervals). Although all local anesthetics block the conduction system through a dose-dependent block of cardiac VG_{Na}, several features of bupivacaine's Na^+ channel blocking abilities may enhance its CVS toxicity. First, bupivacaine exhibits a much stronger binding affinity to resting and inactivated cardiac VG_{Na} compared with that for lidocaine. Second, although all local anesthetics bind to VG_{Na} during systole and subsequently dissociate during diastole, bupivacaine dissociates much slowly compared with lidocaine. Bupivacaine dissociates slowly enough that there is inadequate time during diastole for complete recovery of VG_{Na}, and conduction block accumulates with successive cardiac cycles (7). In contrast, lidocaine completely dissociates with each cardiac cycle, and minimal accumulation of conduction block occurs. Lastly, bupivacaine displays a greater degree of direct myocardial depression compared with that for lidocaine or ropivacaine. Ropivacaine's safer CVS toxicity profile compared with that for bupivacaine stems from a combination of its slightly decreased potency due to its chemical structure (propyl alkyl substitution compared to butyl alkyl substitution on bupivacaine) as well as its formulation as the less cardiotoxic single S-enantiomer.

C. Treatment of Local Anesthetic Systemic Toxicity

LAST is best managed by preventing the occurrence of toxic plasma levels of local anesthetics by using the minimum effective dose required for a specific regional anesthetic technique, vigilance for inadvertent direct intravascular injection, and awareness of the early signs and symptoms of LAST. The basic treatment needed for CNS toxicity is initially supportive. Maintenance of adequate oxygenation and ventilation is mandatory, and if needed, the airway may be secured. Generalized tonic-clonic convulsions rapidly lead to metabolic acidosis, and their associated hypoventilation leads to hypoxemia and hypercapnea, all of which can exacerbate CNS toxicity. Convulsions that persist despite adequate oxygenation and ventilation should be promptly treated with titrated doses of the most readily available sedative hypnotic agent (such as midazolam [0.05 to 0.1 mg/kg] or propofol [0.5 to 1.5 mg/kg]) (8). If convulsions are not readily terminated with appropriate doses of sedative hypnotic agents, a neuromuscular blocker (typically succinylcholine) should be administered to terminate the intense muscular activity and attenuate worsening metabolic acidosis. It should be noted that neuromuscular blockade, however, does not decrease CNS excitation associated with CNS toxicity.

In the event of CVS toxicity, prompt attention should be turned to maintaining adequate oxygenation and, more important, coronary perfusion pressure. Local anesthetics themselves do not irreversibly damage cardiac myocytes. Experimental evidence demonstrates that with adequate coronary perfusion, bupivacaine promptly leaves cardiac tissue with a simultaneous return of normal cardiac function (8). In the event of cardiac arrest due to LAST, standard advanced cardiac life support measures should be instituted with the following modifications: vasopressin is not recommended, smaller initial epinephrine dosing (10 to 100 µg) is preferred, and if ventricular dysrhythmias develop, amiodarone is preferred instead of lidocaine.

Severe bupivacaine-induced CVS toxicity often remains refractory to standard resuscitation efforts. Cardiopulmonary bypass was previously considered the only modality to effectively treat the associated life-threatening malignant dysrhythmias and cardiovascular collapse. However, experimental animal data first demonstrated that intravenous intralipid emulsion (ILE) can significantly attenuate bupivacaine-induced CVS toxicity, followed by numerous case reports of successful rapid resuscitation with ILE administration in cases of severe CVS toxicity from both bupivacaine and ropivacaine (9). ILE has also been used to treat CNS toxicity, and in doing so, it may theoretically prevent progression to CVS toxicity. Although the mechanisms by which ILE reverses severe LAST are not completely understood, the primary mechanism is believed to be related to its ability to extract and partition highly lipid-soluble local anesthetics from affected tissues (myocardium) into a plasma lipid compartment (known as lipid sink). ILE has also been demonstrated to exert direct cardiotonic effects, which contribute to the rapid recovery from CVS toxicity.

D. Neural Toxicity and Myotoxicity

Direct neural toxicity has been described with clinical application of multiple local anesthetic agents (10). Case reports of cauda equina syndrome associated with the administration of high concentrations of lidocaine through spinal microcatheters began to appear in the late 1980s. Subsequent in vitro and in vivo investigations suggested that a combination of maldistribution (pooling) and high doses of local anesthetics led to neurotoxic concentrations localized to the lumbosacral subarachnoid space. Similarly, 2-chloroprocaine was associated with cauda equina syndrome in the 1980s, with the mechanism linked to the preservative used at that time (sodium metabisulfite) when large doses were accidentally administered into the subarachnoid space during attempted epidural administration. Subsequently, 2-chloroprocaine was reformulated as a preservative-free solution.

Transient neurologic symptoms (TNS) are associated with the subarachnoid administration of local anesthetics (most notably lidocaine) and characterized by transient pain or sensory abnormalities in the lower back radiating to the lower extremities and buttocks (10). Additional risk factors for TNS include surgical lithotomy position and ambulatory surgical procedures. Overall, there appears to be a paucity of electrophysiologic evidence to support a direct neurotoxic mechanism for TNS. Furthermore, effective treatment modalities, such as nonsteroidal anti-inflammatory drugs or trigger point injections, indicate a myofascial rather than a neuropathic mechanism for TNS.

Local anesthetics have also been shown to cause direct toxic effects to muscle tissue, leading to destruction of myocytes (11). Despite the predictable nature of muscle damage, local anesthetic myotoxicity is only rarely a clinical problem, as complete muscle regeneration typically occurs within 3 to 4 weeks. Risk factors include potency of the individual local anesthetic agent, direct intramuscular injection, and dose, which is exacerbated with serial or continuous administration. A notable exception to the generally low clinical consequence of local anesthetic myotoxicity is extraocular muscle damage, where there is a reported 0.25% incidence of prolonged extraocular muscle dysfunction (diplopia) after regional anesthesia for ocular surgery.

E. Allergic Reactions

True immune-mediated allergic reactions to local anesthetics are rare, but they occur more commonly, with the vast majority associated with aminoester local anesthetics, most likely due to their metabolism to the pure allergen PABA. Some preparations of aminoamide local anesthetics also contain methylparaben, which has a similar chemical structure to PABA and is the most likely cause of allergic reactions to aminoamide local anesthetics.

V. Local Anesthetic Agents and Their Common Clinical Applications

A. Aminoamide Local Anesthetics
Lidocaine

Lidocaine was the first widely used local anesthetic and remains the most commonly used local anesthetic. It may be used for infiltration, intravenous regional anesthesia (Bier's block), peripheral nerve block, and central neuraxial (subarachnoid and epidural) anesthesia. It is characterized by a rapid to intermediate onset of action and intermediate duration of action for peripheral nerve blocks and epidural anesthesia. Although concerns over TNS have led to decreased use for subarachnoid anesthesia, it remains popular for epidural anesthesia. Lidocaine may be applied topically as a jelly, an ointment, a patch, or in aerosol form to anesthetize the upper airway. Intravenous injections targeting relatively low plasma levels (<5 µg/mL) produce systemic analgesia and have been used as an adjunct to blunt the sympathetic response to laryngoscopy and intubation.

One of its most common uses involves intravenous injection to decrease the discomfort associated with intravenous administration of propofol. Lidocaine infusions have been administered to treat chronic neuropathic pain as well as acute postoperative pain. More recently, lidocaine (5% patch) was U.S. Food and Drug Administration (FDA) approved for the treatment of chronic pain associated with neuropathic postherpetic neuralgia. The patch is a topical delivery system designed to deliver low doses of lidocaine to superficially involved nociceptors in an amount that produces analgesia devoid of sensorimotor block.

Mepivacaine

Mepivacaine has a chemical structure combining the piperidine ring of cocaine with the xylidine ring of lidocaine. It shares a similar clinical profile to lidocaine but with a slightly longer duration of action because it results in less vasodilation. It is relatively ineffective when applied topically. As a spinal anesthetic agent, it appears to have a lower, although not clinically insignificant, incidence of TNS compared with that of lidocaine. Metabolism in the fetus and neonate is prolonged and, therefore, it is not used for obstetric analgesia.

Prilocaine

Prilocaine also has a similar clinical profile to lidocaine and is used for infiltration, peripheral nerve blocks, and spinal and epidural anesthesia. Due to its high clearance, it demonstrates the least systemic toxicity of all the amide local anesthetics and is therefore potentially useful for intravenous regional anesthesia. However, administration of higher doses (>500 to 600 mg) may result in methemoglobinemia. Clinically significant methemoglobinemia may be effectively treated with intravenous administration of methylene blue (1 to 2 mg/kg). Nonetheless, concerns over methemoglobinemia and lack of FDA approval have limited more widespread clinical use.

Bupivacaine

Bupivacaine is a more lipid-soluble, structural homologue of mepivacaine due to a butyl group, rather than a methyl group, on its piperidine ring. Thus, it is characterized by a relatively slower onset compared with that of lidocaine, but it has an extended duration of action. It provides prolonged sensory anesthesia and analgesia that typically outlasts the duration and intensity of its motor block, especially with the use of lower concentrations in continuous infusions. This characteristic has established bupivacaine as the most widely used local anesthetic for labor epidural analgesia and for acute postoperative pain management. Single injections for peripheral nerve block applications may provide surgical anesthesia for up to 12 hours and sensory analgesia lasting as long as 24 hours. It is widely used for subarachnoid anesthesia, typically with duration of action of 2 to 3 hours and, in contrast to lidocaine or mepivacaine, it has rarely been associated with TNS.

Ropivacaine

Ropivacaine is another structural homologue of mepivacaine and bupivacaine, but with a propyl group on its piperidine ring, and it is also formulated as an S-enantiomer. Together, these two characteristics result in clinically equivalent potency for neural blockade, but with a less cardiotoxic profile compared with that for bupivacaine. It has an inherent vasoconstricting effect, which may contribute to its reduced cardiotoxic profile and possibly augment its duration of action. Although there is some evidence to suggest that ropivacaine may produce a more favorable sensorimotor differential block compared with bupivacaine, the lack of equivalent potency hinders true comparisons. Overall, the clinical profile is similar to bupivacaine, taking into account its decreased potency compared with that of bupivacaine.

B. Aminoester Local Anesthetics

Procaine

Procaine was used primarily for infiltration and spinal anesthesia during the first half of the 20th century. Its low potency, relatively slow onset of action (likely due to its high pKa), and short duration of action limit the widespread use of procaine. Concerns regarding TNS with lidocaine prompted a renewed interest in the use of procaine for intermediate duration subarachnoid anesthesia. Despite its lower incidence of TNS compared with that of lidocaine, the increased risk of block failure and associated nausea have limited its clinical utility.

2-Chloroprocaine

Due to its relative low potency and extremely rapid metabolism by plasma cholinesterases, 2-chloroprocaine may be used in relatively higher concentrations (2% to 3%), yet with the lowest potential for systemic toxicity of all the clinically useful local anesthetic agents. Despite its relatively high pKa, the use of relatively higher concentrations results in rapid onset of surgical anesthesia. This characteristic, along with virtually no transmission to the fetus, makes it particularly useful when a rapid onset of surgical epidural anesthesia (i.e., urgent or emergent cesarean delivery) is required. The preservative-free solution of 2-chloroprocaine is gaining increased popularity for ambulatory subarachnoid anesthesia, where a rapid onset of action along with a predictably short duration of action is desired. Furthermore, the use of 2-chlororprocaine has been associated with very low incidence of TNS. Although 2-chloroprocaine has recently been approved for subarachnoid anesthesia in Europe, it has not received FDA approval and its use for this indication in the United States remains off-label.

Tetracaine

Tetracaine is a potent aminoester local anesthetic, characterized by a slow onset and long duration of action. In contrast to bupivacaine, the duration of action of tetracaine is significantly prolonged with the addition of a vasoconstrictor. Due to its slow onset of action and lack of sensorimotor dissociation (resulting in significant motor blockade), it is rarely indicated for epidural anesthesia or peripheral nerve block, and its primary clinical application is for extended duration subarachnoid anesthesia.

Cocaine

Cocaine is the only naturally occurring local anesthetic agent. Current clinical applications for cocaine are largely restricted to topical anesthesia for ear, nose, and throat procedures, where its intense vasoconstriction is clinically useful to reduce bleeding when instrumenting the nasopharynx. Cocaine inhibits the neuronal reuptake of norepinephrine, mediating its neurogenic vasoconstrictive effects. But it can also result in significant cardiovascular side effects, such as hypertension, tachycardia, and dysrhythmias. Concerns regarding its potential for cardiovascular toxicity, along with its potential for diversion and abuse, have markedly limited its clinical use.

Eutectic Mixture of Local Anesthetics

A eutectic mixture of lidocaine and prilocaine, each at a 2.5% concentration, is formulated as viscous liquid (eutectic mixture of local anesthetics [EMLA] cream). This mixture has a lower melting point than either individual local anesthetic, allowing it to exist as oil at room temperature, facilitating its penetration and absorption through dermis. EMLA cream is primarily used to provide dermal analgesia, and it is particularly useful in decreasing the pain associated with venipuncture or placement of a peripheral intravascular catheter. EMLA cream should only be applied to intact skin surfaces as application to breached skin may lead to unpredictably rapid systemic absorption.

References

1. Scholz A. Mechanisms of (local) anaesthetics on voltage-gated sodium and other ion channels. *Br J Anaesth*. 2002;89:52–61.
2. Lambert DH. Clinical value of adding sodium bicarbonate to local anesthetics. *Reg Anesth Pain Med*. 2002;27:328–329.
3. Neal JM. Effects of epinephrine in local anesthetics on the central and peripheral nervous system. *Reg Anesth Pain Med*. 2003;28:124–134.
4. Brummett CM, Williams BA. Additives to local anesthetics for peripheral nerve block. *Int Anesthesiol Clin*. 2011;49:104–116.
5. Rosenberg PH, Veering BT, Urmey WF. Maximum recommended doses of local anesthetics: A multifactorial concept. *Reg Anesth Pain Med*. 2004;29:564–575.
6. Di Gregorio G, Neal JM, Rosenquist RW, et al. Clinical presentation of local anesthetic systemic toxicity: A review of published cases, 1979 to 2009. *Reg Anesth Pain Med*. 2010;35:181–187.
7. Clarkson CW, Hondeghem LM. Mechanisms for bupivacaine depression of cardiac conduction: Fast block of sodium channels during the action potential with slow recovery from block during diastole. *Anesthesiology*. 1985;62:396–405.
8. Weinberg GL. Treatment of local anesthetic systemic toxicity. *Reg Anesth Pain Med*. 2010;35:188–193.
9. Weinberg GL. Lipid emulsion infusion: resuscitation for local anesthetic and other drugs. *Anesthesiology*. 2012;117:180–187.
10. Pollock JE. Neurotoxicity of intrathecal local anaesthetics and transient neurological symptoms. *Best Pract Res Clin Anaesthesiol*. 2003;17:471–484.
11. Zink W, Graf BM. Local anesthetic myotoxicity. *Reg Anesth Pain Med*. 2004;29:333–340.

Questions

1. In a myelinated nerve fiber, local anesthetics slow the rate of cell depolarization and prevent achievement of an action potential by which of the following mechanisms?
   A. Binding to voltage-gated Na^+ channels in the axonal membrane under the myelin sheath
   B. Binding to voltage-gated K^+ channels anywhere in the axonal membrane
   C. Binding to voltage-gated Na^+ channels in the axonal membrane at the nodes of Ranvier
   D. Altering the cell threshold potential such that an action potential is more difficult to achieve

2. When deposited in close proximity to a peripheral nerve, what fraction of the administered local anesthetic reaches the actual neural membrane and can participate in voltage-gated Na^+ channel blockade?
   A. ~2%
   B. ~10%
   C. ~50%
   D. ~99%

3. The pKa of a new, commercially prepared local anesthetic is 8.0; as a result, only a small fraction of the solution exists in lipid-soluble form at physiologic pH. Which of the following maneuvers will increase the lipid-soluble fraction of the solution (thereby improving the speed of onset and quality of conduction block)?
   A. Injecting the local anesthetic solution into infected tissue
   B. Adding 1 mL of sodium bicarbonate to 9 mL of local anesthetic solution
   C. Adding 50 mcg of epinephrine to 10 mL of local anesthetic solution
   D. Injecting the local anesthetic at a rapid rate

4. A 72-year-old, otherwise healthy man is scheduled for an open right thoracotomy and right middle lobectomy for a single cancerous lesion. Preoperatively, the surgeon inquires about alternatives for postoperative regional analgesia and asks specifically which of the following options has the LEAST risk for local anesthetic systemic toxicity:
   A. Thoracic epidural block with 15 mL 0.25% bupivacaine
   B. Multiple intercostal nerve blocks with a total of 15 mL 0.25% bupivacaine
   C. Thoracic epidural block with 10 mL 0.5% bupivacaine
   D. Multiple intercostal nerve blocks with a total of 10 mL 0.5% bupivacaine

5. Due to the topographic arrangement of nerve fibers within the sciatic nerve, an appropriate dose of local anesthetic delivered in close proximity to the nerve will result in sensation loss to the skin on the sole of the foot before the skin on the proximal calf. TRUE or FALSE?
   A. True
   B. False

6. All of the following statements regarding the elimination of aminoamide local anesthetics are true EXCEPT:
   A. Aminoamides are metabolized by cytochrome P-450 pathways in the liver
   B. Renal elimination of unmetabolized aminoamides is limited (<5%)
   C. Plasma cholinesterase deficiency slows the metabolism of aminoamides
   D. Aminoamide metabolites can convert hemoglobin to methemoglobin

7. A 57-year-old female with chronic hepatitis C and cirrhosis requires open reduction and internal fixation of a distal radius fracture. She has normal coagulation function but is hypoalbuminemic. Which of the following statements is TRUE regarding perioperative anesthesia and analgesia with a single-shot infraclavicular block using 30 mL 0.5% ropivacaine?
   A. Hypoalbuminemia lowers her risk of local anesthetic systemic toxicity
   B. Impaired hepatic metabolism lowers her risk of local anesthetic systemic toxicity
   C. Ropivacaine carries a lesser risk of local anesthetic systemic toxicity compared with an equivalent dose of bupivacaine
   D. Adding epinephrine to the ropivacaine solution will prolong the duration of the block

8. A 29-year-old otherwise healthy 90-kg male is scheduled for open repair of a traumatic rotator cuff injury under regional anesthesia with light sedation. Two minutes after receiving an interscalene regional block with 30 mL of 1.5% mepivacaine, he demonstrates a generalized, tonic-clonic seizure. The most appropriate INITIAL step in managing this episode of local anesthetic systemic toxicity is:
   A. Administer 100 mg propofol intravenously to stop the seizure
   B. Provide bag-mask ventilation with 100% oxygen
   C. Administer intralipid emulsion
   D. Perform tracheal intubation with 200 mg propofol and 120 mg succinylcholine

9. Local anesthetics have been associated with all of the following complications EXCEPT:
   A. Direct neural toxicity
   B. Transient impairment of adrenocorticoid release
   C. Direct myocyte toxicity
   D. Allergic reactions

10. A 62-year-old female with severe osteoarthritis is scheduled for a left total knee replacement under regional anesthesia with light sedation. Two minutes after receiving a paravertebral regional block with 30 mL of 0.25% bupivacaine, she demonstrates a ventricular fibrillation. All of the following interventions may be considered in treating her local anesthetic systemic toxicity EXCEPT:
   A. Perform cardiopulmonary bypass
   B. Administer intravenous epinephrine 50 μg
   C. Administer intravenous amiodarone 150 mg
   D. Administer intravenous lidocaine 100 mg

13 Cardiovascular Pharmacology

Kelly A. Linn
Paul S. Pagel

This chapter reviews the cardiovascular pharmacology of medications used to alter hemodynamics during surgery and in the intensive care unit, including endogenous and synthetic catecholamines, sympathomimetics, milrinone, vasopressin, and antihypertensive medications.

I. Catecholamines

The α, β, and dopamine adrenergic receptor subtypes are responsible for mediating the cardiovascular effects of endogenous (epinephrine, norepinephrine, dopamine) and synthetic (dobutamine, isoproterenol) *catecholamines* (Fig. 13-1). These drugs all activate β_1 *adrenoceptors* located on the sarcolemmal membrane of atrial and ventricular myocytes to varying degrees. This β_1 adrenoceptor stimulation causes positive chronotropic (heart rate), dromotropic (conduction velocity), inotropic (contractility), and lusitropic (relaxation) effects. The β_1 adrenoceptor is coupled to a stimulatory guanine nucleotide-binding (G_s) protein that activates the key intracellular enzyme adenylyl cyclase, thereby accelerating the formation of the second messenger *cyclic adenosine monophosphate (cAMP)* from adenosine triphosphate (ATP) (Fig. 13-2). Three major consequences result from activation of this signaling cascade: (a) more calcium (Ca^{2+}) is available for contractile activation; (b) the efficacy of activator Ca^{2+} at troponin C of the contractile apparatus is enhanced; and (c) removal of Ca^{2+} from the contractile apparatus and the sarcoplasm after contraction is accelerated. It should be readily apparent that the first two of these actions produce a direct increase in contractility, whereas the third results in more rapid myocardial relaxation during early diastole. Indeed, treatment of acute or chronic left ventricular (LV) dysfunction is the primary reason for the perioperative use of catecholamines. Notably, how well catecholamines work under these clinical conditions may be affected by the relative density and functional integrity of the β_1 adrenoceptor and its signaling cascade because receptor down-regulation and abnormal intracellular Ca^{2+} homeostasis are characteristic features of heart failure.

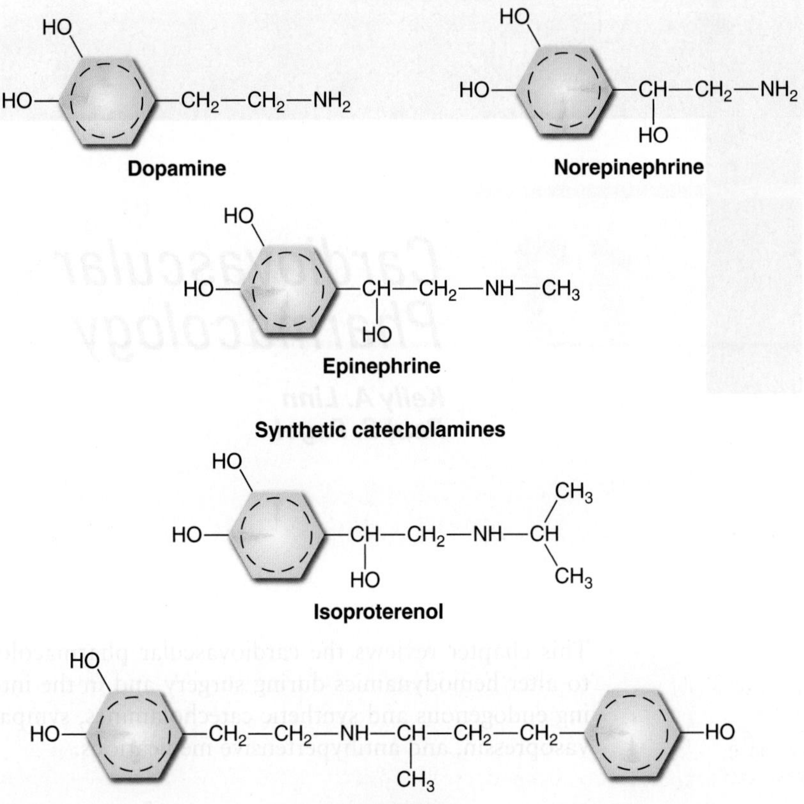

Endogenous catecholamines

Dopamine

Norepinephrine

Epinephrine

Synthetic catecholamines

Isoproterenol

Dobutamine

Figure 13-1   Catecholamine chemical structures.

The circulatory effects of catecholamines in other perfusion territories are dependent on the tissue-specific distribution of α and β adrenoceptor subtypes (Table 13-1). Differences in each catecholamine's chemical structure and its relative selectivity for adrenoceptors also influence the peripheral vascular actions of these medications. This selectivity is often dose related (Table 13-2); dopamine provides a useful pedagogical illustration of this principle. Low doses of this catecholamine predominantly stimulate dopamine subtypes 1 and 2 (DA_1 and DA_2, respectively) receptors, causing arterial vasodilation, but progressively larger doses sequentially activate β_1 and α_1 adrenoceptors, augmenting contractility and causing arterial vasoconstriction, respectively. The α_1 *adrenoceptors* are major regulators of vasomotor tone as a result of their location in arteries, arterioles, and veins. Thus, catecholamines that exert substantial α_1 adrenoceptor agonist activity (e.g., norepinephrine) increase systemic vascular resistance and reduce venous capacitance through arterial and venous vasoconstriction, respectively. The α_1 adrenoceptor-mediated vasoconstriction occurs through phospholipase C-inositol 1,4,5-triphosphate, signaling through an inhibitory guanine nucleotide-binding (G_i) protein (Fig. 13-3). This cascade opens Ca^{2+} channels, releases Ca^{2+} from intracellular stores (sarcoplasmic reticulum and calmodulin), and activates several Ca^{2+}-dependent protein kinases; the sum total of these events causes an increase in intracellular Ca^{2+} concentration and vascular smooth muscle cell contraction. Whereas α_1 adrenoceptors are the major target for catecholamines in cutaneous blood vessels, β_2 *adrenoceptors* predominate in skeletal

? Did You Know

The α_1 adrenoreceptors are major regulators of vasomotor tone, including systemic vascular resistance and venous capacitance.

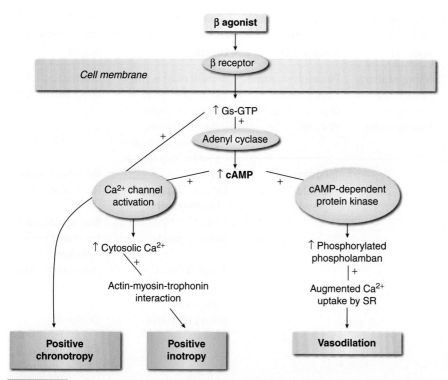

Figure 13-2 Schematic of β adrenergic agonist mechanism of action. (From Gillies M, Bellomo R, Doolan L, et al. Bench-to-bedside review: Inotropic drug therapy after adult cardiac surgery—a systemic literature review. *Crit Care*. 2005;9:266–279, with permission.)

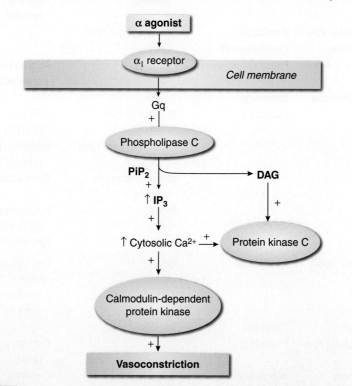

Figure 13-3 Schematic of α adrenergic agonist mechanism of action. (From Gillies M, Bellomo R, Doolan L, et al. Bench-to-bedside review: Inotropic drug therapy after adult cardiac surgery—a systemic literature review. *Crit Care*. 2005;9:266–279, with permission.)

Table 13-1   Adrenergic Receptors: Order of Potency of Agonists and Antagonists

Receptor	Potency[a]	Agonists[b]	Antagonists	Location	Action
α_1	++++ +++ ++ +	Norepinephrine Epinephrine Dopamine Isoproterenol	Phenoxybenzamine[c] Phentolamine[c] Ergot alkaloids[c] Prazosin	Smooth muscle (vascular, iris, radial, ureter, pilomotor, uterus, trigone, gastrointestinal, and bladder sphincters)	Contraction Vasoconstriction
			Tolazoline[c] Labetalol[c]	Brain Smooth muscle (gastrointestinal)	Neurotransmission Relaxation
				Heart Salivary glands	Glycogenolysis Increased force,[d] glycolysis
				Adipose tissue Sweat glands (localized)	Secretion (K^+, H_2O) Glycogenesis
				Kidney (proximal tubule)	Secretion
					Gluconeogenesis Na^+ reabsorption
α_2	++++	Clonidine	Yohimbine	Adrenergic nerve endings	Inhibition norepinephrine release
	+++ ++	Norepinephrine Epinephrine	Piperoxan Phentolamine[c]	Presynaptic—CNS	
	++	Norepinephrine	Phenoxybenzamine[c]	Platelets	Aggregation, granule release
	+	Phenylephrine	Tolazoline[c] Labetalol[c]	Adipose tissue	Inhibition lipolysis
				Endocrine pancreas	Inhibition insulin release
				Vascular smooth muscle	Contraction
				Kidney	Inhibition renin disease
				Brain	Neurotransmission
β_1	++++	Isoproterenol[c]	Acebutolol	Heart	Increased rate, contractility, conduction, velocity
	+++ ++	Epinephrine Norepinephrine	Practolol Propranolol[c]		Coronary vasodilation
	+	Dopamine	Alprenolol[c] Metoprolol Esmolol	Adipose tissue	Lipolysis

Table 13-1　Adrenergic Receptors: Order of Potency of Agonists and Antagonists (*Continued*)

Receptor	Potency[a]	Agonists[b]	Antagonists	Location	Action
β_2	++++	Isoproterenol[b]	Propranolol[c]	Liver	Glycogenolysis, gluconeogenesis
	+++	Epinephrine	Butoxamine		
	+++	Norepinephrine	Alprenolol		
	+	Dopamine	Esmolol	Skeletal muscle	Glycogenolysis, lactate release
			Nadolol		
			Timolol	Smooth muscle (bronchi, uterus, vascular, gastrointestinal, detrusor, spleen capsule)	Relaxation
			Labetalol		
				Endocrine pancreas	Insulin secretion
				Salivary glands	Amylase secretion
DA_1	++++	Fenoldopam		Vascular smooth muscle	Vasodilation
	++	Dopamine	Haloperidol	Renal and mesentery	
	+	Epinephrine	Droperidol		
DA_2	+	Metoclopramide	Phenothiazines		
	++	Dopamine	Domperidone	Presynaptic—adrenergic nerve endings	Inhibits norepinephrine release
	+	Bromocriptine			

CNS, central nervous system; DA, dopamine.
[a]Pluses indicate strength of potency.
[b]Listed in decreasing order of potency.
[c]Nonselective.
[d]β_1 adrenergic responses are greater.

muscle, and activation of this latter adrenoceptor subtype produces arteriolar vasodilation via adenylyl cyclase–mediated signaling.

The actions of specific catecholamines on hemodynamics are summarized in Table 13-3. For example, if a catecholamine acts primarily through the α_1 adrenoceptor (e.g., norepinephrine), an increase in arterial pressure will most likely be observed because enhanced arterial and venous vasomotor tone increases systemic vascular resistance (greater afterload) and augments venous return to the heart (increased preload), respectively. In contrast, a catecholamine with β_1 and β_2 adrenoceptor activity and little effect on the α_1 adrenoceptor (e.g., isoproterenol) would be expected to modestly decrease arterial pressure because reductions in systemic vascular resistance offset increases in cardiac output caused by tachycardia and enhanced myocardial contractility. It is important to note that all catecholamines may cause detrimental increases in myocardial oxygen consumption in patients with flow-limiting coronary artery stenoses and, therefore, contribute to the development of *acute myocardial ischemia*. As a result, the use of catecholamines to support LV function in

(text continues on page 238)

Table 13-2 Inotropic and Vasopressor Drug Names, Clinical Indication for Therapeutic Use, Standard Dose Range, Receptor Binding (Catecholamines), and Major Clinical Side Effects

Drug	Clinical Indication	Dose Range	Receptor Binding				Major Side Effects
			α_1	β_1	β_2	DA	
Catecholamines							
Dopamine	Shock (cardiogenic, vasodilatory) HF Symptomatic bradycardia unresponsive to atropine or pacing	2.0 to 20 μg·kg⁻¹·min⁻¹ (max 50 μg·kg⁻¹·min⁻¹)	+++	++++	++	+++++	Severe hypertension (especially in patients taking nonselective β-blockers) Ventricular arrhythmias Cardiac ischemia Tissue ischemia/gangrene (high doses or due to tissue extravasation)
Dobutamine	Low CO (decompensated HF, cardiogenic shock, sepsis-induced myocardial dysfunction) Symptomatic bradycardia unresponsive to atropine or pacing	2.0 to 20 μg·kg⁻¹·min⁻¹ (max 40 μg·kg⁻¹·min⁻¹)	+	+++++	+++	N/A	Tachycardia Increased ventricular response rate in patients with atrial fibrillation Ventricular arrhythmias Cardiac ischemia Hypertension (especially nonselective β-blocker patients) Hypotension
Norepineph-rine	Shock (vasodilatory, cardiogenic)	0.01 to 3 μg·kg⁻¹·min⁻¹	+++++	+++	++	N/A	Arrhythmias Bradycardia Peripheral (digital) ischemia Hypertension (especially nonselective β-blocker patients)
Epinephrine ▶ VIDEO 13-1 *Anaphylaxis*	Shock (cardiogenic, vasodilatory) Cardiac arrest Bronchospasm/anaphylaxis Symptomatic bradycardia or heart block unresponsive to atropine or pacing	Infusion: 0.01 to 0.10 μg·kg⁻¹·min⁻¹ Bolus: 1 mg IV every 3 to 5 min (max 0.2 mg/kg) IM: (1:1000): 0.1 to 0.5 mg (max 1 mg)	+++++	++++	+++	N/A	Ventricular arrhythmias Severe hypertension resulting in cerebrovascular hemorrhage Cardiac ischemia Sudden cardiac death
Isoproterenol	Bradyarrhythmias (especially torsade des pointes) Brugada syndrome	2 to 10 μg/min	0	+++++	+++++	N/A	Ventricular arrhythmias Cardiac ischemia Hypertension Hypotension

Drug	Clinical use	α_1	β_1	β_2	DA	Dosing	Adverse effects
Phenylephrine	Hypotension (vagally mediated, medication-induced) Increase MAP with AS and hypotension Decrease LVOT gradient in HCM	+++++	0	0	N/A	Bolus: 0.1 to 0.5 mg IV every 10 to 15 min Infusion: 0.15 to 0.75 µg·kg⁻¹·min⁻¹	Reflex bradycardia Hypertension (especially with non-selective β-blockers) Severe peripheral and visceral vasoconstriction Tissue necrosis with extravasation
PDIs							
Milrinone	Low CO (decompensated HF, after cardiotomy)	N/A				Bolus: 50 µg/kg bolus over 10 to 30 min Infusion: 0.375 to 0.75 µg·kg⁻¹·min⁻¹ (dose adjustment necessary for renal impairment)	Ventricular arrhythmias Hypotension Cardiac ischemia Torsade des pointes
Amrinone	Low CO (refractory HF)	N/A				Bolus: 0.75 mg/kg over 2 to 3 min Infusion: 5 to 10 µg·kg⁻¹·min⁻¹	Arrhythmias, enhanced AV conduction (increased ventricular response rate in atrial fibrillation) Hypotension Thrombocytopenia Hepatotoxicity
Vasopressin	Shock (vasodilatory, cardiogenic) Cardiac arrest	V₁ receptors (vascular smooth muscle) V₂ receptors (renal collecting duct system)				Infusion: 0.01 to 0.1 U/min (common fixed dose 0.04 U/min) Bolus: 40-U IV bolus	Arrhythmias Hypertension Decreased CO (at doses >0.4 U/min) Cardiac ischemia Severe peripheral vasoconstriction causing ischemia (especially skin) Splanchnic vasoconstriction
Levosimendan	Decompensated HF	N/A				Loading dose: 12 to 24 µg/kg over 10 min Infusion: 0.05 to 0.2 µg·kg⁻¹·min⁻¹	Tachycardia, enhanced AV conduction Hypotension

α_1 indicates α-1 receptor; β_1, β-1 receptor; β_2, β-2 receptor; DA, dopamine receptors; 0, zero significant receptor affinity; +, through ++++, minimal to maximal relative receptor affinity; N/A, not applicable; IV, intravenous; IM, intramuscular; max, maximum; AS, aortic stenosis; LVOT, LV outflow tract; HCM, hypertrophic cardiomyopathy; and AV, atrioventricular.

From Overgaard CB, Džavík V. Inotropes and vasopressors: review of physiology and clinical use in cardiovascular disease. *Circulation.* 2008;118(10):1047–1056, with permission.

Table 13-3 Dose Schedule and Hemodynamic Effects of the Adrenergic Agonists

Drug Listed from α to β	Dosages		Site of Activity					Hemodynamics (↑ Increase; ↓ Decrease; –, No Change)					
	IV Push Adults	IV Infusion[a]	α₁A	α₁V	β₁	β₂	DA	CO	Inotrop	HR	VR	TPR	RBF
Phenyleph-rine	50–100 µg	a. 10 mg/250 mL b. 40 µg/mL c. 0.15–0.75 µg/kg/min d. 0.15 µg/kg/min	++++	+++++	0	0	0			Reflex Reflex			– ↓
Norepi-nephrine	N/R	a. 4 mg/250 mL b. 16 µg/mL c. 0.01–0.1 µg/kg/min d. 0.1 µg/kg/min	+++	+++	++++	?+	0	–↓	–	↓ Reflex	↑↑↑	↑↑	↓
Epinephrine	0.3–0.5 mL 1:1000 (0.3–0.5 mg) SC—Asthma IV—Anaphy-laxis 5 mL 1:10,000 (0.5 mg) cardiac arrest every 5 min	a. 1 mg/250 mL b. 4 µg/mL 0.01–0.03 µg/kg/min c. 0.03–0.15 µg/kg/min 0.15–0.30 µg/min d. 0.015 µg/kg/min	+ +++ +++++ +	+ +++ +++++ +	++++ ++++ ++++	++++	0	↑–↓	↑–↓	↑ Reflex	↑↑↑	↑↑↑	↓↓
Ephedrine	5–10 mg	N/R ++	+++		++++	+++	↑↑0	↑↑	↑	↑↑	↑	↑	↑

Drug	Dose								
Dopamine[c]	N/R	++	0						
	a. 200 mg/250 mL		↑–	↑–	↑↑	↑↑	↑	↑↑	↓
	b. 800 μg/mL 0.05–5 μg/kg/min		↓↑	↑↑	↑↑	↑	↑	↑↑↑	→↑
	c. 2–10 μg/kg/min 10 μg/kg/min[b]		↑↑	↑↑	↑	↑	↑	↑↑	↑↓
	d. 2 μg/kg/min		↑	↑		↑↑			
Dobutamine[c]	N/R	+	+++						
	a. 250 mg/250 mL	+++++	+++						
	b. 1,000 μg/mL	+++	++						
	c. 2–30 μg/kg/min	++++							
	d. 5 μg/kg/min								
Isoproterenol	0.004 mg (0.2 mL of 0.2 mg/mL solution) Third-degree heart block	0–+	?	++++	++++	+++++	+++++		
	a. 1 mg/250 mL		↑	↑↑	↑	–	→↑	↑	
	b. 4 μg/mL		↑↑	–	↓↑	↑	–↑	↑	
	c. 0.15 μg/kg/min to desired effect		↑↓	↑↑	–	↑↑	↑↑	↑	
	d. 0.015 μg/kg/min		↑	–	↑	↑	–↓	↓	

IV, intravenous; DA, dopamine; CO, cardiac output; Inotrop, contractility; HR, heart rate; VR, venous return (preload); TPR, peripheral resistance (afterload); RBF, renal blood flow; N/R, not recommended.

[a](a) mixture; (b) concentration μg/mL; (c) dose range μg/kg/min; (d) standard rate infusion.

[b]"Rule of six."

[c]Dopamine and dobutamine employ the same doses. Dosage of either may quickly be calculated by multiplying patient's weight (kg) × 6 = mg added to 100 mL D5%W. The number of drops delivered through a calibrated infusor (60 drops = 1 mL) is the number of μg/kg/min infused into the patient. Example: 70 kg × 6 = 420; 420 mg/100 mL = 4,200 μg/kg; 5 μg/kg/min = 5 gtt/min. From Lawson NW, Wallfisch HK. Cardiovascular pharmacology: A new look at the "pressors." In: Stoelting RK, Barash PG, Gallagher TJ, eds. *Advances in Anesthesia*. Chicago: Year Book Medical Publishers; 1986:195, with permission.

patients with coronary artery disease complicated by congestive heart failure requires substantial caution. Thus, it should come as no surprise that a drug that reduces LV afterload, and not one that causes a positive inotropic effect, is usually chosen first to improve cardiac output in a patient with coronary artery disease and heart failure.

A. Epinephrine

Epinephrine is an endogenous catecholamine that exerts its cardiovascular effects by activating *α_1, β_1, and β_2 adrenoceptors*. Epinephrine stimulates β_1 adrenoceptors located on the cell membranes of sinoatrial node cells and cardiac myocytes to produce positive chronotropic and inotropic effects, respectively. Epinephrine-induced activation of β_1 adrenoceptors also enhances the rate and extent of myocardial relaxation, thereby facilitating greater LV filling during early diastole. The combination of these actions on heart rate and LV systolic and diastolic function causes pronounced increases in cardiac output. The tachycardia initially observed during an infusion of epinephrine may be subsequently attenuated as baroreceptor-mediated reflexes are activated. As a result, epinephrine is especially useful for the treatment of *acute LV failure* during cardiac surgery because it predictably increases cardiac output. Epinephrine also enhances cardiac output and oxygen delivery without causing deleterious increases in heart rate in septic, hypotensive patients.

It is important to note that clinical use of epinephrine may be limited because the catecholamine stimulates the development of atrial or *ventricular arrhythmias*. Epinephrine increases conduction velocity and reduces refractory period in the atrioventricular (AV) node, the His bundle, Purkinje fibers, and ventricular muscle. The positive dromotropic effect of epinephrine on AV nodal conduction may cause detrimental increases in ventricular rate in the presence of atrial flutter or fibrillation. Irritability in other parts of the conduction system may also precipitate ventricular arrhythmias, including premature ventricular contractions, ventricular tachycardia, and ventricular fibrillation, especially in the presence of a pre-existing arrhythmogenic substrate (e.g., regional myocardial ischemia or infarction, cardiomyopathy).

Epinephrine causes vasoconstriction of arteriolar vascular smooth muscle in the cutaneous, splanchnic, and renal perfusion territories through its effects at the α_1 adrenoceptor, but the catecholamine also simultaneously produces vasodilation in the skeletal muscle circulation as a result of β_2 adrenoceptor activation. These observations emphasize that the organ-specific distribution of α_1 and β_2 adrenoceptors determines epinephrine's overall effect on blood flow. These effects are also dose dependent: lower doses of epinephrine stimulate β_2 adrenoceptors, causing peripheral vasodilation and modest declines in arterial pressure, but higher doses of the catecholamine activate α_1 adrenoceptors, thereby increasing systemic vascular resistance and arterial pressure. A high density of α_1 adrenoceptors is also present in the venous circulation, and as a result, epinephrine produces venoconstriction and augments venous return. Epinephrine also causes vasoconstriction of the pulmonary arterial tree and increases pulmonary arterial pressures through α_1 adrenoceptor activation. The α_1 and β_2 adrenoceptors exist in the coronary circulation, but these receptor subtypes play minor roles in establishing coronary perfusion during administration of epinephrine. Instead, epinephrine-induced increases in coronary blood flow occur principally because of metabolic autoregulation: increases in myocardial oxygen demand resulting from increases in heart rate, contractility, preload, and afterload are responsible for coronary vasodilation.

Nevertheless, epinephrine may cause epicardial coronary vasoconstriction and reduce coronary blood flow in situations where maximal coronary vasodilation is present (e.g., acute myocardial ischemia distal to a severe coronary stenosis) via direct stimulation of α_1 adrenoceptors.

Prior administration of α or β adrenoceptor antagonists influences the cardiovascular effects of epinephrine. For example, epinephrine causes greater increases in systemic vascular resistance and arterial pressure when administered after the nonselective beta-blocker propranolol because β_2 adrenoceptor-mediated arterial vasodilation no longer opposes α_1 adrenoceptor-induced vasoconstriction. Established beta-blockade also competitively inhibits β_1 adrenoceptor activation by epinephrine, thereby attenuating the positive chronotropic and inotropic effects of the catecholamine. Such a competitive blockade may only be overcome by larger doses of epinephrine. Indeed, the hemodynamic effects of epinephrine may be similar to those the pure α_1 adrenoceptor agonist phenylephrine (see below) in the presence of complete β_1 and β_2 adrenoceptor blockade.

B. Norepinephrine

Norepinephrine is the neurotransmitter that is released from sympathetic nervous system postganglionic neurons. This catecholamine *activates both α_1 and β_1* adrenoceptors similar to epinephrine, but norepinephrine exerts few if any effects on the β_2 adrenoceptor. As a result, norepinephrine enhances myocardial contractility while simultaneously causing *arterial vasoconstriction*. These actions dramatically increase arterial pressure, but cardiac output remains largely unchanged. In contrast, pure α_1 adrenoceptor agonists such as phenylephrine cause predictable, dose-related decreases in cardiac output because simultaneous increases in contractility mediated through the β_1 adrenoceptor do not occur. Unlike epinephrine, norepinephrine does not usually increase heart rate because elevated blood pressure stimulates baroreceptor-mediated reflexes. This action usually balances the direct positive chronotropism of β_1 adrenoceptor activation. In general, greater increases in systemic vascular resistance and diastolic arterial pressure are observed during administration of norepinephrine compared with similar doses of epinephrine. Norepinephrine also causes constriction of venous capacitance vessels through α_1 adrenoceptor stimulation, thereby increasing venous return and augmenting stroke volume.

Norepinephrine is especially useful for treatment of *refractory hypotension* during pathologic conditions in which pronounced vasodilation occurs. For example, norepinephrine increases arterial pressure, cardiac index, and urine output in patients with sepsis. Norepinephrine is also useful for the treatment of *vasoplegic syndrome*, a hypotensive state associated with low systemic vascular resistance that sometimes occurs during prolonged cardiopulmonary bypass in patients undergoing cardiac surgery. Norepinephrine increases coronary perfusion pressure in patients with severe coronary artery disease, but the drug may cause spasm of internal mammary or radial artery grafts used during coronary bypass artery graft (CABG) surgery through α_1 adrenoceptor activation. Norepinephrine is associated with development of ventricular and supraventricular *arrhythmias*, but the potential arrhythmogenic effects of this catecholamine are less than those from epinephrine. As a result, it may be appropriate to substitute norepinephrine for epinephrine when treating cardiogenic shock in the presence of hemodynamically significant atrial or ventricular arrhythmias. Norepinephrine stimulates pulmonary arterial α_1 adrenoceptors and causes dose-related increases in pulmonary arterial pressures that may precipitate right ventricular dysfunction because this chamber is less able to tolerate acute elevations in afterload than the LV. Addition of a selective pulmonary vasodilator such as inhaled nitric oxide may be beneficial to attenuate norepinephrine's actions as a direct pulmonary vasoconstrictor when the drug is used to treat LV dysfunction in patients with pulmonary hypertension. Dose-dependent decreases in hepatic, skeletal muscle, splanchnic, and renal blood flow occur during administration of norepinephrine via α_1 adrenoceptor activation when blood pressure is normal or modestly reduced. But in the presence of profound hypotension (e.g., sepsis), norepinephrine increases perfusion pressure and blood flow to these vascular beds. Nevertheless, sustained reductions in renal and splanchnic blood flow represent a major limitation of prolonged use of norepinephrine.

C. Dopamine

Dopamine is the biochemical precursor of norepinephrine and differentially activates several adrenergic and dopaminergic receptor subtypes in a dose-related manner. Low doses (typically below 3 µg/kg/min) of dopamine selectively increase renal and splanchnic blood flow via activation of *DA_1 receptors* and also reduce norepinephrine release from autonomic nervous system ganglia and adrenergic neurons through a *DA_2 receptor*–mediated mechanism. These combined effects produce a modest decline in arterial pressure. Moderate doses (3 to 8 µg/kg/min) of dopamine activate both α_1 and β_1 adrenoceptors, whereas high doses (in excess of 10 µg/kg/min) almost exclusively act on α_1 adrenoceptors to increase arterial pressure through arteriolar vasoconstriction. However, it is important to realize that this straightforward dose–response description of dopamine pharmacodynamics is overly simplistic because differences in receptor density and regulation, drug interactions, and patient variability cause a broad range of clinical responses to the catecholamine. For example, low doses of dopamine were once thought to provide renal protection through DA_1 receptor–mediated increases in renal blood flow alone. But it is now clear that even low doses of dopamine also stimulate *α_1 and β_1 adrenoceptors*, which may obfuscate the catecholamine's intended dopaminergic effect. Conversely, renal blood flow and urine output may be maintained (and not decreased) during administration of higher doses of dopamine because DA_1 receptors continue to be activated, despite a predominant α_1 adrenoceptor agonist effect. Such varied responses may explain, at least in part, why dopamine fails to consistently provide renal protective effects, despite causing modest increases in renal perfusion and urine output.

Dopamine is often used for inotropic support in patients with acute LV dysfunction. This action occurs as a result of activation of β_1 adrenoceptors. Dopamine also stimulates arterial and venous α_1 adrenoceptors, thereby increasing LV afterload and enhancing venous return, respectively. Thus, dopamine augments arterial pressure. The use of dopamine for the treatment of hypotension associated with depressed contractile function may be limited to some degree in patients with pre-existing pulmonary hypertension or elevated preload. Right atrial, mean pulmonary arterial, and pulmonary capillary occlusion pressures were greater in patients undergoing cardiac surgery after cardiopulmonary bypass who had received dopamine compared with dobutamine, despite producing similar cardiac output. Dopamine may also cause greater increases in heart rate than epinephrine in cardiac surgery patients. Infusion of an arterial vasodilator (e.g., sodium nitroprusside) may be used to mitigate the increases in LV afterload associated with administration of dopamine and, in so doing, may further augment cardiac output. However, administration of an inotrope vasodilator (inodilator), such as milrinone, has largely replaced this "dopamine plus nitroprusside" approach. Like epinephrine and norepinephrine, dopamine *increases myocardial oxygen consumption* and may worsen myocardial ischemia in the presence of hemodynamically significant coronary stenoses.

D. Dobutamine

Dobutamine is a synthetic catecholamine composed of two stereoisomers (negative and positive), both of which stimulate *β adrenoceptors*, whereas these stereoisomers produce opposing agonist and antagonist effects on α_1 adrenoceptors. As a result, dobutamine causes potent β adrenoceptor stimulation, but exerts little or no effect on α_1 adrenoceptors when administered at infusion rates <5 μg/kg/min. As expected, based on this unique adrenergic receptor pharmacology, dobutamine enhances myocardial contractility and modestly reduces arterial vasomotor tone through activation of β_1 and β_2 adrenoceptors, respectively. These properties combine to substantially increase cardiac output in the presence or absence of *LV dysfunction*. Notably, the negative isomer of dobutamine begins to stimulate the α_1 adrenoceptor at infusion rates >5 μg/kg/min, an action that limits the magnitude of β_2 adrenoceptor-mediated vasodilation. This effect preserves LV preload, afterload, and arterial pressure; sustains increases in cardiac output; and may serve to attenuate profound baroreceptor reflex–mediated tachycardia that might otherwise occur. Despite this latter effect, dobutamine often markedly *increases heart rate* by direct chronotropic effects resulting from β_1 adrenoceptor stimulation. Indeed, dobutamine causes significantly higher heart rates than epinephrine at equivalent values of cardiac index in patients after CABG surgery. Dobutamine-induced tachycardia and enhanced contractility directly increase myocardial oxygen consumption and may cause "demand" *myocardial ischemia* in patients with flow-limiting coronary stenoses. The propensity for dobutamine to produce demand myocardial ischemia under such circumstances is the underlying principle behind dobutamine stress echocardiography as a diagnostic tool for the detection of coronary artery disease because regional wall motion abnormalities in the affected coronary perfusion territories occur in response to the transient myocardial oxygen supply–demand mismatch. Conversely, dobutamine may reduce heart rate in patients with decompensated heart failure because increases in cardiac output and systemic oxygen delivery resulting from administration of the drug are capable of decreasing the chronically elevated sympathetic nervous system tone that occurs in heart failure. Dobutamine may also favorably reduce myocardial oxygen consumption in the failing heart because β_2 adrenoceptor activation decreases LV preload and afterload, and consequently, LV end-diastolic and end-systolic wall stress, respectively.

Declines in pulmonary arterial pressures and pulmonary vascular resistance mediated through β_2 adrenoceptor activation occur during administration of dobutamine. This property makes dobutamine a useful inotropic drug to enhance cardiac output in cardiac surgery patients with pre-existing *pulmonary hypertension*. Recall that dopamine, in contrast to dobutamine, activates α_1 adrenoceptors in the pulmonary circulation and venous capacitance vessels, thereby increasing pulmonary arterial pressures and LV preload, respectively. Thus, dobutamine may offer an advantage over dopamine in patients with heart failure accompanied by increased pulmonary vascular resistance and elevated LV filling pressures. Nevertheless, dobutamine-induced pulmonary vasodilation has the potential to increase transpulmonary shunt and cause relative hypoxemia under such conditions. Dobutamine does not activate dopaminergic receptors, but the drug may improve renal perfusion as a result of increases in cardiac output. Despite the aforementioned theoretical beneficial cardiovascular effects of the drug, several clinical trials unfortunately demonstrated that use of dobutamine was linked to an increased incidence of major adverse cardiac events including mortality in patients with heart failure. As a result, the authors no longer recommend the use of dobutamine for inotropic support under these conditions.

E. Isoproterenol

Isoproterenol is a *nonselective β adrenoceptor agonist* synthetic catecholamine that exerts almost no activity at α adrenoceptors. Historically, isoproterenol was used for *"pharmacologic pacing"* because it causes sustained increases in heart rate in patients with symptomatic bradyarrhythmias or AV conduction block (e.g., Mobitz type II second-degree block, third-degree block). Isoproterenol was also used during cardiac transplantation to increase heart rate and augment myocardial contractility in the denervated donor heart. However, use of the catecholamine for these indications has been largely supplanted by transcutaneous or transvenous pacing, especially in view of the drug's propensity to cause untoward supraventricular and ventricular tachyarrhythmias. Isoproterenol was previously used to treat right ventricular dysfunction associated with severe pulmonary hypertension because the drug reduces pulmonary vascular resistance. However, selective inhaled pulmonary vasodilators (e.g., nitric oxide, prostaglandin E_1) are more efficacious and cause fewer adverse effects in this setting as well. The clinical use of isoproterenol may be quite limited at present, but the drug's unique pharmacology compared with that of catecholamines continues to make it worthy of discussion.

Isoproterenol causes β_2 adrenoceptor-mediated arteriolar vasodilation in skeletal muscle and also dilates the renal and splanchnic circulations, thereby reducing systemic vascular resistance. As a result of these peripheral vascular effects, the drug selectively decreases diastolic and mean arterial pressures while systolic arterial pressure is usually maintained. Isoproterenol causes direct positive chronotropic and dromotropic effects through activation of β_1 adrenoceptors, but heart rate also increases because baroreceptor reflexes are stimulated in response to declines in arterial pressure. Isoproterenol is a positive inotrope, but cardiac output may not be reliably increased during the drug's administration because pronounced tachycardia prevents optimal LV filling and β_2 adrenoceptor-mediated venodilation decreases venous return. Dose-related increases in myocardial oxygen consumption occur with isoproterenol accompanied by simultaneous decreases in coronary perfusion pressure and diastolic filling time. These actions may contribute to acute *myocardial ischemia* or subendocardial necrosis, especially in the presence of coronary artery disease.

II. Sympathomimetics

A. Ephedrine

Ephedrine is a sympathomimetic drug that exerts *direct and indirect actions* on adrenoceptors. Transport of ephedrine into α_1 and β_1 adrenoceptor presynaptic terminals *displaces norepinephrine* from the synaptic vesicles. Norepinephrine is then released to activate the corresponding postsynaptic receptors to cause arterial and venous vasoconstriction and increased myocardial contractility, respectively. This indirect effect is the ephedrine's predominant pharmacologic effect, but the drug also directly stimulates β_2 *adrenoceptors*, thereby limiting increases in arterial pressure resulting from α_1 adrenoceptor activation. In this regard, ephedrine's initial cardiovascular effects resemble those of epinephrine because dose-related increases in heart rate, cardiac output, and systemic vascular resistance are observed. However, *tachyphylaxis* to the hemodynamic effects of ephedrine occurs with repetitive administration of the drug because presynaptic norepinephrine stores are rapidly depleted. This tachyphylaxis is not observed with epinephrine because the catecholamine acts directly on α and β adrenoceptors independent of indirect stimulation of norepinephrine release. Notably, drugs that block the ephedrine uptake into adrenergic nerves and those that deplete norepinephrine reserves (e.g., cocaine and reserpine, respectively) predictably attenuate ephedrine's cardiovascular effects. Ephedrine is most often used as an intravenous bolus to treat acute hypotension accompanied by decreases in heart rate.

B. Phenylephrine

The chemical structure of phenylephrine is very similar to epinephrine: the sympathomimetic drug lacks the hydroxyl moiety that is present on the phenyl ring of the endogenous catecholamine. As a result of this minor modification, phenylephrine almost exclusively stimulates α_1 *adrenoceptors* to produce *vasoconstriction*, while exerting little or no effect on β adrenoceptors except when large doses are administered. Unlike ephedrine, phenylephrine is not dependent on presynaptic norepinephrine displacement and, instead, acts directly on the α_1 adrenoceptor to produce its cardiovascular effects. Phenylephrine constricts venous capacitance vessels and causes cutaneous, skeletal muscle, splanchnic, and renal vasoconstriction to increase preload and afterload, respectively. These actions produce dose-related increases in arterial pressure. Decreases in heart rate (mediated by baroreceptor reflex activation) and cardiac output also occur. Phenylephrine increases pulmonary artery pressures through pulmonary arterial vasoconstriction and as a consequence of enhanced venous return. Intravenous boluses or infusions of phenylephrine are most often used intraoperatively for short-term treatment of hypotension resulting from vasodilation. Unlike catecholamines, phenylephrine is *not arrhythmogenic*.

> **? Did You Know**
>
> Phenylephrine stimulates α_1 adrenoreceptors almost exclusively and has little or no effect on β adrenoreceptors.

III. Milrinone

Phosphodiesterases are enzymes that hydrolyze and terminate the intracellular actions of cyclic monophosphate second messengers including cAMP in a variety of tissues. Of most relevance to this chapter, human myocardium contains the type III phosphodiesterase isoenzyme that is bound to the sarcoplasmic reticulum and cleaves active cAMP to its inactive metabolite adenosine monophosphate. Milrinone is a relatively selective bipyridine inhibitor of this cardiac type III phosphodiesterase that preserves intracellular cAMP concentration by preventing the second messenger's degradation. This action increases systolic Ca^{2+} availability by enhancing transsarcolemmal Ca^{2+} influx and Ca^{2+}-induced Ca^{2+} release from the sarcoplasmic reticulum to produce a positive *inotropic effect* independent of the β_1 adrenoceptor. The inhibition of cAMP metabolism by milrinone simultaneously facilitates diastolic Ca^{2+} removal from the sarcoplasm to enhance the rate and extent of myocardial relaxation. This positive lusitropic effect of milrinone may improve diastolic function in patients with heart failure. Milrinone causes potent systemic and pulmonary arterial *vasodilation* mediated by cyclic guanosine monophosphate (cGMP) in vascular smooth muscle. Indeed, milrinone produces greater vasodilation than

> **? Did You Know**
>
> Milrinone increases cardiac contractility by inhibiting cardiac type III phosphodiesterase, the enzyme responsible for the breakdown of cyclic adenosine monophosphate.

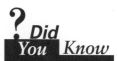

catecholamines, including dobutamine and isoproterenol. The combination of positive inotropic effects and arterial vasodilation increases cardiac output in a dose-related manner, despite declines in preload resulting from dilation of venous capacitance vessels. Mean arterial pressure may be modestly reduced during infusion of the drug unless additional preload is administered.

Milrinone *decreases pulmonary vascular resistance*, and this action may be especially beneficial in patients with pulmonary hypertension who are undergoing cardiac surgery. However, the pulmonary vasodilating properties of milrinone have the potential to increase intrapulmonary shunt and cause arterial hypoxemia. Milrinone causes less pronounced increases in heart rate than catecholamines such as dobutamine, but the phosphodiesterase inhibitor is arrhythmogenic because of its actions on intracellular Ca^{2+} homeostasis. Milrinone also inhibits platelet aggregation without producing thrombocytopenia, blunts the inflammatory cytokine response to cardiopulmonary bypass, and dilates native epicardial coronary arteries and arterial graft conduits. These actions are potentially anti-ischemic in patients with coronary artery disease undergoing CABG surgery.

It is important to recognize that the relative use of milrinone as a positive inotrope may be partially attenuated in the failing heart, but not to the degree that is commonly seen with β_1 adrenoceptor agonists. As a result, the phosphodiesterase inhibitor continues to effectively enhance myocardial contractility in decompensated heart failure, despite the presence of concomitant β_1 adrenoceptor down-regulation. The combination of milrinone and a β_1 adrenoceptor agonist is frequently used to assist weaning from cardiopulmonary bypass in patients with substantially depressed LV systolic function because of the synergistic actions of these drugs on cAMP-mediated intracellular signaling.

IV. Vasopressin

Vasopressin (*antidiuretic hormone*) is a peptide hormone released from the posterior pituitary that regulates water reabsorption in the kidney and exerts potent hemodynamic effects independent of adrenergic receptors. Vasopressin receptors consist of three subtypes (V_1, V_2, and V_3), all of which are five-subunit helical membrane proteins coupled to G proteins. Vasopressin's cardiovascular effects are predominately mediated through V_1 receptors, which are located in the cell membrane of vascular smooth muscle. Activation of the V_1 receptor subtype stimulates phospholipase C and triggers hydrolysis of inositol 4,5-bisphosphate to inositol 1,4,5-triphosphate and diacylglyercol. These second messengers increase intracellular Ca^{2+} concentration and produce contraction of the vascular smooth muscle cell. V_2 receptors are present on renal collecting duct cells, and, when activated, increase reabsorption of free water, whereas the more recently described V_3 receptors are located in the pituitary.

Along with the sympathetic nervous system and renin–angiotensin–aldosterone axis, endogenous vasopressin plays a crucial role in the maintenance of arterial pressure. Exogenous administration of vasopressin does not substantially affect arterial pressure in conscious, healthy patients because activation of central V_1 receptors in the area postrema increases baroreceptor reflex–mediated inhibition of efferent sympathetic nervous outflow that counterbalances the elevated systemic vascular resistance resulting from V_1-induced arterial vasoconstriction. In contrast, vasopressinergic mechanisms are essential for maintaining arterial pressure under conditions in which sympathetic nervous system or renin–angiotensin–aldosterone axis dysfunction is present. Indeed, exogenous administration of vasopressin has been shown to effectively support arterial pressure when a relative vasopressin deficiency exists (e.g., ***catecholamine-refractory hypotension,*** vasodilatory shock, sepsis, cardiac arrest). Angiotensin-converting enzyme inhibitors and angiotensin II receptor blockers used to treat hypertension also affect autonomic nervous system and renin–angiotensin–aldosterone axis function. Intraoperative hypotension that is relatively refractory to administration of catecholamines or sympathomimetics has been repeatedly described in patients who have been treated with these medications.

General or neuraxial anesthesia also reduces sympathetic nervous system tone, resulting in decreased plasma stress hormone concentrations including vasopressin. Under these circumstances, administration of vasopressin activates V_1 vascular smooth muscle receptors and rapidly increases arterial pressure during anesthesia by causing arterial vasoconstriction. Vasopressin therapy has been shown to reduce mortality associated with acute vasodilatory states such as anaphylaxis. In addition, infusion of vasopressin is indicated for the treatment of severe hypotension after prolonged cardiopulmonary bypass in patients who are otherwise unresponsive to phenylephrine or norepinephrine (vasoplegia).

Vasopressin is a useful drug for the treatment of ***sepsis*** and ***cardiac arrest***. Vasodilation that is refractory to fluid resuscitation combined with a relative deficiency of endogenous vasopressin is a characteristic feature of sepsis. Inadequate sympathetic nervous system and renin–angiotensin–aldosterone axis responses to hypotension are also present in sepsis. Administration of vasopressin in the absence or presence of other vasoactive medications often improves hemodynamics and facilitates survival in patients with sepsis. The combined use of vasopressin with other vasoactive medications often reduces the overall dose of vasopressin required to maintain arterial pressure, thereby limiting the adverse effects of vasopressin on organ perfusion. In fact, sustained administration of higher doses of vasopressin may produce mesenteric ischemia, peripheral vascular insufficiency, and cardiac arrest because the drug causes pronounced vasoconstriction of cutaneous, skeletal muscle, splanchnic, and coronary vascular beds concomitant with reduced perfusion of and oxygen delivery to these tissues. Bolus intravenous administration of vasopressin is also used as part of the advanced cardiac life support algorithm for cardiac arrest resulting from ventricular fibrillation, pulseless electrical activity, and asystole.

V. Antihypertensive Medications

A. Beta-Blockers

Many of the cardiovascular actions of *β adrenoceptor antagonists* (beta-blockers) may be anticipated based on the previous discussion of catecholamines. Beta-blockers produce important anti-ischemic effects and are considered a first-line therapy for treatment of patients with ST-segment elevation myocardial infarction in the absence of cardiogenic shock, hemodynamically significant bradyarrhythmias, or reactive airway disease. Indeed, beta-blockers have been repeatedly shown to ***reduce mortality and morbidity*** associated with myocardial infarction in a number of large clinical trials. The most recent American College of Cardiology/American Heart Association guidelines recommend continuation of beta-blockers in patients who are receiving them chronically for established cardiac indications. Beta-blocker initiation should be considered for vascular surgery patients and other patients at high risk of myocardial ischemia who are scheduled to undergo intermediate- or high-risk noncardiac surgery (Table 13.4). Perioperative beta-blocker therapy should

Table 13-4   Recommendations for Perioperative Beta-Blocker Therapy

2007 Perioperative Guideline Recommendations	2009 Perioperative Focused Update Recommendations	Comments
Class I		
1. Beta blockers should be continued in patients undergoing surgery who are receiving beta blockers to treat angina, symptomatic arrhythmias, hypertension, or other ACC/AHA Class I guideline indications. *(Level of Evidence: C)*	1. Beta blockers should be continued in patients undergoing surgery who are receiving beta blockers for treatment of conditions with ACCF/AHA Class I guideline indications for the drugs. *(Level of Evidence: C)*	2007 recommendation remains current in 2009 update with revised wording.
2. Beta blockers should be given to patients undergoing vascular surgery who are at high cardiac risk owing to the finding of ischemia on preoperative testing. *(Level of Evidence: B)*		Deleted/combined recommendation (class of recommendation changed from I to IIa for patients with cardiac ischemia on preoperative testing).
Class IIa		
1. Beta blockers are probably recommended for patients undergoing vascular surgery in whom preoperative assessment identifies coronary heart disease. *(Level of Evidence: B)*	1. Beta blockers titrated to heart rate and blood pressure are probably recommended for patients undergoing vascular surgery who are at high cardiac risk owing to coronary artery disease or the finding of cardiac ischemia on preoperative testing. *(Level of Evidence: B)*	Modified/combined recommendation (wording revised and class of recommendation changed from I to IIa for patients with cardiac ischemia on preoperative testing).
2. Beta blockers are probably recommended for patients in whom preoperative assessment for vascular surgery identifies high cardiac risk, as defined by the presence of more than 1 clinical risk factor.[a] *(Level of Evidence: B)*	2. Beta blockers titrated to heart rate and blood pressure are reasonable for patients in whom preoperative assessment for vascular surgery identifies high cardiac risk, as defined by the presence of more than 1 clinical risk factor.[a] *(Level of Evidence: C)*	Modified recommendation (level of evidence changed from B to C).
3. Beta blockers are probably recommended for patients in whom preoperative assessment identifies coronary heart disease or high cardiac risk, as defined by the presence of more than 1 clinical risk factor,[a] who are undergoing intermediate-risk or vascular surgery. *(Level of Evidence: B)*	3. Beta blockers titrated to heart rate and blood pressure are reasonable for patients in whom preoperative assessment identifies coronary artery disease or high cardiac risk, as defined by the presence of more than 1 clinical risk factor,[a] who are undergoing intermediate-risk surgery. *(Level of Evidence: B)*	2007 recommendation remains current in 2009 update with revised wording.

Table 13-4   Recommendations for Perioperative Beta-Blocker Therapy (*Continued*)

2007 Perioperative Guideline Recommendations	2009 Perioperative Focused Update Recommendations	Comments
Class IIb		
1. The usefulness of beta blockers is uncertain for patients who are undergoing either intermediate-risk procedures or vascular surgery, in whom preoperative assessment identifies a single clinical risk factor.[a] *(Level of Evidence: C)*	1. The usefulness of beta blockers is uncertain for patients who are undergoing either intermediate-risk procedures or vascular surgery in whom preoperative assessment identifies a single clinical risk factor in the absence of coronary artery disease.[a] *(Level of Evidence: C)*	2007 recommendation remains current in 2009 update with revised wording.
2. The usefulness of beta blockers is uncertain in patients undergoing vascular surgery with no clinical risk factors who are not currently taking beta blockers. *(Level of Evidence: B)*	2. The usefulness of beta blockers is uncertain in patients undergoing vascular surgery with no clinical risk factors[a] who are not currently taking beta blockers. *(Level of Evidence: B)*	2007 recommendation remains current in 2009 update.
Class III		
1. Beta blockers should not be given to patients undergoing surgery who have absolute contraindications to beta blockade. *(Level of Evidence: C)*	1. Beta blockers should not be given to patients undergoing surgery who have absolute contraindications to beta blockade. *(Level of Evidence: C)*	2007 recommendation remains current in 2009 update.
	2. Routine administration of high-dose beta blockers in the absence of dose titration is not useful and may be harmful to patients not currently taking beta blockers who are undergoing noncardiac surgery. *(Level of Evidence: B)*	New recommendation

[a]Clinical risk factors include history of ischemic heart disease, history of compensated or prior heart failure, history of cerebrovascular disease, diabetes mellitus, and renal insufficiency (defined in the Revised Cardiac Risk Index as a preoperative serum creatinine of >2 mg/dL).
ACC, American College of Cardiology; AHA, American Heart Association.
From Fleishmann KE, Buller CE, Fleisher LA, et al. 2009 ACCF/AHA focused update on perioperative beta blockade. *JACC.* 2009;54(22): 2102–2128, with permission.

most likely be initiated well before anticipated elective surgery to mitigate the risk of stroke and death that was reported when an arbitrary dose of metoprolol was first initiated on the day of surgery. Beta-blockers are effective for the treatment of *essential hypertension* and also exert useful antiarrhythmic effects, especially in the presence of increased sympathetic nervous system tone associated with surgery or during conditions characterized by elevated levels of circulating catecholamines (e.g., pheochromocytoma, hyperthyroidism). Beta-blockers reduce heart rate, myocardial contractility, and arterial pressure by binding to β_1 adrenoceptors and inhibiting the actions of circulating catecholamines and norepinephrine released from postganglionic sympathetic nerves. The decrease in heart rate produced by beta-blockers also serves to prolong diastole, increase coronary blood flow to the LV, enhance coronary collateral perfusion to ischemic myocardium, and improve oxygen delivery to the coronary microcirculation. These combined effects serve to *reduce myocardial oxygen* demand while simultaneously increasing supply. Beta-blockers have also been shown to inhibit platelet aggregation. This latter action is particularly important during acute myocardial ischemia or evolving myocardial infarction because platelet aggregation at the site of an atherosclerotic plaque may worsen a coronary stenosis or produce acute occlusion of the vessel. Beta-blockers vary in their affinity for and relative selectivity at the β_1 adrenoceptor, while some of these drugs exert "intrinsic sympathetic activity" by acting as partial β adrenoceptor agonists. Nevertheless, all beta-blockers effectively reduce arterial pressure.

Esmolol

Esmolol is a relatively selective *β_1 adrenoceptor blocker*. The chemical structure of esmolol is very similar to that of propranolol and metoprolol, but esmolol contains an additional methylester group that facilitates the drug's rapid metabolism via *hydrolysis* by red blood cell esterases, resulting in an elimination half-life of approximately 9 minutes. The rapid onset and metabolism of esmolol makes the drug very useful for the treatment of acute tachycardia and hypertension during surgery. Esmolol is most often administered as an intravenous bolus, which causes almost immediate dose-related decreases in heart rate and myocardial contractility. Arterial pressure declines as a result of these direct negative chronotropic and inotropic effects. Esmolol is often used to attenuate the sympathetic nervous system response to laryngoscopy, endotracheal intubation, or surgical stimulation, particularly in patients with known or suspected coronary artery disease who may be at risk of myocardial ischemia. Esmolol is also useful for rapid control of heart rate in patients with supraventricular tachyarrhythmias (e.g., atrial fibrillation, atrial flutter). Finally, esmolol effectively blunts the sympathetically mediated tachycardia and hypertension that occur shortly after the onset of seizure activity during electroconvulsive therapy. Because esmolol does not appreciably block β_2 adrenoceptors due to its relative β_1 selectivity, *hypotension* is more commonly observed after administration of this drug compared with other nonselective beta-blockers.

> **? Did You Know**
>
> Esmolol has an elimination half-life of approximately 9 minutes because it is hydrolysed by red cell esterases.

Labetalol

Labetalol is composed of four stereoisomers that *inhibit α and β adrenoceptors* to varying degrees. One of the four stereoisomers is an α_1 adrenoceptor antagonist, another is a nonselective β adrenoceptor blocker, and the remaining two do not appreciably affect adrenergic receptors. The net effect of this mixture is a drug that selectively inhibits α_1 adrenoceptors while simultaneously blocking β_1 and β_2 adrenoceptors in a nonselective manner. The intravenous formulation of labetalol contains a ratio of α_1 to β adrenoceptor blockade of approximately 1:7. Blockade of the α_1 adrenoceptor causes arteriolar vasodilation and decreases arterial pressure through a reduction in systemic vascular resistance. This property makes the drug very useful for the treatment of *perioperative hypertension*. Despite its nonselective beta-blocking properties, labetalol is also a partial β_2 adrenoceptor agonist; this latter characteristic also contributes to vasodilation. Labetalol-induced inhibition of β_1 adrenoceptors decreases heart rate and myocardial contractility. Stroke volume and cardiac output are essentially unchanged as a result of the combined actions of labetalol on α_1 and β adrenoceptors. Unlike other vasodilators, labetalol produces vasodilation without triggering baroreceptor reflex tachycardia because the drug blocks anticipated increases in heart rate mediated through β_1 adrenoceptors. This action may be especially beneficial for the treatment of hypertension in the setting of acute myocardial ischemia. Labetalol is most commonly used for the treatment of perioperative hypertension. Labetalol may also be useful for controlling arterial pressure without producing tachycardia in patients with hypertensive emergencies and those with acute type A aortic dissection. Labetalol has been shown to attenuate the sympathetic nervous system response to laryngoscopy and endotracheal intubation, although the drug's relatively long elimination half-life (approximately 6 hours) limits its use in this setting.

B. Nitrovasodilators

Nitrovasodilators include organic nitrates (e.g., *nitroglycerin*) and nitric oxide (NO) donors (e.g., *sodium nitroprusside*) that release NO through enzymatic sulfhydryl group reduction or through a spontaneous mechanism that occurs independent of metabolism, respectively. Like endogenous NO produced by vascular endothelium, exogenous NO stimulates guanylate cyclase within the vascular smooth muscle cell to convert guanosine triphosphate to cGMP. The second messenger activates a cGMP-dependent protein kinase (protein kinase G) that dephosphorylates myosin light chains and contributes to relaxation of vascular smooth muscle. NO also stimulates Ca^{2+} reuptake into the sarcoplasmic reticulum by activating the sarcoplasmic reticulum Ca^{2+} ATPase through a cGMP-independent mechanism, thereby reducing intracellular Ca^{2+} concentrations and causing relaxation. Finally, NO stimulates potassium (K^+) efflux from the cell by activating the K^+ channel. The net effect of this shift in K^+ balance is cellular hyperpolarization, which closes the voltage-gated Ca^{2+} channel and also facilitates relaxation.

Nitrovasodilators are often used to improve hemodynamics and myocardial oxygen supply–demand relations in patients with *heart failure*. Vasodilation reduces venous return, contributing to declines in left and right ventricular end-diastolic volume, pressure, and wall stress, and also reduces systemic and pulmonary arterial pressures, which decreases left and right ventricular end-systolic wall stress, respectively. These actions combine to *decrease myocardial oxygen consumption*. Simultaneously, nitrovasodilators increase myocardial oxygen supply through direct dilation of epicardial coronary arteries in the absence and presence of flow-limiting stenoses. The reduction in LV end-diastolic pressure observed during administration of nitrovasodilators coupled with coronary vasodilation substantially enhances subendocardial perfusion. The clinical efficacy of nitrovasodilators may display some initial variability between patients, but the cardiovascular effects of these drugs inevitably diminish with prolonged use. Some patients may be relatively resistant to the effects of organic nitrates in the presence of oxidative stress because superoxide anions scavenge NO, cause reversible oxidation of guanylate cyclase, and inhibit aldehyde dehydrogenase. The latter action prevents the release of NO from organic nitrates. A progressive attenuation of hemodynamic responses to nitrovasodilators may develop in other patients as a result of sympathetic nervous system and renin–angiotensin–aldosterone axis activation. This phenomenon (pseudo-tolerance) accounts for the *rebound hypertension* that may be observed after abrupt discontinuation of nitrovasodilator therapy. Inhibition of guanylate cyclase activity is most likely responsible for true tolerance to organic nitrates. A "drug holiday" is a useful strategy for reversing this effect in patients requiring prolonged treatment in the intensive care unit. Administration of *N*-acetylcysteine, a sulfhydryl donor, may also be effective for reversing true tolerance. Notably, prolonged use of organic nitrates may also cause methemoglobinemia, interfere with platelet aggregation, and produce heparin resistance. It is also important to recognize that organic nitrates should also be used with caution in patients receiving phosphodiesterase type V inhibitors (e.g., sildenafil) because NO-induced vasodilation is enhanced, and profound hypotension, myocardial ischemia or infarction, and death may result.

Nitroglycerin

Nitroglycerin *dilates venules* to a greater degree than arterioles. At lower doses, this organic nitrate produces venodilation without causing a significant decrease in systemic vascular resistance. Arterial pressure and cardiac output fall in response to the reduction in preload, despite a modest baroreceptor reflex–mediated increase in heart rate. Nitroglycerin also decreases pulmonary arterial pressures and vascular resistance. At higher doses, nitroglycerin dilates arterioles, reducing LV afterload, causing more pronounced decreases in arterial pressure, and stimulating greater reflex tachycardia. Overshoot hypotension and tachycardia is a particularly common setting of hypovolemia, such as is often observed in patients with poorly controlled essential hypertension and parturients with pregnancy-induced hypertension.

Nitroglycerin improves the balance of myocardial oxygen supply to demand through its actions as a direct *coronary vasodilator* (which increases supply) and its systemic hemodynamic effects (which reduce demand). Nitroglycerin dilates both normal and poststenotic epicardial coronary arteries, enhances blood flow through coronary collateral vessels, and preferentially improves subendocardial perfusion. The drug also inhibits coronary vasospasm and dilates arterial conduits used during CABG surgery. Nitroglycerin *decreases myocardial oxygen* demand by reducing LV preload and, to a lesser extent, afterload, thereby producing corresponding reductions in LV end-diastolic and end-systolic wall stress. These effects are particularly important in patients with acutely decompensated heart failure resulting from *myocardial ischemia*. Based on the aforementioned actions, it should be readily apparent that nitroglycerin is a very effective first-line drug for the treatment of myocardial ischemia, but it is also important to emphasize that caution should be exercised when using nitroglycerin in patients with ischemia who are also *hypovolemic*. Under these circumstances, administration of nitroglycerin may precipitate life-threatening hypotension by compromising coronary perfusion pressure, reducing coronary blood flow despite epicardial vasodilation, and worsening ischemia.

Sodium Nitroprusside

Sodium nitroprusside is an *ultrashort-acting direct NO donor*. It is a potent *venous and arterial vasodilator* devoid of inotropic effects that quickly reduces arterial pressure by decreasing LV preload and afterload. These characteristics make sodium nitroprusside a first-line drug for the treatment of hypertensive emergencies. Sodium nitroprusside may be useful for the treatment of cardiogenic shock because arterial vasodilation improves forward flow by reducing impedance to LV ejection, while venodilation decreases LV filling pressures. Unlike nitroglycerin, sodium nitroprusside is relatively *contraindicated* in patients with acute *myocardial ischemia* because the drug causes abnormal redistribution of coronary blood flow away from ischemic myocardium (coronary steal) by producing greater coronary vasodilation in vessels that perfuse normal myocardium compared with those that supply the ischemic territory.

Baroreceptor reflex–mediated tachycardia is also more pronounced during administration of sodium nitroprusside compared with nitroglycerin because the direct NO donor is a more potent arteriolar vasodilator than the organic nitrate. This *reflex tachycardia* dramatically increases heart rate and myocardial oxygen consumption, thereby exacerbating acute myocardial ischemia. Sodium nitroprusside is often combined with a β_1 adrenoceptor antagonist such as esmolol to decrease arterial pressure, depress myocardial contractility, and reduce ascending aortic wall stress in patients with acute type A aortic dissection until direct surgical control of the injury can be achieved. Clinical use of sodium nitroprusside is limited by its toxic metabolites, which predictably accumulate when administration is prolonged or relatively high doses are used. Metabolism of sodium nitroprusside produces cyanide, which binds with cytochrome C to inhibit aerobic metabolism and cause lactic acidosis. Cyanide derived from sodium nitroprusside metabolism also binds with hemoglobin to form methemoglobin and with sulfur to form thiocyanate. The latter metabolite may accumulate in patients with renal insufficiency and produce neurologic complications including delirium and seizures.

C. Hydralazine

Hydralazine is a *direct vasodilator* that reduces intracellular Ca^{2+} concentration in vascular smooth muscle, at least in part, by activating adenosine triphosphate–sensitive potassium channels. This action produces direct relaxation of small arteries and arterioles in coronary, cerebral, splanchnic, and renal vascular beds, declines in systemic vascular resistance, and decreases in arterial pressure. Left ventricular preload is relatively preserved because hydralazine does not dilate venous capacitance vessels. The primary reduction in afterload stimulates baroreceptor reflex–mediated tachycardia and increases cardiac output. The magnitude of tachycardia observed with administration of hydralazine is often greater than expected based solely on baroreceptor reflexes alone and may instead reflect a direct effect of the drug on other centrally mediated cardiovascular regulatory mechanisms. The pronounced *tachycardia* associated with administration of hydralazine may produce acute myocardial ischemia in patients with critical coronary stenoses based on increases in myocardial oxygen demand and reductions in coronary perfusion pressure. Hydralazine-induced tachycardia responds appropriately to β_1 adrenoceptor antagonists, but caution should be exercised because further declines in arterial pressure may also occur. Hydralazine is commonly used for management of sustained postoperative hypertension in the absence of tachycardia.

D. Calcium Channel Antagonists

Calcium channels are asymmetric biochemical pores consisting of at least four subunits (α_1, α_2/Δ, and β with or without γ) that traverse many biologic membranes. Under quiescent conditions, Ca^{2+} channels are closed, but they may open through a voltage-dependent (requiring cell depolarization) or receptor-operated (activation) mechanism to allow Ca^{2+} entry into the cell or an organelle (e.g., mitochondria, sarcoplasmic reticulum), most often down an electrochemical gradient. Myocardial and vascular smooth muscle cell membranes contain two distinct types of voltage-dependent Ca^{2+} channels that are denoted based on the relative duration of pore opening: T (transient) and L (long). The *L-type Ca^{2+} channel* is the predominant target of all calcium channel antagonists in current clinical use (these drugs do not block the T-type Ca^{2+} channel). There are four major classes of chemically distinct Ca^{2+} channel antagonists: (a) 1,4-dihydropyridines (e.g., nifedipine, nicardipine, clevidipine),

(b) benzothiazepines (diltiazem), (c) phenylalkylamines (verapamil), and (d) diarylaminopropylamine ethers (bepridil). In general, Ca^{2+} channel antagonists produce vasodilation, direct negative chronotropic, dromotropic, and inotropic effects and baroreceptor reflex–mediated increases in heart rate, to varying degrees, depending on each drug's relative selectivity for voltage-gated Ca^{2+} channels in myocardium and vascular smooth muscle. All Ca^{2+} channel antagonists cause greater relaxation of arterial compared with venous vascular smooth muscle. This action reduces LV afterload while preserving preload. Calcium channel antagonists improve myocardial oxygen supply through coronary arterial vasodilation and inhibition of coronary artery vasospasm. In addition to eliciting declines in LV afterload, Ca^{2+} channel antagonists such as diltiazem and verapamil may also reduce myocardial oxygen demand via depression of myocardial contractility and decreases in heart rate mediated by reduced sinoatrial node automaticity and atrioventricular node conduction. However, it is important to note that some dihydropyridine Ca^{2+} channel antagonists may inadvertently increase myocardial oxygen demand as a result of baroreceptor reflex–induced tachycardia, and as a result, may not consistently produce anti-ischemic effects in patients with coronary artery disease. For the sake of brevity, the discussion here is limited to two intravenous dihydropyridines that are commonly used for the treatment of perioperative hypertension.

? Did You Know

All Ca^{2+} channel blockers produce greater relaxation of arterial than venous vascular smooth muscle.

Nicardipine

Nicardipine is a dihydropyridine Ca^{2+} channel antagonist that is highly selective for *vascular smooth muscle*. Nicardipine produces cardiovascular effects that are similar to nifedipine but has a longer half-life than the latter drug. Nicardipine is a *profound vasodilator* because of its pronounced inhibition of Ca^{2+} influx in vascular smooth muscle. Like other dihydropyridine Ca^{2+} channel antagonists, nicardipine preferentially dilates arteriolar vessels, which decreases arterial pressure. In contrast to diltiazem and verapamil, nicardipine does not substantially depress myocardial contractility nor does it affect the rate of sinoatrial node firing. As a result, stroke volume and cardiac output are relatively preserved or may increase. Nicardipine-induced decreases in arterial pressure trigger increases in heart rate through activation of baroreceptor reflexes, but the *tachycardia* observed during administration of nicardipine is less pronounced than typically occurs with sodium nitroprusside at comparable levels of arterial pressure. Nicardipine is also a highly potent *coronary vasodilator* and is often used to dilate arterial grafts during CABG surgery. Because of its relative long half-life, nicardipine is primarily used for treatment of sustained perioperative hypertension and not for acute, often transient, hypertensive episodes that are commonly observed during surgery.

Clevidipine

Clevidipine is a relatively new, *ultrashort-acting* dihydropyridine L-type voltage-gated Ca^{2+} channel antagonist with a plasma half-life of approximately 2 minutes after intravenous administration. Like nicardipine and nifedipine, clevidipine exerts pronounced effects at the less negative resting membrane potentials typically observed in vascular smooth muscle cells, but demonstrates lower potency in cardiac myocytes in which resting membrane potentials are substantially more negative. As a result of these differences in cellular electrophysiology, clevidipine is highly selective for *arterial vascular smooth muscle* and is nearly devoid of negative chronotropic or inotropic effects. This hemodynamic profile may be especially useful for the treatment of hypertension in patients with compromised LV function. Clevidipine causes dose-related arteriolar vasodilation while sparing venous vasomotor tone, thereby reducing systemic vascular resistance and arterial pressure without affecting LV preload. These actions may combine to augment cardiac output. Modest increases in heart rate may also occur during administration of clevidipine as a result of baroreceptor reflex activation. Unlike other short-acting antihypertensive drugs, administration of clevidipine is not associated with the development of tachyphylaxis, and abrupt discontinuation of the drug does not appear to cause rebound hypertension. Because tissue and plasma esterases are responsible for clevidipine metabolism, little to *no accumulation* of the drug occurs even in the setting of hepatic or kidney dysfunction.

Selected Readings

Benham-Hermetz J, Lambert M, Stephens RC. Cardiovascular failure, inotropes and vasopressors. *Br J Hosp Med (Lond).* 2012;73:C74–C77.

Erstad BL, Barletta JF. Treatment of hypertension in the perioperative patient. *Ann Pharmacother.* 2000;34:66–79.

Friederich JA, Butterworth JF 4th. Sodium nitroprusside: Twenty years and counting. *Anesth Analg.* 1995;81:152–162.

Gillies M, Bellomo R, Doolan L, et al. Bench-to-bedside review: Inotropic drug therapy after adult cardiac surgery—a systemic literature review. *Crit Care.* 2005;9:266–279.

Iachini Bellisarii F, Radico F, Muscente F, et al. Nitrates and other nitric oxide donors in cardiology: Current positioning and perspectives. *Cardiovasc Drugs Ther.* 2012;26:55–69.

MacCarthy EP, Bloomfield SS. Labetalol: a review of its pharmacology, pharmacokinetics, clinical uses and adverse effects. *Pharmacotherapy.* 1983;3:193–219.

Overgaard CB, Dzavik V. Inotropes and vasopressors: Review of physiology and clinical use in cardiovascular disease. *Circulation.* 2008;118:1047–1056.

Pagel PS, Warltier DC. Positive inotropic drugs. In: Evers AS, Maze M, Kharasch E, eds. *Anesthetic Pharmacology: Physiologic Principles and Clinical Practice.* 2nd ed. Cambridge, UK: Cambridge University Press; 2011:706–723.

Prlesi L, Cheng-Lai A. Clevidipine: A novel ultra-short-acting calcium antagonist. *Cardiol Rev.* 2009;17:147–152.

Treschan TA, Peters J. The vasopressin system: Physiology and clinical strategies. *Anesthesiology.* 2006;105:599–612.

Questions

1. The α_1 adrenoreceptor-mediated vasoconstriction occurs through what signaling mechanism?
   A. A stimulatory guanine nucleotide-binding (G_s) protein
   B. An inhibitory guanine nucleotide-binding (G_i) protein
   C. An adenosine coupled trans-membrane kinase
   D. A nitric oxide scavenging free radical
   E. None of the above

2. How will the chronic administration of therapeutic doses of propranolol affect the hemodynamic response to intravenous epinephrine?
   A. The heart rate response will be increased
   B. The blood pressure response will be decreased
   C. The systemic vascular resistance response will be increased
   D. The inotropic response will be increased
   E. None of the above

3. Compared with epinephrine at low doses, norepinephrine produces a greater increase in blood pressure because it causes:
   A. A greater increase in cardiac output
   B. A greater increase in cardiac inotropy
   C. A greater increase in systemic vascular resistance
   D. A greater increase in venous return
   E. None of the above

4. Tachyphylaxis to the hemodynamic effects of ephedrine results from:
   A. Depletion of presynaptic norepinephrine stores
   B. Down regulation of postsynaptic adrenoreceptors
   C. Hyperpolarization of the β_1 postganglionic neurons
   D. Increased β_2 adrenoreceptor sensitivity at higher dose levels
   E. None of the above

5. Labetalol decreases systemic vascular resistance by:
   A. Inhibiting α_1 and β_2 receptors
   B. Inhibiting α_1 and β_1 receptors
   C. Inhibiting α_1 and β_1 and β_2 receptors
   D. Inhibiting α_1 and stimulating β_2 receptors
   E. None of the above

6. Unlike nitroglycerine, nitroprusside may be contraindicated in patients with myocardial ischemia because it:
   A. Reduces arterial blood pressure
   B. Reduces systemic venous return
   C. Increases myocardial blood flow to normal myocardium
   D. Produces cyanide and methemoglobin
   E. None of the above

PART C

Technology

14

The Anesthesia Workstation

Naveen Nathan
Tom C. Krejcie

It is common for students, nurses, and physicians in the embryonic phase of their anesthesiology training to be intimidated when confronted by the current iteration of the anesthesia machine, the anesthesia workstation. The sheer number of cables, hoses, knobs, digital displays, and alarms may seem formidable. This chapter aims to deconstruct the anatomy and functionality of the conventional anesthesia workstation and characterize the principles underlying its use.

As a salient and indispensable component of the operating room environment, the anesthesia workstation serves to achieve four goals: 1) provide a reliable mechanism to continually ventilate the anesthetized patient, 2) serve as a source for supplemental O_2, 3) provide a mechanism for the delivery of volatile anesthetic agents, and 4) serve as a monitor and early-warning system for several potential hazards encountered in clinical anesthetic care. Note that a variety of simple tools exist to achieve each of these goals individually (e.g., a bag-valve-mask device [Ambu-bag] may be used to ventilate a patient's lungs and a simple E-cylinder filled with pressurized oxygen may be used to increase the fraction of inspired oxygen [FiO_2]). The anesthesia workstation, however, incorporates and consolidates all of the above goals in a manner that is convenient and allows the anesthesiologist to be more vigilant in performing other equally important facets of anesthetic care. It cannot be overemphasized that this convenience comes at the price of complexity. Many intraoperative crises can be avoided by appreciating the design, functionality, and limitations of modern anesthesia workstations.

I. Functional Anatomy of the Anesthesia Workstation

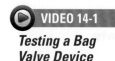

VIDEO 14-1

Testing a Bag Valve Device

In its entirety, the anesthesia workstation encompasses a broad range of equipment, including the anesthesia machine, physiologic monitors, and accessories such as active suction equipment and adjunctive bag-valve-mask device. Patient monitoring and airway management are discussed elsewhere. The remainder of this chapter directs attention specifically to the anesthesia machine. The basic construct of the anesthesia machine is defined by three concepts (Fig. 14-1). The first is a system that originates with a *gas*; typically

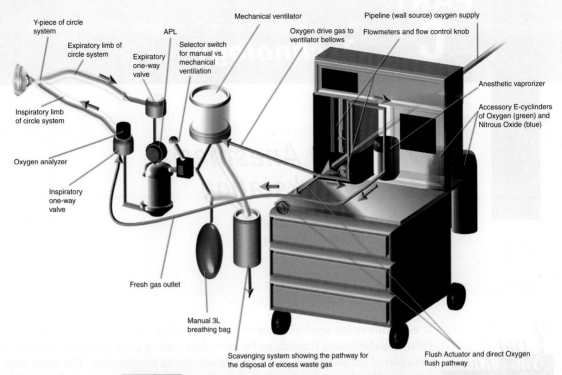

Y-piece of circle system

Expiratory limb of circle system

Expiratory one-way valve

APL

Selector switch for manual vs. mechanical ventilation

Mechanical ventilator

Oxygen drive gas to ventilator bellows

Pipeline (wall source) oxygen supply

Flowmeters and flow control knob

Anesthetic vaprorizer

Accessory E-cyclinders of Oxygen (green) and Nitrous Oxide (blue)

Inspiratory limb of circle system

Oxygen analyzer

Inspiratory one-way valve

Fresh gas outlet

Manual 3L breathing bag

Scavenging system showing the pathway for the disposal of excess waste gas

Flush Actuator and direct Oxygen flush pathway

Figure 14-1 Representation of a typical anesthesia workstation. Arrows indicate direction of oxygen flow. Pipeline sources of air and nitrous oxide are not shown. APL, adjustable pressure-limiting valve.

this is pressurized oxygen/air delivered from a central hospital source, directly into the operating room. A series of *pressure-reducing systems* follows, after which the anesthesiologist directly controls the flow of these gases to achieve the desired flow rate and oxygen concentration that is delivered to the second system. Integrated into this gas delivery design is the anesthetic *vaporizer*, which allows for the administration of volatile anesthetic to the patient.

The system described above converges on the *fresh gas outlet*, which delivers the desired concentrations of gases and volatile anesthetics into the next conceptual framework (system) of the anesthesia machine: the *anesthesia breathing apparatus*. Patient ventilation is achieved through the use of either the automated controlled mechanical ventilator or manually through the breathing bag, both of which are incorporated into a system of corrugated tubes and unidirectional valves known as the *circle system*. This design enables reciprocal inflation and deflation of the patient's lungs with the ventilator or breathing bag. It also incorporates an absorbent compound to neutralize expired carbon dioxide.

Lastly, there must be a mechanism to remove excess gas or pressure from the system. This is accomplished through another structural arrangement, the *scavenging system*. The mechanics, safeguards, and hazards of each of these three systems will be discussed below.

II. Delivery of Gases: High, Intermediate, and Low Pressure Systems

Most anesthesia workstations receive a dual supply of medical-grade gases. Oxygen is delivered at high pressure from the central hospital supply source (liquid oxygen tanks) into the operating room through readily visible green

Table 14-1 Pressure Readings Encountered in an Anesthesia Workstation			
	psi	mm Hg	cm H$_2$O
Anesthesia workstation: High pressure oxygen or air source (a full E cylinder containing 625 L of gas)	**2,200**	113,773	154,675
Anesthesia workstation: High pressure nitrous oxide source (a full E cylinder containing 1,590 L of gas)	**745**	38,528	52,379
Anesthesia workstation: Intermediate pressure oxygen, air or nitrous oxide (inline working pressure within the machine)	**50–55**	2,586	3,515
Typical peak airway pressure during mechanical ventilation of a healthy patient at 6 cc/kg tidal volume and respiratory rate of 10 breaths/min	0.2–0.3	11–18	**15–25**

Note: The most commonly used unit of measurement is indicated in bold text.

hoses, or alternatively, can be delivered from a cylinder (size E) of oxygen attached to the anesthesia machine. Air is color coded in yellow. Note that these color designations apply to medical centers located in the United States and vary internationally. A third supply line of nitrous oxide at high pressure, coded in blue, may also be present, or a backup supply of nitrous oxide stored in an E cylinder attached to the anesthesia machine (1). The delivery of these gases through the anesthesia machine and ultimately to the patient is marked by a progressive, regulated decrement in pressure. Wall source gases are delivered to the anesthesia machine at a pressure of 50 pounds per square inch (psi). E cylinders contain considerably higher pressures but are regulated to 45 psi prior to their interface with the anesthesia machine (1,2). The user further regulates and fine tunes the low-pressure flow of gases to the patient using flow control knobs specific to each gas. Table 14-1 lists pressure readings encountered in the anesthesia workstation.

Pressure gauges reflective of both wall and cylinder sources of medical gases are displayed on the anesthesia machine. The gauges for the central hospital gas source measures the *intermediate* in-line working pressure and typically reads approximately 50 to 55 psi. The most common reason why this pressure reading would decrease is that the hose from the wall source has been disconnected from the anesthesia machine, but it could also result from a complete or partial failure of the central hospital gas source. This pressure gauge reading remains constant through the routine and continuous use of wall source gases even when used at high flow rates. In contrast, the gauges for medical cylinders reflect the *high* internal pressure of the cylinders themselves. A full E cylinder of oxygen or air will contain roughly 625 L of gas at a pressure of 2,200 psi. The pressure will drop proportionately as these gases are used (1–3). If a tank is used to oxygenate the patient at 10 L/min, then it will only last approximately 60 minutes (4). A full tank of nitrous oxide contains 1,590 L of gas at a pressure of 745 psi. Nitrous oxide, in contrast to oxygen and air, exists as a combination of liquid and gas at room temperature due to its physicochemical properties and critical temperature. As a result, continuous use of a nitrous oxide cylinder will *not* result in a pressure drop at the gauge until nearly 75% (1,200 L) of the nitrous oxide in the cylinder has been used. During the routine

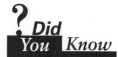
? *Did* You Know

Most operating rooms have reliable piped in oxygen. However, if this should fail, a low pressure alarm will be triggered. The hose should be disconnected and the auxiliary E cylinder of oxygen turned on.

use of the anesthesia machine, the E cylinder sources are kept in the off position as these are intended for use only during central pipeline failure. If such an event occurs, two actions are to be undertaken. First, the central pipeline gas source is disconnected from the anesthesia machine. Second, the E cylinder is turned to the on position so that continued oxygenation and ventilation of the patient may proceed (1–3).

A. Flowmeters

From the flowmeter assembly onward, the anesthesia machine is considered a *low* pressure system. The anesthesiologist may individually manipulate the flow of air, oxygen, and nitrous oxide to achieve flow rates of 0.2 L/min to more than 10 L/min for each gas. The fine control over the flow of these gases is achieved as they pass through specialized, variable orifice glass tubes known as Thorpe tubes. The height of a floating bobbin within the tapered lumen (increasing internal diameter) of these tubes indicates the current flow rate being used (Fig. 14-2). At very low flow rates (0.1 to 0.3 L/min), the passage of gas molecules through the smaller diameter section of these tubes is laminar. Concentric telescoping tubes of gas molecules moving parallel to one another in this fashion are influenced by gas *viscosity*, or, in other words, the frictional properties between the inner surface of an outer layer of gas flow against the outer surface of the inner layer adjacent to it. In contrast, at high flow rates in the large diameter section of the Thorpe tube (5 to 10 L/min), gas flow is turbulent, which is characterized by the

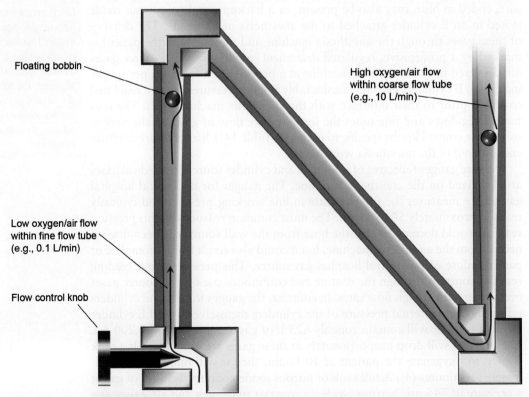

Figure 14-2 A flowmeter assembly and Thorpe tube. The black circle represents the floating bobbin, which indicates the current flow rate being used. Low flows at the narrow end of the tapered glass tube (e.g., 100 cc/min) are characterized as laminar and viscosity dependent. In contrast, high flows at the large diameter end of the tube (e.g., 10 L/min) are turbulent and density dependent.

random trajectory of gas molecules, though en masse there is bulk movement of air in the antegrade direction. In this scenario, flow is significantly affected by gas *density*. Larger gas molecules will result in greater intermolecular collisions and hence greater impedance to gas flow (1,2).

B. Flush Actuator and One-Way Check Valve

Thus far, the discussion of gas delivery from its source to the patient has followed a single path that begins with very high pressures. However, it is ultimately received by the patient's lungs under low pressure conditions within agreeably physiologic limits. Anesthesia machines are equipped with an alternate pathway for oxygen that may expose the patient to the intermediate pressure system. The *flush actuator* permits the application of oxygen flow from the in-line working pressure of 55 psi through the common gas outlet to the patient. Flow rates of oxygen through this alternate pathway that bypasses the flowmeters can range from 35 to 75 L/min. As a matter of perspective, using the flush valve to inflate a patient's lungs exposes the patient to roughly 200 times the typical inflation pressures used during routine mechanical ventilation. One may wonder why this pathway exists at all? Should the patient somehow become disconnected from the anesthesia breathing apparatus during controlled ventilation, the ventilator bellows (or the breathing bag) will immediately deflate as the volume of gas within will be drained into the operating room environment. The flush actuator could be used to rapidly increase the volume of gas in the system, so that normal tidal volumes may resume. This should be undertaken with care and advisably only during the *expiratory* phase of respiration when any excess gas or pressure resulting from the use of the flush valve can be scavenged away from the system (see "Scavenging Systems" later in this chapter). Additionally, the flush valve may be used for more complex ventilation strategies such as high-frequency jet ventilation (1,2).

A further consideration involves the potential presence of a one-way check valve just *upstream* of where the flush actuator joins the fresh gas outlet to the patient. This valve is present on many models of Datex Ohmeda (GE Healthcare Company) brand workstations and allows for the unidirectional flow of gas only in the antegrade route. As a consequence, using the flush valve exposes the patient to *all* of the oxygen flow from the intermediate pressure system. In the absence of this one-way check valve, as is the case in Dräger workstations (Dräger Medical Inc.), some of the oxygen flow from flushing the system may course in a retrograde fashion (Fig. 14-3) (1).

C. Safeguards in the Delivery of Medical Gases

It is imperative that the anesthesiologist verifies the presence of adequate gas supply pressures for both the wall source and the auxiliary E cylinder(s) during the preuse check of the workstation (see "Anesthesia Workstation Preuse Checkout" later in this chapter). Acceptable gas pressure readings, however, still do not guarantee that the *correct* gas is in fact being delivered to the patient. Misconnecting a nitrous oxide wall hose or nitrous cylinder to the noncorresponding interface for oxygen could result in the delivery of a hypoxic gas mixture. Thankfully, modern anesthesia systems help prevent such catastrophic occurrences. Wall source hoses are connected to the back of the anesthesia machine through noninterchangeable fittings, each with a diameter specific to its respective gas (the *diameter index safety system*). Additionally, E cylinders for oxygen, air, and nitrous oxide each have a specific arrangement of two holes that mate with their corresponding pins on the yoke of the anesthesia machine (the pin index safety system) (Fig. 14-4) (1,2).

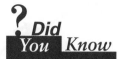
? Did You Know

The oxygen flush actuator ("flush valve") delivers oxygen at high pressure and flow directly to the common gas outlet. Its primary purpose is to enable rapid filling of a deflated rebreathing bag or ventilator bellows.

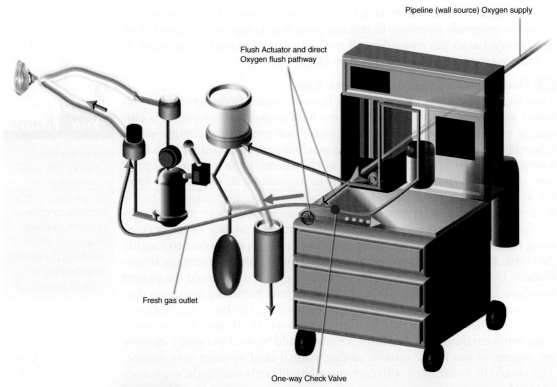

Figure 14-3 Oxygen flush actuator showing how the high pressure (50 pounds per square inch) of oxygen can bypass the flowmeters and be directly administered to the patient. The presence of a one-way check valve (*red dot*) forces all of the high-flow oxygen to course antegrade into the fresh gas outlet (*solid green arrow*). In the absence of such a check valve, some of the oxygen will flow retrograde into the anesthesia machine (*dotted yellow arrow*).

Labels on Figure 14-3:
- Pipeline (wall source) Oxygen supply
- Flush Actuator and direct Oxygen flush pathway
- Fresh gas outlet
- One-way Check Valve

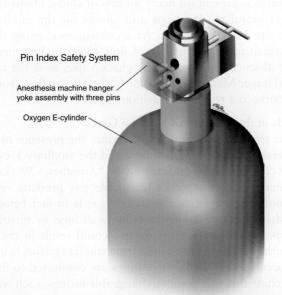

Labels on Figure 14-4:
- Pin Index Safety System
- Anesthesia machine hanger yoke assembly with three pins
- Oxygen E-cylinder

Figure 14-4 Pin index safety system for medical gas cylinders.

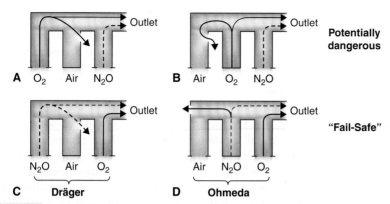

Figure 14-5 Flowmeter sequence—a potential cause of hypoxia. In the event of a flowmeter leak, a potentially dangerous arrangement exists when nitrous oxide is located in the downstream position (**A,B**). The safest configuration exists when oxygen is located in the downstream position (**C,D**). O_2, oxygen; N_2O, nitrous oxide. (From Riutort KT, Eisenkraft JB. The anesthesia workstation and delivery systems for inhaled anesthetics. In: Barash PB, Cullen BF, Stoelting RK, et al., eds. *Clinical Anesthesia*. 7th ed. Philadelphia: Lippincott Williams & Wilkins; 2013:641–696, with permission.)

Additional measures exist to ensure appropriate oxygenation of the patient. Consider the scenario in which a fresh gas mixture of 50% oxygen and 50% nitrous oxide is being used and an isolated drop in oxygen pipeline pressure occurs. The sequence in which these two gases enter the fresh gas main line impacts the resulting gas mixture delivered to the patient. Oxygen is always the last gas to sequentially enter the fresh gas mixture to minimize (but not eliminate) the alteration in inspired oxygen (Fig. 14-5).

Although inspection of the oxygen pipeline pressure gauge, a low O_2 pressure alarm and low fraction of inspired oxygen (FiO_2) concentration alarm would alert the user to the hazardous event described above, a mechanism known as the oxygen *fail-safe system* exists to minimize the decrement in FiO_2. The fail-safe system proportionally decreases the flow of all other gases in use or halts their administration completely when a decline in oxygen pressure occurs. This prevents a disproportionate increase in the relative contribution of fresh gases that do not contribute to the oxygenation of the patient (1–3).

Even under conditions in which the integrity of the oxygen pipeline source is maintained, it would still be possible to deliver a hypoxic fresh gas mixture to a patient. Imagine that oxygen flow is set to 1 L/min and nitrous oxide is delivered concurrently at 4 L/min. In this situation, the consequent FiO_2 would be 20%, less than that of room air. *Proportioning systems* within the flowmeter assembly prevent exactly this type of problem from occurring. One possible design is the use of chain-linked sprockets that unite the control knobs for nitrous oxide and oxygen to each other. The effect imposes limits such that the ratio of nitrous oxide flow to oxygen flow never exceeds 3:1 (an FiO_2 of 25%). Other types of proportioning mechanisms actively reduce nitrous oxide flows when oxygen flows are decreased by the user (1).

Lastly, an *oxygen analyzer* oversees the delivered concentration of oxygen just beyond the fresh gas outlet. Although not a constituent of the anesthesia machine per se, it is a final check on what concentration of oxygen is in fact ultimately being administered to the patient. Although the anesthesiologist

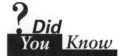

Did You Know

A properly functioning and calibrated oxygen analyzer is a mandatory part of the anesthesia workstation. There are several safeguards in modern machines to prevent delivery of a hypoxic gas mixture to the patient, but the oxygen analyzer is last in line and is the only device that actually measures the concentration.

cannot ascertain the functionality of the oxygen fail-safe system, he or she has an opportunity and a responsibility to certify the functionality of *all* of the safeguards just described (see "Anesthesia Workstation Preuse Checkout" later in this chapter).

D. Anesthetic Vaporizers

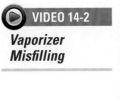

VIDEO 14-2

Vaporizer Misfilling

Commonly used volatile anesthetics are halogenated ether compounds that readily vaporize when exposed to the atmosphere. If kept in a closed container, the space above the liquid will contain molecules of these agents in the vapor state, equilibrating with the liquid surface. The pressure exerted against the walls of the container in this space by the gas-phase molecules is known as *vapor pressure*. At standard temperature and pressure, the measured vapor pressure for volatile anesthetics reflects the unique physicochemical characteristics of these drugs. Vapor pressure, however, is not a static value and will increase if the ambient temperature rises. The temperature at which the kinetic energy of these molecules is sufficient to counterbalance the pressure of the atmosphere (760 mm Hg at sea level) is known as the agent's *boiling point*. At this temperature and beyond, *all* of the liquid agent will readily vaporize into gas (1,2).

Figure 14-6 illustrates how the concept of saturated vapor pressure is exploited to allow safe use of the volatile anesthetics in clinical anesthesia. *Variable bypass vaporizers* are typically installed on most anesthesia machines. They contain an internal reservoir of liquid anesthetic agent that saturates a large wick. Molecules of anesthetic in the gaseous state emanate from this wick to create a saturated vapor pressure within the vaporizing chamber. These vaporizers are referred to as *variable bypass* because when they are not in use, the fresh gas flow of oxygen/air/nitrous oxide "bypasses" these vaporizers and continues onward to the patient. When the control dial of the anesthetic vaporizer is rotated in the counterclockwise direction, it diverts a portion of the carrier gas to the internal vaporizing chamber, where it will incorporate a certain amount of anesthetic gas and then return to join the fresh gas flow where the mixture of anesthetic and oxygen will be delivered to the common gas outlet. The more the dial is turned, the greater amount of anesthetic vapor is incorporated and administered to the patient.

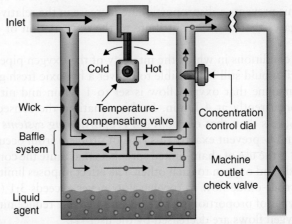

Figure 14-6 Simplified schematic of the GE-Ohmeda Tec Type Vaporizer. Note bimetallic strip temperature-compensating mechanism in the bypass chamber. (From Riutort KT, Eisenkraft JB. The anesthesia workstation and delivery systems for inhaled anesthetics. In: Barash PB, Cullen BF, Stoelting RK, et al., eds. *Clinical Anesthesia*. 7th ed. Philadelphia: Lippincott Williams & Wilkins; 2013:641–696, with permission.)

The transformation of a substance from the liquid state into the gas phase is an endothermic process. It requires energy to make this transition. Yet, most variable bypass vaporizers are not actively heated. Therefore, the energy required to continually vaporize liquid anesthetic into gas comes from the environment, the existing thermal energy of the operating room, and the walls of the vaporizer itself. If the operating room is unusually cold or high fresh gas flow is being used, which requires vaporization of a large volume of anesthetic, the temperature in the vaporizing chamber may drop. Consequently, there will be a predictable and proportional decrease in the vapor pressure of the agent and less anesthetic will be available in the gas state to be delivered to the patient. To allow for changing temperatures in the vaporizing chamber, a bimetallic switch is placed at the interface where fresh gas flow enters the vaporizing chamber. When two metals of differing thermal conductivities are joined together, one will expand or shrink at a rate much different from the other when the local temperature increases or decreases, respectively. The result will create a shearing of one metal against another. When the internal temperature or vapor pressure falls, the bimetallic strip bends and allows more fresh gas flow to enter the vaporizing chamber (Fig. 14-6) (1,2).

E. Desflurane and the Tec-6 Vaporizer

Each variable bypass vaporizer described above is constructed to be agent specific and calibrated to accommodate an individual drug's unique vapor pressure and potency. Currently, these vaporizers are used to deliver isoflurane and sevoflurane.

Desflurane, on the other hand, is a newer volatile anesthetic, which, unlike its predecessors, has a boiling point close to that of room temperature. This prohibits its use in a conventional variable bypass vaporizer. The Tec-6 (GE Healthcare, Little Chalfont, UK) vaporizer is uniquely designed to overcome the challenges posed by desflurane's low boiling point. In this system, a reservoir of liquid desflurane is actively heated to twice its boiling point, generating pure desflurane gas. This gas is then "fuel injected" directly into the fresh gas flow line based on how far the control dial setting is opened. Whereas a conventional variable bypass vaporizer is characterized by two parallel circuits (a bypass pathway and a vaporizing pathway), the Tec-6 is more appropriately described as a *single circuit gas–vapor blender* (Fig. 14-7) (5,6).

III. Anesthesia Breathing Systems

Thus far, this chapter has characterized the confluence of oxygen/air/nitrous oxide and volatile anesthetics on the common fresh gas flow outlet. This section will explain what happens to this fresh gas as it enters the anesthesia breathing system. The *circle system* is the most commonly used design. In this system, a breathing bag (or ventilator bellows) contracts and delivers a tidal volume of gas into a patient's lungs. The patient exhales back into the breathing bag (or ventilator). This to-and-fro reciprocal exchange of gas between the breathing bag/ventilator and the patient's lungs allows for *rebreathing* of exhaled gases (Fig. 14-8). The components of this system are as follows. First, just past the point where the fresh gas flow enters the circle system exists the *one-way inspiratory valve*. This allows for both the delivered tidal volume and fresh gas flow to travel only in the antegrade direction to the patient through a section of corrugated tubing known as the *inspiratory limb*. The inspiratory limb attaches to a *Y-piece* connector, which, in turn, is connected to the patient via a mask, laryngeal mask, or endotracheal tube.

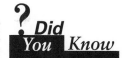

? Did You Know

Anesthetic vaporizers must be filled with the correct agent. Failure to do so could have disastrous consequences. This is particularly true for desflurane, which requires a specially designed heated vaporizer.

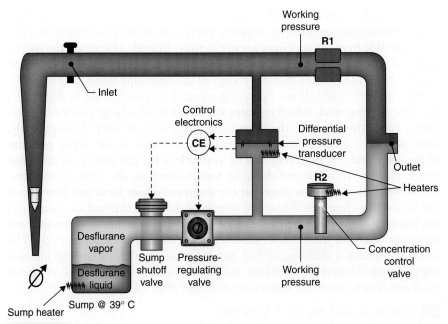

Figure 14-7 Simplified schematic of the Tec-6 desflurane vaporizer. (From Riutort KT, Eisenkraft JB. The anesthesia workstation and delivery systems for inhaled anesthetics. In: Barash PB, Cullen BF, Stoelting RK, et al., eds. *Clinical Anesthesia*. 7th ed. Philadelphia: Lippincott Williams & Wilkins; 2013:641–696, with permission.)

Second, during expiration, the exhaled tidal volume courses out through the Y piece and through the *expiratory limb* of corrugated tubing past the *expiratory one-way valve*. Again, this valve allows for unidirectional flow of expired gases. Between the inspiratory and expiratory valves, flow is unidirectional, as seen in Figure 14-8.

Third, the expired tidal volume may enter two different paths. During manual or spontaneous ventilation, some of the expired volume will pass through the *adjustable pressure-limiting (APL) valve* (commonly referred to as the pop-off valve) and enter the scavenging system or instead go on to reinflate the breathing bag. What fraction of the tidal volume enters scavenging versus reinflates the breathing bag is largely determined by how open or closed the APL valve position might be and the fresh gas flow rate entering the system. Additionally, a positive pressure is needed to exit through the APL valve. Hence, this typically only happens during manual, positive-pressure inspiration or at end exhalation when the breathing bag is full. Analogously, during mechanical ventilation, expired gases will act to reinflate the ventilator bellows. The ventilator contains its own pressure-relief valve, which allows expired gases to enter the scavenging system (discussed later).

Fourth, upon the next inspiratory cycle, another tidal volume enters the inspiratory limb. Prior to doing so, however, this volume of gas must first pass through a canister filled with absorbent material aimed at neutralizing any carbon dioxide. Recall that this is a *circle* system that allows for *rebreathing*. Were it not for the presence of this carbon dioxide absorbent, the patient would ultimately sustain increasing carbon dioxide tension and hypercapnia. The circle system is intrinsically complex. Disadvantages naturally arise from multiple connections and constituent components that may malfunction or be misconnected. Adding to the intricacy is the fact that some components

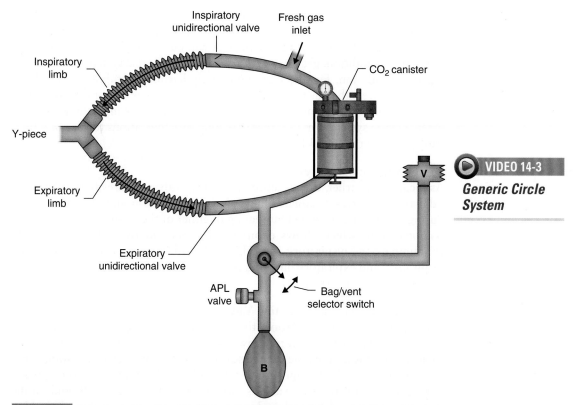

Inspiratory
unidirectional valve

Fresh gas
inlet

CO_2 canister

Inspiratory
limb

Y-piece

Expiratory
limb

Expiratory
unidirectional valve

APL
valve

Bag/vent
selector switch

B

VIDEO 14-3
*Generic Circle
System*

Figure 14-8 Components of the circle breathing system. B, reservoir bag; CO_2, carbon dioxide; V, ventilator; APL, adjustable pressure-limiting (pop-off) valve. (From Riutort KT, Eisenkraft JB. The anesthesia workstation and delivery systems for inhaled anesthetics. In: Barash PB, Cullen BF, Stoelting RK, et al., eds. *Clinical Anesthesia*. 7th ed. Philadelphia: Lippincott Williams & Wilkins; 2013:641–696, with permission.)

are disposable and others are permanent. However, this design is a popular one owing to its allowance for very low fresh gas flows and conservation of anesthetic gases, heat, and humidity (1–3). Several interesting considerations related to the use of the circle breathing system are illustrated below.

A. **Impact of Fresh Gas Flow**

Proper function of the circle system depends significantly on the fresh gas flow rate being delivered from the common gas outlet. If a very high flow (e.g., >10 L/min) enters the circle system and the patient is being mechanically ventilated, there is a risk of trauma to the lungs. This is because the ventilator's automatic pressure relief valve is completely closed during the inspiratory phase (2), and the simultaneous inflow of fresh gas during this short interval can cause a dangerously high increase in the inspiratory pressure.

Additionally, if the fresh gas flow is high (e.g., 10 L/min), virtually *all* of the expired tidal volume will escape through the scavenging system, creating a *nonrebreathing circuit*. This phenomenon can be effectively used at the conclusion of surgery to allow patients to emerge from inhalational anesthesia because there is no rebreathing of exhaled anesthetic gases.

Conversely, if the fresh gas flow into the circle system is too low, this can be problematic. For example, a patient's normal oxygen consumption is approximately 300 mL/min, and this can increase significantly if the patient is hypermetabolic (e.g., fever). If less than the patient's required volume of oxygen is provided, the rebreathing bag (or ventilator bellows) will collapse, and the patient will be unable to breathe. Also, if it is desired to rapidly change the concentration of delivered anesthetic, this will take considerable time at a low flow rate. In addition, gas analyzers attached to the circle system can draw off up to 150 mL/min. Finally, some potentially harmful metabolites of volatile anesthetics are exhaled. Use of extremely low fresh gas flow rates will allow these products to accumulate in the circle system. Under most circumstances when a circle system is in use, there are only rare indications for use of a total fresh gas flow rate of <3 L/min.

B. Unidirectional Valves

As mentioned earlier, the presence of one-way valves ensures that a delivered tidal volume enters a patient's lungs during inspiration and exits the system during expiration. Incompetent seating of either of these valves results in *bidirectional* flow, which allows expired gases, particularly carbon dioxide, to contaminate the inspiratory gas. This carbon dioxide oscillates between the inspiratory and expiratory limb and is therefore immune to the presence of the carbon dioxide absorbent (1).

C. Adjustable Pressure-Limiting Valve

During manual (bag) ventilation, the APL valve is carefully adjusted. It is partially closed off just enough to allow a sufficient tension in the breathing bag to develop. This permits the user to squeeze the bag and reliably insufflate the patient's lungs with an appropriate tidal volume. With practice, one quickly appreciates that if the APL valve is too constricted, pressure will build in the system as evidenced by high pulmonary pressures and a swelling breathing bag. Conversely, an APL valve left completely open will not enable any tension in the circuit to occur. Therefore, the anesthesiologist will not be able to manually deliver a tidal volume to the patient.

When a patient is breathing spontaneously through the circle system, the breathing bag does not require any manual compression by the anesthesiologist. Therefore, the APL valve may remain in the open position to discourage any accumulation of gas and pressure within the system. In some circumstances, such as with a patient who is developing atelectasis, the APL can be adjusted to enable a small amount of continuous positive pressure to develop in the system and expand collapsed alveoli.

D. The Breathing Bag

During the anesthetic management of adult patients, a 3-L breathing bag is typically affixed to the circle system. Smaller volume bags are available for pediatric and neonatal use. Breathing bags are considered high-volume, low pressure systems. Beyond 3 L, the pressure within a breathing bag will rise steeply with increasing volume. However, these bags are designed so that their compliance will actually change at extremes of capacity. This limits the rise in internal pressure that can be attained (1,2).

E. Carbon Dioxide Absorbents

Carbon dioxide absorbents consist of fine, solid phase granules that participate in an acid-base reaction with carbon dioxide. Smaller-sized granules result in greater absorptive capacity, however, this also creates increased resistance to gas flow through the absorbent. The primary purpose of these absorbents is to ultimately convert carbon dioxide into an inert salt, calcium carbonate. Classically, older absorbents such as soda lime consisted of water, calcium hydroxide

Ca(OH)₂, and a more potent base, sodium hydroxide (NaOH). The reaction between soda lime and carbon dioxide proceeded as follows:

1. $CO_2 + H_2O \rightarrow H_2CO_3$ (carbonic acid)
2. $H_2CO_3 + 2NaOH \rightarrow Na_2CO_3$ (sodium carbonate) $+ 2H_2O$
3. $Na_2CO_3 + Ca(OH)_2 \rightarrow 2NaOH + CaCO_3$ (calcium carbonate)

Of note, soda lime also contained small amounts of another reactive base, potassium hydroxide (KOH), which also participated in the above reaction in a manner entirely analogous to sodium hydroxide. Although carbon dioxide absorbents are highly effective at mitigating the risks of hypercapnia in the circle system, they impose their own brand of hazards. Strong bases such as NaOH and KOH are highly reactive, so much so that they react not only with carbon dioxide but also with the volatile anesthetics that must pass through the absorbent. Specifically, the use of sevoflurane with older absorbents has been noted to generate an intense amount of thermal energy, to the point of inciting absorbent canister fires. By-products of anesthetic degradation have also been problematic. Sevoflurane may react with carbon dioxide absorbents to form Compound A, a vinyl ether that could potentially be nephrotoxic. Desflurane, more than any other anesthetic, is also notable for its degradation to carbon monoxide in the presence of desiccated absorbent. All of these untoward effects of anesthetic reactions with carbon dioxide absorbents are augmented when older, dry absorbent is used for prolonged periods under low fresh gas flow conditions (1–3). Modern carbon dioxide absorbents (i.e., Amsorb, Armstrong Medical, Coleraine, Northern Ireland; Drägersorb, Dräger, East Tamaki, New Zealand) have addressed the potential toxicities listed above by completely eliminating the presence of highly reactive bases such as sodium hydroxide. They consist solely of calcium hydroxide and water (7). This results in a somewhat diminished capacity to absorb carbon dioxide. Alternatively, absorbents with a new chemical composition using lithium (Litholyme, Allied Health Care Products, St. Louis, Missouri) are characterized by different chemical reactions with carbon dioxide and greater absorbent capacity.

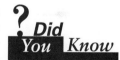

Did You Know

Evidence of exhausted carbon dioxide absorbent includes a change to violet color, attempts by the patient to hyperventilate, and elevated inspired carbon dioxide with capnography.

Continued use of absorbent will eventually extinguish its capacity to absorb any further carbon dioxide. Carbon dioxide absorbents are typically impregnated with an indicator dye that responds to decreasing pH when the absorbent is exhausted. Ethyl violet is most commonly used. This dye imparts a violet hue to the absorbent when it is exhausted.

E. End-Tidal Gas Monitoring, Oxygen Analyzer, and Spirometry

Measurements of respiratory gases and pulmonary volumes are not required components for a functional circle system but they provide valuable added safety. The *oxygen analyzer* sits atop the inspiratory one-way valve. This location for the analyzer is particularly suitable as it will gauge the FiO_2 immediately downstream of the fresh gas flow inlet. The most commonly used analyzers use galvanic cell analysis to measure oxygen. These analyzers measure the current produced as oxygen diffuses across a membrane within, ultimately being reduced to molecular oxygen at the anode of an electrical circuit. The amount of current produced is proportional to the partial pressure of oxygen present (2).

Whereas inspiratory gas analysis focuses on the fraction of inspired oxygen, *expiratory gas analysis* measures and displays the tensions of carbon dioxide and inhaled anesthetics. Most often, a Luer-lock port at the Y-piece connector draws away expired gas at a rate of 50 to 150 mL/min to an independent infrared absorbance analyzer. This device is capable of identifying the presence and concentrations of carbon dioxide, nitrous oxide, and volatile anesthetics (2).

Lastly, the patient's *expired tidal volumes* are typically measured in the expiratory limb just upstream of the expiratory one-way valve. Spirometers use a rotating vane, ultrasound, or a heated wire to measure gas flow and display the values electronically.

G. Mechanical Ventilators

Frequently, a mechanical ventilator is employed to ventilate the patient during anesthesia. This can be done to permit the anesthesiologist to have a "hands-free" method for delivering a reliable volume of ventilation, or it can be a necessity when the patient is paralyzed or has significant lung disease.

Ventilators associated with the anesthesia workstation often use a dual-circuit, gas-driven design (Fig. 14-9). A compressible bellows assembly delivers a volume of gas to the patient. These bellows are compressed through the action of a "drive" gas, which is external to the bellows. Thus, there are *two circuits of gas*: one for the patient's lungs, the other to drive the bellows. The drive gas may either be compressed air, oxygen, or a mixture of the two. If oxygen is used as the drive gas, then any disruption of the central supply of oxygen to the workstation will not only compromise delivery of carrier gas to the fresh gas outlet, but will also render the mechanical ventilator incapable of delivering a tidal volume. Newer anesthesia machines may use a ventilator that incorporates a single-circuit, *piston-driven* design. In such cases, an electrically powered piston delivers a tidal volume to the patient. This of course means that failure of electrical power will incapacitate the ventilator. The latest design for delivery of controlled tidal volumes has been the inclusion of an electrically driven compressor turbine within the inspiratory limb of the circle system (1–3).

Regardless of the mechanism through which the ventilator delivers the proposed tidal volume, there must be a route for the escape of excess gas during expiration. Similar to how the APL valve interfaces with the scavenging system during spontaneous or manual bag ventilation, a dedicated *spill valve* directs excess expiratory gas through this evacuation route during mechanical ventilation (1).

Characterizing the settings of a mechanical ventilator requires defining how each breath is *cycled* and by what measure it is *limited*. Most often, mechanical ventilation is *time cycled*, that is, the selected respiratory rate will define how often the ventilator delivers a breath. Very commonly, mechanical ventilation is *volume limited*, that is, the set tidal volume predicts the maximum volume that will be delivered to the patient. Although defining these two simple parameters should generate a predictable minute ventilation (tidal volume × respiratory rate), the true limitation of this strategy may be governed by a variety of other parameters also under the control of the anesthesiologist. In addition to *tidal volume* and respiratory *rate*, the user customarily predefines the settings for inspiratory *pressure* limit, drive gas *flow* rate, and the *inhale to exhale ratio* prior to initiating controlled mechanical ventilation. An illustrative example follows: a 600-cc tidal volume at a respiratory rate of 10 breaths/min is selected for a healthy patient. The predicted minute ventilation is thus 6 L/min. However, if the inspiratory pressure limit (the peak pulmonary pressure beyond which the ventilator will no longer continue to deliver any further volume) is inadvertently set to a very low threshold, for example 10 cm H_2O,

Ascending Bellows Ventilator

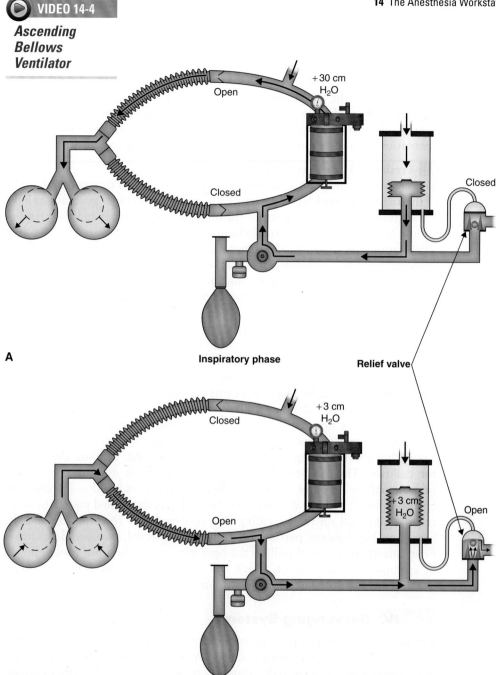

A

Inspiratory phase

Relief valve

B

Expiratory phase late

Figure 14-9 Inspiratory (**A**) and expiratory (**B**) phases of gas flow in a traditional circle system with an ascending bellows ventilator. The bellows physically separates the driving gas circuit from the patient gas circuit. The driving gas circuit is located outside the bellows, and the patient gas circuit is inside the bellows. During inspiratory phase (**A**), the driving gas enters the bellows chamber, causing the pressure within it to increase. This causes the ventilator relief valve to close, preventing anesthetic gas from escaping into the scavenging system, and the bellows to compress, delivering anesthetic gas within the bellows to the patient's lungs. During expiratory phase (**B**), pressure within the bellows chamber and the pilot line decreases to zero, causing the mushroom portion of the ventilator relief valve to open. Gas exhaled by the patient refills the bellows before any scavenging occurs, because a weighted ball is incorporated into the base of the ventilator relief valve. Scavenging occurs only during the expiratory phase, because the ventilator relief valve is only open during expiration. (From Riutort KT, Eisenkraft JB. The anesthesia workstation and delivery systems for inhaled anesthetics. In: Barash PB, Cullen BF, Stoelting RK, et al., eds. *Clinical Anesthesia*. 7th ed. Philadelphia: Lippincott Williams & Wilkins; 2013:641–696, with permission.)

only a small tidal volume will be delivered. In this case, the inspiratory pressure limit serves as the true limitation to minute ventilation.

Additionally, depending on the surgical procedure and the patient's underlying illnesses, the anesthesiologist may select from a variety of profiles that define how the mechanical breath is delivered. These include volume-controlled ventilation, pressure-controlled ventilation, and pressure-support ventilation with or without the inclusion of positive end-expiratory pressure.

H. Fresh Gas Flow Decoupling

This chapter has thus far described the characteristics of a conventional model of the anesthesia workstation. Such classic machines of older generations have a consistent architecture; much of the machinery is external and they require a more hands-on approach to checkout and usage. In contrast, more modern workstations rely heavily on sophisticated, computerized processing. These workstations have automated self-checkouts and often employ an ergonomic design that keeps much of the machine anatomy hidden.

By far the most important feature that many of these new workstations incorporate is the concept of *fresh gas flow decoupling*. Recall how tidal ventilation can become augmented when high fresh gas flows are used during mechanical ventilation in conventional anesthesia machines. This occurs because the fresh gas flow is "coupled" to the circle system during inspiration. Many new workstation designs divorce the fresh gas flow from the circle system during the inspiratory phase, and, as a result, the patient only receives the prescribed tidal volume set by the user. A decoupling valve diverts fresh gas flow typically into the breathing bag during the inspiratory phase. Once expiration commences, fresh gas flow is coupled and the gas within the breathing bag deploys into the circuit, refilling the ventilator bellows. This remarkably different design in the anesthesia workstation virtually eliminates the risk of fresh gas flow–induced volutrauma or barotrauma. The major disadvantage to fresh gas decoupled machines is the reliance imposed on the breathing bag as a fresh gas reservoir. Should the breathing bag become partially or fully disconnected, two problems arise. First, anesthetic gas will pollute the operating room. Second, room air will be entrained into the circuit, which will dilute the intended fraction of oxygen and anesthetic desired for the patient.

IV. Scavenging Systems

The primary determinant of the amount of waste gas scavenged is the fresh gas flow out of the common gas outlet. At very low flow rates, a relatively unchanging volume of gas will constantly oscillate between the patient's lungs and the breathing bag or ventilator, and very little gas will escape through the waste gas scavenging system. At high fresh gas flow rates, excess gas will vent through the scavenging system to prevent a buildup of volume and pressure. Both the mechanical ventilator and the breathing bag are connected to the scavenging terminal through 19-mm hose connectors. During manual or spontaneous ventilation, waste gas is vented through the APL. When the ventilator is in use, waste gas is vented during the expiration and prior to initiation of inspiration. During that interval in the respiratory cycle, after a certain pressure threshold has been reached, typically 2-cm H_2O, the spill valve will open and vent the excess gas into the scavenging hose. From the scavenging terminal, a third hose directs the waste gas out of the operating room and ultimately out of the hospital (Fig. 14-10).

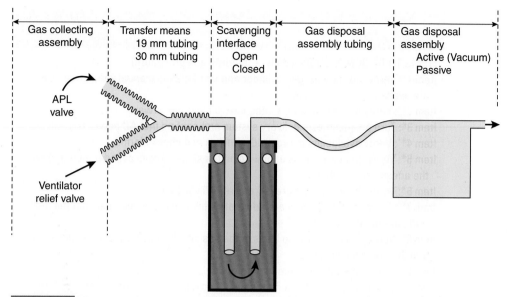

Figure 14-10 Components of a scavenging system. APL, adjustable pressure-limiting valve. (From Riutort KT, Brull SJ, Eisenkraft JB. The anesthesia workstation and delivery systems for inhaled anesthetics. In: Barash PB, Cullen BF, Stoelting RK, et al., eds. *Clinical Anesthesia.* 7th ed. Philadelphia: Lippincott Williams & Wilkins; 2013:641–696, with permission.)

Once waste gas exits the anesthesia workstation, a variety of systems exist to dispose of the waste gases. A defining characteristic of scavenging systems relates to the dynamics of gas flow, which may be either *active* or *passive*. In active systems, negative pressure is applied through the hospital vacuum to facilitate the removal of waste gas. Passive systems rely simply on the small amount of positive pressure generated during exhalation to promote waste gas disposal. Scavenging systems may additionally be defined according to their anatomic design, either open or closed. Closed systems are self-explanatory: a system of hoses evacuates exhaled gas in a contained manner that prohibits the waste gas from entering the operating room. Open systems contain vents in the scavenging reservoir that *do* allow waste gas to *potentially* enter the operating room. At first glance, one may question the merit of an open system, a system that decidedly allows waste gas to contaminate the operating room environment. The following two examples serve to justify how open systems may be intrinsically safer than closed systems.

Think about what might happen if the hose that sends waste gases out of the room becomes occluded. In a closed system, waste gas would accumulate, generating positive pressure that could theoretically be conveyed to the patient. The presence of vents in the scavenging reservoir in an open system, however, would allow this excess pressure to dissipate into the operating room. Consider the opposite problem as well. Perhaps an excessive amount of negative pressure is applied to evacuate waste gas. In such a scenario, too *much* gas is being relieved from the circle system in closed designs. The very same vents described earlier in open systems would entrain room air to accommodate this excessive negative pressure. Closed systems are acceptable for use, but they must retain mechanisms that mitigate the problems illustrated by the above examples. Closed systems harbor positive-pressure and negative-pressure relief valves. The former bleeds open into the operating room when

Table 14-2	Summary of the American Society of Anesthesiologists Preanesthesia Checkout Recommendations

ITEMS TO BE COMPLETED (*, daily; +, before each procedure):

Item 1*: Verify auxiliary oxygen cylinder and self-inflating manual ventilation device are available and functioning.

Item 2*+: Verify patient suction is adequate to clear the airway.

Item 3*: Turn on anesthesia delivery system and confirm that AC power is available.

Item 4*+: Verify availability of required monitors and check alarms.

Item 5*: Verify that pressure is adequate on the spare oxygen cylinder mounted on the anesthesia machine.

Item 6*: Verify that piped gas pressures are ≥50 psi gauge.

Item 7*+: Verify that vaporizers are adequately filled and, if applicable, that the filler ports are tightly closed.

Item 8*: Verify that there are no leaks in the gas supply lines between the flowmeters and the common gas outlet.

Item 9*: Test scavenging system function.

Item 10*: Calibrate, or verify calibration of, the oxygen monitor and check the low oxygen alarm. Verify the function of the carbon dioxide analyzer.

Item 11*+: Verify carbon dioxide absorbent is not exhausted.

Item 12*+: Breathing system pressure and leak testing.

Item 13*+: Verify that gas flows properly through the breathing circuit during both inspiration and exhalation. Check function of one-way valves.

Item 14*+: Document completion of checkout procedures.

Item 15*+: Confirm ventilator settings and evaluate readiness to deliver anesthesia care.

From The American Society of Anesthesiologists. 2008 Recommendations for Preanesthesia Checkout. Available at: www.asahq.org/For-Members/Clinical-Information/2008-ASA-Recommendations-for-PreAnesthesia-Checkout.aspx.

? Did You Know

Like competent pilots before they fly, it is highly recommended that the anesthesiologist perform a thorough check of the anesthesia workstation before use, and for quality control purposes, to document that it was done.

VIDEO 14-5

Water Condensation in Breathing Circuit

excessive pressure accumulates within the scavenging system. Negative-pressure relief valves, on the other hand, respond to excessive negative pressure and evacuate room air to compensate (1–3).

V. Anesthesia Workstation Preuse Checkout

The American Society of Anesthesiologists (ASA) has published, and regularly revises, recommendations for a preuse checkout of the anesthesia workstation. A basic summary of the 15-point checklist is provided in Table 14-2. However, the full, comprehensive elaboration of the checklist can be found at the ASA. Anesthesiologists are advised to follow these recommendations (8,9). Additionally, they are encouraged to become familiar with the manufacturer's operations manual for the specific workstation(s) they intend to use.

References

1. Dorsch JA, Dorsch SE. *A Practical Approach to Anesthesia Equipment*. Philadelphia: Lippincott Williams & Wilkins; 2011.
2. Davey AJ, Diba Ali. *Ward's Anaesthetic Equipment*. 5th ed. Philadelphia: Elsevier; 2005.
3. Brockwell RC, Andrews JJ. Understanding your anesthesia machine. In: Schwartz AJ, ed. *ASA Refresher Courses*. Philadelphia: Lippincott Williams & Wilkins; 2002.
4. Atlas G. A method to quickly estimate remaining time for an oxygen E-cylinder. *Anesth Analg*. 2004;98:1190.

5. Weiskopf RB, Sampson D, Moore MA. The desflurane (Tec 6) vaporizer: Design, design considerations and performance evaluation. *Br J Anaesth.* 1994;72:474.

6. Andrews JJ, Johnston RV Jr, Kramer GC. Consequences of misfilling contemporary vaporizers with desflurane. *Can J Anaesth.* 1993;40:71.

7. Versichelen LF, Bouche MP, Rolly G, et al. Only carbon dioxide absorbents free of both NaOH and KOH do not generate compound-A during in vitro closed system sevoflurane. *Anesthesiology.* 2001;95:750.

8. U.S. Food and Drug Administration. *Anesthesia Apparatus Checkout Recommendations.* Rockville, MD: Author, 1993.

9. The American Society of Anesthesiologists. 2008 Recommendations for Preanesthesia Checkout. Available at: www.asahq.org/For-Members/Clinical-Information/2008-ASA-Recommendations-for-PreAnesthesia-Checkout.aspx.

Questions

1. The most significant drawback of the modern anesthesia workstation is the:
   A. Dependence on a high pressure oxygen source for its operation
   B. Dependence on a source of electricity for its operation
   C. Complexity of its operation
   D. Potential for barotrauma to the lung resulting from use of high fresh gas flows during mechanical ventilation

2. Which of the following pressure values displayed on an E cylinder of oxygen indicates that it is approximately half full?
   A. 1,700 psi
   B. 1,100 psi
   C. 750 psi
   D. 405 psi

3. All of the following are appropriate uses for the flush actuator EXCEPT:
   A. To rapidly deepen the level of anesthesia
   B. To fill an empty rebreathing bag
   C. To fill ventilator bellows during the expiratory phase of ventilation
   D. High frequency jet ventilation

4. If a hospital supply of medical air was accidently connected to the oxygen inlet of the anesthesia workstation, which of the following safety devices would alert the user to the problem?
   A. The oxygen fail-safe alarm
   B. The flowmeter proportioning system
   C. An oxygen analyzer located outside the fresh gas outlet
   D. Activation of the low oxygen pressure alarm

5. Which of the following anesthetics requires active heating of a vaporizer to enable delivery of a precise concentration of gas?
   A. Desflurane
   B. Isoflurane
   C. Sevoflurane
   D. Xenon

6. A patient is anesthetized with 1% isoflurane. He is breathing spontaneously via a circle system with 5 L/min oxygen. The mean airway pressure rises to 20 cm H_2O and the tidal volume falls to 100 mL. The next most appropriate step is to:
   A. Administer a bronchodilator
   B. Institute mechanical ventilation
   C. Decrease the flow rate of oxygen to 2 L/min
   D. Open the APL

7. A healthy, normothermic, 70-kg patient is anesthetized with isoflurane and oxygen via a circle system and breathing at a rate of 16 breaths/min. Which of the following conditions is potentially most hazardous?
   A. Spontaneous ventilation with a total fresh gas flow of 1 L/min
   B. Spontaneous ventilation with a total fresh gas flow of 15 L/min
   C. Mechanical ventilation with a total fresh gas flow of 1 L/min
   D. Mechanical ventilation with a total fresh gas flow of 15 L/min

8. Capnography of a patient's inhaled and exhaled gases shows that the inspired value of carbon dioxide is greater than zero. This could be explained by:
   A. A light violet hue in half of the carbon dioxide canister
   B. The carbon dioxide canister being warm to the touch
   C. Accumulation of Compound A associated with use of sevoflurane
   D. A malfunction of the unidirectional valve in the inspiratory limb of the circle system

9. A patient is attached to a ventilator with a compressible bellows. The flowmeters are set to deliver 2 L/min oxygen and 2 L/min nitrous oxide. The "drive gas" is air. All of the following could indicate a hole in the bellows EXCEPT:
   A. An increase in inspired volume above that preset
   B. An increase in expired volume above that expected
   C. An increase in the oxygen analyzer reading from 50% to 80%
   D. A decrease in the bellows volume at end expiration

10. The ASA recommends that all of the following parameters should be checked before every anesthetic EXCEPT:
    A. Verify patient suction is adequate to clear the airway
    B. Verify that piped gas pressures are ≥50 psi gauge
    C. Breathing system pressure and leak testing
    D. Check function of circle system one-way valves

Standard Anesthesia Monitoring Techniques and Instruments

15

Ryan J. Fink
Jonathan B. Mark

Monitoring of patients during anesthesia begins with a *vigilant anesthesia provider*—visual inspection of chest rise and patient color for ventilation and oxygenation and palpation of the pulse for heart rate and blood pressure estimation. Although technology has enhanced the anesthesia provider's ability to monitor and treat patients during anesthesia and surgery, a vigilant anesthesia provider with good clinical decision-making skills is still required. Standards for basic anesthetic monitoring published by the American Society of Anesthesiologists emphasize the need for a qualified anesthesia provider to be in the room for all anesthetics and monitored anesthesia care (Table 15-1).

I. Basic Anesthesia Monitoring

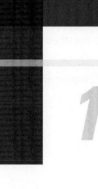

VIDEO 15-1

Monitoring Standards

The "Standards for Basic Anesthetic Monitoring" were first published in 1986 and updated in 2011 (Table 15-1) (1). These standards lay the foundation for the minimal monitoring needed during all anesthesia care, and they begin with the continual presence of a qualified anesthesia provider. Depending on the clinical judgment of this provider, more intensive monitoring may be needed in some cases.

A. Oxygenation

Proper *oxygenation* of the patient is ensured in two ways. During general anesthesia using an anesthesia machine, the provider needs to confirm that there is a sufficient concentration of oxygen being delivered. Most anesthesia machines use a galvanic cell analyzer located in the inspired limb of the anesthesia circuit and are equipped with a low oxygen concentration alarm that will alert the provider to a dangerous hypoxic gas mixture. The oxygen analyzer may require daily calibration and intermittent replacement. If a patient is receiving supplemental oxygen by nasal cannula or facemask during regional anesthesia or monitored anesthesia care, the provider must ensure the proper flow of oxygen from the wall oxygen supply or gas cylinder.

After ensuring sufficient oxygen delivery to the patient or the breathing circuit, oxygenation of the patient's blood must be monitored qualitatively, most

Table 15-1	Summary of the American Society of Anesthesiologists "Standards for Basic Anesthetic Monitoring"

Standard 1
Qualified anesthesia personnel shall be present in the room throughout the conduct of all general anesthetics, regional anesthetics and monitored anesthesia care.

Standard 2
During all anesthetics, the patient's oxygenation, ventilation, circulation and temperature shall be continually evaluated.
   Oxygenation
      Oxygen concentration of the inspired gas
      Observation of the patient's skin and mucous membrane color
      Pulse oximetry
   Ventilation
      Observation of the patient and reservoir bag
      Mechanical ventilation circuit disconnection alarms
      Auscultation of breath sounds
      Continuous end-tidal carbon dioxide measurement
   Circulation
      Continuous ECG display
      Heart rate and blood pressure measured at least every 5 minutes
      Evaluation of the circulation: auscultation of heart sounds, palpation of pulse, pulse plethysmography, pulse oximetry, intra-arterial pressure tracing
   Temperature
      Continual temperature monitoring, when significant changes are anticipated or suspected

ECG, electrocardiogram.
From https://www.asahq.org/For-Members/Standards-Guidelines-and-Statements.aspx.

often via the patient's skin or mucous membrane color, and quantitatively with a *pulse oximeter*. This device has become ubiquitous both inside and outside the operating room because it provides a continuous, noninvasive, and accurate measurement of arterial hemoglobin oxygen saturation.

The pulse oximeter emits two wavelengths of light (red and near infrared) and uses a photo detector to measure the absorbance of oxygenated and deoxygenated hemoglobin in the blood. The oximeter then uses an algorithm to calculate the percentage of the total hemoglobin that exists as oxyhemoglobin, and displays this as the hemoglobin saturation (SpO_2). This monitor must also differentiate the *pulsatile arterial signal* (and thus the *arterial* hemoglobin oxygen saturation) from the nonpulsatile venous (and other tissue) saturation. Although a pulse oximeter is considered to be a continuous monitor, there can still be a significant delay (of up to 15 to 30 seconds) before it alarms to note a decrease in the SpO_2.

The pulse oximeter is an extremely important monitor during anesthesia, and an abnormally low or suddenly decreasing SpO_2 (<90%) triggers the monitor to provide an audible warning alert of impending patient deterioration. However, like any monitor, the pulse oximeter is subject to artifacts and inaccurate readings (Table 15-2). A vigilant anesthesia provider is necessary to determine whether a low SpO_2 on the monitor is artifactual or a real event that necessitates intervention.

Beyond measurement of SpO_2, the pulse oximeter may have other features that are useful during anesthesia. The pulse oximeter *plethysmographic*

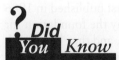
Did You Know

The pulse oximeter has a significant delay (15 to 30 seconds) in the detection of changes in arterial oxygen saturation.

Table 15-2   Limitations of the Pulse Oximeter
Low Blood Flow Conditions (or decrease in arterial pulsatility):
• Hypotension
• Hypothermia causing peripheral vasoconstriction
• High-dose vasopressors
• Cardiopulmonary bypass
Movement Artifacts
• Light anesthesia/no paralysis
• Surgical interference
• Neuromuscular twitch monitor causing motion artifact
• Shivering
Varying Light Absorbance
• Methemoglobinemia
• Carboxyhemoglobinemia
• Methylene blue/Indigo carmine
• Nail polish
• Ambient light

waveform provides a measurement of heart rate (pulse rate) and a crude estimation of blood pressure, because the waveform will appear dampened when there is severe hypotension. Newer generations of pulse oximeters are less influenced by patient motion and other sources of artifact. Some devices measure the concentration of other forms of hemoglobin (i.e., carboxyhemoglobin and methemoglobin) and even measure the total hemoglobin concentration (2). Pulse oximeter waveform analysis may also be used to estimate intravascular volume status and volume responsiveness through analysis of the changes in pulse wave contour during the respiratory cycle. Although the pulse oximeter is mostly used with a finger probe, other probes can be used on the ear, nares, or cheek. Pulse oximeters will not work when there are no arterial pulsations (e.g., on cardiopulmonary bypass), and other techniques must be used, such as reflectance oximetry, which does not depend on arterial pulsations.

B. Ventilation

Ventilation, or the movement of gases between the environment and the alveoli, is another important aspect of a patient's physiology to monitor during anesthesia (Table 15-1). This can be accomplished by visual inspection of chest rise and fall, condensation of airway water vapor in the endotracheal tube or facemask during expiration, or the cyclic filling and emptying of the reservoir bag or ventilator bellows. The anesthesia machine measures tidal volume and respiratory rate and can alarm if these ventilator parameters fall outside a predetermined range.

During general anesthesia, the best monitor for determining adequacy of ventilation is the measurement of *exhaled carbon dioxide (CO_2).* A small sample of respiratory circuit gas is continually removed from the anesthesia breathing circuit for measurement of CO_2 and other gases using an infrared absorption spectrophotometer. The CO_2 concentration is continually displayed as a time-dependent waveform, called a *capnogram* (Fig. 15-1), and is usually reported in millimeters of mercury (mm Hg).

At the beginning of a general anesthetic, a normal-appearing capnogram confirms correct placement of the endotracheal tube in the trachea rather

VIDEO 15-2

Capnogram and Airway Pressure Tracing

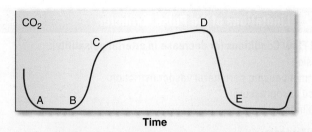

A – B: Initial expiration, mostly dead space with no CO_2
B – C: Exhaled CO_2 begins to reach the analyzer
C – D: Expiratory plateau, alveolar CO_2 being measured
Point D: End-tidal CO_2 measurement taken here
D – E: Inspiration

Figure 15-1   Normal capnogram and phases of the respiratory cycle. (From Connor, CE. Commonly used monitoring techniques. In: Barash P, Cullen B, Stoelting R, et al., eds. *Clinical Anesthesia.* 7th ed. Philadelphia: Wolters Kluwer/Lippincott Williams & Wilkins, 2013:263–285, with permission.)

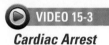

VIDEO 15-3

Cardiac Arrest

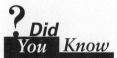

Did You Know

The shape of the capnograph provides important information including the presence of bronchospasm.

than the esophagus. Both the CO_2 value and the shape of the capnogram provide important diagnostic clues about metabolic, respiratory, circulatory, or technical problems with the patient or anesthesia machine (Fig. 15-2 and Table 15-3). For example, a decrease in the end-expiratory or end-tidal CO_2 (ETCO$_2$) indicates a potentially serious problem that must be addressed. Although the most common cause of low ETCO$_2$ is hyperventilation or increased dead space ventilation, a sudden and large decrease may be a sign of a misplaced endotracheal tube or a reduction in lung perfusion resulting from pulmonary embolism, anaphylaxis, or cardiac arrest. Capnography is also an important monitor during regional anesthesia or monitored anesthesia care. Although the CO_2 value measured from a nasal cannula or facemask will likely underestimate the true ETCO$_2$, owing to dilution with room air, a marked change in the capnogram or loss of the waveform entirely provides a prompt alert that there

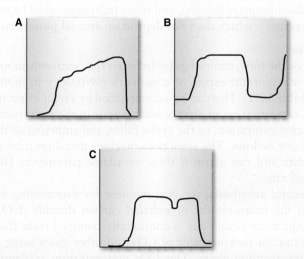

Figure 15-2   Abnormal capnograms. **A:** Steep, prolonged upslope indicating bronchospasm or expiratory airway obstruction. **B:** Increase in the baseline due to rebreathing carbon dioxide (CO_2), such as with an exhausted CO_2 absorbent. **C:** "Curare cleft," which may indicate a patient's attempt at spontaneous ventilation during positive pressure mechanical ventilation.

Table 15-3	Factors that May Change the End-Tidal CO_2 Measurement or Waveform during Anesthesia	
Increases in ETCO$_2$	**Decreases in ETCO$_2$**
Changes in CO$_2$ Production	
Increases in metabolic rate:	Decreases in metabolic rate:
• hyperthermia	• hypothermia
• sepsis	• hypothyroidism
• malignant hyperthermia	
• shivering	
• hyperthyroidism	
Changes in CO$_2$ Elimination	
• hypoventilation	• hyperventilation
• rebreathing	• hypoperfusion
	• pulmonary embolism

ETCO$_2$, end-tidal carbon dioxide; CO$_2$, carbon dioxide.
Adapted from Connor, CE. Commonly used monitoring techniques. In: Barash P, Cullen B, Stoelting R, et al., eds. *Clinical Anesthesia*. 7th ed. Philadelphia: Wolters Kluwer/Lippincott Williams & Wilkins, 2013:263–285, with permission.

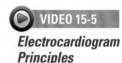
VIDEO 15-4
Hypocarbia Differential Diagnosis

may be severe hypoventilation, apnea, or obstruction of the airway. Particularly in patients who are breathing supplemental oxygen, the capnogram is an early warning that occurs before a low SpO$_2$ is detected by the pulse oximeter.

C. Circulation

A patient's *circulation* is monitored in multiple different ways during anesthesia. *Continuous electrocardiogram (ECG) monitoring* is standard of care in anesthesia and provides continuous important information (Table 15-4), including cardiac rate and rhythm. A wide range of rhythm disturbances may occur during anesthesia, and most all can be detected and diagnosed with a simple three-lead ECG system. However, cardiac ischemia is best detected by monitoring a five-lead ECG and displaying both leads II and V$_5$, a technique that can have a sensitivity of up to 80% (3). V$_5$ is often used instead of the potentially more sensitive medial leads (i.e., leads V$_3$ and V$_4$) (Fig. 15-3), because the latter often interfere with the sterile surgical field. ST-segment depression, or *subendocardial ischemia* (Fig. 15-4), is probably the most common form of perioperative cardiac ischemia, reflecting an oxygen supply–demand mismatch, or *demand ischemia*. However, transmural cardiac ischemia reflected by ECG ST elevations can also be seen in the perioperative setting (Fig. 15-5).

It is important to note that the ECG is only a monitor of cardiac electrical activity and it is possible to have a normal-appearing ECG tracing with little or no cardiac output or blood pressure (i.e., pulseless electrical activity or pulseless

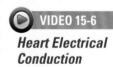
VIDEO 15-5
Electrocardiogram Principles

VIDEO 15-6
Heart Electrical Conduction System

Table 15-4	Goals of Intraoperative Electrocardiogram Monitoring

- Heart rate monitoring
- Detection of arrhythmias and conduction abnormalities
- Detection of myocardial ischemia
- Monitoring pacemaker function or malfunction
- Identification of electrolyte abnormalities

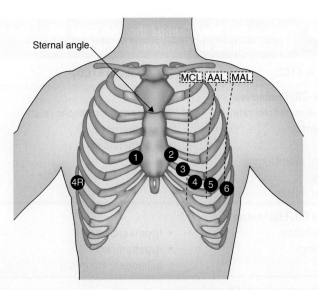

Sternal angle

MCL AAL MAL

Figure 15-3 Precordial electrocardiogram lead placement. V_3 or V_4 may be more sensitive for detecting cardiac ischemia, however V_5 is often used, as it is more likely to avoid the surgical field. MCL, mid-clavicular line; AAL, anterior axillary line; MAL, mid-axillary line. (From Mark JB. *Atlas of Cardiovascular Monitoring*. New York: Churchill Livingstone; 1998, with permission.)

electrical activity arrest). Therefore, other devices are used in the operating room to further assess a patient's circulation. As already mentioned, the pulse oximeter plethysmographic waveform can provide an indication of adequate perfusion to an extremity and displays an additional monitor of pulse rate.

Blood pressure should, at the very least, be monitored every 5 minutes via a noninvasive blood pressure cuff. Automatic blood pressure cuffs differ slightly

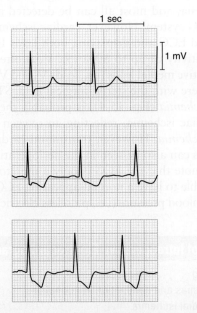

1 sec

1 mV

Figure 15-4 Electrocardiogram changes displaying horizontal or down-sloping ST-segment depression may indicate "demand ischemia." (From Mark JB. *Atlas of Cardiovascular Monitoring*. New York: Churchill Livingstone; 1998, with permission.)

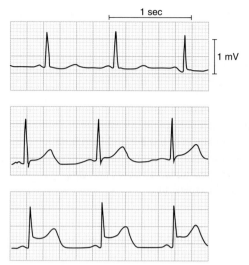

Figure 15-5 Electrocardiogram changes displaying ST-segment elevation, usually the result of coronary artery occlusion. (From Mark JB. *Atlas of Cardiovascular Monitoring.* New York: Churchill Livingstone; 1998, with permission.)

between manufacturers but most commonly use the *oscillometric method.* This method measures the pressure fluctuations that occur with arterial pulsation and usually measure a mean arterial pressure as the pressure at which arterial pulsations are maximal in amplitude (Fig. 15-6). The systolic and diastolic blood pressures are usually determined as the pressure at onset and offset of arterial pulsations sensed by the cuff monitoring system. Some devices, however, use proprietary algorithms to derive the systolic and diastolic pressure values. Given that all electronic monitors can fail or provide spurious values,

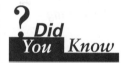

Most noninvasive blood pressure devices use an oscillometric technique, which explains why they are so sensitive to movement artifact.

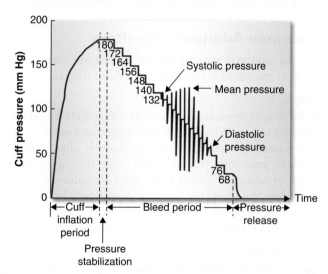

Figure 15-6 Noninvasive blood pressure measurement via the oscillometric method. The cuff is automatically inflated above systolic pressure (no pressure fluctuations present) and then decrementally deflated. Sensors measure the magnitude of the pressure oscillations in the surrounding cuff, which initially increase in magnitude then decrease. Oscillations are analyzed to give the systolic, mean, and diastolic pressure. (From Connor, CE. Commonly used monitoring techniques. In: Barash P, Cullen B, Stoelting R, et al., eds. *Clinical Anesthesia.* 7th ed. Philadelphia: Wolters Kluwer/Lippincott Williams & Wilkins, 2013:263–285, with permission.)

Table 15-5   Major Consequences of Mild Perioperative Hypothermia

- Increased incidence of surgical woud infection
- Increased number of adverse myocardial outcomes
- Increased incidence of ventricular arrhythmias
- Coagulopathy
- Increased intraoperative blood loss
- Increased requirement for allogeneic transfusion
- Increased duration of action of some muscle relaxants
- Postoperative shivering
- Increased duration of post anesthetic care unit stay
- Increased duration of hospital stay

whenever there is concern about the adequacy of the circulation in a patient, the anesthesia provider should feel for a pulse and listen for heart sounds.

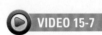

VIDEO 15-7

Temperature Monitoring

D. Temperature

Anesthesia impairs the body's ability to maintain normal body temperature, and *hypothermia* is not only common, but is also associated with adverse outcomes (Table 15-5). On the other hand, although very rare, hyperthermia can alert the provider to rare but serious complications of anesthesia, such as malignant hyperthermia or other metabolic disturbances such as sepsis, thyroid storm, or neuroleptic malignant syndrome. Therefore, *temperature should be monitored during anesthesia* whenever clinically significant changes in body temperature are anticipated or suspected. Several methods, each with their advantages and disadvantages, are available for temperature monitoring (Table 15-6). In general, monitoring of nasopharyngeal or esophageal temperature is preferred, as this reflects the temperature of the major, highly perfused organs.

II. Common Additional Monitors

In addition to the minimal monitoring for anesthesia care previously mentioned, a few other monitors are commonly used during anesthesia.

A. Urine Output

Adequate production of urine is often used as a surrogate marker for adequate perfusion to the rest of the body. Therefore, during major surgery, or even minor surgery of long duration, a urinary (Foley) catheter is often placed to measure urine output. Many anesthesia providers will target 0.5 mg/kg/hr of urine production as a sign of adequate overall body perfusion, although the significance of urine output below this threshold has been questioned. Although urine output is not a good monitor of blood volume, intraoperative oliguria or anuria should be taken seriously and investigated in the context of the overall clinical picture.

B. Neuromuscular Blockade

Pharmacologically induced *muscle paralysis* during anesthesia and major surgery is common, because muscle paralysis facilitates tracheal intubation and may improve operating conditions. The degree of neuromuscular blockade is usually assessed by stimulation of a peripheral nerve and subsequent measurement of the muscle response. Varying sites for measurement are available (Table 15-7) as well as various stimulation patterns (4). Assessment may be visual, tactile, or more accurately measured using a quantitative device such as accelerometry. The most commonly used stimulation pattern is the

Table 15-6 Common Methods for Body Temperature Monitoring during Anesthesia and Potential Advantages and Disadvantages of Each Method

Method	Advantages	Disadvantages	Notes
Skin	Simple, noninvasive	Variable depending on site, and inaccurate; does not correlate well with core temperature	Only use for screening or when others are not available or indicated
Esophageal	Accurate in lower third of esophagus	Only used during general anesthesia and tracheal intubation	Most common
Nasopharyngeal	Accurate when resting on posterior nasopharyngeal wall	Only used during general anesthesia and tracheal intubation	Can cause epistaxis
Tympanic membrane	Correlates well with hypothalamic temp, rapid response time	Risk of tympanic membrane rupture; no continuous reading	Consider in neurologic surgery to estimate brain temperature
Pulmonary artery catheter	Considered a core temperature	Invasive; any complications associated with a pulmonary artery catheter	Thermistor at the tip of the catheter
Bladder	Reasonable accuracy	Slow response time; influenced by urine flow	Not recommended for routine use
Rectal	Reasonable accuracy	Slow response time; influenced by stool	Not recommended for routine use

train-of-four (TOF): Each train consists of four stimuli (T1, T2, T3, T4) applied at 2 Hz (two twitches per second). With increasing nondepolarizing neuromuscular blockade, the "height" or amplitude of the twitch response decreases, and each twitch in the TOF sequence has a smaller height than the one before it. The TOF ratio, which is the ratio of the amplitude of the fourth and first twitches (T4/T1), should be >0.9 at the end of surgery for neuromuscular blockade to be considered fully reversed (Fig. 15-7). Monitoring the level of neuromuscular blockade during anesthesia is important not only for optimizing operating conditions but also for avoiding postoperative weakness.

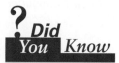

? *Did* *You* *Know*

Postoperative residual neuromuscular blockade is quite common and is associated with postoperative respiratory events.

Table 15-7 Potential Sites for Monitoring Neuromuscular Blockade

Nerve	Muscle
Ulnar	Adductor pollicis
Tibialis posterior	Flexor hallucis brevis
Facial nerve	Orbicularis occuli or corrugator supercilii

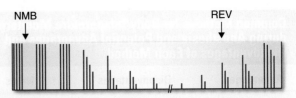

Figure 15-7 Train-of-four monitoring at onset of nondepolarizing neuromuscular blockade (NMB), followed by reversal (REV) with neostigmine.

Residual and often subclinical muscle weakness following reversal of neuromuscular blockade is surprisingly common, and it is a significant contributing factor to postoperative adverse respiratory events (5).

C. Neurologic Monitoring

Monitoring the *electrical activity of the brain* via a processed electroencephalogram (i.e., BIS monitor, Aspect Medical Systems, Norwood, MA) has become a common way to measure the depth of general anesthesia. The *bispectral index (BIS)* is a dimensionless number between 0 and 100, with different ranges purported to correlate with different stages of alertness (Table 15-8). The main goal of the BIS monitor is to decrease the risk of intraoperative awareness, however, studies are conflicting as to the ability of the BIS monitor to accomplish this goal (6,7).

III. Advanced Hemodynamic Monitors

If patient or surgical factors dictate, more advanced monitoring may be needed to deliver safe and effective anesthesia care. The majority of these advanced monitors focus on hemodynamic measurements, including blood pressure, cardiac output, and blood volume. Many of these monitors are considered "invasive" and employ a catheter to be placed within a blood vessel and connected, via a stiff fluid-filled tubing, to an electromechanical transducer, which will produce a waveform. The data derived from these measurements need to be correctly obtained and interpreted, and both the technical and physiologic aspects of the monitor need to be understood. There are two particularly important technical features that must be addressed for accurate monitoring: (a) establishing the appropriate transducer reference level relative to the patient and (b) "zeroing" or balancing the transducer against atmospheric pressure. In most cases, pressure transducers should be placed at a level with the upper border of the heart, which is approximately 5 cm below the sternal

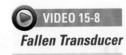
VIDEO 15-8
Fallen Transducer

Table 15-8	Bispectral Index Monitor Values and Corresponding Levels of Sedation and Anesthesia
BIS Number	**Effect**
0	EEG silence
1–40	Deep anesthesia
41–60	Desired range for general anesthesia
61–90	Light anesthesia
91–100	Awake

EEG, electroencephalogram.

Table 15-9	Indications for Intra-arterial Blood Pressure Monitoring
Indication	**Examples**
Rapid changes or extremes in BP expected	• High-risk patients undergoing vascular, trauma, neurologic, cardiac, thoracic operations • Deliberate hyper- or hypotension
Patient intolerance of hemodynamic instability	• Significant cardiac disease or risk of cardiac ischemia • Cerebrovascular disease • Hemodynamically unstable patients (i.e., sepsis)
Patient intolerance of expected respiratory or ventilator changes; impaired oxygenation/ ventilation expected	• Pulmonary comorbidities (i.e., ARDS), severe COPD, or pulmonary hypertension • One-lung ventilation
Expected metabolic abnormalities	• Anticipated large intravascular volume shifts • Expected acid-base abnormalities (i.e., sepsis, hemorrhage)
Miscellaneous	• Failure of or inability to obtain indirect blood pressure measurement • Determination of volume responsiveness from systolic pressure or pulse pressure variation • Need to obtain multiple arterial blood gas samples

BP, blood pressure; ARDS, acute respiratory distress syndrome; COPD, chronic obstructive pulmonary disease.

border in a supine patient. To zero or balance the transducer, it is exposed to atmospheric pressure by opening an adjacent stopcock, exposing the transducer to atmospheric pressure, and then pressing the monitor "zero" control (or its equivalent), which thereby assigns atmospheric pressure a value of zero. All monitored intravascular pressures are subsequently measured in reference to ambient atmospheric pressure.

A. Invasive Monitoring of Systemic Blood Pressure

Invasive blood pressure measurement with an *intra-arterial catheter* is commonly performed for certain patient, surgical, or anesthetic reasons (Table 15-9). The radial artery is the most commonly used site, although ulnar, brachial, axillary, femoral, or dorsalis pedis arteries may also be used. For an individual patient, the anesthesia provider needs to assess whether the benefits of having an arterial line outweigh the risks (Table 15-10).

A normal intra-arterial waveform is shown in Figure 15-8A. The measurements obtained include the systolic blood pressure at the peak of the upstroke, diastolic blood pressure at the nadir, and mean arterial pressure. In addition, the dicrotic notch can often be seen after the systolic peak, during the down stroke, and represents the pressure reflection from closure of the aortic valve (arrow in Fig. 15-8A). *Overdamping* of the waveform (Fig. 15-8B) attenuates the peaks and troughs and is commonly caused by air bubbles or blood clots in the catheter or tubing. This results in underestimation of the true arterial systolic blood pressure. *Underdamping* of the pressure waveform is also possible (Fig. 15-8C) and is a result of the dynamic response characteristics of the fluid-filled catheter tubing system. An underdamped arterial pressure

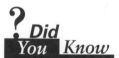

? Did You Know

Invasive blood pressure monitoring is subject to artifacts, including under- and overdamping.

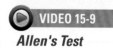

VIDEO 15-9

Allen's Test

Table 15-10   Risks of Intra-arterial Catheter Placement
Bleeding Complications: • Hemorrhage, hematoma
Vascular Complications: • Ischemia, thrombosis, embolism, aneurysm, fistula formation
Other: • Nerve damage/injury • Skin necrosis • Infection • Misinterpretation of data

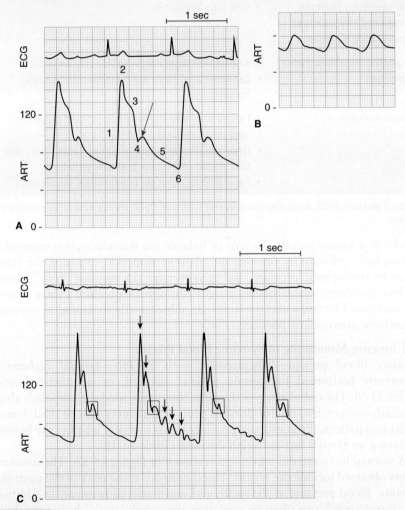

Figure 15-8 Arterial pressure waveforms. **A:** Normal arterial blood pressure tracing. 1, systolic upstroke; 2, systolic peak; 3, systolic decline; 4, dicrotic notch (*red arrow*) indicating closure of the aortic valve; 5, diastolic run-off; 6, end-diastolic pressure. **B:** Overdamped waveform, characterized by a prolonged upstroke, loss of the dicrotic notch, and loss of fine detail. **C:** An underdamped waveform, characterized by systolic pressure overshoot and additional small, nonphysiologic pressure waves (*arrows*) that distort the waveform and make it hard to discern the dicrotic notch (*boxes*). ART, arterial line pressure scale; ECG, electrocardiogram. (From Mark JB. *Atlas of Cardiovascular Monitoring.* New York: Churchill Livingstone; 1998, with permission.)

Table 15-11   Common Indications for Central Venous Catheterization

- Administration of drugs/solutions
  - Vasopressor/inotropic drugs
  - Parenteral nutrition
  - Long-term infusions
- Patient factors
  - Poor peripheral IV access
  - Pulmonary artery catheter or temporary pacemaker placement
- Surgical factors
  - Need for large volume administration, transfusion
- Central venous pressure monitoring

IV, intravenous.

waveform will cause overestimation of true arterial systolic pressure. Owing to these common artifacts, the mean arterial blood pressure is the most reliable measurement for most monitoring purposes. Before treating abnormal blood pressure, the anesthesia provider should quickly assess whether the tracing appears to be under- or overdamped. In addition, the provider should check that the transducer is at the correct level and confirm the abnormal pressure by comparison with a noninvasive blood pressure measurement.

B. Central Venous Pressure Monitoring

Central venous catheterization and monitoring of *central venous pressure (CVP)* remains a common procedure during anesthesia, especially for patients who undergo high-risk surgical procedures. Indications for central venous catheter placement and well-recognized complications can be found in Tables 15-11 and 15-12, respectively. Multiple sites are available for central venous access, but the most common include the internal jugular (usually the right), subclavian, or femoral veins.

CVP monitoring can occur when a central line is in place. The normal CVP waveform consists of three peaks (a, c, v) and two descents (x, y) (Fig. 15-9 and Table 15-13). For many years, the CVP was thought to reflect the overall "volume status" of a patient. If the CVP was low, the patient was hypovolemic

Table 15-12   Common Complications of Central Venous Catheterization

- **Bleeding**
  - Adjacent arterial injury
  - Hematoma formation
  - Airway compromise
  - Cardiac tamponade
- **Pneumothorax, hemothorax, or chylothorax**
- **Nerve injury**
- **Infection**
  - Bacteremia, sepsis
  - Endocarditis
- **Venous thromboembolism**
- **Venous (and paradoxical) air embolism**

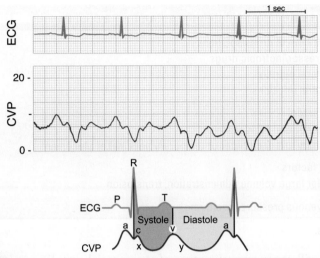

Figure 15-9 Normal central venous pressure (CVP) waveform, showing the timing of waveform components in relation to the electrocardiogram (ECG). See Table 15-13 for descriptions of the peaks and descents. (From Mark JB. *Atlas of Cardiovascular Monitoring.* New York: Churchill Livingstone; 1998, with permission.)

and required fluid administration, and conversely, if the CVP was high, the patient was volume overloaded and required diuresis. However, this physiologic reasoning has proven invalid in clinical practice, owing to the many factors that confound accurate and reproducible measurement and interpretation of CVP, including the complex nonlinear relation between cardiac chamber pressure and volume (8,9). For patients with relatively normal heart function undergoing noncardiac surgery, following the *change* in CVP resulting from a fluid bolus may be more useful than single pressure measurements. Although CVP has its limitations as an assessment of intravascular volume, the CVP waveform can provide additional information to help diagnose other conditions (Table 15-14).

Table 15-13	Physiologic Basis of a Normal Central Venous Pressure Waveform	
Waveform Component	**Cardiac Cycle Phase**	**Causative Mechanical Event**
a wave	End diastole	Atrial contraction; end-diastolic atrial kick that loads the right ventricle through the open tricuspid valve
c wave	Early systole	Isovolumetric ventricular contraction, closure of tricuspid valve
x descent	Mid-systole	Atrial relaxation and descent of the base of the heart
v wave	Late systole	Venous filling of the right atrium, tricuspid valve closed
y descent	Early diastole	Blood flow from the right atrium to right ventricle after tricuspid valve opens

Table 15-14	Abnormalities of the Central Venous Pressure Waveform	
Condition	**Change in Central Venous Pressure Waveform**	**Reason for Change**
Atrial fibrillation	• a wave disappears • c wave becomes more prominent	• No atrial contraction • Atrial volume is greater at end diastole and onset of systole
Junctional rhythm	• Tall cannon a wave	• Atrial contraction occurs during ventricular systole, when the tricuspid valve is closed
Tricuspid regurgitation	• Broad, tall systolic c–v wave	• Abnormal systolic filling of the right atrium through the incompetent valve

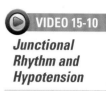

VIDEO 15-10

Junctional Rhythm and Hypotension

C. Pulmonary Artery Catheter

The *pulmonary artery catheter (PAC), or Swan-Ganz catheter,* is a balloon-tipped catheter that is advanced and blood flow directed through the right atrium, tricuspid valve, right ventricle, pulmonic valve, and finally into the pulmonary artery. PAC monitoring has been widely used by anesthesia providers and critical care physicians caring for acutely and severely ill patients because of its ability to continually monitor a number of important hemodynamic variables (Table 15-15). However, the PAC is not without its risks, which include those for central venous catheterization (Table 15-12) as well as additional potential complications specifically related to the PAC (Table 15-16). Currently, PAC monitoring is mainly reserved for patients undergoing complicated cardiac operations and critically ill patients requiring advanced cardiopulmonary support therapies.

During flotation of a PAC through the right heart chambers, typical pressure waveforms are recorded as the catheter tip traverses the right side of the heart (Fig. 15-10). Occasionally, distinguishing right ventricular from pulmonary artery pressure is difficult, but careful examination of the diastolic portion of these two pressure waveforms clarifies the different locations of the catheter tip. During diastole, filling of the right ventricle results in a pressure increase in that chamber, while diastolic flow from the pulmonary artery toward the lung results in a pressure decrease (Fig. 15-10, red arrows).

Table 15-15	Standard Variables Measured with a Pulmonary Artery Catheter

- **Intracardiac pressures**
  - Central venous pressure/right atrial pressure
  - Right ventricular pressure
  - Pulmonary artery pressure
  - Pulmonary artery wedge pressure/left atrial pressure
- **Cardiac output**
- **Mixed venous oxygen saturation**
- **Core body temperature**

Table 15-16   Complications of Pulmonary Artery Catheterization

- Atrial and ventricular dysrhythmias, including ventricular fibrillation
- Right bundle-branch block
- Pulmonary infarction
- Pulmonary artery rupture
- Misinterpretation of derived data

Advancing the balloon-tipped PAC further into the pulmonary artery will allow the catheter to "wedge" and record the *pulmonary artery wedge pressure*, or *pulmonary artery occlusion pressure*. The pulmonary artery wedge pressure provides an indirect measurement of *left atrial pressure*, and the wedge waveform is a slightly delayed and damped reflection of left atrial pressure.

D. Noninvasive Cardiac Output and Volume Assessment

Given the complications and complexity associated with the PAC, a number of minimally invasive cardiac output monitors have been developed (Table 15-17). These monitors use a range of fundamental technologies (ultrasound, indicator dilution, pulse contour analysis) to provide estimates of cardiac output, stroke volume, and other derived parameters, such as the variation in pulse pressure during the respiratory cycle. Many of these monitors provide "dynamic" indicators of a patient's volume status by measuring changes that occur during the respiratory cycle in a patient who is receiving positive pressure mechanical ventilation. Thus, they are specifically designed to be used intraoperatively for patients under general anesthesia. These dynamic variables have been shown to be superior to static indices such as CVP in predicting volume responsiveness, thereby providing a clinically useful guide to perioperative fluid administration (10).

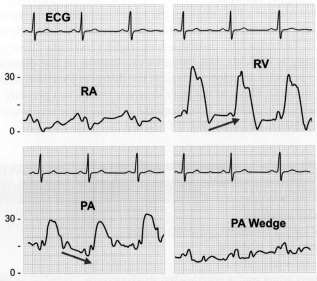

Figure 15-10 Pulmonary artery catheter waveforms as the tip of the catheter advances through the cardiac chambers. The *red arrows* highlight the different pattern of diastolic pressure in the right ventricle (RV) and pulmonary artery (PA). ECG, electrocardiogram; RA, right atrium; PA Wedge, pulmonary artery wedge pressure. (From Mark JB. *Atlas of Cardiovascular Monitoring.* New York: Churchill Livingstone; 1998, with permission.)

Table 15-17   **Noninvasive Cardiac Output Monitors**
• Esophageal Doppler
• Carbon dioxide rebreathing systems
• Indicator dilution methods
• Thoracic bioimpedance

• Pulse contour analysis
   • Invasive (i.e., arterial line required)
   • Noninvasive (i.e., finger cuff)

E. Transesophageal Echocardiography

Transesophageal echocardiography (TEE) has been used for many years in cardiac surgery, but its use has expanded to include other major operations (i.e., abdominal transplant, major vascular surgery). TEE is really a diagnostic tool as well as a monitoring modality, and it can provide accurate information about volume status, ventricular and valvular function, and a wide range of other cardiac conditions. In current anesthesiology practice, diagnostic TEE is generally used by physicians specifically trained and credentialed in its use. There are simpler disposable TEE monitors available for limited monitoring, and in the future their perioperative use may increase.

Basic anesthesia monitoring is required to safely administer anesthetic care. More advanced monitoring may be required, depending on the clinical situation, including patient and surgical factors. There are a wide array of monitors available for use, and over time, the specialty of anesthesiology has seen a trend toward use of less-invasive monitors that often rely on complex algorithms. Despite these sophisticated monitors, a competent and vigilant anesthesia provider is absolutely essential to choose and use these monitors correctly.

References

1. American Society of Anesthesiologists. Standards for Basic Anesthetic Monitoring. Available at: https://www.asahq.org/For-Members/Standards-Guidelines-and-Statements.aspx.
2. Berkow LL, Rotolo SS, Mirski EE. Continuous noninvasive hemoglobin monitoring during complex spine surgery. *Anesth Analg.* 2011;113(6):1396–1402.
3. London MJ, Hollenberg M, Wong MG, et al. Intraoperative myocardial ischemia: Localization by continuous 12-lead electrocardiography. *Anesthesiology.* 1988;69(2):232–241.
4. Fuchs-Buder T, Schreiber J-U, Meistelman C. Monitoring neuromuscular block: An update. *Anaesthesia.* 2009;64(Suppl 1):82–89.
5. Murphy GS, Szokol JW, Marymont JH, et al. Residual neuromuscular block and adverse respiratory events. *Anesth Analg.* 2008;107(5):1756.
6. Avidan MS, Zhang L, Burnside BA, et al. Anesthesia awareness and the bispectral index. *N Engl J Med.* 2008;358(11):1097–1108.
7. Myles PS, Leslie K, McNeil J, et al. Bispectral index monitoring to prevent awareness during anaesthesia: The B-Aware randomised controlled trial. *Lancet.* 2004;363(9423): 1757–1763.
8. Marik PE, Cavallazzi R. Does the central venous pressure predict fluid responsiveness? An updated meta-analysis and a plea for some common sense. *Crit Care Med.* 2013; 41(7):1774–1781.
9. Marik PE, Baram M, Vahid B. Does central venous pressure predict fluid responsiveness? A systematic review of the literature and the tale of seven mares. *Chest.* 2008;134(1):172–178.
10. Marik PE, Cavallazzi R, Vasu T, et al. Dynamic changes in arterial waveform derived variables and fluid responsiveness in mechanically ventilated patients: A systematic review of the literature. *Crit Care Med.* 2009;37(9):2642–2647.

Questions

1. Which two wavelengths are employed by the pulse oximeter?
   A. Red and near infrared
   B. Red and infrared
   C. Infrared and blue
   D. Near infrared and blue
   E. None of the above

2. A sudden large decrease in the end-tidal carbon dioxide concentration most likely indicates:
   A. Hypovolemia
   B. Hypothermia
   C. Sepsis
   D. Pulmonary embolism
   E. None of the above

3. Which two leads of the electrocardiogram provide a sensitivity of 80% for the detection of myocardial ischemia?
   A. Leads I and II
   B. Leads I and V_5
   C. Leads II and V_5
   D. Leads II and V_3
   E. None of the above

4. When an electromechanical transducer is zeroed, the actual pressure it is measuring is:
   A. Zero pressure
   B. Ambient atmospheric pressure
   C. The pressure of the fluid in the attached monitoring catheter
   D. The pressure of the fluid in the transducer flush system
   E. None of the above

5. The x descent of the central venous pressure trace is caused by:
   A. The opening of the tricuspid valve
   B. Isovolumetric ventricular contraction
   C. The descent of the base of the heart
   D. Atrial diastasis
   E. None of the above

Clinical Practice
of Anesthesia

16 *Preoperative Evaluation and Management*

Natalie F. Holt

Preoperative evaluation of the patient by an anesthesiologist is a cornerstone of perioperative patient care. The main purpose is to obtain information about a patient's medical, surgical, and anesthetic history and to perform a focused physical examination that will help determine whether the patient is in optimum medical condition to proceed with the planned procedure. It has become clear that increased efficiency can be achieved when need-based preoperative laboratory and other diagnostic tests are ordered by an anesthesiologist in a dedicated preoperative evaluation clinic, rather than by surgeons or primary care doctors. Anesthesia preoperative clinics can also help enhance operating room efficiency by reducing day-of-surgery cancellations or delays due to incomplete workups. In addition, anesthesia preoperative clinics benefit patients by providing education and counseling, as well as pharmacologic preparation, when necessary, to reduce anxiety or prevent known complications such as postoperative nausea and vomiting.

I. Approach to the Patient

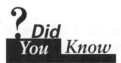

Age alone is not a factor in determining ASA physical status. An ambulatory, fit, cognitively aware 80 year old patient with moderate hypertension is ASA PS 2.

Key elements of the preanesthetic evaluation include a review of (a) the planned surgical procedure and its indication; (b) the patient's present and past medical history; (c) current medications and drug allergies; (d) social history, including use of alcohol, tobacco, or illicit drugs; (e) response to previous anesthetics; and (f) performance of a focused physical examination (Table 16-1). By convention, anesthesiologists use the American Society of Anesthesiologists' (ASA) physical status classification system to summarize the health status of the patient (Table 16-2). Information obtained during the preoperative evaluation guides the development of an anesthetic and postoperative pain management plan. Most preanesthetic clinics use standardized evaluation templates to guide patient evaluations; use of these forms also increases reporting consistency and limits the risk of missing information. The growing use of electronic medical records is also helping to maximize consistency in preanesthetic evaluation.

Table 16-1   Components of the Preanesthetic Evaluation

I. Review of planned surgical procedure and its indication

II. Review of systems
  a. Head, ears, eyes, throat (glaucoma, dental care, implanted jewelry)
  b. Cardiovascular (exercise tolerance, angina, dyspnea on exertion, hypertension)
  c. Vascular (peripheral vascular, aneurysm)
  d. Pulmonary (smoking, COPD, asthma)
  e. Gastrointestinal (reflux, obstruction)
  f. Hepatic (liver disease, alcohol abuse)
  g. Endocrine (diabetes, thyroid disease)
  h. Renal (chronic kidney disease, dialysis)
  i. Genitourinary (benign prostatic hypertrophy, hematuria)
  j. Musculoskeletal (rheumatoid arthritis)
  k. Neurologic (neuropathy, stroke, seizure)
  l. Psychiatric (bipolar disorder, substance abuse)
  m. Other (dermatologic diseases, chronic pain, etc.)

III. Medication history

IV. Drug/latex allergies (including reactions, if known)

V. Social history
  a. Tobacco use—past and present
  b. Alcohol use
  c. Illicit substance use

VI. Past surgeries and anesthetics (including complications, personal and familial)

VII. Physical examination
  a. Vital signs: blood pressure, heart rate, temperature
  b. Heart
  c. Lungs
  d. Neurologic examination: peripheral neuropathies, asymmetries
  e. Airway: oral aperture, Mallampati score, dentition, thyromental distance, neck range of motion

VIII. Laboratory tests (blood, ECG, chest x-ray) as needed based on history and physical examination

COPD, chronic obstructive pulmonary disease; ECG, electrocardiogram.

A. Planned Surgery and Its Indication

The planned surgical procedure is an important determinant of the type of anesthesia that will be required for the procedure and the expected level of postoperative pain. The planned procedure also dictates the anticipated patient positioning, blood loss, and monitoring requirements. Understanding the indication for the procedure is important for establishing the risk of postoperative complications. Procedures performed for urgent conditions (e.g., small bowel obstruction, limb ischemia) are associated with an increased risk of perioperative morbidity and mortality.

B. Present and Past Medical History

Medical history is best addressed using a systems-based approach. A useful way to screen for occult cardiovascular disease is to inquire about the patient's

Table 16-2	American Society of Anesthesiologists' (ASA) Physical Status Classification System
ASA Physical Status Classification	
1	Normal healthy person
2	Mild systemic disease that results in no functional limitation
3	Severe systemic disease that results in functional limitation
4	Severe systemic disease that causes a constant threat to life
5	Moribund patient not expected to live without the planned surgery
6	Brain-dead person whose organs are being removed for donation
E	Qualifier used for emergency procedures

Modified from American Society of Anesthesiologists: New classification of physical status. *Anesthesiology.* 1963;24:111.

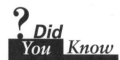

? Did You Know

Routine referral of presurgical patients to an internist to be "cleared for surgery" is an unnecessary expenditure. The competent anesthesiologist should only request consultation when it is felt the patient is in need of additional evaluation or treatment prior to surgery.

ability to exercise at 4 metabolic equivalents (METs) without dyspnea, chest pain, or lightheadedness (Table 16-3). An example of an activity that uses about 4 METs is climbing 1 to 2 flights of stairs. Pulmonary evaluation should take into account a history of asthma or recent upper respiratory infection (URI) and signs and symptoms suggestive of obstructive sleep apnea (OSA). Asthma or recent URI may predispose the patient to bronchospasm with airway instrumentation, and OSA may signal difficulty with ventilation and the need for increased respiratory monitoring postoperatively. When the review of systems reveals signs and symptoms suggestive of an undiagnosed or uncontrolled medical condition, the patient should be referred to his or her primary care practitioner for further evaluation and management. Whether this workup needs to be completed prior to surgery is at the discretion of the anesthesiologist and surgeon and is often dependent on the urgency and severity of the planned surgical procedure.

Table 16-3	Metabolic Equivalents for Common Physical Activities	
Metabolic Equivalents	**Examples**
1	Watching television
		Eating, dressing
		Walking on level ground at 2 to 3 mph
∨	Doing light housework (e.g., dusting)
4	Climbing a flight of stairs
		Walking on level ground at 4 mph
∨	Doing heavy chores (e.g., scrubbing floors)
>10	Playing strenuous sports (e.g., tennis)

Adapted from Fleisher LA, Beckman JA, Brown KA, et al. American College of Cardiology American Heart Association Task Force on Practice Guidelines; American Society of Echocardiography. ACC/AHA 2007 guidelines on perioperative cardiovascular evaluation and care for noncardiac surgery. *J Am Coll Cardiol.* 2007;50(17):e170.

C. Current Medications and Drug Allergies

Review of current medications, including over-the-counter and herbal or complementary drugs, is an essential component of the preanesthetic assessment, as many drugs used in the perioperative period have important interactions with commonly prescribed pharmaceuticals. Consideration should be given to discontinuation of some drugs with known interactions with anesthetics prior to surgery (e.g, monoamine oxidase inhibitors), but it may be appropriate to continue some drugs into the operative period despite known interactions (e.g., antihypertensives). Additionally, some medications with known rebound side effects when withdrawn abruptly (e.g., propranolol, clonidine) should be continued or tapered slowly prior to surgery.

Cardiovascular Medications

Patients on chronic beta-blocker therapy should continue their medications perioperatively, as abrupt withdrawal may precipitate angina, ischemia, or dysrhythmias. Whether to initiate beta-blocker treatment in patients with known coronary artery ischemia on preoperative stress testing who are scheduled for vascular or other high-risk surgery is a point of much controversy. Too rapid initiation of beta-blocker therapy increases the risk of perioperative bradycardia, hypotension, and stroke. Patients who take centrally acting sympatholytics, such as clonidine, may experience rebound hypertension with abrupt discontinuation. Therefore, it is recommended that these drugs be continued in patients who take them chronically.

There are conflicting results from randomized trials as to whether calcium channel–blocking drugs increase the risk of surgical bleeding; however, it is generally agreed that calcium channel blockers may be continued perioperatively. In the context of major surgery, angiotensin converting enzyme (ACE) inhibitors and angiotensin II receptor blocking drugs (ARBs) have been associated with refractory intraoperative hypotension. For this reason, they are generally discontinued the night prior to surgery, with the caveat that patients who normally take these drugs may be somewhat more prone to postoperative hypertension as a result of their discontinuation. Diuretics are also generally discontinued the night prior to surgery to avoid intravascular volume depletion prior to major surgery where fluid shifts are expected. For more minor procedures, it is probably okay to continue ACE inhibitor, ARBs, and diuretics throughout the perioperative period.

There is evidence that the use of perioperative 3-hydroxy-3-methyl-glutaryl-coenzyme A reductase inhibitors (known as statins) reduces cardiovascular morbidity and mortality, especially for patients undergoing vascular surgery. Therefore, it is recommended that statins be continued perioperatively, and consideration should be given to initiating statin therapy in patients with cardiac risk factors who will be undergoing vascular surgery.

Endocrine Medications

Patients who take glucocorticoids should continue these medications perioperatively. Patients who are on a chronic dose equivalent to prednisone ≥5 mg/day are at risk of adrenal suppression and may require supplemental glucocorticoid administration perioperatively. Table 16-4 summarizes an approach to glucocorticoid supplementation in these patients.

The management of patients with diabetes should be individualized. However, in general, oral hypoglycemic drugs and short-acting insulin preparations should be withheld on the morning of surgery. Intermediate or long-acting insulin preparations should be administered in a reduced dose on the day of

Table 16-4	An Approach to Perioperative Corticosteroid Coverage
For minor surgeries, take usual morning steroid dose. No supplementation is needed.	
For moderate surgeries, take usual morning steroid dose. Administer 50 mg hydrocortisone IV prior to induction and 25 mg IV every 8 hours for 24 hours.	
For major surgeries, take usual morning steroid dose. Administer 100 mg IV hydrocortisone IV prior to induction, and 50 mg IV every 8 hours for 24 hours.	

IV, intravenous.

surgery. Metformin is associated with an increased risk of lactic acidosis in the context of severe dehydration; therefore, most clinicians discontinue its use a full 24 hours prior to surgery. Table 16-5 presents general guidelines for the perioperative management of oral hypoglycemic drugs and insulin in diabetic patients.

Women who take oral contraceptives or hormone replacement therapy are at increased risk for venous thrombosis, owing to the estrogen content in these medications. Therefore, consideration should be given to discontinuing these medications 4 to 6 weeks preoperatively for surgeries associated with a high risk of venous thromboembolism.

Psychotropic Medications
Although many psychotropic medications have interactions with anesthetic and analgesic agents, most are continued in the perioperative period, owing to the potential consequences of withdrawing these agents in patients with serious mood disorders. Tricyclic antidepressants may cause QT_c prolongation and are associated with anticholinergic effects that may be exacerbated by drugs used during anesthesia. Nonselective monoamine oxidase inhibitors (MAOI), such as phenelzine and tranylcypromine, though rarely used today, pose a special concern in the context of anesthesia. They inhibit the breakdown of monoamine neurotransmitters including dopamine, serotonin, epinephrine, and norepinephrine. In patients taking MAOI, coadministration of indirect acting sympathomimetic agents such as ephedrine may cause

? Did You Know

The manifestations of severe hypoglycemia can be masked during general anesthesia. While it is desirable to keep blood glucose at near normal levels during anesthesia, the consequences of over treatment with insulin are significant. Frequent perioperative measurement of blood glucose is indicated.

Table 16-5	Guidelines for the Perioperative Management of Patients with Diabetes
Schedule as first case of the day to avoid prolonged fasting, if possible.	
Hold oral hypoglycemic drugs on the day of surgery; hold metformin for 24 hours prior to surgery.	
Continue usual insulin regimen through the evening prior to surgery.	
For patients with type 1 diabetes, administer half the usual dose of intermediate or long-acting insulin on the morning of surgery; for patients with insulin pumps, continue infusions on a basal rate. Begin a dextrose-containing insulin infusion upon arrival in surgical suite.	
For patients with type 2 diabetes, administer one-third to two-thirds the usual dose of intermediate or long-acting insulin on the morning of surgery, depending on the patient's usual morning fasting blood glucose measurements.	
Measure blood glucose level every 1 to 2 hours during surgery.	

a hypertensive crisis. In addition, concomitant administration of drugs with anticholinergic properties, such as meperidine and dextromethorphan, may cause *serotonin syndrome,* a condition marked by agitation, hyperthermia, and muscular rigidity and caused by an excess of serotonergic activity in the central nervous system.

Mood stabilizing agents, antipsychotics, antianxiety medications, and antiseizure drugs may be continued perioperatively. However, if patients are taking medications with a narrow therapeutic window, such as lithium and valproate, perioperative monitoring of drug blood levels may be appropriate, as drug absorption may be affected by surgery.

Drugs Affecting Platelet Function

Aspirin irreversibly inhibits the platelet cyclooxygenase (COX) enzyme, which is responsible for prostaglandin and thromboxane production. Among its many effects, aspirin inhibits platelet aggregation. For this reason, aspirin is widely used for prevention of clotting in patients at risk for cardiovascular disease, as well as those with a history of angina, myocardial infarction, stroke, and peripheral vascular disease. Daily aspirin therapy is also necessary for patients with coronary artery stents to prevent in-stent thrombosis. In the context of surgery, however, decreased platelet aggregation predisposes patients on aspirin to increased surgical bleeding. Therefore, decisions about perioperative aspirin use must weigh the risk of perioperative hemorrhage against that of cardiovascular complications. It is generally agreed that aspirin should be withheld for 7 to 10 days prior to surgeries where bleeding would have catastrophic consequences (e.g., intracranial, intraocular, middle ear, and intramedullary spine surgeries).

Platelet P2Y12 receptor blockers (e.g., clopidogrel, ticlopidine, prasugrel, ticagrelor) are another class of antiplatelet agents commonly used in patients following an ischemic cerebrovascular event (e.g., acute myocardial infarction) or in patients who have undergone coronary artery stent implantation. Combined use of aspirin and a platelet P2Y12 receptor blocker markedly reduces the risk of in-stent thrombosis in patients with vascular stents. The optimal duration of dual antiplatelet therapy in these patients is unknown; most guidelines recommend that patients who have drug-eluting coronary stents remain on dual antiplatelet therapy for 1 year. If discontinued perioperatively, these medications should be resumed as soon possible. It is suggested clopidogrel and ticagrelor should be stopped 5 days, prasugrel 7 days, and ticlopidine 10 days preoperatively.

It is generally recommended that nonsteroidal anti-inflammatory agents such as ibuprofen and naproxen be discontinued for a period of 3 to 5 days preoperatively, owing to their effect on platelet aggregation. Patients are advised to use acetaminophen as the pain reliever of choice preoperatively, as it has no effect on platelet function.

Oral Anticoagulants

Oral anticoagulants include warfarin, which blocks the production of vitamin K–dependent clotting factors, direct thrombin inhibitors, such as dabigatran, and direct Xa inhibitors, such as rivaroxaban and apixaban. Because the half-life of warfarin is long, it is recommended that warfarin be stopped 5 days prior to elective surgery. When there is a desire to minimize the duration that the patient is without anticoagulation, bridging therapy may be used. This generally involves the administration of low molecular weight heparin, which is usually given via subcutaneous injection and typically commences 3 days prior to surgery, with the last dose administered 24 hours before the start of the procedure. Dabigatran is used primarily to prevent stroke in patients with atrial fibrillation. It has a half-life of about 12 hours in patients with normal renal function, but in patients with kidney disease, its half-life can be more than 24 hours. In patients with normal renal function, dabigatran should be stopped 1 to 2 days prior to surgery; in patients with a creatinine clearance of <50 mL/min, it should be stopped 3 to 5 days prior to surgery. Rivaroxaban and apixaban are less dependent on renal function for clearance and may be stopped 1 to 2 days prior to surgery. Because of their relatively short half-life, bridging therapy is not usually required for the direct thrombin and Xa inhibitors.

Opioids and Medications Used to Treat Addiction

Patients who take opioids for chronic pain should continue these medications perioperatively and often benefit from a pain management plan that includes multimodal treatments such as intraoperative ketamine infusions and regional anesthetic techniques. Patients recovering from opioid or alcohol addiction are sometimes prescribed partial opioid agonists, such as buprenorphine, or opioid antagonists such as naltrexone. These drugs are helpful in addiction recovery because they block the euphoric effects associated with opioid use; however, in the context of surgery, they also interfere with the pain-relieving properties of legitimately administered opioids. As a result, the preferred approached is to discontinue these drugs prior to surgery. This should be performed in consultation with the patient's primary care physician, recognizing that there is an increased risk of relapse during this period of drug holiday.

Herbal or Complementary Supplements

Owing to concerns about their purity and the potential for adverse effects, it is safest to advise that all herbal or complementary drugs be discontinued 1 week prior to surgery. Specific supplements have been associated with particular complications. For example, garlic, ginger, and ginseng may increase bleeding risk. Table 16-6 summarizes the potential side effects of common herbal supplements.

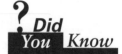

Perioperative pain control in patients taking opioids on a chronic basis requires careful planning. Typically these patients are tolerant to opioids and may require extremely high doses of opioids to be rendered comfortable. Concomitant use of regional anesthesia techniques is beneficial.

Drug Allergies

Information about drug allergies should be elicited during the preanesthetic interview. It has been reported that 5% to 10% of the population has a penicillin allergy; however, based on prior studies, the majority of these patients (80% to 90%) do not have a true penicillin allergy. Signs and symptoms suggestive of true type 1 immunoglobulin-E–mediated allergy include urticaria, angioedema, and wheezing. Although the potential for cross-reactivity exists between allergy to penicillin and the cephalosporins because of the common β-lactam ring, only about 2% of patients with a documented penicillin allergy will have an allergic reaction to a cephalosporin. Patients should also be asked about a history of allergy to latex, as this allergy requires advance preparation of the operating suite with latex-free equipment.

D. Social History

It is useful to inquire about patients' tobacco, alcohol, and illicit drug habits, as patients who abuse these substances have an increased risk of complications, including postoperative withdrawal. Smoking is also associated with an increased risk of perioperative respiratory complications, including airway hyperreactivity. In patients in whom a strong suspicion of substance abuse is suspected, urine drug screening on the day of surgery may be indicated.

Table 16-6	Perioperative Effects of Common Herbal Supplements
Name	**Perioperative Effects**
Echinacea	Hepatotoxicity; allergic reactions
Ephedra	Enhanced sympathomimetic effects with other sympathomimetic agents, dysrhythmias
Feverfew	Inhibits platelet activity
Garlic	Inhibits platelet aggregation
Ginkgo	Inhibits platelet activating factor
Ginseng	Hypoglycemia; inhibits platelet aggregation and coagulation cascade
Kava	Hepatotoxicity, decreased MAC
Licorice	Increased blood pressure, hypokalemia
St. John's wort	Inhibits serotonin, norepinephrine, and dopamine reuptake; induction of cytochrome P450 enzyme, leading to increased drug metabolism
Vitamin E	Increased bleeding when taken with other anticoagulant or antithrombotic medications

MAC, minimum alveolar concentration.
Adapted from ASA Physician Brochure "What You Should Know About Your Patients' Use of Herbal Medicines and Other Dietary Supplements," 2003. www.ASAhq.org. Available at: https://ecommerce.asahq.org/p-147-what-you-should-know-about-herbal-and-dietary-supplement-use-and-anesthesia.aspx.

E. Response to Prior Anesthetics

The preanesthetic interview should include a discussion of any personal or familial history of complications related to anesthesia. Patients should be queried about a personal history of difficult tracheal intubation, prolonged postoperative nausea or vomiting, difficulty associated with spinal anesthesia, and so forth. Each of these scenarios may have important implications for planning an upcoming anesthetic. *Malignant hyperthermia* is a rare but potentially life-threatening anesthetic-triggered disorder of skeletal muscle metabolism that is often inherited in an autosomal dominant fashion. Patients heterozygous or homozygous for the atypical plasma cholinesterase gene may describe prolonged hospital stays or ventilator dependence after brief surgical procedures. Advanced planning for these patients is a must.

F. Focused Physical Examination

Components of the physical examination of main interest to the anesthesiologist involve the neurologic system, heart, lungs, and airway. Notation of blood pressure and heart rate is useful in screening for undiagnosed or poorly treated hypertension. Auscultation of the heart may reveal murmurs suggestive of cardiac valve abnormalities that require further workup prior to surgery. Wheezing, rhonchi, or other abnormal lung sounds may require follow-up with a chest x-ray or indicate patients who may benefit from pretreatment with bronchodilators or steroids. In patients with a history of congestive heart failure, wheezing may also be indicative of decompensation. It is also important to note pre-existing neuropathies, central nervous system deficits, and skeletal muscle weakness, as these affect the ability to position patients intraoperatively and may affect the decision to perform neuraxial or regional anesthetic blockade.

Evaluation of the neck and oral airway helps to determine the potential for difficult ventilation or tracheal intubation and, therefore, preferred methods of

Table 16-7	Modified Mallampati Airway Classification
Class	**Direct Visualization**
I	Soft palate, uvula, tonsillar pillars
II	Soft palate, upper portion of the uvula
III	Soft palate
IV	Only hard palate

Modified from Mallampati RS, Gatt SP, Gugino LD, et al. A clinical sign to predict difficult tracheal intubation. A prospective study. *Can Anaesth Soc J.* 1985;32:429.

perioperative airway management. Basic components of the airway examination include measurement of the oral aperture, Mallampati score, thyromental distance, range of neck motion, as well as examination of dentition and neck circumference. The *Mallampati score* evaluates the size of the tongue in relation to the oral cavity, and the test is performed by having the patient protrude the tongue while keeping his or her head in a neutral position. The anesthesiologist then grades the view on a 4-point scale based on visualization of the uvula and the soft and hard palate (Table 16-7). Thyromental distance is measured from the tip of the chin (mentum) to the thyroid cartilage, while the patient's head is maximally extended. A thyromental distance less than 6 cm is suggestive of possible difficult intubation. The patient should also be asked to extend the neck as far as possible (normal is 35 degrees). Significant limitation of neck extension is also a risk factor for difficult intubation. Preoperative evaluation of dentition is important to determine the presence of prosthetics that should be removed prior to anesthesia and to identify pre-existing loose, chipped, or fractured teeth that might later be erroneously attributed to airway manipulation.

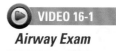

VIDEO 16-1

Airway Exam

II. Evaluation of the Patient with Known Systemic Disease

A. Cardiovascular Disease

Cardiac Risk Assessment

Cardiovascular complications are a significant source of perioperative morbidity and mortality. Therefore, identifying patients at risk for these complications and finding ways to mitigate these risks preoperatively is a major objective of the preanesthetic workup. The risk of a perioperative major adverse cardiac event (MACE) or death is related to patient factors and the planned surgery. Several validated risk prediction tools have been developed to estimate risk. The *Revised Cardiac Risk Index* is among the most popular. Based on a retrospective review of over 4,000 patients presenting for noncardiac surgery, this index identified six independent predictors of cardiac complications: history of ischemic heart disease; history of congestive heart failure; history of cerebrovascular accident; preoperative insulin-requiring diabetes; creatinine >2.0 mg/dL; and those presenting for high-risk surgery (intraperitoneal, intrathoracic, or suprainguinal vascular surgery). Two newer risk tools have been created by the American College of Surgeon's National Surgical Quality Improvement Program (NSQIP). These incorporate additional patient factors such as age and functional status. NSQIP has used the information from these tools to create calculators that estimate the risk of MACE and death based on the value of the input variables (www.riskcalculator.facs.org and http://www.surgicalriskcalculator.com/microcardiacarrest).

In patients with known coronary artery disease, cerebrovascular or peripheral artery disease, significant arrhythmias, or structural heart disease, a preoperative resting 12-lead electrocardiogram (ECG) provides a point of comparison by which to determine changes in the postoperative period. Preoperative ECG abnormalities such as bundle branch block and pathological Q waves may be poor prognostic indicators, but results from observational trials are mixed. In general, the best available evidence suggests that preoperative noninvasive stress testing should be reserved for patients with cardiac risks factors who demonstrate poor (<4 METS) or unknown functional capacity and are undergoing anything other than low risk surgery (MACE risk ≥1%). Regarding the decision to undertake coronary revascularization before surgery, the Coronary Artery Revascularization Prophylaxis (CARP) trial was the first large, randomized study designed to evaluate whether prophylactic coronary revascularization prior to major vascular surgery reduced perioperative cardiac events relative to optimal pharmacologic management. The main finding was no difference in all-cause mortality at a median follow-up of 2.7 years. A secondary finding was no difference in the incidence of postoperative myocardial infarction. A criticism that has been rendered against the CARP trial was that selection criteria resulted in the exclusion of too many high-risk patients. However, for the majority of patients, current evidence supports pharmacologic optimization as the best cardiac risk reduction strategy prior to surgery. The 2014 American College of Cardiology/American HeartAssociation "Perioperative Cardiovascular Evaluation and Management of Patients Undergoing Noncardiac Surgery" guideline presents an algorithmic approach to perioperative cardiac assessment aimed at helping clinicians in the evaluating of these patients (Fig. 16-1).

? Did You Know

When patients present for surgery and are either taking anti-platelet therapy, or have a CIED in place, there should be communication between the anesthesiologist, surgeon, and cardiologist well in advance of surgery. Waiting until the last minute will be an inconvenience to everyone, and could invoke unnecessary costs.

Figure 16-1 Stepwise Approach to Perioperative Cardiac Assessment for Coronary Artery Disease. The American College of Cardiology/American Heart Association (ACC /AHA) guideline calls for stepwise cardiac risk assessment involving consideration of the patient's cardiac risk factors, functional capacity, and the planned surgical procedure. If the surgery is an emergency, it should proceed and cardiac risk be mitigated with appropriate intraoperative monitoring and pharmacologic techniques. If surgery is non-emergent and an acute coronary syndrome (e.g., unstable angina) is identified, surgery should be delayed and the patient should receive appropriate medical treatment. In general, during preanesthetic evaluation, all patients should receive a cardiac risk assessment using a validated risk tool (RCRI or NSQIP risk calculator). If the risk of MACE is ≥1% and the patient's functional capacity is ≥4 METS, no further testing is indicated. If, however, the risk of MACE is ≥1% and the patient's functional capacity is < METS or unknown, pharmacological stress testing should be considered. If the result is abnormal, consideration may be given to PCI or CABG. Pharmacological stress testing is not advised for patients undergoing low risk surgery (MACE <1%). In addition, pharmacological stress testing should only be undertaken if it is expected to change management. An alternative to stress testing is guideline-directed medical therapy, e.g. beta blockers and statins. (Modified from Fleisher LA, Fleischmann KE, Auerbach AD, et al. 2014 ACC/AHA Guideline on Perioperative Cardiovascular Evaluation and Management of Patients Undergoing Noncardiac Surgery: A Report of the American College of Cardiology/American Heart Association Task Force on Practice Guidelines. *J Am CollCardiol*. 2014;():. doi:10.1016/j.jacc.2014.07.944. Available at http://content.onlinejacc.org/article.aspx?articleid=1893784. Page 30 of 105) ACS, acute coronary syndrome; CABG, coronary artery bypass graft; CAD, coronary artery disease; CPG, clinical practice guideline; GDMT, guideline-directed medical therapy; MACE, major adverse cardiac event; MET, metabolic equivalent; NSQIP, National Surgical Quality Improvement Program; PCI, percutaneous coronary intervention; RCRI, Revised Cardiac Risk Index.

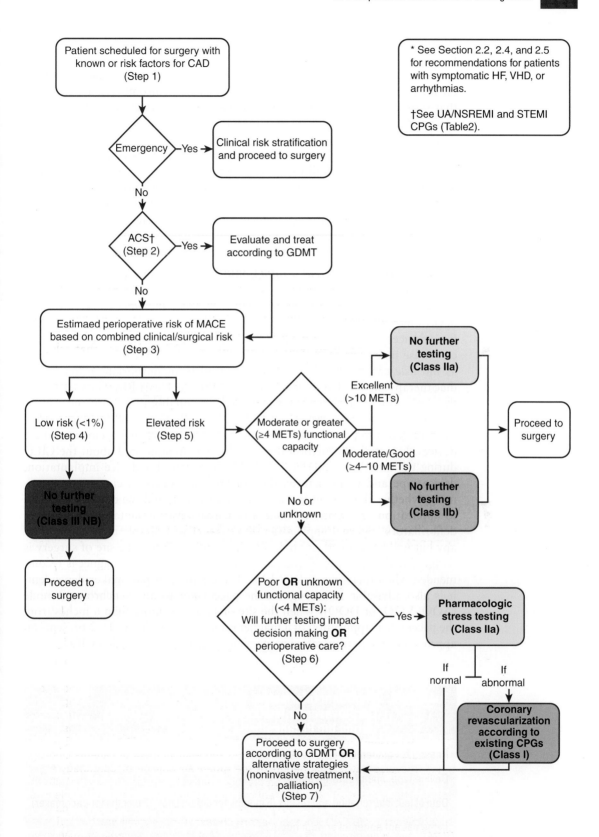

Perioperative Coronary Stents

Patients with indwelling coronary stents, especially those that have been inserted recently, present a treatment dilemma, as these patients are frequently on lifelong antiplatelet therapy to prevent in-stent thrombosis. Information that should be obtained during the preanesthetic interview includes the type of stent, time since placement, and input from the consulting cardiologist as to whether antiplatelet therapy can be discontinued in the perioperative period. Current recommendations from the American Heart Association/American College of Cardiology call for postponing elective surgery for a minimum of 4 weeks after placement of a bare-metal stent and 12 months after placement of a drug-eluting stent (Figure 16-2). However, recent evidence suggests the risk of adverse events after placement of a drug-eluting stent may stabilize after 6 months. Whenever possible, dual antiplatelet therapy, or at least aspirin, should be continued throughout the perioperative period.

Patients with Cardiovascular Implantable Electronic Devices

Patients with cardiovascular implantable electronic devices (CIEDs) are presenting for surgery with increasing frequency, as the indications for these devices increase and the population ages. *Electromagnetic interference* (EMI) from devices in the operating suite, most commonly monopolar electrocautery, can cause malfunction of these devices. Specifically, EMI may be interpreted as intrinsic cardiac activity and thereby lead to inappropriate antitachycardiac therapy (defibrillation or pacing). In 2011, the Heart Rhythm Society and the ASA published a consensus statement in collaboration with the American Heart Association, American College of Cardiology, and Society of Thoracic Surgeons to provide guidance on the perioperative management of these devices. Essential information that should be communicated about the CIED during the anesthetic interview includes the reason for device implantation, device type and manufacturer, date of last interrogation, current programming, whether the patient is pacemaker dependent, and the device's response to application of a magnet (Table 16-8). For most implantable cardioverter defibrillators, external application of a magnet will disable tachycardic therapy but will have no effect on pacemaker settings. When the site of surgery is within 6 inches (15 cm) of the pacemaker, application of a magnet is recommended when there is a risk of EMI. If the patient is pacemaker dependent, it is also advisable to reprogram the pacemaker to an asynchronous mode (AOO, VOO, or DOO). When the site of surgery is more than 6 inches from the pacemaker, application of a magnet is unnecessary. Figure 16-2 presents an approach to the perioperative management of the patient with a CIED.

Table 16-8	Important Information to be Determined about Cardiovascular Implantable Electronic Devices during the Preanesthetic Evaluation
Reason for placement	
Device type, manufacturer, model	
Date of last interrogation and results (6 months for defibrillator, 12 months for pacemaker)	
Is the patient pacemaker dependent?	
Device programming and response to magnet	

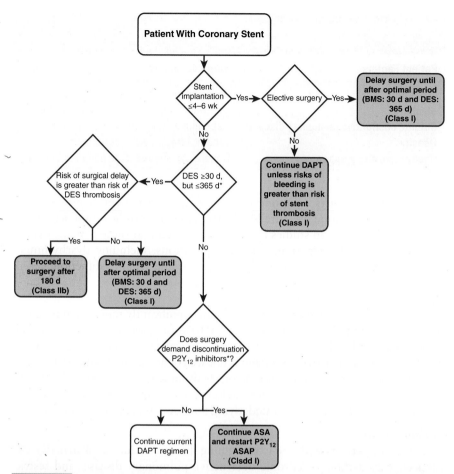

Figure 16-2 Proposed algorithm for antiplatelet management in patients with percutaneous coronary intervention and noncardiac surgery. Elective surgery should be delayed until 30 days after placement of a BMS and 365 days after placement of a DES. DAPT therapy should be continued in the perioperative period unless the risk of surgical bleeding outweighs the risk of stent thrombosis; at minimum, aspirin should be continued in the perioperative period. If $P2Y_{12}$-inhibitor therapy is discontinued, it should be reinitiated as soon as possible after surgery. In patients with a DES ≥30 days but ≤365 days post-implantation, consideration may be given to proceeding with surgery, if the risk of surgical delay is deemed greater than the risk of DES thrombosis. (Modified from Fleisher LA, Fleischmann KE, Auerbach AD, et al. 2014 ACC/AHA Guideline on Perioperative Cardiovascular Evaluation and Management of Patients Undergoing Noncardiac Surgery: A Report of the American College of Cardiology/American Heart Association Task Force on Practice Guidelines. *J Am CollCardiol.* 2014;():. doi:10.1016/j.jacc.2014.07.944. Available at http://content.onlinejacc.org/article.aspx?articleid=1893784. Page 52 0f 105) ASA, aspirin; ASAP, as soon as possible; BMS, bare-metal stent; DAPT, dual antiplatelet therapy; DES, drug-eluting stent; PCI, percutaneous intervention.

Hypertension

Induction of anesthesia results in sympathetic stimulation that manifests as a rise in blood pressure of about 20 to 30 mm Hg and heart rate of about 15 to 20 beats per minute. This response is exaggerated in patients with pre-existing hypertension, especially those who are untreated or poorly controlled with medications. Patients with undiagnosed hypertension are also more likely to exhibit intraoperative blood pressure lability. Whether to postpone elective surgery in patients with poorly controlled hypertension is controversial.

Table 16-9	Potential Risk Factors for Perioperative Pulmonary Complications	
Patient Factors	**Surgical Factors**
Older age	Incisions close to the diaphragm (e.g.,
Smoking	thoracic, upper abdominal procedures,
Chronic obstructive pulmonary disease	abdominal aortic aneurysm repair)
Obesity	Longer duration procedures
Obstructive sleep apnea	General (vs. neuraxial, regional) anesthesia

Some anesthesiologists postpone elective surgery in patients who exhibit a sustained systolic blood pressure of >200 mm Hg or diastolic blood pressure of >110 mm Hg, based on studies that have suggested that these patients experience a greater risk of perioperative complications, including dysrhythmias, myocardial ischemia, neurologic complications, and renal dysfunction.

B. Pulmonary Disease

Postoperative pulmonary complications occur significantly more often than cardiac complications in an estimated 5% to 10% of surgeries. The risk of their occurrence is related to both patient and surgical factors (Table 16-9). What constitutes a pulmonary complication is not well defined, but it is generally taken to mean any clinically significant pulmonary dysfunction that adversely affects a patient's clinical course. This includes atelectasis, pneumonia, prolonged mechanical ventilation, exacerbation of underlying lung disease, and bronchospasm.

Patient Factors

As expected, patients with pre-existing lung disease, including obstructive diseases such as asthma or chronic obstructive pulmonary disease, and restrictive diseases such as pulmonary fibrosis, have an increased risk of pulmonary complications compared with healthy adults. Evidence is conflicting as to the magnitude of this increased risk, and, in general, there is no level of pulmonary dysfunction for which elective surgery is contraindicated, so long as the patient is medically optimized.

Smoking

Tobacco and nicotine increase sputum production, reduce ciliary function, stimulate the cardiovascular system, and increase carboxyhemoglobin levels. Although smoking cessation for as little as 2 days decreases carboxyhemoglobin levels and improves mucociliary clearance, most studies suggest it takes at least 8 weeks of smoking cessation to reduce the rate of postoperative pulmonary complications.

Obstructive Sleep Apnea

OSA is a syndrome marked by periodic upper airway obstruction during sleep, which leads to oxygen desaturation and carbon dioxide retention, sleep deprivation, and daytime somnolence. The prevalence of OSA is estimated to be 9% in women and 24% in men, and most patients with the condition are undiagnosed. Patients with OSA are particularly susceptible to the respiratory depressant effects of inhaled anesthetics and opioids and, therefore are more likely to suffer critical respiratory events, including unplanned postoperative hypoxemia and tracheal reintubation. For this reason, screening for OSA is an important part of the preanesthetic examination. There are a

Table 16-10	Factors Associated with an Increased Risk of Obstructive Sleep Apnea

Historical Features
History of apparent obstruction during sleep
Observed pauses in breathing during sleep
Snoring
Awakens from sleep with a choking sensation
Daytime somnolence

Clinical Signs and Symptoms
Body mass index >25 kg/m^2
Neck circumference >17 inches (men) and >16 inches (women)
Craniofacial abnormalities affecting the airway
Anatomical nasal obstruction
Tonsils nearly touching midline

From Practice Guidelines for the Perioperative Management of Patients with Obstructive Sleep Apnea. American Society of Anesthesiologists. *Anesthesiology.* 2006;104:1081–1093.

number of screening tools used to evaluate for the presence of OSA, including the Berlin questionnaire, the STOP-Bang screening tool, and one published by the American Society of Anesthesiologists. Symptoms suggestive of OSA include a history of snoring, daytime sleepiness, and headaches. Physical signs include body mass index >25 kg/m^2, neck circumference >17 inches in men or >16 inches in women, and tonsillar hyperplasia (Table 16-10). Potential consequences of OSA include difficult airway management, systemic and pulmonary hypertension, cardiac dysrhythmias, and coronary artery disease. Preoperative use of continuous positive airway pressure or noninvasive positive pressure ventilation may improve the patient's preoperative condition and reduce perioperative complications. Postoperatively, these patients may require monitoring in a setting with continuous pulse oximetry. If outpatient surgery is planned, discharge should be delayed until postoperative respiratory function has returned to baseline. When possible, it is useful to minimize the use of opioids in favor of nonnarcotic analgesics.

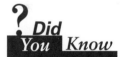

? Did You Know

A women who is 5 ft tall and weighs 200lb has a BMI = (200/2.2)/(60/39.4)2 = 39.2 kg/m^2

Surgical Factors
The site of surgery is the most important factor related to the risk of developing pulmonary complications postoperatively. Patients having thoracic and upper abdominal surgeries are far more likely to suffer pulmonary complications relative to those having lower abdominal or extremity procedures. Abdominal aortic aneurysm repair, head and neck surgery, and neurosurgical procedures are also associated with a higher risk of pulmonary complications relative to other surgeries. This is related mostly to effects on the muscles of the upper airway, accessory respiratory muscles, and diaphragmatic function. Duration of surgery is also important, with longer procedures leading to a higher risk of complications. Relative to neuraxial or regional anesthesia, general anesthesia is associated with a higher rate of clinically significant pulmonary complications.

C. Endocrine Disease
Diabetes Mellitus
Diabetes is the most common endocrinopathy, affecting nearly 10% of the population. Patients with diabetes have an accelerated rate of atherosclerosis and are susceptible to microvascular complications that manifest as

retinopathy, neuropathy, cerebrovascular, peripheral vascular, and kidney disease. Autonomic neuropathy may predispose those with diabetes to intraoperative hemodynamic instability. Gastroparesis makes the risk of pulmonary aspiration relatively more likely. Poorly controlled diabetic patients are also at greater risk of developing postoperative infections.

A number of factors, including preoperative fasting and the surgical stress response, result in large swings in blood glucose levels perioperatively, which make tight glucose control extremely challenging. Overly aggressive glycemic control introduces the risk of life-threatening hypoglycemia, which can go unrecognized under anesthesia. Therefore, in general, guidelines recommend a perioperative glycemic target between 140 and 180 mg/dL. Regarding preoperative management of oral hypoglycemics and insulin regimens, recommendations vary by institution. Table 16-5 presents a suggested approach.

Thyroid and Parathyroid Disorders

Both hypothyroidism and hyperthyroidism have important anesthetic implications; therefore, screening for these conditions should be conducted during the preanesthetic interview. Hypothyroidism is more common in women; signs and symptoms include bradycardia, cold intolerance, hypoventilation, and hyponatremia. Hyperthyroidism is marked by tachycardia, tremor, weight loss, and heat intolerance. Patients may also exhibit dysrhythmias such as atrial fibrillation. In symptomatic patients, it may be prudent to delay elective surgery. In addition, thyroid masses may cause distortion of upper airway anatomy. A computed tomography scan of the neck is often useful to evaluate the upper airway and identify signs of tracheal deviation or compression.

Hyperparathyroidism is a fairly common condition that increases in incidence with age. Symptoms include weight loss, polydipsia, hypertension, heart block, lethargy, bone pain, kidney stones, and constipation. In patients with suspected hyperparathyroidism, preoperative determination of serum calcium concentration is prudent.

Adrenal Disorders

Pheochromocytoma, though rare, should be considered in any patient who relates a history of refractory hypertension, often combined with headache and intermittent tachycardia. In these patients, preoperative pharmacologic preparation (alpha-blockers followed by beta-blockers) as well as appropriate volume loading is important to reduce intraoperative hemodynamic instability. Use of invasive cardiovascular monitoring may be indicated.

Adrenal suppression should be considered in any patient who has taken steroids chronically in a dose equivalent to prednisone ≥5 mg/day for at least 1 month within 6 to 12 months of surgery. Regimens for steroid supplementation perioperatively vary by institution. For minor surgeries, supplementation is rarely needed. For major procedures, one option is to administer 100 mg of hydrocortisone intravenously prior to induction of anesthesia, then 50 mg intravenously every 8 hours for 24 hours.

Other Organ Systems and Conditions

Patients with *rheumatoid arthritis (RA)* have a higher risk of cardiovascular disease compared with the general population. In addition, they are prone to cervical joint instability, which must be taken into consideration during intubation. Patients are often maintained on long-term glucocorticoid therapy and may require supplementation perioperatively. Biologic agents used to treat

RA may adversely affect the immune response and may predispose patients to perioperative infectious complications and poor wound healing. However, stopping these medications prior to surgery increases the likelihood of RA flares. Patients with significant osteoarthritis or osteoporosis should be positioned with care, as should patients with indwelling artificial joints.

Various neurologic conditions have implications for anesthesia and surgery. For patients with a history of seizures, antiepileptic medications should be continued in the perioperative period and drug levels should be carefully monitored, as surgery and no food by mouth status may affect drug absorption and metabolism. Patients with Parkinson's disease have an increased risk of orthostatic hypotension, aspiration, and postoperative pulmonary complications. Drugs used to treat Parkinson's disease should be continued perioperatively in an attempt to reduce symptom exacerbation. Patients with a history of stroke are at increased risk of perioperative stroke. Patients with spinal injury and denervation, such as quadriplegia, are at risk for hyperkalemia and cardiac arrest if given succinylcholine.

Clinical features suggestive of liver disease include a history of heavy alcohol use, hepatitis, illicit drug use, or sexual promiscuity. Signs on examination include increased abdominal girth, spider telangiectasias, jaundice, gynecomastia, and splenomegaly. Signs of renal disease may be difficult to identify on examination but include hypertension, edema, and lethargy. Of note, patients who are dialysis dependent should ideally be dialyzed as soon prior to surgery as feasible (usually the day before surgery) to optimize preoperative fluid and electrolyte status.

III. Perioperative Laboratory Testing

There is no benefit to "routine" preanesthetic laboratory testing in patients presenting for elective surgery. Furthermore, this approach is extremely inefficient. Routine preoperative testing has been estimated to cost $3 billion per year. Owing to the intrinsic characteristic of screening tests, especially when a panel of tests is ordered, there is a high likelihood that one result will return as abnormal. However, in a person with no risk factors, this result is more likely to be a false positive than a true positive. The ASA "Statement on Routine Preoperative Laboratory and Diagnostic Screening" (2008) supports this view.

Nevertheless, selective preanesthetic laboratory testing is appropriate for some patients, based on their medical conditions, symptomatology elicited on interview, and the nature of the planned surgery. Table 16-11 summarizes the general principles of preoperative laboratory testing in patients undergoing elective noncardiac surgery.

IV. Preparation for Anesthesia

A. Fasting Guidelines

Preoperative fasting is the mainstay of preparation for anesthesia and is designed mainly for minimizing the risk of pulmonary aspiration of gastric contents. Pulmonary aspiration is estimated to occur in 1 in 3,000 to 1 in 6,000 elective anesthetics, but up to 1 in 600 emergency anesthetics. Risk factors for aspiration include emergency surgery, obesity, difficult airway, reflux, hiatal hernia, and inadequate anesthesia. The ASA has developed the "Practice Guidelines for Preoperative Fasting and Pharmacologic Intervention for Prevention of Perioperative Aspiration" (Table 16-12). These guidelines advise that clear liquids should be stopped at least 2 hours prior to surgery, breast

Table 16-11	General Principles on Preoperative Testing in Adults Undergoing Elective Noncardiac Surgery
Factor	**Comment**
ASA physical status	ASA PS 1 patients generally do not require preoperative testing before low or intermediate risk surgeries
Pregnancy testing	Should be carried out in female patients of reproductive age unless patient has had hysterectomy or is confirmed to be postmenopausal
Pulmonary function testing	Is performed prior to lung resection and most cardiac surgeries. May be indicated if patient has significant pulmonary morbidity (e.g., morbid obesity, chronic lung disease, unexplained dyspnea)
Chest x-ray	Only indicated for patients with a history of significant lung or cardiac disease, malignancy, or radiation to the chest. No need to repeat if one has been completed within 12 months, results were within normal limits, and there has been no change in clinical status.
Serum chemistries, complete blood count, coagulation profile	No need to repeat within 1 month if results are within normal limits, there has been no change in clinical status, and the patient is not on an anticoagulant or antiplatelet agent (e.g., warfarin, clopidogrel)
Cataract surgery, endoscopy procedures, other low-risk surgeries	Blood tests, ECG, chest x-ray are generally not indicated unless the patient's clinical history or physical examination warrants specific cause for concern

ASA, American Society of Anesthesiologists; PS, physical status; ECG, electrocardiogram.

milk at least 4 hours, and nonhuman milk and solids at least 6 hours before surgery. Examples of clear liquids include water, tea, black coffee, and fruit juices without pulp. Fried or fatty foods should be stopped at least 8 hours prior to surgery, as these require longer gastric emptying times.

B. **Pharmacologic Agents to Reduce the Risk of Pulmonary Aspiration**
Routine use of drugs to prevent pulmonary aspiration is not advised, but they are effective when used in patients with risk factors for pulmonary

Table 16-12	Summary of Fasting Guidelines as Prophylaxis for Pulmonary Aspiration
Ingested Substance	**Minimum Fasting Period (hours)**
Clear liquids (water, carbonated beverages, tea, black coffee)	2
Breast milk	4
Infant formula	6
Nonhuman milk	6
Light meal (toast, clear liquids)	6
Heavy meal (fatty foods)	8

From ASA Practice Guidelines for Preoperative Fasting and the Use of Pharmacologic Agents to Reduce the Risk of Pulmonary Aspiration: Application to Healthy Patients Undergoing Elective Procedures. *Anesthesiology.* 2011;114:495–511.

Table 16-13	Drugs Used to Reduce the Risk of Pulmonary Aspiration		
Drug	**Onset**	**Effect**	**Comment**
Antacids (e.g., sodium citrate, aluminum or magnesium hydroxide, calcium carbonate)	15–30 min	Raise gastric pH	Nonparticulate antacids (sodium citrate) do not cause pulmonary damage if aspirated, in contrast to particulate antacids (calcium carbonate, aluminum hydroxide)
Histamine-2 receptor antagonists (e.g., ranitidine, famotidine)	60 min	Reduce gastric volume Increase gastric pH	
Proton pump inhibitors (e.g., omeprazole, pantoprazole)	30 min	Reduce gastric acid secretion Reduce gastric volume	Block proton pump on gastric parietal cells
Prokinetic agents (e.g., metoclopramide)	15–30 min	Increase gastric motility Increase gastroesophageal sphincter tone	Useful for patients with known or suspected large gastric volume or delayed gastric emptying, such as obese patients, parturients, and diabetics Contraindicated in patients with a known bowel obstruction and should be used with caution in the elderly, because they are more likely to experience side effects such as confusion and drowsiness

aspiration. Several agents with varying mechanisms of action are available (Table 16-13).

V. Preoperative Medication

A number of medications may be used prior to anesthetic induction to help reduce the patient's anxiety about anesthesia, improve conditions for intubation, reduce complications such as nausea and vomiting, and improve postoperative pain control.

A. Benzodiazepines

In many cases, patient education and informed consent conducted during the preanesthetic interview replaces the need for pharmacologic anxiolysis prior to anesthetic induction. However, benzodiazepines are useful for producing moderate sedation and reducing anxiety, as well as providing some degree of anterograde amnesia. Midazolam is commonly used, owing to its rapid onset of action (1 to 2 minutes) and relatively short half-life (1 to 4 hours). It can be administered orally as a fluid or in a "lollipop" sponge as well as intravenously.

B. Antihistamines

Diphenhydramine is a histamine-1 antagonist that has sedative, antiemetic, and anticholinergic properties. Although still used in some conscious sedation protocols, it is rarely used as premedication, owing to its long half-life (3 to 6 hours), which tends to prolong recovery times. Diphenhydramine, along with a histamine-2 antagonist and steroids, may be given to patients with a history of latex allergy, chronic atopy, or patients undergoing procedures requiring administration of radiocontrast dye as prophylaxis against allergic reactions.

C. Antisialogogues

It is often helpful to administer an anticholingeric agent to reduce upper airway secretions when a fiberoptic-assisted tracheal intubation is expected. Glycopyrrolate is a potent antisialagogue and produces less tachycardia compared to scopolamine or atropine. In addition, glycopyrrolate does not cross the blood–brain barrier; therefore, it does not have central nervous system side effects.

D. Antiemetics

The prophylactic administration of antiemetic agents is not a cost-effective strategy. However, selective premedication of patients with a history of postoperative nausea and vomiting (PONV) and those with risk factors for PONV (females, history of motion sickness, those undergoing gynecologic, ophthalmologic, or cosmetic procedures) may be of benefit. Agents used for this purpose include serotonin antagonists such as ondansetron, phenothiazines such as perphenazine, butyrophenones such as droperidol, and antihistamines such as dimenhydrinate. These drugs are best administered just prior to the end of surgery for optimal onset of action. The exception is scopolamine, an anticholinergic drug with antiemetic properties. It is routinely applied as a transdermal patch prior to induction, and it is especially useful in patients with a history of motion sickness.

E. Pre-emptive Analgesia

Pre-emptive analgesia involves the administration of analgesics prior to an expected noxious stimulus. It is becoming more widely appreciated that this strategy may not only help improve postoperative pain control but also prevent central sensitization that is responsible for the development of chronic pain syndromes. Examples of pre-emptive analgesia include the use of neuraxial techniques (with or without concomitant use of general anesthesia), infiltration with local anesthetics, and the administration of intravenous agents such as ketamine or opioids. Gabapentin or pregabalin may also be administered orally for this purpose.

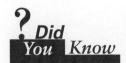

VI. Antibiotic Prophylaxis

Antibiotics are administered prior to surgical procedures in order to prevent surgical site infections (SSI), which occur in 2% to 5% of surgical patients. Documentation of the administration of antibiotic prophylaxis is a commonly used process measure by which anesthesia departments and hospitals are evaluated (e.g., Surgical Care Improvement Program, Joint Commission). Surgical wounds are classified into four categories based on the degree of expected microbial contamination: clean, clean-contaminated, contaminated, and dirty. Although there is a moderate correlation between wound classification and SSI risk, other factors are also important. These include length of surgery, health status of the patient, and operative technique.

The microbial flora associated with SSIs vary based on surgical procedure and have also changed over time. For clean wounds, SSIs are usually caused by gram-positive skin flora such as *Staphylococcus aureus, Staphylococcus epidermidis,* and streptococcal species. For clean-contaminated wounds, gram-negative organisms are more commonly involved. In recent years, the proportion of SSIs caused by gram-negative bacteria has decreased. *S. aureus* is currently the most common cause of SSIs, accounting for about 30% of SSIs. Methicillin-resistant *S. aureus* (MRSA) species are isolated from about half of these cases. In addition, fungi such as *Candida albicans* have been isolated from SSIs with growing frequency.

Cefazolin, a first-generation cephalosporin, is the most commonly used antibiotic for prophylaxis against SSIs. It has coverage against gram-positive cocci (except *Enterococcus*) as well as many gram-negative organisms such as *Escherichia coli, Proteus,* and *Klebsiella.* For most adults, an initial dose of 2 g is advised; 3 g is recommended for patients weighing ≥120 kg, and weight-based dosing is used for pediatric patients. Clindamycin or vancomycin is recommended in patients with a true immunoglobulin-E mediated β-lactam antibiotic allergy. For patients known to be colonized with MRSA, a single dose of vancomycin may also be added preoperatively, as cefazolin does not cover MRSA. Antibiotic infusions should be administered within 1 hour of incision, with the exception of vancomycin and fluoroquinolones, which may be administered within 2 hours of incision. Infusions should be completed prior to incision and prior to the inflation of surgical tourniquets. Intraoperative redosing of antibiotics is recommended at intervals of approximately 2 drug half-lives. Redosing is also recommended in surgeries where blood loss is excessive (>1,500 mL) and when duration of drug half-life is shortened, such as through drug-drug interaction or in the setting of extensive burns. In general, antibiotics initiated solely for the purpose of prophylaxis against SSI need only be given intraoperatively; they should certainly be discontinued within 24 hours of surgery. There is no need to continue antibiotic prophylaxis based on the presence of indwelling catheters or surgical drains.

Colonization with *S. aureus,* which usually occurs in the nose, occurs in about 25% of the population and is a risk factor for SSI. For this reason, preoperative screening and eradication of *S. aureus* has been recommended as a means to reduce the rate of SSI, especially in high-risk groups such as cardiac and orthopedic surgery patients. Mupirocin is an intranasal ointment used to treat MRSA colonization. When used preoperatively, it is generally administered 5 days prior to surgery. Although some studies have suggested that its use is potentially beneficial, its widespread application is controversial, in part because of concerns over the development of antimicrobial resistance.

Suggested Readings

American Society of Anesthesiologists: New classification of physical status. *Anesthesiology.* 1963;24:111.

American Society of Anesthesiologists Task Force on Preanesthesia Evaluation. Practice advisory for preanesthesia evaluation. An updated report by the ASA task Force on preanesthesia evaluation. *Anesthesiology.* 2012;116:1.

Benarroch-Gampel J, Sheffield KM, Duncan CB, et al. Preoperative laboratory testing in patients undergoing elective, low-risk ambulatory surgery. *Ann Surg.* 2012;256:518.

Fleisher LA, Fleischmann KE, Auerbach AD, et al. 2014 ACC/AHA Guideline on Perioperative Cardiovascular Evaluation and Management of Patients Undergoing Noncardiac Surgery: A Report of the American College of Cardiology/American Heart Association Task Force on Practice Guidelines. *J Am CollCardiol.* 2014;64(22):2373. doi:10.1016/j.jacc.2014.07.944.

Mallampati RS, Gatt SP, Gugino LD, et al. A clinical sign to predict difficult tracheal intubation. A prospective study. *Can Anaesth Soc J.* 1985;32:429.

Practice guidelines for preoperative fasting and the use of pharmacologic agents to reduce the risk of pulmonary aspiration: application to healthy patients undergoing elective procedures. American Society of Anesthesiologists. *Anesthesiology.* 2011;114:495.

Practice guidelines for the perioperative management of patients with obstructive sleep apnea. American Society of Anesthesiologists. *Anesthesiology.* 2014;120:268–286.

Qaseem A, Snow V, Fitterman N, et al. Risk assessment for and strategies to reduce perioperative pulmonary complications for patients undergoing noncardiothoracic surgery: A guideline from the American College of Physicians. *Ann Intern Med.* 2006;14:575.

Sebranek JJ, Kopp Lugli A, Coursin DB. Glycaemic control in the perioperative period. *Br J Anaesth.* 2013;111:18.

Stone ME. Salter B. Fischer A. Perioperative management of patients with cardiac implantable electronic devices. *Br J Anaesth.* 2011;107(Suppl 1):i16.

Questions

1. A 79-year-old man is scheduled for a transurethral prostatectomy. His only limitation for moderate exercise is an arthritic shoulder. His only current symptoms are those related to prostatic hypertrophy. Past medical history includes glaucoma and hypertension. Medications include aspirin 70 mg/day, timolol eye drops every day, and lisinopril 10 mg every day. An electrocardiogram 8 months ago showed sinus bradycardia. Heart rate 60, blood pressure 150/90, weight 200 lb, hemoglobin 14 g/dL. According to the ASA classification system, he would be classified as physical status:
   A. I
   B. II
   C. III
   D. IV

2. Which of the following classes of drugs must be discontinued prior to elective surgery?
   A. Monoamine oxidase inhibitors (e.g., phenelzine)
   B. Beta-blockers (e.g., metoprolol)
   C. α_2 adrenergic agonists (e.g., clonidine)
   D. None of the above

3. Discontinuation of daily aspirin therapy (80 mg) is most appropriate prior to which of the following surgical procedures?
   A. Laparoscopic cholecystectomy
   B. Craniotomy for resection of a meningioma
   C. Simple mastectomy
   D. Vaginal hysterectomy

4. A patient who has been abusing opioids for many years is scheduled for elective total knee replacement. All of the following are appropriate for use in the perioperative period EXCEPT:
   A. Spinal anesthesia
   B. Continuous epidural anesthesia
   C. General anesthesia followed by patient-controlled opioid analgesia
   D. Avoidance of all opioids

5. When examining the patient preoperatively, all of the following are good predictors of a potentially difficult oral tracheal intubation EXCEPT:
   A. With the patient's mouth open and the tongue protruded, the soft palate can be seen, but not the uvula
   B. Body weight in excess of 300 lb
   C. A thyromental distance of 5 cm with the next extended
   D. Limited neck extension

6. When evaluating a patient preoperatively for noncardiac surgery, which of the following is considered a major risk factor for cardiovascular complications in the perioperative period?
   A. Insulin dependent diabetes mellitus
   B. Angina at rest
   C. Morbid obesity
   D. A blood pressure >180/110 mm Hg

7. A patient has a cardiac pacemaker implanted on the left anterior chest. Which of the following would place the patient at greatest risk for malfunction of the pacemaker?
   A. Use of a nerve stimulator to assist with placement of a right axillary block
   B. Use of bipolar cautery during a craniotomy
   C. Use of monopolar cautery for excision of a lipoma from the upper back
   D. Use of monopolar cautery for transurethral resection of the prostate

8. It is recommended that the perioperative blood glucose level of diabetic patients be maintained in what range?
   A. 70–100 mg/dL
   B. 100–140 mg/dL
   C. 140–180 mg/dL
   D. 180–200 mg/dL

9. Perioperative concerns for the patient with severe rheumatoid arthritis include all of the following EXCEPT:
A. Predisposition to malignant hyperthermia
B. Suppressed adrenal cortical response to stress
C. Cervical spine instability during airway manipulation
D. Higher than normal risk of cardiovascular disease

10. Recommendations for perioperative administration of cefazolin include all of the following EXCEPT:
A. Administer only to patients undergoing intra-abdominal procedures
B. Administer by intravenous infusion within 1 hour prior to surgical incision
C. Repeat administration during surgery at intervals approximating 2 half-lives of the drug
D. Dosing need not be continued postoperatively as prophylaxis against infection when intravascular catheters or surgical site drains are in place

17 Coexisting Diseases Impacting Anesthetic Management

Gerardo Rodriguez

Many conditions impact anesthetic management. Some are rare and are unlikely to be encountered during an anesthesiologist's career. It is essential to always investigate thoroughly how to properly manage a rare disorder. When encountering a patient with an uncommon condition, it is advisable to review sources detailing each topic.

I. Duchenne Muscular Dystrophy

Duchenne muscular dystrophy is an X-linked disorder leading to a loss of functional dystrophin, a protein integral to muscle membrane cytoskeleton stability. It presents in childhood and is characterized by proximal muscle weakness and painless muscle atrophy in boys. Serum creatine kinase levels are used for screening in newborns and assessment of muscle degeneration. Patients succumb to cardiopulmonary complications by middle age.

Cardiomyopathy and rhythm disorders are common. Surveillance with electrocardiography and echocardiography, and treatment with angiotensin-converting enzyme inhibitors and beta-blockers are routine. Dysrhythmias should be periodically assessed with Holter monitoring.

Recurrent pneumonia occurs due to poor cough effort and inadequate secretion clearance. Derangements in gastric motility result in delayed gastric emptying.

A. Management of Anesthesia

Gastric dysmotility increases the risk of aspiration. Succinylcholine is contraindicated due to risk of hyperkalemia and rhabdomyolysis. Prolonged muscle relaxation may occur with nondepolarizing agents. Potent volatile anesthetics should be used with caution, since exposure may trigger rhabdomyolysis and cardiac complications. Postoperative ventilatory support may be needed especially if there is poor preoperative pulmonary function (1).

? Did You Know

In Duchenne muscular dystrophy, succinylcholine is contraindicated due to risk of hyperkalemia and rhabdomyolysis.

II. The Myotonias

Myotonic dystrophy is an autosomal dominant disorder caused by gene mutations that lead to RNA toxicity, ion channel dysfunction, and myotonias, or impaired skeletal muscle relaxation. Progressive muscle wasting with weakness combined with multisystem involvement characterizes this disorder. Myotonic dystrophy is divided into two chief genetic entities. Myotonic dystrophy type 1 (DM1), the predominant major type, is subdivided into congenital, child, and adult onset. Myotonic dystrophy type 2 is rare, with a highly variable, late adult onset presentation.

Adult onset DM1, the most common subtype, is characterized by muscle weakness, myotonias, and cataracts. Facial, neck, and distal limb weakness progress to muscle wasting, immobility, and bulbar palsies. Respiratory dysfunction is compounded by aspiration and respiratory muscle weakness.

Functional and anatomical brain dysfunction is manifested by cognitive dysfunction and diffuse white matter atrophy. Systolic and diastolic cardiac failure are complicated by conduction defects, such as atrioventricular conduction blocks and tachyarrhythmias. *Sudden cardiac death* due to dysrhythmias is common. Gastrointestinal signs include constipation and diarrhea. Impaired endocrine function results in hypothyroidism and insulin resistance. Treatment is primarily supportive.

A. Management of Anesthesia

Cardiopulmonary abnormalities, muscle weakness, and clinical myotonia are the primary causes of perioperative risk in adult onset DM1, regardless of anesthetic technique. Sedatives should be used with caution due to potential exaggerated response to their respiratory depression side effects. Succinylcholine should be avoided due to its potential to trigger a severe myotonic muscle contraction. Both nondepolarizing and reversal agents may exacerbate muscle weakness and should be avoided. Respiratory insufficiency can occur. Transcutaneous pacing pads should be considered.

There is potential for prolonged labor, postpartum hemorrhage, and congenital myotonic dystrophy of the neonate.

III. Familial Periodic Paralysis

Channelopathies are a heterogenous group of defects in ion channel function that result in a spectrum of anomalies. Familial periodic paralysis is a subgroup of inherited defects comprising hyperkalemic and hypokalemic periodic paralysis.

A. Hyperkalemic Periodic Paralysis

Hyperkalemic periodic paralysis is an autosomal-dominant inherited disease characterized by episodes of hyperkalemia-related muscle weakness and myotonia. The episodes are triggered by transient hyperkalemia from exercise, fasting, or consumption of potassium-rich foods.

B. Hypokalemic Periodic Paralysis

Hypokalemic periodic paralysis, the most common periodic paralysis disease, is an autosomal-dominant disease characterized by recurrent episodes of hypokalemia-related flaccid paralysis, lasting hours to days. Respiratory insufficiency and cardiac arrhythmias can occur during acute attacks. Chronic proximal myopathy is a common outcome in many cases.

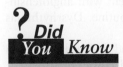

Did You Know

Hypokalemic periodic paralysis is the most common periodic paralysis disease, characterized by recurrent episodes of hypokalemia-related flaccid paralysis, which can last hours to days.

C. Management of Anesthesia

Potassium homeostasis is the goal of perioperative management. Electrolyte levels should be monitored and corrected with an emphasis on avoiding metabolic states or medications that may alter serum potassium levels, either directly or indirectly. Nondepolarizing muscle relaxants are best avoided due to unpredictable patient sensitivities. Succinylcholine should be avoided, because it may cause transient hyperkalemia (2).

IV. Myasthenia Gravis

Myasthenia gravis (MG) is a neuromuscular autoimmune disease characterized by skeletal muscle weakness worsened by exertion and improved with rest. Extraocular muscles are affected primarily, with less frequent impact on limb and respiratory muscles strength.

The etiology is a decrease in the number of functional postsynaptic, acetylcholine receptors (AChR) in the neuromuscular junction available for acetylcholine binding. Direct antibody receptor blockade, increased antibody-mediated receptor turnover, and postsynaptic membrane complement–mediated injury can contribute to AChR decline. Abnormal thymus tissue is frequently involved.

Signs include ptosis, blurred vision, diplopia, dysphagia, dysarthria, and generalized limb weakness. *Myasthenic crisis* is a progression to severe muscle weakness and respiratory failure, usually requiring ventilatory support. Cardiac abnormalities include bundle branch blocks, atrial fibrillation, and focal myocarditis.

Transient neonatal myasthenia is known to occur in newborns of women with active MG, with feeding problems and respiratory distress immediately postpartum. Edrophonium testing is used to diagnosis MG with high sensitivity. Serologic testing, tomographic imaging, and electrophysiological testing comprise a comprehensive MG workup. Treatment is aimed at both symptom management and immunomodulation.

Acetylcholinesterase inhibitors, such as pyridostigmine, minimize MG symptoms by increasing the acetylcholine available at neuromuscular junction sites. Excessive drug administration can result in severe cholinergic side effects, or *cholinergic crisis*, characterized by hypersalivation, abdominal cramping, bradycardia, and weakness. Plasmapheresis and intravenous immunoglobulin can provide short-term relief. Chronic therapy includes steroids and nonsteroidal immunosuppressants. *Thymectomy* is recommended for MG patients with thymomas (3).

A. Myasthenic Syndrome (Lambert-Eaton Syndrome)

Lambert-Eaton myasthenic syndrome (LEMS) is an autoimmune, neuromuscular disorder of transmission mediated by antibodies to voltage-gated calcium channels at the presynaptic, motor nerve terminal, resulting in acetylcholine release reduction. It is characterized by proximal limb weakness, autonomic dysfunction such as dry mouth, and diminished deep tendon reflexes. In contrast to MG, exercise in LEMS might suddenly improve symptoms. LEMS is a paraneoplastic condition, often associated with small cell lung cancer. Increasing presynaptic, neurotransmitter release with 3,4-diaminopyridine is considered the mainstay of treatment.

V. Guillain-Barre Syndrome (Polyradiculoneuritis)

Guillain-Barre syndrome (GBS) is an autoimmune disorder characterized by the acute or subacute onset of ascending skeletal muscle weakness or paralysis of the legs occurring in the context of a viral or bacterial infection. This inflammatory, multifocal demyelinating disease usually produces varying

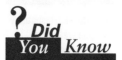
? Did You Know
Myasthenia gravis is caused by a decrease in the number of functional postsynaptic, acetylcholine receptors in the neuromuscular junction available for acetylcholine binding.

? Did You Know
The newborn of a mother with myasthenia gravis can suffer from a condition known as transient neonatal myasthenia, which may present with feeding problems and respiratory distress at birth.

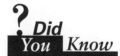
? Did You Know
The Lambert-Eaton myasthenic syndrome is associated with small cell lung cancer and, in contrast to myasthenia gravis, exercise might improve the muscle weakness-related symptoms.

degrees of autonomic dysfunction. Respiratory muscle weakness is common during severe cases of GBS. Treatment is primarily supportive (4).

A. Management of Anesthesia

Multifocal demyelination and muscle disuse atrophy in GBS prohibit the use of succinylcholine due to the risk of life-threatening hyperkalemia. Expected muscle relaxation from nondepolarizing agents may be highly variable and unpredictable and should be avoided. Autonomic nervous system lability is common, which can result in hyperdynamic and hypodynamic responses to stimuli or transient preload changes, respectively; therefore, hemodynamic support should be judicious.

VI. Central Nervous System Diseases

A. Multiple Sclerosis

Multiple sclerosis (MS) is an inflammatory multifocal demyelinating disorder caused by autoimmune neurodegenerative changes leading to progressively irreversible neurologic deficits. The clinical course is characterized by subacute, relapsing–remitting changes that correlate to activated T-cell blood–brain barrier penetration with subsequent multifocal gray and white matter demyelination and edema (Fig. 17-1).

MS has a peak incidence at age 20 to 40 years. Signs and symptoms can be vague or specific, usually determined by the neurologic site focally affected.

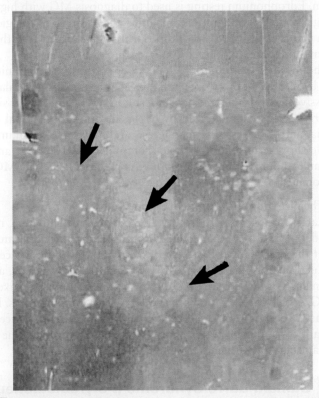

Figure 17-1 The subcortical white matter of a patient with multiple sclerosis showing multiple, small, irregular, partially confluent areas of demyelination (*arrows*). Normal intact myelin stains blue in this Luxol fast blue–stained section. (From Rubin R, Strayer DS, Rubin E. *Rubin's Pathology.* 6th ed. Philadelphia: Wolters Kluwer Health/Lippincott Williams & Wilkins, 2011, with permission.)

Symptoms include headache, fatigue, and depression. Sensory symptoms such as numbness and paresthesias are common. Partial paralysis of the lower limbs is a common motor symptom that usually correlates to anterior column spinal cord lesions. Visual loss, diplopia, nystagmus, and papillary abnormalities reflect cranial nerve involvement. Diagnosis is based on history and clinical examination with reliance on magnetic resonance imaging to characterize demyelinating, often clinically silent, focal lesions. Cerebral spinal fluid may demonstrate intrathecal immunoglobulin production.

Management strategies are evolving to target acute relapse and symptomatic control. Corticosteroids can hasten acute clinical recovery. Plasma exchange removes harmful antibodies to treat relapses. Interferon-beta and glatiramer acetate block antigen presentation to minimize relapsing–remitting events. Mitoxantrone, an antineoplastic agent, reduces lymphocyte counts to delay progression to secondary degenerative phase. Symptomatic management is usually determined by the diffuse nature of MS. Severe fatigue is common and should be treated promptly with central nervous system stimulants, such as amantadine. Routine depression screening and early treatment are important given the propensity to affect quality of life in this disease. Spasticity treatment requires both physical therapy and antispasticity medications. Intrathecal baclofen pump implantation is reserved for severe cases. Pain is usually due to varied factors, such as neuropathic pain, indirect pain from MS, and treatment-related pain. As a result, pain management is multimodal, potentially involving antiepileptics, tricyclic antidepressants, nonsteroidal anti-inflammatory drugs (NSAIDs), and antispastic agents.

> **? Did You Know**
>
> In multiple sclerosis, pain is caused by a variety of mechanisms; therefore, the best treatment is using multimodal analgesia.

B. Epilepsy

Epilepsy is a disorder characterized by sudden, unprovoked, and recurrent seizures. A seizure is a neurologic symptom characterized by a transient attack of rhythmic electroneuronal discharges, resulting in altered consciousness and disturbances in brain function. Seizures can be provoked by factors such as metabolic derangements, or unprovoked, by intrinsic brain disease.

Epilepsies and seizures are mostly clinical diagnoses with reliance on history, physical examination, laboratory testing, electroencephalography, and neuroimaging. Investigating the paroxysmal event, triggers, and recurrence potential helps exclude or confirm the diagnosis.

Epilepsies are broadly divided into *focal* and *generalized*. In focal epilepsies, usually localized pathologic conditions, such as brain tumors, lead to focal cortical discharges that can generalize and recruit other cortical regions. In generalized epilepsies, diffuse cortical discharges develop, affecting the cortex and bilaterally. *Grand mal seizure* is the most recognized type of generalized epilepsy. It is characterized by a loss of consciousness followed by several minutes of a *tonic phase* of body stiffening, followed by a *clonic phase* of repetitive contractions, and ending in a prolonged *postictal phase* of lethargy and return of consciousness. During the tonic phase, breath-holding, incontinence, tongue biting, tremors, and sinus tachycardia may occur. Trauma, aspiration pneumonia, and arrhythmias may also occur during these seizures. Benzodiazepines or propofol can be used to terminate seizure activity. Ventilatory support may be needed. *Status epilepticus* is a potentially fatal convulsive disorder marked by serial tonic–clonic phases occurring without return of consciousness. Untreated, hyperpyrexia, hypoxia, and shock can develop acutely. Multiple precipitating risk factors exist, including brain tumor and drug intoxication. Treatment goals should be supportive care, seizure termination, and prevention. Endotracheal intubation should be performed for airway protection. Intravenous phenytoin can be used for seizure recurrence prophylaxis. Refractory seizures may require benzodiazepine or propofol infusion; general anesthesia may even be necessary (5).

C. Alzheimer's Disease

Dementia is an irreversible, chronic, neurodegenerative disease marked by a constant decline in cognitive function, affecting memory, behavior, and executive function that, over time, degrades daily activities and social interaction. *Alzheimer's disease (AD)* is the most common cause of dementia. Senile plaques and neurofibrillary tangles are the hallmarks of AD. Acetylcholinesterase inhibitors (AChEIs) are considered the first line of pharmacotherapy to treat the central cholinergic deficiency-related cognitive decline in AD. Side effects from cholinergic stimulation during AChEI therapy include hypotension, bradycardia, and bronchoconstriction. Drug interactions with AChEI and muscle relaxants may result in prolonged paralysis with succinylcholine and resistance to muscle relaxation with *N*-methyl-D-aspartates (6).

D. Parkinson's Disease

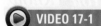

VIDEO 17-1

Parkinson's Disease

Parkinson's disease (PD) is a neurodegenerative movement disorder marked by an acetylcholine–dopamine imbalance caused by loss of dopamine-producing cells within the substantia nigra. It is a clinical diagnosis confirmed by motor and nonmotor features in the absence of a pertinent drug history. Common motor features of PD are "pill-rolling" tremors at rest, rigidity, bradykinesia, postural instability, flexed posture, or incapacity to move. Nonmotor features include cognitive impairment, neuropsychiatric disorders, sensory disturbances, sleep disorders, and autonomic dysfunction.

Medical management is determined by factors such as age of onset, symptom fluctuations, dopamine responsiveness, and end-stage disease. *Levodopa* remains the most effective form of oral therapy for motor symptoms. It is highly metabolized and can cause nausea and hypotension. Long-term levodopa use can result in confusion, dyskinesia, and poor symptom relief. Hepatic metabolism and peripheral side effects are commonly reduced by combining levodopa with carbidopa, a *decarboxylase inhibitor*. Pramipexole, ropinirole, and bromocriptine are *dopamine agonists* used when levodopa response decreases. Side effects include hallucinations and confusion. Selegiline and rasagiline are *monoamine oxidase-B inhibitors* used to augment dopamine concentrations. *Deep brain stimulation* via implanted generator electrodes is a surgical treatment option.

VIDEO 17-2

Parkinson's Disease and Deep Brain Stimulation

VII. Inherited Disorders

A. Malignant Hyperthermia

VIDEO 17-3

Malignant Hyperthermia

Malignant hyperthermia (MH) is an autosomal dominant, hypermetabolic disorder triggered by halogenated volatile anesthetics and succinylcholine. The principal diagnostic features of MH are unexplained hypercapnia, tachycardia, muscle rigidity, acidosis, hyperthermia, and hyperkalemia. The disorder is variable in its presentation. A ryanodine receptor (RYR) gene mutation is the etiology in the majority of cases. Precipitation of MH in genetically susceptible patients occurs when the RYR, a type of calcium channel located in the sarcoplasmic reticulum membrane, is activated during an exposure to a triggering agent, resulting in a tremendous release of intracellular calcium within skeletal muscle.

Detection and treatment are critical for survival. If MH is suspected, triggering agents should be discontinued immediately. Dantrolene should be administered intravenously, with an initial dose of 2.5 mg/kg, with repeat dosing as needed. MH can be lethal if untreated. Rhabdomyolysis and hyperkalemia should be managed with volume resuscitation and diuresis. Cooling should be instituted immediately with monitoring for coagulopathy. Ventilatory support should be maintained until the patient is stabilized. Once stabilized, the Malignant Hyperthermia Association of the United States hotline should be contacted. Recurrence of MH is possible and patients should be monitored for up to 72 hours.

The in vitro contracture test is used to analyze the presence of muscle fiber contraction during halothane and caffeine exposure. It is the standard for diagnosis of MH susceptibility. Genetic testing may be pursued with appropriate counseling for patients about the implications of testing results. MH-susceptible patients planning to undergo surgery should have a thoroughly purged anesthesia machine available for use, whether or not the patient is to receive a general anesthetic. Triggering agents should be avoided. Total intravenous general anesthesia should be considered if regional anesthesia is not possible (7).

B. Porphyria

Porphyrias are a group of enzyme deficiencies that result in heme and P450 cytochrome biosynthesis impairment and a concomitant accumulation of harmful metabolites. *Acute intermittent porphyria (AIP)* is among the most severe of the porphyrias. It is a deficiency in porphobilinogen deaminase that leads to nonspecific neuropsychiatric and abdominal complaints. Symptoms include severe abdominal pain, vomiting, seizures, tachycardia, and generalized weakness. Triggers include infection, fasting, ethanol, and medications, including barbiturates, etomidate, and phenytoin. Treatment of symptoms entails the discontinuation of triggers and infusion of hemin. Liver transplantation is reserved for AIP patients with severe, recurrent attacks (Fig. 17-2).

C. Cholinesterase Disorders

Pseudo-cholinesterase (PChE) deficiency is an inherited or acquired disorder that results in an inability to efficiently metabolize specific ester substrates. Prolonged paralysis after an anesthetic procedure using succinylcholine usually reveals this deficiency. Delayed metabolism is also seen with use of

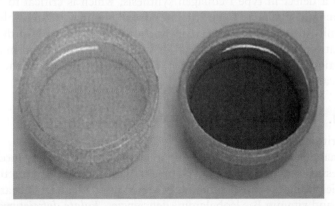

Figure 17-2 Urine from a patient with porphyria cutanea tarda (*right*) and from a patient with normal porphyrin excretion (*left*). (From Champe PC, Harvey RA, Ferrier DR. *Biochemistry.* 4th ed. Philadelphia: Wolters Kluwer Health/Lippincott Williams & Wilkins, 2008, with permission.)

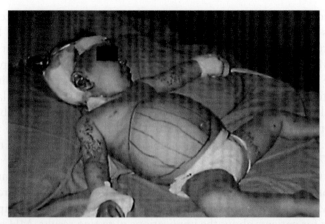

Figure 17-3 A 25-month-old child with von Gierke disease. Note the hepatomegaly and eruptive xanthomas on the arms and legs. The child is in the third percentile for height and weight, indicating a failure to thrive. (From Lieberman MA, Ricer R. *Lippincott's Illustrated Q&A Review of Biochemistry*. Philadelphia: Wolters Kluwer Health/Lippincott Williams & Wilkins, 2010, with permission.)

mivacurium, cocaine, chloroprocaine, procaine, and tetracaine. Deficiency of this hepatic esterase can be due to PChE gene mutations or systemic disease, such as severe liver disease, renal failure, carcinomas, and severe malnutrition. PChE activity and dibucaine inhibition testing can be used to identify individuals at high risk for prolonged paralysis following succinylcholine administration.

D. Glycogen Storage Diseases
Glycogen storage diseases (GSD) are a rare group of inherited disorders of glycogen production and metabolism that result in excess glycogen storage. Hypoglycemia, metabolic ketoacidosis, and infiltrative organ dysfunction are common among most types of GSD. There are numerous types of GSD, each with a unique set of characteristics based on factors such as enzyme mutation and clinical features (Fig. 17-3, Table 17-1).

E. Osteogenesis Imperfecta
Osteogenesis imperfecta (OI) is an inherited connective tissue disorder that produces a defect in type I collagen synthesis, which is critical to bone and tissue strength. Pediatric bone fractures from minimal trauma, blue sclera, and a family history of OI are usually adequate for diagnosis. Cardiovascular manifestations of OI include arterial dissections and aortic and mitral valve regurgitation. Several types of OI exist, classified by type, inheritance pattern, and clinical features.

VIII. Anemias

A. Nutritional Deficiency Anemias
Nutritional deficiency anemias are due to an insufficiency of any food component necessary for growth and development, with complex vitamin B and iron deficiencies being the most common. Megaloblastic anemia is a characteristic of folate and vitamin B_{12} (cobalamin) deficiencies. *Folate deficiency* is associated with malnutrition, chronic alcohol abuse, and medications that interfere with folate metabolism. Clinically evident *cobalamin deficiency* presents with signs of demyelinating disease. Features include peripheral neuropathy with

Table 17-1	Types of Glycogen Storage Diseases	
Type	**Enzyme Mutation**	**Clinical Features**
Type I (von Gierke disease)	Glucose-6-phosphatase deficiency	Hypoglycemia, acidosis, and seizures
Type II (Pompe disease)	Lysosomal acid glucosidase deficiency	Infantile; cardiac infiltrative cardiomyopathy
Type III (Forbes or Cori disease)	Glycogen debranching enzyme deficiency	Hepatomegaly, muscle weakness, and cardiomyopathy
Type IV (Andersen disease)	Branching enzyme deficiency	Hepatosplenomegaly, cirrhosis, cardiomyopathy, hypotonia, and failure to thrive
Type V (McArdle disease)	Muscle glycogen phosphorylase deficiency	Rhabdomyolysis and myoglobinuria after exercise or succinylcholine
Type VI (Hers disease)	Hepatic phosphorylase deficiency	Benign; mild hypoglycemia, hepatomegaly
Type VII (Tarui disease)	Muscle phosphofructokinase deficiency	Muscle cramps, exercise intolerance, and episodic myoglobinuria
Type IX	Hepatic glycogen phosphorylase kinase deficiency	Hypotonia, short stature, and exertional myoglobinuria
Type XI (Fanconi-Bickel syndrome)	Glucose transporter enzyme deficiency	Hepatomegaly, fasting hypoglycemia, short stature, and proximal renal tubular acidosis
Type 0	Hepatic glycogen synthase deficiency	Severe fasting ketotic hypoglycemia, short stature, seizures, and severe developmental delay

lower extremity loss of proprioception and vibratory sensation. Clinically evident cobalamin deficiency is most often due to *pernicious anemia*, an autoimmune loss of intrinsic factor from gastric parietal cells needed for cobalamin binding. Nitrous oxide exposure can interfere with cobalamin metabolism in susceptible patients. *Iron deficiency* leads to a microcytic, hypochromic anemia, associated with poor iron intake, impaired iron absorption, chronic blood loss, or systemic inflammation. Treatment for all three nutritional deficiency anemias entails supplementation and reversal of contributing causes.

B. Hemolytic Anemias

Hemolytic anemias are any inherited or acquired anemias caused by hemolysis of red blood cells (RBCs). The common presenting features of all hemolytic anemias are jaundice, splenomegaly, increased reticulocyte count, and hyperbilirubinemia. *Hereditary spherocytosis* is an inherited disorder characterized by fragile, spherical RBCs that are prone to rupture during transit and spleen sequestration. Another manifestation is cholelithiasis. Treatment recommendations include splenectomy, antipneumococcal vaccination presplenectomy, and prophylactic cholecystectomy.

Immune hemolytic anemias can be caused by autoimmunity, alloimmunity, and drug reactions. *Autoimmune hemolytic anemias (AIHA)* can be caused primarily, usually idiopathic, or secondarily, which is divided into warm and cold agglutinin diseases. Warm AIHA can be caused by leukemias, lymphomas, scleroderma, and rheumatoid arthritis. Cold AIHA can be triggered by infections and cold temperature exposure. *Drug-induced immune hemolysis anemias* can be subdivided into type II and type III hypersensitivity reactions. Penicillin and α-methyldopa can result in a type II reaction, where the drug binds to RBCs, triggering antibody-mediated destruction. Drugs known to potentially trigger a type III immune complex reaction include cephalosporins, hydrochlorothiazides, isoniazid, and tetracycline. Hemolytic disease of the newborn, or Rh incompatibility, is the most recognized example of an *alloimmunity hemolytic disease.*

C. Glucose-6-phosphate Dehydrogenase Deficiency

Glucose-6-phosphate dehydrogenase (G6PD) is an ubiquitous, X-linked maintenance enzyme present in RBCs and other cell types, which is essential to the pentose phosphate pathway that generates nicotinamide adenine dinucleotide phosphate for oxidative stress resistance. An acute, nonimmune hemolytic anemia reaction to ordinary infections, medications, or fava bean ingestion may be the presenting sign of G6PD deficiency. Aminoester local anesthetics and nitroprusside may trigger *methemoglobinemia* in patients with G6PD deficiency.

D. Hemoglobinopathies

Hemoglobinopathies are a group of predominantly genetic RBC diseases caused by aberrant hemoglobin production. Sickle cell disease and thalassemia are the most clinically relevant hemoglobinopathies. *Sickle cell disease (SCD)* is caused by an autosomal recessive β-globin gene defect that leads to structurally abnormal hemoglobin, called hemoglobin-S (HbS). RBCs affected with HbS have a propensity for "sickling" and for premature destruction. SCD produces acute and chronic multisystem complications. Acute, painful, and life-threatening attacks of SCD, called *sickle cell crisis*, can occur spontaneously or be triggered by systemic stressors, such as dehydration, hypoxia, and infections.

Manifestations of sickle cell crisis include vaso-occlusive crisis, acute chest syndrome, splenic sequestration crisis, and aplastic crisis. Sickled RBCs clump together to obstruct capillaries and cause painful tissue ischemia and infarction, called a *vaso-occlusive crisis.* This is the most common complication of SCD. Treatment consists of intravenous opioids, fluid replacement, and blood transfusion. Acute chest syndrome is a life-threatening manifestation of SCD, where pulmonary inflammation or infection triggers localized pulmonary infarctions that progress to death without appropriate supportive therapy. Clinical signs include acute dyspnea, chest pain, cough, and hypoxia. Aggressive fluid therapy, intravenous opioids, and exchange transfusion should be instituted promptly. Severe hypoxia may require ventilatory support. *Splenic sequestration crisis* is an acute splenic enlargement from sequestered abnormal RBCs, resulting in severe abdominal pain, anemia, and hypotension. Treatment is mainly supportive with fluid therapy and blood transfusion. Parvovirus B19 infection, a predominantly pediatric disease, can trigger an *aplastic crisis* in adults with SCD, characterized by profound depression of erythropoiesis resulting in life-threatening anemia.

Prophylactic treatment in SCD with oral penicillin, pneumococcal vaccination, and hydroxyurea is intended to reduce infections and recurrence of sickle cell crises.

Thalassemia is a diverse group of autosomal recessive disorders caused by insufficient α- or β-globin synthesis. The β-thalassemias in order of clinical severity include thalassemia major, thalassemia intermedia, and thalassemia minor. *Thalassemia major* usually presents by early childhood with anemia and failure to thrive. In time, young adult survivors go on to develop severe anemia, hypertrophic facial and long bone deformities, and secondary multi-organ dysfunction from severe transfusion-related hemochromatosis. Cardiac siderosis can lead to congestive heart failure and arrhythmias. Extensive endocrine dysfunction can present as hypopituitarism, hypothyroidism, hypoparathyroidism, diabetes, and adrenal insufficiency. Infections are common due to secondary immunodeficiency of hemochromatosis, blood-borne infections, and splenomegaly. Primary treatment includes periodic blood transfusions and iron chelating therapy.

IX. Collagen Vascular Diseases

A. Rheumatoid Arthritis

Rheumatoid arthritis (RA) is a chronic, autoimmune disease marked by systemic inflammation that primarily affects peripheral synovial joints, leading to symmetric painful arthritis. Eventual joint deformity, cartilage erosion, and ankylosing, or joint stiffening, develop in patients. *Atlantoaxial subluxation* is a common occult radiographic finding. Clinical signs of prolonged joint involvement, synovial fluid analysis, imaging, the presence of RA serology markers, such as rheumatoid factor, and nonspecific inflammatory markers, such as erythrocyte sedimentation rate and C-reactive protein, support the diagnosis. Extra-articular involvement is common and unpredictable. Chronic inflammation likely contributes to accelerated atherosclerotic disease, myocarditis, pericarditis, and valvulopathies. Ischemic heart disease is the most common cause of death. Rheumatoid lung disease can manifest as pleurisy, pulmonary nodules, interstitial lung disease, and pulmonary hypertension. Rheumatoid vasculitis can cause widespread organ injury, specifically renal failure and ischemic stroke.

Therapeutics for RA are broadly divided into NSAIDs, corticosteroids, disease-modifying antirheumatic drugs (DMARDs), and biologic DMARDs. *Prednisone* is used during flare-ups or until DMARD therapy is optimized. Despite the risks of long-term corticosteroid use, many RA patients remain on chronic prednisone therapy. *Methotrexate* is the mainstay drug of DMARD therapy. Drug-induced interstitial lung disease is a known risk of methotrexate in RA therapy. Other DMARDs include leflunomide, hydroxychloroquine, and sulfasalazine. Biologic DMARDs are intended to target cell surface molecules and cytokines to block the inflammation cascade. Infection and hypersensitivity reactions are the most serious complications associated with DMARD therapy (8).

B. Systemic Lupus Erythematosus

Systemic lupus erythematosus (SLE) is an autoimmune disorder in which immune complexes formed by autoantibodies and soluble antigens, also known as *type III hypersensitivity*, deposit in various organs, producing inflammation and tissue injury. Clinical features of SLE and detection of antinuclear antibody most often confirm diagnosis.

The presenting time course and symptoms are variable. Myalgias and fatigue are common symptoms. A photosensitive "butterfly rash" over the malar eminence is characteristic of SLE. Most patients experience mild to severely debilitating polyarthritis. Lupus glomerulonephritis, if untreated, can lead to end-stage renal disease and death. Pericarditis and pleuritis are common manifestations of SLE. Vascular occlusive disease may present with Raynaud's phenomenon, acute ischemic stroke, or myocardial infarction.

Current treatment options have reduced morbidity and mortality. Corticosteroids and hydroxychloroquine are first-line therapies for acute flare-ups. Inflammation, chronic pain, and arthralgias are usually controlled with NSAIDs. Potent immunosuppressive agents, such as cyclophosphamide or mycophenolate, are used to treat severe glomerulonephritis.

C. Systemic Sclerosis

Systemic sclerosis (SSc), or scleroderma, is a rare autoimmune disorder marked by destructive, multisystem microvasculopathy, and organ fibrosis. Skin thickening is the most obvious physical sign, whereas Raynaud's phenomenon is usually the presenting sign associated with scleroderma. Traditionally, the presence of CREST syndrome (*C*alcinosis, *R*aynaud's phenomenon, *E*sophageal dysmotility, *S*clerodactyly, *T*elangiectasia) has been used for diagnosis. Quality-of-life optimization, organ injury prevention, and delay of disease progression are the focuses of treatment. Painful ischemic digits are treated with calcium channel blockers, stress management, and cold temperature avoidance. Active skin disease can be treated with immunosuppressants, such as mycophenolate or cyclophosphamide. Corticosteroids for skin disease should be avoided, because they can lead to a scleroderma renal crisis, manifested by acute hypertension and oliguric renal failure. The most common problem in scleroderma is gastrointestinal dysfunction. Dysphagia, esophageal dysmotility, esophageal strictures, gastroesophageal reflux, and delayed gastric emptying are treated with proton pump inhibitors and prokinetics. Myocarditis and conduction abnormalities are usually silent. Calcium channel blockers and other vasodilators may be used to preserve cardiac function. Lung disease is the primary cause of death in scleroderma.

D. Inflammatory Myopathies

Inflammatory myopathies are a rare group of muscle disorders typified by muscle inflammation and weakness. *Dermatomyositis (DM)* and *polymyositis (PM)* are the predominant subtypes of inflammatory myopathies. Both conditions are considered autoimmune disorders, with an acute to subacute presentation usually after a systemic infection. Presenting features of PM include muscle pain and weakness that typically affects muscles of the proximal limbs, posterior neck, pharynx, and larynx. Ocular muscles are spared. DM has a similar presentation, except that onset can be more severe with additional dermal features: heliotropic eyelid discoloration, periorbital edema, and erythematous scaly rash involving the face and the extensor surface of limbs. Muscle necrosis and inflammatory cells on muscle tissue biopsy confirms diagnosis. Complications of both PM and DM include cardiomyopathy, respiratory insufficiency, dysphagia, and aspiration pneumonia.

X. Skin Disorders

A. Epidermolysis Bullosa

Epidermolysis bullosa (EB) is a group of rare, acquired, and inherited skin disorders that result in epidermal fragility due to abnormalities in basement membrane integrity within skin and mucosa. Shear stress across skin can result in epidermal layer detachment and painful, bullae formation. Multiorgan dysfunction, such as cardiomyopathy, may develop depending on EB subtype. Esophageal strictures can be disabling, leading to malnutrition and dysphagia.

Patients with EB are at risk for secondary bacterial infection and squamous cell carcinoma (9).

B. Pemphigus Vulgaris

Pemphigus vulgaris (PV) is an autoimmune skin disorder that results in keratinocytes adhesion loss due to antibodies directed at desmoglein-1 and -3. The disorder is characterized by painful, epidermal blistering that develops immediately after minimal skin rubbing. This hypersensitivity reaction can be triggered by many medications, such as angiotensin-converting enzyme inhibitors, nifedipine, and penicillin. Painful, oral lesions are common. Corticosteroids are effective therapy for PV.

References

1. Segura LG, Lorenz JD, Weingarten TN, et al. Anesthesia and Duchenne or Becker muscular dystrophy: Review of 117 anesthetic exposures. *Paediatr Anaesth.* 2013;23(9):855–864.
2. Bandschapp O, Iaizzo PA. Pathophysiologic and anesthetic considerations for patients with myotonia congenita or periodic paralyses. *Paediatr Anaesth.* 2013;23(9):824–833.
3. Blichfeldt-Lauridsen L, Hansen BD. Anesthesia and myasthenia gravis. *Acta Anaesthesiol Scand.* 2012;56(1):17–22.
4. Turakhia P, Barrick B, Berman J. Pre-operative management of the patient with chronic disease: Patients with neuromuscular disorder. *Med Clin North Am.* 2013;97(6):1015–1032.
5. Shorvon S. The historical evolution of, and the paradigms shifts in, the therapy of convulsive status epilepticus over the past 150 years. *Epilepsia.* 2013;54(6):64–67.
6. Seitz DP, Shah PS, Herrmann N, et al. Exposure to general anesthesia and risk of Alzheimer's disease: A systematic review and meta-analysis. *BMC Geriatr.* 2011;11:83.
7. Stowell KM. DNA testing for malignant hyperthermia: The reality and the dream. *Anesth Analg.* 2014;118(2):397–406.
8. Samanta R, Shoukrey K, Griffiths R. Rheumatoid arthritis and anaesthesia. *Anaesthesia.* 2011;66(12):1146–1159.
9. Nandi R, Howard R. Anesthesia and epidermolysis bullosa. *Dermatol Clin.* 2010;28(2):319–324.

Questions

1. Which of the following is a common finding in patients with Duchenne muscular dystrophy?
   A. Distal muscle atrophy
   B. Resistance to succinylcholine
   C. Cardiomyopathy
   D. Gastric hypermotility

2. A 30-year-old full-term parturient with myasthenia gravis presents for an elective cesarean section. Which of the following conditions may occur in the immediate postpartum period?
   A. Respiratory distress
   B. Weakness with tensilon testing
   C. Hypersalivation
   D. Seizure

3. A 16-year-old male with a family history of malignant hyperthermia is undergoing an inguinal hernia repair. The patient inadvertently receives succinylcholine during general anesthesia. Which of the following is the most appropriate management?
   A. Administer dantrolene immediately
   B. Terminate the surgery
   C. Monitor for hypermetabolism
   D. Institute therapeutic hypothermia

4. Which of the following drugs is prolonged in pseudocholinesterase deficiency?
   A. Lidocaine
   B. Bupivicaine
   C. Ropivicaine
   D. Tetracaine

5. A 20-year-old male with sickle cell disease develops acute chest pain and cough 1 hour after a splenectomy. Which of the following is the most appropriate initial management?
   A. Computed tomography pulmonary angiogram
   B. Aggressive fluid therapy
   C. NSAIDs
   D. Heparin

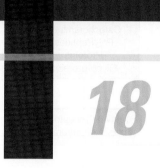

18 *Endocrine Function*

Shamsuddin Akhtar

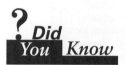

I. Integrated Physiology

Hormones play an essential role in maintaining homeostasis (1–4). Hormones are divided chemically either into steroids or nonsteroids. Steroid hormones are lipophilic and able to cross the cell membrane to act directly on cytoplasmic pathways (Fig. 18-1). They are transported in the plasma bound to specific globulins, albumin, and other plasma proteins and have longer half-lives (hours to even days).

Nonsteroid hormones include catecholamines, peptides, proteins, or glycoproteins. They are hydrophilic and thus unable to cross the cell membrane and require specific cell membrane receptors to exert their effect. These hormones are typically not bound to plasma proteins, have fast onset of actions (minutes), have shorter half-lives (minutes), and are metabolized quickly. Some hormones are secreted continuously, whereas others are secreted in a pulsatile manner (cortisol).

II. Hypothalamus–Pituitary Complex

In conjunction with the hypothalamus, the *pituitary gland* is considered a master endocrine gland. Input from various regions of the brain is relayed to specific nuclei in the hypothalamus, which secretes specific releasing factors or hormones that regulate pituitary function (4). The pituitary gland is composed of two parts: the anterior and posterior pituitary.

A. Anterior Pituitary

The anterior pituitary is responsible for producing six hormones that subsequently affect thyroid, adrenal cortex, gonads, and mammary glands. The production and release of anterior pituitary hormones is controlled by *releasing hormones* (e.g., thyroid-stimulating releasing hormone), which are produced by the hypothalamus. The anterior pituitary hormones are then released into the systemic circulation and exert their effects on their target organs (Fig. 18-2).

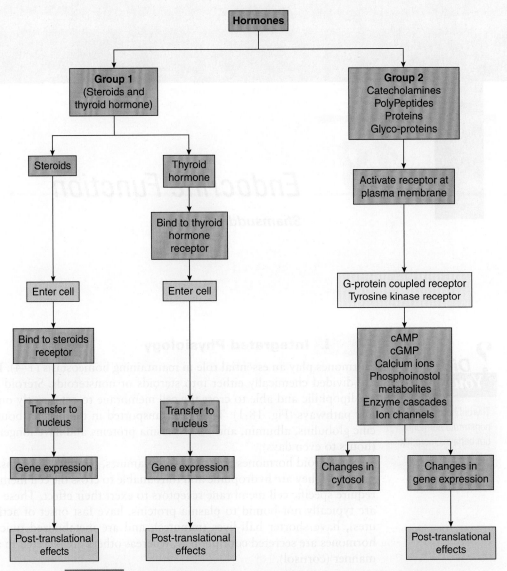

Figure 18-1 Integrated physiology of steroid and nonsteroid hormones.

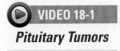

VIDEO 18-1

Pituitary Tumors

In addition, excessive secretion of growth hormone (GH), usually from a pituitary adenoma, results in acromegaly. Acromegaly occurs after excess GH is produced *before* epiphyseal closure. In the setting of excess GH, gigantism occurs *after* epiphyseal closure. Acromegaly is seen much more frequently (Table 18-1).

B. Posterior Pituitary
Posterior pituitary gland is an extension of the hypothalamus. It produces two hormones: *oxytocin* and *vasopressin* (*antidiuretic hormone*, ADH) (Fig. 18-2) (1).

Diabetes Insipidus
Deficiency of vasopressin (*central diabetes insipidus [DI]*) or resistance to its effect (nephrogenic DI) causes an inability to absorb water in the renal tubules

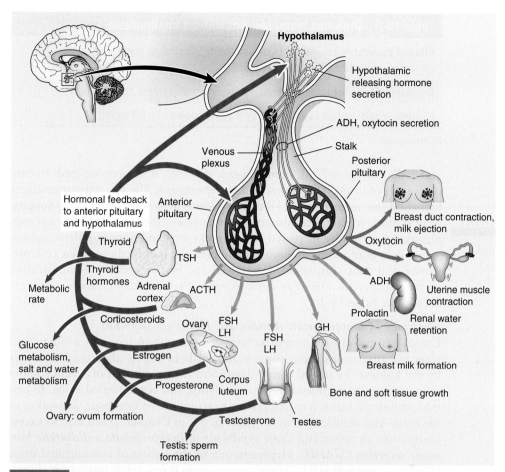

Figure 18-2 Hypothalamus, pituitary gland, and endocrine target organs. (This chapter will focus on hypothalamus, pituitary gland, and the target organs thyroid gland, adrenal gland, parathyroid gland, and the pancreas. For additional information regarding other target endocrine organs, the reader is referred to reference 4.) (From Turbow SD, Patterson BC. Hypothalamic and pituitary disorders. In: Felner EI, Umpierrez GF, eds. *Endocrine Pathophysiology*. Philadelphia: Wolters Kluwer Health/Lippincott Williams & Wilkins; 2014:17, with permission.)

Table 18-1   Anesthetic Problems Associated with Acromegaly
Hypertrophy of skeletal, connective, and soft tissues
Enlarged tongue and epiglottis (upper airway obstruction)
Increased incidence of difficult intubation
Thickening of the vocal cords (hoarseness; consider awake tracheal intubation)
Paralysis of the recurrent laryngeal nerve (stretching)
Dyspnea or stridor (subglottic narrowing)
Peripheral nerve or artery entrapment
Hypertension
Diabetes mellitus

From Endocrine function. In: Barash PG, Cullen BF, Stoelting RK, eds., et al. *Handbook of Clinical Anesthesia*. 7th ed. Philadelphia: Wolters Kluwer/Lippincott Williams & Wilkins; 2013.

Table 18-2	Diabetes Insipidus: Anesthesia Implications

Clinical picture: Hypovolemia, hyperosmolality, electrolyte disturbances, hypotension, and cardiac dysrhythmias

Treatment: Fluids (hypotonic saline), electrolyte replacement as indicated

Pharmacologic: vasopressin 0.1–0.2 U/hr IV, desmopressin 0.3 mg/kg IV

IV, intravenous.

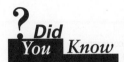

? Did You Know

Certain medications cause nephrogenic diabetes insipidus (e.g., lithium).

and collecting ducts (2,3). In *neurogenic diabetes*, desmopressin leads to concentration of urine. This is not seen in *nephrogenic* DI. The patient produces liters of dilute urine per day. DI can develop acutely after intracranial surgery, head trauma, intracranial tumors, and infections. If the water loss is not supplemented, either by increased water intake or exogenous supplementation, severe dehydration, hyperosmolality, hypernatremia, cardiovascular collapse, stupor, and coma can result. Central DI can be managed by administration of the vasopressin analogue desmopressin. Perioperative considerations are detailed in Table 18-2.

Syndrome of Inappropriate Antidiuretic Hormone Secretion

Excess vasopressin (or inappropriate vasopressin) secretion is a ubiquitous response after trauma and surgery and leads to excess absorption of water by the kidneys. Increased water absorption causes dilution of serum sodium (hyponatremia), decreased serum osmolality, and concentrated urine. In certain pathologic states (i.e., congestive heart failure or cirrhosis), activation of the renin–angiotensin system (2) (see Fig. 5-7 in Chapter 5) can lead to excess vasopressin secretion and cause *syndrome of inappropriate antidiuretic hormone secretion (SIADH)*. Hyponatremia in the setting of concentrated urine strongly suggests SIADH. Typical management is free water restriction, diuretics, and control of any precipitating condition. Severe hyponatremia, levels <115 to 120 mEq/L, is a medical emergency. It causes mental status changes and may require hypertonic saline for correction. Perioperative considerations are detailed in Table 18-3.

? Did You Know

The thyroid gland secretes three hormones: thyroxine (T_4), triiodothyronine (T_3), and calcitonin (involved in calcium homeostasis).

III. Thyroid Gland

The thyroid gland is one of the largest endocrine glands. *Thyroxine (T_4)* and *triiodothyronine (T_3)* are under tight control of thyroid-stimulating hormone (TSH) from the pituitary gland (Fig. 18-3) (3).

A. Thyroid Hormone Metabolism

Tyrosine and iodine are needed to form T_4 and T_3 (Fig. 18-3). Absorbed iodine is converted to iodide and transported and concentrated in thyrocytes.

Table 18-3	Syndrome of Inappropriate Antidiuretic Hormone Secretion: Anesthesia Implications

Clinical picture: Hyponatremia, increased urinary sodium and osmolarity. Serum sodium <115 mEq/L leads to seizures.

Treatment: Restrict IV fluids, diuresis, use normal or hypertonic saline and correct serum Na^+ concentrations slowly (<12 mEq/24 hr).

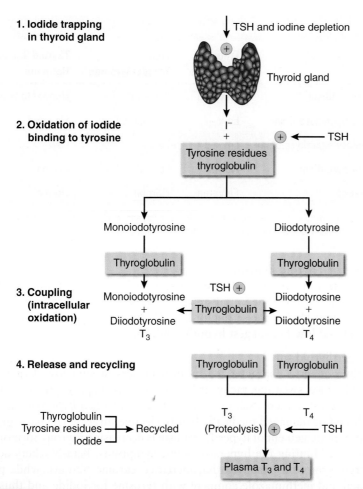

1. Iodide trapping in thyroid gland

TSH and iodine depletion

(+)

Thyroid gland

2. Oxidation of iodide binding to tyrosine

I⁻
+   (+) ← TSH

Tyrosine residues thyroglobulin

Monoiodotyrosine   Diiodotyrosine

Thyroglobulin   Thyroglobulin

3. Coupling (intracellular oxidation)

Monoiodotyrosine   TSH (+)   Diiodotyrosine
+   ← Thyroglobulin →   +
Diiodotyrosine   Diiodotyrosine
T_3 T_4

4. Release and recycling

Thyroglobulin   Thyroglobulin

Thyroglobulin ⎫
Tyrosine residues ⎬ → Recycled
Iodide ⎭

T_3 T_4
(Proteolysis) (+) ← TSH

Plasma T_3 and T_4

Figure 18-3 Thyroid hormone biosynthesis consists of four stages: (1) organification, (2) binding, (3) coupling, and (4) release. TSH, thyroid-stimulating hormone; T_3, triiodothyronine; T_4, thyroxine. (From Schwartz JJ, Akhtar S, Rosenbaum SH. Endocrine function. In: Barash PG, Cullen BF, Stoelting RK, et al., eds. *Clinical Anesthesia*. 7th ed. Philadelphia: Wolters Kluwer Health/Lippincott Williams & Wilkins; 2013:1327, with permission.)

Tyrosine, which is attached to thyroglobulin, is then iodinated by a complex process to yield T_3 and T_4 (Fig. 18-3). T_4 is converted in the peripheral tissues to T_3. T_4 feeds back to the pituitary and hypothalamus and decreases the secretion of TSH, which then leads to a decrease in T_4. T_4 and T_3 are lipophilic and are 99.8% bound to albumin, thyroxine-binding globulin, and prealbumin. It is the free hormone that exerts a biologic effect. T_4 and T_3 are metabolized in the liver, kidney, and many other tissues. Glucocorticoids, dopamine, somatostatin, and stress decrease TSH secretion.

B. Physiologic Effects of Thyroid Hormone

T_3 and T_4 increase oxygen consumption of target organs. Thyroid hormones increase carbohydrate, fat, and protein metabolism and are essential for normal growth. They increase cardiac output by increasing heart rate and myocardial contraction and enhance the effect of circulatory catecholamines. Thyroid hormones have marked effects on brain and enhance catecholamine effect on the reticular activating system.

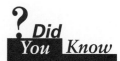

? *Did* *You* *Know*

Twenty times more T_4 is produced by the thyroid gland than T_3. However, T_3 is the more active form and produces the preponderance of clinical effects.

Table 18-4 Tests of Thyroid Function	Free Thyroxine	Free Triiodothyronine	Thyroid Stimulating Hormone
Hyperthyroidism	Elevated	Elevated	Normal to Low
Primary hypothyroidism	Low	Normal to Low	Elevated
Secondary hypothyroidism	Low	Low	Low
Sick euthyroidism	Normal	Low	Normal
Pregnancy	Elevated	Normal	Normal

From Endocrine function. In: Barash PG, Cullen BF, Stoelting RK, eds., et al. *Handbook of Clinical Anesthesia*. 7th ed. Philadelphia: Wolters Kluwer/Lippincott Williams & Wilkins; 2013.

C. Tests of Thyroid Function

Abnormalities in thyroid function are seen in both thyroid and nonthyroid diseases (Table 18-4). The initial step is to measure TSH and free T_4 (fT_4) (3). Extremely low TSH in the setting of high fT_4 suggests hyperthyroidism, while high TSH and low fT_4 suggest hypothyroidism.

D. Hyperthyroidism

Hyperthyroidism is characterized by nervousness, weight loss, hyperphagia, heat intolerance, sweating, tachycardia, and increase in pulse pressure (because of vasodilation). Patients who present with uncontrolled *hyperthyroid symptoms* should be managed medically before elective surgery. The basic principle of medical management of hyperthyroidism is decreasing thyroid hormone production and blunting the hyperadrenergic symptoms. Beta-blockers decrease adrenergic symptoms (tachycardia, increased cardiac output), while propylthiouracil and methimazole compete with tyrosine for iodide and thus block T_3 and T_4 production. In acute situations, exogenous iodine can be administered, which depresses thyroid hormone production. After adequate control of hyperthyroid symptoms, surgical excision of the thyroid gland can be performed. Radioactive iodine ablates the thyroid gland and leads to a progressive loss of function. Loss of thyroid function is replaced with exogenous levothyroxine. Acute thyroid storm is a medical emergency. Patients can present with or develop it intraoperatively. Management of thyrotoxicosis is detailed in Table 18-5.

E. Hypothyroidism

Patients with *hypothyroidism* present with peripheral vasoconstriction, poor mentation, cold intolerance, and weight gain. Hypothyroidism is treated with exogenous levothyroxine. Patients with *severe hypothyroidism* should be treated prior to elective procedures. In this situation, T_3 can be used, which has a faster onset of action. These patients are exquisitely sensitive to sedative medications and can quickly develop cardiorespiratory collapse. Management of myxedema coma requires inotropic agents, administration of intravenous T_4 or T_3, fluids, hydrocortisone, and respiratory support (Table 18-5).

F. Anesthetic Priorities in Thyroid Surgery

General anesthesia with an endotracheal tube is used for thyroid surgery (2,3). Anesthesiologists may encounter unexpected difficult airway in 5% to 8% of cases. Retrosternal thyroid behaves as an anterior mediastinal mass,

Table 18-5 Perioperative Thyroid Emergencies (Thyrotoxicosis and Myxedema Coma)

Management of Thyroid Storm

IV fluids
Sodium iodide: 250 mg orally or IV every 6 hr
Propylthiouracil: 200–400 mg orally or via nasogastric tube every 6 hr
Hydrocortisone: 50–100 mg IV every 6 hr
Propranolol: 10–40 mg orally every 4–6 hr or esmolol (titrate)
Cooling blankets and acetaminophen: 12.5 mg IV of meperidine every 4–6 hr may be used to treat or prevent shivering
Diltiazem: Congestive heart failure with atrial fibrillation and rapid ventricular response

Management of Myxedema Coma

Tracheal intubation and controlled ventilation of the lungs as needed
Levothyroxine: 200–300 mg IV over 5–10 min
Cortisol: 100 mg IV and then 25 mg IV every 6 hr
Fluid and electrolyte therapy as guided by serum electrolyte measurements
Warm environment to conserve body heat

IV, intravenous.
From Endocrine function. In: Barash PG, Cullen BF, Stoelting RK, eds., et al. *Handbook of Clinical Anesthesia.* 7th ed. Philadelphia: Wolters Kluwer/Lippincott Williams & Wilkins; 2013, with permission.

and special consideration should be kept in mind (see Chapter 34). *Recurrent laryngeal nerve injury* is a distinct possibility, leading to airway compromise after surgery (see Chapter 20) (Table 18-6). Tracheal compression due to hematoma or tracheomalacia (after excision of a large thyroid) is an emergency (see Chapter 20). Hypocalcemia due to hypoparathyroidism can develop within 24 to 96 hours after surgery.

VI. Adrenal Gland
A. Adrenal Cortex
The adrenal gland is composed of two parts: the outer cortex and the inner medulla. The cortex is divided into three zones—the *zona glomerulosa*, *zona fasciculata*, and *zona reticularis*—which produce *mineralocorticoids*,

Table 18-6 Complications of Thyroid Surgery

Thyroid storm: should be distinguished from malignant hyperthermia, pheochromocytoma, and inadequate anesthesia; it most often develops in undiagnosed or untreated hyperthyroid patients because of the stress of surgery.

Airway obstruction: Hematoma in the neck or trachomalacia causing airway obstruction.

Recurrent laryngeal nerve damage: hoarseness may be present if the damage is unilateral, and aphonia may be present if the damage is bilateral.

Hypoparathyroidism: symptoms of hypocalcemia develop within 24 to 48 hours and include laryngospasm.

CT, computed tomography.
From Endocrine function. In: Barash PG, Cullen BF, Stoelting RK, eds., et al. *Handbook of Clinical Anesthesia.* 7th ed. Philadelphia: Wolters Kluwer/Lippincott Williams & Wilkins; 2013.

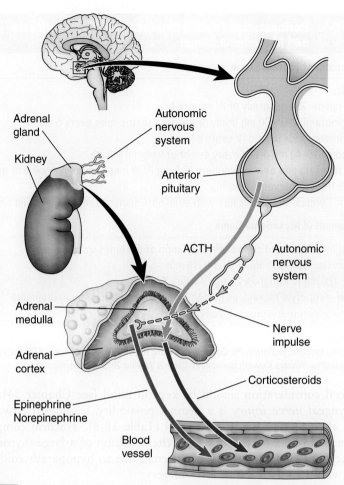

Figure 18-4 The hypothalamic–pituitary axis controls many of the functions of the normal adrenal gland. The cortex is responsive to corticotropin, while the medulla is under control of the autonomic nervous system. (From Hammel JA, Umpierrez GE. Adrenal gland disorders. In: Felner EI, Umpierrez GF, eds. *Endocrine Pathophysiology*. Philadelphia: Wolters Kluwer Health/Lippincott Williams & Wilkins; 2014:480.)

glucocorticoids, and androgens, respectively (Fig. 18-4) (4–6). The precursor of all steroid hormones is cholesterol, which is converted to pregnenolone in the mitochondria and transported to the cytoplasm and converted by various enzymes into specific steroid hormones.

Physiologic Effects of Glucocorticoids

Glucocorticoid production and secretion is controlled by *corticotropin* from the pituitary gland. Glucocorticoids increase protein catabolism, glycogenolysis, and gluconeogenesis and have an anti-inflammatory and anti-insulin effect. They are required for glucagon and catecholamines to have their metabolic effects, normal vascular reactivity, neurologic function, and water excretion. Glucocorticoids also decrease eosinophils and basophils but increase neutrophils, platelets, and red blood cells (3).

VIDEO 18-2

Cushing Syndrome

Glucocorticoid Excess (Cushing Syndrome)

Glucocorticoid excess leads to *Cushing syndrome*. This excess can be due to either an increase in corticotropin (corticotropin dependent) or increased

Table 18-7	Manifestations of Excess Glucocorticoid in Patient Adrenalectomy (Cushing Syndrome)
Manifestations of Glucocorticoid Excess	
Truncal obesity and thin extremities (reflects redistribution of fat and skeletal muscle wasting) Osteopenia Hyperglycemia Hypertension (fluid retention) Emotional changes Susceptibility to infection	

From Endocrine function. In: Barash PG, Cullen BF, Stoelting RK, eds., et al. *Handbook of Clinical Anesthesia*. 7th ed. Philadelphia: Wolters Kluwer/Lippincott Williams & Wilkins; 2013.

production by the adrenal gland (corticotropin independent). Corticotropin-dependent production, also called *Cushing disease* (for historical reasons), can be caused by corticotropin-secreting tumors of the anterior pituitary. Ectopic corticotropin produced by other tumors (e.g., the lung) can lead to Cushing syndrome. Causes of corticotropin-independent glucocorticoid excess include glucocorticoid secreting tumors of the adrenal gland, hyperplasia of the adrenal gland, or prolonged exogenous administration of glucocorticoids. As expected, because of the catabolic effects of glucocorticoids, patients with Cushing syndrome have significant glucose intolerance and develop diabetes and muscle atrophy. They retain water and develop hypertension. They also develop osteoporosis, central distribution of fat, and classic truncal obesity and may also manifest psychological complaints. Anesthetic implications for patients with Cushing syndrome undergoing an adrenalectomy are detailed in Table 18-7.

Glucocorticoid Deficiency (Addison's Disease/Addisonian Crisis)
Glucocorticoid deficiency can occur because of primary adrenal failure or lack of sufficient corticotropin from the pituitary gland. Patients may present with nonspecific symptoms (chronic fatigue, muscle weakness, anorexia, weight loss, nausea, vomiting, diarrhea). *Chronic adrenal insufficiency* is diagnosed by determining the plasma cortisol response to a corticotropin stimulation test. *Addison's disease* is treated with daily exogenous glucocorticoids and mineralocorticoids. *Acute adrenal insufficiency (Addisonian crisis)* frequently presents with hypotension, decreased consciousness, and shock and requires intravenous hydrocortisone. Perioperative implications for patients with Addisonian crisis are detailed in Table 18-8.

Table 18-8	Adrenal Insufficiency (Addison's Crisis): Anesthesia Implications
Clinical picture: In Addisonian crisis, recurrent hypotension requiring multiple doses of vasopressors, hypovolemia, hypokalemia, and hyponatremia. In chronic Addison's disease due to primary adrenal insufficiency, hyperpigmentation is seen.	
Treatment: Hydrocortisone 100 mg IV, then 100 mg every 8 hr or by continuous infusion.	

IV, intravenous.

Table 18-9 Comparative Pharmacology of Corticosteroids

	Anti-inflammatory*	Mineralocorticoid*	Approximate Equivalent Dose (mg)	Plasma Half-Life (min)	Duration of Action (hr)
Short Acting					
Cortisol (hydrocortisone)	1.0	1.0	20	90	8–12
Prednisone	4.0	0.25	5.0	60	12–36
Methylprednisolone	5.0	+/−	4.0	180	12–36
Long Acting					
Dexamethasone	30	+/−	0.75	200	36–54

*The glucocorticoid and mineralocorticoid properties are considered to be equivalent to one.
From Endocrine function. In: Barash PG, Cullen BF, Stoelting RK, eds., et al. *Handbook of Clinical Anesthesia*. 7th ed. Philadelphia: Wolters Kluwer/Lippincott Williams & Wilkins; 2013 and Felner EI, Umpierrez GE. *Endocrine Pathophysiology*. Philadelphia: Lippincott Williams & Wilkins; 2014:480.

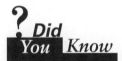

Did You Know

The "Rule of Fives": Prednisone is five times more potent than cortisone; dexamethasone is five times more potent than prednisone.

Exogenous Glucocorticoid Therapy

Anesthesiologists should be familiar with the different preparations of synthetic steroids that are used therapeutically (Table 18-9). Dexamethasone, betamethasone, and triamcinolone have no mineralocorticoid activity and are typically used for their anti-inflammatory properties. Fludrocortisone has 12 times more mineralocorticoid activity than anti-inflammatory activity and is used to supplement mineralocorticoid activity in adrenal deficiency. Cortisol, hydrocortisone, and cortisone have equal mineralocorticoid and glucocorticoid activity. *Prednisone* and *methylprednisone* are typically used for immunologic and inflammatory diseases.

Steroid Replacement during the Perioperative Period

One of the major consequences of administering exogenous steroids is suppression of the *hypothalamic–pituitary axis (HPA)* (2,3,7). Suppression of the HPA is unlikely to develop in a patient who has received <1 week of lower-dose exogenous steroid therapy. Patients who receive >1 to 3 weeks of steroid therapy can be considered to have a suppressed HPA, especially if they are consuming more than 15 mg/day of prednisolone (or equivalent doses of other steroids). It can take up to 6 to 9 months for the HPA to normalize. If patients do not receive steroid supplementation in the perioperative period, they can present in Addisonian crisis. Patients who receive ≤5 mg/day of prednisolone usually do not require additional supplementation if they have taken their usual morning dose prior to surgery. Perioperative supplementation of steroids is based on expected physiologic stress induced by surgery (7). For high-risk surgeries, 300 mg of hydrocortisone, divided into three doses in 24 hours is recommended, while for low-risk surgeries, 25 mg at induction, followed by 100 mg in the next 24 hours may be sufficient (Table 18-10).

Physiological Effects of Aldosterone

Aldosterone is predominantly controlled by *angiotensin II*, corticotropin, and serum potassium (see Fig. 5-7 in Chapter 5). Mineralocorticoids, predominantly aldosterone, are responsible for sodium and water absorption to maintain adequate intravascular volume. Decreased intravascular volume leads to a decrease in afferent arteriolar pressures in the nephron. This is sensed by the

Table 18-10	Supplemental Steroid Coverage
Physiologic (low-dose approach): Cortisol 25 mg IV before induction of anesthesia followed by a continuous infusion (100 mg IV over 24 hr)	
Supraphysiologic: Cortisol 200–300 mg IV in divided doses on the day of surgery	

IV, intravenous.
From Endocrine function. In: Barash PG, Cullen BF, Stoelting RK, eds., et al. *Handbook of Clinical Anesthesia.*
7th ed. Philadelphia: Wolters Kluwer/Lippincott Williams & Wilkins; 2013.

juxtaglomerular apparatus, which secretes renin. *Renin* converts circulating angiotensinogen to angiotensin I, which is further converted to angiotensin II by angiotensin-converting enzyme in the lungs. Angiotensin II is a potent stimulus for aldosterone secretion. Aldosterone acts on the distal renal tubules and promotes sodium and water absorption, which leads to restitution of intravascular volume (see Fig. 5-7 in Chapter 5). Sodium is exchanged for potassium or hydrogen ions in the distal tubules.

Mineralocorticoid Excess
Mineralocorticoid (aldosterone) excess leads to sodium absorption and potassium or hydrogen ion *excretion* in renal tubules (*Conn syndrome*). This causes hypertension, muscle weakness (due to contractile dysfunction of the skeletal muscle), polyuria, tetany, and hypokalemic alkalosis. Aldosterone excess can be broadly classified as primary or secondary hyperaldosteronism. In primary hyperaldosteronism, high levels of aldosterone are caused by increased production by the adrenal cortex. Aldosterone excess can be a result of primary adrenal disease (Conn syndrome), adrenal hyperplasia, adrenal adenoma or carcinoma, or a genetic disorder involving corticotropin. Renin activity is typically depressed. In secondary hyperaldosteronism, which is commonly seen in heart failure, cirrhosis, and nephrosis, aldosterone excess is caused by an increase in renin. The kidneys in these conditions sense a low intravascular volume and trigger increased renin release, which ultimately leads to increased angiotensin II production and aldosterone secretion. Patients retain sodium and water to compensate for low intravascular volume and developed significant edema (Table 18-11).

B. **Adrenal Medulla**
Adrenal medulla predominantly produces *epinephrine* and small amounts of *norepinephrine* and *dopamine*. All three catecholamines are derived from the amino acid tyrosine. Adrenal phenylethanolamine N-methyltransferase is induced by glucocorticoids; thus, glucocorticoids are intricately involved in catecholamine production and function. Epinephrine and norepinephrine

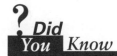

? *Did* **You** *Know*

Only the brain and adrenal gland have the specific enzyme phenylethanolamine N-methyltransferase, which can convert norepinephrine to epinephrine.

Table 18-11	Hyperaldostonerism (Conn Syndrome): Anesthesia Implications
Clinical picture: Hypertension, hypokalemia, hypernatremia, hypomagnesaemia, hypervolemia, and suppression of plasma–renin axis. Hypokalemic effect on non-depolarizing neuromuscular blockers.	
Treatment: Potassium-sparing diuretics, and potential depression of pituitary–adrenal axis by etomidate.	

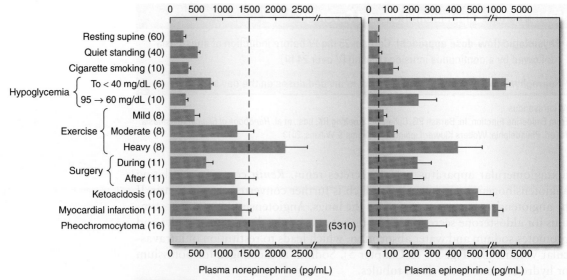

Figure 18-5 Norepinephrine and epinephrine levels in human venous blood in various physiologic and pathologic states. Note that the horizontal scales are different. The numbers to the left in parentheses are the numbers of subjects tested. In each case, the vertical dashed line identifies the threshold plasma concentration at which detectable physiologic changes are observed. (From Barrett KE, Barman SM, Boitano S, Brooks H. Ganong's Review of Medical Physiology. 24th Edition. New York: McGraw Hill Professional, 2012.)

levels are significantly increased during and after surgery (Fig. 18-5) (8). Catecholamines have a very short half-life (2 minutes) and are metabolized to *vanillylmandelic acid*, metanephrines, or normetanephrine and excreted in the urine (Fig. 18-6). Adrenal medulla also secretes opioids, adenosine triphosphate, and adrenomedullin (a vasodepressive polypeptide).

Pheochromocytoma

Pheochromocytoma is a rare tumor of the adrenal gland that produces norepinephrine. Patients present with sustained or paroxysmal hypertensive attacks. Because of enhanced vasoconstriction, patients are significantly volume depleted. Diagnosis is established by measuring free catecholamines and vanillylmandelic acid in 24-hour urine samples. Patients with pheochromocytoma are managed medically before elective surgery. The basic principle of medical management of pheochromocytoma is decreasing catecholamine production (metyrosine) and blunting the hyperadrenergic symptoms. Initially, *alpha-blockers* are used (phenoxybenzamine, α_1 antagonists) followed by *beta-blockers* (labetalol, metoprolol). Beta-blockers should be used in conjunction with alpha-blockers, as predominant beta-blockade can lead to unopposed alpha effect of catecholamines and worsen hypertension (8). Surgery is usually curative. Anesthetic implications for patients with pheochromocytoma are detailed in Table 18-12.

V. Calcium Homeostasis

Calcium is found in plasma in three states: bound to albumin (50%), bound to phosphate, bicarbonate, and citrate (5% to 10%), and free ionized calcium (40% to 45%) (Fig. 18-7) (3). It is the *ionized calcium* that plays a

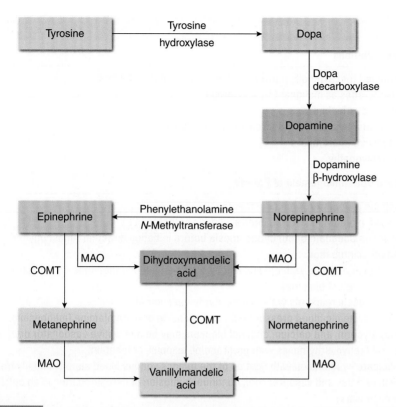

Figure 18-6 Synthesis and metabolism of endogenous catecholamines. COMT, catechol-O-methyltransferase; MAO, monoamine oxidase. (From Schwartz JJ, Akhtar S, Rosenbaum SH. Endocrine function. In: Barash PG, Cullen BF, Stoelting RK, et al., eds. *Clinical Anesthesia*. 7th ed. Philadelphia: Wolters Kluwer Health/ Lippincott Williams & Wilkins; 2013:1327, with permission.)

critical role in regulating muscle contraction, coagulation, neurotransmitter release, and second messenger intracellular functions. Ionized calcium is tightly regulated and is affected by pH and temperature, which affect its binding to albumin. Alkalosis causes a decrease in ionized calcium, while acidosis causes an increase in ionized calcium. *Parathyroid hormone (PTH)*

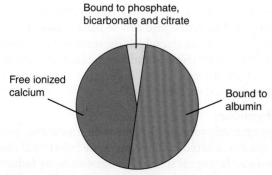

Figure 18-7 Calcium is found in plasma in three states: bound to both albumin and phosphate, as well as ionized calcium.

Table 18-12   Pheochromocytoma
Manifestations
Sustained (occasionally paroxysmal) hypertension (headaches)
Masquerades as malignant hyperthermia
Cardiac dysrhythmias
Orthostatic hypotension (decreased blood volume)
Congestive heart failure
Cardiomyopathy
Anesthetic Management of Patients
Continue preoperative medical therapy
Invasive monitoring (arterial central venous catheter, TEE)
Ensure an adequate depth of anesthesia before initiating direct laryngoscopy for tracheal intubation
Maintain anesthesia with opioids and a volatile anesthetic that does not sensitize the heart to catecholamines
Select muscle relaxants with minimal cardiovascular effects
Control systemic blood pressure with nitroprusside or phentolamine (magnesium, nitroglycerin, and calcium channel blockers may be alternative vasodilator drugs)
Control tachydysrhythmias with propranolol, esmolol, or labetalol
Anticipate hypotension with ligation of the tumor's venous blood supply (initially treat with IV fluids and vasopressors; continuous infusion of norepinephrine is an option if necessary)

IV, intravenous; TEE, transesophageal echocardiography.
From Endocrine function. In: Barash PG, Cullen BF, Stoelting RK, eds., et al. *Handbook of Clinical Anesthesia*. 7th ed. Philadelphia: Wolters Kluwer/Lippincott Williams & Wilkins; 2013.

is secreted by the parathyroid glands and is intricately involved in regulation of plasma calcium (Fig. 18-8).

A. Hyperparathyroidism
Excess PTH leads to *hypercalcemia* and presents with polyuria, polydipsia, generalized muscle weakness, fatigability, peptic ulceration, constipation, and psychiatric complaints. Hyperparathyroidism is diagnosed by increased plasma levels of PTH and hypercalcemia. Secondary hyperparathyroidism is a compensatory increase in PTH and is seen in conditions that cause either hypocalcemia or hyperphosphatemia (e.g., chronic renal failure). In hyperparathyroidism, treatment of hypercalcaemia is of primary concern. Hydration with intravenous normal saline is the first step, followed by loop diuretics. Calcitonin inhibits PTH secretion and can be used for the first 24 to 48 hours. Mithramycin and bisphosphonate, which decrease bone resorption, may have to be used. Severe hypercalcaemia should be treated prior to elective surgery. Surgical excision of parathyroid gland is curative. Anesthetic implications of hypocalcaemia are detailed in Table 18-13.

B. Hypoparathyroidism
Patients with *hypoparathyroidism* present with numbness, paresthesia, muscle cramps and spasms, altered mental status, or behavioral disturbances and rarely with seizures or laryngeal stridor. Congestive heart failure and hypotension can also occur. Hypocalcaemia in the setting of low PTH confirms the diagnosis. Patients are treated with exogenous calcium, vitamin D analogues,

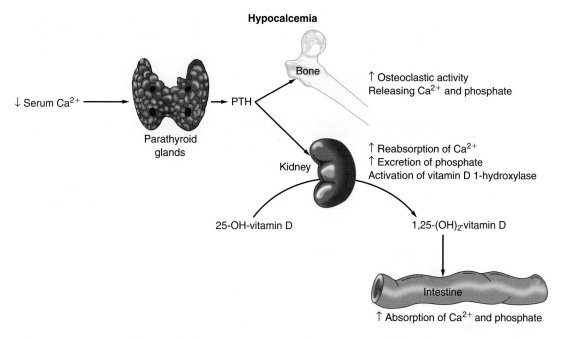

Hypocalcemia

↓ Serum Ca^{2+} ⟶ Parathyroid glands ⟶ PTH

Bone
↑ Osteoclastic activity
Releasing Ca^{2+} and phosphate

Kidney
↑ Reabsorption of Ca^{2+}
↑ Excretion of phosphate
Activation of vitamin D 1-hydroxylase

25-OH-vitamin D   1,25-(OH)$_2$-vitamin D

Intestine
↑ Absorption of Ca^{2+} and phosphate

Hypercalcemia

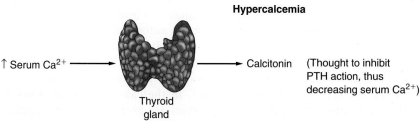

↑ Serum Ca^{2+} ⟶ Thyroid gland ⟶ Calcitonin   (Thought to inhibit PTH action, thus decreasing serum Ca^{2+})

Figure 18-8 Parathyroid hormone (PTH) and vitamin D metabolism and action. 25-OH, 25-hydroxycholecalciferol; 1,25-(OH)$_2$, 1,25-dihydroxycholecalciferol. (From Schwartz JJ, Akhtar S, Rosenbaum SH. Endocrine function. In: Barash PG, Cullen BF, Stoelting RK, et al., eds. *Clinical Anesthesia*. 7th ed. Philadelphia: Wolters Kluwer Health/Lippincott Williams & Wilkins; 2013:1327, with permission.)

and, in severe cases, intravenous calcium infusion. Clinical manifestations of hypocalcaemia are detailed in Table 18-14.

C. Anesthetic Implications of Parathyroid Surgery

General anesthesia with endotracheal tube or a laryngeal mask airway can be used for parathyroid surgery. Regional anesthesia can be used for minimally invasive parathyroidectomies. *Recurrent laryngeal nerve injury* is a distinct possibility, leading to airway compromise after surgery (see Chapter 20).

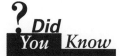
?Did You Know

Propofol can interfere with rapid PTH assay and should not be used 15 minutes prior to measurement of PTH levels.

Table 18-13 **Hyperparathyroidism: Anesthesia Implications**
Clinical picture: Hypercalcemia, hypophosphatemia, hypovolemia, cardiac dysrhythmias, and pathologic fractures.
Treatment: Correct hypercalcemia (preop Ca^{++} >14 mEq/L) may require fluids, diuretics, dialysis, and medications (calcitonin, mithramycin, bisphosphonates, or glucocorticoids). Neuromuscular blockers may have variable effect due to hypercalcemia. Follow electrocardiogram for signs of Ca^{++} levels.

Table 18-14   Hypoparathyroidism: Clinical Manifestations
Neuronal irritability
Skeletal muscle spasms
Congestive heart failure
Prolonged Q-T interval on the electrocardiogram

From Endocrine function. In: Barash PG, Cullen BF, Stoelting RK, eds., et al. *Handbook of Clinical Anesthesia.* 7th ed. Philadelphia: Wolters Kluwer/Lippincott Williams & Wilkins; 2013.

Hypocalcaemia due to *hypoparathyroidism* can develop and may require intravenous calcium supplementation.

VI. Diabetes Mellitus

A. Physiology

Diabetes mellitus affects millions of individuals worldwide. It is considered primarily a dysfunction of glucose metabolism as a result of either absolute or relative deficiency (lack of affect) of insulin on the tissues (3,10). Insulin is produced in the pancreas by the β *cells in the islets of Langerhans.* Factors that increase insulin secretion include increased levels of plasma glucose, gastrointestinal hormones (incretin hormones), autonomic stimulation (vagal and β adrenergic), α blockade, and nitric oxide. Hypoglycemia and hypokalemia decrease insulin secretion. Insulin is metabolized in the liver and kidneys.

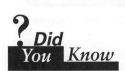
? Did You Know

All tissues do not require insulin for glucose entry (e.g., brain, liver, reticuloendothelial cells).

The principal effect of insulin is to increase glucose uptake in insulin-sensitive cells (skeletal and adipose tissue). In the case of absolute absence or lack of effective insulin, lipids and proteins are broken down to produce glucose, and as a byproduct, ketones (ketoacids) are generated.

Insulin secretion or action is opposed by counter-regulatory hormones (glucagon, glucocorticoids, catecholamines, growth hormone) and cytokines, which are typically released under stress (trauma, surgery, sepsis) and lead to stress-induced hyperglycemia. Hyperglycemia (defined as >180 mg/dL) leads to osmotic diuresis and fluid and electrolyte disturbances. Diabetes is associated with micro- and macrovascular diseases, neuropathy, nephropathy, retinopathy, impaired wound healing, and deficient immunocompetence.

B. Classification

Diabetes is classified into four broad categories: type 1, type 2, gestational diabetes, and diabetes due to other causes (Table 18-15) (3,9). *Type 1 diabetes* results from an absolute lack of insulin, typically due to autoimmune destruction of the islets of Langerhans. It presents early in life and requires exogenous insulin. These patients are also prone to diabetic ketoacidosis.

Type 2 diabetes accounts for 90% of all patients with diabetes. They are typically older and obese and have developed resistance to the effects of insulin. Initially, hyperglycemia causes a compensatory increase in insulin production. As disease progresses, many patients subsequently require exogenous insulin to control hyperglycemia.

C. Diagnosis

A fasting blood glucose of <100 mg/dL is considered normal, while a fasting glucose of >126 mg/dL on two occasions confirms the diagnosis of diabetes (Table 18-15) (9,10). Patients with fasting glucose between 101 and 125 mg/dL

Table 18-15   Diabetes Mellitus Classification and Diagnosis
Classification
Type 1 (Insulin Dependent) Childhood onset Thin Prone to ketoacidosis Always requires exogenous insulin
Type 2 (Noninsulin Dependent) Maturity onset Obese Not prone to ketoacidosis May be controlled by diet or oral hypoglycemic drugs
Gestational Diabetes May presage future type 2 diabetes mellitus
Diabetes from Other Causes Pancreatic surgery Chronic pancreatitis Endocrine diseases (pheochromocytoma, acromegaly, Cushing disease, exogenous steroids) Treatment of HIV/AIDS
Diagnosis
Hemoglobin A1$_c$ ≥6.5% Fasting plasma glucose ≥126 mg/dL (7.0 mmol/L) 2-hour plasma glucose ≥200 mg/dL (11.1 mmol/L) Random plasma glucose ≥200 mg/dL (11.1 mmol/L) in a patient with symptoms of hyperglycemia

From Endocrine function. In: Barash PG, Cullen BF, Stoelting RK, eds., et al. *Handbook of Clinical Anesthesia.* 7th ed. Philadelphia: Wolters Kluwer/Lippincott Williams & Wilkins; 2013.

are considered *prediabetics*. An abnormal glucose tolerance test or severe hyperglycemia (>200 mg/dL) in the presence of classic symptoms of hyperglycemia also fulfills the criteria of diabetes (3,9). A hemoglobin A1c level of >6.5 strongly supports the diagnosis of diabetes and requires confirmation.

D. Treatment

Type 1 diabetics require *insulin* and can be managed with long-acting insulin, with intermittent shorter-acting insulin, or with an insulin pump. Type 2 diabetics can be initially managed with diet and exercise. *Oral hypoglycemics* that increase insulin secretion (sulfonylureas), decrease hepatic glucose production (biguanides), increase peripheral insulin sensitivity (glitazones), or enhance or mimic the action of gastrointestinal hormones that increase insulin secretion, may be used in combination with exogenous insulin to control hyperglycemia.

E. Anesthetic Management

Diabetes is associated with micro- and macrovascular disease, neuropathy, nephropathy, retinopathy, and impaired wound healing (2,3). These patients are particularly prone to coronary artery disease, cerebrovascular disease,

Table 18-16	Diabetes Mellitus Preoperative Evaluation
History and physical examination (detect symptoms of cerebrovascular disease, coronary artery disease, peripheral neuropathy)	
Laboratory tests (electrocardiography; blood glucose, creatinine, and potassium levels; urinalysis [glucose, ketones, albumin])	
Evidence of stiff joint syndrome difficult-to-perform laryngoscopy	
Evidence of cardiac autonomic nervous system neuropathy (resting tachycardia, orthostatic hypotension)	
Evidence of vagal autonomic nervous system neuropathy (gastroparesis slows emptying of solids [metoclopramide may be useful] but probably not clear fluids)	
Autonomic neuropathy predisposes the patient to intraoperative hypothermia	

From Endocrine function. In: Barash PG, Cullen BF, Stoelting RK, eds., et al. *Handbook of Clinical Anesthesia.* 7th ed. Philadelphia: Wolters Kluwer/Lippincott Williams & Wilkins; 2013.

and peripheral vascular disease. They have a higher incidence of perioperative major adverse cardiovascular events. Management of an oral hypoglycemic and insulin regimen is of particular concern in the perioperative period, as non per os status significantly impacts exogenous glucose consumption (Table 18-16). Oral hypoglycemics are not administered on the day of surgery and withheld until the patient resumes eating. The insulin regimen has to be modified in the perioperative period. Initially, tight glucose control was advocated by some experts. However, because of the significantly increased risk of *hypoglycemia* and no significant benefit of tight glucose control (<110 mg/dL) when compared with modest control (140 to 180 mg/dL), tight glucose control is no longer advocated. It is now recommended to keep the glucose levels <180 mg/dL perioperatively. Frequent glucose monitoring is recommended to prevent inadvertent hypoglycemia (Table 18-17).

F. Diabetic Emergencies

Severe hypoglycemia (blood glucose <60 mg/dL) requires a rapid response (3,9). Anesthetic drugs and adjuvants (e.g., beta-blockers) can obscure the signs of a hypoglycemic reaction (Table 18-17).

Two other life-threatening emergencies specifically related to diabetes are also encountered in these patients. Lack of insulin leads to poor utilization of glucose by insulin-dependent tissues, and the body responds by generating alternative sources of energy. Breakdown of lipids leads to formation and accumulation of ketoacids, which causes severe metabolic acidosis in the setting of hyperglycemia. This condition is called *diabetic ketoacidosis* and it is a metabolic emergency (Table 18-17). It carries a significant mortality if not recognized and treated promptly. Basically, diabetic ketoacidosis is managed by brisk fluid administration and exogenous insulin therapy.

Severe hyperglycemia (>600 mg/dL) *without* ketoacidosis can also occur (*hyperglycemic hyperosmolar state* or *hyperglycemic nonketotic coma*). This typically occurs in older patients who have some insulin that blunts fat breakdown and formation of ketones. Though metabolic acidosis due to ketoacids does not occur, osmotic diuresis, fluid and electrolyte disturbances, and severe hyperosmolarity lead to altered mental status and to coma. Treatment is hydration and insulin therapy. Diabetic ketoacidosis and hyperosmotic

Table 18-17	Diabetic Emergencies

Hypoglycemia

Clinical picture: Alert patient (blood glucose <60 mg/dL) to comatose patient (blood glucose <40 mg/dL). Seizures can present will severe hypoglycemia (blood glucose <30 mg/dL).

Treatment: Moderate to severe hypoglycemia: Dextrose 25 g IV (1 amp $D_{50}W$) follow with D_5W or $D_{10}W$. Continue to monitor and treat blood glucose until >100 mg/dL. If no IV, glucagon 1 mg intramuscular

Under Manifestations of Nonketotic Hyperosmolar Coma

Clinical picture: Altered mental status, delirium, coma, seizures, dehydration.

Treatment: Significant fluid and electrolyte replacement, insulin therapy (regular insulin); hemodynamic instability and decreased airway reflexes may be present.

Manifestations of Hyperosmolar Nonketotic Coma

Elderly patients with impaired thirst mechanism
Minimal or mild diabetes
Profound hyperglycemia (>600 mg/dL)
Absence of ketoacidosis
Hyperosmolarity (seizures, coma, venous thrombosis)

Manifestations of Diabetic Ketoacidosis

Metabolic acidosis
Hyperglycemia (300–500 mg/dL)
Dehydration (osmotic diuresis and vomiting)
Hypokalemia (manifests when acidosis is corrected)
Skeletal muscle weakness (hypophosphatemia with correction of acidosis)

Management of Diabetic Ketoacidosis

10 U IV of regular insulin followed by a continuous IV infusion (insulin in U/hr = blood glucose/150)
IV fluids (isotonic) as guided by vital signs and urine output (anticipate a 4- to 10-L deficit)
10–40 mEq/hr IV of potassium chloride when urine output exceeds 0.5 mL/kg/hr
Glucose 5% 100 mL/hr when serum glucose concentration decreases <250 mg/dL
Consider IV sodium bicarbonate to correct pH below 6.9

IV, intravenous.
From Endocrine function. In: Barash PG, Cullen BF, Stoelting RK, eds., et al. *Handbook of Clinical Anesthesia.* 7th ed. Philadelphia: Wolters Kluwer/Lippincott Williams & Wilkins; 2013, with permission.

hyperglycemic state should be treated prior to elective surgery. Anesthetic implications of diabetic emergencies are detailed in Table 18-17.

VII. Endocrine Response to Surgery

Trauma, surgery, and psychological stress elicit a generalized activation of the neuroendocrine system (3,10). Plasma levels of catecholamines, vasopressin, cortisol, and glucagon go up significantly. This leads to hypertension, tachycardia, fluid retention, and stress-induced hyperglycemia. Protein breakdown is significant after surgery and trauma. Concurrently, endogenous endorphins are released to counteract the stress response, pain, and some of the hyperadrenergic effects of the postoperative states. General anesthesia with regional anesthesia can blunt this stress response to a variable extent perioperatively.

Insulin resistance is seen for up 10 to 14 days following major surgery; therefore, the patient may require a higher dose of insulin than they received preoperatively. Finally, excellent pain control can also assist in blunting some aspects of the stress response and help in early recovery.

References

1. Barret KE, Boitano S, Barman SM, et al. Basic concepts of endocrine regulation. In: *Ganong's Review of Medical Physiology.* 24th ed. New York: McGraw-Hill; 2012: 299–306.
2. Russell TW. Endocrine disease. In: Hines RL, Marschall KE, eds. *Stoelting's Anesthesia and Co-existing Disease.* 6th ed. Philadelphia: Elsevier; 2012:376–406.
3. Schwartz J, Akhtar S, Rosenbaum SH. Endocrine function. In: Barash PG, Cullen BF, Stoelting RK, et al., eds. *Clinical Anesthesia.* 7th ed. Philadelphia: Lippincott Williams & Wilkins; 2013:1326–1372.
4. Felner EI, Umpierrez GE. *Endocrine Pathophysiology.* Philadelphia: Lippincott Williams & Wilkins; 2014:480.
5. Molina PE. Adrenal gland. In: *Endocrine Physiology.* 4th ed. New York: McGraw-Hill; 2013:49–72.
6. White BA, Portfield SP. The adrenal gland. In: *Endocrine and Reproductive Physiology.* 4th ed. Philadelphia: Elsevier; 2013:147–176.
7. Coursin DE, Wood KE. Corticosteroid supplementation for adrenal insufficiency. *JAMA.* 2002;287:236–240.
8. Deegnan RJ, Furman WR. Cardiovascular manifestations of endocrine dysfunction. *J Cardiothorac Vasc Anesth.* 2011;25:705–720.
9. Inzucchi SE. Diabetes facts and guidelines 2011–2012. For hardcopy email YDCbooklets @ironmountain.com. For PDF version http://endocrinology.yale.edu/patient/314_50135_YaleNationalF.pdf.
10. Akhtar S, Barash, PG, Inzucchi SE. Perioperative hyperglycemia: Scientific principles, clinical applications. *Anes Analg.* 2010;110:478–497.

Questions

1. Hypoglycemia in the anesthetized patient:
   A. Is easily recognized under general anesthesia.
   B. Is confused for "light anesthesia."
   C. Is defined as a blood sugar <80 mg/dL.
   D. Rarely presents in patients with renal failure and diabetes.

2. Which of the following increases ionized serum Ca^{++}?
   A. Increase serum albumin
   B. Respiratory alkalosis
   C. Acute hypomagnesemia
   D. Hyperphosphatemia

3. Which of the following is the most potent anti-inflammatory corticosteroid?
   A. Cortisol
   B. Prednisone
   C. Dexamethasone
   D. Triamcinolone

4. Which of the following is the most potent mineralocorticoid?
   A. Cortisol
   B. Prednisone
   C. Dexamethasone
   D. Triamcinolone

5. You evaluate a 65-year-old male in the preanesthesia who is scheduled for a laparoscopic cholecystectomy. He has a history of diabetes mellitus (metformin), hypertension (hydrochlorothiazide), atrial fibrillation (amiodarone), and depression (sertraline). He notes a 20-pound weight gain and muscle weakness. His laboratory work documents markedly elevated thyroid-stimulating hormone. Which drug is most likely to account for this finding?
   A. Metformin
   B. Hydrochlorothiazide
   C. Sertraline
   D. Amiodarone

6. In the preanesthesia clinic, you see the following patient. Which of the following thyroid function test panel results belong to this patient?

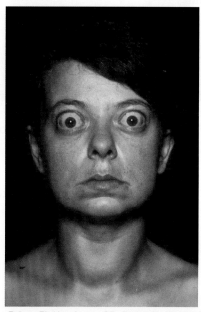

(From Felner EI, Umpierrez GE. *Endocrine Pathophysiology.* Philadelphia: Lippincott Williams & Wilkins; 2014:480.)

	Free Thyroxine (T₄)	Free Triiodothyronine (T₃)	Thyroid-Stimulating Hormone
A.	↑	↑	↓
B.	↓	↓	↓
C.	→	↓	→
D.	↑	→	→

7. Patients with mild to moderate hypothyroidism:
   A. Can be safely anesthetized without preoperative thyroid supplement.
   B. Are very sensitive to the sedative effects of anesthetics.
   C. Who have coronary artery disease require urgent thyroid replacement.
   D. Are a significant risk of requiring postoperative ventilatory support.

8. A 45-year-old female presents to the pre-anesthesia clinic with the following sestamibi scan. Based on the scan, which of the following is the appropriate surgical procedure?

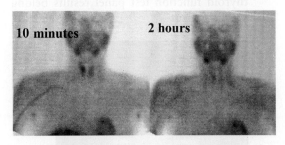

10 minutes   2 hours

A. This is a normal scan; no operation is indicated
B. Thyroidectomy
C. Right parathyroidectomy
D. Combined subtotal right thyroidectomy and parathyroidectomy

9. A 35-year-old male type 1 diabetic is in the postanesthetic care unit following a lumbosacral fusion. He has a seizure with a blood glucose 35 mg/dL and elevated serum ketones. Of the following, which is the most likely cause of these biochemical abnormalities?
A. Insulinoma
B. Hyperinsulinism
C. Adrenal Insufficiency
D. Hyperthyroidism

10. A 40-year-old female presents for a thyroidectomy for Graves' disease. Her preoperative preparation should include:
A. Administration of potassium iodide plus propranolol for 10 days
B. A 1-week course of thyroxine (T_4)
C. A three-day course of propylthiouracil
D. Iodine-131 treatment

19

General Anesthesia

Mark C. Norris
Roya Saffary

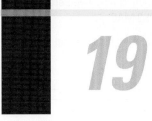

VIDEO 19-1

General Anesthesia: An Example

The operating room is a complex environment full of bright lights, sharp instruments, and elaborate equipment, with people speaking a strange language (Table 19-1). Modern surgery can remove, repair, or even replace almost every body part. Anesthesia makes these interventions possible, but anesthesia itself can be complicated and overwhelming. This chapter follows a "typical" patient through the planning and conducting of a general anesthetic, highlighting many of the decisions involved. This chapter's purpose is to demystify anesthetic care and provide a basic understanding of the steps involved in planning and conducting a safe procedure.

I. Purpose/Goals of an Anesthetic

A. What Is Anesthesia?

General anesthesia is a process whereby the patient is rendered unconscious in a reversible, controlled manner. Anesthetics induce unconsciousness by binding to specific receptors throughout the brain, brainstem, and spinal cord. Emerging evidence suggests that anesthetics interrupt the neural networks that underlie consciousness. General anesthetics also produce *immobility*. Although anesthetics most likely make patients unconscious by acting on the brain, immobility appears to result from effects on the brainstem.

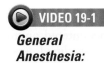

? Did You Know

Anesthetics most likely produce unconsciousness by acting on the brain. However, immobility appears to result from their effects on the brainstem.

Some operations require skeletal muscle relaxation. Complete muscle paralysis can produce immobility in response to surgical stimulation, although paralysis without unconsciousness can lead to awareness with recall, an uncommon but potentially horrifying complication. In addition, muscle relaxation provides optimal conditions for endotracheal intubation and improves surgical exposure during intra-abdominal and intrathoracic procedures. Although a patient may not move, the body can mount a robust *sympathetic response* to surgical stimulation with hypertension, tachycardia, and tachypnea. The last element of general anesthesia aims at controlling these changes. Some drugs provide all of the elements of anesthesia, while others have more specific roles. Table 19-2 shows the actions of some commonly used anesthetic drugs.

Table 19-1	Common Anesthesia-Related Terms and Acronyms
Term/Acronym	**Definition**
MAC	Minimum alveolar concentration: The concentration of inhaled anesthetic that will keep half the patients immobile in response to surgical stimulation. Ninety-five percent of patients will be immobilized at 1.3 MAC.
MAC	Monitored anesthesia care: Monitoring plus varying amounts of sedation.
TIVA	Total intravenous anesthesia
GA	General anesthesia
Reversal	A combination of anticholinesterase and anticholinergic drugs used to terminate the effect of certain paralytic drugs
LMA	Laryngeal mask airway
ET tube	Endotracheal tube
TOF	Train-of-four: a measurement of the degree of neuromuscular blockade
PACU	Postanesthesia care unit (or recovery room)

B. Who Gives Anesthesia?

There are a variety of medical professionals who will be encountered on an anesthesia rotation (Table 19-3). These people are known as *qualified anesthesia care providers*. They have different backgrounds and training and may work alone or as part of an anesthesia care team.

C. What Are the Risks of Anesthesia?

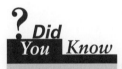

Most anesthesia consent forms include a list of possible complications. Some of these, such as sore throat and postoperative nausea or vomiting, are common but transient. Others, such as dental damage or corneal abrasion, are less common but self-limited or repairable. A few, including awareness, brain damage, or death, are rare but catastrophic. About 1 in 10,000 patients will have awareness during anesthesia. Patients with a previous episode of *awareness* with recall are at increased risk of this complication after a subsequent anesthetic (1). Death solely due to anesthesia is very rare, occurring in fewer than 1 in 100,000 anesthetics.

Awareness during anesthesia is rare, occurring in about 1 in 10,000 cases.

II. Preoperative Evaluation

A. Patient Assessment

Surgery stresses the body, and anesthetics have significant physiologic effects. Therefore, before giving any anesthetic, the anesthesiologist evaluates the patient, looking for problems that might increase risk. This assessment requires knowledge of the patient's past and current medical and surgical conditions. The preoperative evaluation may be completed in person by the anesthesiologist, by a nurse in a preoperative clinic or via a phone interview, or by the patient via a web-based questionnaire. In many centers, healthy patients presenting for outpatient surgery and any patient needing emergency surgery may be evaluated on the day of the operation.

Table 19-2   Actions of Commonly Used Anesthetic Drugs

Drug	Amnesia/ Unconsciousness	Immobility	Muscle Relaxation	Suppression of Sympathetic Reflexes
Potent inhaled agents (isoflurane, sevoflurane, desflurane)	+++	+++	+ (Dose-dependent muscle relaxation. Unacceptably low blood pressure can accompany profound relaxation.)	+ (Dose-dependent. Isoflurane and desflurane can initially produce tachycardia.)
Nitrous oxide	+/– (Not potent enough to produce anesthesia but can supplement the potent agents.)	+/–	–	+
Intravenous anesthetics (propofol, barbiturates, benzodiazepines, ketamine)	+++	+++	–	+/– (Some efficacy at higher doses)
Paralytics (succinylcholine, atracurium, rocuronium, vecuronium)	–	–	+++	–
Opioids (fentanyl, remifentanil, hydromorphone, etc.)	– (Do not produce unconsciousness or immobility but potentiate the effects of inhaled and intravenous anesthetics.)	–	– (fentanyl and remifentanil can cause chest wall rigidity)	++ (Longer acting opioids can also provide postoperative analgesia)
Sympatholytic Drugs (labetalol, esmolol, metoprolol)	–	–	–	++ (No analgesic effects, but can blunt the hemodynamic response to surgical stimulation)

+ (weak effect), ++ (moderate effect), +++ (strong effect), – (no effect).

The preanesthetic evaluation begins with the chief complaint. In this case, what surgery is needed and why. Although this information should be available in the medical record, confirming the site and side of surgery directly with the patient is an important safeguard against wrong-site, wrong-side surgery. Next the patient's age, height, and weight are reviewed. Extremes in any of these values can present unique concerns (see Chapters 28 and 33). Reviewing the patient's surgical history can alert the anesthesiologist to significant medical problems. Questions about previous anesthetics can help prepare for a difficult airway, postoperative nausea and vomiting, and other possible complications.

Table 19-3	Who's Who in the Operating Room		
Qualified Anesthesia Providers	Training	Role	Professional Organization
Anesthesiologist (MD/DO)	Bachelor's degree + medical school + 1-year internship + 3-year residency ± 1- or 2-year fellowship	Can personally provide anesthesia care or "medically direct" up to four qualified anesthesia providers or two trainees	American Society of Anesthesiologists (www.asahq.org)
Nurse anesthetist (CRNA)	Bachelor's degree in nursing (BSN), at least 1-year critical care nursing experience + 2- or 3-year nurse anesthesia program	Depending on the state, may personally provide anesthesia care, may be supervised by a physician (i.e., a surgeon), or may be medically directed by an anesthesiologist as a member of the anesthesia care team	American Association of Nurse Anesthetists (www.aana.com)
Anesthesiologist assistant (AA)	Bachelor's degree + 2- or 3-year master's of medical science program	AAs only work under the medical direction of an anesthesiologist as a member of the anesthesia care team	American Academy of Anesthesiologist Assistants (www.anesthetist.org)

Even if a patient has never had anesthesia, the family history might reveal malignant hyperthermia, pseudo-cholinesterase deficiency, or other heritable problems. The anesthesiologist also checks the patient's medications and allergies and asks targeted questions about the patient's medical problems and systems review.

On the day of surgery, the anesthesiologist reviews the patient's history and conducts a focused physical examination with emphasis on the heart, lungs, airway, and, if regional anesthesia is planned, the site of the regional anesthetic. Most patients need only this focused history and physical examination before undergoing anesthesia. Some, because of coexisting diseases, and others, because of the proposed surgery, will need additional evaluation.

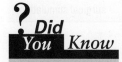

?Did You Know

The duration of required fasting (NPO) before an anesthetic depends on the type of food or liquid ingested. For clear liquids, it is as short as 2 hours, but for fatty foods, it is at least 8 hours.

B. Anesthetic Plan

Anesthesia is often viewed as "putting the patients to sleep." However, there are multiple ways to provide an anesthetic. Choosing the best approach requires an understanding of each patient, his or her medical history, and the proposed procedure. Ideally, an anesthetic should produce the minimum physiologic trespass, optimal surgical conditions, and a comfortable and expeditious recovery.

C. Nil Per Os Status

General anesthesia and sedation place patients at risk for regurgitation and aspiration of gastric contents. This complication can produce problems ranging from mild *chemical pneumonitis* and pneumonia to death (see Chapter 40). To minimize this risk, a patient should fast before an elective anesthetic. The

Table 19-4 Duration of Preoperative Fasting	
Duration of Fasting	**Type of Food or Fluid**
≥2 hr	Clear liquids
≥4 hr	Breast milk
≥6 hr	Infant formula Light meal Nonhuman milk
≥8 hr	Fried or fatty food

From Practice guidelines for preoperative fasting and the use of pharmacologic agents to reduce the risk of pulmonary aspiration: Application to healthy patients undergoing elective procedures: An updated report by the American Society of Anesthesiologists Committee on Standards and Practice Parameters. *Anesthesiology.* 2011;114:495–511, with permission.

duration of fasting (nil per os [NPO]) depends on the type of food or liquid ingested (Table 19-4). Despite these NPO guidelines, patients may take oral medications with a sip of water on the day of surgery (see Chapter 16).

There are exceptions to these rules. Emergency surgeries must begin regardless of the duration of fasting. Trauma patients, those in severe pain, and those with nausea and vomiting or intestinal obstruction may have full stomachs regardless of how long they have been NPO. For these patients, the anesthesiologist may choose a *"rapid sequence"* induction to quickly secure the airway and minimize the risk of aspiration. Also, due to the physiologic changes of pregnancy, parturients are treated as having a full stomach regardless of their last food or liquid intake (see Chapter 31).

D. Informed Consent

The last step in the preoperative evaluation is obtaining informed consent, which should be targeted to the patient's specific risks and concerns. Disclose pertinent risks and allow the patient to ask questions. In some cases (i.e., minors), a legal guardian or medical proxy will give consent. Regardless, it is important for the patient to understand and agree with the anesthetic plan. Rarely, in a life-threatening emergency, anesthesia and surgery may proceed without informed consent.

E. Premedication

Many patients are anxious when they are getting ready to have surgery. A thorough preoperative consultation with an anesthesiologist is the best way to relieve a patient's anxiety (2). In addition, patients sometimes receive a small dose of intravenous benzodiazepine (i.e., midazolam) for additional anxiolysis before entering the operating room. Midazolam should be used carefully. Oversedated patients may not cooperate with moving and positioning in the operating room. In outpatient settings, even small doses of midazolam can delay discharge. The elderly are especially sensitive to its sedating effects.

III. Intraoperative Management

Although complications can occur at any time during an anesthetic, *induction* and *emergence* are especially fraught. During induction, the anesthesiologist administers drugs that render the patient unconscious and have significant cardiac and respiratory effects. Anesthetics can lower the patient's blood pressure by dilating arteries and (mostly) veins, depressing cardiac function, or both.

Unconscious patients have diminished upper airway muscle tone, which can obstruct breathing. Many anesthetics act at the brainstem to decrease respiratory drive. Paralytic agents directly affect respiratory muscles. The anesthesiologist gauges and mitigates these effects with careful monitoring and appropriate interventions.

A. Monitoring

Because most anesthetics depress cardiorespiratory function and surgery can increase heart rate and blood pressure, anesthesiologists use both noninvasive and invasive methods to monitor the patient. The most important of these monitors are looking at the patient to help assess oxygenation and perfusion, listening to breath sounds to detect airway problems, bronchospasm, and pulmonary edema, and touching the patient's skin for clues about perfusion and body temperature.

Routine noninvasive monitors include electrocardiogram, blood pressure, pulse oximetry, capnography, and temperature. The electrocardiogram provides information about cardiac rate and rhythm and may detect myocardial ischemia. Blood pressure can vary depending on the depth of anesthesia, the degree of surgical stimulation, and the patient's volume status. Pulse oximetry provides critical information about the adequacy of oxygenation and detects the presence of pulsatile blood flow. Capnometry and capnography detect the presence and adequacy of ventilation. Lastly, changes in body temperature occur routinely during anesthesia, and hypo- and hyperthermia are possible.

When paralytic agents are used during an anesthetic, neuromuscular function should be evaluated with a **twitch monitor**. This device consists of a pair of electrodes placed over a motor nerve (usually the ulnar or facial nerve). The electrodes are connected to a device that delivers a reproducible electrical stimulus. The most commonly used stimulus pattern is called a train-of-four (TOF), consisting of four equal pulses delivered at half-second intervals. In patients with normal neuromuscular function, these four pulses will elicit four equal muscular twitches. Stimulating the ulnar nerve will trigger finger flexion and thumb adduction. If the electrodes are on the facial nerve, the orbicularis oculi muscle causes the patient to wink. During onset of muscle paralysis, all four twitches will decrease at the same time and may completely disappear. As the effects of the nondepolarizing muscle relaxant begin to wane, the twitches reappear in a different pattern. Initially, only the first twitch appears. As neuromuscular function recovers further, the other twitches reappear. However, the first twitch (T1) is stronger than the subsequent twitches. The ratio of the fourth twitch (T4) to T1 is a measure of neuromuscular function. When T4:T1 is ≥0.9, the patient should be able to breathe normally and have intact upper airway reflexes (see Chapter 11). Incomplete recovery of neuromuscular function is common and is associated with hypoxemia, airway obstruction, and an increased risk of postoperative pulmonary complications (3).

Some operations risk major blood loss. Hemodynamically unstable patients can be sensitive to the effects of anesthetic drugs. In these situations, the anesthesiologist may choose invasive methods such as intra-arterial catheters for blood pressure monitoring, central venous or pulmonary artery catheters to follow changes in blood volume and cardiac output, and transesophageal echocardiography to evaluate cardiac filling and function.

B. Time Out

Wrong-site, wrong-side, and wrong-patient surgeries still occur. A universal protocol has been developed by the Joint Commission on Accreditation of Healthcare Organizations and numerous professional organizations to help prevent these

? *Did*
You Know

Using a train-of-four stimulus pattern during the onset of muscle paralysis with a nondepolarizing agent, all four twitches decrease or disappear at the same time. However, as the muscle relaxant effects wear off, the twitches reappear gradually beginning with only one twitch.

SURGICAL SAFETY CHECKLIST (FIRST EDITION)

World Health Organization

Before induction of anaesthesia ▶▶▶▶▶▶▶▶ Before skin incision ▶▶▶▶▶▶▶▶▶▶▶▶ Before patient leaves operating room

SIGN IN

☐ PATIENT HAS CONFIRMED
• IDENTITY
• SITE
• PROCEDURE
• CONSENT

☐ SITE MARKED/NOT APPLICABLE

☐ ANAESTHESIA SAFETY CHECK COMPLETED

☐ PULSE OXIMETER ON PATIENT AND FUNCTIONING

DOES PATIENT HAVE A:

KNOWN ALLERGY?
☐ NO
☐ YES

DIFFICULT AIRWAY/ASPIRATION RISK?
☐ NO
☐ YES, AND EQUIPMENT/ASSISTANCE AVAILABLE

RISK OF >500ML BLOOD LOSS
(7ML/KG IN CHILDREN)?
☐ NO
☐ YES, AND ADEQUATE INTRAVENOUS ACCESS AND FLUIDS PLANNED

TIME OUT

☐ CONFIRM ALL TEAM MEMBERS HAVE INTRODUCED THEMSELVES BY NAME AND ROLE

☐ SURGEON, ANAESTHESIA PROFESSIONAL AND NURSE VERBALLY CONFIRM
• PATIENT
• SITE
• PROCEDURE

ANTICIPATED CRITICAL EVENTS

☐ SURGEON REVIEWS: WHAT ARE THE CRITICAL OR UNEXPECTED STEPS, OPERATIVE DURATION, ANTICIPATED BLOOD LOSS?

☐ ANAESTHESIA TEAM REVIEWS: ARE THERE ANY PATIENT-SPECIFIC CONCERNS?

☐ NURSING TEAM REVIEWS: HAS STERILITY (INCLUDING INDICATOR RESULTS) BEEN CONFIRMED? ARE THERE EQUIPMENT ISSUES OR ANY CONCERNS?

HAS ANTIBIOTIC PROPHYLAXIS BEEN GIVEN WITHIN THE LAST 60 MINUTES?
☐ YES
☐ NOT APPLICABLE

IS ESSENTIAL IMAGING DISPLAYED?
☐ YES
☐ NOT APPLICABLE

SIGN OUT

NURSE VERBALLY CONFIRMS WITH THE TEAM:

☐ THE NAME OF THE PROCEDURE RECORDED

☐ THAT INSTRUMENT, SPONGE AND NEEDLE COUNTS ARE CORRECT (OR NOT APPLICABLE)

☐ HOW THE SPECIMEN IS LABELLED (INCLUDING PATIENT NAME)

☐ WHETHER THERE ARE ANY EQUIPMENT PROBLEMS TO BE ADDRESSED

☐ SURGEON, ANAESTHESIA PROFESSIONAL AND NURSE REVIEW THE KEY CONCERNS FOR RECOVERY AND MANAGEMENT OF THIS PATIENT

THIS CHECKLIST IS NOT INTENDED TO BE COMPREHENSIVE. ADDITIONS AND MODIFICATIONS TO FIT LOCAL PRACTICE ARE ENCOURAGED.

Figure 19-1 World Health Organization Surgical Safety Checklist. Available at: http://www.who.int/patientsafety/safesurgery/tools_resources/SSSL_Checklist_final Jun08.pdf?ua=1.

errors. Although each institution will have its own version of the *universal protocol*, three elements remain standard. First, a preprocedure verification confirms the patient's identity, the type of surgery, and the site or side of the procedure. Second, the physician performing the surgery or procedure places a clearly visible, distinctive marking on the site of incision. Lastly, a "time out" occurs immediately before beginning the procedure to confirm that steps one and two have been performed correctly and the incision is about to occur at the correct site and side.

The World Health Organization (WHO) has developed a checklist, "The WHO Surgical Safety Checklist" (Fig. 19-1), for use in operating rooms worldwide to increase safety and reliability. Implementation of this checklist decreases surgery complications by more than one-third and deaths by almost half (4). Many hospitals have expanded their universal protocol to include some iteration of this surgical safety checklist. There are two key elements that help ensure successful use of the universal protocol and the surgical safety checklist. First, everyone in the operating room stops whatever they are doing and actively participates. Second, *anyone* in the room can stop the process and voice questions or concerns.

C. Induction

General anesthesia begins with induction. Babies and small children commonly undergo an inhalation induction (see Chapter 33). Here, the patient breathes increasing amounts of anesthetic through a facemask until he or she becomes unconscious. This approach avoids the need for intravenous access while the child is awake. Inhalation induction can also be used in adults. It may be chosen for patients who are needle phobic or those with poor peripheral venous access.

Table 19-5	Induction Agents		
Agent	**Advantages**	**Disadvantages**	**Comments**
Propofol	• Rapid onset • Short duration • Rapid recovery • No residual effects	• Burns on injection • Hypotension • Can cause respiratory depression, especially when given with opioids • Not an analgesic	Most commonly used induction agent
Methohexital	• Rapid onset • Short duration	• Postoperative nausea and vomiting more likely vs. propofol • Contraindicated in patients with acute intermittent porphyria	Often used to induce anesthesia for electroconvulsive shock treatment
Etomidate	• Minimal hemodynamic effects	• Adrenal suppression • May increase mortality	
Ketamine	• Minimal hemodynamic depression (releases catecholamines) • Maintains respiration and airway reflexes • Has analgesic effects	• Dysphoria and hallucinations • Hypertension and tachycardia	

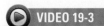

VIDEO 19-2

Drawing Medication From A Vial

Because intravenous induction is rapid and reliable, it is the more common choice for older children and adults. The anesthetist usually injects a combination of drugs chosen to quickly anesthetize the patient and provide optimal conditions for airway management and surgery. Today, propofol is the most commonly used intravenous induction agent. This drug has a rapid onset (<60 seconds). Small doses provide sedation and anxiolysis. Larger doses cause loss of consciousness. The patient will remain unconscious for 3 to 5 minutes after an induction dose of propofol. Other induction agents include methohexital, etomidate, and ketamine (Table 19-5).

Propofol often burns when injected and does a poor job of blunting the hemodynamic responses to painful stimuli like endotracheal intubation. Intravenous lidocaine can dull the burning and limit the blood pressure and heart rate response to laryngoscopy and intubation. Fast-acting opioids like fentanyl, sufentanil, or remifentanil also are effective at blocking the cardiovascular responses to laryngoscopy and surgery. Less commonly, *β-adrenergic blocking drugs* also can be used for this purpose.

VIDEO 19-3

Torn Endotracheal Tube Cuff

Some operations require endotracheal intubation and skeletal muscle relaxation. In commonly used doses, propofol does not induce skeletal muscle relaxation. So, after the patient loses consciousness, the anesthetist will often inject a paralytic agent (Table 19-6). These drugs act at the neuromuscular junction to produce muscle weakness or total paralysis.

Agent	Mechanism of Action	Onset	Duration	Side Effects	Comments
Succinylcholine	Depolarizing[a]	Rapid: 30–60 sec	Short: 10–15 min Can cause prolonged blockade if given as an infusion, in repeat doses, or to patients with atypical or absent pseudo-cholinesterase	• Tachycardia • Bradycardia • Myalgia • Hyperkalemia • Rhabdomyolysis • Malignant hyperthermia • Increased intraocular pressure	Almost never used in children
Pancuronium	Nondepolarizing[b]	4–5 min	75–90 min	• Hypertension • Tachycardia	
Vecuronium	Nondepolarizing[b]	3 min	30–45 min		Duration may increase with repeat doses in patients with renal failure
Rocuronium	Nondepolarizing[b]	1–2 min	30–45 min		
Cisatracurium	Nondepolarizing[b]	2–3 min	45 min		Self-destructs in plasma (Hoffman elimination)

Table 19-6   Muscle Relaxants

[a]Depolarizing muscle relaxants produce noncompetitive neuromuscular blockade. Their actions cannot be reversed by anticholinesterases.
[b]Nondepolarizing muscle relaxants produce competitive neuromuscular blockade. Their residual actions can be reversed by an anticholinesterase.

D. Airway

Anesthetics impair respiration in many ways. Sedatives like midazolam and propofol relax oropharyngeal muscles and can produce airway obstruction, especially in patients with obstructive sleep apnea. Opioids, like fentanyl, and potent inhaled agents, like sevoflurane, depress the ventilatory response to carbon dioxide. Patients who receive propofol and fentanyl often stop breathing altogether. Potent inhaled agents may also obliterate the respiratory response to hypoxemia. *Paralytic drugs*, such as succinylcholine and rocuronium, relax oropharyngeal muscles, impair airway protective reflexes, and can paralyze respiratory muscles. For these reasons, the anesthetist must be ready to assist or control the patient's breathing.

Because of these effects on the airway and respiration, patients usually breathe 100% oxygen for a few minutes before induction of anesthesia. This step, used to replace the nitrogen in a patient's lungs with oxygen, is called *preoxygenation* or *denitrogenation*. This extra oxygen in the patient's lungs helps maintain oxygenation of the blood during the periods of apnea and airway obstruction that can occur during induction of anesthesia. In normal circumstances, the anesthetist will allow 3 minutes for complete denitrogenation. However, in emergencies, four tidal breaths of 100% oxygen will suffice.

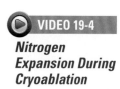

VIDEO 19-4

Nitrogen Expansion During Cryoablation

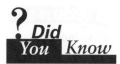

?Did You Know

Preoxygenation is also referred to as denitrogenation because the administration of 100% oxygen causes the nitrogen in the lungs to be completely replaced by oxygen.

If induction of anesthesia merely causes airway obstruction, chin lift and jaw thrust maneuvers may open the airway and allow spontaneous ventilation to resume. If respiration is significantly depressed or the patient is apneic, the anesthetist must begin providing artificial respirations. Initially, the facemask and breathing bag attached to the anesthesia machine are used. An oral or nasal airway may be inserted to help relieve upper airway obstruction and improve ventilation. A *supraglottic airway* or an endotracheal tube provides a hands-free airway and allows assisted or controlled ventilation. The most commonly used supraglottic airway is the laryngeal mask airway (LMA). This device sits in the posterior pharynx and separates the larynx from the rest of the upper airway. It can be used in spontaneously breathing patients, and, in certain circumstances, to provide controlled ventilation.

Endotracheal (ET) tubes are inserted through the larynx and into the trachea. Most ET tubes used in adults have a cuff at their tracheal end to separate the lungs from the pharynx. This cuff allows positive pressure ventilation and can protect the lungs against aspiration of gastric contents.

For many surgeries, either the LMA or the ET tube can be safely used. Advantages of the LMA include:

- It can be inserted without using paralytic agents
- It can be inserted blindly
- It is unlikely to damage teeth, gums, or vocal cords
- It is less likely than an ET tube to cause hoarseness, coughing, sore throat, or laryngospasm
- It is less stimulating than an ET tube so less anesthesia is required to put it in or keep it in.

The main advantage of the ET tube is that it allows higher inflation pressures during controlled ventilation.

E. The Anesthesia Record

Medical students and others with no formal training often performed early anesthetics. Complications were routine and mortality was all too common. In 1895, one such medical student was Harvey Cushing (later a well-known neurosurgeon). Cushing hoped that by keeping a record of the drugs he used and the patient's pulse and respirations, he would learn from his mistakes and administer anesthetics more safely. From Cushing's idea came the modern anesthesia record. Today's anesthesia record contains far more information but still serves much the same purpose as in Cushing's time.

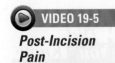

VIDEO 19-5

Post-Incision Pain

F. Maintenance

The *maintenance* phase of the anesthetic begins after induction when the airway is secured. The anesthetist may use various intravenous or inhaled agents to keep a patient unconscious throughout surgery. Most often, a balanced combination of intravenous and inhaled drugs provides the elements of general anesthesia (Table 19-7). Sometimes, only inhaled agents are used (Table 19-7). In other situations, the anesthetist might only use a total intravenous anesthetic.

The goal of anesthesia is to ensure unconsciousness and amnesia, immobility, muscle relaxation, and blunted sympathetic reflexes. Both propofol, if given as a continuous infusion, and the potent inhaled agents provide amnesia and block purposeful movement in response to surgical stimulation.

Paralytic agents (muscle relaxants) produce immobility (Table 19-6). However, paralytic agents do not produce unconsciousness or amnesia and, if used

Table 19-7	Inhaled Anesthetics
Agent	**Comment**
Desflurane	Most insoluble of the potent agents. Most rapid wake up. Pungent aroma can irritate airway. Causes sympathetic stimulation during induction.
Isoflurane	Most potent and most soluble of the currently used agents. Slowest emergence, especially after longer cases. Pungent aroma. Can cause tachycardia during induction.
Nitrous oxide	Not potent enough to produce anesthesia on its own. Often used in combination with other potent agents.
Sevoflurane	Pleasant aroma. Good choice for inhalation induction. No sympathetic stimulation.

improperly, can leave the patient awake but paralyzed. Intra-abdominal and intrathoracic surgeries often require skeletal muscle relaxation for optimal operating conditions. Muscle relaxants are useful in this situation but must be titrated carefully. Not enough and the surgeon may have difficulty exposing the operative site or the patient may cough or move during a delicate part of the procedure. Give too much and the patient may still be paralyzed at the end of the surgery. The anesthesiologist decides how much muscle relaxant to give by following the TOF. A patient with two or three of the four twitches should be adequately relaxed for most operations but not so paralyzed that the neuromuscular blocking drug cannot be reversed at the end of the surgery.

Opioids are commonly given during general anesthesia (Table 19-8). They decrease the dose of potent inhaled agent (or propofol) needed to keep the patient unconscious and immobile. They also help minimize the cardiac depression associated with these drugs. During induction, isoflurane and desflurane

Table 19-8	Opioids		
Opioid	**Onset**	**Duration**	**Comment**
Remifentanil	Rapid	Brief	Rapidly hydrolyzed by nonspecific esterases. Does not accumulate even with prolonged administration.
Fentanyl	1–2 min (maximum effect within 30 min)	15–20 min	Small doses have a short duration because they are rapidly redistributed from central to peripheral tissues. Larger doses or repeat injection causes accumulation of drug in the peripheral tissues producing longer duration of analgesia.
Hydromorphone	15–30 min (maximum effect may not occur for up to 150 min)	Duration 3–5 hr	

often produce tachycardia. Small intravenous doses of opioid can block this effect. Lastly, intraoperative opioids may provide *postoperative analgesia* but may cause respiratory depression, nausea, and vomiting. Paradoxically, intraoperative opioids may increase postoperative pain (5).

Surgical stimulation can produce hypertension and tachycardia, even when a patient is adequately anesthetized. Because some patients may not tolerate this increased cardiac workload, the anesthetist often tries to minimize these sympathetic responses by deepening the anesthetic with a potent agent, or by injecting intravenous opioids. In some situations, the anesthesiologist may numb the affected area with a peripheral nerve block or the surgeon may inject local anesthetic directly into the operative site. Lastly, sympathetic blocking drugs such as labetalol, esmolol, or metoprolol can blunt these hemodynamic responses and may decrease postoperative pain compared with the more commonly used opioids (6).

G. Fluid Management

Almost all patients receiving general anesthesia will have at least one intravenous catheter inserted. This catheter is used both to give medications and to infuse fluids (see Chapter 23). Most patients need only enough fluids to keep their intravenous catheters patent. However, many surgeries cause significant bleeding. Trauma victims also may suffer considerable blood loss even before arriving in the operating room. These patients need additional intravenous fluid.

The most commonly used intravenous fluids are called *crystalloids*. These fluids are isotonic solutions formulated to mimic the body's electrolyte composition. Crystalloids are inexpensive and do not require special storage. Although crystalloids can be life-saving when given to a patient suffering significant bleeding, they are inefficient volume expanders. Crystalloids are isotonic, but they are hypo-osmolar. Only about one-third of infused crystalloid stays within the vascular system. The remainder leaks out of the vasculature and causes interstitial edema throughout the body.

An alternate class of fluids, *colloids* contains protein (albumin) or starch to maintain osmotic pressure within the blood vessels. Colloids are better volume expanders than crystalloids, but they are expensive and have undesirable side effects (e.g., platelet inhibition and possible renal toxicity). Despite years of study, colloids have never been shown to improve outcome compared with the less-expensive but less-efficient crystalloids. As long as volume status is maintained, most patients can tolerate a remarkable degree of anemia. However, some will require blood and blood products (see Chapter 24).

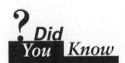

?Did You Know

Crystalloids are isotonic, but they are also hypo-osmolar. Only about one-third of infused crystalloid stays within the vascular system with the remainder leaking into the tissues.

H. Temperature

Anesthesia impairs the body's ability to maintain temperature. After induction, core temperature drops as body heat transfers to peripheral tissues. Anesthetics lower the temperature at which peripheral blood vessels constrict in response to cold. In addition, the operating room environment offers several avenues for heat loss: *radiation, conduction, convection, and evaporation*. Patients lose most heat through radiation from their exposed skin to the surrounding cold environment. Conductive heat loss occurs through contact between the patient and the cold operating room table, other equipment, and to the air layer surrounding the skin. The body loses heat through convection when this warmed air circulates away from the patient and more heat transfers to the new layer of colder air. Evaporation from skin and respiratory mucosa also drains heat from the body. Together, these events cause core body temperature to decrease about 1 degree shortly after induction of anesthesia. Body temperature will continue to fall for the next 3 to 5 hours until a new equilibrium is established.

There are many ways to help maintain the patient's temperature. Prewarming can help prevent the initial redistribution of heat from core to periphery. Warming the operating room is another option. This step is often taken for especially vulnerable patients like small children and trauma victims. However, an operating room that is warm enough for patient comfort is often too warm for the surgical team. One of the most effective ways to maintain a patient's body temperature is with a forced-air warming blanket. These devices blow warmed air across the patient's skin, helping to prevent conductive and convective heat loss. These devices do not prevent the initial redistribution of body heat and can burn the patient's skin if misused. Radiant heat lamps can be helpful, especially when caring for infants and small children.

I. Emergence

As surgery winds down, anesthesiologists prepare the patient for emergence. They review the patient's hemodynamics and temperature, evaluate the degree of residual neuromuscular blockade, and ensure adequate analgesia for the transition to recovery. At the end of the anesthetic, the patient must be hemodynamically stable and normothermic. Hypothermia can increase oxygen consumption, impair hemostasis, and delay emergence. The unstable patient is better left intubated, ventilated, and sedated until his or her vital signs are normal.

If the patient has received a nondepolarizing muscle relaxant (Table 19-6), the anesthetist will use an anticholinesterase to reverse residual neuromuscular blockade (see Chapter 11). TOF monitoring can help determine the amount of anticholinesterase needed. Sometimes, the patient is profoundly paralyzed at the end of surgery (no twitches after TOF stimulation). Anticholinesterase medications will not adequately reverse this degree of paralysis. These patients should remain intubated and ventilated until spontaneous recovery from the paralytic drug begins.

In addition to assessing the patient's readiness for emergence, the anesthetist begins to decrease or discontinue any intravenous or inhaled anesthetics. The timing of these changes depends on the type of drugs given and the duration of their administration. For example, remifentanil is rapidly broken down by plasma esterases. Its action terminates promptly and predictably no matter how long the anesthetic. On the other hand, isoflurane and sevoflurane are fat soluble and accumulate in the patient's adipose tissues (isoflurane more so than sevoflurane). With these drugs, the longer the anesthetic, the longer the emergence. The anesthetist uses his or her knowledge of the drug kinetics to time the end of the anesthetic.

Removing the endotracheal tube (extubation) is the trickiest part of the emergence process. Before the patient can be extubated, he or she must have reestablished adequate ventilation and respiration. In addition, the patient must have appropriate protective airway reflexes. Some patients can be extubated "deep" before protective airway reflexes have fully recovered, as long as they are ventilating adequately and the anesthetist is prepared to help maintain an open airway. Others should remain intubated until they are awake and can follow commands. Risks of extubating too soon include airway obstruction, aspiration, and *laryngospasm*. Delaying extubation too long can cause hypertension and tachycardia, increased intracranial pressure, and bleeding,

Table 19-9	The I-PASS Mnemonic	
I	Illness severity	• Stable, "watcher," unstable
P	Patient summary	• Summary statement • Events leading to admission • Hospital course • Assessment • Plan
A	Action list	• To do list • Timeline and ownership
S	Situation awareness and contingency planning	• Know what is going on • Plan for what might happen
S	Synthesis by receiver	• Receiver summarizes what was heard • Asks questions • Restates key action items

Modified from Starmer AJ, Spector ND, Srivastava R, et al. I-PASS, a mnemonic to standardize verbal handoffs. *Pediatrics.* 2012;129:201–205.

especially in patients who have undergone surgery about the head and neck. Once the patient is extubated and ventilating adequately, it is time to go to the recovery room or postanesthesia care unit (PACU).

IV. Postoperative Care

Once the patient arrives in the PACU, the anesthetist must safely transfer care to the recovery room nurse. This transfer of care, or handoff, requires clear and effective communication between health care providers. Lapses in communication during patient care handoffs can lead to errors and harm. Mnemonics have been developed to try to standardize handoff communication. Two such mnemonics are I-PASS (Table 19-9) and ISBAR (*I*ntroduction, *S*ituation, *B*ackground, *A*ssessment, and *R*esponse). A key part of these structured communication tools is the response. The person assuming care for the patient (i.e., the PACU nurse) responds to the person transferring care (i.e., the anesthetist) to confirm that he or she heard and understands the relayed information. As with the "WHO Safe Surgery Checklist," using a structured handoff tool can improve patient safety (7).

V. Summary

Although the drugs and techniques may differ from anesthetist to anesthetist, some things remain constant with all anesthetics. The anesthesiologist and anesthetist strive to guide the patient's safe passage through the surgical experience by understanding the patient's medical and surgical history. They use their knowledge of physiology and pharmacology to plan and conduct a safe and effective anesthetic. Throughout the perioperative period, they maintain constant vigilance to ensure the patient's well-being.

References

1. Aranake A, Gradwohl S, Ben-Abdallah A, et al. Increased risk of intraoperative awareness in patients with a history of awareness. *Anesthesiology.* 2013;119:1275–1283.

2. Egbert LD, Jackson SH. Therapeutic benefit of the anesthesiologist–patient relationship. *Anesthesiology.* 2013;119:1465–1468.
3. Murphy GS, Brull SJ. Residual neuromuscular block: Lessons unlearned. Part I: Definitions, incidence, and adverse physiologic effects of residual neuromuscular block. *Anesth Analg.* 2010;111:120–128.
4. de Vries EN, Prins HA, Crolla RM, et al. Effect of a comprehensive surgical safety system on patient outcomes. *N Engl J Med.* 2010;363:1928–1937.
5. Guignard B, Bossard AE, Coste C, et al. Acute opioid tolerance: Intraoperative remifentanil increases postoperative pain and morphine requirement. *Anesthesiology.* 2000;93:409–417.
6. Collard V, Mistraletti G, Taqi A, et al. Intraoperative esmolol infusion in the absence of opioids spares postoperative fentanyl in patients undergoing ambulatory laparoscopic cholecystectomy. *Anesth Analg.* 2007;105:1255–1262.
7. Starmer AJ, Sectish TC, Simon DW, et al. Rates of medical errors and preventable adverse events among hospitalized children following implementation of a resident handoff bundle. *JAMA.* 2013;310:2262–2270.

Questions

1. A man presents to the emergency room with right lower-quadrant pain. He is diagnosed with acute appendicitis. During the preoperative evaluation, he states that he ate half a sandwich 2 hours ago. How should you proceed?
   A. Cancel the surgery and inform the surgical team that the patient has to be NPO for 8 hours before surgery.
   B. Proceed with surgery because it was only half a sandwich and the risk of aspiration is therefore low.
   C. Proceed with surgery because this is an emergency and the NPO status does not matter.
   D. Proceed with surgery because this is an emergency, but perform rapid sequence induction to minimize the risk of aspiration.

2. Immediately after induction of general anesthesia, the decrease in the patient's temperature is due to:
   A. The low room temperature in the operating room
   B. Evaporation
   C. Heat conduction
   D. Heat redistribution

3. You are administering an anesthetic for an abdominoplasty (tummy tuck). The surgeon requests a deep extubation to prevent "bucking" and potential dehiscence of the surgical wound. Which of the following is correct regarding the criteria for deep extubation?
   A. The surgeon's request is appropriate and in the best interest of the patient; therefore, no further criteria are necessary.
   B. Criteria for deep extubation include easy intubation, easy mask ventilation, and absence of risk factors for aspiration.
   C. The main criterion is the patient's preference after being informed of the risks and benefits.
   D. Deep extubation can be performed once any residual neuromuscular blockade is reversed.

4. You are on call and a 24-year-old gunshot victim is brought to the operating room. The surgeon states that he has to perform an emergent laparotomy to determine the source of bleeding. The patient is not intubated, and the blood pressure is 68/36 mm Hg with a heart rate in the 120s. How would you induce the patient?
   A. Perform a standard induction with propofol. If the hypotension worsens, treat the patient with phenylephrine.
   B. Use etomidate for induction because it causes less hypotension than propofol.
   C. The patient will not tolerate any induction agent, so just intubate the trachea.
   D. Stabilize the patient first. Once the blood pressure approaches normal, proceed with induction.

5. You are asked to obtain informed consent from a patient for an elective cholecystectomy the following day. When meeting the patient, you find him to be confused about the plan and he repeatedly refers to the hospital as his house. His nurse states that she just met the patient for the first time and that the nurse on the previous shift has already left. What do you do next?
   A. Explain the risks and benefits of the anesthetic plan to the patient and obtain his consent.
   B. Call the nearest relative and obtain consent from him or her.
   C. Discuss the patient's mental status with the primary team and determine if he is competent to sign the consent.
   D. Cancel the case.

20 Airway Management

Ron O. Abrons
William H. Rosenblatt

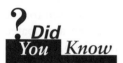
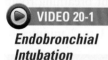
I. Airway Anatomy

The term *airway* refers to the upper airway—consisting of the nasal and oral cavities, pharynx, larynx, trachea, and principal bronchi. The laryngeal skeleton houses and protects the vocal folds, which extend in an anterior–posterior plane from the thyroid cartilage to the arytenoid cartilages. The cricothyroid membrane is an important, externally identifiable structure. In an adult, it typically is identified 1 to 1.5 fingerbreadths below the laryngeal prominence (thyroid notch) (Fig. 20-1).

The signet ring–shaped cricoid cartilage is located at the base of the larynx, suspended by the underside of the cricothyroid ligament. Inferiorly, the trachea measures approximately 15 cm and ends at the carina where it bifurcates into the principal bronchi. Aspirated materials, as well as a deeply inserted *endotracheal tube (ETT)*, tend to gain entry into the right principal bronchus due to its size and less acute angle of divergence from the midline.

There are three clinically important neural innervations of the upper airway. The glossopharyngeal nerve (cranial nerve IX) supplies sensory innervation to the base of the tongue, rostral surface of the epiglottis, and pharynx. The superior laryngeal nerve (branch of vagus nerve X) supplies sensation from the underside of the epiglottis to the surface of the vocal cords and motor innervation to the cricothyroid muscle. The recurrent laryngeal nerve, also a branch of the vagus nerve (cranial nerve X), supplies motor innervation to the remaining muscles of the larynx and sensation to the mucosal surface of the larynx and trachea (Table 20-1; Fig. 20-2).

II. Patient History and Physical Examination

Airway management always begins with a thorough airway-relevant history, including a search for documentation of airway-related events during previous anesthetics. Signs and symptoms related to potentially difficult airway management including aspiration risk should be sought (Table 20-2), as many congenital and acquired syndromes are associated with difficult airway management (Table 20-3).

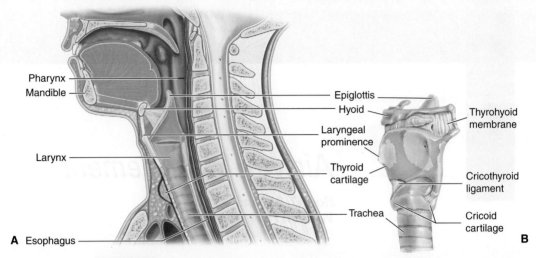

Pharynx
Mandible
Larynx

A   Esophagus

Epiglottis
Hyoid
Laryngeal prominence
Thyroid cartilage
Trachea

Thyrohyoid membrane
Cricothyroid ligament
Cricoid cartilage

B

Figure 20-1 Sagittal view of upper airway anatomy (**A**) and lateral view of laryngeal skeleton (**B**). (From Moore KL, Agur AMR, Dalley AF. *Clinically Oriented Anatomy.* 7th ed. Philadelphia: Wolters Kluwer Health; 2013, with permission.)

Table 20-4 lists the commonly documented airway examination features. Historically, airway assessment has been synonymous with evaluation for the ease of **direct laryngoscopy (DL)**, with the endpoint being the anticipated degree of laryngeal visualization (e.g., Mallampati score) (Fig. 20-3). Unfortunately, efforts to identify attributes that place patients at high risk for difficult laryngoscopy have been only modestly successful (Table 20-5) (1).

III.   Clinical Management of the Airway

A.   Preoxygenation

Preoxygenation (also termed *denitrogenation*) should be practiced in all cases when time allows. Under ideal conditions, a healthy patient breathing room air (fraction of inspired oxygen [FiO_2] = 0.21) will experience oxyhemoglobin desaturation to a level of <90% after approximately 1 to 2 minutes of

Table 20-1A Innervation of the Laryngotracheal Airway		
Nerve	**Motor**[a]	**Sensory**[a]
Glossopharyngeal nerve (cranial nerve IX)	None	Posterior 1/3 of tongue Epiglottis (rostral) Pharynx
Vagus nerve—recurrent laryngeal nerve (cranial nerve X)	Larynx (except cricothyroid)	Larynx: mucosal surface Trachea: mucosal surface
Vagus nerve—internal branch of the Supersior Laryngeal Nerve (cranial nerve X)	None	Epiglottis (dorsal) Vocal cords
Vagus nerve—external branch of the Supersior Laryngeal Nerve (cranial nerve X)	Cricothyroid	None

[a]Predominant action.

Table 20-1B Muscles of the Larynx (Innervation and Action)

Muscle	Innervation	Main Action(s)
Cricothyroid	External laryngeal nerve (from CN X)	Stretches and tenses vocal ligament
Thyro-arytenoid[a]	Recurrent laryngeal nerve (from CN X)	Relaxes vocal ligament
Posterior crico-arytenoid	Recurrent laryngeal nerve (from CN X)	Abducts vocal folds
Lateral crico-arytenoid	Recurrent laryngeal nerve (from CN X)	Adducts vocal folds (interligamentous portion)
Transverse and oblique arytenoids[b]	Recurrent laryngeal nerve (from CN X)	Adduct arytenoid cartilages (adducting intercartilaginous portion of vocal folds, closing posterior rima glottidis)
Vocalis[c]	Recurrent laryngeal nerve (from CN X)	Relaxes posterior vocal ligament while maintaining (or increasing) tension of anterior part

From Moore KL, Agur AMR, Dalley AF. *Clinically Oriented Anatomy.* 7th ed. Philadelphia: Wolters Kluwer Health; 2013:Table 8-5, with permission.

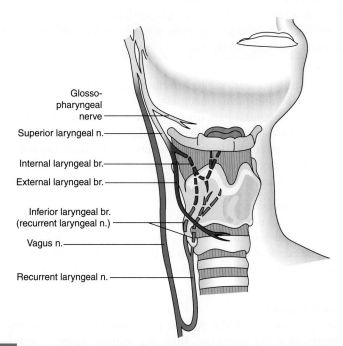

Glosso-pharyngeal nerve
Superior laryngeal n.
Internal laryngeal br.
External laryngeal br.
Inferior laryngeal br. (recurrent laryngeal n.)
Vagus n.
Recurrent laryngeal n.

Figure 20-2 Laryngeal innervation. The dashed lines are nerve branches within the laryngeal-tracheal tree from the branches of the glossopharyngeal and vagus cranial nerves. (From Rosenblatt WH, Sukhupragarn W. Airway management. In: Barash PG, Cullen BF, Stoelting RK, et al., eds. *Clinical Anesthesia.* 7th ed. Philadelphia: Lippincott Williams & Wilkins; 2013:790, with permission.)

Table 20-2   Conditions with Airway Management Implications
Increased Risk of Difficult Laryngoscopy, Mask Ventilation, or Supraglottic Airway Ventilation

History of failed or traumatic airway management
    Dental damage or prolonged airway soreness after a previous anesthetic
History of head/neck surgery or radiation therapy
Various congenital and acquired syndromes (Table 20-3)
Supraglottic pathology
    Obstructive sleep apnea
    Lingual tonsil hyperplasia
Acute airway pathology
    Airway cyst or tumor
    Airway bleeding
    Stridor
Cervical spine disease or limited range of motion
Temporomandibular joint disease

Increased Aspiration Risk
Recent meal Acute trauma Acute gastrointestinal pathology Acute narcotic therapy Significant gastroesophageal reflux Current intensive care unit admission Pregnancy (gestational age ≥12 weeks) Immediate postpartum (before second postpartum day) Systemic disease associated gastroparesis: diabetes mellitus, collagen vascular disease, advanced Parkinson disease

VIDEO 20-2
Vocal Cord Polyp Ball-Valve Effect

VIDEO 20-3
Temporomandibular Joint Assessment

apnea. In the same patient, several minutes of preoxygenation with 100% oxygen (O_2) via a tight-fitting facemask may support ≥8 minutes of apnea before desaturation occurs. Patients with pulmonary disease, obesity, or conditions affecting metabolism frequently evidence desaturation sooner, owing to increased O_2 extraction, decreased functional residual capacity, or right-to-left transpulmonary shunting. The most common reason for suboptimal preoxygenation is a loose-fitting mask, which allows entrainment of room air.

B. Facemask Ventilation
The anesthesia facemask is gently held on the patient's face with the thumb and first finger of the left hand, leaving the right hand free for other tasks. Air leak around the edges of the mask can be prevented by gentle downward pressure. A two-handed grip or an elastic "mask strap" may be used to complement the left-hand grip.

C. Patient Positioning
Appropriate positioning of the patient is paramount for delivering *positive pressure ventilation* via facemask. With the patient supine, "ramped" or in reverse Trendelenburg position, the neck is flexed by 35 degrees and the head extended by 15 degrees. This *sniffing position* improves mask ventilation by anteriorizing the base of the tongue and the epiglottis.

Dentures left in place may improve the mask seal for an edentulous patient. The advantage of this must be weighed against the risk of denture

Table 20-3   Syndromes Associated with Difficult Airway Management

Pathologic Condition	Features Affecting Airway Management
Congenital	
Pierre Robin syndrome	Micrognathia, macroglossia, glossoptossis, cleft soft palate
Treacher Collins syndrome	Malar and mandibular hypoplasia, microstomia, choanal atresia
Down syndrome	Macroglossia, microcephaly, cervical spine abnormalities
Klippel-Feil syndrome	Congenital fusion of cervical vertebrae, decreased cervical range of motion
Cretinism	Macroglossia, compression or deviation of larynx/trachea by goiter
Cri du chat syndrome	Micrognathia, laryngomalacia, stridor
Acquired Infections	
Epiglottitis	Epiglottal edema
Croup	Laryngeal edema
Papillomatosis	Obstructive papillomas
Intraoral/retropharyngeal abscess	Airway distortion/stenosis, trismus
Ludwig angina	Airway distortion/stenosis, trismus
Arthritis	
Rheumatoid arthritis	Restricted cervical spine mobility, atlantoaxial instability
Ankylosing spondylitis	Ankylosis/immobility of cervical spine and temporomandibular joints
Tumors	
Cystic hygroma, lipoma, adenoma, goiter	Airway distortion or stenosis
Carcinoma of tongue/ larynx/thyroid	Airway distortion or stenosis, fixation of larynx or adjacent tissues
Trauma	
Head/facial/cervical spine	Airway edema or hemorrhage, unstable facial or mandibular fractures, intralaryngeal damage
Miscellaneous Conditions	
Morbid obesity	Short, thick neck, large tongue and obstructive sleep apnea are likely
Acromegaly	Macroglossia, prognathism
Acute burns	Airway edema, bronchospasm, decreased apnea tolerance

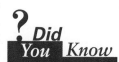

VIDEO 20-4

Bronchospasm Under Anesthesia

displacement or damage. Dentures should be removed after the airway is secured.

D. Difficult Mask Ventilation

Table 20-6 describes five independent clinical predictors for difficult mask ventilation (2). Normally, no more than 20 to 25 cm water (H_2O) pressure in the anesthesia circuit (created by squeezing the reservoir bag) is needed to inflate the lungs. If more pressure is required to produce adequate lung inflation, the anesthesiologist should re-evaluate the situation. This includes adjusting the mask fit, seeking aid with the mask hold, or considering adjuncts such as oral and nasal airways. Oral and nasal airways can bypass obstruction by creating an artificial passage through the pharynx and hypopharynx. Nasal airways are less likely to stimulate cough, gag, or vomiting in the lightly anesthetized patient but more likely to cause epistaxis, thus typically avoided in patients at high risk for nasal bleeding.

? Did You Know

The leading cause of airway obstruction during induction of anesthesia is the tongue.

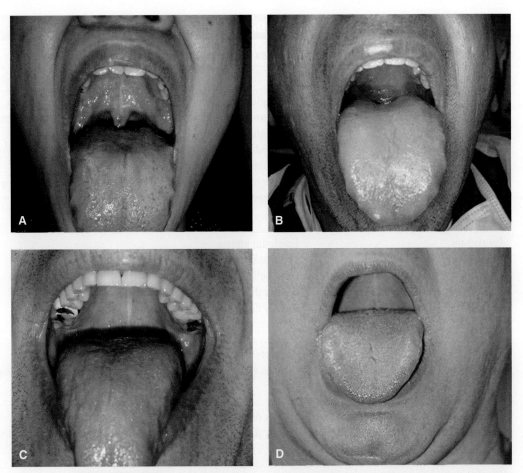

Figure 20-3 Mallampati/Samsoon-Young classification of the oropharyngeal view. **A:** Class I: Uvula, faucial pillars, soft palate visible. **B:** Class II: Faucial pillars, soft palate visible. **C:** Class III: Soft and hard palate visible. **D:** Class IV: Hard palate visible only (added by Samsoon and Young). (From Rosenblatt WH, Sukhupragarn W. Airway management. In: Barash PG, Cullen BF, Stoelting RK, et al., eds. *Clinical Anesthesia.* 7th ed. Philadelphia: Lippincott Williams & Wilkins; 2013:775, with permission.)

Obstruction to mask ventilation may be caused by *laryngospasm,* a local reflex closure of the vocal folds. Laryngospasm may be triggered by a foreign body (e.g., oral or nasal airway), saliva, blood, or vomitus touching the glottis. It may also result from pain or visceral stimulation. Management of laryngospasm consists of removing the offending stimulus (if identified), administering oxygen with continuous positive airway pressure, deepening the plane of the anesthesia, and, if other maneuvers are unsuccessful, using a rapid-acting muscle relaxant (3).

E. Supraglottic Airways

Airway devices that isolate the airway above the vocal cords are referred to as *supraglottic airways* (SGAs). These may be advantageous in patients with reactive airway disease as they lead to less reversible bronchospasm than endotracheal tubes. A wide variety of SGA devices are currently available. The original SGA, the laryngeal mask airway (LMA), is composed of a perilaryngeal mask and an airway barrel. The mask has an inflatable cuff, which fills the hypopharyngeal space, creating a seal that allows positive pressure ventilation with up to 20 cm H_2O pressure.

Table 20-4	Physical Examination Features with Airway Management Implications
Physical Examination Feature	**Significance**
Mouth opening	Difficult blade insertion/tongue displacement if limited
Jaw protrusion	Difficult tongue displacement if limited
Dentition	Obstructed view (if large central incisors), increased risk of dental trauma (if poor or restored dentition), difficult mask ventilation (if edentulous)
Retrognathia	Difficult tongue displacement
Thyromental distance	Reflects neck mobility and degree of retrognathia
Mallampati grade	Describes the relationship between mouth opening, tongue size, and pharyngeal space
Presence of beard	Difficult mask seal
Airway pathology	Potential for difficult mask ventilation (obstructive masses/tissue, atypical facial contours) and laryngoscopy (friable tissue, atypical or absent landmarks, and limited mouth opening, jaw protrusion, tongue displacement, and neck mobility)

▶ **VIDEO 20-5**

Torus Mandibularis

Table 20-5	Summary of Pooled Sensitivity and Specificity of Commonly Used Methods of Airway Evaluation	
Examination	**Sensitivity (%)**	**Specificity (%)**
Mouth opening	46	89
Thyromental distance	20	94
Mallampati classification	49	86

From Shiga T, Wajima Z, Inoue T, et al. Predicting difficult intubation in apparently normal patients: A meta-analysis of bedside screening test performance. *Anesthesiology.* 2005;103:429.

Table 20-6	Independent Risk Factors for Difficult Mask Ventilation
Risk Factors	**Odds Ratio**
Presence of a beard	3.18
Body mass index >26 kg/m^2	2.75
Lack of teeth	2.28
Age >55 yrs	2.26
History of snoring	1.84

From Langeron O, Masso E, Huraux C, et al. Prediction of difficult mask ventilation. *Anesthesiology.* 2000;92:1229.

The manufacturer recommends that the clinician choose the largest size LMA that fits comfortably within the oral cavity. For use, the LMA mask is completely deflated. The patient's neck is extended and the superior surface of the mask is placed against the hard palate. Force is applied by the index finger in an upward direction toward the top of the patient's head, and the mask is allowed to follow the palate into the pharynx and hypopharynx. Next, the LMA is inflated to the minimum pressure that allows ventilation to 20 cm H_2O without an air leak. The intracuff pressure should never exceed 60 cm H_2O and should be periodically monitored if nitrous oxide is used. When an adequate seal cannot be obtained with 60 cm H_2O cuff pressure, the LMA's positioning or sizing should be re-evaluated. Light anesthesia and laryngospasm also may contribute to poor seal.

Positive-pressure ventilation can be used safely with the LMA (4). There is no difference in gastric inflation with positive pressure ventilation (<17 cm H_2O) when compared with the LMA and ETT (5). With the classic LMA, tidal volumes should be limited to 8 mL/kg and airway pressure to 20 cm H_2O.

If at any time regurgitated gastric contents are noted in the LMA barrel, the LMA should be left in place. The patient is placed in a Trendelenburg position, 100% oxygen is administered, and the LMA barrel is suctioned.

Supraglottic Airways Removal
SGAs should be removed either when the patient is deeply anesthetized or after protective reflexes have returned and the patient is able to open his or her mouth on command. Many clinicians remove the LMA fully inflated so that it acts as a "scoop" for secretions above the mask, bringing them out of the airway.

Contraindications to Supraglottic Airways Use
The primary contraindication to elective use of a SGA is the clinical scenario where there is an increased risk of gastric contents aspiration (Table 20-2). Other contraindications include high airway resistance, glottic or subglottic airway obstruction, and limited mouth opening (<1.5 cm) (6).

Complications of Supraglottic Airways Use
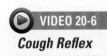
Cough Reflex

Apart from gastroesophageal reflux and aspiration, reported complications include laryngospasm, coughing, gagging, and other events characteristic of airway manipulation. The incidence of SGA-induced postoperative sore throat varies from 4% to 50% and is highly dependent on the study methods. No single device shows a consistently lower rate of dysphagia, though all appear to be better than tracheal intubation in this regard (7). Rare reports exist of nerve injury associated with SGA use.

Second-Generation Supraglottic Airways
Many modern SGAs now incorporate a second lumen, which, when properly placed, sits within the upper esophagus. Second-generation SGAs tend to allow higher airway positive pressure than the first-generation SGAs (≥40 cm H_2O), as well as passive (regurgitation) and active (gastric tube insertion) emptying of the stomach.

F. Tracheal Intubation
Direct Laryngoscopy
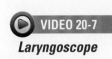
Laryngoscope

The ultimate goal of direct laryngoscopy is to produce a direct line of sight from the operator's eye to the larynx. The view of the larynx is generally described in terms of the Cormack-Lehane grade (grades 1 to 4), which correlate with

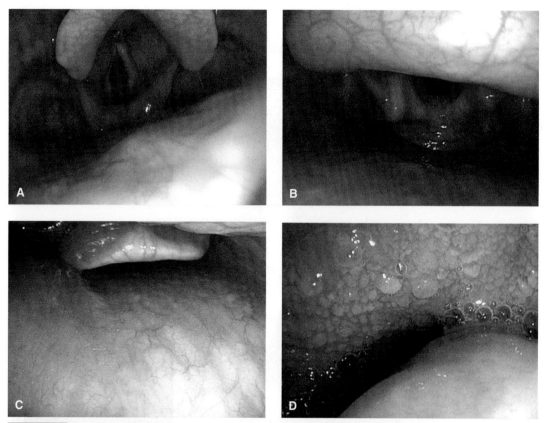

increasingly difficult intubation (Fig. 20-4). No single preoperative measure is adequate to predict difficulty of DL. Unanticipated failure of DL is primarily a problem of tongue displacement, and lingual tonsil hyperplasia is the most commonly undiagnosed cause of unanticipated difficult DL (Fig. 20-5).

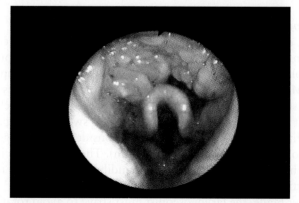

⏵ VIDEO 20-8

Tonsil Size Classification

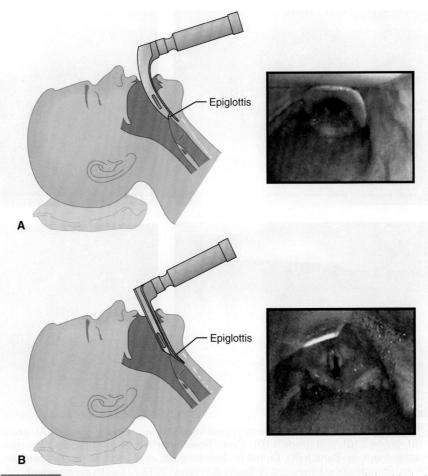

Figure 20-6 **A:** When a curved laryngoscope blade is used, the tip of the blade is placed in the vallecula, the space between the base of the tongue and the pharyngeal surface of the epiglottis. **B:** The tip of a straight blade is advanced beneath the epiglottis. (From Rosenblatt WH, Sukhupragarn W. Airway management. In: Barash PG, Cullen BF, Stoelting RK, et al,, eds. *Clinical Anesthesia.* 7th edition. Philadelphia: Lippincott Williams & Wilkins; 2013:775, with permission.)

? Did You Know

Application of the Miller blade stimulates the vagus cranial nerve (X), while the Macintosh blade stimulates the glossopharyngeal cranial nerve (IX). Thus, there is a greater risk of bradycardia with the Miller blade.

Direct Laryngoscope Blades

Two blades, each with a unique manner of application, are in common use. The *Macintosh* (curved) *blade* is used to displace the epiglottis out of the line of sight by placement in the vallecula and tensing of the glossoepiglottic ligament. The *Miller* (straight) *blade* reveals the glottis by compressing the epiglottis against the base of the tongue (Fig. 20-6). Both blades include a flange along the left side of their length, which is used to sweep the tongue to the left. As a generalization, the Macintosh blade is considered advantageous there is little room to pass an ETT (e.g., small mouth). The Miller blade is considered superior in the patient who has a small mandibular space, large incisors, or a large epiglottis.

With either blade, the laryngoscopist must strive to avoid rotating the wrist and laryngoscope handle in a cephalad direction, bringing the blade against the upper incisors. Extending either blade style too deeply can bring the tip of the blade to rest under the larynx itself, so that forward pressure lifts the airway from view. If a satisfactory laryngeal view is not achieved, the BURP maneuver may be applied. In this maneuver, the larynx is displaced (B) backward, (U) upward, and (R) to the right, using pressure (P) over the cricoid cartilage (8).

A variety of methods can be used to verify that the tracheal tube has been successfully placed into the larynx and trachea. These methods include seeing humidity in the tracheal tube, chest rise and fall, full return of the tidal volume during expiration, auscultation of breath sounds, and detection of sustained end-tidal carbon dioxide.

Airway Bougies

Airway bougies are low-cost adjuncts that can aid with intubation when a poor laryngeal view (Cormack-Lehane grade 3 or 4) is obtained. These semiflexible stylets can be blindly manipulated under the epiglottis and into the trachea. The operator often feels "clicks" as the bougies' tip passes over the tracheal rings. An ETT is then "threaded" over the bougie and into the trachea.

Optical Stylets

Optical stylets incorporate both optical and light source elements into a single stylet-like stainless steel shaft.

Videolaryngoscopy

Videolaryngoscopy (VL) mimics the actions of a traditional laryngoscope but, by placing an imaging device toward the distal end of a laryngoscope blade, removes the need for a direct line of sight to the glottis. The first widely available videolaryngoscope was the Glidescope, which has a 60-degree angulated blade. The "channel configuration" VLs incorporate a semicircular channel alongside the optical elements. These scopes have an anatomic shape with a near right angle between the handle-oral segment and the pharyngeal-hypopharyngeal segment. The channels are aligned with the laryngoscopic view so that, once the glottis is visualized, a preloaded, lubricated tube is advanced through the channel.

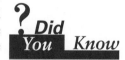

The American Society of Anesthesiologists (ASA) Difficult Airway Taskforce recommends that a videolaryngoscope be available as a first attempt or rescue device for all patients being intubated (9). VL improves the ability to visualize the larynx, and intubation success approaches 97% to 98%. An added benefit is decreased cervical motion when compared with DL, which appears to be more pronounced with the channeled devices.

? Did You Know

As many as 96% of failed attempts at intubation with direct laryngoscopy can be rescued with a videolaryngoscope.

G. Control of Gastric Contents

Risk of Aspiration

Preventing pulmonary *aspiration* of gastric contents is a primary concern during airway management. Altered physiologic states (e.g., pregnancy and diabetes mellitus) and gastrointestinal pathology (e.g., bowel obstruction and peritonitis) adversely affect the rate of gastric emptying, thereby increasing aspiration risk. Clear liquids can be administered to children and adults up to 2 and 3 hours, respectively, prior to anesthesia without increased risk for regurgitation and aspiration (10). The ASA recommends a fasting period of 4 hours for breast milk and 6 hours for nonhuman milk, infant formula, and a light solid meal.

Reduction of gastric acidity can be achieved with the aid of H_2 receptor antagonists and proton pump inhibitors, which also reduce gastric volume. Sodium citrate oral solution increases gastric pH (more alkaline) and is best administered within 1 hour preoperatively. A nasogastric tube can be used to reduce gastric volume prior to anesthesia in patients at hight risk of regugitation.

Rapid-Sequence Induction

Rapid sequence induction (RSI) is indicated when aspiration of gastric contents poses a significant risk. The goal of RSI is to gain control of the airway in the shortest amount of time after the ablation of protective airway reflexes with the induction of anesthesia. In the RSI technique, an intravenous anesthetic induction agent is administered and immediately followed by a rapidly acting neuromuscular blocking drug. Laryngoscopy and intubation are performed as soon as muscle relaxation is confirmed. *Cricoid pressure* is employed (Sellick's maneuver), which entails the downward displacement of the cricoid cartilage against the vertebral bodies in an attempt to ablate the esophageal lumen. The effectiveness of cricoid pressure is in question, as it may make laryngoscopy more difficult. Historically, face mask ventilation is not undertaken prior to intubation, but little evidence supports this. Many practicing clinicians have abandoned these latter two practices in lieu of no evidence-based support.

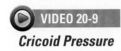

VIDEO 20-9

Cricoid Pressure

H. Intubating Supraglottic Airways

A variety of SGAs specifically designed to facilitate intubation are available. These SGAs are inserted using a similar technique to the classic LMA and other supraglottic airways. Once seated, the mask is inflated and ventilation is attempted. After adequate ventilation is achieved, an ETT, is advanced through the barrel of the LMA. Although the Fastrach LMA excels at blind intubation, a fiberscope should be used with the other varieties. Once intubation is achieved and confirmed, an intubating SGA may be removed, leaving the ETT in place.

I. Extubation of the Trachea

Criteria for routine postsurgical extubation are outlined in Table 20-7. After the patient is asked to open his or her mouth, a suction catheter is used to remove supraglottic secretions or blood. The airway pressure is allowed to rise to 5 to 15 cm of H_2O to facilitate a "passive cough," and the ETT is removed

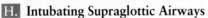

Table 20-7 Criteria for Routine "Awake" Postsurgical Extubation
Subjective clinical criteria:
Breathing spontaneously
Following commands
Five-second sustained head lift
Intact gag reflex
Airway clear of debris
Adequate pain control
Minimal end expiratory concentration of inhaled anesthetics
Objective criteria:
Vital capacity: $\geq$10 mL/kg
Peak voluntary negative inspiratory pressure: $\geq$20 cm H_2O
Tidal volume >6 cc/kg
Sustained tetanic contraction (5 s)
T1/T4 ratio >0.7

Table 20-8	Complications of Tracheal Extubation
Respiratory drive failure (e.g., residual anesthetic)	
Hypoxia (e.g., atelectasis)	
Upper airway obstruction (e.g., edema, residual anesthetic/reduced upper airway tone)	
Vocal fold–related obstruction (e.g., laryngospasm, vocal cord paralysis)	
Tracheal obstruction (e.g., subglottic edema)	
Bronchospasm (airway irritation from endotracheal tube)	
Aspiration (from decreased gag and swallow reflexes)	
Hypertension	
Increased intracranial pressure	
Increased ocular pressure	
Increased abdominal wall pressure (risk of wound dehiscence)	

after the cuff (if present) is deflated (4). If coughing or straining is contraindicated or hazardous (e.g., in the presence of an increased intracranial pressure), extubation may be performed with the patient in a surgical plane of anesthesia and breathing spontaneously ("deep" extubation). Deep extubation is helpful if, for example, a laryngoscopy is required after a thyroidectomy to view vocal cord function. There are three requirements for deep extubation: (a) excellent mask fit and ventilation during induction, (b) no surgical procedure within the airway, and (c) absence of a full stomach. Extubation of the trachea has its own set of potential complications and may prove more perilous than the act of intubation (Table 20-8).

Difficult Extubation

Airway obstruction is a common cause of extubation failure. Incomplete recovery from neuromuscular relaxation, aspirated blood, and edema of the uvula, soft palate, tongue, and structures of the glottis all may contribute to the obstruction (11). Laryngospasm upon ETT removal may also cause extubation failure and accounts for 23% of all critical postoperative respiratory events in adults (3). Unilateral vocal cord paralysis may result from trauma to the recurrent laryngeal nerve during surgery in the neck. Airway obstruction can occur if the contralateral nerve has been damaged previously. Transient vocal cord and swallowing dysfunction has been demonstrated in absence of injury, placing even healthy patients at risk of aspiration after general anesthesia.

Pharmacologic agents used during the maintenance and emergence phases of the anesthetic also may affect the success of extubation. Though low concentrations of potent inhalation anesthetics (e.g., 0.2 minimal alveolar concentration) do not alter the respiratory response to carbon dioxide, they may blunt hypoxic drive. Opiates, and to a lesser extent benzodiazepines, affect both hypercarbic and hypoxic respiratory drives. Some nondepolarizing muscle relaxants may also reduce the hypoxic ventilatory drive.

Identification of Patients at Risk for Complications at Time of Extubation

All patients should be evaluated for the potential of difficult extubation just as they are evaluated for potential difficult intubation. A number of well-known clinical situations may place patients at increased risk for difficulty

Table 20-9   Clinical Situations Presenting Increased Risk for Complications at Time of Extubation

Edema (local, generalized, or angioneurotic)	Airway narrowing
Thyroid surgery	Risk of recurrent laryngeal nerve injury
Laryngoscopy (diagnostic)	Edema, laryngospasm (especially after biopsy)
Uvulopalatoplasty	Palatal and oropharyngeal edema
Obstructive sleep apnea	Upper airway obstruction
Carotid endarterectomy	Wound hematoma, glottic edema, nerve palsies
Maxillofacial trauma	Laryngeal fracture, mandibular/maxillary wires
Cervical vertebrae decompression/fixation	Supraglottic and hypopharyngeal edema
Anaphylaxis	Laryngotracheal narrowing
Hypopharyngeal infections	Laryngotracheal narrowing
Hypoventilation syndromes	Residual anesthetic, central sleep apnea, myasthenia gravis, morbid obesity, severe chronic obstructive pulmonary disease
Hypoxemic syndromes	Ventilation–perfusion mismatch, increased oxygen consumption, impaired alveolar oxygen diffusion, severe anemia
Inadequate airway-protective reflexes	Increased aspiration risk

VIDEO 20-10

Anaphylaxis

with oxygenation or ventilation at the time of extubation (Table 20-9). Management strategies range from continued ventilation to the preparation of standby reintubation equipment to the active establishment of a bridge or guide for reintubation or oxygenation. A number of obturators, which may be left in the airway for extended periods, are available for use in trial extubation. These devices are generally referred to as airway exchange catheters (AECs). The success of first-pass reintubation is significantly higher, and the incidence of hypoxia is lower, in patients with a retained exchange catheter (12). AECs have been associated with significant morbidity, including loss of airway control, mucosal trauma, pneumothorax, esophageal intubation, and death.

J. The Difficult Airway Algorithm
The American Society of Anesthesiologists Difficult Airway Algorithm
Difficult and failed airway management accounts for 2.3% of anesthetic deaths in the United States. The ASA defines the difficult airway as the situation in which the "conventionally trained anesthesiologist experiences difficulty with intubation, mask ventilation or both" and has designed the *difficult airway algorithm* (ASA-DAA, Fig. 20-7) to address such a scenario (10).

Entry into the algorithm begins with the evaluation of the airway, which should direct the clinician to enter the ASA-DAA at one of its two root points: awake intubation (Fig. 20-7 Box A) or intubation attempts after the induction

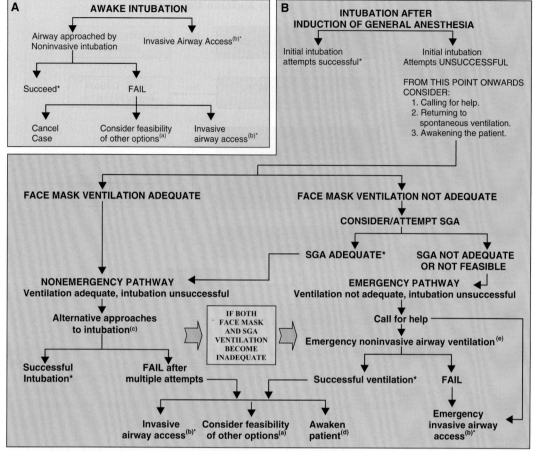

*Confirm ventilation, tracheal intubation, or SGA placement with exhaled CO_2.

a. Other options include (but are not limited to): surgery utilizing face mask or supraglottic airway (SGA) anesthesia (e.g., LMA, ILMA, laryngeal tube), local anesthesia infiltration or regional nerve blockade. Pursuit of these options usually implies that mask ventilation will not be problematic. Therefore, these options may be of limited value if this step in the algorithm has been reached via the Emergency Pathway.

b. Invasive airway access includes surgical or percutaneous airway, jet ventilation, and retrograde intubation.

c. Alternative difficult intubation approaches include (but are not limited to): video-assisted laryngoscopy, alternative laryngoscope blades, SGA (e.g., LMA or ILMA) as an intubation conduit (with or without fiberoptic guidance), fiberoptic intubation, intubating stylet or tube changer, light wand, and blind oral or nasal intubation.

d. Consider re-preparation of the patient for awake intubation or canceling surgery.

e. Emergency non-invasive airway ventilation consists of a SGA.

Figure 20-7 The American Society of Anesthesiologists difficult airway algorithm. **A:** Awake intubation. **B:** Intubation after induction of general anesthesia. (From Apfelbaum JL, Hagberg CA, Caplan RA, et al; American Society of Anesthesiologists Task Force on Management of the Difficult Airway. Practice guidelines for management of the difficult airway: an updated report by the American Society of Anesthesiologists Task Force on Management of the Difficult Airway. *Anesthesiology.* 2013 Feb;118(2):251-70, with permission.)

of general anesthesia (Fig. 20-7 Box A). Awake intubation is chosen when difficulty is anticipated that will place the patient's life in jeopardy, while the airway management after induction is chosen when an uncorrectable situation is not expected.

The Airway Approach Algorithm

This has been further delineated in a preoperative decision tree by Rosenblatt (13) known as the *airway approach algorithm (AAA)*. Figure 20-8 outlines

Airway Approach Algorithm

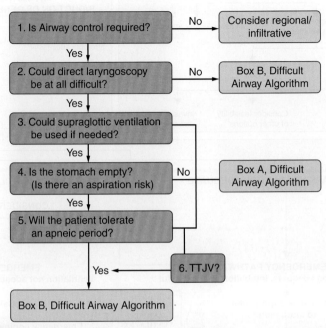

Figure 20-8 The airway approach algorithm: A decision tree approach to entry into the American Society of Anesthesiologists difficult airway algorithm. TTJV, transtracheal jet ventilation. (From Rosenblatt WH, Sukhupragarn W. Airway management. In: Barash PG, Cullen BF, Stoelting RK, et al., eds. *Clinical Anesthesia.* 7th ed. Philadelphia: Lippincott Williams & Wilkins; 2013:788, with permission.)

the AAA, a simple one-pathway algorithm for entering the ASA-DAA, which follows five steps:

1. *Is airway control necessary?* Can regional or infiltrative anesthesia be applied?
2. *Could tracheal intubation be (at all) difficult?* Based on the airway evaluation.
3. *Can supraglottic ventilation be used if needed?* If both intubation and ventilation may be difficult, an awake intubation is chosen (Fig. 20-7A).
4. *Is there an aspiration risk?* The patient at risk for aspiration is not a candidate for elective SGA use. If intubation is also evaluated to be difficult, Figure 20-7A is chosen.
5. *Will the patient tolerate an apneic period?* Should intubation fail and SGA ventilation is inadequate, will the patient rapidly desaturate? If so, awake intubation is the better choice (Fig. 20-7A).

The ASA-DAA becomes truly useful with the unanticipated difficult airway. When initial attempts fail, the airway is supported via mask ventilation. Then, if needed, the clinician may turn to the most convenient or appropriate technique for establishing tracheal intubation. The number of laryngoscopy attempts should be limited (14). This is because soft tissue trauma can result from multiple laryngoscopies, which may diminish the efficacy of a rescue facemask or supraglottic ventilation. When mask ventilation fails, the algorithm suggests supraglottic ventilation via an SGA. Should SGA ventilation fail to sustain the patient adequately, the emergency pathway is entered

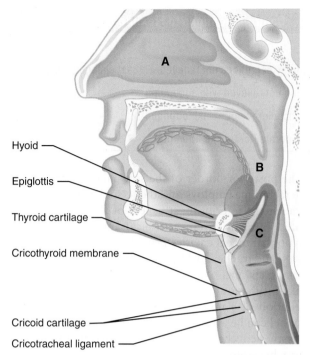

Hyoid

Epiglottis

Thyroid cartilage

Cricothyroid membrane

Cricoid cartilage

Cricotracheal ligament

Figure 20-9 Areas of local anesthetic delivery for awake airway management: The nasal cavity/nasopharynx (**A**), pharynx/base of tongue (**B**), hypopharynx, and (**C**) larynx/trachea.

and the ASA-DAA suggests the use of transtracheal oxygenation or a surgical airway.

K. Awake Airway Management

Awake airway management provides maintenance of spontaneous ventilation and airway protection in the event that the airway cannot be secured rapidly. A sedative agent can be used during awake intubation, but the clinician must remember that producing obstruction or apnea in the difficult airway patient can be devastating. Administration of an antisialagogue, commonly atropine or glycopyrrolate, is important to the success of awake intubation techniques as even small amounts of liquid can obscure the objective lens of indirect optical instruments (e.g., flexible or rigid intubating scope, videolaryngoscope). Vasoconstriction of the nasal passages is also required for instrumentation of this part of the airway.

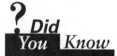

Elective awake intubation is relatively contraindicated by patient refusal, inability to cooperate (e.g., child, profound mental retardation, intoxication), or allergy to local anesthetics.

Local anesthetics are a cornerstone of awake airway control techniques (see Chapter 12). Both topical anesthesia and injected nerve block techniques are commonly used to blunt airway reflexes and provide analgesia. This chapter focuses on the noninvasive options.

The clinician directs local anesthetic therapy to three anatomic areas: the nasal cavity/nasopharynx, the pharynx/base of tongue, and the hypopharynx/larynx/trachea (Fig. 20-9). Cotton-tipped applicators soaked in local anesthetic are passed along the lower border of the middle turbinate of the nasal cavity until the posterior wall of the nasopharynx is reached. They are left in place for 5 to 10 minutes.

The glossopharyngeal nerve can be blocked as its branches transverse behind the palatoglossal folds. These folds are seen as soft tissue ridges that

Table 20-10   Contraindications to Flexible Scope Intubation

Hypoxia

Significant airway secretions not relieved with antisialagogues and suction

Airway bleeding not relieved with suctioning

Local anesthetic allergy (for awake attempts)

Inability to cooperate (for awake attempts)

extend from the posterior border of the soft palate to the base of the tongue. A noninvasive technique employs anesthetic-soaked cotton-tipped applicators positioned against the inferior-most aspect of the folds and left in place for 5 to 10 minutes. In many instances topical application of anesthetics in the pharyngeal/hypopharyngeal cavities provides adequate analgesia of the hypopharynx, larynx, and trachea. Additional anesthetic agents can also be injected down the working channel of a flexible intubation scope.

When awake intubation fails, the clinician has a number of options. They include cancellation of a nonemergent surgical case until specialized equipment or personnel can be arranged for a return to the operating room, the use of regional anesthetic techniques, or, if demanded by the situation, a surgical airway (e.g., tracheostomy).

VIDEO 20-11

Tracheostomy Intubation

L. The Flexible Intubation Scope in Airway Management

The *flexible intubation scope* is the most versatile tool available in situations when it is difficult, or dangerous, to create a line of sight to the glottis. The scope allows a practitioner to maneuver past many pathologic airway obstructions as well as normal anatomy that cannot be manipulated safely (e.g., the unstable or fixed cervical spine). Unlike the other devices used to intubate the trachea, the flexible intubation scope also allows visualization of structures below the level of the vocal folds. This is helpful in characterizing subglottic pathology as well as verifying tracheal tube placement. The choice of oral or nasal intubation is based on clinical requirements, surgical needs, operator experience, and other intubation techniques available if flexible scope intubation fails. Contraindications to flexible scope-aided intubation are relative (Table 20-10). Although flexible scope-aided intubation is a versatile and vital

Table 20-11   Common Reasons for Failure of Flexible Scope Intubation

Lack of provider experience

Failure to adequately dry the airway: Antisialagogue underdose, rushed technique

Failure to adequately anesthetize the airway (awake patient)

Nasal cavity bleeding: Inadequate vasoconstriction/lubrication, rushed technique

Obstructing base of tongue: Insufficient tongue displacement (may require jaw thrust/tongue extrusion)

Hang-up: Endotracheal tube/scope diameter ratio too large

Flexible scope fogging: Suction or oxygen not attached to working channel, cold bronchoscope

Table 20-12   Criteria for Use of an Emergent Invasive Airway

When all five criteria are met, an emergent invasive airway is indicated:
Cannot intubate
Cannot ventilate
Cannot awaken patient
Supraglottic airway has failed
Clinically significant hypoxemia

technique, there are several pitfalls. Table 20-11 lists the most common reasons for failure.

M. The Supraglottic Airways in the Failed Airway
Failed intubations and failed mask ventilation can be rescued with SGA insertion. The major disadvantage of the SGAs in resuscitation is the lack of mechanical protection from regurgitation and aspiration, which is a secondary concern in the face of life threatening hypoxemia.

N. Transtracheal Procedures
When intubation and mask and SGA ventilation fail, airway access via the extrathoracic trachea may be warranted (Table 20-12). These techniques range from minimally invasive (e.g., retrograde wire aided intubation and percutaneous translaryngeal jet ventilation) to surgical (e.g., cricothyrotomy and open tracheostomy). Although these techniques are beyond the scope of this chapter, it is important to be aware of their presence at the terminal end of the DAA.

Although the ASA's Taskforce on the difficult airway has given the medical community an immensely valuable tool in the approach to the patient with the difficult airway, the ASA's algorithm must be viewed as a starting point only. Judgment, experience, the clinical situation, and available resources all affect the appropriateness of the chosen pathway through, or divergence from, the algorithm. When managing the difficult airway, flexibility, not rigidity, prevails.

> **? Did You Know**
>
> The clinician does not need to be expert in all the airway equipment and techniques. No one device can be considered superior to another for all tasks. A broad range of approaches should be mastered so that the failure of one does not preclude safe airway management and emergency rescue.

References

1. Shiga T, Wajima Z, Inoue T, et al. Predicting difficult intubation in apparently normal patients: A meta-analysis of bedside screening test performance. *Anesthesiology.* 2005; 103:429.
2. Langeron O, Masso E, Huraux C, et al. Prediction of difficult mask ventilation. *Anesthesiology.* 2000;92:1229.
3. Hagberg CA, ed. *Benumof's Airway Management: Principles and Practice.* Philadelphia, PA: Mosby; 2007.
4. Idrees A, Khan FA. A comparative study of positive pressure ventilation via laryngeal mask airway and endotracheal tube. *J Pak Med Assoc.* 2000;50:333.
5. Brimacombe JR, Brain AI, Berry AM, et al. Gastric insufflation and the laryngeal mask. *Anesth Analg.* 1998;86:914.
6. Brimacombe JR. Advanced uses: Clinical situations. In: Brimacombe JR, Brain AIJ, eds. *The Laryngeal Mask Airway. A Review and Practical Guide.* London: Saunders; 2004:138.
7. Turkstra TP, Smitheram AK, Alabdulhadi O, et al. The Flex-Tip™ tracheal tube does not reduce the incidence of postoperative sore throat: A randomized controlled trial. *Can J Anaesth.* 2011;58:1090.

8. Ulrich B, Listyo R, Gerig HJ, et al. The difficult intubation: The value of BURP and 3 predictive tests of difficult intubation. *Anaesthesist.* 1998;47:45.
9. Practice guidelines for management of the difficult airway. *Anesthesiology.* 2013;118(2): 251–270.
10. Practice guidelines for preoperative fasting and the use of pharmacologic agents to reduce the risk of pulmonary aspiration. Application to healthy patients undergoing elective procedures. *Anesthesiology.* 2011;114:495.
11. Cook TM, Woodall N, Frerk C. Fourth National Audit Project. Major complications of airway management in the UK: Results of the Fourth National Audit Project of the Royal College of Anaesthetists and the Difficult Airway Society. Part 1: Anaesthesia. *Br J Anaesth.* 2011;106(5):617–631.
12. Mort TC. Emergency tracheal intubation: Complications associated with repeated laryngoscopic attempts. *Anesth Analg.* 2004;99:607.
13. Rosenblatt W. The airway approach algorithm. *J Clin Anesth.* 2004;16:312.
14. Mort TC. Continuous airway access for the difficult extubation: The efficacy of the airway exchange catheter. *Anesth Analg.* 2007;105:1357.

Questions

1. The positive predictive value of the Mallampati score to predict a difficult laryngoscopy is approximately:
   A. 20% to 30%
   B. 40% to 50%
   C. 60% to 70%
   D. 80% to 90%

2. Which of the following cannot be given to an infant *within* 6 hours of an elective general anesthetic?
   A. Breast milk
   B. Carbonated soda
   C. Gelatin water
   D. Light solid meal

3. Following a thyroidectomy, a patient is noted to speak with a newly acquired hoarseness. Which of the following is consistent with a recurrent laryngeal nerve injury?
   A. Lack of adduction of the ipsilateral vocal cord
   B. Lack of abduction of the ipsilateral vocal cord
   C. Loss of sensory innervation above the vocal cords
   D. Paralysis of the cricothyroid muscle

4. Which of the following is a contraindication to awake fiber optic endotracheal intubation?
   A. Lingual tonsil
   B. Hypercarbia
   C. Secretions
   D. Intoxicated patient

5. A patient (body mass index 29) is scheduled for a laparoscopic cholecystectomy, in whom you do not anticipate a difficult laryngoscopy. After administering propofol (200 mg) and rocuronium (50 mg), you cannot ventilate or visualize the larynx (after three attempts). According to the ASA difficult airway algorithm, your next management step is:
   A. Call for help
   B. Return to spontaneous ventilation
   C. Awaken the patient
   D. Insert LMA

6. A 70-year-old male receives atenolol 50 mg each morning for treatment of hypertension. Two hours after receiving his morning dose, he is scheduled to undergo an emergency appendectomy. You plan to use a rapid sequence induction with propofol and succinylcholine (Mallampati 1 airway). As you are ready to start induction of anesthesia, you note the heart rate is 50 beats per minute. The preferred method of laryngoscopy is use of a:
   A. Miller 3
   B. Macintosh 3
   C. Fiberoptic laryngoscopy
   D. All of the above

7. Which of these variables has the highest risk for difficult mask ventilation?
   A. History of snoring
   B. Body mass index >26
   C. Presence of a beard
   D. Age >55 years

8. As compared to preoxygenation with FiO_2 = 1.0 for 5 minutes, preoxygenation with FiO_2 = 0.21 for 5 minutes and a tight fitting facemask results in desaturation:
   A. Two times faster
   B. Four times faster
   C. Ten times faster
   D. Clinically irrelevant difference

9. A 70-year-old male has clinically significant hemoptysis. The surgeon prefers doing a fiberoptic bronchoscopy via an endotracheal tube. Which of the following approaches to primary securing of the airway is relatively contraindicated?
   A. Retrograde wire intubation
   B. Esophageal-tracheal combitube
   C. Intubating LMA
   D. Fiberoptic bronchoscopy

10. The maximal recommended intracuff pressure for a number 4 LMA is:
    A. 10 cm H_2O
    B. 20 cm H_2O
    C. 60 cm H_2O
    D. None; a volume of 25 cc is inserted regardless of cuff pressure

21

Regional Anesthesia

Alexander M. DeLeon
Yogen G. Asher

I. General Principles and Equipment

Surgeons and patients often prefer regional anesthetic techniques due to their associated decreases in perioperative pain and improved discharge times. A regional block can be used in conjunction with general anesthesia to reduce the need for opioids, which cause nausea and sedation. Although these blocks require technical finesse, knowledge of the indications, contraindications, side effects, complications, as well as the pharmacology of local anesthetics is necessary to make decisions regarding which patients should receive a block.

A. Setup and Monitoring

Peripheral nerve blocks are often performed preoperatively outside the operating room. The nerve block can be placed and have time to take effect prior to the patient entering the operating room. Monitors such as pulse oximetry, continuous electrocardiogram, and blood pressure cuffs should be applied to all patients undergoing a peripheral nerve block. A "block cart" should be in the immediate vicinity and contain airway equipment as well as emergency supplies.

B. Peripheral Nerve Stimulators

Motor nerves can be identified with the use of peripheral nerve stimulators with or without ultrasound imaging. The lower the current required to stimulate a specific motor response (<0.5 mA) indicates close proximity of the tip of an insulated stimulating needle to a nerve. Longer duration impulses (>0.3 ms) are more likely to cause pain by stimulating sensory nerves, while shorter duration impulses (0.1 ms) cause significantly less discomfort because the motor component of the nerve is primarily stimulated.

C. Ultrasound Guidance

The prevalence of ***ultrasound guidance*** has increased the popularity of regional anesthesia. Ultrasound allows for the visualization of nerve structures, vascular structures, and local anesthetic spread. Ultrasound guidance has not definitively been proven to be safer or more effective, yet evidence is emerging

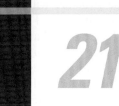

? Did You Know

Ultrasound guidance has not definitively been proven to be safer or more effective, yet evidence is emerging showing that ultrasound allows for faster onset, lower doses of local anesthetics, and fewer needle passes.

395

showing that ultrasound allows for faster onset, lower doses of local anesthetics, and fewer needle passes (1). To obtain the optimal view of a target nerve, a basic understanding of ultrasound physics is useful.

Ultrasound beams are sound waves beyond the threshold of hearing (>20,000 MHz). *Acoustic impedance* is the quality of structures allowing for visualization using ultrasound. Differences in acoustic impedance of a structure relative to its surrounding tissue dictate whether the structure will be visible. Certain structures are more likely to attenuate an ultrasound beam. For example, ultrasound waves pass easily through blood vessels (i.e., minimal attenuation), compared with bone and air, which cause of great degree of attenuation.

Probes differ in frequency ranges. Higher frequency probes have less penetration but greater resolution and are useful for superficial structures, including most peripheral nerves. Lower frequency probes are useful for deeper structures such as the heart.

Once the appropriate depth is set when viewing an ultrasound image, the *gain* can be adjusted to brighten or darken the image. Color flow Doppler can help to identify blood vessels due to the turbulent nature of blood flow toward and away from the probe.

When orienting the needle to the probe, two different techniques have been defined: in plane versus out of plane (Fig. 21-1). The benefit of an in-plane approach is that it allows for the entire needle, including the tip, to be visualized at all times.

D. Other Related Equipment

Insulated needles must be used when nerve stimulation is desired. Needles designed for peripheral nerve blocks are usually short beveled to decrease

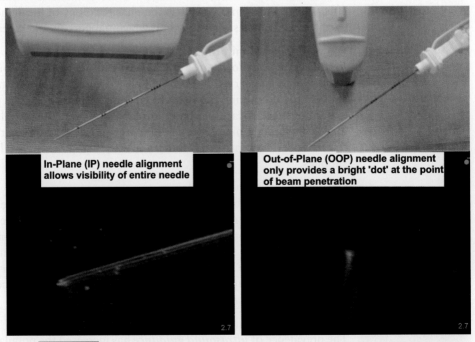

In-Plane (IP) needle alignment allows visibility of entire needle

Out-of-Plane (OOP) needle alignment only provides a bright 'dot' at the point of beam penetration

Figure 21-1 In-plane versus out-of-plane approaches. (From Tsui BCH, Rosenquist RW. Peripheral nerve blockade. In: Barash PG, Cullen BF, Stoelting RK, et al., eds. *Clinical Anesthesia*. 6th ed. Philadelphia: Wolters Kluwer Health/Lippincott Williams & Wilkins; 2009:959, with permission.)

the likelihood of injuring nerves and vascular structures, in contrast to long-beveled needles intended for intramuscular injections. Although a standard insulated needle can be seen with ultrasound, specifically produced hyperechoic needles are considerably easier to view.

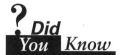

II. Avoiding Complications

Complications from peripheral nerve blocks can be divided into four categories: *local anesthetic toxicity, nerve injury*, infections, and damage to adjacent structures. Local anesthetic systemic toxicity is discussed in Chapter 12. Techniques to reduce the risk of local anesthetic systemic toxicity include reducing the dose to the lowest effective dose, intermittent aspiration during injection to ensure that the needle tip has not entered a blood vessel, the addition of intravascular markers such as epinephrine combined with the local anesthetic, and maintaining communication with the patient to assess for symptoms of local anesthetic systemic toxicity (e.g., metallic taste in mouth, ringing in the ears).

Avoidance of nerve injury can theoretically be reduced with ultrasound imaging, yet ultrasound has not been conclusively shown to reduce such complications. Infectious complications can be minimized with sterile technique such as a sterile sheath used to cover the ultrasound probe. Damage to associated structures can be minimized through identification of such structures (e.g., pleura, blood vessels).

Other complications such as hematoma formation can be minimized by avoidance of trauma to blood vessels and performing regional anesthesia in coagulopathic patients.

III. Specific Techniques for the Head, Neck, Upper Extremities, and Trunk

A. Head and Neck
Head and neck blocks can be used for a variety of procedures including carotid endarterectomy, awake craniotomy, and plastic and maxillofacial surgeries. Only a few landmark-based techniques will be discussed here.

Supraorbital and Supratrochlear Nerve Blocks
The ophthalmic division of the trigeminal nerve (V1) supplies the supraorbital and supratrochlear nerves, which provide sensory innervation to the anterior scalp. The supraorbital nerve can be blocked by injecting local anesthetic near the supraorbital foramen above the eyebrow. The supratrochlear nerve can be blocked by extending this injection medially approximately 1 cm.

Infraorbital Block
The infraorbital block is useful for providing analgesia after cleft lip repair. This terminal branch of the maxillary division of the trigeminal nerve (V2) can be blocked by injecting local anesthetic near the infraorbital foramen inferior to the eye.

Superficial Cervical Plexus Block
The ventral rami of the C2-4 form the superficial and deep cervical plexuses. The superficial cervical plexus comprises four nerves (supraclavicular, transverse cervical, greater auricular, and lesser occipital) and can be located posterolateral to the sternocleidomastoid at the level of the cricoid cartilage. The greater auricular and lesser occipital nerves provide sensory innervation to the lateral and posterolateral scalp, respectively.

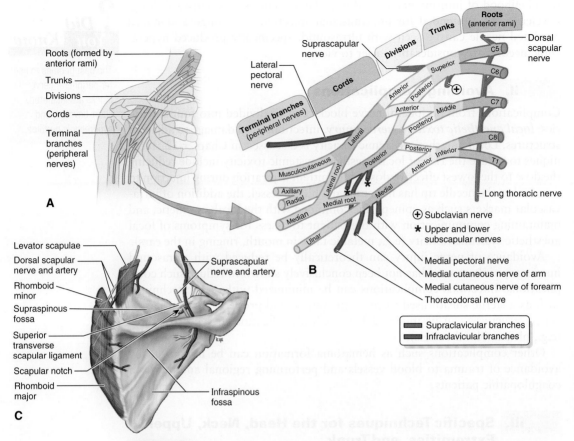

Greater Occipital Nerve Block

To provide analgesia for the posterior scalp, the greater occipital nerve (dorsal rami C2) can be blocked along the superior nuchal line lateral to the occipital protuberance and adjacent (typically medial) to the occipital artery.

B. Brachial Plexus Blockade

The brachial plexus consists of spinal roots C5-T1 with a variable contribution from C4 and T2. There are four major approaches to blockade of the brachial plexus: interscalene, supraclavicular, infraclavicular, and axillary (Fig. 21-2).

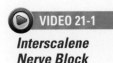

*Interscalene
Nerve Block*

Interscalene Block

The primary use of the interscalene block is for shoulder surgery (e.g., total shoulder arthroplasty, rotator cuff repair, arthroscopic shoulder surgery). The interscalene approach targets the nerves of the upper brachial plexus (C4-7). Inferior nerve roots of the brachial plexus (C8-T1) are least likely to be blocked (Fig. 21-2).

Known side effects of the interscalene block include phrenic nerve paralysis, Horner's syndrome, and recurrent laryngeal nerve paralysis. Phrenic nerve paralysis has been reported in up to 100% of patients, yet with the introduction of ultrasound, the incidence has been reduced considerably to as low as 13% (2,3). Horner's syndrome results from blockade of the cervical

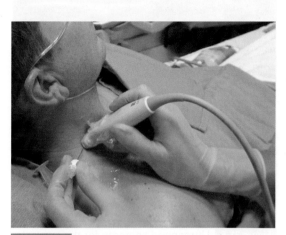

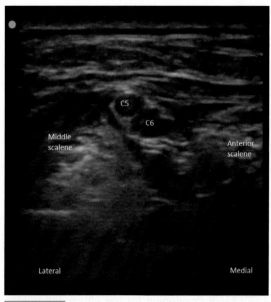

Figure 21-3 Positioning for the ultrasound-guided interscalene block. Patient is seated at 70 to 90 degrees. The ultrasound probe is placed at the level of the cricoid cartilage (C6) in the transverse plane with a slightly downward angle.

Figure 21-4 Ultrasound anatomy for the interscalene block. The C5-6 nerve roots can been seen between the anterior and middle scalene muscles.

sympathetic chain, as seen in up to half of patients who receive interscalene blocks. The incidence of hoarse voice from recurrent laryngeal nerve block is on the order of 10% to 20%.

The interscalene approach targets the level of the distal roots or proximal trunks of the brachial plexus. Two of the primary nerves of the shoulder derived from the C5-6 nerve roots, suprascapular nerve and axillary nerve, are blocked by this approach. The supraclavicular nerve (C4), which provides the cutaneous innervation for the top of the shoulder, is often blocked by the interscalene approach.

In order to perform an ultrasound-guided interscalene block, the patient is positioned in a near-seated position of 70 to 90 degrees (Fig. 21-3). Ultrasound scanning with a high-frequency probe (7 to 10 MHz) begins above the midpoint of the clavicle where the subclavian artery is located. The nerves of the brachial plexus will be located lateral to the subclavian artery and should be traced to the level of the cricoid cartilage, which corresponds to the level of the C6 vertebrae. The needle is inserted posterior to the ultrasound probe for the in-plane approach (Fig. 21-4).

When performing a landmark-based interscalene block, the interscalene groove should be palpated lateral to the clavicular head of the sternocleidomastoid at the level of the cricoid cartilage (C6). The needle should be advanced 60 degrees to the sagittal plane until motor response is obtained at the deltoid, biceps, or triceps at <0.5 mA.

Supraclavicular Block
The supraclavicular block is indicated for elbow, wrist, and hand surgery. The supraclavicular block can also be used for shoulder surgery. But it tends to miss the C4 distribution and may require a superficial cervical plexus block if anesthesia of the top of the shoulder is needed. The supraclavicular block targets the distal trunks and divisions (Fig. 21-2).

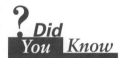

? *Did* *You Know*

The introduction of ultrasound-guided needle placement has reduced the incidence of phrenic nerve blockade from nearly 100% to as low as 13% during interscalene block.

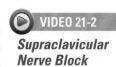

VIDEO 21-2

Supraclavicular Nerve Block

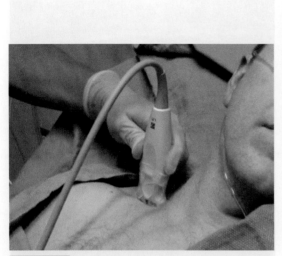

Figure 21-5 Positioning for the ultrasound guided supraclavicular block.

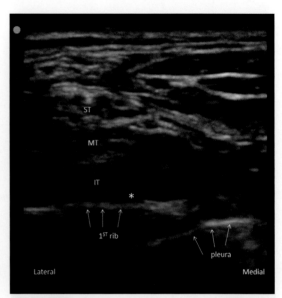

Figure 21-6 Ultrasound anatomy for the supraclavicular block. ST, superior trunk; MT, middle trunk; IT, inferior trunk; SA, subclavian artery. The asterisk (*) signifies the "corner pocket" injection target.

Side effects are similar to the interscalene block. Phrenic nerve paralysis is possible, although it occurs about half as often as with an interscalene block. Pneumothorax is possible, but it is less common when ultrasound is used.

To perform an ultrasound-guided supraclavicular block, ultrasound scanning begins with a high-frequency ultrasound probe at the midpoint of the clavicle with the ultrasound probe angled vertically, similar to the start of the interscalene block (Fig. 21-5). The brachial plexus appears as a bundle of "grapes" lateral and superficial to the subclavian artery (Fig. 21-6). The target location for the needle tip is posterior and slightly lateral to the subclavian artery and has been described as the "corner pocket" location (4).

Due to the risk of pneumothorax being as high as 6% with the landmark technique, other blocks such as the axillary or infraclavicular block have replaced the supraclavicular block when ultrasound is not available (5).

Infraclavicular Block

The infraclavicular block can be used interchangeably with the supraclavicular block for wrist and hand surgery but spares the C5-6 distribution necessary for shoulder surgery. Compared with the supraclavicular block, the infraclavicular block has virtually no risk of phrenic nerve paralysis and can be used in patients with pre-existing lung disease. The infraclavicular block targets the level of the medial, lateral, and posterior cords (Fig. 21-2).

When performing an ultrasound-guided infraclavicular block, scanning should begin in the parasagittal plane medial to the coracoid process and inferior to the clavicle (Fig. 21-7). The axillary artery is located deep to the pectoralis major and minor muscles. The target is the posterior cord, which is immediately deep to the subclavian artery (Fig. 21-8).

A landmark-based technique can be alternatively used. The needle insertion site is immediately inferior to the clavicle, 1 to 2 cm medial to the coracoid process. The needle angle is perpendicular to the skin with a slight (15 to

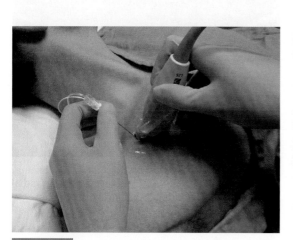

Figure 21-7 Positioning and needle placement for the ultrasound-guided infraclavicular block.

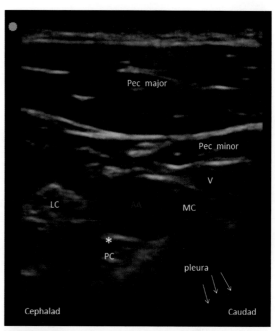

Figure 21-8 Ultrasound anatomy for the infraclavicular block. LC, lateral cord; PC, posterior cord; MC, medial cord; AA, axillary artery; V, subclavian vein. The asterisk (*) signifies the injection target.

30 degree) caudad angle. The desired endpoints are either extension of the hand- or elbow-indicated posterior cord stimulation or flexion at the fingers, indicating medial cord stimulation. Biceps flexion indicates lateral cord stimulation and has been associated with a high failure rate of the block (6).

Axillary Block
The axillary block is a more distal approach to the brachial plexus when compared with the infraclavicular and supraclavicular blocks. The axillary block is performed at the level of the terminal branches of the brachial plexus (Fig. 21-2). The musculocutaneous, median, ulnar, and radial nerves are blocked, although the musculocutaneous nerve may require a separate injection. Given that the terminal branches are individually visible when using ultrasound, the axillary block can be used as a rescue block when a particular distribution is missed with an infraclavicular or supraclavicular block (Figs. 21-9 and 21-10). The musculocutaneous nerve terminates as the lateral cutaneous nerve of the forearm and may be missed by the axillary block. For this reason, a separate injection targeting the musculocutaneous nerve may be necessary for surgery involving the lateral wrist.

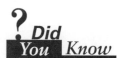

The musculocutaneous nerve terminates as the lateral cutaneous nerve of the forearm and may be missed by the axillary block.

C. Terminal Upper Extremity Nerve Blocks
The terminal branches of the brachial plexus can be blocked individually using more distal approaches. The use of ultrasound to specifically target terminal branches with the axillary approach has made the use of distal rescue blocks less common. Specific circumstances can make these blocks ideal, such as a patient requiring a rescue block from an inadequate supraclavicular block who cannot abduct his or her arm.

Using ultrasound, the median nerve can be blocked at the antecubital fossa. The median nerve appears as a hypoechoic structure medial to the brachial

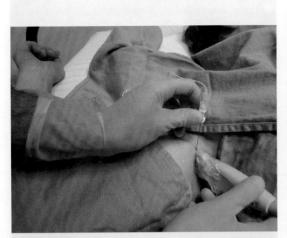

Figure 21-9   Positioning and needle placement for the ultrasound-guided axillary block.

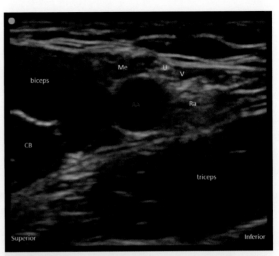

Figure 21-10   Ultrasound anatomy for the axillary block. Me, median nerve; U, ulnar nerve; Ra, radial nerve; AA, axillary artery; CB, coracobrachialis.

artery. The radial nerve can be located on the anterior surface of the elbow, 1 to 2 cm lateral to the biceps tendon, and appears hypoechoic, similar to the median nerve. Nerve stimulation can be used to confirm identification by eliciting a radial nerve response such as wrist or finger extension. The ulnar nerve can be localized at the midforearm. The nerve will appear hyperechoic, just medial to the pulsating ulnar artery.

D. Intravenous Regional Anesthesia

Commonly known as a *Bier block*, the *intravenous regional anesthesia (IVRA)* duration of action is mainly limited by a patient's ability to tolerate tourniquet pain. Therefore, IVRA is indicated for surgeries lasting approximately 40 minutes or less that do not require a block for postoperative analgesia. IVRA is commonly used for carpal tunnel releases, trigger finger releases, and wrist arthroscopy.

An intravenous (IV) line is placed at a distal location of the operative hand. A double tourniquet is placed on the upper arm with the proximal and distal tourniquets clearly identified. An elastic bandage is then used to exsanguinate the arm followed by inflation of the distal tourniquet to 250 mm Hg. Next, the proximal tourniquet is inflated followed by deflation of the distal tourniquet. The elastic bandage is removed and a dose of 3 mg/kg of lidocaine is then injected. The IV is removed prior to surgery.

The patient will often begin to complain of dull tourniquet pain between 20 and 40 minutes after tourniquet inflation. Treatment of tourniquet pain may require inflation of the distal tourniquet followed by deflation of the proximal tourniquet. If surgery is completed prior to 20 minutes, the tourniquet should remain inflated until at least 20 minutes have passed due to the association with toxic intravenous concentration of local anesthetic when tourniquets are released after less than 20 minutes. If a patient begins to experience symptoms of local anesthetic systemic neurotoxicity (e.g., tinnitus, perioral numbness), the tourniquet should be reinflated and deflated in a cyclic manner until symptoms no longer occur with deflation. After 45 minutes, the tourniquet can be released with minimal risk of systemic neurotoxicity.

E. Intercostal Nerve Blocks

Intercostal nerve blocks are useful in an array of acute or chronic pain settings from rib fractures to zoster. The intercostal nerve travels in between the internal and innermost intercostal muscles and lies inferior to the intercostal artery and vein, which are inferior and deep to the rib. Due to the proximity to these vessels and high rate of vascular uptake of local anesthetic, patients should be adequately monitored for local anesthetic systemic toxicity.

F. Paravertebral Nerve Blocks

Bounded medially by the intervertebral foramina and lateral spine, anteriorly by the parietal pleura, and posteriorly by the superior costotransverse ligament, the thoracic paravertebral space houses the spinal nerve root as it splits into dorsal and ventral rami. It is contiguous medially with the epidural space via foramina, laterally to the intercostal nerve and vessels, and the cephalo–caudad paravertebral spaces (Fig. 21-11). When unilateral analgesia is desired (e.g., for breast or thoracic surgery), local anesthetic can be injected via one large volume injection or multiple smaller volume injections at adjacent levels. When performed under ultrasound guidance, the parietal pleura appears to be "pushed down" by the spread of local anesthetic during injection. Potential complications include pneumothorax, epidural or intrathecal spread of local anesthetic, bleeding, and infection.

G. Transversus Abdominis Plane Block

In the anterior abdomen, deep to a fascial plane that lies between the transversus abdominis and internal oblique muscles, there is a network of terminal branches of the ventral rami of the T7-L1 nerve roots and their communicating nerves (Fig. 21-12). The plane extends medially to the rectus sheath,

 VIDEO 21-3

Ultrasound-Guided Transversus Abdominis Plane (TAP) Block

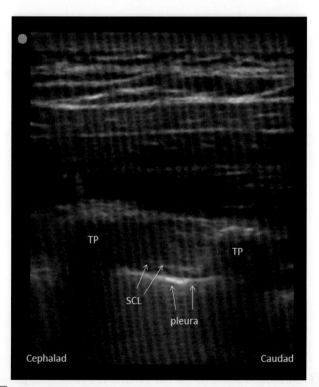

Figure 21-11 Ultrasound anatomy for the paravertebral block. The probe is oriented in the parasagital plane at the T2-3 level, 5 cm lateral to midline.

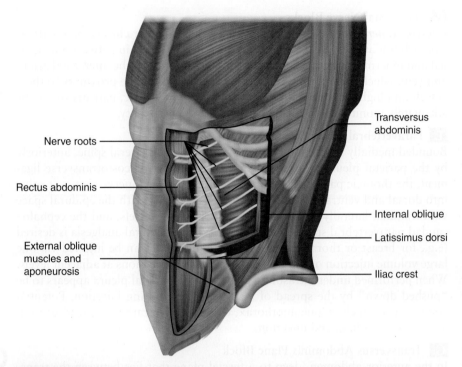

Nerve roots

Rectus abdominis

External oblique
muscles and
aponeurosis

Transversus
abdominis

Internal oblique

Latissimus dorsi

Iliac crest

Figure 21-12 Anatomy for the transversus abdominis plane block. The nerves (T7-L1) are located in the fascial layer between the internal oblique and the transversus abdominis muscles.

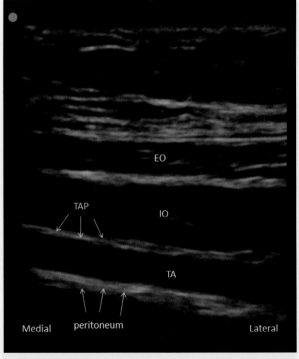

Figure 21-13 Ultrasound anatomy for the transversus abdominis plane block. EO, external oblique; IO, internal oblique; TA, transversus abdominis. The TAP label indicates the injection target.

laterally to the latissimus dorsi, cranially to the rib cage, and caudally to the iliac crest. Injection of local anesthetic at this location provides analgesia to the abdominal wall and skin and can be useful following or preceding laparoscopic or umbilical surgery. This block is most often performed under ultrasound guidance, shown in Figure 21-13 lateral to the rectus sheath in the T10 dermatome. Care must be taken not to traverse the peritoneum, which lies deep to the transversus muscle.

H. Inguinal Nerve Block

The ilioinguinal and iliohypogastric nerves are also located in the transversus plane in the anterior abdomen, which originate from L1. Injection around these nerves can facilitate analgesia following inguinal or scrotal surgery when combined with the genitofemoral nerve block. Optimal image view is obtained when the probe is aligned on an axis between the anterior superior iliac spine and umbilicus. Lateral injection can be preferred to avoid incidental peritoneal injury. Doppler can be useful in avoiding inadvertent vascular injection as small vessels often lie adjacent to these nerves.

I. Penile Nerve Block

Derived from the pudendal nerve, the dorsal penile nerves (S2-4) supply sensory innervation to the tip and shaft of the penis, making the penile block useful for distal urologic surgery such as circumcision. The nerves are located deep to Buck's fascia and lateral to the dorsal arteries, which are in turn lateral to the deep dorsal vein. After careful aspiration, local anesthetic is injected in two separate injections at the base of the penis. Often, epinephrine is omitted from the injection to reduce concern for distal ischemia.

IV. Anatomic Considerations for Lower Extremity Blockade

Blockade of the lumbar and sacral plexuses can be used for surgical anesthesia or analgesia of the lower extremities. When compared with neuraxial anesthesia, lower extremity peripheral nerve blocks provide prolonged analgesia without side effects such as hypotension, urinary retention, and contralateral muscle weakness. Due to the anatomic separation between the lumbar and sacral plexuses, a single injection cannot provide complete anesthesia of the entire lower extremity.

A. Lumbar Plexus

The lumbar plexus is formed from the ventral rami of nerve roots of T12 and L1-4 bilaterally, and gives rise to six major nerves: the femoral, obturator, lateral femoral cutaneous, ilioinguinal, iliohypogastric, and genitofemoral nerves (Fig. 21-14).

The femoral nerve (L2-4) is the largest nerve of the lumbar plexus. It provides the primary innervation to the knee and can be used for postoperative analgesia for total knee arthroplasty, anterior cruciate ligament repair, as well as surgery involving the patellar tendon. The femoral nerve sends motor branches to the quadriceps muscles and provides the cutaneous innervation for the anterior thigh and knee. The femoral nerve is located approximately 1 to 2 cm lateral to the femoral artery at the level of the inguinal crease. The terminal branch of the femoral nerve is the saphenous nerve, which innervates the skin of the medial knee, calf, and ankle. The saphenous nerve follows the femoral artery laterally and crosses the artery in the adductor canal and continues medially to the artery proximal to the knee.

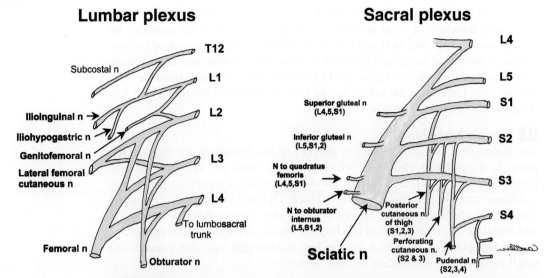

Figure 21-14 Anatomy of the lumbar and sacral plexuses. (From Tsui BCH, Rosenquist RW. Peripheral nerve blockade. In: Barash PG, Cullen BF, Stoelting RK, et al., eds. *Clinical Anesthesia*. 6th ed. Philadelphia: Wolters Kluwer Health/Lippincott Williams & Wilkins; 2009:983, with permission.)

The obturator nerve (L2-4) supplies the cutaneous innervation to the medial thigh and knee. The motor innervation of adductors of the leg (adductor longus, gracilis, adductor brevis, and pectineus) is to a variable extent supplied by the obturator nerve. The medial knee can be supplied by articular braches of the obturator nerve. The obturator nerve courses from the medial border of the psoas major muscle then courses along the lateral wall of the pelvic cavity toward the obturator canal.

The genitofemoral nerve (L1-2) supplies the cremaster muscle and skin over the scrotum in men and the anterior part of the labium majorus and mons pubis in women. The lateral femoral cutaneous nerve (L2-3) supplies the cutaneous innervation to the lateral thigh.

B. Sacral Plexus

The anterior rami of S1-4 join the lumbosacral trunk after exiting the sacral foramina toward the sacral plexus. Various nerves are derived from the sacral plexus including the pudendal nerve, gluteal nerves, and pelvic splanchnic nerves, yet the nerves most relevant to lower extremity surgery are the sciatic nerve and the posterior cutaneous nerve of the thigh (Fig. 21-14).

The sciatic nerve (L4-S3) passes through the sciatic notch, anterior to the piriformis muscle, and then travels lateral and deep to the biceps femoris tendon at the gluteal crease. At this level, the nerve is located between the ischial tuberosity and the greater trochanter of the femur. As the nerve approaches the popliteal fossa, the two components—tibial (medial) and peroneal (lateral)—separate at a variable distance from the knee. The common peroneal nerve terminates as the superficial peroneal, deep peroneal, and lateral sural nerves in the foot and primarily innervates the dorsal surface of the foot as well as the dorsiflexors of the foot. The tibial nerve terminates as the posterior tibial nerve and the medial sural nerve. The tibial nerve innervates the plantar flexors of the foot, including the gastrocnemius, soleus, popliteus, and plantaris muscles.

The nerves at the ankle derived from the sciatic nerve include the posterior tibial, superficial peroneal, deep peroneal, and sural. The saphenous nerve is the only nerve at the ankle that is a branch of the femoral nerve. The posterior tibial nerve branches into the calcaneal, medial plantar, and lateral plantar nerves. The posterior tibial nerve provides motor innervation (plantar flexors), cutaneous innervation (plantar surface of the foot), and bony innervation to the foot. The deep peroneal nerve provides cutaneous innervation to the web space between the first and second toe and terminates as the second, third, and forth dorsal interosseous nerves. The superficial peroneal nerve provides the cutaneous innervation to the dorsum of the foot except for the lateral aspect of the dorsum, which is supplied by the sural nerve. The saphenous nerve supplies the cutaneous innervation to the medial ankle and foot.

V. Specific Techniques for the Lower Extremities

A. Psoas Compartment Block

The *psoas compartment block* is useful for unilateral hip or anterior leg surgery in combination with sciatic nerve block and is often performed with guidance of a nerve stimulator to obtain a quadriceps twitch response. This response is often obtained when a 100-mm insulated block needle is inserted 1 to 2 cm deep to the L4 (sometimes L3) transverse process. Due to the concern of hematoma, retroperitoneal bleeding, or epidural spread, careful consideration and monitoring in addition to an experienced practitioner are mandatory for safe and effective completion of this advanced block.

B. Femoral Nerve Block

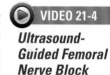

VIDEO 21-4

Ultrasound-Guided Femoral Nerve Block

The femoral nerve can be blocked at the level of the inguinal crease with or without ultrasound guidance. With the patient in the supine position, the femoral artery pulse is palpated. The needle insertion site for the landmark approach is 1 to 1.5 cm lateral to the femoral pulse with a slight cephalad trajectory of about 30 degrees. The goal is to obtain a patellar or quadriceps response at <0.5 mA.

When performing the *femoral nerve block* with ultrasound, the femoral artery is visualized at the inguinal crease. The femoral nerve appears as a hyperechoic triangular structure lateral to the artery (Fig. 21-15). Nerve stimulation can be used in combination with ultrasound to confirm a patellar or quadriceps response.

C. Saphenous Nerve Block

A *saphenous nerve block* can be performed for anesthesia of the medial calf and ankle. The saphenous nerve block can be performed at the midthigh level using ultrasound guidance. The femoral artery becomes the descending genicular artery as it follows its course along the thigh. Initially, the saphenous nerve is lateral to the artery and transitions to medial in the mid- to distal thigh. Using ultrasound, the nerve can be visualized as a hyperechoic structure anterior and medial to the femoral artery, deep to the sartorius muscle (Fig. 21-16).

D. Lateral Femoral Cutaneous and Obturator Nerve Blocks

The frequency for which lateral femoral cutaneous and obturator nerve blocks are performed is relatively low, given that knee surgery does not typically require blockade outside the femoral and sciatic distributions. Detailed descriptions of these blocks can be found in a comprehensive regional text.

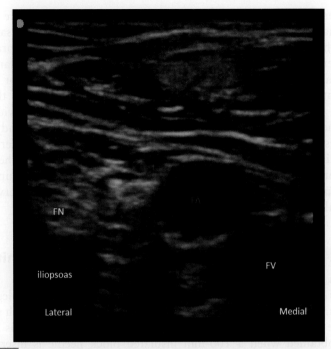

Figure 21-15 Ultrasound anatomy for the femoral nerve block. FN, femoral nerve; FA, femoral artery; FV, femoral vein.

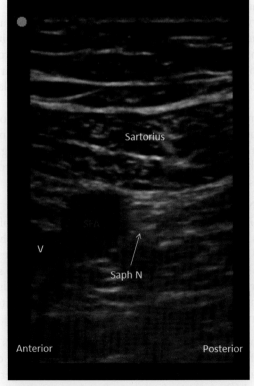

Figure 21-16 Ultrasound anatomy for the midthigh saphenous nerve block. SFA, superficial femoral artery.

E. Sciatic Nerve Block

The *sciatic nerve block* provides complete anesthesia to the ankle and foot when combined with a saphenous nerve block. Surgeries such as mid- and hind foot fusions, open reductions and internal fixations of ankle fractures, Achilles tendon repairs, and total ankle arthroplasties can all be performed with sciatic–saphenous nerve anesthesia with minimal intraoperative sedation required.

Classically the gluteal approach (Labat) has been used, but with the popularity of ultrasound and the ease of visualization of the sciatic nerve at the level of the gluteal crease, more distal approaches have come into favor. The landmarks for the gluteal approach include an oblique line from the posterior superior iliac spine to the greater trochanter of the femur with the patient in a semiprone position with the hip and knee flexed and the operative side up. A second line from the greater trochanter of the femur to the sacral hiatus is drawn. A third line, perpendicular to the first line, will cross the second line at the approximate needle entry point (Fig. 21-17).

An ultrasound-guided subgluteal approach can be performed with the patient either lateral or prone. Either a high-frequency probe or a lower-frequency probe can be used. Many high-frequency probes penetrate up to 6 cm, and thus the vast majority of sciatic nerves may be visible with a high-frequency probe, reducing the need to switch probes between various blocks. The nerve is visualized slightly deep and lateral to the biceps femoris muscle (Fig. 21-18). A nerve stimulator can be used to confirm proper identification of the sciatic nerve. A plantar flexion motor response in the foot indicates that the medial (tibial) component of the nerve is being stimulated. A dorsiflexion (common peroneal) or an eversion (superficial peroneal) response indicates the lateral components of the nerve are being stimulated. An inversion response is considered optimal and signifies that both components (tibial and peroneal) are being stimulated. Regardless of stimulation, local anesthetic spread should be visualized surrounding both components of the sciatic nerve.

The popliteal block is a distal sciatic block performed proximal to the popliteal fossa. The nerve may be more superficial with the distal approaches, yet if the block is attempted distal to the bifurcation of the tibial and peroneal

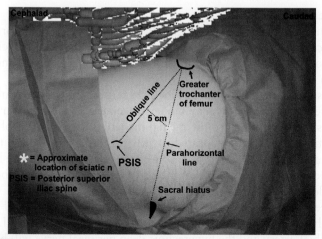

Figure 21-17 Surface anatomy for the gluteal (Labat) approach to the sciatic nerve. (From Tsui BCH, Rosenquist RW. Peripheral nerve blockade. In: Barash PG, Cullen BF, Stoelting RK, et al., eds. *Clinical Anesthesia*. 6th ed. Philadelphia: Wolters Kluwer Health/Lippincott Williams & Wilkins; 2009:994, with permission.)

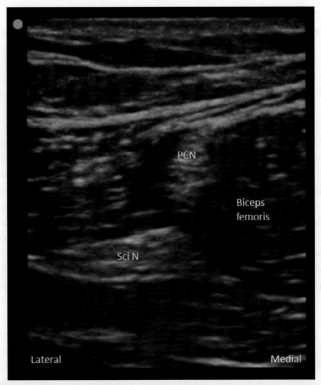

Figure 21-18   Ultrasound anatomy for the infragluteal sciatic nerve block. SciN, sciatic nerve; PCN, posterior cutaneous nerve of the thigh.

nerves, one of the two components may be missed. Blocking approximately 10 to 15 cm proximal to the popliteal crease usually ensures that the two components have joined. A simple technique to locate the sciatic nerve for a distal (popliteal) approach is to begin by visualizing the popliteal artery at the popliteal fossa. The tibial nerve will be located superficial and slightly lateral to the artery and appears hyperechoic. The tibial nerve can then be traced proximally, and the peroneal nerve can be seen joining the tibial component.

F. Ankle Block
Surgery on the distal foot, including bunion surgeries, can be performed with *ankle block* anesthesia. Many clinicians considered the ankle block to be a "field" block in the past, but the use of ultrasound has made ankle block anesthesia more precise.

The posterior tibial nerve can be blocked using a high-frequency ultrasound probe. The medial malleolus may hinder placement of the ultrasound probe. Scanning slightly proximal to the medial malleolus avoids this problem. The posterior tibial nerve will be located slightly posterior and deep to the posterior tibial artery (Fig. 21-19). The needle can be placed out of plane beginning either superior or inferior to the probe. A nerve stimulator can be used to confirm identification of the nerve with toe flexion.

The deep peroneal nerve block can be performed at the level of a line between the upper borders of the medial and lateral malleoluses. Locate the anterior tibial artery and the hyperechoic deep peroneal nerve will be lateral.

The superficial peroneal nerve and saphenous nerves are blocked with a subcutaneous local anesthetic ring circumferentially around the ankle at the upper border of the medial and lateral malleoluses. The sural nerve is blocked

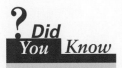

? Did You Know

Many clinicians formerly considered the ankle block to be a "field" block, but the use of ultrasound has made ankle block anesthesia more precise.

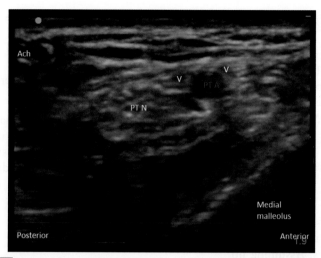

Figure 21-19   Ultrasound anatomy for the posterior tibial nerve at the level of the medial malleolus. Ach, Achilles tendon; PTN, posterior tibial nerve; PTA, posterior tibial artery; V, vein.

by injection of local anesthetic in the space posterior to the lateral malleolus and anterior to the calcaneus.

References

1. Liu SS, Ngeow JE, Yadeau JT. Ultrasound-guided regional anesthesia and analgesia: A qualitative systematic review. *Reg Anesth Pain Med.* 2009;34(1):47–59.
2. Renes SH, Rettig HC, Gielen MJ, et al. Ultrasound-guided low-dose interscalene brachial plexus block reduces the incidence of hemidiaphragmatic paresis. *Reg Anesth Pain Med.* 2009;34(5):498–502.
3. Urmey WF, Talts KH, Sharrock NE. One hundred percent incidence of hemidiaphragmatic paresis associated with interscalene brachial plexus anesthesia as diagnosed by ultrasonography. *Anesth Analg.* 1991;72(4):498–503.
4. Soares LG, Brull R, Lai J, et al. Eight ball, corner pocket: The optimal needle position for ultrasound-guided supraclavicular block. *Reg Anesth Pain Med.* 2007;32(1):94–95.
5. Brown DL, Cahill DR, Bridenbaugh LD. Supraclavicular nerve block: anatomic analysis of a method to prevent pneumothorax. *Anesth Analg.* 1993;76(3):530–534.
6. Rodriguez J, Barcena M, Alvarez J. Restricted infraclavicular distribution of the local anesthetic solution after infraclavicular brachial plexus block. *Reg Anesth Pain Med.* 2003;28(1):33–36.

Questions

1. An ultrasound-guided interscalene block is performed using 25 mL of 0.5% bupivacaine with a 22-gauge short-bevel stimulating needle. Which of the following side effects or complications is MOST likely to occur?
   A. Pneumothorax
   B. Hemidiaphragmatic paresis
   C. Horner's syndrome
   D. Recurrent laryngeal nerve blockade

2. An otherwise healthy 54 year old male patient is scheduled for a wrist arthroscopy estimated to take 2.5 hours. Assuming no contraindications to regional anesthesia, which of the following blocks would be best to offer to the patient?
   A. IV regional (Bier block) with 0.5% lidocaine
   B. IV regional (Bier block) with 0.5% bupivacaine
   C. Interscalene block
   D. Supraclavicular block

3. Which of the following nerves is originally derived from the sacral plexus?
   A. Tibial and common peroneal neves
   B. Obturator nerve
   C. Lateral femoral cutaneous nerve
   D. Femoral nerve

4. A patient is undergoing a sciatic block via gluteal (Labat) approach under the guidance of a peripheral nerve stimulator. Which if the following is the ideal motor response of the ipsilateralfoot, indicating both components of the sciatic nerve are being stimulated?
   A. Dorsiflexion
   B. Eversion
   C. Inversion
   D. Plantar flexion

Patient Positioning and Potential Injuries

Mary E. Warner

The single most important principle of patient positioning is "to do no harm." Anesthesiologists often reduce or eliminate the ability of patients to sense the positions in which they have been placed for procedures by giving amnesic, analgesic, and anesthetic drugs. Thus, it is the responsibility of anesthesiologists, as well as other members of the surgical team, to ensure that patients are not placed into positions that may harm them.

I. Anesthesia and Sedation: So Different than Regular Sleep

Many of us develop mild symptoms of *perioperative neuropathy* or soft tissue injury when sleeping naturally. We may awaken from sleep with tingling in an ulnar nerve distribution. The buttock soft tissues may become painful and awaken us when we have fallen asleep while sitting on long air flights. Our awakening allows us to both consciously or unconsciously move and reduce the tissue stretch and compression forces that caused our symptoms.

Anesthetized or sedated patients usually have their ability to sense sufficiently blunted by drugs to hinder them from awaking or moving. Prolonged immobilization of impacted tissues leads to the development of interstitial edema and inflammation. These two factors exacerbate stretch and compression forces and, over a sufficient period of time, may cause ischemia and more significant tissue damage. The loss of ability of anesthetized or sedated patients to respond to painful stimuli by moving is a major factor in perioperative position problems and for this reason anesthesiologists are taught basic position issues in their training.

Not all patient positioning problems involve mechanical forces on tissues. Although these tend to be the most common, other positioning issues may result in patient harm. For instance, anesthetized patients may be placed in head-elevated positions (e.g., for shoulder surgery) and could have decreased perfusion pressures in the brain if blood pressure measured at the level of the upper arm (i.e., with a standard blood pressure cuff) is not sufficient to

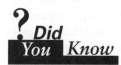

? Did You Know

Gravity reduces blood pressure. Patients with a reasonable, but low, pressure measured in the arm may potentially have ischemia in an elevated head or lower extremity.

413

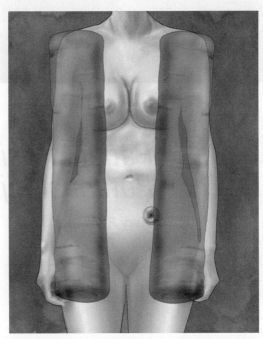

Figure 22-1 Soft tissues can be compressed and even become ischemic if there is too much pressure on them for long periods of time. This figure illustrates how chest rolls may compress the lateral aspects of large breasts or a stoma in prone-positioned patients.

drive blood flow up to the brain and overcome the hydrostatic pressure gradient between the elevated head and upper extremity. Similarly, anesthetized patients may be placed into lithotomy positions in which the legs are elevated higher than the level of blood pressure measurement by inflatable cuff in the upper extremity. Although the patient's blood pressure may be "normal" at the level of the upper extremity, it may be insufficient to pump blood upward against gravity to the elevated lower extremities. The resulting ischemia may cause hypoxic tissue damage and clinical *compartment syndrome*.

Perioperative positioning problems have not been well studied. In many cases, etiologic factors are not well defined or known, although many have been proposed. Although some etiologies are clear (e.g., direct compression of a stoma in a prone-positioned patient that causes ischemia to the externalized stomal tissues), others are not as evident (Fig. 22-1). For example, many plaintiff experts in malpractice legal cases have pronounced that inappropriate patient positioning by anesthesiologists has caused perioperative ulnar neuropathy. Although there is little doubt that direct pressure on ulnar nerves can cause ischemic neuropathy, in many cases it is well documented that the anesthesiologists diligently placed their patients into positions that would avoid direct pressure on their ulnar nerves. Despite this deliberate, presumably preventive approach to patient positioning, patients have developed perioperative ulnar neuropathy.

Why would this happen? Most patients who develop perioperative ulnar neuropathy do not become symptomatic until 2 to 5 days after their procedures (1). However, direct compression to nerves should cause immediate ischemia and symptoms of neuropathy. Thus, it appears that factors beyond intraoperative positioning may be at play. Further, recent findings suggest that a number of patients with new-onset ulnar neuropathy have systemic

? Did You Know

It is overly simplistic to assume all perioperative neuropathy is due to direct compression of the nerve. Other factors, such as inflammation may also be involved.

lymphatic microvasculitis of their peripheral nerves, which is treatable with corticosteroids (2). These findings suggest that the perioperative inflammatory response associated with most surgical procedures may be a factor in the development of what initially appeared to be a simple isolated peripheral nerve injury.

There is much more to learn about positioning problems, and simple etiologic assumptions may not be correct until scientifically proven. This chapter explains the mechanisms of soft tissue injury and common perioperative soft tissue injuries, cognizant that etiologic factors and appropriate preventive measures may not be known at this time.

II. Mechanisms of Soft Tissue Injury

Tissue stretch and compression are commonly considered to be associated with positioning-related problems in anesthetized or sedated patients. The perioperative period anatomic considerations include stretch and compression.

A. Stretch

Nerves are typically well vascularized by short nutrient arteries that divide and anastomose upon and within them. These effectively are the structures of a nerve's vasa nervosum (Fig. 22-2). In peripheral nerves, these minute arteries profusely anastomose to form an unbroken intraneural net. This net rarely leaves any particular segment of a peripheral nerve dependent on a single vessel for nutrient support. This net is not seen as commonly in central nerve tissue.

Stretch of nerve tissue, especially to more than 5% of resting length, may kink or reduce the lumens of feeding arterioles and draining venules (3). This phenomenon can lead to direct ischemia from reduced arteriole blood flow; indirect ischemia from venous congestion, increased intraneural pressure, and the need for high driving pressures of arteriolar blood flow; or both. Prolonged periods of ischemia may cause transient or permanent nerve injury. The lack of extensive vascular nets in central nervous tissue suggests that less stretch may be tolerated.

Soft tissues generally are less susceptible to stretch injury than nervous tissue. They are often more compliant and elastic, and many peripheral soft tissues do not need the same level of blood flow as nervous tissue. Nonetheless, prolonged stretch of any soft tissue may result in ischemia and tissue injury. Unique perioperative patient positions may increase the risk of soft tissue stretch (e.g., prone positions and their impact on breast tissue) (Fig. 22-1).

B. Compression

Direct pressure on soft and nerve tissues may reduce local blood flow and disrupt cellular integrity, resulting in tissue edema, ischemia, and, if prolonged, necrosis. The impact is especially damaging to ischemic-susceptible soft tissues (e.g., stomas associated with gastrointestinal diversions into cutaneous stomas) (Fig. 22-1).

III. Common Perioperative Neuropathies

A. Upper Extremity Neuropathies

Ulnar Neuropathy

Ulnar neuropathy is the most common perioperative neuropathy (4). There are a number of factors that may be associated with ***ulnar neuropathy***, including direct extrinsic nerve compression (often on the medial aspect of the elbow),

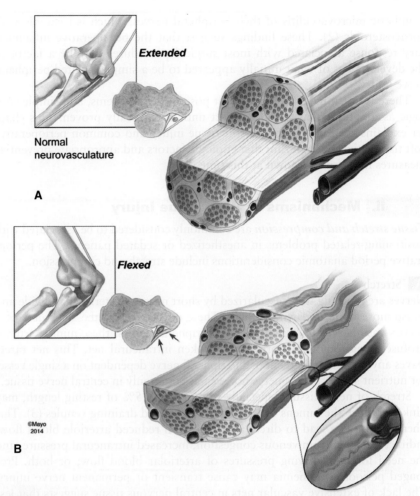

Figure 22-2 Effect of tissue stretch and compression on nerve vasa nervosum. This example shows potential ulnar nerve injury with elbow flexion. **A:** Extended elbow and relaxed ulnar nerve, noting patent perforating arterioles and venules. **B:** Flexed elbow, noting that stretch of the penetrating arterioles and venules from elongation of the ulnar nerve or compression by the cubital tunnel retinaculum can lead to vessel kinking and result in reduced arteriole blood flow from outside to inside the nerve (causing direct ischemia) and venous congestion from reduced venule outflow as vessel exits the nerve (leading to indirect ischemia). Prolonged ischemia can lead to nerve injury.

intrinsic nerve compression (associated with prolonged elbow flexion), and inflammation. Key points of interest are:

- *Timing of postoperative symptoms:* Most develop during the postoperative, not the intraoperative, period. There are good data that most surgical patients who develop ulnar neuropathy experience their first symptoms at least 24 hours postoperatively. This suggests that the mechanism of acute injury occurs primarily outside the operating room setting. Parenthetically, medical patients also develop ulnar neuropathies during hospitalization.
- *Impact of elbow flexion:* The ulnar nerve is the only major peripheral nerve in the body that always passes on the extensor side of a joint, in this case, the elbow. All other major peripheral nerves primarily pass on the flexion side of joints (e.g., median and femoral nerves). This anatomic difference may play

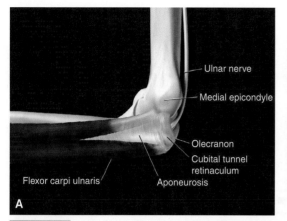 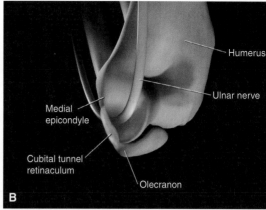

Figure 22-3 **A:** The ulnar nerve of the right arm passes distally behind the medial epicondyle and underneath the aponeurosis that holds the two heads of the flexor carpi ulnaris together. The proximal edge of the aponeurosis is sufficiently thick in 80% of men and 20% of women to be distinct anatomically from the remainder of the tissue. It is commonly called the cubital tunnel retinaculum. **B:** Viewed from behind, the cubital tunnel retinaculum intrinsically compresses the ulnar nerve when the elbow is progressively flexed beyond 90 degrees and the distance between the olecranon and the medial epicondyle increases.

a role in some perioperative ulnar neuropathies. In general, peripheral nerves begin to lose function and develop foci of ischemia when they are stretched >5% of their resting lengths. Elbow flexion, particularly >90 degrees, stretches the ulnar nerve. Prolonged elbow flexion and stretch of the ulnar nerve can result in sufficient ischemic areas to cause symptoms in awake and sedated patients and potential long-lasting damage in all patients.

- *Anatomy and elbow flexion:* Prolonged elbow flexion of >90 degrees increases intrinsic pressure on the nerve and may be as important an etiologic factor as prolonged extrinsic pressure (5,6). The ulnar nerve passes behind the medial epicondyle and then runs under the aponeurosis that holds the two muscle bodies of the flexor carpi ulnaris together. The proximal edge of this aponeurosis is sufficiently thick, especially in men, to be separately named the ***cubital tunnel retinaculum***. This retinaculum stretches from the medial epicondyle to the olecranon. Flexion of the elbow stretches the retinaculum and generates high pressures intrinsically on the nerve as it passes underneath (Figs. 22-3 and 22-4).

- *Forearm supination and ulnar neuropathy:* Supination of the forearm and hand does not, by itself, reduce the risk of ulnar neuropathy. The action of forearm supination occurs distal to the elbow. Supination is typically used when positioning arms on arm boards or at patients' sides because of the impact it has on humerus rotation. That is, supination is uncomfortable for most patients, and they will externally rotate their humerus to increase comfort. It is this external rotation of the humerus that lifts the medical aspect of the elbow, including the ulnar nerve, from directly resting on the table or arm-board surface. This rotation helps reduce extrinsic pressure on the ulnar nerve.

- *Outcomes of ulnar neuropathy:* Forty percent of sensory-only ulnar neuropathies resolve within 5 days; 80% resolve within 6 months. Few combined sensory and motor ulnar neuropathies resolve within 5 days; only 20% resolve within 6 months, and most result in permanent motor dysfunction and pain. The motor fibers in the ulnar nerve are primarily located in its middle. Injury to those fibers likely is associated with a more significant

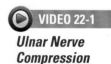

VIDEO 22-1

Ulnar Nerve Compression

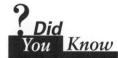

? *Did You Know*

Ulnar neuropathy manifested by sensory loss only has a good prognosis. Most resolve spontaneously within a few days or months.

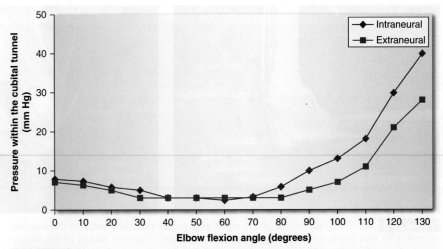

Figure 22-4 Pressure within the cubital reticulum at the elbow escalates once the angle of elbow flexion reaches and exceeds 90 degrees. (From Gelberman RH, Yamaguchi K, Hollstien SB, et al. Changes in interstitial pressure and cross-sectional area of the cubital tunnel and of the ulnar nerve with flexion of the elbow. An experimental study in human cadavera. *J Bone Joint Surg.* 1998;80(4):492–501, with permission.)

ischemia or pressure insult to all of the ulnar nerve fibers, and recovery may be prolonged or not possible.

Brachial Plexopathies

Brachial plexopathies occur most often in patients undergoing sternotomy. The risk for this plexopathy in patients undergoing sternotomy is particularly high in those with internal mammary artery mobilization. This finding is presumed to be associated with excessive concentric retraction on the chest wall and potential compression of the plexus between the clavicle and rib cage or stretch of the plexus. Otherwise, patients in prone and lateral positions have a higher risk of developing this problem than those in supine positions. Key points of interest are:

- *Brachial plexus entrapment:* There are many problems that can occur to the plexus in prone and laterally positioned patients. For example, the brachial plexus can become entrapped between compressed clavicles and the rib cage. Special attention should be given to altering positions that might exacerbate this potential problem.
- *Prone positioning:* In prone-positioned patients, it is prudent to tuck the arms at the side if at all possible; many patients have somatosensory-evoked potential changes when their arms are abducted (e.g., a "surrender" position).
- *Anatomy of shoulder abduction:* Abduction of the shoulder >90 degrees places the distal plexus on the extensor side of the joint and potentially stretches the plexus (Fig. 22-5). Therefore, it is best to avoid abduction >90 degrees, especially for extended periods.

Median Neuropathies

Median neuropathies primarily occur in men between the ages of 20 and 40 years. These men often have large biceps and reduced flexibility (e.g., as in the case of weightlifters). The large biceps and reduced flexibility tend to prevent complete extension at the elbow. This chronic limitation in range of motion results in shortening of the median nerve over time. *Median neuropathies* typically involve motor dysfunction and do not resolve readily. In fact, up

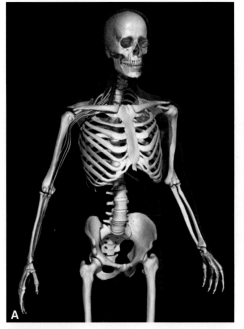
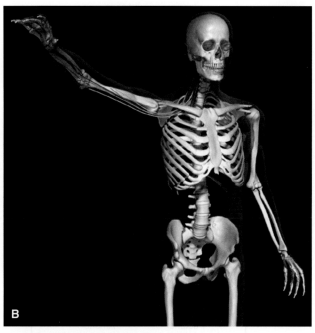

Figure 22-5 **A:** The neurovascular bundle to the upper extremity passes on the flexion side of the shoulder joint when the arm is at the side or abducted <90 degrees. **B:** Abduction of the arm beyond 90 degrees transitions the neurovascular bundle to where it now lies on the extension side of the shoulder joint. Progressive abduction >90 degrees increases stretch on the nerves at the shoulder joint.

to 80% of median neuropathies with motor dysfunction are sustained 2 years after the initial onset. Key points of interest are:

- *Stretch of a nerve:* As mentioned previously, nerves become ischemic when stretched >5% of their resting length. This amount of stretch tends to kink penetrating arterioles and exiting venules, both of which decrease perfusion pressure.
- *Arm support:* When these men are subsequently anesthetized, their arms may be fully extended at the elbow and placed on arm boards or at the patients' sides. This full extension of the elbow stretches chronically contracted median nerves and promotes ischemia, often at the level of the elbow. Thus, it is important to support the forearm and hand to prevent full extension in men who have large, bulky biceps and who cannot fully extend their elbows because of a lack of flexibility.

Radial Neuropathies
Radial neuropathies occur more often than median neuropathies. The radial nerve appears to be injured by direct compression (in contrast to the median nerve being injured primarily by stretch). The important factor appears to be compression of the nerve in the midhumerus region, where it wraps posteriorly around the bone (Fig. 22-6). *Radial neuropathies* tend to have a better chance of recovery than ulnar or median neuropathies. Approximately half get better within 6 months, and 70% appear to resolve completely within 2 years. Key points of interest are:

- *Surgical retractors:* A case series reported several radial neuropathies associated with compression of the radial nerve by the vertical bars of upper

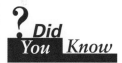

? **Did You Know**

Muscular men with large biceps are susceptible to median nerve injury if the arm is fully extended during surgery.

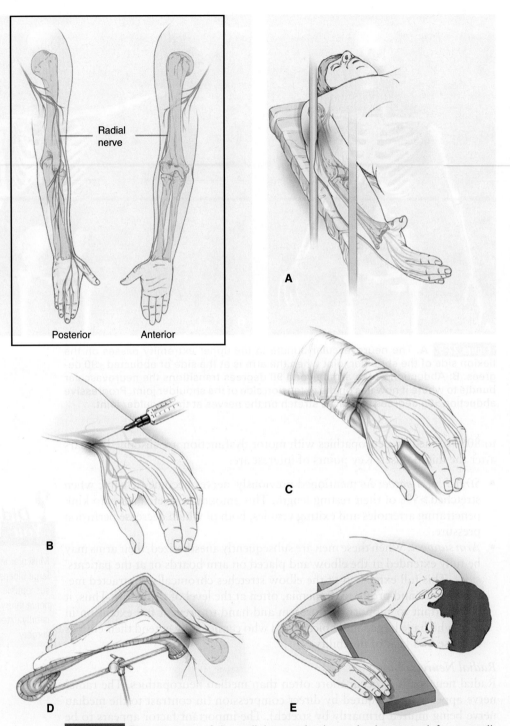

Figure 22-6 The anatomy of the radial nerve is shown in the upper left corner, illustrating how it wraps around the midhumerus. Reported mechanisms of perioperative injury include (**A**) compression by surgical retractor support bar; (**B**) direct needle trauma at the wrist; (**C**) compressive tourniquet effect by a draw sheet at the wrist; (**D**) impingement by an overhead arm board; (**E**) compression in the midhumerus level as the arm supports much of the weight of the upper extremity.

abdominal retractor holders. These vertical support bars reportedly impinged the arms (Fig. 22-6A).

- *Lateral positions:* The radial nerve may be impinged by overhead arm boards when they protrude into the midhumerus soft tissue (Fig. 22-6D).
- *An unsupported arm:* Anecdotal reports discuss compression on the nerve in the midhumerus when the elbow of a fixated arm (at the patient's side or on an arm board) slips, loses support, and the weight of the upper extremity is supported by the midhumerus (Fig. 22-6E).

B. Lower Extremity Neuropathies

Although common peroneal and sciatic neuropathies have the most impact on ambulation, the most common perioperative neuropathies in the lower extremities involved the obturator and lateral femoral cutaneous nerves. Key points of interest are:

- *Obturator neuropathy:* Hip abduction >30 degrees results in significant strain on the obturator nerve (7). The nerve passes through the pelvis and out the obturator foramen. With hip abduction, the superior and lateral rim of the foramen serves as a fulcrum (Fig. 22-7). The nerve stretches along its full length and is also compressed at this fulcrum point. Thus, excessive hip abduction should be avoided whenever possible. With obturator neuropathy, motor dysfunction is common. Thankfully, it is usually not painful, but it can be crippling. Approximately 50% of patients who have motor dysfunction in the perioperative period will continue to have it 2 years later.
- *Later femoral cutaneous neuropathy:* Prolonged hip flexion >90 degrees increases ischemia on fibers of the lateral femoral cutaneous nerve. One-third of this nerve's fibers pass through the inguinal ligament as they pass into the thigh (Fig. 22-8). Hip flexion >90 degrees results in lateral displacement of the anterior superior iliac spine and stretch of the inguinal ligament. The penetrating nerve fibers are compressed by this stretch and, with time, become ischemic and dysfunctional. The lateral femoral cutaneous nerve carries only sensory fibers, so there is no motor disability when it is injured. However, patients with this perioperative neuropathy can have disabling pain and dysesthesias of the lateral thigh. Approximately 40% of these patients have dysesthesias that last longer than 1 year.

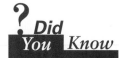

Great care must be exercised when placing the hip in unusual positions. Excessive flexion or abduction can injure the lateral femoral cutaneous or obturator nerves respectively.

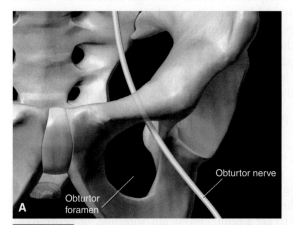
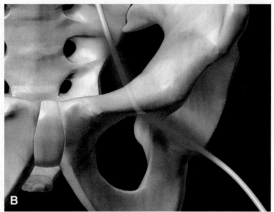

Obturtor nerve

Obturtor foramen

A   B

Figure 22-7 **A:** The obturator nerve passes through the pelvis and exits out the superior and lateral corner of the obturator foramen as it continues distally down the inner thigh. **B:** Abduction of the hip stretches the obturator nerve and can provoke ischemia, especially at the exit point of the obturator foramen. The point serves as a fulcrum for the nerve during hip abduction.

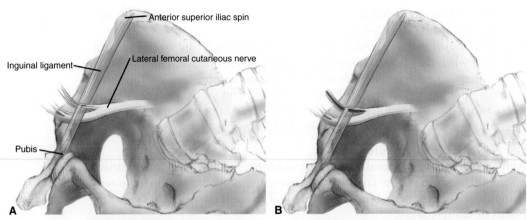

Figure 22-8 **A:** Approximately one-third of the lateral femoral cutaneous nerve fibers penetrate the inguinal ligament as the nerve passes out of the pelvis and distally into the lateral thigh. **B:** Hip flexion, especially when >90 degrees, leads to stretch of the inguinal ligament as the ilium is displaced laterally. This stretch causes the intraligament pressure to increase and compresses the nerve fibers as they pass through the ligament.

- *Peroneal neuropathy:* It appears that most peroneal neuropathies are associated with direct pressure of the lateral leg, just below the knee, where the peroneal nerve wraps around the head of the fibula. Leg holders, ranging from "candy cane" leg holders to various leg holders or "crutches" that hold the leg and foot, can impinge on the nerve as it wraps around the head of the fibula. The result can be devastating, with prolonged foot drop and difficulty ambulating.

IV. Practical Considerations for Perioperative Peripheral Neuropathies

There are some practical considerations that should be taken to prevent perioperative peripheral neuropathies. These include:

- Use padding to distribute compressive forces. Although there are few studies that demonstrate generous padding can impact the frequency or severity of perioperative neuropathies, it makes sense to distribute the point of pressure. Juries find the use of padding to be a positive step in medicolegal actions.
- Position joints to avoid excessive stretching, recognizing that stretch of any nerve >5% of its resting length over a prolonged period results in varying degrees of ischemia and dysfunction.

What the next step is if a patient develops a peripheral neuropathy depends on the type of neuropathy:

- If the loss is sensory only, it is reasonable to follow up with the patient daily for up to 5 days. Many sensory deficits in the immediate postoperative period will resolve during this time. If the deficit persists for longer than 5 days, it is likely that the neuropathy will have an extended impact. It is appropriate at that point to get a family physician, internist, or neurologist involved to provide long-term care.
- If the loss is motor only or combined sensory and motor, it would be prudent to get a neurologist involved early. These patients likely have a significant neuropathy and will need prolonged postoperative care.

V. Unique Positioning Problems with Catastrophic Results

A. Spinal Cord Ischemia with Hyperlordosis

This rare event occurs when patients undergoing pelvic procedures (e.g., prostatectomy) are placed in a *hyperlordotic position*, with >15 degrees of hyperflexion at the L2-3 interspace. This results in spinal cord ischemia, infarction, and devastating neurologic deficit. Magnetic resonance imaging detects this best. Operating room tables made in the United States are designed to limit hyperlordosis in supine patients, even when the table is maximally retroflexed with the kidney-rest elevated. In almost all reported cases, the table has been maximally retroflexed, the kidney-rest has been elevated, and towels or blankets have been placed under the lower back to promote further anterior or forward tilt of the pelvis (to improve vision of deep pelvic structures). In general, anesthesiologists should not allow placement of materials under the lower back for this purpose.

B. Thoracic Outlet Obstruction

Thoracic outlet obstruction is a rare event that occurs when patients with this syndrome are positioned prone or, less commonly, laterally. In almost all reported cases, the shoulder has been abducted >90 degrees. In that position, the vasculature to the upper extremity is either compressed between the clavicle and rib cage or between the anterior and middle scalene muscle bodies. This entrapment of the vasculature leads to upper extremity ischemia. When prolonged, the results range from minor disability to severe tissue loss that requires forequarter amputation. Simple preoperative questions such as "Can you use your arms to work above your head for more than a minute?" can elicit a history of thoracic outlet obstruction and reduce the risk of this potentially devastating complication.

C. Steep Head-Down Positions

As surgeons gain experience with new technologies (e.g., robotics for pelvic procedures), they often request steep head-down positions. These positions can be associated with cephalad shifting of anesthetized patients on operating room tables. Patients often are fixated to these tables with draw sheets and other retaining devices (e.g., shoulder braces). Cephalad shifting can lead to *cervical plexopathies* from stretch and subclavian vessel obstruction from compression. Although intracranial pressure also increases, it rarely results in a negative outcome. However, orofacial edema requires careful attention as it may compromise the airway. There are reports of patients sliding off operating room tables when they are placed in steep head-down positions and not secured to the beds. The resulting cervical spine and cerebral injuries have been devastating to both patients and members of the surgical team.

D. Steep Head-Up Positions

Although it is customary to think of use of this position for sitting craniotomies, the most common use of the steep head-up position is the *"beach chair" position* used for many shoulder surgeries. In addition to the well-known risk of venous air embolism in the craniotomy patient, this position can have considerable hemodynamic impact, specifically on systemic blood pressure and cerebral blood pressure (8). In addition, a number of severe brachial and cervical plexopathies have been reported. It appears that at least some of these

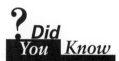

? Did You Know

Significant complications are associated with the sitting position for craniotomy, but also for shoulder surgery—such as cervical plexopathy.

plexopathies have been associated with nerve stretch or compression when patients have their heads fixated laterally during procedures.

E. Soft Tissue Problems

Skin and soft tissues are particularly vulnerable to sustained pressure, resulting in ischemia. Although there are many examples of this, several related to the prone position deserve special mention. Tissues in direct contact with rolls that extend from the shoulder girdle across the chest and to the pelvis may become ischemic with prolonged pressure (Fig. 22-1). There are multiple cases of women who have large breasts that developed severe ischemia of one or both breasts because they had been pushed in between chest rolls. The lateral pressure was sufficient to cause necrosis and sloughing. In most of these reported cases, the women subsequently underwent mastectomies. Similarly, ostomies have developed ischemia from pressure after they were placed in direct contact with these rolls.

VI. Summary

There are many ways for anesthetized patients to be harmed due to perioperative positioning. These include the use of positions that apply damaging mechanical forces to soft tissues and peripheral nerves. Unique positions may also impair normal physiologic function and need to be considered for every patient, especially those in any position other than level supine positions. The understanding of the etiologic factors that result in positioning problems is rudimentary at this time. There may be nonpositioning issues such as perioperative systemic inflammatory responses that contribute significantly to these problems. Nonetheless, careful assessment of individual patients and their ability to be positioned comfortably awake before anesthetized for surgical procedures is important to reduce the risk of complications associated with perioperative positioning.

References

1. Warner MA, Warner DO, Matsumoto JY, et al. Ulnar neuropathy in surgical patients. *Anesthesiology.* 1999;90:54–59.
2. Staff NP, Engelstad J, Klein CJ, et al. Post-surgical inflammatory neuropathy. *Brain.* 2010;133:2866–2880.
3. Warner MA. Patient positioning and related injuries. In: Barash PG, Cullen BF, Stoelting RK, et al., eds. *Clinical Anesthesia.* 7th ed. Philadelphia: Wolters Kluwer Health/Lippincott Williams & Wilkins; 2013:803–823.
4. American Society of Anesthesiologists Task Force on the Prevention of Perioperative Neuropathies. Practice guidelines for the prevention of perioperative neuropathies. *Anesthesiology.* 2000;92:1168–1182.
5. Contreras MG, Warner MA, Charboneau WJ, et al. Anatomy of the ulnar nerve at the elbow: Potential relationship of acute ulnar neuropathy to gender differences. *Clin Anat.* 1998;11:372–378.
6. Gelberman RH, Yamaguchi K, Hollstien SB, et al. Changes in interstitial pressure and cross-sectional area of the cubital tunnel and of the ulnar nerve with flexion of the elbow. An experimental study in human cadavera. *J Bone Joint Surg.* 1998;80(4):492–501.
7. Litwiller JP, Wells RE, Halliwill JR, et al. Effect of lithotomy positions on strain of the obturator and lateral femoral cutaneous nerves. *Clin Anat.* 2004;17:45–49.
8. Lee LA, Caplan RA. APSF workshop: Cerebral perfusion experts share views on management of head-up cases. *APSF Newslett.* 2009–10;24(4):45–48.

Questions

1. Which of the following statements is TRUE?
   A. In the seated position, the blood pressure measured in the brain is the same as in the arm.
   B. In the seated position, the blood pressure measured in the brain is higher than in the arm.
   C. In the lithotomy position, the blood pressure measured in the leg is less than in the arm.
   D. In the lithotomy position, the blood pressure measured in the leg is higher than in the arm.

2. A patient awakens from general anesthesia experiencing numbness and tingling is his fourth and fifth fingers. Which of the following factors is LEAST likely to cause this complication?
   A. A malfunctioning blood pressure cuff on that arm
   B. Trauma associated with starting an intravenous line in the antecubital fossa
   C. Prolonged flexion of the elbow at >90 degrees
   D. Microvasculitis and the perioperative inflammatory response

3. Damage to the interior fibers of the ulnar nerve is likely to result in:
   A. Primarily a sensory deficit that usually resolves in 5 days
   B. Primarily a sensory deficit that usually resolves in 6 months
   C. A motor deficit that usually resolves in 6 months
   D. A combined motor and sensory deficit that will likely be permanent

4. Brachial plexopathy is LEAST likely to occur following:
   A. Thyroidectomy
   B. Sternotomy and internal mammary artery mobilization
   C. Rotator cuff repair of the shoulder
   D. Lumbar spine fixation in the prone position with the arms abducted

5. Characteristics of median nerve injury include all of the following EXCEPT:
   A. It is usually due to excessive stretch of the nerve.
   B. It is likely to resolve in 4 weeks.
   C. It is common in men with large biceps.
   D. It is usually associated with full extension of the arm on an arm board.

6. A postoperative sensory deficit involving the lateral thigh without an associated motor deficit in that extremity suggests neuropathy of which of the following nerves:
   A. Sciatic
   B. Obturator
   C. Lateral femoral cutaneous
   D. Peroneal

7. A patient underwent a 5-hour facial plastic surgical procedure under general anesthesia with arms at his side. The first postoperative day he complained of numbness in the fourth and fifth digits of his right hand, but no loss of motor function. The most appropriate next step is to:
   A. Observe the patient daily for 5 days for signs of resolution of the neuropathy
   B. Institute physical therapy
   C. Obtain an electromyography study
   D. Send the patient to a neurologist

8. Asking patients whether they can work for more than 1 minute with their arms extended above their heads might be useful to determine whether they are at risk for which of the following anesthetic complications associated with prone positioning:
   A. Radial nerve motor deficit
   B. Ulnar nerve sensory deficit
   C. Compression of the C6 nerve root
   D. Thoracic outlet syndrome

9. When a patient is placed in the prone position, all of the following structures are at risk for pressure injury EXCEPT:
   A. A colostomy stoma
   B. The femoral artery
   C. Female breasts
   D. Male genitalia

23

Fluids and Electrolytes

Elizabeth E. Hankinson
Aaron M. Joffe

I. Acid–Base Interpretation and Treatment

A. Overview of Acid–Base Equilibrium

Precise regulation of *blood pH* is necessary for maintaining physiologic homeostasis. Outside of the normal physiologic range (7.35 to 7.45), vital functions such as oxygen transport, organ perfusion, and cellular metabolism may become impaired. At extremes of pH (<6.8 or >7.8), basic cellular processes are so impaired as to be incompatible with life.

The body is presented with significant acid and alkali loads daily, largely a consequence of nutrient intake and cellular metabolism. Nonetheless, the blood pH remains stable through buffering of *hydrogen ions (H⁺)* in the blood, their excretion by the kidneys (see Chapter 5), and elimination of *carbon dioxide (CO₂)* by the lungs (see Chapter 2). The amount of H⁺ in the blood is determined by the ratio of CO_2 and *bicarbonate* (hydrogen carbonate, HCO_3^-) as represented by the *Henderson-Hasselbalch equation:*

$$H^+ = (24 \times PCO_2)/HCO_3^- \qquad \text{(Eq. 23-1)}$$

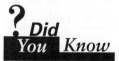

Accumulation of H⁺ or HCO_3^- due to exhaustion of body buffers or dysregulation by the kidneys results in *metabolic* disturbances, whereas high or low arterial CO_2 results from *respiratory* disturbances. Note the semantic difference between an "*–emia*" and an "*–osis.*" *Acidemia* and *alkalemia* refer to a low or high blood pH, respectively. *Acidosis* or *alkalosis* refers to the primary processes responsible for the alterations in pH (Fig. 23-1). Only one *–emia* can ever be present at one time, while more than one *–osis* can coexist.

B. Metabolic Acidosis

Primary *metabolic acidosis* is characterized by an arterial pH <7.35 and HCO_3^- <22 mEq/L and occurs as a result of either accumulation of H⁺ or a loss of HCO_3^-. The nature of the acidosis can be further characterized by the presence or absence of a greater than expected concentration of unmeasured anions (high gap or normal gap, respectively). Because the plasma normally

427

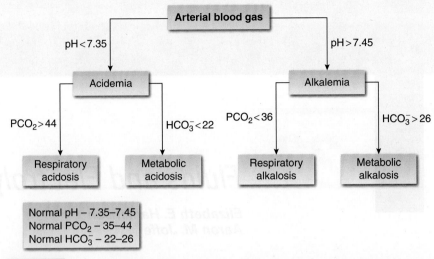

Figure 23-1 Derangements in acid–base status can be derived from arterial blood gas analysis by first determining acidemia or alkalemia from the pH, and then assessing the respiratory and metabolic components of the derangement from the PCO_2 and HCO_3^- values (see text and Table 23-6 for details). PCO_2, partial pressure of carbon dioxide; HCO_3^-, hydrogen carbonate.

contains more unmeasured anions than cations, an *anion gap (AG)* in the 6 to 11 mEq/L range is normally present. Calculation of the AG is determined with the following equation:

$$AG = Na^+ - (Cl^- + HCO_3^-)$$ (Eq. 23-2)

where Na^+ is the sodium ion and Cl^- is the chloride ion.

An elevated AG develops when an acid accumulates and then dissociates into a proton (H^+) and the unmeasured anion (UA^-). The proton is titrated by HCO_3^-, decreasing its concentration, while the UA^- remains in the plasma. Because neither the Na^+ nor Cl^- change, the AG increases (Eqs. 23-2 and 23-3):

$$H^+ + HCO_3^- \rightarrow H_2O + CO_2$$ (Eq. 23-3)

The most common causes of *high AG metabolic acidosis (HAGMA)* include ketoacidosis, uremia, lactic acidosis, and a variety of toxins including methanol, salicylates, paraldehydes, and ethylene glycol (Table 23-1).

Table 23-1   Causes of Metabolic Acidosis
High Anion Gap
Ketones—diabetic, starvation
Uremia
Lactate—sepsis, hypovolemia, congestive heart failure
Toxins—methanol, ethylene glycol, paraldehydes, salicylates, isoniazid
Nonanion Gap
Hyperchloremia (excessive saline administration)
Renal tubular acidosis
Gastrointestinal losses (diarrhea, ileostomy)

Nonanion gap metabolic acidosis (NAGMA) results when HCO_3^- is lost from the gastrointestinal tract or kidneys or due to an inability of the kidneys to excrete protons. Because electroneutrality is maintained by Cl^- retention, the AG remains unchanged. The most common causes of NAGMA are excessive administration of 0.9% NaCl solution, diarrhea, and renal tubular acidosis (Table 23-1).

Treatment of metabolic acidosis should be directed toward correcting the underlying cause. For example, in the case of a NAGMA due to 0.9% NaCl administration, the Cl^- load can be reduced with balanced lactate solutions for resuscitation or by adding 150 mL of 8.4% $NaHCO_3$ to a 1,000-mL bag of 5% dextrose in water. Antidiarrheal medications can be given, and in cases of severe diarrhea where HCO_3^- losses are significant, administration of sodium bicarbonate can be considered. Treatment for HAGMA is based on the underlying cause. *Ketoacidosis* should be treated with insulin therapy, and *lactic acidosis* is treated with oxygenation, resuscitation, and cardiovascular support. Treatment of lactic acidosis with sodium bicarbonate is not recommended unless pH is <7.15 and the patient is clinically deteriorating (1,2).

C. Metabolic Alkalosis
Metabolic alkalosis is characterized by an arterial pH >7.45 (alkalemia) and HCO_3^- >26 mEq/L. This disorder results from a net gain of HCO_3^- or loss of H^+ ions. The kidney has a tremendous ability to excrete HCO_3^-, so metabolic alkalosis must not only be generated but also maintained, usually by obligatory $NaHCO_3^-$ reabsorption in the proximal tubule in the setting of hypovolemia. Severe hypokalemia from any cause may also lead to HCO_3^- retention. Loss of H^+ ions usually results from significant vomiting or renal excretion, as suggested by a history of vomiting or diuretic use. Urine electrolytes (notably urine Cl^-) are used to further characterize the metabolic alkalosis. Low urine Cl^- is considered saline responsive, whereas normal or high urine Cl^- is saline unresponsive. The most common causes of metabolic alkalosis are listed in Table 23-2.

Treatment of metabolic alkalosis is based on correcting the underlying cause. Saline responsive metabolic alkalosis should receive resuscitation with sodium and potassium chloride to enable to kidneys to resume HCO_3^- excretion.

D. Respiratory Acidosis
Respiratory acidosis is defined as an arterial pH <7.35 and partial pressure of CO_2 (PCO_2) >44 mm Hg. An increase in CO_2 will result in more H^+ ions, decreasing the pH (Eq. 23-3). Arterial CO_2 levels reflect the balance between CO_2 production via cellular respiration and its excretion through alveolar ventilation. It should be noted that increased production alone would rarely be

Table 23-2 Causes of Metabolic Alkalosis

Low Urine Cl⁻ (Saline Responsive)	Normal or High Urine Cl⁻ (Saline Unresponsive)
Vomiting	Primary aldosteronism
Nasogastric suctioning	Renal failure
Hypokalemia	Cushing syndrome
Diuretic use	Hypomagnesemia

Table 23-3   Causes of Respiratory Acidosis

Decreased CO_2 Elimination

Pulmonary disease (acute respiratory distress syndrome, pneumonia)
Airway obstruction (laryngospasm, asthma, obstructive sleep apnea)
Central nervous system depression (opioids, anesthetics)
Neuromuscular weakness (amyotrophic lateral sclerosis, Guillain-Barre syndrome, residual drug-induced paralysis)

Increased CO_2 Production

Laparoscopy
Exhausted soda lime
Sepsis
Fever
Hyperthyroidism
Overfeeding
Malignant hyperthermia
Neuroleptic malignant syndrome

Increased Inspired CO_2

Exhausted soda lime (circle breathing system)

the cause of respiratory acidosis, as healthy spontaneously breathing individuals have the ability to increase their alveolar ventilation. The most common causes of respiratory acidosis are listed in Table 23-3. Respiratory acidosis can be further classified as acute or chronic based on the presence and extent of renal compensation (see below).

Treatment of respiratory acidosis relies on identification of the underlying cause. The most common interventions include supporting increased alveolar ventilation by institution of noninvasive or invasive mechanical ventilation or reversal of respiratory depressant medications. Avoiding high carbohydrate foods and providing sedative medications will decrease metabolic CO_2 production. Sodium bicarbonate is not recommended, as it offers no proven benefit and can worsen the hypercapnea by producing more CO_2 (Eq. 23-3).

E. Respiratory Alkalosis

Respiratory alkalosis is defined as an arterial pH >7.45 and PCO_2 <36 mm Hg. Because arterial partial pressure of CO_2 ($PaCO_2$) is inversely proportional

Table 23-4   Causes of Respiratory Alkalosis

Pain

Hyperventilation

Pregnancy

Hypoxia

Central nervous system disease

Medications

Liver disease

Table 23-5   Physiologic Compensation for Acid–Base Disturbances

Primary Disorder	Disturbance	Compensation
Metabolic alkalosis	↑ HCO_3	PCO_2 ↑ 0.5–0.7 mm Hg per 1 mEq/L ↑ HCO_3^-
Metabolic acidosis	↓ HCO_3	PCO_2 ↓ 1.2 mm Hg per 1 mEq/L ↓ HCO_3^-
Respiratory alkalosis		
Acute	↓ PCO_2	HCO_3^- ↓ 2 mEq/L per 10 mm Hg ↓ PCO_2
Chronic	↓ PCO_2	HCO_3^- ↓ 5–6 mEq/L per 10 mm Hg ↓ PCO_2
Respiratory acidosis		
Acute	↑ PCO_2	HCO_3^- ↑ 1 mEq/L per 10 mm Hg ↑ PCO_2
Chronic	↑ PCO_2	HCO_3^- ↑ 4–5 mEq/L per 10 mm Hg ↑ PCO_2

HCO_3^-, hydrogen carbonate; PCO_2, partial pressure of carbon dioxide.

to alveolar ventilation, respiratory alkalosis results from low $PaCO_2$ due to inappropriate alveolar hyperventilation. Equation 23-3 demonstrates that a decrease in CO_2 results in fewer H^+ ions and therefore an increase in pH. The most common causes of respiratory alkalosis are listed in Table 23-4. Treatment is to identify the underlying cause and provide appropriate treatment.

F. Physiologic Compensation of Acid–Base Disorders

Primary metabolic disorders lead to *respiratory compensation* and vice versa. Respiratory compensation is quite swift. Rapid increases in alveolar ventilation can normalize pH in a matter of minutes. Conversely, *metabolic compensation* for respiratory disorders takes hours to days, as it requires the kidneys to alter plasma HCO_3^- levels. Most compensatory responses are quite effective, although respiratory compensation for metabolic alkalosis requires alveolar hypoventilation to increase PCO_2, but it is limited to a maximum of 75% due to the resulting hypoxemia that occurs. A list of the normal compensatory responses expected for the acid–base disturbances is provided in Table 23-5.

II. Practical Approach to Acid–Base Interpretation

Arterial blood gas (ABG) analysis is primarily used to assess adequacy of gas exchange and oxygen delivery. It is the most frequently ordered test in anesthetized and critically ill patients to guide ventilation and treatment, and it provides data including pH, arterial partial pressure of oxygen (PaO_2), $PaCO_2$, and HCO_3^-. Analysis of these values can be used to determine whether an acid–base disturbance exists, what the disturbance is, and its possible etiologies. Thus, the understanding and ability to quickly analyze ABG data are crucial for every anesthesiologist.

A simple acid–base disorder, typically one of the metabolic or respiratory disturbances occurring in isolation, is the most common clinical presentation. However, critically ill patients can have multiple acid–base disorders. Physiologic compensation is never complete, thus the pH will never be completely normal in a simple acid–base disorder. However, in the presence of

Table 23-6   Step-wise Approach to Arterial Blood Gas Analysis

Step 1: Examine the pH to determine whether academia or alkalemia is present:
If the pH is <7.35 a primary acidemia present
If the pH is >7.45 a primary alkalemia is present

Step 2: Examine the $PaCO_2$ to determine if the primary disturbance is respiratory or metabolic:
If acidemia present: $PaCO_2$ >40 mm Hg = respiratory acidosis; $PaCO_2$ <40 mm Hg = metabolic acidosis (proceed to Step 3)
If alkalemia present: $PaCO_2$ >40 mm Hg = metabolic alkalosis; $PaCO_2$ <40 mm Hg = respiratory alkalosis (proceed to Step 4)

Step 3 (acidemia only): Calculate the anion gap (AG):
$AG = Na^+ - (Cl^- + HCO_3^-)$; If AG >11 then a "high anion gap metabolic acidosis" is present (see Table 23-1)

Step 4: Determine if appropriate compensation is present to assess whether the disturbance is acute or chronic:
See Table 23-5

Step 5: Determine likely etiologies of the acid–base disturbance:
See Tables 23-1, 23-2, 23-3, and 23-4

$PaCO_2$, arterial partial pressure of carbon dioxide; Na, sodium; Cl, chlorine; HCO_3^-, hydrogen carbonate.

multiple acid–base disturbances, the pH can normalize or reach life-threatening extremes.

Arterial blood gas analysis is best approached systematically to ensure rapid and precise interpretation. One common, step-wise method is based on the Henderson-Hasselbalch equation and analyzes the pH, $PaCO_2$, HCO_3^-, AG, and presence of compensation (Table 23-6).

A typical perioperative clinical scenario illustrating the application of this step-wise method is shown below.

Clinical Scenario: Arterial Blood Gas Interpretation

A 52-year-old morbidly obese diabetic female presents to the operating room for emergent debridement of a necrotizing soft tissue infection of her left foot, with the following preoperative ABG (room air):

ABG: pH 7.10, $PaCO_2$ 28 mm Hg, PaO_2 88 mm Hg, HCO_3^- 11 mEq/L, Na^+ 136 mEq/L, K^+ 5.5 mEq/L, Cl^- 99 mEq/L, lactate 14 mmol/L
Step 1: because the pH is <7.35, acidemia is present
Step 2: because the $PaCO_2$ is <40, a primary metabolic acidosis is present
Step 3: because the anion gap is [136 − (99 + 11)] 26, a "high anion gap" metabolic acidosis is present
Step 4: because the $PaCO_2$ is appropriately decreased (HCO_3^- is 13 mEq/L below the normal of 24 mEq/L; 13 × 1.2 mm Hg = 15.6 mm Hg; 28 + 15.6 = 43.6 mm Hg), a compensated metabolic acidosis is present
Step 5: The patient has a severe soft tissue infection and systemic sepsis, with impaired tissue oxygen use resulting in anaerobic metabolism and accumulation of lactic acid, leading to a compensated, high anion gap, metabolic acidosis.

III. Physiology of Fluid Management

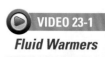
VIDEO 23-1
Fluid Warmers

The kidneys play several key roles in maintaining homeostasis in the human body. In addition to maintaining normal acid–base status, the kidneys must regulate total body water and solute because daily intake of each is variable. Improper regulation can result in too little body water (cellular dehydration) or too much (tissue edema). Similar regulation occurs when patients have no oral intake and instead are receiving intravenous fluid (i.e., water with dissolved solute). A thorough knowledge of how administered fluids are distributed among the various body compartments, as well as their individual components, is essential. Intravenous fluid should be considered like any other pharmaceutics insofar as there are specific indications and clinical contexts that determine proper fluid therapy. For example, patients residing in the intensive care unit or presenting to the operating room may have low extracellular fluid volume, cellular dehydration, or both as a result of major trauma, hemorrhage, prolonged fasting or malnutrition, or protracted vomiting or diarrhea. Both the choice of fluid composition and its infusion rate are dictated accordingly, in this case, most likely high-volume resuscitation with isotonic crystalloid. The anesthesiologist must take into account such clinical contexts and pathophysiologies when tailoring fluid management for a given patient.

A. Body Fluid Compartments

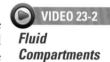
VIDEO 23-2
Fluid Compartments

Total body water (TBW) is estimated to comprise 60% and 50% of the lean body mass of adult males and females, respectively. TBW is distributed throughout various body compartments with roughly 66% making up the *intracellular fluid (ICF)* and 33% making up the *extracellular fluid (ECF)*. ECF is further divided into interstitial fluid and plasma, which account for approximately 24% and 8% of the TBW, respectively (Fig. 23-2). Thus, for an adult male weighing 70 kg, the TBW is estimated to be 42 L. Of this amount, only 3.5 L is plasma, with the remainder of the circulating blood volume being red blood cells (see also Chapter 3).

Distribution of TWB in a 70 Kg adult male

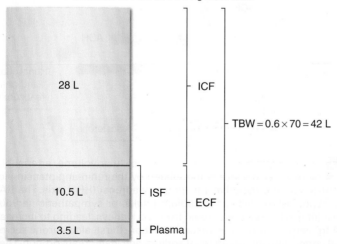

Figure 23-2 The approximate distribution of total body water (TBW) in the various body compartments is shown for a 70-kg adult male. ICF, intracellular fluid; ECF, extracellular fluid; ISF, interstitial fluid.

B. Regulation of Extracellular Fluid Volume

The control of ECF concentration and volume is important for cellular function, transfer of molecules between ICF and ECF, and maintenance of circulating blood volume. Normal serum osmolarity is 285 to 295 mOsm/L and is calculated from measured concentrations of sodium, glucose, and urea (blood urea nitrogen [BUN]) as follows:

$$\text{Serum osmolarity} = (2 \times Na^+) + (\text{Glucose}/18) + (\text{BUN}/2.8) \quad (\text{Eq. 23-4})$$

It should be noted, however, that a difference exists between *osmolarity* (the concentration of particles dissolved per unit of serum volume) and *tonicity* (the effective osmolarity that can exert an osmotic force across a membrane). Tonic molecules (e.g., Na^+) are considered "effective osmoles" because they do not move freely across a membrane. They are able to cause water movement down a concentration gradient. In contrast, because urea freely diffuses across biologic membranes and distributes itself throughout the total body water, it is not *tonic*. Thus, under conditions of relative normoglycemia, the major contributor to serum osmolarity and tonicity is the Na^+ concentration.

The concentration and volume of the ECF are maintained by both thirst and the hormonal actions of the *renin-angiotensin-aldosterone system (RAAS)* and *antidiuretic hormone (ADH)* on the kidneys, which alter the amount of Na^+ and water excreted in urine. ADH is released (i.e., nontonic release) from the posterior pituitary in response to small changes (2% to 3%) in serum tonicity or >10% decreases in effective circulating volume. The RAAS is activated

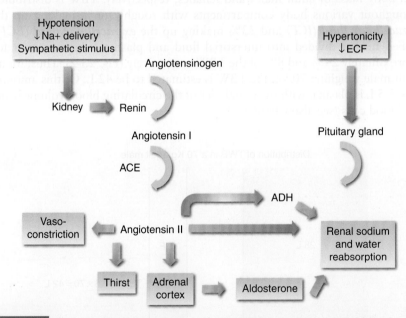

Figure 23-3 Neurohormonal regulation of extracellular volume, arterial blood pressure, and sodium/water balance is modulated by the renin-angiotensin-aldosterone system (RAAS) and the hypothalamic-pituitary-adrenal (HPA) axis. The RAAS is activated by hypotension, decreased sodium intake, or sympathetic nervous system activity, resulting in the release of renin from the kidneys, leading to increased angiotensin II. Angiotensin II promotes vasoconstriction, thirst, aldosterone secretion from the adrenal cortex, and increased renal sodium and water reabsorption. The HPA axis secretes antidiuretic hormone (ADH) in response to increased plasma osmolarity, decreased extracellular fluid (ECF), or decreased plasma angiotensin and leads to increased renal free water absorption in the kidneys and further vasoconstriction. ACE, angiotensin converting enzyme.

by hypotension, the sympathetic nervous system, and decreased Na^+ delivery to the kidneys (Fig. 23-3). The end result is increased thirst (increased water intake), increased renal retention of Na^+ and water, and vasoconstriction, all of which act to maintain effective circulating volume and perfusion of vital organs.

C. Distribution of Infused Fluids

There are two types of fluids commonly used for intravenous administration that are categorized by their ability to diffuse through a semipermeable membrane: *crystalloids* and *colloids*. Crystalloids readily diffuse across a semipermeable membrane, whereas colloids do not. Crystalloids are generally a base of sterile water in which various electrolytes are dissolved. They may be further categorized by their tonicity relative to serum: *hypotonic*, *isotonic*, and *hypertonic* solutions. The composition of several commonly used intravenous solutions is presented in Table 23-7.

Renal excretion notwithstanding, the tonicity of a given crystalloid will determine across which body compartments the solution will initially distribute. Hypotonic and isotonic solutions generally equilibrate across TBW and ECF, respectively. An estimation of the initial volume distribution following the rapid infusion of 1,000 mL of various crystalloids and colloids is presented in Table 23-8.

Traditional teaching is that colloids are unable to move across an intact endothelial barrier and therefore remain entirely within the plasma. Additionally, the maintenance of normal plasma colloid oncotic pressure allows for maximal reabsorption of interstitial fluid back into the vascular tree on the venular side of the microcirculation (see Chapter 3). Consequently, it has long been taught that three or four times as much crystalloid must be administered as colloid to achieve the same plasma volume expansion. However, this is not supported by current evidence. Most studies report a volume equivalence of colloid to isotonic crystalloid less than two to one (see below).

Table 23-7	Composition of Common Intravenous Solutions					
Solution	pH	Osmolarity (mMol/L)	K$^+$ (mEq/L)	Na$^+$ (mEq/L)	Cl$^-$ (mEq/L)	Other Additives
0.9% NS	4.5–7	308		154	154	
0.45% NS	4.5–7	154		77	77	
D5W	5.0	278				Dextrose
Ringer's lactate	6–7.5	273	4	130	109	Lactate, calcium
Plasmalyte	6.5–7.6	294	5	140	98	Acetate, gluconate, magnesium
Albumin 5%	6.9	300		145	145	
Albumin 25%	6.9	1500		145	145	
HES 450/0.7 (Hespan)	5.9	309		154	154	
HES 130/0.4 (Voluven)	4–5.5	309		154	154	

K$^+$, potassium; Na$^+$, sodium; Cl$^-$, chlorine; D5W, 5% dextrose in water; NS, normal saline.

Table 23-8	Comparison of Body Compartment Distribution of 1,000 mL Intravenous Fluid		
Hypotonic	**Isotonic**	**Hypertonic**	**Colloids**
Dextrose 5% water	0.9% normal saline	3% NaCl	Blood
0.45% normal saline	Ringer's lactate		Albumin
	Plasmalyte		
Distribution	**Distribution**	**Distribution**	**Distribution**
ICF—650 mL	ICF—None	ICF—None	ICF—None
ISF—250 mL	ISF—750 mL	ISF—None	ISF—None
IVF—100 mL	IVF—250 mL	IVF—1,000 mL	IVF—>1,000 mL

ICF, intracellular fluid; ISF, interstitial fluid; IVF, intravascular fluid.

IV. Fluid Replacement Therapy

Maintenance of sufficient intravascular volume to support organ perfusion is the chief goal of perioperative fluid administration. Perioperative intravascular volume depletion (i.e., *hypovolemia*) is common for various reasons, including prolonged preoperative starvation (NPO) status, sepsis, hyperthermia, chronic diuretic use, uncontrolled hyperglycemia, vomiting, and diarrhea. Hypovolemia results in organ hypoperfusion, tissue hypoxia, acidosis, and arterial hypotension. Replacing any existing fluid deficit and administering maintenance intravenous fluids to achieve normovolemia both promote adequate organ perfusion pressure and tissue oxygenation, thereby improving surgical outcomes (3,4). Although hypovolemia is often the main concern perioperatively, excessive fluid administration leading to volume overload has been shown to increase postoperative complications. *Hypervolemia* increases the risk for bowel edema, nausea, vomiting, pulmonary edema, and decompensated heart failure. Thus, obtaining a detailed history and accurate preoperative assessment of volume status (see below) are important factors when managing fluid perioperatively.

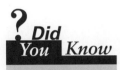

Did You Know

Maintenance of sufficient intravascular volume to support organ perfusion, tissue oxygenation, and aerobic metabolism is the chief goal of perioperative fluid administration.

A. Maintenance Requirements for Water, Sodium, and Potassium

Under normal physiologic conditions, the average adult loses approximately 1,500 mL of water daily from perspiration, respiration, feces, and urine. Sodium and potassium losses are minimal and replacement is roughly 1 mmol/kg daily. Generally these daily water and electrolyte requirements are easily achieved with oral intake. However, various disease states alter normal electrolyte balance, resulting in severe abnormalities, and can pose great challenges to perioperative fluid administration.

B. Glucose Requirements and Dextrose

Blood glucose is under tight hormonal control, such that a healthy adult is capable of maintaining normal blood glucose levels for weeks without caloric intake. Thus, blood glucose is not routinely monitored in healthy adults, nor are dextrose-containing fluids routinely administered. However, patients with insulin-dependent diabetes mellitus are susceptible to both *hypoglycemia* and *hyperglycemia*; therefore, blood glucose should be carefully monitored in these patients perioperatively. In addition, infants younger than 6 months old have limited glycogen stores, are susceptible to hypoglycemia after short periods of fasting, and typically receive dextrose-containing fluids perioperatively.

C. Surgical Fluid Requirements

Traditional teaching surrounding the estimation of perioperative fluid deficit and the calculation of maintenance intravenous fluid has relied upon a seminal 1957 study by Holliday and Segar that generated the often-quoted "4-2-1 rule" of maintenance fluid management based on body weight (i.e., hourly hypotonic fluid requirement is 4 mL/kg for the first 10 kg, 2 mL/kg for the second 10 kg, and 1 mL/kg for all remaining kilograms) (5). However, application of this method fails to account for a number of physiologic factors and can lead to hypervolemia and hyponatremia that are associated with increased postoperative complications, including longer hospital stay, pulmonary edema, pneumonia, and ileus. Thus, current practice is to use isotonic solutions for maintenance fluid, with superior outcomes demonstrated for balanced electrolyte solutions over normal saline.

Despite numerous studies, controversy still exists over optimal perioperative fluid management. However, recent studies have demonstrated improved outcomes when fluid therapy is based on specific clinical criteria. Notably, consensus guidelines from the Enhanced Recovery Partnership recommend the use of *goal-directed fluid management* for patients who are acutely ill, undergoing major surgery, or have comorbidities that warrant cardiac output monitoring, but not for patients undergoing low-risk surgery (6). However, evidence does not support a single, specific hemodynamic goal or method of measurement. Furthermore, intraoperative maintenance fluids should be limited to 2 mL/kg/hr (including drug infusions). Postoperatively, intravenous fluids should be limited and oral hydration resumed as soon as possible.

V. Colloids, Crystalloid, and Hypertonic Solutions

The ideal resuscitative fluid would have a similar composition to plasma, have predictable and reliable effects on circulating blood volume, be free of undesired side effects, be inexpensive, and lead to improvements in patient-centered outcomes (morbidity, mortality, or length of stay). However, as one might expect, such a fluid does not exist, thus, the ongoing controversy between crystalloid and colloid solutions. The most commonly used resuscitation fluids are isotonic salt solutions and colloids, whose compositions are listed in Table 23-7.

A. Physiology and Pharmacology

The efficacy of any intravenous fluid in expanding the plasma volume is dependent on the proportion of administered fluid that remains in the intravascular space. Traditionally, net transcapillary fluid flux within the extracellular fluid space—from plasma to interstitial fluid—is described by the *Starling equation:*

$$F = Kf^* \left([Pc - Pt] - \sigma[\pi c - \pi i]\right), \qquad \text{(Eq. 23-5)}$$

where F is the net fluid movement between compartments, Kf is a filtration coefficient, Pc is the capillary hydrostatic pressure, Pt is the tissue hydrostatic pressure, σ is the reflection coefficient (a measure of leakiness to a particular substance), πc is the capillary oncotic pressure, and πi the interstitial oncotic pressure.

Based on the traditional Starling equation (described in detail in Chapter 3), fluid moves from the plasma to the interstitium at the arteriolar level driven by the dominant hydrostatic pressure gradient. On the venular side of the circulation, the colloid oncotic pressure within the vasculature promotes fluid reabsorption back into circulation (see Fig. 3-18). In order to exploit these basic physiologic mechanisms, hypertonic salt and colloidal solutions were introduced into clinical practice.

However, in clinical practice, volume expansion as a result of administered intravenous resuscitative fluids cannot be reliably predicted by the traditional Starling equation. This is especially true in states of inflammation, physiologic stress, and shock, in which capillary permeability is altered. In these situations, intravascular fluid loss (including both crystalloid and colloid solutions) to the interstitium is greater than would be expected. This signals the emerging importance of multiple capillary components (e.g., endothelial glycocalyx, capillary basement membrane, and extracellular matrix) in driving diffusion physiology, as well as highlights the importance of the lymphatic circulation in returning interstitial fluid to the intravascular compartment. Thus, the actual volume equivalence of colloids to crystalloids observed in clinical practice is actually closer to two to one rather than the predicted three or four to one (7).

B. Clinical Implications of Choosing Crystalloid a Colloid

The debate over crystalloid and colloid fluid administration is long-standing, and an overwhelming number of studies in the literature have compared their benefits and liabilities. For example, crystalloid resuscitation is generally associated with greater weight gain, which itself is associated with various negative clinical outcomes. However, this association is not causation and the literature still lacks strong evidence supporting one fluid type over the other. Studies suggest, however, that there are subsets of patients in whom the use of albumin and synthetic colloids appears to confer a worse outcome. Table 23-9 summarizes selected literature comparing clinical outcomes with colloid and crystalloid resuscitation. Additional characteristics should also factor into the decision. Crystalloids are inexpensive, nonallergenic, and do not inhibit coagulation. However, their administration results in tissue edema, leading to gut flora translocation, poor wound healing, impairment of alveolar gas exchange, limited intravascular volume expansion, and metabolic derangements. Conversely, colloids are expensive, allergenic, and linked to renal failure and coagulopathy, and their theoretic benefit of remaining in the intravascular space is not supported by evidence.

C. Implications of Crystalloid and Colloid Solutions on Intracranial Pressure

Based on the discussion above, it could be expected that colloid solutions increase *intracranial pressure (ICP)* less than crystalloid, thus improving outcomes in *traumatic brain injury (TBI)* patients. This theory, however, assumes ideal physiologic conditions in which the *blood–brain barrier* remains intact. Unfortunately, as demonstrated in the SAFE trial (Table 23-9), this theory does not hold true clinically, and TBI patients resuscitated with colloids demonstrated increased mortality. A subgroup analysis of the SAFE trial further indicated that albumin resuscitation in TBI patients is associated with significantly higher ICPs in the first week postinjury than for those receiving crystalloids. The mechanism is not fully elucidated, but it is thought to involve a disruption in the blood–brain barrier, resulting in colloid leaking into brain parenchyma and rebound intracranial hypertension. Thus, colloid administration should be avoided in patients with suspected or known TBI.

D. Clinical Implications of Hypertonic Fluid Administration

Hypertonic fluids commonly used in clinical practice include hypertonic saline and mannitol. Hypertonic saline is most commonly used to treat symptomatic hyponatremia, whereas hypertonic mannitol is used primarily to reduce

? Did You Know

Hypertonic crystalloids can be administered in smaller volumes than isotonic crystalloids to achieve the same effect in intravascular fluid expansion, making hypertonic solutions attractive for use in low-resource settings such as military combat care.

Table 23-9   Summary of Literature Comparing Colloid and Crystalloid as Primary Resuscitative Fluids

Cochrane Injuries Group Albumin Reviewers. Human albumin administration in critically ill patients: Systematic review of randomised controlled trials. *BMJ.* 1998;317(7153):235–240.	• Albumin increased overall rate of death in patients with hypovolemia, burns, hypoalbuminemia
Finfer S et al. A comparison of albumin and saline for fluid resuscitation in the intensive care unit. *N Engl J Med.* 2004;350(22):2247–2256.	• No statistically significant difference in 28-day mortality • Subgroup analysis showed increased rates of death at 2 years with the use of colloid in TBI but decreased risk of death at 28 days in severe sepsis
Mybergh JA et al. Hydroxyethyl starch or saline for fluid resuscitation in intensive care. *N Engl J Med.* 2012;367(20):1901–1911.	• Mortality higher in HES group but not statistically significant • AKI higher in Saline group • Need for RRT higher in HES group • HES was associated with significantly more adverse events
Bayer O et al. Effects of fluid resuscitation with synthetic colloids or crystalloids alone on shock reversal, fluid balance, and patient outcomes in patients with severe sepsis; a prospective sequential analysis. *Crit Care Med.* 2012;40(9):2543–2551.	• PRAC concluded that the benefits of HES no longer outweighed the risks, and it was withdrawn from the market in Europe • FDA recommends HES not be used in critically ill patients or those with pre-existing renal dysfunction
Perel P, Roberts I, Ker K. Colloids versus crystalloids for fluid resuscitation in critically ill patients. *Cochrane Database Syst Rev.* 2013;2:CD000567.	• Time to shock reversal was equal in both groups • Similar in-hospital mortality, total LOS, and ICU LOS • HES and gelatin were independent risk factors for AKI • Crystalloid volume equivalence 1.4:1 with HES; 1.1:1 with gelatin • Fluid balance more negative in crystalloid group by HD 5
Surviving Sepsis Guidelines 2013—review and update (2).	Authors' conclusion: "As colloids are not associated with an improvement in survival and are considerably more expensive than crystalloids, it is hard to see how their continued use in clinical practice can be justified." • Crystalloids supported as primary resuscitative fluid for severe sepsis and septic shock • Use of HES for fluid resuscitation in severe sepsis and septic shock not supported • Albumin resuscitation for severe sepsis and septic shock supported when patients require substantial amounts of crystalloids

TBI, traumatic brain injury; HES, hydroxyethyl starch; RRT, renal replacement therapy; PRAC, Pharmacovigilance Risk Assessment Committee; FDA, Food and Drug Administration; LOS, length of stay; AKI, acute kidney injury; HD, hospital day.

increased ICP. Theoretically, administration of a hypertonic fluid creates a large osmotic gradient between ECF and ICF, drawing interstitial fluid into the intravascular space. The rapid increase in intravascular volume is the rationale behind giving hypertonic salt solutions for volume resuscitation. Initial successful studies of low-volume, hypertonic saline resuscitation in hemorrhagic shock were conducted in military environments where medical supply weight is of significant importance. Subsequent trials in civilian settings comparing hypertonic saline to isotonic fluid for resuscitation in trauma patients are sparse in number but have failed to show significant clinical improvement and, in fact, may worsen outcomes.

Hypertonic mannitol is used as a temporizing measure to decrease ICP until the primary pathology can be addressed. Mannitol remains intravascular and rapidly decreases ICP by drawing fluid into the intravascular space from brain interstitium and parenchyma. Additionally, mannitol inhibits reabsorption of free water and sodium in the kidneys, resulting in a rapid and large volume diuresis. However, a recent meta-analysis reviewing the studies comparing hypertonic saline and mannitol for treatment of elevated ICP concludes that hypertonic saline may be superior (8). Unfortunately, only limited trials exist assessing long-term neurologic outcomes and adverse events associated with hypertonic saline administration, warranting further investigation.

VI. Fluid Status: Assessment and Monitoring

A. Conventional Clinical Assessment

Hypovolemia, defined as inadequate circulating blood volume, results from either volume depletion (ECF sodium deficit) or dehydration (ECF water deficit). Prolonged hypovolemia increases patient morbidity and mortality, yet can be rapidly corrected with fluid resuscitation. However, evidence also demonstrates poor patient outcomes with excessive fluid administration. Although the goal of fluid management and resuscitation is to maintain an effective circulating volume, many of the conventional metrics used to assess volume status do not accurately reflect intravascular volume. Table 23-10 lists the most commonly used noninvasive tools for clinical assessment of volume status.

Physical examination findings and body weight changes are all potentially useful tools in the assessment of volume status. Caution must be used in their application, however, as concomitant pharmacotherapy (e.g., beta-blockade,

Table 23-10   Conventional Methods of Volume Assessment
Physical Examination
Jugular venous distension
Skin turgor, dry mucous membranes, dry axilla
Inspiratory crackles
Tissue edema
S3 heart sound
Capillary refill
Vital signs (including orthostatic changes)
Body weight changes
Fluid intake/output balance
Laboratory Values
Hematocrit
Serum sodium
Serum blood urea nitrogen (BUN)
Serum creatinine
Urine electrolytes
Acid–base status

diuretics), comorbid conditions (congestive heart failure, chronic hepatic or renal impairment), and interobserver bias can limit the use of these clinical signs. Similarly, laboratory values, including serum electrolytes, BUN, and creatinine, are important components of volume assessment, but premorbid states can complicate their interpretation. Despite these limitations, tachycardia, oliguria, and eventually hypotension are normal physiologic responses to intravascular volume depletion. Considered together in the appropriate clinical setting, these signs frequently indicate hypovolemia and warrant an isotonic crystalloid fluid bolus challenge for both diagnostic and therapeutic purposes. Initially, a 20 to 30 mL/kg fluid bolus should be administered. Serial reassessment of vital signs and laboratory values is essential to evaluate the progress of resuscitation efforts and determine whether hypovolemia is indeed the underlying problem and if further resuscitation is indicated.

B. Intraoperative Clinical Assessment

Although physical examination and laboratory assessment also play a role in the evaluation of volume status in the operating room, the increased acuity and frequent changes in intravascular volume in this setting make invasive measures of volume status of paramount importance. Static measures of volume status that are used intraoperatively include central venous pressure, pulmonary artery occlusion pressure, and inferior vena cava diameter. Once thought to be highly accurate measurements of intravascular volume status, recent evidence has shown these static measurements to be neither accurate measures of intravascular volume nor accurate predictors of fluid responsiveness. Coupled with the fact that these measures are heavily influenced by mechanical ventilation and perturbations in cardiac function, they have fallen out of favor as primary measures of volume status.

Dynamic measures of volume status, however, take into account fluctuations of the cardiopulmonary system across a period of time and have been shown to be more accurate for predicting fluid responsiveness (see Chapter 15). One increasingly popular dynamic measure that has been shown to be useful is *pulse pressure variation (PPV)*, the variation in pulse pressure with the respiratory cycle. PPV is easily obtained from an arterial blood pressure waveform, provided the patient is mechanically ventilated and in sinus rhythm (Fig. 23-4). PPV is

?Did You Know

Static measures of intravascular volume status, such as central venous pressure, do not adequately account for cardiovascular and pulmonary fluctuations over time. In contrast, dynamic measures, such as pulse pressure variation, may more accurately predict patients who will respond to volume resuscitation.

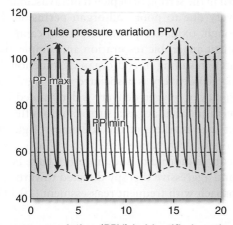

Figure 23-4 Pulse pressure variation (PPV) is identified on the arterial blood pressure waveform by first determining the maximum pulse pressure (PP$_{max}$) and the minimum pulse pressure (PP$_{min}$), and then comparing their difference to the mean pulse pressure, as described in Equation 23-6.

Table 23-11   Markers of Tissue Perfusion and Organ Dysfunction

Markers of End Organ Dysfunction

Hypoxemia: PiO_2/FiO_2 ratio <300
Oliguria: urine output <0.5 kg/hr × 2 hr despite fluid resuscitation
Serum creatinine increase >0.5 mg/dL
Coagulopathy: INR >1.5 or PTT >60 seconds
Thrombocytopenia: platelet count <100,000 platelets/µL
Hyperbilirubinemia: total serum bilirubin >4 mg/dL
Ileus

Evidence of Tissue Hypoperfusion

Base deficit >2 mEq/L
Lactate >2.5 mmol/L
Capillary refill >2 seconds
Cold mottled skin
Mixed venous oxygen saturation <65%
Central venous oxygen saturation <70%

PiO_2, partial pressure of inspired oxygen; FiO_2, fraction of inspired oxygen; INR, international normalized ratio; PTT, partial thromboplastin time; O_2, oxygen.

calculated as a percentage, as shown in Equation 23-6, with values >12% over at least three respiratory cycles predictive of both hypovolemia and fluid responsiveness:

$$PPV = (PP_{max} - PP_{min}/PP_{mean}) \times 100 \qquad (Eq. 23-6)$$

Both PPV and the related measure of stroke volume variation (SVV) have been shown to be highly predictive of responsiveness to fluid resuscitation (9), an important observation because up to 50% of hypovolemic patients may not respond to fluid resuscitation. That PPV and SVV may accurately identify those patients who will benefit from volume repletion makes them both valuable clinical tools.

C. Oxygen Delivery as a Goal of Management

The primary concern in the setting of depleted intravascular volume is impaired tissue oxygen delivery due to poor end-organ perfusion. If this impairment becomes severe enough, oxidative phosphorylation cannot occur, and tissues must rely on inefficient anaerobic respiration and simple glycolysis for energy production, ultimately resulting in end-organ dysfunction. Furthermore, prolonged impaired oxygen delivery is associated with significant morbidity and mortality. The adequacy of oxygen delivery is determined by measuring markers of end-organ perfusion that act as a surrogate for effective circulating volume. Commonly utilized markers of the adequacy of global tissue perfusion as well as signs of organ dysfunction are listed in Table 23-11. Over the past decade, improvements in morbidity and mortality have been attributed to the adoption of early and aggressive therapy directed toward such markers, using an algorithmic approach with frequent reassessment (10,11).

VII. Electrolytes

A. Physiologic Role of Electrolytes

The body's primary electrolytes (sodium, potassium, calcium, magnesium, phosphate, and chloride) are critical components of physiologic homeostasis.

Table 23-12	Clinical Manifestations of Electrolyte Abnormalities
Hyponatremia	**Hypernatremia**
Cerebral edema	Weakness
Impaired thermoregulatory control	Lethargy, seizures, coma
Lethargy, coma, seizures	Demyelinating lesions
Nausea	Intracerebral or subarachnoid hemorrhage
Reflex impairments	
Hypokalemia	**Hyperkalemia**
Muscle weakness	Severe muscle weakness
Respiratory failure	Ascending paralysis
Rhabdomyolysis	Cardiac conduction abnormalities
Ileus	ECG changes
Cardiac arrhythmias	Cardiac arrhythmias
ECG changes	
Nephrogenic diabetes insipidus	
Hypomagnesemia	**Hypermagnesemia**
Tremors, tetany, convulsions	Nausea
Arrhythmias	Flushing
ECG changes	Decreased deep tendon reflexes
	Hypotension
	Bradycardia
	Somnolence, coma
Hypocalcemia	**Hypercalcemia**
Tetany	Weakness
Anxiety, depression	Anxiety, depression
Papilledema	Constipation, nausea
Seizures	Dehydration
Hypotension	Cardiac conduction abnormalities

ECG, electrocardiogram.

In the ionized form in which they exist in both ICF and ECF, these electrolytes create electrical and osmotic gradients that are tightly regulated and essential to many of the body's core functions. Abnormalities of serum electrolyte levels in the perioperative and critical care setting can lead to severe perturbations in physiologic function. Clinical manifestations of these various abnormalities are shown in Table 23-12.

B. Sodium

Sodium is the most prevalent electrolyte in the ECF. Abnormalities of serum sodium are most often due to some form of abnormal renal water regulation. Loss of water by the kidneys or in the gastrointestinal tract, lack of oral intake (typically in the setting of an impaired thirst mechanism), or administration of hypertonic salt solutions may all lead to *hypernatremia*. Clinical manifestations of hypernatremia are varied. Correction of hypernatremia can be achieved with 0.9% saline, 0.45% saline, or 5% dextrose in water, depending on the cause and level of sodium elevation. Great care should be taken to avoid rapid overcorrection of the serum sodium in cases of chronic hypernatremia. Except in emergent circumstances, hypernatremia should not be corrected more quickly than ~0.7 mEq/hr, to avoid fluid shifts that can lead to life-threatening cerebral edema.

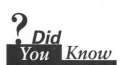
Did You Know

Too rapid correction of both hypernatremia or hyponatremia—particularly when chronic—can result in central nervous system dysfunction, including cerebral edema and central pontine myelinolysis.

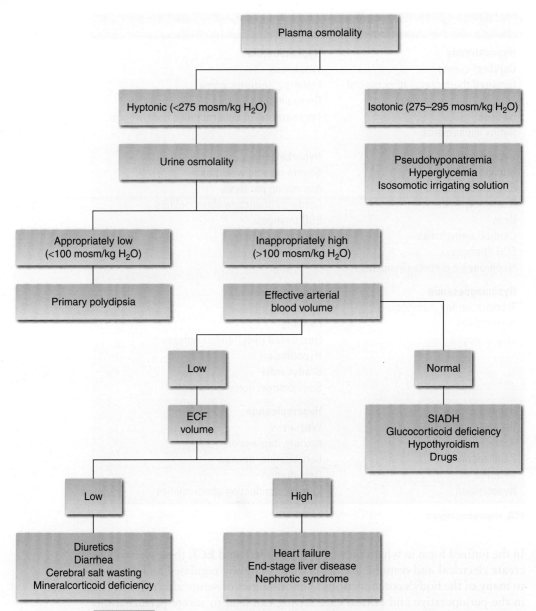

Figure 23-5 Potential etiologies of hyponatremia can be identified with an algorithm that uses serum osmolarity, urine osmolarity, intravascular fluid volume, and extracellular fluid volume. ECF, extracellular fluid; SIADH, syndrome of inappropriate antidiuretic hormone secretion.

The differential diagnosis of *hyponatremia* is presented in Figure 23-5. Clinical manifestations can be mild to severe, and at its extreme, cerebral edema, coma, or seizures may develop. As a general rule, patients cannot become more hyponatremic than they already are if hypotonic fluid is not administered. Thus, fluid restriction to an amount less than the previous day's urine output is a reasonable initial measure. In cases of symptomatic hyponatremia (severely altered mentation or seizures), correction with hypertonic saline is recommended. Overzealous correction, however, as with the irreversible and devastating neurologic injury of central pontine myelinolysis, can result from too rapid correction of the serum sodium.

Serum potassium	Typical ECG appearance	Possible ECG abnormalities
Mild (5.5–6.5 mEq/L)	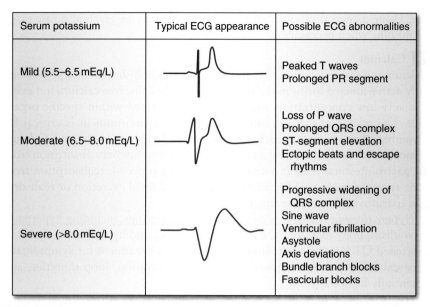	Peaked T waves Prolonged PR segment
Moderate (6.5–8.0 mEq/L)		Loss of P wave Prolonged QRS complex ST-segment elevation Ectopic beats and escape rhythms
Severe (>8.0 mEq/L)		Progressive widening of QRS complex Sine wave Ventricular fibrillation Asystole Axis deviations Bundle branch blocks Fascicular blocks

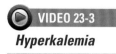

VIDEO 23-3

Hyperkalemia

Figure 23-6 As hyperkalemia progresses from mild to severe, the electrocardiogram tracing evolves in a predictable fashion and may include abnormal T waves, ST segments, QRS duration, and characteristic dysrhythmias.

C. Potassium

Abnormalities in potassium concentration hold great clinical significance, as *hyperkalemia* may result in severe life-threatening cardiac conduction abnormalities (Fig. 23-6). Its differential diagnosis includes renal insufficiency or failure, metabolic acidosis, severe tissue injury or rhabdomyolysis, iatrogenic oversupplementation, or drug effect (succinylcholine, nonselective beta-blockers). Symptomatic hyperkalemia is often not present until serum levels are >6.5 mEq/L, and its treatment should initially include administration of parenteral calcium as a cardiac membrane stabilizer. Reduction in the serum potassium level can be achieved by administration of a combination of dextrose and insulin (the latter forces uptake of potassium into cells), sodium bicarbonate if the patient is acidemic (potassium is forced into cells in exchange for H^+ ion to achieve pH balance), or treatment with furosemide or β-agonists. Ultimately, none of these mechanisms lowers total body potassium definitively, as this requires either potassium-binding resins (e.g., Kayexalate) or hemodialysis.

Hypokalemia may be seen in the setting of excessive diuresis or in patients with renal artery stenosis or hyperaldosteronism. Clinically, the condition may also lead to cardiac dysrhythmias, and early electrocardiogram (ECG) findings include blunted T waves and the presence of U waves. Treatment includes potassium supplementation and correction of the underlying condition. Serum potassium does not accurately reflect changes in total body potassium stores, which are equal to ~50 mEq/kg. Depending on the patient's size, it will take 150 to 300 mEq of exogenous potassium to raise the serum potassium 1 mEq/L. However, potassium supplementation is commonly given orally or intravenously in 10, 20, 40 or 80 mEq aliquots. Intravenous potassium is toxic and extremely painful and must be diluted prior to administering. Hypokalemia is rarely life-threatening, and thus standard practice for intravenous potassium replacement is not to exceed 10 mEq/hr using a peripheral intravenous line. Using a central venous catheter, however, it may be given at a rate up to 40 mEq/hr when necessary.

D. Calcium

Calcium is a divalent cation that exists in both albumin-bound and physiologically active ionized forms in the serum. Within the cells, free calcium ion exists at a very low concentration and is mostly sequestered within specific organelles. The release of calcium into the intracellular environment is critical for a number of cell-signaling pathways and second messenger systems. Calcium homeostasis is maintained by a complex system that involves absorption from the gastrointestinal tract (a vitamin D–regulated process), reabsorption from bone stores (parathyroid hormone function), and renal excretion or reabsorption (parathyroid hormone function).

Hypercalcemia is seen in a number of clinical settings, including hyperparathyroidism, bony metastases, thiazide diuretic use, and hypervitaminosis D. A shortened QT interval is a common ECG finding. Treatment for symptomatic hypercalcemia includes aggressive saline administration, loop diuretics, and potentially hemodialysis.

Hypocalcemia may be secondary to hypoparathyroidism, renal failure, vitamin D deficiency, tumor lysis syndrome, and alkalosis. An important perioperative cause is massive blood transfusion, as the citrate anticoagulant in transfused blood products will bind calcium and deplete levels in the serum. Treatment includes calcium supplementation and treatment of the underlying cause. When assessing serum calcium levels, bear in mind that total calcium levels are affected by serum albumin, such that low serum albumin will result in low total calcium levels. To correct for this, simply measure the ionized calcium levels.

E. Magnesium

Magnesium is the second most important physiologically active divalent cation next to calcium. Magnesium is a critical component of nucleic acid structure and is an important cofactor for numerous enzymatic functions. It also plays a role in the maintenance of normal serum levels of other electrolytes. *Hypermagnesemia* may be seen in cases of hemolysis, tumor lysis, renal insufficiency, or in severe burns or trauma. In minor cases, symptoms are similar to hypercalcemia. However, if serum levels continue to rise, this may result in progressive atrioventricular block and cardiac arrest. Treatment includes parenteral calcium supplementation as a membrane stabilizer and hemodialysis to definitively decrease serum magnesium levels.

Hypomagnesemia may occur due to renal losses, chronic diarrhea, alcoholism, diuresis, nutritional deficiency, or in cases of refeeding syndrome. Symptoms are similar to those for hypocalcemia. ECG findings may include a wide QRS or long QT segment. Treatment of the underlying condition is key. It is also important to note that repletion of magnesium is essential in order to adequately maintain normal serum potassium and calcium levels.

References

1. Boyd JH, Walley KR. Is there a role for sodium bicarbonate in treating lactic acidosis from shock? *Curr Opin Crit Care.* 2008;14(4):379–383.
2. Dellinger RP, Levy MM, Rhodes A, et al. Surviving Sepsis Campaign: International guidelines for management of severe sepsis and septic shock: 2012. *Crit Care Med.* 2013;41(2):580–637.

3. Joshi GP. Intraoperative fluid restriction improves outcome after major elective gastro-intestinal surgery. *Anesth Analg.* 2005;101(2):601.
4. Chappell D, Jacob M, Hofmann-Kiefer K, et al. A rational approach to perioperative fluid management. *Anesthesiology.* 2008;109(4):723.
5. Holiday MA, Segar WE. The maintenance need for water in parenteral fluid therapy. *Pediatrics.* 1957;19(5):823–832.
6. Mythen MG, Swart M, Acheson N, et al. Perioperative fluid management: Consensus statement from the enhanced recovery partnership. *Periop Med.* 2012;1:2.
7. Woodcock TE, Woodcock TM. Revised Starling equation and the glycocalyx model of transvascular fluid exchange: An improved paradigm for prescribing intravenous fluid therapy. *Br J Anesth.* 2012;108(3):384–394.
8. Kamel H, Navi BB, Nakagawa K, et al. Hypertonic saline versus mannitol for the treatment of elevated intracranial pressure: A meta-analysis of randomized clinical trials. *Crit Care Med.* 2011;39(3):554–559.
9. Marik PE. Techniques for Assessment of Intravascular Volume in Critically Ill Patients. *J Intens Care Med.* 2009;24:329.
10. Rivers E, Nguyen B, Havstad S, et al. Early goal directed therapy in the treatment of severe sepsis and septic shock. *N Engl J Med.* 2001;345:1368–1377.
11. The ProCESS Investigators, Yealy DM, Kellum JA, Huang DT, et al. A randomized trial of protocol-based care for early septic shock. *N Engl J Med.* 2014;370(18):1683–1693.

Questions

1. In the presence of an acute acid–base disorder, which of the following statements describes the typical time course of physiologic compensation to maintain normal pH?
   A. Both respiratory compensation for primary metabolic disorders, and renal compensation for primary respiratory disorders require hours to days.
   B. Renal compensation for primary respiratory disorders can occur within minutes; respiratory compensation for primary metabolic disorders requires hours to days.
   C. Both respiratory compensation for primary metabolic disorders, and renal compensation for primary respiratory disorders can occur within minutes.
   D. Respiratory compensation for primary metabolic disorders can occur within minutes; renal compensation for primary respiratory disorders requires hours to days.

2. A 47-year-old otherwise healthy female is undergoing a laparoscopic cholecystectomy for symptomatic cholelithiasis. She is receiving general endotracheal anesthesia (oxygen, air, sevoflurane, rocuronium, fentanyl) with mechanical ventilation via a circle system. An ABG shows pH 7.26, $PaCO_2$ 61 mm Hg, PaO_2 267 mm Hg, HCO_3^- 25 mEq/L. All the following clinical conditions could explain her acid–base disturbance EXCEPT:
   A. Abnormally low minute ventilation due to a restrictive lung defect caused by insufflation of the abdominal cavity
   B. Prolonged orogastric tube suctioning
   C. Untreated and previously undiagnosed hyperthyroidism
   D. Exhausted soda lime

3. All of the following intravenous solutions are isotonic EXCEPT:
   A. Ringer's lactate
   B. 25% albumin
   C. Plasmalyte
   D. 0.9% normal saline

4. Despite the long-standing debate between crystalloid and colloid solutions for perioperative fluid repletion, several characteristics of each fluid type are generally agreed upon. For example, crystalloids are more allergenic than colloids. TRUE or FALSE?
   A. True
   B. False

5. Infants under the age of 6 months are at risk of hypoglycemia with prolonged fasting periods. TRUE or FALSE?
   A. True
   B. False

6. A 36-year-old male is undergoing an emergent exploratory laparotomy for a single, low-caliber gunshot wound to the anterior abdomen (entry wound in right-upper quadrant, no exit wound). The patient is receiving general endotracheal anesthesia (oxygen, sevoflurane, vecuronium, fentanyl) with mechanical ventilation and has two large-bore peripheral intravenous catheters and a radial artery catheter. His electrocardiogram demonstrates sinus tachycardia (126 beats per minute). His arterial pressure tracing indicates a maximum pulse pressure at a blood pressure of 97/61 mm Hg and a minimal pulse pressure at a blood pressure of 80/50 mm Hg. His mean pulse pressure is 34 mm Hg. What is his pulse pressure variation?
   A. 7%
   B. 10%
   C. 12%
   D. 18%

7. A 66-year-old male with a 2-day history of nausea, vomiting, and recent acute epigastric pain is scheduled for emergent exploratory laparotomy to repair a perforated duodenal ulcer. His past medical history is notable for chronic alcoholism and type 2 diabetes. Preoperative blood chemistry demonstrates a serum osmolarity of 280 mOsm/L and the following electrolytes: Na^+ 125 mEq/L, K^+ 3.5 mEq/L, Cl^- 99 mEq/L, and HCO_3^- 30 mEq/L. Which of the following is the MOST LIKELY etiology of his hyponatremia?
   A. Hyperglycemia
   B. Syndrome of inappropriate antidiuretic hormone
   C. Primary polydipsia
   D. Heart failure

8. In the presence of acute hyperkalemia (K^+ >5.5 mEq/L), which of the following electrocardiogram finding is MOST LIKELY to appear first?
   A. Prolonged QRS complex
   B. Peaked T waves
   C. Ventricular fibrillation
   D. Asystole

9. In the presence of hypoalbuminemia, measuring the ionized calcium level is a better indicator of body calcium homeostasis than is the total calcium level. TRUE or FALSE?
   A. True
   B. False

10. A 77-year-old otherwise healthy woman is undergoing an elective posterior spinal decompression, instrumentation, and fusion at levels T9-L1 for symptomatic spinal stenosis. She is receiving general endotracheal anesthesia with mechanical ventilation. Arterial blood gas (ABG) results demonstrate: pH 7.51, $PaCO_2$ 29 mm Hg, PaO_2 197 mm Hg, HCO_3^- 23 mEq/L. Which of the following is the MOST LIKELY interpretation of this ABG?
    A. Acute metabolic acidosis
    B. Chronic respiratory alkalosis
    C. Acute metabolic alkalosis
    D. Acute respiratory alkalosis

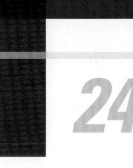

24

Blood Therapy

Louanne M. Carabini
Glenn Ramsey

Blood component therapy is the mainstay of treatment for hemorrhagic shock, acute or chronic anemia, and acquired or congenital disorders in hemostasis. Anesthesiologists serve a unique role as perioperative physicians frequently charged with the management of patients suffering acute blood loss or coagulopathy. Therefore, it is important to understand the physiologic principles of oxygen delivery and hemostasis, the risks and safety precautions associated with blood-product transfusion, and the pharmacology of anticoagulants, antithrombotics, and procoagulant medications.

I. Blood-Product Transfusion

A. Component Therapy and Indications for Transfusion

Blood-product transfusion is conventionally performed with individual component therapy targeted to replace the specific deficiencies at hand. Whole fresh blood is occasionally used for critical bleeding at field hospitals for the military, but it is difficult to store and inefficient. Most patients require only a single blood component or a combination of selected components. For example, red blood cells (RBC) are needed to treat anemia with evidence of tissue hypoxia, whereas plasma is used to treat coagulopathy and factor deficiencies. Separating blood transfusion into component therapies allows for targeted efficient treatment while also minimizing the risks of transfusion reactions and transfusion transmitted infection.

Packed red blood cells (PRBCs) are the most common blood product transfused worldwide, with over 13 million units administered annually in the United States (1). A unit of PRBCs is obtained from a single donor and consists of about 300 mL, with a hematocrit of approximately 70% and only about 20 to 30 mL of plasma. One unit of PRBCs generally increases the patient's hemoglobin concentration by 1 g/dL. Table 24-1 presents the blood component storage and preparation details.

The simplest indications for PRBC transfusion are acute blood loss or anemia with evidence of inadequate oxygen delivery to the tissues. Patients suffering

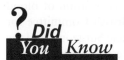

? Did You Know

There are few, if any, indications for transfusion of whole blood. Transfusion of separated blood components, such as RBCs or plasma, allows for targeted treatment and saves a precious resource.

Table 24-1	Blood Component Storage and Preparation	
Component	Average Volume per Dose	Comments
PRBCs	300 mL	1–6°C for 21–35 days or up to 42 days with adenine added to citrate, dextrose, and phosphate preservative
FFP	250 mL	<–20°C for up to 1 year
Platelets, whole blood derived	50 mL/bag pooled to usual dose 4–6 bags	20–24°C for 5 days
Platelets, apheresis	300 mL	20–24°C for 5 days
Cryoprecipitate	15 mL/bag pooled to usual dose of 4–6 bags	<–20°C for up to 1 year

PRBCs, packed red blood cells; FFP, fresh frozen plasma.

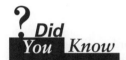

? Did You Know

There is no general rule regarding the minimum hemoglobin at which patients should be transfused. The trigger for transfusion should be individualized for each specific patient.

hypovolemic shock secondary to critical bleeding clearly require resuscitation with PRBCs, but they may also require treatment of dilutional coagulopathy and thrombocytopenia. Typically, the hemoglobin transfusion threshold for active bleeding in hemodynamically unstable patients is higher (hemoglobin goals of >8.0 g/dL) to allow for reserve during active bleeding. Transfusion for major bleeding should also include replacement of coagulation factors and platelets with consideration given to administration of medications and strategies for blood conservation.

The transfusion threshold for hemodynamically stable patients with anemia has been the topic of many review articles and original studies for over two decades. The controversy stems around the balance of the benefits of RBC treatment for anemia versus the risks of transfusion. Most international guidelines, including the AABB, formerly the American Association of Blood Banks, the American Society of Anesthesiologists, the British Committee for Standards in Haematology (BCSH), the Society for Thoracic Surgeons, and the Society of Cardiovascular Anesthesiologists, agree that restrictive transfusion practices are indicated for most hemodynamically stable trauma, perioperative, and critically ill patients (2). There are a few circumstances, such as severe sepsis, acute myocardial ischemia, and acute neurologic injury, where higher transfusion triggers are indicated to maximize oxygen delivery to end organs under stress. Otherwise, hemodynamically stable patients without evidence of tissue hypoxia (elevated lactate levels, low central venous oxygen saturation) generally tolerate hemoglobin levels as low as 7.0 g/dL with compensatory mechanisms to increase cardiac output and oxygen extraction at the tissue level. Figure 24-1 describes a suggested clinical algorithm adapted from the BCSH guidelines for management of anemia and RBC transfusion (2,3).

Fresh frozen plasma (FFP) contains all the clotting factors, fibrinogen, and plasma proteins from whole blood donation or apheresis. The volume of 1 unit of FFP is approximately 300 mL, with physiologic levels of stable clotting factors and approximately 70% of labile factors VIII and V. The most common indications for FFP are treatment of dilutional coagulopathy and factor deficiency. The recommended dose is 10 to 15 mL/kg. Other indications for FFP include replacement of antithrombin in cases of long-term heparin use or as a second-line agent for warfarin reversal.

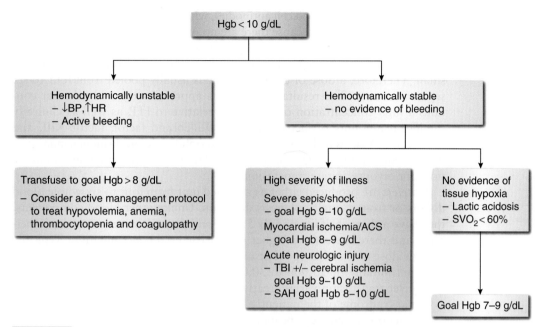

Figure 24-1 Suggested algorithm for red blood cell transfusion in hemodynamically stable and unstable patients. Stable angina and history of cardiovascular disease do not require transfusion thresholds greater than 7.0 g/dL. BP, blood pressure; HR, heart rate; ACS, acute coronary syndrome; TBI, traumatic brain injury; SAH, subarachnoid hemorrhage. (From Retter A, Wyncoll D, Pearse R, et al. Guidelines on the management of anaemia and red cell transfusion in adult critically ill patients. *Br J Haematol.* 2013;160(4):445–464, with permission.)

FFP contains the antibodies to blood type antigens and must therefore be compatible when transfused. Table 24-2 presents the FFP compatibility profiles as they compare with RBC component compatibility. The ABO blood system is the major carbohydrate-derived blood-borne antigen system that produces naturally occurring immunoglobulin-M (IgM) antibodies without the need for RBC exposure. Thus, ABO incompatibility for PRBCs or plasma-containing components carries significant risk of acute hemolytic transfusion reactions (discussed in depth below). Type AB plasma is the universal FFP donor as it does

▶ **VIDEO 24-1**

Blood Transfusion Compatibility

Table 24-2	ABO Blood Group Prevalence and Blood Component Compatibility		
Recipient Blood Type	**Prevalence in U.S. Population (%)**	**PRBC Compatibility**	**FFP/Cryoprecipitate Compatibility**
A	40	A or O donor	A or AB donor
B	16	B or O donor	B or AB donor
AB	4	Universal recipient	Universal donor Only receive AB plasma
O	45	Universal donor only receive O blood	Universal recipient

PRBCs, packed red blood cells; FFP, fresh frozen plasma.

not contain any ABO blood cell antibodies, while type O patients are the universal recipient for plasma because there are no A or B antigens in type O blood.

Cryoprecipitate (sometimes called simply cryo) is produced after a controlled thaw and centrifuge of frozen plasma. The yield from 1 unit of FFP is small. Therefore, a dose of cryoprecipitate is usually pooled from four to six separate donors. The resultant product is approximately 100 mL that contains a high concentration of fibrinogen relative to FFP, as well as clinically significant amounts of factor VIII, von Willebrand factor, factor XIII, and fibronectin. Von Willebrand disease, hemophilia, hypofibrinogenemia, and disseminated intravascular coagulopathy (DIC) are the most common indications for cryoprecipitate transfusion.

Platelets are produced either as a pooled unit from four to six whole blood donors or from a single apheresis donation. Unlike other blood components, they have a short shelf life of only 5 days, and they are stored at room temperature and therefore carry a higher risk of bacterial contamination. Typically a single dose of platelets (pool or apheresis) is expected to increase the platelet count initially by 25,000 to 30,000 per microliter. However, the response to platelet transfusion varies greatly depending on the indication, acuity, and systemic syndrome of the patient.

Platelet transfusion may be indicated when platelets are decreased as a result of dilution, bleeding, destruction, or sequestration. Transfusion thresholds for thrombocytopenia depend on whether the patient has clinical signs of bleeding or whether bleeding or the risk of bleeding involves the limited intraorbital, intracranial, or neuraxial spaces. In such instances, the transfusion threshold is <100,000 per microliter. Otherwise, for surgical patients where bleeding is anticipated and prophylaxis is desired, the threshold is generally <50,000 per microliter. Patients without clinical signs of bleeding are not at risk of spontaneous hemorrhage until the platelet count drops to <10,000 per microliter. Platelet transfusion may also be necessary for patients with qualitative deficiencies that are acquired or congenital. Commonly acquired platelet dysfunction occurs with extracorporeal circulation, such as cardiopulmonary bypass, or with medications or systemic illnesses, such as liver disease and uremia.

II. Blood Compatibility

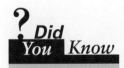
? Did You Know

In an emergency, when a bleeding patient's blood type is not known and there is no time to perform a crossmatch, it is best to transfuse type O Rh-negative blood.

RBC compatibility testing consists of typing for ABO and Rh(D), screening the plasma for non-ABO antibodies, and crossmatching prospective RBC units. Group O, A, and B persons have naturally occurring strong plasma anti-A and/or anti-B to the antigen(s) they lack, and RBC units must be ABO compatible to avoid hemolytic transfusion reactions. D-negative persons can easily make anti-D when exposed to D-positive RBCs and should normally receive D-negative RBCs. This is especially important for girls and young women to avoid risk of hemolytic disease of the newborn in future D-positive fetuses. One to 2% of all patients, and 5% to 20% of multitransfused patients have non-ABO hemolytic alloantibodies to Rh and other blood group antigens. These antibodies must be identified so that RBC units negative for the target antigens can be given to avoid hemolysis. After these "type and screen" tests, donor RBC units are crossmatched for the patient, either by computer confirmation or, if significant antibodies are present, by serological crossmatching of plasma versus donor RBCs. Compatibility testing routinely takes 45 to 60 minutes or longer if RBC alloantibodies, warm (IgG), or cold (IgM) autoantibodies are present. If RBCs must be given emergently before testing is completed, uncross-matched group O RBCs (D-negative for girls and young women) are the best choice, after weighing the risk of non-ABO hemolytic RBC antibodies. In an emergency, as a guide to help remember that group O is a "universal donor," think of the "O" in donor.

III. Blood Administration

Before transfusion, it is mandatory that the blood bank's transfusion *tag* on the blood unit be carefully checked against the blood *bag* and the patient's *wristband* identification to avoid a hemolytic reaction from administering the wrong blood or component. All blood components must be administered through a 150- to 260-μm blood filter to prevent clots from entering the patient's bloodstream. Products should be infused within 4 hours of issuance from the blood bank. A blood warmer should be used in rapid large-volume transfusions to avoid hypothermia and may be recommended for transfusing RBCs to patients with cold autoantibodies.

IV. Transfusion Reactions

With over 20 million blood components transfused annually, the risks of transfusion are relatively rare, with an overall incidence of 0.24% or 2.4 reactions per 1,000 units transfused (1). More than half of these reactions are mild, febrile nonhemolytic reactions or mild to moderate allergic reactions. However, the overall incidence of transfusion reactions is likely underreported and significantly higher than published. Transfusion reactions are often organized by pathophysiology into immune-mediated or nonimmune-mediated reactions. The latter include transmission of infection (e.g., hepatitis C) or metabolic derangements associated with massive transfusion (e.g., hyperkalemia). Table 24-3 summarizes many of the reported noninfectious adverse effects of transfusion, but the following sections will focus on some of the most clinically significant reactions.

Hemolytic transfusion reactions result from intravascular or extravascular hemolysis of endogenous and transfused RBCs, typically when the recipient expresses antibodies to blood-borne antigens within the donor product. This reaction is acute and severe when transfusion involves the naturally occurring IgM anti-A and anti-B antibodies to the ABO blood cell antigens. Acute hemolytic transfusion reactions (AHTR) are rare and almost always result from clerical errors with blood sampling, typing, crossmatch, or erroneous administration of an inappropriate blood product to the wrong patient. Rarely, transfusion of incompatible plasma can also result in acute hemolysis (Table 24-2) (4).

Vigilance for the diagnosis of AHTR must remain high because many of the signs and symptoms can be masked during general anesthesia. Responsive patients may complain of itching, chest pain, or abdominal discomfort. Vital signs become unstable, with diffuse bradykinin and histamine release leading to fever, hypotension, tachycardia, and bronchospasm. AHTRs are best treated with supportive care after discontinuing all blood-product transfusions and initiating investigation into the etiology of the incompatibility. The mortality from AHTR remains high, accounting for up to 26% of the transfusion-related fatalities reported to the U.S. Food and Drug Administration from 2008 to 2012. Patients may progress to multiorgan system failure from systemic shock, DIC, acute renal failure, and obstructive hepatic dysfunction (5).

? Did You Know

Acute hemolytic transfusion reactions most often result from errors made by medical personnel. It is critical that blood donors and recipients be properly identified and all labels on blood products be properly matched to those individuals.

Table 24-3   Noninfectious Transfusion Reactions

Adverse Reaction	Incidence[a]	Notes
Overall	1:400	
All life-threatening	1:66,000	
Immune-Mediated Reactions		
Febrile Nonhemolytic reaction	1:950	
Mild–moderate allergic reactions	1:1500	
Anaphylaxis	1:43,000	IgA deficiency increases risk
PRBC		Washing may avoid reaction
FFP and platelets		More prevalent with plasma products
Hemolytic transfusion reaction acute	1:125,000	ABO incompatibility
Delayed	1:21,000	Alloantibodies to minor RBC antigens
Transfusion-related immuno-modulation	See text	
Alloimmunization	1:8000	Risk increases with number of units
Transfusion-related acute lung injury	1:64,000	Higher risk with plasma products
Graft versus host disease	1:931,000	Reduced risk with irradiation
Nonimmune Mediated		
Transfusion-associated circulatory overload	1:13,800	Higher risk in critically ill patients
Metabolic derangements		Hyperkalemia, hypocalcemia, hypothermia, iron overload

IgA, immunoglobulin-A; PRBCs, packed red blood cells; FFP, fresh frozen plasma.
[a]Reactions per components transfused. Frequencies are from the 2011 National Blood Collection and Utilization Survey.

Delayed hemolytic transfusion reactions (DHTR) often occur days after blood-product administration and are typically less severe, presenting with progressive anemia, jaundice, and hemoglobinuria in the absence of hemodynamic instability. DHTR results from a humoral reaction to antigens in transfused blood products in recipients with a history of alloimmunization to antigens such as Rh, Kell, Kidd, Duffy, among others. *Alloimmunization* occurs with pregnancy or exposure to blood-product transfusion as the recipient develops antibodies to blood-borne antigens. This puts these patients at risk for future hemolytic transfusion reactions and emphasizes the importance of antibody screen and complete crossmatch prior to nonemergency transfusion.

Transfusion-related immunomodulation (TRIM) was originally described in the 1970s when it was observed that patients who received transfusion were less likely to reject solid organ transplants. The exact mechanism of immunomodulation is not clear. But it likely relates to the adverse pro-inflammatory effects of biologic response modifiers (lipid breakdown products, chemokines, leukotrienes) included in blood-product components as well as the anti-inflammatory cell-mediated response of white blood cells included in blood component transfusions containing plasma. TRIM presumably occurs with every transfusion but may be limited with leukoreduction or irradiation. Recent reviews in transfusion medicine point to the adverse immune response as the etiology for morbidity and mortality with liberal transfusion strategies (4).

Transfusion-related acute lung injury (TRALI) remains one of the leading causes of transfusion-associated fatalities. The National Heart, Lung, and Blood Institute's diagnostic criteria require acute, noncardiogenic pulmonary edema with bilateral infiltrates and a ratio of arterial partial pressure of oxygen to the inspired concentration of oxygen of <300 (e.g., 200/0.75) temporally related to transfusion. Blood products with high plasma content are responsible for the majority of the cases of TRALI, which can be explained by two suggested pathophysiologic mechanisms.

The most likely cause involves antineutrophil (anti-HNA) or anti-HLA antibodies formulated in multiparous female donors during a past pregnancy. In fact, the United Kingdom significantly decreased their incidence of TRALI with the limitation of plasma products to male-only donors. The second commonly discussed "two hit hypothesis" for TRALI implicates the role of pro-inflammatory biologic response modifiers released in stored blood products that activate primed neutrophils in the recipient. Both pathophysiologic mechanisms result in breakdown of the capillary alveolar membrane, interstitial pulmonary edema, and microscopic alveolar hemorrhage, all of which lead to acute lung injury. The treatment for TRALI focuses on supportive care and lung protective low tidal volume mechanical ventilation as the low pressure pulmonary edema does not generally respond to diuretic therapy.

Transfusion-associated circulatory overload (TACO) involves high-pressure cardiogenic pulmonary edema frequently associated with large volume or rapid transfusion. It is not an immune-mediated response and occurs more frequently in critically ill patients or those with a history of cardiovascular comorbidities. These patients develop hypoxemia secondary to ventilation perfusion mismatch and intrapulmonary shunt. Furthermore, patients may express a high level of brain natriuretic peptide in response to ventricular distension. Typically, TACO responds to diuretic treatment and pulmonary alveolar recruitment (4).

Transfusion-transmitted infections have been a focus of transfusion medicine research for several decades, which has resulted in a significant decrease in the rate of infection for recipients of allogeneic transfusion. The greatest fear among blood transfusion recipients usually concerns the highly publicized viral infections such as hepatitis C and human immunodeficiency virus (HIV). However, these are actually a rare result of blood-product transfusion because of the increased sensitivity of donor screening tests now available and a short window of time between donor infection and seroconversion. In contrast, transfusion transmission of hepatitis B remains high due to the higher prevalence of the disease in the population and the long window of time during which infected donor units cannot be identified. Table 24-4 summarizes the residual risk of transfusion transmission for the most commonly reported infections.

V. Perioperative Alternatives to Transfusion

The risks of transfusion are indisputable. Even 1 unit of PRBCs can significantly increase perioperative morbidity. Fortunately, there are some blood conservation strategies to minimize allogenic RBC transfusion. However, each of these methods has advantages and risks that must be carefully weighed.

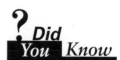

? Did You Know

Only in unusual circumstances is it appropriate to transfuse an anemic patient prior to elective surgery. The cause for anemia should be found and the patient treated. Alternatives to transfusion, such as perioperative cell salvage, should be considered.

Table 24-4 Residual Risk of Transfusion-Transmitted Infections		
Infection	Residual Risk	Window Period and Comments
Viral Infections		
Human immunodeficiency virus	1:1,860,800	9.1-day window
Hepatitis C	1:1,657,700	7.4-day window
Hepatitis B	1:366,500	38-day window
West Nile virus	Rare	11 cases reported from 2003–2010
Cytomegalovirus—all donors	1–3%	
Leuko-reduced products	0.023%	
Bacterial Contamination—all types	1:3,000	
Packed red blood cells	1:35,000	Lower risk than platelet concentrates
Platelets	1:15,000	Apheresis decreases risk

Factors to consider in this decision include patient characteristics, such as blood type, the presence of antibodies, or a preference not to receive blood, as well as the risk for blood loss during the surgical procedure and the risks of specific blood conservation technologies.

Preoperative anemia is an independent risk factor for perioperative blood transfusion, morbidity, and mortality. Thus, strategies to increase the patient's hemoglobin concentration prior to surgery should be considered for all elective cases. There should be a thorough preoperative diagnostic workup for the cause of the anemia and, if indicated, aggressive treatment of an iron deficiency or replacement of vitamin deficiencies (e.g., vitamin B_{12} or folic acid). With a longer lead time before surgery for diagnosis and treatment of anemia, fewer patients require perioperative transfusion (6).

Erythropoietin is the most common erythropoiesis-stimulating agent (ESA) approved for use in patients with end-stage renal disease, presurgical anemia, and chemotherapy or malignancy-associated anemia. Erythropoietin increases RBC production in the bone marrow. However, it carries a significant risk of venous and arterial thromboembolism, especially in patients who cannot receive deep vein thrombosis chemoprophylaxis. The literature supports the use of ESAs as part of a blood-conservation protocol, especially in conjunction with preoperative autologous donation (6).

Autologous blood donation (collection and saving of the patient's own blood for later use) reduces several of the risks associated with allogenic blood transfusion, including viral infection and immune reactions such as TRALI and alloimmunization. However, preoperative autologous donation has not been shown to reduce perioperative allogenic transfusion due to the resultant lower preoperative hemoglobin concentration. Autologous blood donation still carries the risks associated with clerical error, bacterial contamination, and storage lesions. Furthermore, there is significant waste associated with the procedure as the donors are not screened thoroughly and unused donations cannot be used for other people. Certain patients may be candidates for autologous transfusion if they have rare antibodies to blood antigens or they refuse allogenic transfusion and are at risk for significant surgical blood loss (7).

Acute normovolemic hemodilution involves the removal of 2 or 3 units of whole blood with volume replacement with intravenous fluids immediately preincision. The blood is typically stored in the operating room but may be preserved for 24 hours prior to reinfusion. This results in the patient losing blood at a lower hematocrit during surgery and for the patient to be resuscitated with autologous whole fresh blood after the majority of surgical blood loss has resolved. This method is very efficacious in young healthy patients who can tolerate intraoperative anemia without risk of end-organ hypoxia or for patients who have a higher risk of transfusion reactions from allogenic blood products (7).

Perioperative blood salvage with intraoperative "cell saver" technology or postoperative intracompartment cell salvage is the most commonly used and efficacious method for perioperative blood conservation. Especially in orthopedic surgery for total knee arthroplasty and hip replacement, perioperative cell salvage has significantly decreased patient risk for blood transfusion. Postoperative cell salvage is generally limited to orthopedic surgery as mediastinal cell salvage after cardiac and thoracic surgery has been associated with worse postoperative bleeding and morbidity.

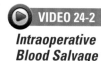

VIDEO 24-2

Intraoperative Blood Salvage

Intraoperative RBC salvage systems typically involve three phases, all of which must be run by trained operators to optimize RBC return and minimize risks. Shed blood is first anticoagulated and collected with limited variable suctioning to minimize the detrimental effects of sheer forces. Inefficient collection may increase the risk of hemolysis. Suction of wounds contaminated with frank infection, ruptured tumor sections, amniotic fluid, metal, or pharmaceutical compounds may increase the risks associated with cell salvage. Generally, leucodepletion filters limit the white blood cells and contaminants, including tumor cells and amniotic fluid contents, from entering the collection chamber. Thus, intraoperative cell salvage systems remain acceptable in obstetrics, as well as any procedures with anticipated blood loss >1,500 mL. Meta-analysis of studies using cell salvage in urologic and gynecologic cancer surgery demonstrates that it is safe and is not associated with additional risk of tumor recurrence or metastasis. Risks associated with reinfusion of salvaged RBCs include air embolism and hemolysis. But these risks are minimal when the system is used properly and still negligible when compared with the risk of allogeneic blood transfusion.

Overall, perioperative blood salvage is cost-efficient, low risk, and clinically effective at reducing the need for RBC transfusion. It is particularly important when considering use of perioperative blood conservation strategies for patients with rare blood antibodies and those who are Jehovah's Witnesses, who generally refuse any transfusion when RBCs have been removed from the body. Often Jehovah's Witness patients will accept RBC salvage if the salvaged blood remains in continuity with the patient. This is easily established with a primed venous line attached to the reinfusion bag of the cell savage system (7).

Blood substitutes are an attractive alternative to transfusion, eliminating many of the risks associated with RBC administration. There are no compounds currently approved for human use, although this is an active field of research. Unfortunately, blood substitutes containing recombinant hemoglobin molecules have been associated with hypertension and renal and liver dysfunction, while substitutes containing perfluorocarbon compounds, which increase the fraction of dissolved oxygen, commonly cause thrombocytopenia. Hopefully, further studies will provide an efficient low-risk alternative blood substitute (6).

Platelet Function

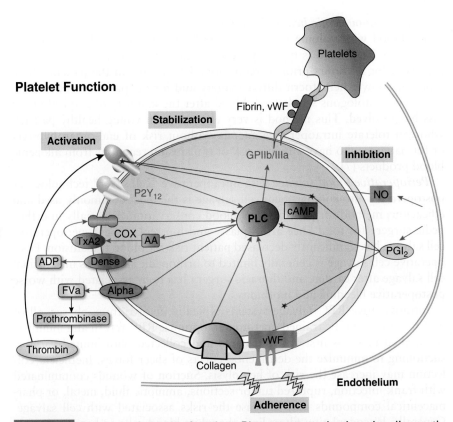

Figure 24-2 Diagram of platelet function. *Blue arrows:* activating signaling pathways. *Red lines:* inhibiting signaling pathways. *Double triangles:* surface receptors. *Green arrows:* secretion. *Dashed arrows:* clotting-factor cascade. Adherence: *Yellow lightning bolts:* injury. vWF: von Willebrand factor. Activation: PLC: phospholipase C. Alpha: alpha granules. Dense: dense granules. TxA_2: thromboxane A_2. COX: cyclo-oxygenase. ADP: adenosine diphosphate. FVa: activated factor V. $P2Y_{12}$: ADP receptor. Not all activation elements are shown. Stabilization: GPIIb/IIIa: glycoprotein IIb/IIIa. Inhibition: NO: nitric oxide. PGI_2: prostaglandin I_2 (prostacyclin). cAMP: cyclic adenosine monophosphate. Targets of antiplatelet medications (*blue*): COX: aspirin and nonsteroidal anti-inflammatory drugs. P_2Y_{12}: clopidogrel class. cAMP: dipyridamole class. GPIIb/IIIa: abciximab class.

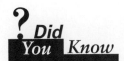

? Did You Know

The process of coagulation is complex, involving numerous components and interactive processes. If time permits, the cause for unusual bleeding should be carefully elucidated and therapy precisely targeted. In an emergency, "shotgun" therapy with fresh frozen plasma or platelets may be necessary.

VI. Primary Hemostasis

Figure 24-2 shows the three general phases of platelet function: adherence, activation, and stabilization. When the blood vessel is injured, platelets adhere via surface receptors to underlying collagen and to von Willebrand factor (vWF) on endothelium or in a blood clot. These engaged receptors set off signaling pathways mediated via phospholipase C (PLC) to cause platelet activation. In the activation phase, platelets secrete numerous agents to stimulate other platelets, including calcium (Ca^{++}), adenosine diphosphate (ADP), and serotonin released from dense granules, and thromboxane A_2 produced from arachidonic acid via the cyclo-oxygenase pathway. The outer platelet membrane has receptors for these agonists, including the $P2Y_{12}$ receptor for ADP and for thrombin, setting off further internal signaling via PLC. Activated platelets also release α-granules containing activated factor V for the coagulation cascade, and they change shape from round to flat and spiky. Finally, in stabilization, PLC mediates "inside-out" signaling to activate the surface receptor for

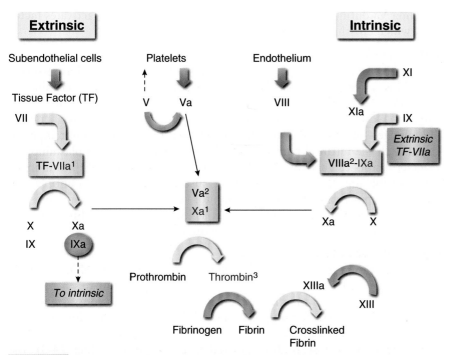

Figure 24-3 Extrinsic and intrinsic pathways for coagulation cascade. *Gray arrows: secretion. Red:* vitamin K–dependent enzymes. *Blue arrows:* activation by thrombin. *Solid boxes:* enzymes with cofactors, Ca++, and platelet-membrane phospholipid. Inhibition: [1]tissue factor pathway inhibitor; [2]activated protein C; [3]antithrombin.

fibrin and vWF binding. Other activated platelets crosslink to fibrin and vWF at these sites, creating the platelet-fibrin plug (8).

A. Secondary Hemostasis

Classically, the coagulation cascade is subcategorized into (a) the *extrinsic pathway,* activated by tissue factor (TF) from cells outside a disrupted blood vessel; (b) the *intrinsic pathway,* involving only plasma factors; and (c) the *common pathway,* fed by both the intrinsic and extrinsic to form thrombin, then fibrin (Fig. 24-3). However, the extrinsic and common pathways also amplify the intrinsic pathway. Each of these three pathways has a central enzyme complex with four parallel elements: a plasma enzyme, a cofactor (mostly cell or platelet derived), the Ca++ ion, and a phospholipid (PL) platform provided in vivo by the platelet membrane.

The extrinsic pathway activates factor X to Xa via the extrinsic "ten-ase," comprising enzyme factor VIIa (activated by TF), its cofactor TF, Ca++, and PL. The intrinsic pathway activates Xa with the intrinsic ten-ase, containing enzyme IXa, cofactor VIIIa, Ca++, and PL. In the common pathway, the Xa enzyme formed by these processes combines with cofactor Va, Ca++, and PL to form prothrombinase. Prothrombin is then converted to thrombin, which in turn converts fibrinogen to the end product fibrin.

When thrombin is formed, it also amplifies the intrinsic VIIIa to IXa ten-ase: thrombin activates VIIIa and XIa, which produces IXa. The extrinsic ten-ase also makes some IXa for the intrinsic ten-ase. Thrombin amplifies its own prothrombinase by activating some plasma Va. However, platelets provide most of the Va by taking up plasma factor V, converting it to Va, and then secreting Va during platelet activation. Finally, thrombin also activates factor XIII, which crosslinks and stabilizes the fibrin clot (8).

B. Fibrinolysis

Fibrin is broken down by plasmin after the need for hemostasis has resolved. Plasmin is activated from plasminogen in several ways: (a) tissue plasminogen activator (tPA) from endothelial cells cleaves to plasminogen and is itself activated by plasmin; (b) urokinase from the endothelium and kidney activates plasminogen; (c) factor IXa and the contact factors XIIa and kallikrein, associated with the intrinsic pathway, activate a minor fraction of plasminogen. Contact factors can activate XIa during *in vitro* testing (partial thromboplastin time) but not *in vivo*. Fibrinolysis is also regulated. The α_1-antiplasmin and thrombin-activated fibrinolysis inhibitor (TAFI) inhibit plasmin. TAFI and plasminogen activation inhibitor-1 (PAI-1) interfere with tPA function, and PAI-1 promotes clearance of tPA and urokinase.

C. Regulation of Hemostasis

Platelet activation is physiologically inhibited by nitric oxide (NO) and prostaglandin I_2 (PGI_2) secreted by endothelial cells. NO stimulates a pathway leading to inhibition of the thromboxane A_2 receptor. PGI_2 binds to a platelet receptor, which signals for suppression of vWF adherence, PLC function, and thromboxane A_2 activation.

Secondary hemostasis is also regulated at several junctures (Fig. 24-3). Tissue factor pathway inhibitor, secreted by endothelial cells and facilitated by its cofactor protein S, dampens functions of extrinsic TF-VIIa ten-ase and the common pathway Xa. Antithrombin, particularly when bound to heparin, inhibits thrombin and all the other enzyme factors.

Activated protein C cleaves extrinsic VIIIa and common-pathway Va. Protein C is activated by protein C-ase, comprising the enzyme thrombin, a cofactor thrombomodulin secreted by endothelial cells, Ca^{++}, and PL.

VII. Pharmacology

Anticoagulant and antiplatelet medications target various points within the hemostatic pathways. Antiplatelet medications prevent platelet activation and aggregation, while anticoagulant medications inhibit coagulation factor activation at various points within secondary hemostasis. Table 24-5 outlines the specific targets inhibited by each drug along with some details about monitoring their effect and drugs that can be used in the event of bleeding emergencies.

Antiplatelet therapy is the mainstay of treatment for cerebrovascular and cardiovascular disease. Aspirin is an irreversible inhibitor of cyclo-oxygenase, thereby preventing the synthesis of thromboxane, a major stimulant for platelet activation. The second most commonly used class of antiplatelet medications includes clopidogrel and ticlopidine, $P2Y_{12}$ receptor antagonists, which result in a decreased expression of the glycoprotein IIb/IIIa receptors on the surface of activated platelets, thereby inhibiting platelet adhesion and aggregation. Finally, the direct glycoprotein IIb/IIIa receptor antagonists—abciximab and eptifibatide—prevent platelet aggregation by inhibiting the crosslink of fibrinogen. These agents are only available for intravenous administration and are primarily used in treatment of acute coronary syndrome.

Unfractionated heparin is one of the oldest and most commonly used medications for anticoagulation, especially for emergency treatment of pulmonary embolism, myocardial infarction, vascular thrombosis, or cardiopulmonary

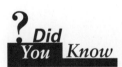

? Did You Know

Use of low-dose aspirin is ubiquitous among patients because it is an effective prophylaxis against myocardial infarction. It acts by irreversibly inhibiting cyclo-oxygenase and impairing platelet aggregation. It should be discontinued more than a week before intraocular or intracranial surgery to reduce the risk of devastating hemorrhage.

Table 24-5   Anticoagulant and Anti-Platelet Medications

Medication	Trade Name	Target/MOA	Monitor Test	Antidote
Anticoagulants				
Heparin		Antithrombin enhanced activity	aPTT or ACT	Protamine
LMWHs				
Enoxaparin	Lovenox	Factor Xa inhibition	Anti-Xa	Protamine has limited effect
Fondaparinox	Arixtra	Factor Xa inhibition	Anti-Xa	None
Argatroban	Acova	DTI	ACT	None
Bivalirudin	Angiomax	DTI	aPTT or ECT	None but rapid metabolism
Warfarin	Coumadin	Vitamin K antagonist	INR	Vitamin K or PCC
NOAC				
Apixaban	Eliquis	Factor Xa inhibition	none	Limited evidence but
Rivaroxaban	Xarelto	Factor Xa inhibition		PCCs are first line
Dabigatran	Pradaxa	DTI		
Anti-Platelet Drugs				
Aspirin		COX inhibition	Platelet assay	Platelet transfusion
Clopidogrel	Plavix	P_2Y_{12} antagonist	P_2Y_{12} assay	Platelet transfusion
Abciximab	ReoPro	Monoclonal antibody to GPIIb/IIIa	aPTT or ACT	None

LMWHs, low molecular weight heparins; MOA, mechanism of action; COX, cyclo-oxygenase; DTI, direct thrombin inhibitor; NOAC, new oral anticoagulants; aPTT, activated thromboplastin time; ACT, activated clotting time; ECT, ecarin clotting time; INR, international normalized ratio; PCC, prothrombin complex concentrate.

bypass. It acts by improving the affinity of antithrombin for thrombin, thereby inhibiting the final step of secondary hemostasis. The therapeutic effects of heparin primarily inhibit the intrinsic and common coagulation pathway and can be monitored with the activated partial thromboplastin time or the activated clotting time. However, it is a large molecule with significant risks of heparin-induced thrombocytopenia (HIT), a disorder characterized by microvascular thrombosis secondary to platelet-activating IgG antibodies to the heparin and platelet factor 4 complexes. Low molecular weight heparins such as enoxaparin and fondaparinox, inhibit the activation of factor X as a means of preventing thrombin formation and hemostasis. They are smaller molecules with longer half-lives making them less likely to cause HIT and suitable for intermittent therapeutic dosing that does not require an infusion. Parenteral direct thrombin inhibitors such as argatroban and bivalirudin bind to free thrombin preventing ongoing hemostatic activity. They are primarily indicated for patients with HIT or those with a heparin allergy and can be monitored with activated clotting times (8).

Warfarin is a classic oral anticoagulant medication clinically used for treatment and prophylaxis in patients at high risk for stroke or venous thromboembolism such as those with a hypercoagulable disorder (i.e., lupus anticoagulant, factor V Leiden, antithrombin deficiency) or a history of deep vein thrombosis, pulmonary embolism, heart valve replacement, or atrial fibrillation. Mechanistically, it is a vitamin K antagonist that prevents the hepatic synthesis of vitamin K–dependent coagulation factors, including factors II, VII, IX, and X. Incidentally, it also prevents the synthesis of protein C, a natural anticoagulant with a short half-life. Therefore, patients initiated on warfarin treatment will be hypercoagulable for the first 1 to 2 days until the available supply of factors is depleted. The effective concentration of warfarin is highly variable between patients and commonly affected by food and drug interactions. Regular monitoring is necessary and facilitated by the international normalized ratio (INR), a hemostatic assay designed to normalize the prothrombin time across different laboratories for patients with a combined deficiency of factors II, VII, IX, and X. For patients on warfarin therapy who experience a bleeding emergency, the warfarin should be reversed with vitamin K supplementation or prothrombin complex concentrates (PCCs). FFP is the second-line therapy indicated for warfarin reversal if PCCs are not available (8).

The new oral anticoagulants (NOACs) include dabigatran, a direct thrombin inhibitor, and rivaroxaban or apixaban, direct factor Xa antagonists. This class of anticoagulants is very popular for patients at risk of venous thromboembolism or stroke related to atrial fibrillation because of their rapid onset, simple dosing, and lack of need for regular laboratory monitoring secondary to a high degree of bioavailability and no significant drug or food interactions. However, there is currently little evidence regarding the best method for drug effect reversal in the setting of emergency surgery or critical bleeding. The most recent recommendations dictate waiting four to five half-lives of a NOAC prior to elective procedures, including neuraxial anesthesia, and longer for patients with renal insufficiency. In the case of an emergency, PCCs are likely the best therapeutic agent for reversal given their composition. Table 24-6 outlines the pharmacokinetics and pharmacodynamics of warfarin versus the NOACs (9).

Hemostatic medications serve an integral role in blood conservation and the medical management of hemorrhage by promoting the formation and

Table 24-6	Oral Anticoagulant Medications			
	Warfarin	**Dabigatran**	**Apixaban**	**Rivaroxaban**
Target	Vitamin K	Thrombin	Factor Xa	Factor Xa
Time to peak	72–96 hr	1–2 hr	3 hr	2.5–4 hr
Half-life	40 hr	9–13 hr	8–15 hr	7–11 hr
Dose	2–10 mg	150 mg	5 mg	20 mg
Frequency	Daily or qod	Once or twice daily	Twice daily	Daily
Metabolism	None	Renal excretion	Hepatic	Hepatic
Drug interactions	CYP2C9	Few	CYP3A4	CYP3A4

qod, every other day.

stabilization of blood clots. There are several mechanistic targets for procoagulant agents from the initiation of primary hemostasis to the activation of clotting factors. However, it is imperative that these agents target only the site of vascular injury as systemic activation of hemostatic pathways can lead to catastrophic arterial and venous thromboembolism.

Desmopressin (1-deamino-8-D-argenine vasopressin [DDAVP]) is a synthetic analogue of vasopressin with a diversity of clinical hemostatic effects, some of which are still poorly understood. DDAVP is clinically indicated for treatment and prophylaxis of bleeding in patients with platelet dysfunction, often related to hemophilia and von Willebrand disease, as it facilitates the cleavage of factor VIII and vWF to increase the activity of both factors, thereby improving platelet function. Additionally, DDAVP provides a modest decrease in bleeding associated with major surgery such as spinal fusion, revision orthopedic procedures, and high-risk cardiac surgery, without a significant increased risk of thromboembolism. Other adverse effects of DDAVP include hyponatremia and resultant cerebral edema, but this is clinically rare in the adult population (6).

Antifibrinolytics prevent the dissolution of established blood clots, thereby improving vascular integrity at the site of injury and decreasing bleeding. There are two types of antifibrinolytics. Aprotinin is a serine protease inhibitor that directly inhibits plasmin. It is not available in the United States because a large randomized trial demonstrated an association between use of aprotinin and increased morbidity and mortality. However, it has been proven to be effective at decreasing blood loss and transfusion requirements for patients undergoing high-risk surgery and is currently approved for use in Canada and Europe (6).

The lysine analogue antifibrinolytics, including epsilon-aminocaproic acid (EACA) and tranexamic acid (TXA), inhibit the cleavage of plasminogen to plasmin. They are less potent than aprotinin and in comparative trials less effective, but the incidence of thromboembolism and adverse effects from TXA and EACA are minimal, making them an attractive option for prophylaxis in patients at risk for major bleeding. Large clinical trials in trauma patients, as well as many studies in cardiac and orthopedic surgical patients, have documented the clinical use of these medications especially when used prophylactically (6).

Factor concentrates provide the substrates for the secondary hemostasis phase of the clotting cascade without the transfusion risks associated with plasma administration. Concentrates can be delivered individually when indicated, for example, factor VIII concentrates in classic hemophilia or in complexes with multiple factors in PCCs of various compositions. Recombinant activated factor VII is currently approved for treatment of hemophilia in patients with inhibitors to factors VIII or IX. However, it is more commonly used for hemostasis in patients suffering critical bleeding (6).

PCCs have different compositions, but generally include varied amounts of three to four factor concentrates, including factors II, IX, X, and sometimes VII. For most of the PCCs, these factors are administered inactive and complexed with an anticoagulant such as antithrombin, protein C, or heparin, making the overall therapy less likely to cause unwanted thromboembolism. PCCs are currently indicated for treatment of hemophilia patients with inhibitors to specific factor concentrates. However, they are more frequently used as the first-line reversal agents for warfarin and the NOACs in cases of critical bleeding. It is important to recognize that these medications carry a risk of arterial and venous thromboembolism and are contraindicated in patients with suspicion of having DIC, a systemic disorder of uncontrolled hemostasis with microvascular clotting, coagulation factor, and platelet consumption that may progress to multiorgan system failure and massive hemorrhage.

References

1. Whitaker BI. *The 2011 National Blood Collection and Utilization Survey Report.* Bethesda, MD: U.S. Department of Health and Human Services with the AABB; 2011.
2. Carson JL, Grossman BJ, Kleinman S, et al. Red blood cell transfusion: A clinical practice guideline from the AABB. *Ann Intern Med.* 2012;157(1):49–58.
3. Retter A, Wyncoll D, Pearse R, et al. Guidelines on the management of anaemia and red cell transfusion in adult critically ill patients. *Br J Haematol.* 2013;160(4):445–464.
4. Hendrickson JE, Hillyer CD. Noninfectious serious hazards of transfusion. *Anesth Analg.* 2009;108(3):759–769.
5. Bolton-Maggs PH, Cohen H. Serious hazards of transfusion (SHOT) haemovigilance and progress is improving transfusion safety. *Br J Haematol.* 2013;163(3):303–314.
6. Goodnough LT, Shander A. Current status of pharmacologic therapies in patient blood management. *Anesth Analg.* 2013;116(1):15–34.
7. Ashworth A, Klein AA. Cell salvage as part of a blood conservation strategy in anaesthesia. *Br J Anaesth.* 2010;105(4):401–416.
8. De Caterina R, Husted S, Wallentin L, et al. General mechanisms of coagulation and targets of anticoagulants (Section I). Position paper of the ESC Working Group on Thrombosis—Task Force on Anticoagulants in Heart Disease. *Thromb Haemost.* 2013;109(4):569–579.
9. Levy JH, Key NS, Azran MS. Novel oral anticoagulants: Implications in the perioperative setting. *Anesthesiology.* 2010;113(3):726–745.

Questions

1. As a result of trauma a 60-year-old patient is undergoing an emergent leg amputation in the hospital. An indication for transfusion of whole blood is:
   A. A hemoglobin level of <5 g/dL
   B. A blood pressure of <70/50 mm Hg for 10 minutes
   C. Ongoing blood loss exceeding 8,000 mL
   D. None of the above

2. A otherwise healthy 25-year-old woman is admitted to the hospital with clinical and radiographic signs of appendicitis. Workup yields the following data: blood pressure 115/85 mm Hg, heart rate 110, temperature 39°C, white blood cell count 12,000, hemoglobin 7.5 g/dL, urinalysis normal. The most appropriate next step is:
   A. Proceed urgently to perform an appendectomy
   B. Administer erythropoietin and then proceed to surgery
   C. Transfuse 2 units of PRBCs and then proceed to surgery
   D. Delay surgery for 24 hours to determine the cause of the anemia

3. All of the following are indications for transfusion of fresh frozen plasma EXCEPT:
   A. Dilutional coagulopathy
   B. A deficiency of coagulation factors
   C. Hypovolemia with a normal hemoglobin
   D. Bleeding due to a warfarin overdose

4. The recommended indications for platelet transfusion include all of the following EXCEPT:
   A. Patient having intraocular surgery; platelet count 75,000 per microliter
   B. Asymptomatic patient; platelet count 25,000 per microliter
   C. Patient scheduled for resection of abdominal aortic aneurysm; platelet count 40,000 per microliter
   D. Patient scheduled for resection of intracranial meningioma; platelet count 80,000 per microliter

5. A 25-year-old man is seriously hemorrhaging secondary to trauma. Until his blood type can be identified, which of the following would be the BEST choice of blood for transfusion until type-specific blood is available?
   A. Type O Rh-positive
   B. Type A Rh-negative
   C. Type B Rh-negative
   D. Type AB Rh-negative

6. Which of the following is a sign of an acute hemolytic transfusion reaction during general anesthesia?
   A. Tachycardia
   B. Hypotension
   C. Bleeding
   D. All of the above

7. Which of the following is the most common infection transmitted by blood transfusion?
   A. *Escherichia coli*
   B. Hepatitis B
   C. Hepatitis C
   D. Human immunodeficiency virus

8. For most patients undergoing major surgical procedures associated with significant blood loss, the overall most efficacious alternative to RBC transfusion is:
   A. Blood salvage with "cell saver" technology
   B. Autologous blood donation
   C. Acute normovolemic hemodilution
   D. Perfluorocarbon blood substitutes

9. What coagulation factor is responsible for conversion of fibrinogen to fibrin?
   A. Tissue factor (TF)
   B. Factor VIII
   C. Thrombin
   D. Factor XIII

10. All of the following statements about aspirin are true EXCEPT:
    A. It inhibits cyclo-oxygenase
    B. It prevents synthesis of thromboxane
    C. It interferes with platelet activation
    D. Its effect is readily reversible

25 Ambulatory Anesthesia, Monitored Anesthesia Care, and Office-Based Anesthesia

Meghan E. Rodes
Shireen Ahmad

The most recent update available from the Centers for Disease Control and Prevention regarding Ambulatory Surgery in the United States from 2006 indicates that outpatient surgery visits in the United States increased from 20.8 million visits in 1996 to 34.7 million in 2006. Additionally, the proportion of outpatient surgeries has increased from one-half to two-thirds of all surgeries over the same time period (1). The most common ambulatory procedures performed were endoscopy and cataract surgery, both typically performed under *monitored anesthesia care (MAC)*. Therefore, it is important for anesthesiologists to be able to formulate an appropriate anesthetic plan. This includes an expeditious return of consciousness without significant side effects, thereby allowing the timely discharge of patients undergoing ambulatory procedures. This chapter will discuss the principles applied in MAC, the techniques and common medications used in *ambulatory anesthesia*, and a brief introduction to office-based anesthesia.

I. Monitored Anesthesia Care

A. Terminology

According to the American Society of Anesthesiologists (ASA) position statement, MAC is a specific anesthesia service for a diagnostic or therapeutic procedure and does not describe the continuum of depth of sedation (2). Indications for MAC include the type of procedure, the patient's clinical condition, and the potential need to convert to a general or regional anesthetic (2). Furthermore, it includes all aspects of anesthetic care, including a preprocedure visit, intraprocedure care, and postprocedure recovery management (2).

The anesthesia provider must be prepared and qualified to convert to general anesthesia if necessary (3). If the patient loses consciousness and the ability to respond purposefully, the anesthesia care is a general anesthetic, irrespective of whether airway instrumentation is required (2). ASA standard monitoring, which includes electrocardiography (ECG), pulse oximetry, noninvasive blood pressure, and more recently end-tidal carbon dioxide ($ETCO_2$) monitoring, must be used for every anesthetic including MAC.

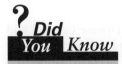

B. Preoperative Assessment

Patients scheduled for MAC should receive a *preoperative assessment* similar to any other preoperative patient. MAC is unique in that it also requires an element of cooperation on the part of the patient. It is important for the patient to accept the possibility to some degree of awareness during the procedure, to tolerate positioning required for surgery, and in some instances, to be able to communicate with the surgeon or proceduralist.

C. Techniques of Monitored Anesthesia Care

Successful MAC involves the use of combinations of anesthetic agents. Typically, a combination of a sedative hypnotic and an analgesic agent is used in dosages that vary depending on the goals of the anesthetic and the requirements of the procedure. Medications with minimal side effects and short duration of action are preferable in ambulatory anesthesia, where efficiency and rapid recovery are highly desirable.

D. Pharmacologic Basis of Monitored Anesthesia Techniques: Optimizing Drug Administration

Pharmacokinetics and pharmacodynamics are important to consider when selecting medications for any anesthetic. Simply defined, pharmacokinetics is what the body does to the drug, as opposed to pharmacodynamics, which is the effect of the drug on the body (4). Knowledge of this information is essential in order to select the appropriate medications for specific procedures and individual patients. Many anesthetic drugs are administered as a bolus. However, it is generally preferable to deliver the drugs in smaller doses or as titratable infusions that allow the maintenance of a suitable therapeutic level of drug in the patient, thereby enhancing safety (5). Furthermore, patients require smaller amounts of drug during infusions compared with bolus dosing, which affects both recovery time and resource utilization (6). A more thorough discussion of the principles of pharmacokinetics and pharmacodynamics can be found in Chapter 7.

E. Distribution, Elimination, Accumulation, and Duration of Action

Elimination Half-life

Elimination half-life is the time taken for a drug to lose half of its pharmacologic or physiologic activity. It is significant only if elimination is the exclusive route for the decline in plasma drug concentration. Therefore, this parameter is only useful in single compartment models, which do not typically apply to the human body.

Context-sensitive Half-time

The *context-sensitive half-time* is a more relevant parameter, and it is defined as the time required for plasma drug concentration to decrease by 50% after discontinuing an infusion of a specific duration (Fig. 25-1) (7). At the beginning of an infusion, plasma drug levels are decreased primarily by distribution to other body compartments as opposed to elimination. After the infusion is discontinued, drug that has been distributed to other compartments will return to the central plasma compartment for elimination. Factors that affect context-sensitive half-time include elimination mechanisms and propensity for distribution. A lipophilic drug, such as fentanyl, is much more likely to be transported into the tissues and to re-emerge into the plasma compartment after the infusion is stopped, resulting in a prolonged context-sensitive half-time. This phenomenon is unlike that of remifentanil, which is rapidly hydrolyzed by plasma

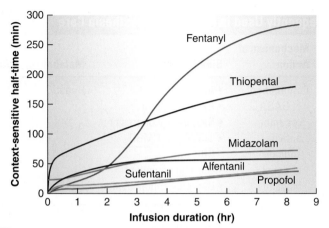

Figure 25-1 Context-sensitive half-time as a function of infusion duration. These data were generated from the computer model of Hughes et al. It can be seen that the context-sensitive half-time of propofol demonstrates a minimal increase as the duration of the infusion increases. Also note that for infusions of short duration, sufentanil has a shorter half-time than alfentanil. (From Hillier SC, Mazurek MS, Havidich, JE. Monitored anesthesia care. In: Barash PG, Cullen BF, Stoelting RK, et al. *Clinical Anesthesia,* 7th ed. Philadelphia: Lippincott Williams & Wilkins, 2013:827.)

esterases and has a smaller amount of drug available for transport into tissues and a significantly shorter context-sensitive half-time.

How Does the Context-sensitive Half-time Relate to the Time of Recovery?
Context-sensitive half-time merely refers to the time it takes for the plasma concentration to decline by 50% after terminating an infusion. It may not have a direct correlation with the time required for an individual patient to awaken or recover from the infusion, which is a function of the time it takes for the drug to clear the brain compartment to a sufficient level to allow arousal.

Effect-site Equilibration
The delay between drug administration and effect reflects the effect-site equilibration. It is important to observe the effects of the drugs prior to the administration of repeated doses to avoid oversedation.

F. Drug Interactions in Monitored Anesthesia Care
Because there is no intravenous agent that provides all of the desired qualities in an anesthetic, namely anxiolysis, amnesia, analgesia, and anesthesia, multiple medications are often combined to produce these characteristics. These agents potentiate one another. Therefore, it is important to administer smaller doses of each medication when they are given in combination with one another. This synergism applies not only to desired therapeutic effects of medications, but also to potentially dangerous side effects of these drugs.

G. Specific Drugs Used during Monitored Anesthesia Care
This section presents a brief description of the drugs most commonly used in MAC. For a more in-depth discussion of these medication classes, please refer to their dedicated chapters (see Chapters 9 and 10). Table 25-1 provides a succinct profile of several drugs commonly used in MAC.

Propofol
Propofol is a short-acting, intravenous, sedative-hypnotic agent and is one of the most ubiquitous anesthetic drugs across all types of anesthesia. It is used

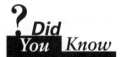

Context-sensitive half-time merely refers to the time it takes for the plasma concentration to decline by 50% after terminating an infusion.

Table 25-1   Profile of Drugs Frequently Used in Monitored Anesthesia Care

Drug	Route of Administration	Mechanism of Action	Side Effects	Metabolism	Antagonist
Propofol	IV	Potentiation of GABA receptor activity, sodium channel blockade	• Antiemetic • Bronchodilator • Respiratory depression • ↓ SVR, BP, CMRO$_2$, CBF, ICP • Burning sensation • Bacterial contamination	Hepatic	None
Midazolam	IV IM PO	Enhancement of GABA	• ↓ CMRO$_2$, CBF • Anticonvulsant	Hepatic	Flumazenil
Fentanyl	IV transmucosal neuraxial	Opioid receptor agonist	• Respiratory depression • ↓ HR, CBF • Delayed gastric emptying • Urinary retention • Nausea/vomiting	Hepatic	Naloxone
Ketamine	IV IM PO	NMDA antagonist	• ↑ CMRO$_2$, CBF, ICP, IOP, HR, BP • Secretions • Hallucinations	Hepatic	None
Dexmedetomine	IV	Alpha$_2$ agonist	• ↓ CMRO$_2$, CBF, HR, BP	Hepatic	None

IV, intravenous; IM, intramuscular; PO, by mouth; NMDA, N-methyl-D-aspartate; GABA, γ-aminobutyric acid; SVR, systemic vascular resistance; CMRO$_2$, cerebral metabolic rate for oxygen; ICP, intracranial pressure; IOP, intraocular pressure; CBF, cerebral blood flow; HR, heart rate; BP, blood pressure.

for induction and maintenance of general anesthesia, for procedural sedation, and as a sedative for mechanically ventilated patients in the intensive care unit. Propofol has multiple mechanisms of action, including potentiation of γ-aminobutyric acid (GABA) receptor activity and sodium channel blockade. It has a favorable side-effect profile, possesses antiemetic and bronchodilator properties, and has a short context-sensitive half-time that is minimally affected by the duration of infusion. In addition to its desired therapeutic effects, propofol also decreases systemic vascular resistance, blood pressure (BP), cerebral metabolic rate for oxygen (CMRO$_2$), cerebral blood flow (CBF), and intracranial pressure (ICP) and produces respiratory depression. Propofol is metabolized by the liver and excreted by the kidneys. Propofol is associated with a burning sensation at the injection site. However, a small dose of lidocaine alone or combined with propofol is the most effective strategy to attenuate this effect (8). Because propofol is prepared in a lipid emulsion, this presents the risk of bacterial contamination if the drug is not discarded within 6 hours of being withdrawn from the vial. Additionally, propofol contains an egg phospholipid as an emulsifier and should be avoided in patients with egg allergies.

Fospropofol

Fospropofol is a water-soluble prodrug form of propofol. It is metabolized by alkaline phosphatases to its active metabolite, propofol, and therefore has a

? Did You Know

Propofol is a short-acting, intravenous, sedative-hypnotic agent and is one of the most ubiquitous anesthetic drugs across all types of anesthesia.

slower onset. Potential advantages over propofol include less chance of bacterial contamination, less pain on injection, and lower risk of hyperlipidemia associated with long-term administration. Although fospropofol has been approved by the U.S. Food and Drug Administration for use during MAC, there are limited data on the safety and efficacy of the drug, and it is not commonly used in clinical practice at this time.

Benzodiazepines

Benzodiazepines, most commonly midazolam, are used prior to induction of most anesthetics to provide anxiolysis and amnesia. The therapeutic effects of midazolam are related to the enhancement of the effect of GABA on its receptors. The effects of benzodiazepines on the body include minimal respiratory depression when used alone and decreased $CMRO_2$ and CBF, with no effect on ICP. Benzodiazepines are also potent anticonvulsants and may be used to treat status epilepticus and seizures related to local anesthetic toxicity or alcohol withdrawal. Midazolam is metabolized by the liver and subsequently excreted by the kidneys. In addition to the intravenous route, it can be administered intramuscularly, intranasally, or orally. The oral dose of midazolam is much higher than the intravenous dose due to poor oral bioavailability. Although midazolam has a short elimination half-life, larger doses may be associated with delayed emergence. For this reason, it is typically used in small doses at the beginning of an anesthetic to facilitate patient comfort through anxiolysis and amnesia, while sedation is maintained with a drug that has a more favorable recovery profile, such as propofol. Benzodiazepines offer an advantage over propofol, in that there is a specific benzodiazepine antagonist, flumazenil. However, the effects of midazolam frequently outlast the dose of flumazenil, resulting in resedation.

Opioids

The analgesia during MAC is typically provided by the injection of local anesthetic at the surgical site. However, opioids, most commonly fentanyl, are administered for additional analgesia and to improve the patient's comfort. Opioids are administered by various routes, including oral, intramuscular, subcutaneous, transmucosal, neuraxial, and most commonly in anesthesia, intravenous. The mechanism of action of opioids is through an agonist action at specific opioid receptors in the central and peripheral nervous systems, decreasing the transmission of pain signals. Potential side effects of opioids include bradycardia, a dose-dependent respiratory depression, decreased CBF, delayed gastric emptying, increased urinary sphincter tone leading to failure to void, and most commonly, nausea and vomiting. Additionally, it is possible to induce skeletal muscle rigidity when large doses of opioids are administered rapidly. Chest wall rigidity can be severe enough to make ventilation difficult and, therefore, large doses should be avoided. It is also important to note that opioids alone do not provide amnesia.

Opioids are metabolized by the liver and excreted mainly in the urine. The differences in lipid solubility within this class of drugs account for varying pharmacokinetic profiles of individual opioids. Like benzodiazepines, opioids also have a specific antagonist. Naloxone can be given to reverse the respiratory effects of opioids. But it should be used judiciously due to the potential adverse side effects such as tachycardia and hypertension, as well as pulmonary edema.

Ketamine

Ketamine is a phencyclidine derivative that produces intense analgesia and amnesia. Although small doses are often used as an adjunct in MAC, larger

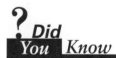

? Did You Know

Benzodiazepines are also potent anticonvulsants and may be used to treat status epilepticus and seizures related to local anesthetic toxicity or alcohol withdrawal.

? Did You Know

Intravenous opioid administration may induce skeletal muscle rigidity and chest wall rigidity that can be severe enough to make ventilation difficult when large doses are administered rapidly.

? Did You Know

Opioids alone do not provide amnesia.

? Did You Know

Naloxone can precipitate tachycardia and hypertension when given to reverse the respiratory effects of opioids.

doses can be used to induce general anesthesia. Its primary mechanism of action is antagonism at the *N*-methyl-D-aspartate receptor. Ketamine can be administered by oral, intramuscular, or intravenous routes. Ketamine has bronchodilator properties, making it beneficial in asthmatic patients. It has minimal effect on respiration, in contrast to other intravenous sedatives and opioids. In addition to its therapeutic effects, ketamine is also associated with increased $CMRO_2$, CBF, ICP, and stimulation of the sympathetic nervous system, resulting in increased heart rate (HR) and BP. For these reasons, ketamine may be a poor choice in patients with increased ICP or intraocular pressure and patients with coronary artery disease. Ketamine may have a paradoxical cardiac effect in patients with disease states associated with catecholamine depletion (e.g., septic shock), resulting in direct myocardial depression. Ketamine may also produce increased secretions, which are often managed with administration of an antisialagogue. The incidence of hallucinations with ketamine is minimized by administration of a benzodiazepine. Ketamine is metabolized in the liver to norketamine, which has approximately one-fifth the potency of ketamine and may contribute to lingering effects.

? *Did You Know*

Ketamine and dexmedetomidine are the only drugs in the analgesic sedative armamentarium that do not suppress ventilatory drive.

Dexmedetomidine

Dexmedetomidine is an intravenous selective α_2 receptor agonist that can be used to provide sedation. Its major benefit is that it has little effect on respiratory drive when used alone. Dexmedetomidine has no intrinsic amnestic properties. Side effects of dexmedetomidine include decreased $CMRO_2$ and CBF, as well as a combination of decreased sympathetic outflow and increased vagal activity, commonly precipitating hypotension and bradycardia, which can be profound. Dexmedetomidine is extensively metabolized in the liver and excreted by the kidneys.

Amnesia during Sedation with Dexmedetomidine or Propofol

Because dexmedetomidine has no amnestic properties, it must be supplemented with a drug such as propofol or midazolam if amnesia is desirable.

H. Patient-controlled Sedation and Analgesia

Patient-controlled analgesia (PCA) is a familiar concept for management of postoperative pain. PCA has a favorable safety profile compared with intermittent larger boluses of analgesics as well as increased patient satisfaction with pain control compared with medical-provider analgesic administration. Patient-controlled sedation has been shown to be effective for use during procedural sedation (9). The cumbersome nature of the PCA pump and set up as well as a decreased margin of safety when dealing with anesthetic doses of medications rather than analgesic doses are the major limiting factors.

I. Respiratory Function and Sedative Hypnotics

Many of the medications referred to above are associated with dose-dependent adverse respiratory effects, which include direct respiratory depression, suppression of normal airway reflexes, and an increase in upper airway resistance.

Sedation and the Upper Airway

Successful ventilation requires coordination of all parts of the airway from the oropharynx to the muscles of the thorax. The upper airway is particularly susceptible to the effects of anesthetic drugs. Although this may not be a major concern for the young, healthy patients with normal airway anatomy and respiratory function, significant ventilatory problems may be encountered in the patient with pre-existing lung or airway disease.

Sedation and Protective Airway Reflexes

Intact upper airway reflexes are necessary to safeguard against pulmonary aspiration. Unfortunately, many anesthetic drugs have an adverse effect on these protective upper airway reflexes. Caution must be exercised in patients at risk for aspiration and protection of the airway with an endotracheal tube should be considered, regardless of the procedure.

Sedation and Respiratory Control

The negative pulmonary effects of anesthetic agents are potentiated when they are used in combination with one another due to a synergistic effect. Therefore, smaller doses must be used with combinations of the agents, and patients must be closely monitored for adverse effects.

J. Supplemental Oxygen Administration

It is not uncommon for mild hypoventilation and hypoxemia to occur during administration of anesthetic medications. Although this is typically treated with supplemental oxygen administration, there is no substitute for close monitoring of the patient to ensure a patent airway. Although $ETCO_2$ monitoring became an ASA standard monitor in 2011, it has been shown to be a poor indicator of ventilation in the sedated, spontaneously breathing patient.

K. Monitoring during Monitored Anesthesia Care

Standards for Basic Anesthetic Monitoring

The ASA standards for basic anesthetic monitoring apply to every anesthetic delivered by an anesthesia provider, regardless of anesthetic type, patient condition, and duration or urgency of procedure (10). These standards require that qualified anesthesia personnel must be present in the room throughout the course of all anesthetics and that there is continual evaluation of oxygenation, ventilation, circulation, and temperature. Oxygenation is most commonly monitored by pulse oximetry. For all general anesthetics delivered with an anesthesia machine, an in-line (within the breathing circuit) oxygen analyzer is required to detect unsafe low levels of inspired oxygen.

Capnography is used to monitor ventilation when an endotracheal tube or laryngeal mask airway is in place. But it is not quantitatively accurate when measured with a nasal cannula. Alarms must be in place to detect the absence of $ETCO_2$ or a disconnection in components of the breathing system. Circulation is monitored by continuous ECG and pulse oximetry. BP and HR are evaluated at a minimum of 5-minute intervals. Temperature must be monitored when clinically significant changes in body temperature are intended, anticipated, or suspected.

Communication and Observation

There is no substitute for a meticulous, focused, and attentive anesthesia provider. Although basic monitors are applied for all anesthetics, sight and sound are also important tools for the assessment of clinical condition, particularly during MAC.

Preparedness to Recognize and Treat Local Anesthetic Toxicity

Because sedation is often provided as an adjunct to regional, neuraxial, or local anesthesia, it is important for the anesthesia provider to be aware of toxic dose ranges of local anesthetics. He or she must be able to recognize the signs and symptoms of local anesthetic toxicity and to be prepared to treat them in an expeditious fashion.

Symptoms of local anesthetic toxicity often begin with numbness of the tongue or perioral area and a metallic taste in the mouth. As the concentration of local anesthetic in the central nervous system increases, patients may report tinnitus or restlessness. This may progress to slurred speech and muscle twitching, which often signal an impending seizure. Sedation may mask these early signs of local anesthetic toxicity. The side effects of sedation, such as hypercarbia and acidemia, result in increased CBF. An increase in the ionized form of the local anesthetic may also aggravate the central nervous system toxicity by crossing the blood brain barrier more easily. In the worst case scenario, cardiovascular collapse may occur. The anesthesia provider must be vigilant and prepared to respond quickly once local anesthetic toxicity is manifested.

L.   Depth of Sedation and Analgesia

Anesthesiologists are trained to provide all types of anesthesia. Nonanesthesiologists are able to plan and provide only minimal or moderate levels of sedation and are not trained to provide a general anesthetic, which could inadvertently result from deep sedation. However, because nonanesthesiologists have become involved in administering sedation, the ASA has developed practice guidelines to delineate four levels of sedation: minimal sedation, moderate sedation, deep sedation, and general anesthesia. The spectrum of anesthetic depth is fluid, meaning there are no concrete demarcations between levels of sedation and the level of sedation intended may differ from the level of sedation achieved from time to time. Table 25-2 defines each of the four levels on the continuum of depth of sedation, as developed by the ASA (11).

Table 25-2 lists observations regarding patient responsiveness, airway, spontaneous ventilation, and cardiovascular function for each of the four levels of sedation. The goal is for the provider to have early recognition of a patient progressing to a deeper level of sedation than intended, and to take action accordingly to return the patient to the planned level of sedation.

Table 25-2	Continuum of Depth of Sedation: Definition of General Anesthesia and Levels of Sedation/Analgesia			
	Minimal Sedation, Anxiolysis	**Moderate Sedation/Analgesia "Conscious Sedation"**	**Deep Sedation/ Analgesia**	**General Anesthesia**
Responsive-ness	Normal response to verbal stimulation	Purposeful response to verbal or tactile stimulation	Purposeful response following repeated or painful stimulation	Unarousable even with painful stimulus
Airway	Unaffected	No intervention required	Intervention may be required	Intervention often required
Spontaneous ventilation	Unaffected	Adequate	May be inadequate	Frequently inadequate
Cardiovascular Function	Unaffected	Usually maintained	Usually maintained	May be impaired

From American Society of Anesthesiologists. Continuum of depth of sedation, definition of general anesthesia and levels of sedation/analgesia. 2009. www.asahq.org.

II. Ambulatory Anesthesia

A. Place, Procedures, and Patient Selection

Complex ambulatory procedures have become increasingly common due to advances in surgical techniques. Thus, the anesthesiologist will find it necessary to adapt anesthetic plans to provide adequate anesthesia while minimizing adverse side effects and allowing timely discharge. Ambulatory surgeries can be done in a setting as basic as a physician office, in a freestanding ambulatory surgery center, or in a hospital. One advantage of an outpatient site is that costs are generally much lower than in the hospital. Turnaround time is also frequently improved in an ambulatory center, which may also be partially financially motivated or incentivized. Generally, cases tend to be of a more routine nature and are often limited in spectrum, also increasing efficiency.

A commonly held misconception is that *ambulatory surgery* is only for healthy, ASA physical status (PS) I and II patients. More recently, however, ASA PS III and IV patients have been cared for successfully in ambulatory centers, provided their comorbidities are stable and optimized. Appropriate procedure selection is important for the success of ambulatory surgery. Only those types of surgery that are associated with a relatively low risk of postoperative complications and minimal postoperative care, including infrequent attention from a medical provider, are good choices.

Ideally, procedures should be of short duration. If longer procedures are to be done, as well as those on complex patients who might need longer postoperative monitoring, they should be scheduled earlier in the day. Premature and young infants require up to 12 hours of postoperative monitoring for apnea, and longer if an apneic event occurs. Age extremes alone are not a sufficient reason to avoid surgery in an ambulatory center. However, it should be noted that medications are often more slowly metabolized in the elderly, so anesthetic plans need to be modified accordingly.

Uncomplicated obesity is also not necessarily a risk factor for poor outcome, but it may be associated with an increased risk for obstructive sleep apnea (OSA), which is associated with a higher rate of respiratory complications. The ASA has published specific guidelines pertaining to perioperative management of ambulatory surgery patients with OSA. Regardless of age and comorbidities, all patients who undergo ambulatory surgery should have a responsible adult escort them home and assist with postoperative care for the first 24 hours when needed.

B. Preoperative Evaluation and Reduction of Patient Anxiety

Preoperative screening is an important tool to reduce adverse outcomes on the day of surgery. This screening typically involves a complete medical history, including surgeries, difficulties with anesthesia in the past, current medications, and allergies. This is also the appropriate occasion to iterate preoperative fasting and medication instructions and postoperative plans for transportation by a responsible adult.

Upper Respiratory Tract Infection

Adults with an active *upper respiratory infection (URI)* should not undergo elective surgery. In fact, elective surgery should be delayed until at least 6 weeks after an acute URI. The recommendations for children are different, mainly due to the fact that children have URIs much more frequently than adults, and delaying surgery may only result in perpetual cancellations due to subsequent URIs. Most anesthesiologists would proceed with

Table 25-3	American Society of Anesthesiologists Fasting Guidelines for Elective Surgery	
Substance	**Fasting Time**	**Examples**
Clear liquids	2 hours	Water, transparent juice, coffee/tea without additives
Breast milk	4 hours	
Infant formula	6 hours	
Light meal	6 hours	Dry toast
Fatty meal	8 hours	Fried food, butter, cream

From American Society of Anesthesiologists Committee. Practice guidelines for preoperative fasting and the use of pharmacologic agents to reduce the risk of pulmonary aspiration: Application to healthy patients undergoing elective procedures: an updated report by the American Society of Anesthesiologists Committee on Standards and Practice Parameters. *Anesthesiology.* 2011;114:495–511.

surgery if a patient appears well, is afebrile, and is breathing and eating normally.

Restriction of Food and Liquids Prior to Ambulatory Surgery

The ASA has established practice guidelines for preoperative fasting, which are listed in Table 25-3 (12). These guidelines allow a light meal up to 6 hours prior to elective surgery (8 hours for fatty meals) and clear liquids (liquids one can see through, without cream or other additives) up to 2 hours in advance. It is particularly important that patients take all regular medications prior to surgery, with few exceptions.

Anxiety Reduction

Probably the most effective and undervalued anxiety reducer is a preoperative visit with an anesthesiologist. Other methods of anxiolysis include preoperative education, instructions, and medication. For children, parental presence may be of benefit, as well as an involvement of a child life specialist and distraction techniques, in addition to medications.

C. Managing the Anesthetic: Premedication

Premedication is often not very different from one setting to the next. But in the ambulatory arena, careful selection of the agent and dose is important to facilitate timely discharge from the facility.

Benzodiazepines

Midazolam is the most commonly used benzodiazepine for the purpose of anxiolysis. Due to a synergistic effect with other anesthetic agents, it may delay emergence or discharge following very short procedures. Therefore, it is important to assess whether the patient requires or desires preoperative sedation. In addition to its anxiolytic properties, midazolam also has the benefit of inducing amnesia. These effects on memory are independent of the sedation. A patient may appear completely awake yet have no recollection of events at a later time.

Opioids and Nonsteroidal Analgesics

In addition to the analgesic effects of opioids, they are often administered during an anesthetic as part of preprocedural sedation and as a strategy to decrease the hemodynamic response to sympathetic stimulation (e.g., laryngoscopy, intubation, or surgical incision). The addition of nonsteroidal anti-inflammatory drugs (NSAIDs), such as ketorolac and ibuprofen or acetaminophen (exact mechanism of action unknown), may also help modulate pain through alternative pathways. These drugs effectively decrease the amount of opioid analgesics required, thereby reducing the adverse side effects related to opioid administration.

D. Intraoperative Management: Choice of Anesthetic Method
Anesthetic Options
The anesthetic choices for ambulatory surgery include general anesthesia, regional or neuraxial anesthesia, MAC, and local anesthesia. Regional and local anesthetic techniques have the potential benefit of requiring minimal sedation. In some situations, the type of surgery dictates the choice of anesthetic, while in other situations, a discussion between patient, surgeon, and anesthesiologist may help to determine the most appropriate choice for the individual patient, procedure, or surgeon. In an ambulatory setting, the recovery time is an important element in determining the most appropriate anesthetic choice (Fig. 25-2).

Regional Techniques
The regional anesthetic techniques frequently used in ambulatory surgery include neuraxial anesthesia, peripheral nerve blocks (PNBs), intravenous regional anesthesia, and local anesthetic infiltration or field blocks. Although the duration of most local anesthetics is relatively short, the duration of analgesia can be prolonged with the use of a long-acting PNB or catheter, which can provide postoperative analgesia as well.

Spinal Anesthesia
Spinal anesthesia is an appropriate choice for surgery on the lower extremities, pelvis, or lower abdomen. The use of a short-acting local anesthetic will result

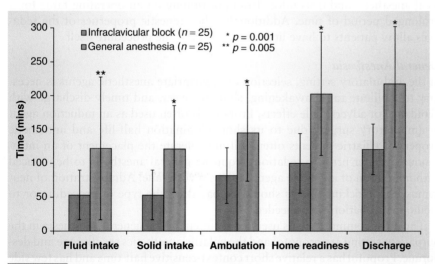

Figure 25-2 Recovery was faster when an infraclavicular brachial plexus block with a short-acting local anesthetic was used, compared with general anesthesia and wound infiltration for outpatients undergoing hand and wrist surgery. Times are calculated from the end of anesthesia. (From Lichtor, JL. Ambulatory anesthesia. In: Barash PG, Cullen BF, Stoelting RK, et al. *Clinical Anesthesia,* 7th ed. Philadelphia: Lippincott Williams & Wilkins, 2013:852.)

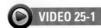

VIDEO 25-1

*Hypotension
after Spinal
Anesthesia*

in rapid recovery of motor and sensory function and can shorten the time to discharge. Postspinal headache is not a common complication when smaller gauge needles are used.

Epidural and Caudal Anesthesia

Epidural anesthesia usually involves the introduction of a catheter into the epidural space, which may be placed preoperatively and injected with local anesthetic just prior to surgery. Doses of local anesthetic can be repeated intermittently or the catheter can be connected to an infusion for longer surgeries. Caudal anesthesia is a form of epidural anesthesia often performed in children for surgery in the lower abdomen and involves local anesthetic injection into the caudal canal. It is frequently used in conjunction with general anesthesia because children cannot generally tolerate the needle insertion. Caudal anesthesia allows surgery to be performed with minimal perioperative opioids. Postoperative analgesia may last for several hours based on the choice of medication and dose administered.

Nerve Blocks

PNBs are associated with reduced pain, nausea, and vomiting and increased patient satisfaction. The use of PNBs for certain painful procedures, such as shoulder surgery, allows these procedures to be performed in the ambulatory setting. The discomfort after painful ambulatory orthopedic procedures is often routinely managed with a continuous infusion of local anesthetic around the nerves supplying the surgical site. However, it is necessary to provide a detailed postoperative instruction program if patients are discharged home with drug infusions and indwelling catheters. A more in-depth discussion of regional anesthesia can be found in Chapter 21.

Sedation and Analgesia

Intravenous sedation is a common adjunct to local anesthesia for a variety of reasons. The analgesic agents decrease the pain during the initial injection of local anesthetic and discomfort from positioning on an operating table for a prolonged period of time. Additionally, the amnestic properties of the sedatives allow patients to have little recollection of the procedure itself.

General Anesthesia

In the ambulatory setting, selection of appropriate anesthetic agents is necessary to facilitate rapid awakening, short recovery, and timely discharge with avoidance of adverse side effects. Propofol is often used as an induction agent in ambulatory surgery due to its short elimination half-life and antiemetic property. Pediatric patients often will not tolerate the placement of an intravenous catheter prior to sedation, requiring general anesthesia to be induced with inhalation of a volatile agent such as sevoflurane. Administration of neuromuscular blocking agents should be based on the type of procedure or to facilitate intubation when needed.

The most common agents used for maintenance of general anesthesia in the outpatient setting are propofol and the volatile anesthetics sevoflurane and desflurane. Propofol has a relative short context-sensitive half-time and has few side effects. The volatile agents are associated with a rapid induction and rapid recovery, which are conducive to the ambulatory setting. Nitrous oxide, while more rapid in recovery than sevoflurane or desflurane, may be associated with a higher incidence of postoperative nausea and vomiting (PONV), making it a poor choice for the ambulatory patient.

E. Management of Postanesthesia Care

Many potential postoperative adverse events or complications can be anticipated and prevented. Patient selection plays a major role in planning a successful ambulatory surgical experience. Patients who are expected to have postoperative difficulties are not good candidates for ambulatory surgery. The careful selection and titration of anesthetic agents have a significant impact on recovery. The most common causes of delayed recovery are pain, nausea, and sedation due to residual anesthetic effect. The early identification of these complications and effective management are paramount in facilitating discharge. A more thorough discussion of this topic can be found in Chapter 39, but will be addressed briefly below.

Reversal of Drug Effect

It may occasionally become necessary to administer agents to reverse the respiratory depression or sedation associated with opioids or benzodiazepines, respectively. Caution is advised when using these antagonists because they also have serious side effects and should be administered only when absolutely necessary and only in small incremental doses.

Nausea and Vomiting

PONV is a primary cause of delayed discharge and in rare cases may require admission to the hospital. In addition, PONV has a negative impact on patient satisfaction and quality of recovery. Factors predictive of PONV include female gender, history of PONV or motion sickness, nonsmoking, and certain types of surgery such as head and neck, breast, and laparoscopy. The risk factors have an additive effect: the greater the number of risk factors present, the greater the risk of PONV. Unfortunately, many anesthetic agents may contribute to PONV. Volatile anesthetics, nitrous oxide, and opioids all have emetogenic effects (Fig. 25-3). However, there are several antiemetics available for prevention and treatment that are not sedating and are suitable in the outpatient setting. The most commonly used antiemetics are selective serotonin antagonists, such as ondansetron.

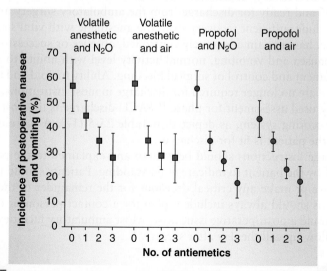

Figure 25-3 Postoperative nausea and vomiting (PONV) is least after a propofol anesthetic with air. Illustrated is the incidence of PONV when different anesthetics and different numbers of prophylactic antiemetic treatments are administered. (From Lichtor, JL. Ambulatory anesthesia. In: Barash PG, Cullen BF, Stoelting RK, et al. *Clinical Anesthesia,* 7th ed. Philadelphia: Lippincott Williams & Wilkins, 2013:854.)

Other drugs include dopamine antagonists, antihistamines, and anticholinergics. Dexamethasone is also commonly used for PONV prevention and treatment. It has been shown to improve quality of recovery and has recently been shown to have little effect on glucose regulation in healthy patients undergoing surgery (13,14). The most effective method to prevent PONV is to identify patients at greatest risk and to employ a combination of preventive medication strategies, including the use of anesthetics with antiemetic properties, in addition to minimizing the exposure to agents known to contribute to PONV.

Pain
A multimodal approach to analgesic management is generally the most effective. The multimodal approach involves the concomitant use of analgesic agents with different mechanisms of action, an opioid sparing effect, and results in fewer deleterious side effects associated with opioids. The most commonly used adjuncts include the NSAIDs ketorolac and ibuprofen as well as acetaminophen.

Preparation for Discharging the Patient
Standardized criteria are used to determine when a patient can safely transition through recovery and finally be discharged home. Although most patients who receive general anesthesia require a period in the phase I postanesthesia care unit (PACU), most patients receiving MAC are ready for phase II PACU immediately following surgery. Some patients who receive general anesthesia may be sufficiently recovered at the end of surgery to bypass the phase I PACU. This rapid movement to phase II is called *fast tracking*. One recent study demonstrated significantly shortened recovery duration by eliminating phase I PACU after general anesthesia (based on standardized criteria), without any change in patient outcome (15). The modified Aldrete scoring system is frequently used to assess suitability for phase I PACU discharge, and it is depicted in Table 25-4 (16). A score of at least 9/10 is required for discharge to phase II.

In most institutions, a score of nine or more is needed for transfer into the next phase of recovery. Additional criteria exist to determine when patients are "street fit" and ready for discharge from the ambulatory surgery area. These criteria include sufficient recovery from the anesthetic with vital signs similar to baseline, having pain adequately controlled, absence or successful management of nausea and vomiting, normal activity level with ability to ambulate, and assessment and control of surgical bleeding. Ability to void and to tolerate oral intake are no longer required for discharge in most institutions. The most commonly used assessment for phase II PACU discharge is the postanesthetic discharge scoring system, as depicted in Table 25-5 (17). A score of 9 or 10 indicates the patient is fit for discharge.

Discharge instructions should be written and explained to the patient and signed off by the patient to indicate understanding. Patients should be advised not to drive or make any critical decisions for the remainder of the day. The instructions should always include a plan for a contact person or emergency facility should a postoperative issue arise. Most ambulatory facilities also conduct a follow-up call the day after surgery.

III. Office-based Anesthesia
Office-based anesthesia involves anesthesia provided at a location other than a hospital or freestanding surgical facility. The major incentives for office-based procedures are the financial benefits and convenience to the surgeon

Table 25-4	Postanesthesia Care Unit Recovery and Discharge Criteria, Modified Aldrete Score	
Parameter	**Description of Patient**	**Score**
Activity level	Moves all extremities voluntarily/on command	2
	Moves 2 extremities	1
	Cannot move extremities	0
Respirations	Breathes deeply and coughs freely	2
	Is dyspneic, with shallow, limited breathing	1
	Is apneic	0
Circulation	BP within 20 mm Hg greater than preanesthetic level	2
	BP 20–50 mm Hg greater than preanesthetic level	1
	BP greater than 50 mm Hg above preanesthetic level	0
Consciousness	Is fully awake	2
	Is arousable on calling	1
	Is not responding	0
Oxygen saturation as determined by pulse oximetry	>90% breathing room air	2
	Requires supplemental oxygen to maintain level >90%	1
	Has level <90% with oxygen supplementation	0

From Vasanawala M, Macario A, Canales M. Some common problems in the postanesthetic care unit. *Contemp Surg.* 2000;56:691–700.

Table 25-5	Postanesthetic Discharge Scoring System	
Parameter	**Value**	**Score**
Vital signs	BP and pulse within 20% of preop	2
	BP and pulse within 20–40% of preop	1
	BP and pulse greater than 40% different from preop	0
Activity	Steady gait, no dizziness or meets preop level	2
	Requires assistance	1
	Unable to ambulate	0
Nausea and vomiting	Minimal/treated with oral medication	2
	Moderate/treated with parenteral medication	1
	Severe/continues despite treatment	0
Pain	Controlled with oral analgesics and acceptable to patient	2
	Uncontrolled or unacceptable to patient	1
Surgical bleeding	Minimal/no dressing changes	2
	Moderate/up to two dressing changes required	1
	Severe/more than three dressing changes required	0

From Chung F, Chan V, Ong D. A postanesthetic discharge scoring system for home readiness after ambulatory surgery. *J Clin Anesth.* 1995;7:500–506.

Table 25-6   Patients Not Suitable for Office-Based Anesthesia

Cardiac conditions:	Pulmonary conditions:	Central nervous system:
• Activity level <4 mets • Unstable angina • MI: 0–3 months • MI: 3–6 months, must have evaluation by cardiologist before surgery • Severe cardiomyopathy • Poorly controlled hypertension • Internal defibrillator or pacemaker • Heart transplant recipient/candidate	• Obstructive sleep apnea • Severe chronic obstructive pulmonary disease • Airway abnormality • Previous difficult intubation • Asthma: <6 months since last emergency department visit/acute exacerbation • Lung transplant recipient/candidate	• Multiple sclerosis • Stroke <6 months prior • Para/quadriplegia • Seizure disorder • Psychological instability • Dementia with disorientation
Renal:	**Hepatic:**	**Endocrine:**
• Creatinine >2 mg/dL • End-stage renal disease on dialysis • On special diet due to renal disease • Kidney transplant candidate	• Elevated bilirubin or transaminases • Liver transplant candidate	• Morbid obesity with BMI >35 • Poorly controlled diabetes mellitus • Hemoglobin A1c >8 • Type 1 diabetes mellitus
Hematologic:	**Musculoskeletal:**	**Other:**
• Sickle cell disease • Anticoagulant therapy • Von Willebrand disease • Hemophilia	• History of malignant hyperthermia • Myasthenia gravis • Muscular dystrophy or myopathy	• Alcohol/substance overuse • No adult escort

MI, myocardial infarction; BMI, body mass index.
Adapted from Ahmad S. Office based—is my anesthetic care any different? Assessment and management. *Anesthesiol Clin.* 28;2010:369–384.

and patient. A potential disadvantage of being remote from a hospital may be the lack of assistance in the event of an emergency. Because the concept of office-based anesthesia is fairly new, there are not significant amounts of long-term data on outcomes. In fact, some states still do not have regulations or mandatory reporting of adverse events for office-based anesthesia. Current studies and review of closed claims data seem to indicate increased risk with an office-based anesthetic. Problems range from inadequate equipment, monitoring, and evaluation to poor preparation and response to events. Almost half of the adverse events reported in office settings were classified as preventable.

A. Patient Selection and Preoperative Management

Thoughtful selection and preoperative evaluation are essential in order to optimize the patient prior to an office-based surgery. Patients with significant comorbidities who are at risk for anesthetic or surgical complications are not appropriate candidates for office-based procedures. Table 25-6 provides criteria for patients who may not be appropriate for an office-based procedure (18).

Careful selection of the procedures to be performed in the office setting is also necessary. Longer surgical procedures have a greater likelihood of postoperative complications and need for hospital admission. Many facilities plan to have procedures completed by early afternoon to provide for complete recovery prior to discharge from the facility.

B. Equipment

Office surgery locations must be equipped appropriately. It is mandatory that all machines be current, in functioning order, and serviced on a regular basis.

Total intravenous anesthesia (TIVA) must be employed unless a scavenging system for waste anesthetic gases is in place. All ASA standard monitors are required, including pulse oximetry, BP, continuous ECG, capnography, and ability to measure temperature. A selection of suitable airway equipment is needed, including various oxygen delivery devices from nasal cannula to bag and mask, intubation equipment, emergency airway supplies, and suction capability. An oxygen supply (including backup tanks) must be present. Emergency medications and a crash cart, including a defibrillator, are essential.

C. Safety and Organization

In addition to having proper equipment, policies must be developed and training for the correct use of the equipment must be conducted regularly. Each facility must have a medical director who is in charge of delineating responsibilities of each staff member. At least one member of the staff must be advanced cardiovascular life support certified and must remain present until all patients have been discharged from the facility. Plans for management of emergency situations, such as loss of power or oxygen supply, equipment malfunction, cardiac arrest, suspected malignant hyperthermia, and fire, must be developed. It is important to establish a relationship with a hospital in the event there is a need for transfer to a tertiary care center.

D. Anesthetic Management

Similarly to ambulatory anesthesia, the choice of anesthetic in the office setting is based on the need to facilitate rapid discharge and minimize adverse side effects. Cost of anesthetic equipment and medications must be considered. The details regarding these anesthetic agents have been reviewed elsewhere in the chapter.

IV. Conclusion

The same standards for preoperative evaluation and preparation, intraoperative monitoring, and postoperative care must be maintained regardless of the patient, setting, or type of anesthetic to be administered. Policies and procedures must be in place to ensure a minimum standard of care across all anesthetizing locations. All persons providing sedation or anesthesia must be trained in the use of drugs, recognition and management of their adverse side effects, and emergency procedures to rescue patients experiencing a level of sedation deeper than what is intended. The ideal analgesic or anesthetic agents are those that are inexpensive and free from adverse side effects. The duration of action of medications used in any individual anesthetic should be based on the nature of the procedure and the setting. Follow-up of patients and outcomes will allow this specialty to continually increase patient safety and satisfaction.

References

1. Centers for Disease Control and Prevention. Ambulatory Surgery in the United States. 2006. Available at http://www.cdc.gov/nchs/data/nhsr/nhsr011.pdf.
2. American Society of Anesthesiologists. Position on monitored anesthesia care. 2008. Available at www.asahq.org.
3. American Society of Anesthesiologists. Distinguishing monitored anesthesia care ("MAC") from moderate sedation/analgesia (Conscious sedation). 2013. Available at www.asahq.org.
4. Benet LZ. Pharmacokinetics: Basic principles and its use as a tool in drug metabolism. In: Mitchell JR, Horning MG, eds. *Drug Metabolism and Drug Toxicity*. New York: Raven Press, 1984:199.

5. Miner JR, Huber D, Nichols S, et al. The effect of the assignment of a pre-sedation target level on procedural sedation using propofol. *J Emerg Med*. 2007;32:249–255.

6. Ausems ME, Vuyk J, Hug CC, et al. Comparison of a computer-assisted infusion versus intermittent bolus administration of alfentanil as a supplement to nitrous oxide for lower abdominal surgery. *Anesthesiology*. 1988;68:851–861.

7. Bailey JM. Context-sensitive half-times: What are they and how valuable are they in anaesthesiology? *Clin Pharmacokinet*. 2002;41:793–799.

8. Jalota L, Kalira V, George E, et al. Prevention of pain on injection of propofol: Systematic review and meta-analysis. *BMJ*. 2011;342:d1110.

9. Mazanikov M, Udd M, Kylanpaa L, et al. Patient-controlled sedation for ERCP: A randomized, double-blind comparison of alfentanil and remifentanil. *Endoscopy*. 2012; 44(5):487–492.

10. American Society of Anesthesiologists. Standards for basic anesthetic monitoring. 2011. Available at www.asahq.org.

11. American Society of Anesthesiologists. Continuum of depth of sedation, definition of general anesthesia and levels of sedation/analgesia. 2009. www.asahq.org.

12. American Society of Anesthesiologists Committee. Practice guidelines for preoperative fasting and the use of pharmacologic agents to reduce the risk of pulmonary aspiration: Application to healthy patients undergoing elective procedures: an updated report by the American Society of Anesthesiologists Committee on Standards and Practice Parameters. *Anesthesiology*. 2011;114:495–511.

13. De Oliveira GS Jr, Ahmad S, Fitzgerald PC, et al. Dose ranging study on the effect of preoperative dexamethasone on postoperative quality of recovery and opioid consumption after ambulatory gynaecological surgery. *Br J Anaesth*. 2011;107(3):362–371.

14. Murphy GS, Szokol JW, Avram MJ, et al. The effect of single low-dose dexamethasone on blood glucose concentrations in the perioperative period: A randomized, placebo-controlled investigation in gynecologic surgical patients. *Anesth Analg*. 2014; 118(6):1204–1212.

15. Apfelbaum JL, Walawander CA, Grasela TH, et al. Eliminating intensive postoperative care in same-day surgery patients using short-acting anesthetics. *Anesthesiology*. 2002;97:66–74.

16. Vasanawala M, Macario A, Canales M. Some common problems in the postanesthetic care unit. *Contemp Surg*. 2000;56:691–700.

17. Chung F, Chan V, Ong D. A post anesthetic discharge scoring system for home readiness after ambulatory surgery. *J Clin Anesth*. 1995;7:500–506.

18. Ahmad S. Office based—is my anesthetic care any different? Assessment and management. *Anesthesiol Clin*. 2010;28:369–384.

Questions

1. Monitored anesthesia care (MAC) is defined as:
   A. A level of sedation for a patient undergoing a procedure
   B. A specific anesthesia service for a diagnostic or therapeutic procedure
   C. A type of anesthesia requiring fewer monitors than general anesthesia
   D. Twilight anesthesia

2. Which one of the following is needed for preoperative assessment for a patient scheduled for MAC?
   A. NPO time
   B. Complete history
   C. Airway assessment
   D. All of the above are required

3. Which one of the following monitors is NOT required for provision of MAC?
   A. Pulse oximetry
   B. End-tidal carbon dioxide
   C. Electrocardiography
   D. All of the above monitors are required

4. Context-sensitive half-time refers to:
   A. When to discontinue an infusion of medication
   B. The time taken for a drug to lose half of its pharmacologic or physiologic activity
   C. The amount of time it takes for a patient to awaken from a sedative infusion
   D. The time it takes for the plasma concentration to decline by 50% after discontinuing an infusion

5. All of the following medications provide amnesia EXCEPT:
   A. Propofol
   B. Midazolam
   C. Dexmedetomidine
   D. Ketamine

6. Which of the following medications is NOT associated with respiratory depression when given in sedative/analgesic doses?
   A. Fentanyl
   B. Propofol
   C. Ketamine
   D. All of the above cause respiratory depression

7. Which of the following properties is NOT associated with opioids?
   A. Amnesia
   B. Analgesia
   C. Respiratory depression
   D. Nausea

8. According to the ASA fasting guidelines for elective surgery, the fasting time for breast milk is:
   A. 2 hours
   B. 4 hours
   C. 6 hours
   D. 8 hours

9. Which of the following would prevent discharge after ambulatory surgery?
   A. Pain controlled with oral medication
   B. Uncontrolled nausea
   C. Minimal bleeding at surgical site
   D. Inability to urinate after general anesthesia

10. Which of the following is a goal of an ambulatory anesthetic?
    A. Minimize use of medications with poor side effect profile
    B. Facilitate rapid emergence and awakening
    C. Use of alternative analgesics to decrease opioid requirement
    D. All of the above are goals of an ambulatory anesthetic

26 Spine and Orthopedic Anesthesia

Yulia Ivashkov
Armagan Dagal

I. Preoperative Assessment

Orthopedic spine and extremity surgeries are generally classified as intermediate-risk surgery, although major spine surgery or more limited procedures in patients with pre-existing medical conditions (e.g., hip arthroplasty in the elderly) can significantly increase perioperative risk. The purpose of the preoperative assessment includes the identification and optimization of modifiable risk factors, explanation of the risks, and formulating the best possible anesthetic plan for the patient. In addition to the standard preoperative assessment (see Chapter 16), focused orthopedic evaluation should include:

- Airway and cervical spine assessment (e.g., rheumatoid arthritis, osteoarthritis, and ankylosing spondylitis could result in limited neck motion, atlantoaxial instability, or limited mouth opening due to the involvement of the temporomandibular joint).
- Assessment of respiratory system (e.g., scoliosis-induced restrictive chest defects, impaired diaphragm function due to spinal cord injury).
- Assessment of cardiovascular system. Fitness level is the deciding criteria for the need for further assessment. Spine and orthopedic surgery patients may have limited exercise tolerance due to other reasons (pain) and therefore complicate this assessment.
- Assessment of neurologic status, including existing neurologic deficiencies and active range of motion and strength of extremities.
- Assessment of pain and psychological burden in order to establish realistic postoperative expectations for pain and function.
- Review of past medical, surgical, and anesthetic history, allergies, and current medications with special attention to chronic opioid use and disease modifying drugs such as steroids, methotrexate, and nonsteroidal anti-inflammatory drugs.
- Hematologic profile and anticoagulant or antiplatelet drug use. Management of anemia and modification or discontinuation of the drugs affecting coagulation will likely be required.

- Assessment and improvement of nutritional status (e.g., serum albumin concentration).
- Planning for the postoperative care transition, intensity of care, and eventual discharge destination.

II.   Surgery to Spine

A.   Spinal Cord Injuries

The incidence of *traumatic spinal cord injury* (TSCI) and its average patient age are increasing, with falls now being the most common overall cause of such injuries. Injury most commonly affects the cervical column (57.4%), followed by thoracic (21.5%) and lumbosacral (13.8%) levels. The initial trauma can result in irreversible neuronal damage (primary injury) that is "complete" (no spinal cord function distal to the injury) or "incomplete" (partial function distal to the injury) and is only modifiable by prevention. *Secondary injury* starts within minutes and is exacerbated by inflammation and edema, leading to further ischemia and neurologic deterioration. Focused medical care aims to limit its extent with careful coordinated management strategies (1). The American Spinal Injury Association score is used to classify the neurologic injury severity (Table 26-1). Incomplete neurologic injuries are eight times more common than complete injuries and may have a variety of presentations (Table 26-2).

Hemodynamic Management

Hypotension is common after TSCI and may be associated with intravascular volume depletion, tension pneumothorax, pericardial tamponade, and neurogenic shock. *Neurogenic shock* is characterized by hypotension with or without bradycardia due to loss of sympathetic tone when the injury occurs at the level of T6 and above. Maintaining mean arterial blood pressure at 85 to 90 mm Hg with the help of intravenous volume expansion, vasopressors, and inotropes is required for the optimization of spinal cord perfusion. Chronotropic agents or cardiac pacing may be required for the treatment of associated bradycardia.

Decompressive Surgery

Decompression of the injured spinal cord and stabilization of the spinal column is generally required after TSCI. It follows the initial resuscitation and surgical management of other immediate life-threatening conditions such

Table 26-1	American Spinal Injury Association (ASIA) Spinal Cord Injury Classification	
Grade	Type of Injury	Description
A	Complete	No motor or no sensory function in S4-5
B	Incomplete	No motor or sensory function preserved below the level of injury including S4-5
C	Incomplete	Motor and sensory function is preserved below the level of injury (motor strength <3/5 in half of the major muscles)
D	Incomplete	Motor and sensory function is preserved below the level of injury (motor strength ≥3/5 in half of the major muscles)
E	Normal	Motor and sensory functions are intact

Table 26-2	Incomplete Spinal Cord Injury Syndromes
Type	**Description**
Central cord syndrome	Common in elderly with hyperextension injury Motor dysfunction in upper extremities greater than lower extremities Sensory dysfunction below the injury Bladder dysfunction
Anterior cord syndrome	Anterior spinal artery or anterior cord injury Motor function, pain, and temperature sensation impairment Two-point discrimination and proprioception remains intact
Brown-Sequard syndrome	Typically due to penetrating trauma Section of lateral half of the spinal cord Ipsilateral loss of motor and proprioception Contralateral loss of pain and temperature
Posterior cord syndrome	Loss of touch, proprioception, and vibration with intact motor function
Cauda equina syndrome	Injury below the conus medullaris—below L2 Perineal numbness, urinary retention, fecal incontinence Lower extremity weakness

as traumatic brain injury or intra-abdominal hemorrhage. When performed within 24 hours of injury, it is shown to improve neurologic recovery sixfold.

B. Scoliosis

Scoliosis is defined as an abnormal lateral curvature of the spinal column in the coronal plane. It is frequently accompanied by a rotation deformity (Table 26-3). Its severity is assessed by the measurement of Cobb's angle (Fig. 26-1). Despite the application of a brace, progression of the curve to a Cobb's angle >45 degrees generally requires surgery to stop further deterioration. When

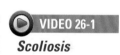

VIDEO 26-1

Scoliosis

Table 26-3	Etiology of Scoliosis	
Idiopathic (80%)	Infantile: 0–3 years old Juvenile: 4–10 years old Adolescent: 11–18 years old	
Congenital	VATER syndrome	
Neuromuscular	Muscular dystrophies Poliomyelitis Cerebral palsy Spina bifida Friedreich ataxia Neurofibromatosis	
Neural	Syringomyelia Chiari malformation	
Syndromic	Marfan syndrome Neurofibromatosis	

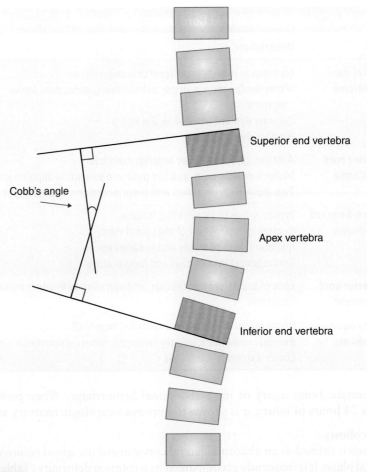

Superior end vertebra

Cobb's angle

Apex vertebra

Inferior end vertebra

Figure 26-1 Cobb's angle is the angle between the two lines drawn **(1)** parallel to the superior border of the superior end vertebra and the **(2)** inferior border of the inferior end vertebra.

untreated, progressive scoliosis may lead to severe back pain, restrictive ventilatory defects, hypoxia, hypercarbia, and pulmonary hypertension.

C. Degenerative Vertebral Column Disease

Adult degenerative spine disease is a major cause of chronic pain and disability. *Spondylolysis* refers to a radiculopathy or myelopathy resulting from osteophyte formation and intervertebral disc disease. It is found in about 6% of adults, is twice as common in males, and usually occurs bilaterally near L5. Its etiology is uncertain (>50% due to repetitive spine trauma), and it is generally managed nonoperatively. *Spondylolisthesis* refers to a loss of vertebral alignment as a result of forward displacement of one vertebra over another and most commonly affects the lumbosacral region. Management is generally conservative (physical therapy, multimodal analgesia, and epidural steroid injections), although progressive myelopathy, neuropathy, or loss of bowel or bladder control are all indications for surgical decompression with or without fusion.

D. Anesthesia for Spine Surgery

Spine surgery is required for the correction of vertebral column deformities and for decompression of nerves and spinal cord due to impingement from diseases of the disc, bone, tumors, and trauma.

Airway

Cervical spine instability requires measures to minimize neck movement during tracheal intubation. All airway instruments and techniques can potentially cause movement in the cervical spine, but these are typically negligible. Thus, when carefully performed, no single technique has been shown superior in terms of neurologic outcomes. TSCI patients who require tracheal intubation in urgent or emergent circumstances and in the absence of other difficult airway issues can generally be safely managed with rapid sequence induction with bimanual cricoid pressure (see Chapters 20 and 32) and manual inline cervical spine stabilization (so that the front of the cervical collar can be temporarily removed to facilitate laryngoscopy). Video laryngoscopy may provide less neck movement and can be used for tracheal intubations in both awake and unconscious patients, particularly those with features predicting difficult laryngoscopy (e.g., large neck circumference, limited mouth opening). Fiberoptic intubation is theoretically associated with minimal cervical spine movement. "Awake" fiberoptic intubation is typically reserved for those with a predicted difficult intubation where maintenance of spontaneous breathing would be advantageous.

> **? Did You Know**
>
> In patients with cervical spine instability, no single airway management technique has been shown superior in preventing rare, tracheal intubation-related spinal cord injury.

Positioning

Most spine surgery patients require prone positioning, although certain cervical or thoracic anterior cord lesions may require supine or lateral positioning, respectively. The sitting position is preferred for some high posterior cervical surgeries. All such positioning requires careful attention to details of patient anatomy, vascular access lines, and monitoring equipment. This is facilitated by adequate numbers of personnel and proper equipment training for safety (Figs. 26-2 and 26-3).

The endotracheal tube and all vascular access lines should be secured adequately before turning from the supine to another position. A soft bite block will prevent tongue or endotracheal tube biting. Special spine tables allow the prone abdomen to hang free and reduce intraoperative bleeding by minimizing compression of abdominal contents (and attendant increases in vena cava and epidural venous pressure) as well as facilitating positive pressure ventilation. Slight reverse Trendelenburg tilt also limits the venous back pressure and bleeding. Foam or gel-based face pillows or Mayfield pins are used to provide pressure-free positioning of the face, with the neck in a neutral position to prevent neurologic injury.

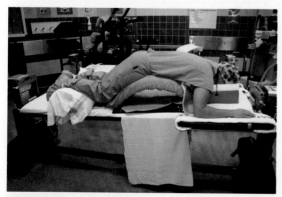
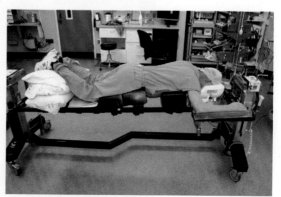

Figure 26-2 Prone positioning on Wilson frame (**left**) and Jackson table (**right**) with foam pillow and Prone View head rest, respectively.

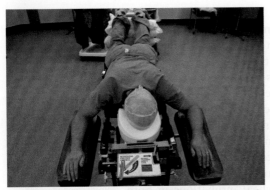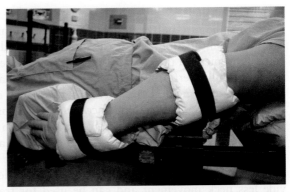

Figure 26-3 Correct placement of the arms in prone position. Arms can be positioned either in swimmer position (**left**) or tucked at the sides (**right**), with the axillae and ulnar grooves free from direct pressure and the wrists and elbows padded.

Monitoring and Access

In addition to standard American Society of Anesthesiologists monitors, an arterial catheter provides continuous blood pressure monitoring and facilitates blood sampling in selected cases of anticipated hemodynamic instability or large blood loss. At least two peripheral intravenous lines are ideal due to the restricted intraoperative extremity access that occurs with cervical spine procedures with arms tucked at the sides. Central venous catheterization may be helpful for resuscitation and aspiration of intracardiac air if an air embolism occurs.

Anesthetic Technique

General anesthesia is required for most spine procedures. Because volatile anesthetics have variable effects on evoked potential monitoring of spinal cord function, total intravenous anesthesia is usually preferred in such cases, either alone or in combination with a low dose (<1% minimum alveolar concentration) volatile agent (Table 26-4).

Table 26-4	Commonly Used Anesthetic Agents in Spine Surgery		
		Primary Anesthetic Dosing	**Adjunct Dosing**
Inhalational Agents	Desflurane	4.5–6% expired concentration	2–3% expired concentration
	Sevoflurane	1.5–2% expired concentration	0.5–1% expired concentration
Intravenous Agents	Propofol	100–150 µg/kg/min	50–75 µg/kg/min
	Ketamine	2–3 mg/kg/hr (may be higher in children)	0.5–2 mg/kg/hr for more potent adjunct Reduce to 8 mg/hr for postop analgesia start 45 min before the end of surgery
	Dexmedetomidine	NA	0.2–0.4 µg/kg/hr (low dose)
	Remifentanil	NA	0.1–0.4 µg/kg/min

NA, not applicable.

Table 26-5	Intraoperative Neurophysiologic Monitoring Modalities	
Monitoring Modality	**Monitored Region of the Cord**	**Significance**
SSEP	Only measures dorsal ascending column	Amplitude reduction >50% or increased latency >10%
tcMEP	Motor descending tracts	Amplitude reduction >50%
EMG	Nerve roots and peripheral nerves	Impingement on a nerve root by an instrument will cause immediate motor activity

SSEP, somatosensory evoked potentials; tcMEP, transcranial motor evoked potentials; EMG, electromyelography.

E. Spinal Cord Monitoring

Intraoperative neurophysiologic monitoring of motor or sensory-evoked potentials in the central nervous system is used during spinal surgery to detect unintended spinal cord injury. It is also used to guide surgical and medical interventions to avoid permanent neurologic injury. Multimodal neurophysiologic monitoring (Table 26-5) is sensitive and specific to detect intraoperative neurologic injury, but evidence that it reduces the incidence of new or worsening neurologic deficits is weak (2).

Management of Acute Evoked Potential Signal Changes

If an acute change in neurophysiologic monitoring is detected, the following steps should be taken to identify its cause and reverse the abnormality:

- Rule out surgical and equipment-related factors; communicate with the surgeon and neuromonitoring team.
- Reposition the patient (maintain natural alignment of spinal column).
- Correct hypotension, metabolic abnormalities, severe anemia, and hypo- or hyperthermia.
- Raise mean arterial blood pressure >85 mm Hg to increase spinal cord perfusion.
- Turn off inhalation agent and switch to total intravenous anesthesia.
- Consider steroid infusion.

F. Blood Loss Prevention Strategies

Blood loss can be significant during spine surgery, with up to 80% of patients requiring an intraoperative transfusion. Perioperative blood loss and blood transfusion have potential negative consequences. Thus, various techniques have been proposed to minimize blood loss and blood product transfusion in this setting (3).

Preoperative Hemoglobin Optimization

Preoperative hemoglobin levels of 12 g/dL for females and 13 g/dL for males serve as thresholds for anemia that generally require further attention in the preoperative period. Laboratory evaluation, diagnosis, and treatment of existing anemia should occur before elective orthopedic procedures through correction of nutritional deficiencies, use of recombinant human erythropoietin, and oral or intravenous iron supplementation.

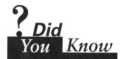

? Did You Know

Prior to the advent of modern neurophysiologic monitoring of spinal cord function with motor- or sensory-evoked potentials, intraoperative assessment of spinal cord function was performed by the "wake-up test," transiently reducing anesthetic depth during the surgical procedure to observe patient extremity movement in response to verbal commands.

Antifibrinolytics

Tranexamic acid is the most common lysin analogue used as an antifibrinolytic to decrease perioperative blood loss and transfusion requirements through the inhibition of clot degradation. Its use is contraindicated in cases of known allergy, history of thromboembolic disease, and pre-existing seizure disorders. Potential adverse effects include thromboembolic events, seizures, and vision changes. The recommended dosing regimen is a 1-g bolus over 10 minutes following by an infusion of 1 g over 8 hours.

Cell Saver

Evidence supports the use of intraoperative washed erythrocyte salvage in spine surgery, as autologous retransfusion significantly lowers donor blood transfusion rates. Its use is controversial, however, during cancer surgery, bacterial infections, wound irrigation with antibiotics, and concurrent use of topical hemostatic agents.

G. Visual Loss After Spine Surgery

Perioperative visual loss (POVL) is a potentially devastating complication that can occur following spine surgery. Its incidence ranges from 0.03% to 0.2%, and it has several different types, presentations, and etiologies (Table 26-6).

The following management strategies have been suggested for prevention of POVL in spine surgery patients with the risk factors noted in Table 26-6 (4):

- POVL should be discussed as part of the preoperative informed consent.
- Continuous blood pressure monitoring (arterial line) is required.
- The neck should be placed in a neutral position, and the head should be level with or higher than the heart to minimize venous congestion.
- Use of large volume crystalloids should be avoided.
- For prolonged operations, consideration should be given for staging the surgery.

H. Venous Air Embolism

Venous air embolism (VAE) results from entrainment of ambient air into the venous circulation through intraosseous vessels or open epidural veins at the

Table 26-6	Perioperative Visual Loss			
	CRAO	**AION**	**PION**	**CB**
Onset	Immediate	First 48 hr	Immediate	Immediate
Site	Unilateral	Frequently bilateral	Mostly bilateral	Bilateral
Potential causes	Direct pressure Emboli Hypotension	History of peripheral vascular disease Hypotension Male more often than females Long surgery Massive blood loss and large volume shifts Large volume crystalloid use	Venous congestion Anemia	Emboli Hypotension Anemia

CRAO, central retinal artery occlusion; AION, anterior ischemic optic neuropathy; PION, posterior ischemic optic neuropathy; CB, cortical blindness.

Table 26-7	Intraoperative Venous Air Embolus Presentation and Management
Presentation	Sudden reduction ETCO$_2$ Hypercarbia (increased PaCO$_2$) Hypoxemia Hypotension Tachyarrhythmias Elevated CVP or distended neck veins Cardiac murmur, respiratory wheeze Cardiac arrest (>5 mL/kg air accumulation)
Management	Stop operating Stop inhalational anesthetics including N$_2$O FiO$_2$ 100% Prevent further emboli Flood the field with fluid Advance the central line intracardiac and attempt to aspirate if in situ Level the table Turn the patient to left lateral decubitus position CPR—fluid boluses, hemodynamic agents
Monitoring	Along with standard ASA monitoring requirements consider precordial or transesophageal Doppler

ETCO$_2$, end-tidal carbon dioxide; PaCO$_2$, arterial carbon dioxide partial pressure; CVP, central venous pressure; N$_2$O, nitrous oxide; FiO$_2$, fraction of inspired oxygen; CPR, cardiopulmonary resuscitation; ASA, American Society of Anesthesiologists.

surgical site. When air accumulation in the right heart reaches a critical level to impact right ventricular output, cardiovascular collapse may occur. The risk of VAE is increased with hypovolemia, hypotension, and spontaneous ventilation and is decreased with positioning to allow epidural veins to remain below the heart level. The presentation and management of VAE are summarized in Table 26-7.

I. Postoperative Care
One in five spine surgery patients will develop immediate postoperative complications. Independent risk factors include male sex, advanced age, surgical approach (combined anterior and posterior approach being associated with the highest complication rates), and pre-existing comorbidities. Hospital mortality rates are 0.2% to 0.5% and are associated most often with concomitant congestive heart failure, liver disease, coagulopathy, neurologic disorders, renal disease, electrolyte imbalances, and pulmonary circulatory diseases.

Decision to Extubate
Anterior cervical fusion surgeries carry the particular risk of hematoma and edema formation up to 36 hours after surgery and tracheal extubation. This may lead to postoperative airway compromise and the need for emergent reintubation. There are no uniformly accepted criteria to guide extubation decisions. Potential risk factors for postoperative reintubation include advanced age, the American Society of Anesthesiologists' class, extent of the procedure and its duration, administered fluid volume, blood loss >300 mL, combined anterior and posterior surgery, and previous spine surgery.

Pain Management

Postoperative pain is a major concern following spine surgery and is frequently complicated by preoperative chronic pain, long-term opioid use, and related psychosocial issues. *Multimodal analgesic management* is recommended in such patients. Combining analgesics with different mechanisms of action such as acetaminophen, nonsteroidal anti-inflammatory drugs, gabapentin, dexamethasone, ketamine, and lidocaine facilitates early mobilization, reduces opioid consumption, and improves patient satisfaction (5).

J. Neuroaxial Anesthesia for Spine Surgery

Neuroaxial (spinal subarachnoid or epidural) anesthesia may be used for lumbar or lower thoracic microdiscectomy or laminectomy surgery that is limited to one or two levels. It has the potential to reduce intraoperative blood loss through the combined effects of sympathetic blockade (leading to vasodilation and relative hypotension) and maintenance of spontaneous ventilation (which lowers intrathoracic ventilation pressures and reduces congestion of the epidural veins). Neuroaxial anesthesia also provides postoperative analgesia and can reduce opioid requirements, nausea and vomiting, urinary retention, and headaches. Intraoperative and postoperative epidural analgesia for major spine surgery has been shown to provide better pain control, less bleeding, and lower surgical stress response compared with general anesthesia and systemic opioid analgesia.

III. Anesthesia for Extremity Surgery

Orthopedic extremity surgery is extremely common. It is performed for both elective and emergent indications and takes place in both inpatient and ambulatory outpatient settings. Furthermore, such surgery spans the age range from newborn (e.g., congenital hip dysplasia) to the elderly (e.g., traumatic hip fracture), as well as the spectrum of concurrent medical morbidities from the healthy professional athlete to a debilitated nursing facility resident. In addition, the following statements generally apply to anesthesia for extremity orthopedic surgery:

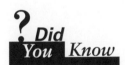

Did You Know

Regional anesthesia, using both single-shot and indwelling catheter techniques, is increasingly common for both inpatient and outpatient orthopedic extremity surgery. It is used not only for intraoperative anesthesia but also for the many benefits of prolonged postoperative analgesia.

- Many orthopedic procedures can potentially use regional anesthesia techniques for intraoperative anesthesia, postoperative pain control, and joint rehabilitation.
- Prevention of positioning-related complications, such as nerve and soft tissue injuries, requires procedural knowledge and meticulous vigilance.
- Significant blood loss can occur and requires familiarity with blood loss–reducing techniques, such as tourniquet use, cell savers, and antifibrinolytics, transfusion triggers, and transfusion-related complications.
- Prolonged immobilization following surgery, particularly involving the knee, hip, or pelvis, is associated with increased risk of deep venous thrombosis and thromboembolism. Conversely, thromboembolism prophylaxis may interfere with regional anesthesia techniques.

A. Choice of Anesthetic Technique

Many orthopedic surgical procedures are well suited for regional anesthesia, the general details of which are described in Chapter 21. Potential clinical benefits of regional anesthesia particular to orthopedic surgery include prolonged analgesia that facilitates joint rehabilitation and increases patient satisfaction. It can also decrease opioid analgesic use, postoperative nausea and vomiting,

Table 26-8 General Considerations for Specific Surgical Procedures

Type of Surgery	Positioning	Anesthetic	Tourniquet	Blood Loss
Total shoulder arthroplasty	Lateral decubitus or beach chair	GA/interscalene block	–	Moderate
Arthroscopic shoulder surgery	Beach chair	GA/interscalene block	–	Minimal
Total elbow arthroplasty	Supine or lateral	GA/supraclavicular, infraclavicular, or axillary nerve block	+	Limited
Elbow arthroscopy	Prone with sandbags under antecubital fossa	GA/supraclavicular, infraclavicular, or axillary nerve block	+/–	Minimal
Total hip arthroplasty, open	Fracture table, lateral	GA/neuraxial/psoas block	–	Moderate
Nondisplaced hip fractures	Fracture table, supine	GA/neuraxial	–	Limited
Total knee arthroplasty	Supine, possible hip bump	GA/neuraxial/sciatic and femoral nerve blocks	+	Moderate
Knee arthroscopy	Supine with operative thigh placed against an arthroscopy post	GA/neuraxial/sciatic and femoral nerve blocks	+/–	Minimal

GA, general anesthesia.

cognitive impairment, immunosuppression, and duration of recovery room stay. Thromboembolism reduction may occur with regional anesthesia and result from diminished sympathetic tone that enhances blood flow and prevents venous stasis. Risks of regional anesthesia include local anesthetic toxicity, hematoma formation, bleeding, nerve damage, and infection. With the introduction of ultrasound-guided techniques, both single-shot and indwelling catheter techniques (that enable prolonged analgesia and facilitate functional therapy) have become more safe, efficient, and desirable anesthetic choices.

Alternatively, general anesthesia can be used for virtually any orthopedic extremity procedure and may be required for prolonged procedures, those involving unique positioning, and those performed on torso anatomy. In some cases, combined general and regional anesthesia may be indicated to achieve both ideal operative conditions and postoperative analgesia. The final choice of anesthetic technique should be tailored to the individual patient's needs based on specific medical conditions, comorbidities, age, type of surgery, and both the surgeon's and patient's preferences (Table 26-8).

IV. Surgery to the Upper Extremities

Regional anesthesia is an excellent choice for anesthesia and postoperative analgesia for upper extremity surgery from the shoulder to the fingers (6). Ultrasound guidance may be particularly advantageous for peripheral upper extremity blocks targeting nerves in close proximity to large vascular structures and the lung (e.g., supraclavicular, infraclavicular, and interscalene blocks). However, some surgical factors (bilateral procedures or prolonged surgery) and patient factors (severe obstructive sleep apnea, pre-existing neurologic deficits, impaired cognition, or failed regional block) may require general anesthesia.

A. Surgery to the Shoulder and Upper Arm

Common shoulder and upper arm procedures include arthroplasty, arthroscopy, subacromial decompression, rotator cuff repair, repair of fracture, and frozen shoulder manipulation. Lateral decubitus and beach chair positions are commonly used with either pharmacologic neuromuscular paralysis or a motor block that facilitates arm traction. Significant blood loss may occur because tourniquet use is not feasible, so careful hemodynamic monitoring is required and serial hemoglobin measurement may be necessary (Table 26-9; Figs. 26-4 and 26-5). Such surgery can be performed under general anesthesia or regional anesthesia (interscalene block).

B. Surgery to the Elbow

Surgeries involving the elbow can be done with either open (e.g., total elbow replacement, fracture repair) or endoscopic (elbow arthroscopy) techniques. Minimally invasive surgery and advances in sedation practices have resulted in an increased ability to perform most elbow surgeries on an ambulatory basis with an emphasis on fast recovery and excellent analgesia. Such surgeries can be performed under general anesthesia or regional anesthesia (supraclavicular or interscalene block).

Table 26-9 Comparison of Different Specialized Surgical Positioning

Surgical Positioning	Body Position	Operative Extremity Position	Positioning-specific Pressure Points	Advantages and Risks
Lateral decubitus (UE, LE)	Lateral, torso stabilized with bean bag or braces	Vertical or on an arm support	Axillary roll to prevent axillary neurovascular compression	Good surgical view Risk of traction arm injury and challenging in obese patients
Beach chair (UE)	Sitting with hips flexed to 45–90 degrees, knees flexed to 30 degrees	On a Mayo stand or mounted arm positioner	Head holder may cause lesser occipital and greater auricular nerve injuries	Easy surgical access but negative pressure gradient between the surgical site and the heart. Risk of hypotension/ bradycardia with possible cerebral ischemia
Fracture table (LE)	Supine or lateral	In a traction device	Perineal post may compress perineal anatomy	Easy C-arm access; risk of traction and pressure-related nerve injuries

UE, upper extremity surgery; LE, lower extremity surgery.

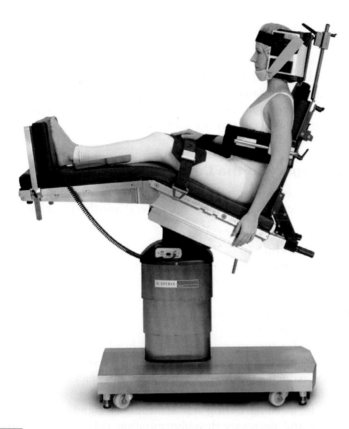

Figure 26-4 Beach chair surgical positioning. (Courtesy of STERIS Corporation, Mentor, OH.)

C. Surgery to the Wrist and Hand

A majority of distal arm and hand procedures are performed on an outpatient basis with regional anesthesia. Axillary, supraclavicular, or infraclavicular blocks can all be used, but axillary block is often favored to avoid potential (albeit low) risk of pneumothorax. For hand surgery, specific ulnar, median, or

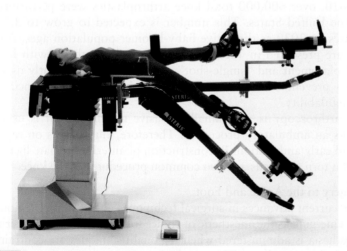

Figure 26-5 Positioning on a fracture table. (Courtesy of STERIS Corporation, Mentor, OH.)

radial nerves can be targeted and blocked, often more distally in the extremity than the classic nerve plexus blocks. Brief surgery below the elbow can also be performed with intravenous regional anesthesia (Bier block) that is simple to perform and has rapid onset and a high success rate. Tourniquet pain with Bier block can be alleviated with use of a double-cuff tourniquet. However, the Bier block provides no postoperative analgesia at the surgical site upon tourniquet release, unlike direct nerve or plexus blocks.

V. Surgery to the Lower Extremities

As with upper extremity orthopedic surgery, lower extremity procedures can be performed under regional anesthesia, general anesthesia, or their combination (7).

A. Surgery to the Hip

In 2010, 258,000 people aged 65 and older were admitted for hip fractures and 332,000 total hip arthroplasties were performed in the United States, making this one of the most common surgical procedures. Three main types of hip fractures based on anatomical location are *intracapsular, intertrochanteric, and subtrochanteric.*

Intracapsular fracture may cause femoral head ischemia if displaced and often requires hemiarthroplasty. Other types of fractures could be treated with closed or open reduction with percutaneous screws placement or intramedullary nail.

Reduction in bleeding during hip arthroplasty significantly shortens the operating time and decreases thromboembolism risk. Therefore, controlled hypotensive epidural anesthesia technique may be an option with a hemodynamic goal to maintain a mean arterial blood pressure of 60 mm Hg, in the absence of contraindications sometimes seen in this age group (e.g., cerebrovascular disease). With spinal subarachnoid anesthesia, a purposeful unilateral block (either hyperbaric or hypobaric spinal) may offer better hemodynamic stability and early recovery. Surgical cement use is common and its implications are described below.

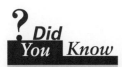

? Did You Know

As the active baby-boomer generation ages, it is anticipated that 3.5 million total knee replacements will be performed annually by 2030.

B. Surgery to the Knee

As of 2010, over 600,000 total knee arthroplasties were performed annually in the United States. This number is expected to grow to 3.5 million procedures by 2030 as the active baby-boomer population ages. Anesthetic options are presented in Table 26-8. Neuraxial anesthesia with indwelling catheter placement and "single-shot" techniques are frequently used. These may also prevent tourniquet-related pain that has been associated with hypercoagulability.

Knee arthroscopy is a minimally invasive technique that is usually performed as an ambulatory procedure. Therefore, emphasis is on rapid emergence and early ambulation. Reconstruction of anterior cruciate ligament and repair of a torn meniscus are also common procedures of the knee.

C. Surgery to the Ankle and Foot

With the current advances in surgical techniques and sedation, regional anesthesia is emerging as the anesthetic of choice for foot and ankle surgeries. General anesthesia is administered when regional techniques are contraindicated or for lengthy procedures. The anesthetic management options for the most common foot and ankle surgeries are presented in Table 26-10.

Table 26-10   Anesthetic Management of Common Foot and Ankle Procedures

Procedure	Tourniquet Placement	Sciatic (popliteal) + Saphenous Block + Sedation	Sciatic (popliteal) Block + GA	NA	Ankle Block	Sciatic + Femoral Blocks
Forefoot: Hallux valgus, hammer toes	Ankle	+	+/–	+/–	+	–
Midfoot: Lisfranc fracture Transmetatarsal amputations	Ankle/calf	+	+	+	+/–	+
Hindfoot	Thigh	+/–	+	+	–	+[a]
Ankle	Thigh	–	+	+	–	+[a]

GA, general anesthesia; NA, neuroaxial anesthesia.
[a]Femoral + high sciatic nerve blocks are generally needed for thigh tourniquet pain relief.

VI. Postoperative Regional and Multimodal Analgesia

With regional anesthesia, the pain pathways are blocked at the level of spinal cord and nerve roots, nerve plexus, or peripheral nerve, providing excellent analgesia and facilitating both rapid recovery and functional physical therapy. Multimodal analgesic agents similar to those described previously for spine surgery should also be included in the postoperative care plan to provide comprehensive postoperative analgesia care, particularly for those patients with chronic pain or substance abuse disorders.

VII. Pediatric Orthopedic Surgery

Anesthetic management of pediatric orthopedic patients encompasses general pediatric anesthesia considerations (see Chapter 33), but in the specific orthopedic context of traumatic injury, cancer, and unique disease states such as congenital disorders. Fractures, scoliosis, joint abnormalities, clubfoot, and syndactyly can require surgical repair in childhood and demand special anesthetic considerations. Positioning can be challenging due to muscle contractures (cerebral palsy) and bone abnormalities (osteogenesis imperfecta). This is also true in other conditions associated with cervical spine instability (Down syndrome), limited neck range of motion (achondroplasia), and cardiac defects (Marfan syndrome). Children with Charcot-Marie-Tooth disease, Duchenne muscular dystrophy, and myotonia dystrophica are prone to succinylcholine-induced hyperkalemia, rhabdomyolysis, and malignant hyperthermia. In addition, pediatric patients present unique challenge to using regional anesthesia, which may need to be performed under general anesthesia or deep sedation. The same peripheral nerve blocks used in adults with ultrasound guidance can generally be used in children (8).

VIII. Other Considerations and Complications

A. Tourniquet Management
The use of a pneumatic tourniquet placed proximal to the surgical site and inflated to suprasystemic pressure minimizes blood loss and facilitates surgery by creating a bloodless field. Potential complications can be local, related to

Table 26-11	Systemic Manifestations with Pneumatic Tourniquet Use			
Tourniquet	Hemodynamic Changes	Hematologic Changes	Temperature Changes	Respiratory Changes
Inflation	Increase in core blood volume, CVP, PVR, BP, HR	Systemic hypercoagulation	Increase of core temperature	Increase in RR due to tourniquet pain
Deflation	Temporary decrease of CVP, HR, possible arrhythmias	Temporary increase in thrombolytic activity	Decrease of core temperature	Increase in end-tidal CO_2 due to reperfusion of ischemic tissue

CVP, central venous pressure; PVR, peripheral vascular resistance; BP, blood pressure; HR, heart rate; RR, respiratory rate; CO_2, carbon dioxide.

tissue pressure and ischemia, or systemic (Table 26-11). Extremity exsanguination prior to tourniquet inflation is performed by elevation of the limb or by compression with an elastic bandage to create a bloodless surgical field. Appropriate cuff sizing (cuff width 20% greater than limb diameter) and thorough padding help to reduce local tissue injury. Maximal duration of tourniquet time is not well defined, although 2 hours is generally considered safe to avoid distal tissue ischemia. If surgery duration requires extended tourniquet time, the tourniquet can be briefly deflated for 5 to 10 minutes before reinflation. The inflation pressure should not exceed 100 mm Hg above the systolic pressure for the upper extremity or above 150 mm Hg for the lower extremity. However, higher pressure may be needed in morbidly obese patients to prevent arterial inflow.

B. Fat Embolus Syndrome

Subclinical fat embolism is common with long bone fractures or major joint prostheses. But when it is significant, it manifests as *fat embolism syndrome* (FES), which is a potentially lethal condition. The prevailing pathogenesis theory of FES involves the increase in intramedullary pressure as a result of traumatic swelling, hematoma formation, or expansion with bone cement. When intramedullary pressure exceeds venous pressure, fat globules are forced into the venous circulation. Another theory suggests that fat globules are formed in the blood as a response to acute changes in fatty acid metabolism. Fat macroemboli can cause mechanical obstruction to pulmonary (and occasionally systemic) blood flow and damage capillary endothelium in the lungs and central nervous system. Major criteria for FES diagnosis include pulmonary manifestations (hypoxia, pulmonary edema, and adult respiratory distress syndrome), neurologic impairment ranging from confusion or lethargy to seizures and coma, and petechia on the conjunctiva and upper trunk. Minor diagnostic criteria include fever, tachycardia, fat globules in sputum and urine, and decreased platelets and hematocrit. Early recognition is essential for therapeutic success. Treatment options include early fracture stabilization and aggressive cardiovascular and pulmonary supportive therapy.

C. Methyl Methacrylate

Polymethyl methacrylate is an acrylic bone cement used for securely binding prosthetic devices to bone during joint arthroplasties. Cement expansion during the hardening process may cause an increase in intramedullary pressure followed by systemic embolization of polymer, bone marrow, or air. Although volatile *methylmethacrylate monomer* can cause direct systemic toxic effects, the deleterious hemodynamic changes most likely result from embolism. Prevention includes surgical precautions such as creating vent holes or avoiding cement overpressurization as well as maintaining normovolemia.

D. Venous Thromboembolism and Antithrombotic Prophylaxis

The incidence of *deep venous thrombosis* can be as high as 60% after major orthopedic procedures if thromboprophylaxis is not used (9). Although often asymptomatic, it can lead to venous thromboembolism and pulmonary embolism. The incidence of venous thromboembolism is especially high after lower extremity fractures and joint replacements. Mechanical (sequential compression devices), pharmacologic, and ancillary (early mobilization) options can be employed for thromboprophylaxis. Pharmacologic methods include low molecular-weight heparin, unfractionated heparin, or other anticoagulants such as fondaparinux or vitamin K inhibitors. Various evidence-based guidelines for *thromboprophylaxis* have been introduced by the American Association of Orthopedic Surgeons, the American College of Chest Physicians, and the National Institute of Clinical Excellence, most of which recommend a combination of pharmacologic and mechanical prophylaxis measures.

Prophylactic anticoagulation (e.g., warfarin for atrial fibrillation) can interfere with regional anesthesia use for orthopedic surgery due to the potenial risk of hematoma formation and permanent neurologic damage. Although the actual incidence of neurologic impairment as a result of this complication is unknown and likely low, the American Society of Regional Anesthesia and Pain Medicine has published evidence-based guidelines for regional anesthesia in patients receiving antithrombotic therapy (10).

? Did You Know

The incidence of deep venous thrombosis after major orthopedic procedures can be as high as 60%, highlighting the importance of perioperative antithrombotic prophylaxis with mechanical, pharmacologic, or other techniques.

References

1. Walters BC, Hadley MN, Hurlbert RJ, et al. Guidelines for the management of acute cervical spine and spinal cord injuries. American Association of Neurological Surgeons, Congress of Neurological Surgeons. *Neurosurgery.* 2013;60(Suppl 1):1–259.
2. Malhotra NR, Shaffrey CI. Intraoperative electrophysiological monitoring in spine surgery. *Spine.* 2010;35(25):2167–2179.
3. Elgafy H1, Bransford RJ, McGuire RA, et al. Blood loss in major spine surgery: Are there effective measures to decrease massive hemorrhage in major spine fusion surgery? *Spine.* 2010;35(9 Suppl):S47–S56.
4. Practice advisory for perioperative visual loss associated with spine surgery: An updated report by the American Society of Anesthesiologists Task Force on Perioperative Visual Loss. *Anesthesiology.* 2012;116:274–285.
5. Rajpal S, Gordon DB, Pellino TA, et al. Comparison of perioperative oral multimodal analgesia versus IV PCA for spine surgery. *J Spinal Disor Tech.* 2010;23(2):139–145.
6. Srikumaran U, Stein BE, Tan EW, et al. Upper-extremity peripheral nerve blocks in the perioperative pain management of orthopaedic patients: AAOS exhibit selection. *J Bone Joint Surg Am.* 2013;95(24):e197(1–13).
7. Memtsoudis SG, Sun X, Chiu YL, et al. Perioperative comparative effectiveness of anesthetic technique in orthopedic patients. *Anesthesiology.* 2013;118(5):1046–1058.
8. DeVera HV, Furukawa KT, Matson MD, et al. Regional techniques as an adjunct to general anesthesia for pediatric extremity and spine surgery. *J Pediatr Orthop.* 2006; 26(6):801–804.
9. Geerts WH, Bergqvist D, Pineo GF, et al. Prevention of venous thromboembolism: American College of Chest Physicians evidence-based clinical practice guidelines (8th edition). *Chest.* 2008;133(6 Suppl):381S–453S.
10. Horlocker TT, Wedel DJ, Rowlingson JC, et al. Executive summary: Regional anesthesia in the patient receiving antithrombotic or thrombolytic therapy: American Society of Regional Anesthesia and Pain Medicine evidence-based guidelines (third edition). *Reg Anesth Pain Med.* 2010;35(1):102–105.

Questions

1. Secondary injury to the spinal cord following traumatic spinal cord injury can result from which of the following?
   A. Local postinjury inflammatory response
   B. Tissue edema in the spinal cord and surrounding structures
   C. Spinal cord ischemia
   D. All of the above

2. Neurogenic shock following traumatic spinal cord injury occurs in which of the following clinical settings?
   A. T4 vertebral burst fracture with no motor or sensory deficit
   B. L1 vertebral burst fracture with complete motor or sensory deficit distal to the injury
   C. T4 vertebral burst fracture with complete motor or sensory deficit distal to the injury
   D. C7 spinous process fracture with no motor or sensory deficit

3. An otherwise healthy 24-year-old female is undergoing posterior spinal instrumentation (rodding) and fusion in the prone position for an acute, American Spinal Injury Association class D traumatic fracture of T8 and T9 sustained in a 10-foot fall from a ladder, with no associated traumatic injuries. She is receiving general anesthesia with sevoflurane 0.7 minimum alveolar concentration (MAC) and continuous remifentanil infusion. Intraoperative somatosensory-evoked potential monitoring reveals new, acute increases in signal latency and decreases in signal amplitude associated with surgeon placement of the stabilizing rods. Appropriate next steps include all of the following EXCEPT:
   A. Communicate the observed changes with the surgeon
   B. Increase the sevoflurane concentration to 1.5 MAC
   C. Ensure that the mean arterial pressure is >85 mm Hg
   D. Consider converting the general anesthetic technique to total intravenous anesthesia

4. An 83-year-old woman with symptomatic spinal stenosis from T6-12 is scheduled for posterior decompression with multilevel instrumentation (rodding) and fusion. Due to previous spine surgery as a young adult, the procedure is anticipated to take 8 hours and involve significant blood loss and large volume shifts associated with crystalloid and blood product administration. Which of the following steps would you take with respect to the potential complication of perioperative visual loss (POVL)?
   A. Perform a careful visual acuity assessment and discuss the potential complication of POVL with the patient during the preanesthetic visit
   B. Discuss preoperatively with the surgeon the potential steps to prevent POVL, including possible staging of the surgical procedure and the use of Mayfield pins to immobilize the head and neck intraoperatively (to prevent pressure on the prone patient's face)
   C. Place an arterial line for careful and continuous intraoperative blood pressure monitoring
   D. All of the above

5. Which of the following statements is true regarding venous air embolism (VAE) occurring intraoperatively during spine surgery in a prone patient receiving general anesthesia with an endotracheal tube?
   A. VAE is accompanied by a sudden decrease in expired carbon dioxide
   B. VAE can be immediately treated by raising the surgical site to a level above the right heart
   C. VAE can be immediately treated by turning the patient to the right lateral decubitus position
   D. The hemodynamic effects of VAE result from air accumulation in the left heart

6. Potential beneficial effects of regional anesthesia or analgesia in patients undergoing orthopedic extremity surgery include all of the following EXCEPT:
   A. Reduced perioperative opioid analgesic consumption
   B. Postoperative analgesia that facilitates immediate joint rehabilitation and physical therapy
   C. Reduced intraoperative surgical bleeding due to increased sympathetic tone
   D. Possible reduced risk of postoperative thromboembolism

7. Regional anesthesia for arthroscopic rotator cuff repair is best accomplished with which of the following nerve plexus blocks?
   A. Infraclavicular block
   B. Interscalene block
   C. Intravenous regional (Bier) block
   D. Axillary block

8. **All of the following statements regarding tourniquet management for extremity surgery are correct EXCEPT:**
   A. For the upper extremity, tourniquet pressure should generally not exceed systolic pressure by more than 100 mm Hg
   B. Tourniquet inflation time should never exceed 2 hours
   C. For the lower extremity, tourniquet pressure should generally not exceed systolic pressure by more than 150 mm Hg
   D. Morbidly obese patients may require a higher tourniquet pressure than non-obese patients

9. A 75-year-old otherwise healthy woman is undergoing hip arthroplasty for a recent femoral neck fracture under spinal subarachnoid anesthesia with light sedation, with nasal prong oxygen at 2 L/min. During placement of the femoral prosthesis, she becomes acutely confused, agitated, and her pulse oximetry reading falls from 99% to 72%. This clinical picture is highly suggestive of fat embolus syndrome.
   A. True
   B. False

10. **An otherwise healthy 65-year-old male is scheduled to undergo surgical repair of a severe hallux valgus deformity (bunion) on his right foot. Appropriate anesthetic options include all of the following EXCEPT:**
    A. Ankle block
    B. General anesthesia
    C. Combined sciatic-popliteal nerve block and saphenous nerve block
    D. Femoral nerve block

27 Anesthesia for Laparoscopic and Robotic Surgeries

Adriana Dana Oprea

Laparoscopic surgical techniques have significant benefits over the traditional open approach, including smaller incisions, decreased postoperative pain, faster recovery time, and reduced chance of blood transfusion and wound infection. Potential disadvantages include higher risk of inadvertent vascular and major organ puncture during placement of the access ports as compared with the traditional open approach. Recently, robot-assisted laparoscopy has been introduced to address some of the disadvantages of laparoscopy, including surgeon fatigue, hand tremor, poor ergonomics, and difficult visualization and manipulation of instruments while retaining all the advantages of laparoscopic techniques (1). Specific disadvantages pertain to the quality and consistency of data connection between the surgeon and the robot and to the high cost of robot-assisted procedures. This chapter reviews laparoscopic and robot-assisted laparoscopic techniques, their physiologic impact on the patient, and the essential perioperative management strategies for patients undergoing these procedures.

I. Surgical Techniques

Laparoscopic surgery has four basic steps: gaining access to the peritoneal cavity, establishing the pneumoperitoneum, the surgical procedure, and the closure. Prior to peritoneal access, the stomach and bladder are decompressed in order to minimize the likelihood of bowel or bladder injury. Then, access can be established using two accepted techniques: an open approach (*Hasson*) or a closed approach (*Veress* needle). The Hasson technique uses a small incision performed anywhere on the abdomen but is most commonly done peri-umbilically, followed by placement of the trocar through that incision and insufflation of the abdomen. The Veress needle technique uses blind passage of the needle through the skin into the peritoneal cavity, followed by insufflation. The Veress needle technique is preferred in patients without intra-abdominal adhesions or umbilical hernias and has a higher risk of organ puncture compared with the Hasson approach. After accessing the peritoneal cavity, it is

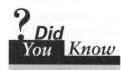

? Did You Know

Did you know that the Hasson technique is preferred to the Veress needle technique in patients with abdominal adhesions?

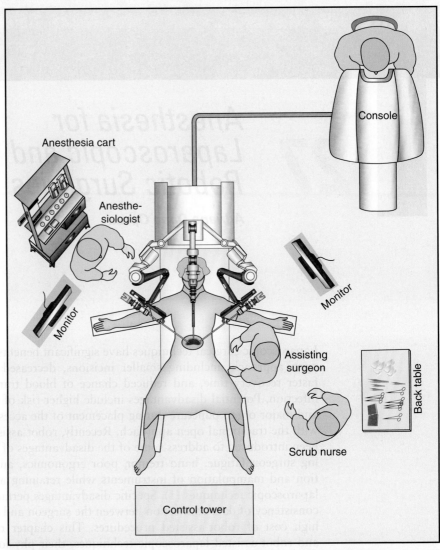

Figure 27-1 Layout of the operating room during robotic surgery. (From Joshi GP, Cunningham A. Anesthesia for laparoscopic and robotic surgeries. In: Barash PG, Cullen BF, Stoelting RK, et al., eds. *Clinical Anesthesia*. 7th ed. Philadelphia: Lippincott Williams & Wilkins; 2013:1260, with permission.)

slowly insufflated with *carbon dioxide (CO₂)* until the intra-abdominal pressure reaches 10 to 15 mm Hg and the abdominal wall is sufficiently distended to allow the surgical procedure. The laparoscopic camera is introduced into the abdomen and, under the visual guidance it provides, additional ports are placed with trocars as needed for the other instruments required for surgery. For robot-assisted procedures, access to the peritoneal cavity is obtained with either technique, followed by laparoscopic exploration of the cavity, placement of the robotic instruments in the peritoneum, positioning of the robot, and then attachment of the robotic arms to the instruments (Fig. 27-1). The surgeon is seated at a console separate from the operating table, and his or her hand movements are computer translated into the movement of the

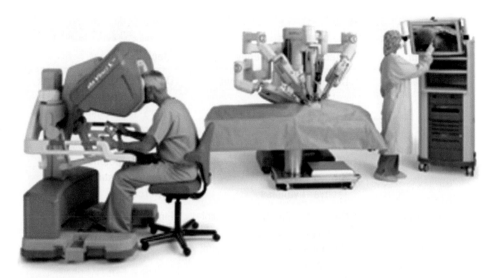

Figure 27-2 A control console where the surgeon is stationed and operates the robotic arms and camera. (© 2012 Intuitive Surgical, Inc., with permission.)

robotic arms and instruments (Fig. 27-2). Following the surgical procedure, the abdominal entry sites are closed.

II. Physiologic Effects

A. Systemic Cardiovascular Effects

Cardiovascular changes during laparoscopy become apparent when the *intra-abdominal pressure* exceeds 10 mm Hg, resulting from the combination of increased intra-abdominal pressure, CO_2 absorption, general anesthesia, and patient positioning. *Cardiac output decreases* due to decreased venous return, which is secondary to the increased intra-abdominal pressure, causing inferior vena cava compression and pooling of blood in the lower extremities. Systemic vascular resistance increases secondary to the catecholamine release stimulated by the absorbed CO_2 and to the release of vasopressin and activation of the renin-angiotensin system caused by the pneumoperitoneum. In addition, during the insufflation phase of laparoscopy, stretching of the peritoneum stimulates a *vagal reflex* and may cause bradycardia or even asystole. These changes occur in the first minutes after establishing the pneumoperitoneum. Subsequently, both cardiac output and systemic vascular resistance normalize within 10 to 15 minutes. When steep Trendelenburg positioning is required, as it is for robot-assisted radical prostatectomies, it increases venous return and cardiac output, thereby opposing the changes due to pneumoperitoneum. In contrast, reverse Trendelenburg and lithotomy positioning further decrease cardiac output by further impairing venous return.

B. Regional Perfusion

Pneumoperitoneum induces a modest *splanchnic hyperemia* due to the vasodilating effects of the absorbed CO_2. In contrast, pneumoperitoneum *decreases renal blood flow*, glomerular filtration rate, and urine output by up to 50%. Cerebral blood flow increases during pneumoperitoneum due to an increase in arterial carbon dioxide partial pressure ($PaCO_2$). This may be a transient

Table 27-1	Physiologic Changes during Laparoscopy	
System	**Effects of Laparoscopy**	**Mechanism**
Cardiac	Decreased cardiac output	Decreased preload (venous return) due to increased intra-abdominal pressure
	Increased systemic vascular resistance and blood pressure	Hypercarbia Hormones (vasopressin, renin-angiotensin system)
	Bradyarrhythmias	Vagal stimulation
	Tachyarrhythmias	Hypercarbia
Respiratory	Decreased thoracic and respiratory compliance	Elevation of the diaphragm due to pneumoperitoneum
	Decreased functional residual capacity	
	Atelectasis	
	Increased peak airway pressures	
	Hypercarbia	Absorption of carbon dioxide Ventilation/perfusion mismatch
Renal	Decreased renal perfusion, urine output, and glomerular filtration rate	Increased intra-abdominal pressure
Regional circulation	Increased intracerebral and intraocular pressure	Hypercarbia
	Modest splanchnic hyperemia	

effect if normocarbia is re-established by increasing minute ventilation appropriately. However, if steep Trendelenburg is employed, it increases intraocular pressure and could further increase intracranial pressure (2). Clearly, patients at risk for *cerebral hypertension* and those with poorly controlled *glaucoma* may not be appropriate candidates for this positioning (Table 27-1).

C. Respiratory Effects
Intra-abdominal insufflation elevates the diaphragm, causing a *decrease* in *thoracic* and *respiratory compliance* and in functional residual capacity. These changes lead to atelectasis unless countered by positive end-expiratory pressure and periodic recruitment maneuvers. General anesthesia and the combined respiratory effects of pneumoperitoneum increase mismatching of ventilation and perfusion, and through that mechanism decreases PaO_2 (3). Postoperative pulmonary function tests demonstrate a reduction in one-second forced expiratory volume (FEV_1) and forced vital capacity (FVC) (Table 27-1).

III. Anesthetic Management

A. Patient Selection
Patients with cardiac disease, especially severe valvular heart, may not tolerate the cardiovascular effects of pneumoperitoneum. Similarly, morbidly obese patients, patients with severe chronic obstructive pulmonary disease, and those with severe cardiac disease may not be able to compensate for the *steep Trendelenburg* position often required for some laparoscopic or robotic-assisted

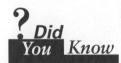

Did You Know

Did you know that the pneumoperitoneum induced for laparoscopy decreases respiratory compliance and functional residual capacity and worsens pulmonary perfusion and ventilation matching?

procedures. For routine laparoscopic cholecystectomy, obesity and even morbid obesity do not seem to increase the rate of significant complications (4).

B. Induction of Anesthesia and Airway Management

Regional or local anesthesia may be adequate for procedures performed
quickly and with low intra-abdominal pressure (<10 to 15 mm Hg) and only
mild degrees of Trendelenburg. However, *general endotracheal anesthesia* is
most often required for laparoscopic procedures because of the discomfort
from the pneumoperitoneum and the required ventilator support. Virtually
any well-managed anesthetic induction technique is acceptable, but propofol may be the preferred agent for its antiemetic properties (5). Like regional
and local anesthesia, use of a laryngeal mask airway instead of endotracheal
intubation is reserved for patients undergoing short procedures requiring low
insufflation pressures and minimal Trendelenburg.

C. Maintenance of Anesthesia

Because neuromuscular relaxation is required to limit the insufflating pressure in the abdomen, the maintenance anesthetic usually includes an inhaled
anesthetic to ensure full unconsciousness. *Nitrous oxide* is usually avoided
given the risk of worsening postoperative nausea and vomiting (PONV) and
its potential for diffusing into the bowel, worsening surgical conditions. Total
intravenous anesthesia can be used if the risk of PONV is significant. But the
remote risk of patient awareness may be higher than when an inhaled agent is
used with monitored exhaled gas analysis. Controlled *normocapnic ventilation* with positive end-expiratory pressure is required for most laparoscopic
and robot-assisted procedures to counter the respiratory impact of the pneumoperitoneum and positioning.

Monitoring other than the American Society of Anesthesiologists standards
for general anesthesia should be dictated by the each patient's comorbidities.
Because of the extremes of positioning and case duration sometimes required,
adequate padding of the ulnar and common peroneal nerves, appropriate positioning of the arms and padding of the shoulders to avoid *brachial plexus
injury*, and *safety belt* securing of the patient to the operating room table must
be confirmed prior to incision. If the Trendelenburg or reverse Trendelenburg
position is required, it should be achieved slowly to allow for management of
hemodynamic changes or migration of the endotracheal tube. Prior to emergence, antiemetic medications should be administered because the incidence of
PONV after laparoscopic procedures is high.

IV. Pain Prevention

Pain after laparoscopy procedures is *far less* than after comparable procedures performed through open laparotomy. However, the insertion sites of the
instruments are painful, and CO_2 insufflation and residual pneumoperitoneum
cause diaphragmatic irritation, leading to referred pain to the shoulder (6).
Local anesthetic infiltration is beneficial at the insertion sites and has very few
potential complications. Narcotic doses can be limited if they are combined
with other analgesics including nonsteroidal anti-inflammatories (NSAIDs).
Prior to administering an NSAID, the surgical team should be consulted to
confirm there is no unreasonable risk of bleeding from the NSAID's antiplatelet effect. Rarely would more invasive pain therapy such as regional block be
required for adequate pain relief except in patients with chronic pain problems
or chronic narcotic use.

V. Intraoperative Complications

A. Cardiopulmonary Complications

Hypotension is quite common during the initial insufflation of the peritoneum due to reduce cardiac output secondary to decreased venous return. Less commonly, a vagal response to stretching of the peritoneum causes significant bradycardia and very *rarely asystole*. Hypertension or tachycardia can result from hypercarbia-induced catecholamine release or, more commonly, inadequate anesthesia. All of these changes in hemodynamics are readily managed with routine measures and should be quite transient. However, profound, persistent hypotension or cardiovascular collapse can occur very rarely and should prompt an urgent search and treatment of other etiologies, including excessive intra-abdominal pressure, *CO_2 embolism*, and *pneumothorax* (Table 27-2). Although pneumoperitoneum and Trendelenburg positioning increase ventilation and perfusion mismatching, significant hypoxia is uncommon during controlled ventilation with supplemental oxygen unless the patient has pre-existing pulmonary disease. Should hypoxia persist despite administration of 100% oxygen, positive end-expiratory pressure, and alveolar recruitment maneuvers, the intra-abdominal pressures should be lowered and other potential etiologies investigated, including endobronchial intubation, pulmonary aspiration, and pneumothorax.

B. Surgical Complications

Carbon Dioxide Extravasation

Subcutaneous emphysema is one of the most common complications of extraperitoneal insufflation of CO_2. This complication is more likely to occur when five or more ports are used for the laparoscopic procedure, during procedures longer than 3.5 hours with intra-abdominal pressures >15 mm Hg, and with improper position of the cannulas. It should be suspected by a rise in end-tidal CO_2 of more than 25% or to more than 50 mm Hg occurring after end-tidal CO_2 has already plateaued. It is confirmed by the presence of crepitus (Table 27-3).

Subcutaneous emphysema can extend into the thorax or mediastinum, as *capnothorax* and *capnomediastinum*, and in the upper torso or neck as

? Did You Know

Did you know that subcutaneous emphysema with CO_2 is common after laparoscopy and can extend all the way to the neck with potential post extubation airway compromise?

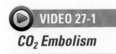

VIDEO 27-1

CO_2 Embolism

Table 27-2	Cardiovascular Complications of Laparoscopy
Complication	**Mechanism**
Hypotension	Decreased venous return
Hypertension	Hypercarbia Neurohumoral factors
Bradyarrhythmias	Vagal reaction to peritoneal stretching
Tachyarrhythmias	Hypercarbia
Cardiovascular collapse	Arrhythmias (tachy/bradyarrhythmias) Blood loss Gas embolism Capno/pneumothorax Capnopericardium Cardiac ischemia Excessive intra-abdominal pressure Hypercapnia Deep anesthesia

Table 27-3   Complications of Pneumoperitoneum

Complication	Mechanism	Diagnosis	Management
CO$_2$ subcutaneous emphysema	Extraperitoneal insufflation in subcutaneous, preperitoneal, or retroperitoneal tissue Extension of extraperitoneal insufflation	Sudden rise in ETCO$_2$ Crepitus If postoperatively, signs of hypercarbia (increased heart rate, blood pressure), somnolence	Deflation of the abdomen
Capnothorax	Tracking of insufflated CO$_2$ around the aortic, caval, and esophageal hiatuses of the diaphragm into the mediastinum with subsequent rupture into the pleural space Tracking of CO$_2$ through diaphragmatic defects Diaphragmatic injury when inserting the laparoscopic needle	High index of suspicion (subcutaneous emphysema of the neck), site of surgical procedure Increased airway pressure Decreased SaO$_2$ Increased ETCO$_2$ Bulging hemidiaphragm If tension capnothorax, hypotension, decreased ETCO$_2$, and cardiovascular collapse Confirmation by chest x-ray	Discontinuation of N$_2$O Hyperventilation Apply PEEP
Capnomediastinum Capnopericardium	Same as for capnothorax	Hemodynamic changes Confirmation by chest x-ray	Deflation of the abdomen Supportive treatment Hyperventilation
Endobronchial intubation	Cephalad migration of the carina	Steep increase in peak airway pressure Decrease in SaO$_2$	Reposition of endotracheal tube
Gas embolism	Placement of the Veress needle into a blood vessel Passage of CO$_2$ into the abdominal wall and peritoneal vessels	Hypoxemia Hypotension Decreased ETCO$_2$ Arrhythmias or right heart strain on ECG	Deflation of the abdomen Supportive treatment/cardiovascular resuscitation Hyperventilation

CO$_2$, carbon dioxide; N$_2$O, nitrous oxide; PEEP, positive end-expiratory pressure; SaO$_2$, oxygen saturation; ETCO$_2$, end-tidal carbon dioxide; ECG, electrocardiogram.

well as toward the groin. Treatment should include deflation of the abdomen and reinflation at lower pressures with confirmation of correct cannula positioning. The presence of subcutaneous emphysema in the neck should raise the question of a possible capnothorax, especially if airway pressures are increased or arterial saturation decreased. Unlike an intraoperative pneumothorax, which presents with increased PaCO$_2$ and decreased end-tidal CO$_2$, a capnothorax presents with both increased (Table 27-3). If blood pressure is well maintained, capnothorax can be treated conservatively by deflation of the abdomen. In the event of a tension capnothorax, as evidenced by tracheal deviation and hypotension, the tension should be vented by a needle thoracostomy and continued mechanical ventilation with positive end-expiratory pressure. Capnopericardium and capnomediastinum are rare complications of laparoscopy, diagnosed by chest x-ray, and treated by deflation of the abdomen and supportive treatment during spontaneously resolution.

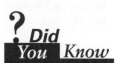

Did You Know

Did you know that Capnopericardium and capnomediastinum are rare complications of laparoscopy, diagnosed by chest X-ray, and treated by deflation of the abdomen and supportive treatment during spontaneous resolution.

Carbon Dioxide Embolization

CO_2 intravascular embolization is a serious but *rare complication* of laparoscopy, usually the consequence of direct insufflation of CO_2 into a vessel or, alternatively, into a solid organ with subsequent intravascular migration. Due to the high blood solubility of CO_2, relatively large amounts of it can be absorbed by the blood and eliminated by the lungs. Thus, a small volume of embolized CO_2 may have no apparent impact except an increase in the end-tidal CO_2. However, a large bolus can impede venous return to the heart, distend the right atrium and ventricle, and produce *cardiovascular collapse*. The acute increase in the right atrial pressure can lead to paradoxical embolism through a foramen ovale and the potential for neurologic injury. A large intravascular CO_2 embolism should be suspected when sudden, severe hypotension is accompanied by a marked decrease in end-tidal CO_2 occurring during insufflation (Table 27-3). Treatment should include immediate cessation of insufflation and deflation of the abdomen, placement of the patient in a head-down, left *lateral decubitus position*, which limits migration of the embolus into the pulmonary artery, hyperventilation in order to speed the elimination of CO_2, and hemodynamic support including cardiac massage if indicated.

Other Surgical Complications

The other most common surgical complications include direct injury to vascular structures and the bowel and bladder occurring during trocar or Veress needle placement. Major *vascular injuries* have a low incidence of 0.02% to 0.03% but can be catastrophic when a trocar is placed into the aorta, vena cava, or iliac vessels causing *massive bleeding*. When a major vessel injury occurs, the trocar should be left in place to tamponade bleeding while the surgical team opens the abdomen to control the damage. Bowel and major organ injuries occur in up to 0.4% of laparoscopy cases and are the result of trocar misplacement. Most of the injuries involve the stomach, duodenum, and small and large bowel. Prior abdominal surgery leading to adhesions is a definite risk factor, and most of the bowel injuries go unrecognized until the postoperative period when the patient develops peritonitis.

C. Hypothermia

Severe hypothermia is a significant risk during laparoscopy because, in addition to the usual mechanisms of heat loss during anesthesia (convection, conduction, radiation, and evaporation), insufflation of cold CO_2 (at 23°C) causes additional heat loss. This loss can be limited by restricting CO_2 flow and leakage and by forced warm air heating of the patient's upper and lower body.

D. Complications Related to Positioning

Nerve and tissue injuries are serious and preventable complication of positioning, especially in patients undergoing robotic-assisted laparoscopy in steep Trendelenburg positioning. Cephalad slippage of the patient can injure nerves and soft tissues by causing pressure points or tissue stretch. If shoulder restraints are used to stabilize the patient, they can apply stretch to the *brachial plexus*. In addition, over the course of hours, steep Trendelenburg can lead to severe head, neck, and facial swelling, resulting in postextubation airway compromise or in very rare cases blindness due to optic nerve ischemia. Chapter 22 provides a detailed discussion of these risks and preventive measures.

VI. Postoperative Considerations

Complete clearance of intra-abdominal CO_2 may require longer than 1 hour, and during that time patients may experience severe shoulder pain referred

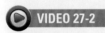

? **Did You Know**

Did you know that in the event that a trocar punctures a major vessel that it should be left in place to help tamponade the bleeding while the abdomen is open and the vessel repaired.

▶ **VIDEO 27-2**

Esophageal Bougie

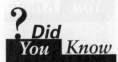

? **Did You Know**

Did you know that cephalad slippage of the patient during steep Trendelenburg can result in movement of the endotracheal tube into the right main stem bronchus?

? **Did You Know**

Did you know that steep Trendelenburg positioning has been associated with blindness due to optic nerve ischemia?

from diaphragmatic irritation. However, most patients tolerate laparoscopy quite well except those with limited pulmonary reserve or patients with prior diaphragmatic paralysis. These patients may require postoperative respiratory support until the intra-abdominal CO_2 is resorbed fully and pain control is optimized. Postoperative hemorrhage is rare but should be suspected when there is hemodynamic instability, a distended abdomen, or an unexpectedly low hematocrit.

VII. Ambulatory Laparoscopic Procedures

Due to the low complication rate and potential for early ambulation, most uncomplicated laparoscopic procedures (cholecystectomy, gynecologic procedures) in patients with no or very well-controlled comorbidities can be performed on an *outpatient basis* (7). Postoperative hospital admission in these patients is rarely needed unless complicated by persistent postoperative nausea and vomiting or inadequate pain control. Safety of outpatient laparoscopic bariatric surgery is controversial because of the high incidence of sleep apnea and postoperative surgical complications. Robot-assisted procedures for radical cancer surgery require postoperative admission hospital because of their duration and extensive fluid shifts.

VIII. Summary

Laparoscopic and robot-assisted procedures have several advantages over the traditional, open approach, including early mobilization, shorter length of hospital stay, and quicker recovery. The hemodynamic and respiratory consequences of the pneumoperitoneum required for these procedures are generally well tolerated except in patients with severe heart or pulmonary disease. General anesthesia is required for the majority of these procedures to ensure adequate ventilation and prevent the pain from peritoneal distension. The majority of complications due to laparoscopy result from insufflation pressures higher than 15 mm Hg or improper placement of trocars. The former complications can be managed most often by decreasing the intra-abdominal pressure, while the latter may require open laparotomy if the trocar has injured a vital organ or major vessel. However, on the whole, laparoscopic techniques have been proven safe and highly effective in reducing surgical morbidity and speeding recovery.

References

1. Liu JJ, Maxwell BG, Panousis P, et al. Perioperative outcomes for laparoscopic and robotic compared with open prostatectomy using the National Surgical Quality Improvement Program (NSQIP) database. *Urology*. 2013;82(3):579–583.
2. Hsu RL, Kaye AD, Urman RD. Anesthetic challenges in robotic-assisted urologic surgery. *Rev Urol*. 2013;15(4):178–184.
3. Grabowski JE, Talamini MA. Physiological effects of pneumoperitoneum. *J Gastrointest Surg*. 2009;13(5):1009–1016.
4. Afaneh C, Abelson J, Rich BS, et al. Obesity does not increase morbidity of laparoscopic cholecystectomy. *J Surg Res*. 2014;19(2):491–497.
5. Vaughan J, Nagendran M, Cooper J, et al. Anaesthetic regimens for day-procedure laparoscopic cholecystectomy. *Cochrane Database Syst Rev*. 2014;1:CD009784.
6. Donatsky AM, Bjerrum F, Gogenur I. Surgical techniques to minimize shoulder pain after laparoscopic cholecystectomy. A systematic review. *Surg Endosc*. 2013;27(7):2275–2282.
7. Vaughan J, Gurusamy KS, Davidson BR. Day-surgery versus overnight stay surgery for laparoscopic cholecystectomy. *Cochrane Database Syst Rev*. 2013;7:CD006798.

Questions

1. What is the recommended initial intra-abdominal insufflation pressure for laparoscopy?
   A. 5–10 mm Hg
   B. 10–15 mm Hg
   C. 15–20 mmHg
   D. 20–25 mmHg
   E. None of the above

2. What are the regional perfusion effects of intra-abdominal CO_2 insufflation?
   A. Splanchnic, renal, and cerebral perfusion increase
   B. Splanchnic, renal, and cerebral perfusion decrease
   C. Splanchnic and cerebral perfusion increase while renal perfusion decreases
   D. Splanchnic and renal perfusion decrease while cerebral perfusion increases
   E. None of the above

3. Sudden hypotension and a marked decrease in end-tidal CO_2 during insufflation of the peritoneum with CO_2 would most likely indicate?

4. Shoulder pain after laparoscopy is likely the result of?
   A. Excessive abduction of the arm during surgery
   B. Brachial plexus injury from shoulder restraints used during steep Trendelenburg
   C. Diaphragmatic irritation
   D. Deltoid injury from arm restraints
   E. None of the above

5. Hypothermia is a significant risk during laparoscopy because of?
   A. Large fluid replacement requirements
   B. Room temperature insufflating gas
   C. Evaporative losses from the peritoneum
   D. Convection losses from the distended abdomen
   E. None of the above

A. A severe vagal reflex
B. A capnothorax
C. A pneumothorax
D. A CO_2 embolism
E. None of the above

28 Anesthetic Considerations for Patients with Obesity, Hepatic Disease, and Other Gastrointestinal Issues

Sundar Krishnan

I. Obesity

Obesity is commonly defined by the patient's body mass index (BMI). The number of obese (BMI >30 kg/m^2) and morbidly obese (BMI >40) patients undergoing surgical procedures is steadily increasing. These patients are at increased risk for various complications, leading to increased morbidity and mortality.

A. Pathophysiology

Respiratory System

Patients with truncal obesity have reduced ventilatory compliance, tidal volume, functional residual capacity (FRC), and vital capacity. As a result, they can become hypoxic much more rapidly than normal patients. Additionally, the impact of positioning and surgery on lung function is exaggerated because of limited baseline function and the effects of a large abdomen on diaphragmatic position and movement, causing FRC to fall below closing capacity. Resultant small airway closure leads to atelectasis and further hypoxemia.

The metabolic activity of fat and supportive tissues increases oxygen consumption and carbon dioxide (CO_2) production in obese patients. This is compensated for with increased minute ventilation and cardiac output. Due to the aforementioned mechanical limitations, patients may be unable to increase tidal volume at times of increased oxygen need and must rely on tachypnea to improve minute ventilation.

Obstructive sleep apnea (OSA), characterized by recurrent episodes of upper airway obstruction during sleep, occurs in up to 70% of morbidly obese patients undergoing bariatric surgery and is a risk factor for adverse perioperative outcomes. Airway obstruction occurs due to growth of adipose tissue in oral and pharyngeal structures. *Obesity hypoventilation syndrome (OHS)* or Pickwickian syndrome is seen in 5% to 10% of patients with OSA, characterized by daytime hypercapnia and hypoventilation and sleep disordered breathing. Patients with OHS are at increased risk for sedative- and opioid-related ventilatory impairment because of upper airway obstruction, depressed

? Did You Know

Obese patients become hypoxic rapidly and can tolerate only brief periods of apnea, such as that associated with airway manipulation.

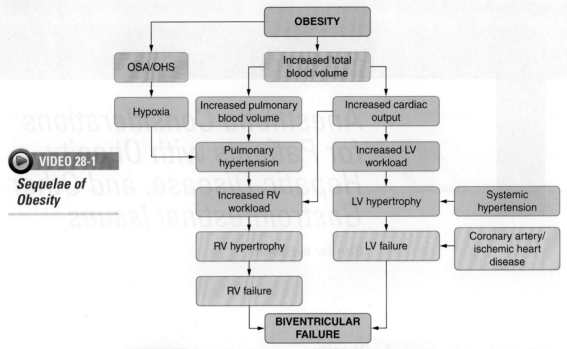

VIDEO 28-1

Sequelae of Obesity

Figure 28-1 Interrelationship of cardiovascular and pulmonary sequelae of obesity. OSA, obstructive sleep apnea; OHS, obesity hypoventilation syndrome; LV, left ventricular; RV, right ventricular. (From Bucklin BA, Fernandez-Bustamante A. Anesthesia and obesity. In: Barash PG, Cullen BF, Stoelting RK, et al. *Clinical Anesthesia*, 7th ed. Philadelphia: Lippincott Williams & Wilkins, 2013:1278.)

central respiratory drive, and impaired lung mechanics. Over the long term, OSA and OHS lead to polycythemia, systemic and pulmonary hypertension, left ventricular hypertrophy, cardiac dysrhythmias, right heart strain, and cor pulmonale (Fig. 28-1).

Cardiovascular System

Obesity is associated with an increase in blood volume, although the weight-based blood volume is reduced (from 70 mL/kg in lean individuals to 50 mL/kg in obese patients). As noted, obese patients are at higher risk for hypertension, left ventricular hypertrophy, diastolic dysfunction, and heart failure. The combination of dyslipidemia, diabetes, and hypertension predisposes obese patients to atherosclerosis and hence coronary and cerebrovascular disease. Obesity also predisposes to a hypercoagulable state because of increased levels of procoagulant factors and decreased fibrinolysis.

Gastrointestinal System

Aspiration risk associated with obesity is discussed later. Obesity-associated liver disease includes fatty infiltration (nonalcoholic fatty liver disease), inflammation (nonalcoholic steatohepatitis), focal necrosis, and cirrhosis. Obese patients are also at risk for cholelithiasis, particularly after intestinal bypass surgery.

Endocrine and Metabolic Systems

Obese patients often exhibit *metabolic syndrome*, which is a combination of risk factors (abdominal obesity, hypertension, dyslipidemia, and insulin resistance or impaired glucose tolerance). This increases their risk for cardiovascular-related morbidity and mortality, type 2 diabetes, polycystic ovary syndrome, nonalcoholic fatty liver disease, cholelithiasis, and a proinflammatory state.

B. Pharmacologic Principles

Drug dosing in obesity is affected by multiple factors, including increased total body fat, reduced total body water, altered protein binding, increased blood volume and cardiac output, increased lipid concentrations in blood, organomegaly, enhanced phase II reactions (glucuronidation and sulfation), and drug absorption in fat stores.

Drugs that are mainly distributed to lean tissues (e.g., nondepolarizing neuromuscular blocking agents) should be dosed based on the *lean body weight* (LBW ≈ ideal body weight [IBW] × 1.2). Although initial doses for lipophilic drugs (e.g., benzodiazepines, barbiturates) have to be based on LBW as well, maintenance doses should be based on *total body weight (TBW)* because of the significantly increased volume of distribution. Multiple doses of lipophilic drugs lead to accumulation in fat stores, causing a prolonged response as the drug is released back into circulation.

In morbidly obese patients, it is more appropriate to use LBW rather than TBW for induction of general anesthesia with propofol. Studies have shown that dosing based on LBW in morbidly obese patients resulted in similar doses and similar times to loss of consciousness when compared to nonobese control patients with dosing based on TBW. However, TBW-based dosing accurately predicted the volume and clearance of propofol, suggesting the use of TBW as the dosing scalar when administering maintenance infusions of propofol.

The principles for administration of commonly used perioperative drugs in obese patients are listed in Table 28-1. It must be noted that the dose–response relationships for most drugs in obese patients have not been completely elucidated. For inhaled anesthetics, the longer time constants for equilibrium with fat along with poor perfusion of fat tissue counteract the effect of increased fat mass on uptake. As a result, obesity does not influence induction times and only modestly affects the wake-up time with the inhaled anesthetics in routine clinical practice, especially in surgeries lasting <4 hours.

C. Preoperative Evaluation

Preoperative evaluation should include assessment of the risk of airway management difficulties, vascular access options, identification of relevant comorbidities, and education of the patient regarding the perioperative anesthetic plan.

There is a high prevalence of *difficult airways* in obese patients due to a large tongue, perimandibular and nuchal fat tissue, and redundant pharyngeal soft tissue. OSA independently correlates with difficult mask ventilation. Difficult intubation rates in obese patients range from 5% to 15% and up to 21% in patients with OSA. Male sex, neck circumference, and Mallampati score have been shown to predict difficult intubation in obese patients, although these results are inconsistent across multiple studies and the positive predictive value for such factors is low. Laryngoscopic view is improved in morbidly obese patients with the use of a video laryngoscope. The ramped position, as described later, also improves laryngoscopic view.

Preoperative evaluation for OSA and initiation of continuous positive airway pressure (CPAP) at home is recommended. In the absence of a formal preoperative sleep study, tools like the *STOP-BANG* questionnaire help identify patients with OSA. The questionnaire consists of questions on *S*noring, *T*iredness, *O*bserved apnea, high blood *P*ressure, *B*MI >35, *A*ge >50, *N*eck circumference >40 cm, and male *G*ender, with positive answers to three or more questions suggesting a higher risk for OSA.

Table 28-1	Principles for Administration of Common Perioperative Drugs in Obese Patients	
Drug	**Initial Dosing Based on**	**Remarks**
Thiopental	LBW	Increased cardiac output in obese patients results in lower peak arterial concentration, resulting in more rapid awakening.
Propofol	LBW	TBW-based dosing should be used for continuous infusions and maintenance dosing.
Etomidate	LBW	
Benzodiazepines	TBW	Longer duration of action due to increased volume of distribution. Higher initial doses may be necessary to achieve adequate sedation, resulting in prolonged sedation.
Dexmedetomidine	TBW	Short-acting sedative infusion that does not cause respiratory depression. Useful for awake fiberoptic intubation and as an anesthetic adjunct. However, bradycardia and hypotension can be significant.
Fentanyl	LBW	Clearance increases with LBW. Dosing based on TBW overestimates dose requirements in obese patients. Titrate doses to clinical response.
Sufentanil	LBW	Increased volume of distribution and elimination half-life because of high lipophilicity.
Remifentanil	LBW	Rapid hydrolysis in plasma and tissues. Dosing by TBW will result in increased incidence of side effects.
Succinylcholine	TBW	Lower doses will result in poor intubating conditions due to increased extracellular volume and increased activity of pseudocholinesterase activity in obese patients. Low incidence of myalgia in obese patients.
Vecuronium	LBW	Dosing by TBW results in prolonged duration of action. Repeat doses should be based on neuromuscular monitoring.
Rocuronium	LBW	Faster onset and prolonged duration of action when dosed by TBW. Repeat doses should be based on neuromuscular monitoring.
Atracurium	LBW	
Cisatracurium	LBW	Dosing by TBW results in prolonged duration of action, while dosing by IBW may result in decreased duration of action.
Pancuronium	BSA	Airway and respiratory derangements in obese patients make this long-acting neuromuscular blocker undesirable.
Sugammadex	IBW + 40%	Not available in the United States as of 2014.
Neostigmine	TBW, not exceeding 5 mg	Prolonged time to adequate reversal (TOF ratio 0.9), up to four times slower than for nonobese patients (26 min vs. 7 min).
Heparin	LBW	Dose response in obese is not established. Obese patients have a higher risk of deep venous thrombosis and pulmonary embolism perioperatively than nonobese patients.

LBW, lean body weight; TBW, total body weight; IBW, ideal body weight; TOF, train of four.

Preoperative assessment of obese patients should include an evaluation of common *comorbidities* (systemic or pulmonary hypertension, diabetes, OSA, ischemic heart disease, heart failure). Preoperative medical management of the comorbidities, when possible, may help reduce the perioperative risk. Patients with OSA should be educated about the use of perioperative CPAP.

D. Intraoperative Considerations

Equipment and Positioning

Whenever possible, patients should position themselves on the operating table. In extreme cases, a mechanical lifting device may be required to move the patient. Although most operating room tables are capable of handling moderately obese patients, specially designed tables are required for surgery in the extremely obese. Well-padded sleds or arm boards are often required to position the arms. For surgeries that require tilting or turning of the table, strapping or taping the patient to the table along with stiffened "bean bags" can prevent accidental falls. Gel and foam pads should be used to support pressure points and prevent peripheral neuropathy and skin breakdown. The supine position is associated with reduction in lung volumes and hypoxemia, and venous return may be impeded through caval compression. In the prone position, emphasis should be placed on free abdominal wall movement, with support for the chest wall and the pelvis. Shoulder bars may cause injury to the brachial plexus if incorrectly placed. The Trendelenburg position causes the highest degree of respiratory compromise with a decrease in FRC and lung compliance. Lateral positioning and the sitting position allow the weight of the abdominal fat to fall away from the chest and diaphragm (Fig. 28-2).

Effect of position on lung volumes

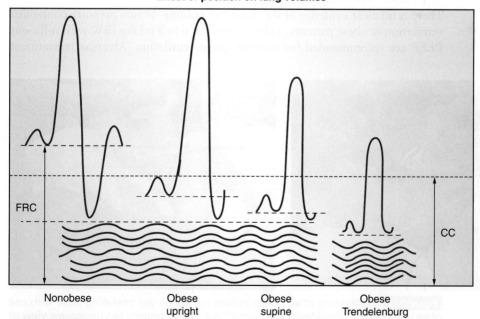

| Nonobese | Obese upright | Obese supine | Obese Trendelenburg |

Figure 28-2 Effects of obesity, positioning, and anesthesia on lung volumes. FRC, functional residual capacity; CC, closing capacity; CV, closing volume; RV, residual volume. (From Bucklin BA, Fernandez-Bustamante A. Anesthesia and obesity. In: Barash PG, Cullen BF, Stoelting RK, et al. *Clinical Anesthesia*, 7th ed. Philadelphia: Lippincott Williams & Wilkins, 2013:1277.)

Monitoring and Vascular Access

Noninvasive monitoring of blood pressure overestimates the blood pressure in a large proportion of obese patients because of *inappropriate cuff size* and the conical shape of the arm. Also, recording times may be prolonged, leading to delayed recognition of a change in blood pressure. Although the use of the forearm for blood pressure measurement may be adequate, use of invasive monitoring should be considered, especially in the presence of comorbid conditions. Peripheral venous access can also be challenging and may require ultrasound guidance.

Airway Management

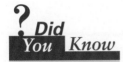

In order to reduce the incidence and impact of aspiration, antacids, prokinetics, H2 receptor antagonists or proton-pump inhibitors should be administered prior to induction in patients with an identifiable risk of aspiration (discussed later). Although cricoid pressure is reasonable, the risk of aspiration should be weighed against the risk of worsened view during laryngoscopy.

With induction of anesthesia in the supine position, obese patients experience a further reduction of FRC, and oxygen saturation may fall rapidly. Maneuvers that prolong safe apnea times during induction include preoxygenation with 100% oxygen, use of a 25- to 30-degree reverse Trendelenburg or semisitting beach-chair position, application of 10 cm H_2O CPAP during preoxygenation, and positive end-expiratory pressure (PEEP) during mask ventilation. The head-up position also minimizes the risk of passive regurgitation.

Placing the obese patient in a *ramped position* can be beneficial for laryngoscopy and intubation. It can be achieved with towels or folded blankets under the patient's shoulders and head or with a commercially available device. The head, shoulders, and upper body are elevated above the chest, with the goal of elevating the external auditory meatus to the level of the anterior chest wall (Fig. 28-3).

Mechanical Ventilation

There is no clear evidence of the benefit of volume- versus pressure-controlled ventilation in obese patients. Tidal volumes of 6 to 8 mL/kg IBW with sufficient **PEEP** are recommended for intraoperative ventilation. Alveolar recruitment

? *Did You Know*

The best position for inducing anesthesia in obese patients is a semisitting position using a ramp to place the patient's ears at the level of the anterior chest wall.

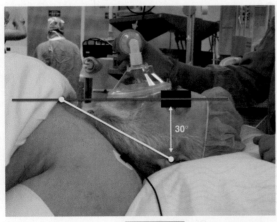 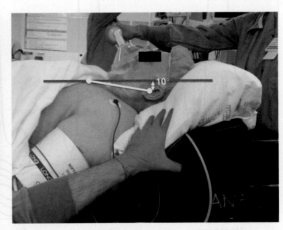

Figure 28-3 Positioning of an obese patient supine on the operating table with use of an upper body (shoulder/head) "ramp" will likely enhance laryngoscopic view of the vocal cords and facilitate tracheal intubation. The goal of such positioning is to bring a line drawn between the external auditory meatus and the sternal notch (*yellow line*) into a position parallel to the horizontal plane (*red line*). Standard supine positioning (*left*) demonstrates a 30° difference between these two lines, whereas proper ramp positioning (*right*) has reduced this angle to only 10°.

maneuvers and subsequent application of moderate PEEP (10 cm H_2O) helps prevent atelectasis, particularly in patients undergoing laparoscopic surgery. Reduced ventilatory compliance can cause high airway pressures, making it difficult to maintain plateau pressures <30, especially with pneumoperitoneum during laparoscopic surgeries. High airway pressures can cause barotrauma and hypotension. Hypercapnia might have to be tolerated. However, hypercapnia can result in a further increase of pulmonary vascular resistance in patients with pre-existing pulmonary hypertension.

Fluid Management
Obese patients may suffer increased perioperative blood loss because of technical difficulties with surgical exposure. It can also be difficult to estimate fluid balance, adequacy of peripheral perfusion, and blood loss. Measurement of urine output, venous pressures, and acid–base balance may be indicated.

Emergence
Precautions similar to induction should be observed. Patients should be extubated when neuromuscular blockade has been completely reversed (ideally assessed quantitatively) and the patient is awake and positioned in a semi-sitting or reverse Trendelenburg position, with *CPAP* maintained to prevent alveolar derecruitment. Postoperative lung function is improved with application of CPAP immediately after extubation.

Monitored Anesthesia Care and Sedation
Procedural sedation of the obese patient is not to be taken lightly. There should be close monitoring of respiratory function because of pre-existing respiratory compromise, increased risk of respiratory depression with sedation, and the potential for difficult mask ventilation and intubation. The presence of OSA increases the risk of perioperative hypoxemia and the requirement of airway interventions during sedation. Dexmedetomidine is a selective α_2-adrenergic agonist that provides sedation without respiratory depression. However, its clinical use can be limited because of hemodynamic instability.

E. Regional Anesthesia
The 2006 American Society of Anesthesiologists' (ASA) practice guidelines for management of patients with OSA recommend that regional analgesic techniques be considered to reduce or eliminate the requirement for systemic opioids. However, excessive sedation used to perform or manage the regional anesthetic may negate the advantages.

Neuraxial Techniques
Spinal or epidural placement in the *sitting position* allows for easier identification of the vertebral midline. Ultrasound can be used to identify the spinous processes and to reduce the number of needle passes. When longer needles are used, a careful assessment of the midline will avoid injury. Epidural placement can be challenging because of the loss of resistance felt in fat planes and difficulties in predicting the depth of the epidural space. There is a higher initial failure rate for epidural catheters in obese laboring patients than in lean patients.

During spinal anesthesia, local anesthetics and opioids can have an exaggerated cephalad spread because of (a) decreased cerebrospinal fluid volume due to fatty tissue spread into the intervertebral foramina and engorged epidural veins (due to elevated venous pressures) and (b) head-down positioning of the vertebral column due to large buttocks. A ramp under the chest elevates the cervical and thoracic spine, limiting cephalad spread of hyperbaric local anesthetic.

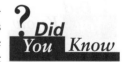

? Did You Know

When placing a spinal or epidural needle in the obese patient, it is best done with the patient sitting up.

Peripheral Nerve Blocks

Local anesthetic dosing for peripheral nerve blocks in obese patients should be based on IBW, rather than TBW, to avoid systemic toxicity. Obese patients suffer a higher rate of block failure than nonobese patients, particularly with epidural, paravertebral, continuous supraclavicular, and superficial cervical blocks. Although the use of ultrasound may improve the success rate and reduce procedure time, ultrasound imaging in obese patients can be suboptimal due to an increased number of reflective surfaces and greater depth to the structures. Retraction and taping of the excessive soft tissue away from the procedural site allow for sterile preparation and easier access to insertion sites.

F. Anesthesia for Bariatric Surgery

Surgical treatment of obesity is generally considered if BMI is >40 kg/m^2 (or BMI >35 kg/m^2 with obesity-related comorbidities) and the patient is unable to maintain weight loss with medical management. All of the intraoperative recommendations noted previously should be considered (e.g., positioning, padding, extubation, etc.). Continuation of home CPAP therapy in the immediate postoperative period, along with a semiupright position, aids in maintaining oxygenation after surgery. Postoperative nausea and vomiting can cause disruption of gastric repair. In addition to antiemetics, adequate fluid replacement reduces postoperative nausea and vomiting in bariatric surgery patients. An *opioid-sparing* postoperative analgesia strategy includes local anesthetic wound infiltration, intravenous acetaminophen, nonsteroidal anti-inflammatory drugs, and thoracic epidural infusion of local anesthetics. Implementation of bariatric clinical care pathways improves patient care and reduces cost.

G. Postoperative Management, Critical Care, and Resuscitation

In addition to challenges with airway, vascular access, and positioning and pharmacologic differences similar to those in the intraoperative period, postoperative care in obese patients presents a unique set of problems. Special beds and lifts are often required to move obese patients, and radiologic imaging can be problematic. Morbidly obese patients are at increased risk for prolonged mechanical ventilation and intensive care unit (ICU) stay, as well as mortality related to these events. Mobilization, incentive spirometry, noninvasive positive airway pressure, and judicious handling of analgesia and sedation are required to prevent reintubation in the postanesthesia care unit and in the ICU. Pulse oximetry monitoring and CPAP therapy should be continued on the surgical floor, especially in patients with OSA.

Postoperative anticoagulation for a prolonged period (e.g., heparin 5,000 to 7,500 U three times daily for 10 days) is helpful to prevent deep vein thrombosis and pulmonary embolism in morbidly obese patients. Early, high-protein, hypocaloric enteral feeding provides an anabolic advantage, reduces infectious complications, and reduces ICU stays in obese patients. Frequent repositioning of the patient, use of pressure-relief mattresses, and early mobilization will prevent decubitus ulcers. Appropriate antibiotic dosing and redosing, prevention of hyperglycemia, and maintenance of arterial and tissue oxygenation are required to prevent surgical site infections in obese patients.

Should cardiopulmonary resuscitation be required, chest compressions may be ineffective in morbidly obese patients. Repeat defibrillation shocks may be necessary because of the higher transthoracic impedance. Although airway management by conventional means can be challenging, surgical access

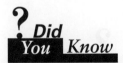

Did You Know

Tracheal intubation of the obese patient in the intensive care unit is to be avoided unless necessary. The patient will generally be better off if other modalities of treatment are used.

through a thick neck can be extremely difficult, requiring expert practitioners; it should be considered only as a final option.

II. Hepatic Disease

Patients with hepatic disease present for hepatic and nonhepatic surgery. The anesthesiologist must be familiar with the unique pathophysiology of cirrhosis and portal hypertension. Comprehensive anesthesia textbooks should be consulted for a more thorough discussion of hepatic anatomy and physiology relevant to anesthesia.

A. Assessment of Hepatic Function
Hepatic function includes bile production, protein synthesis, regulation of glucose metabolism, lipid and protein metabolism, hematopoiesis, and drug and metabolite clearance. Clinical evidence of liver disease can be subtle. Risk factors (alcoholism, illicit drug use, sexual promiscuity, blood transfusions) provide clues to possible hepatic disease. Signs and symptoms often include loss of appetite, malaise, pruritus, abdominal pain, indigestion, jaundice, and changes in urine or stool color. Patients with advanced disease may have ascites, spider angiomas, and encephalopathy.

Standard liver function tests provide information about hepatocyte integrity, cholestasis, and hepatic synthetic function, while other tests evaluate the extent and nature of hepatic injury. Table 28-2 lists the various tests commonly used to evaluate the liver.

B. Hepatic and Hepatobiliary Diseases
Drug toxicity and infection are the most common causes of acute liver disease, which can either progress to acute liver failure, resolve spontaneously, or progress into chronic liver failure. Other causes include alcoholic hepatitis, nonacetaminophen drug toxicity, and pregnancy-related hepatic diseases. Chronic liver disease is usually a consequence of chronic viral hepatitis, alcoholic liver disease, or nonalcoholic fatty liver disease. Chronic liver disease can lead to portal hypertension, cirrhosis, and malignancy.

C. Cirrhosis and Portal Hypertension
Recurrent episodes of inflammation cause hepatic parenchymal necrosis and fibrosis, leading to cirrhosis. The resistance to blood flow through the hepatic capillary bed increases, causing *portal hypertension*. Systemic manifestations of cirrhosis and portal hypertension are listed in Table 28-3.

Hemostasis
Laboratory tests in cirrhotic patients often show alterations in the procoagulant system. However, the anticoagulant system is also altered. Hence, tests of coagulation should be interpreted carefully. Patients may also have dysfibrinogenemia. Thrombocytopenia develops as a result of decreased production and increased splenic sequestration. Fibrinolysis may occur in cirrhotic patients because of decreased clearance of tissue plasminogen activator.

Cardiac
Cirrhosis and portal hypertension cause an increased production of vasodilators, usually causing a *hyperdynamic circulation* with high cardiac output and low systemic vascular resistance. Systolic blood pressure is often <100 mm Hg. A large amount of blood is sequestered in the splanchnic bed, causing a decreased effective circulating volume.

Table 28-2   Liver Function Tests

Function	Test	Remarks
Hepatocyte integrity	AST	Formerly, SGOT. Produced in the liver, heart, skeletal muscle, kidney, brain, and red blood cells.
	ALT	Formerly, SGPT. Produced in the liver.
	LDH	Also increased with hemolysis, rhabdomyolysis, tumor necrosis, myocardial infarction.
	GST	Released from cells in the centrilobular region (zone 3). Sensitive marker of centrilobular necrosis in the early stages. Short plasma half-life (30 min).
Synthetic function	Albumin	Protein loss through the gastrointestinal tract and kidneys and increased catabolism can also cause hypoalbuminemia. Long half-life (2–3 wk).
	PT/INR	Both bile salt-mediated vitamin K absorption and hepatic synthesis of coagulation factors are necessary to maintain normal PT/INR. Short half-life of factor VII (4–6 hr) makes PT/INR a sensitive indicator of acute liver disease.
	Ammonia	Markedly elevated in patients with hepatic encephalopathy, when hepatic urea synthesis is disrupted.
Excretory function	Alkaline phosphatase	Present in biliary canaliculi, bone, intestine, liver, and placenta. Lacks specificity for hepatobiliary disease.
	GGT	Elevated in hepatobiliary disease, closely tracks alkaline phosphatase in timeline. Most sensitive laboratory marker of biliary tract disease, but not specific.
	5′ NT	Elevations are specific to hepatobiliary obstruction.
	Bilirubin	Product of heme catabolism. Indirect (unconjugated) hyperbilirubinemia happens in prehepatic disease, while direct (conjugated) hyperbilirubinemia is present in intra- or extrahepatic bile duct obstruction. Hepatic disease causes elevation of both kinds of bilirubin.

AST, aspartate aminotransferase; ALT, alanine aminotransferase; LDH, lactate dehydrogenase; GST, glutathione S-transferase; SGOT, serum glutamic-oxaloacetic transaminase; SGPT, serum glutamic-pyruvic transaminase; PT/INR, prothrombin time/international normalized ratio; GGT, γ-glutamyl transferase; 5′ NT, 5′-nucleotidase.

Renal

Cirrhosis causes an activation of the sympathetic, renin–angiotensin–aldosterone, and vasopressin systems and salt and water retention. Patients are at risk of renal hypoperfusion due to decreased effective circulating volume, systemic hypotension, diuresis, gastrointestinal bleeding, and diarrhea as well as other renal insults, including drug-related nephrotoxicity, sepsis, and immune complex–related nephropathies. Hepatorenal syndrome is an extreme manifestation of the systemic circulatory derangement in cirrhosis.

Pulmonary

Ascites and pleural effusion can cause ventilation–perfusion mismatch in cirrhotic patients due to restriction of lung expansion and atelectasis. Portal hypertension also causes hepatopulmonary syndrome (liver dysfunction, unexplained hypoxemia, and intrapulmonary vascular dilatation causing right-to-left shunting) and portopulmonary hypertension (pulmonary hypertension with no other known cause in patients with portal hypertension).

Table 28-3	Clinical Manifestations of Cirrhosis and Portal Hypertension
Cardiovascular	Hyperdynamic circulation Low systemic vascular resistance Low systemic systolic blood pressure Systolic and diastolic dysfunction Reduced effective circulating volume
Pulmonary	Decreased functional residual capacity Restrictive ventilation due to ascites and pleural effusion Hepatopulmonary syndrome Portopulmonary hypertension
Gastrointestinal	Ascites Esophageal varices Hemorrhoids Gastrointestinal bleeding
Renal	Salt and water retention Decreased renal function Hepatorenal syndrome
Hematologic	Anemia Coagulopathy Thrombocytopenia Spontaneous bacterial peritonitis
Metabolic	Sodium, potassium, calcium, and magnesium abnormalities Hypoalbuminemia Hypoglycemia
Neurologic	Hepatic encephalopathy

Encephalopathy

Hepatic encephalopathy is related to the amount of hepatic parenchymal damage and shunting of portal venous blood into the systemic circulation. Gastrointestinal bleeding, increased oral protein intake, dehydration, infections, and worsening liver function can precipitate this condition. Neurologic signs include altered mental status with fluctuating neurologic signs of asterixis and hyperreflexia, along with characteristic high-voltage, slow-wave activity on electroencephalography. Treatment includes supportive care, amelioration of the precipitating cause, and oral lactulose or neomycin to decrease the intestinal ammonia production.

Ascites

Portal hypertension, hypoalbuminemia, lymphatic fluid seepage from the diseased liver, and renal fluid retention are all implicated in the development of cirrhotic ascites. Treatment includes salt restriction, diuretics, paracentesis, and, occasionally, a transjugular intrahepatic portosystemic shunting (TIPS) procedure. It is recommended that large-volume (>5 L) ascitic fluid drainage should be accompanied with albumin replacement (6 to 8 g/L). Patients with ascites can commonly develop spontaneous bacterial peritonitis due to bacterial translocation from the bowel flora.

Table 28-4	Modified Child-Pugh Score		
	Points[a]		
Presentation	**1**	**2**	**3**
Albumin (g/dL)	>3.5	2.8–3.5	<2.8
Prothrombin time			
Seconds prolonged	<4	4–6	>6
International normalized ratio	<1.7	1.7–2.3	>2.3
Bilirubin (mg/dL)[b]	<2	2–3	>3
Ascites	Absent	Slight to moderate	Tense
Encephalopathy	None	Grades I–II	Grades III–IV

[a]Class A = 5–6 points; B = 7–9 points, C = 10–15 points. Perioperative mortality: Class A: 10%, B: 30%, C: >80%.
[b]For cholestatic diseases, assign 1, 2, and 3 points for bilirubin <4, 4–10, and >10 mg/dL, respectively.
From Kamath PS. Clinical approach to the patient with abnormal liver test results. *Mayo Clin Proc.* 1996; 71:1089, with permission.

Varices

Esophageal varices develop as portosystemic shunts because of portal hypertension. They can cause massive bleeding, leading to hypovolemia from blood loss and hepatic encephalopathy from the intestinal nitrogen load from blood breakdown. Treatment includes supportive care, endoscopic sclerotherapy, electrocoagulation or banding, medical therapy (vasopressin, somatostatin, or propranolol), and balloon tamponade. Anesthetic challenges include the full stomach, fragile physiology, acute hypovolemia, and encephalopathy.

D. Preoperative Evaluation

Preoperatively, the severity of liver disease and the risk of surgery can be estimated using the modified *Child-Pugh* and MELD (model for end-stage liver disease) scoring systems. The Child-Pugh score is described in Table 28-4. The MELD score ranks patients according to their risk of death from liver disease, based on a logarithmic calculation of creatinine, bilirubin, and the international normalized ratio of the prothrombin time.

On preoperative evaluation, minor, asymptomatic elevations of liver function tests are most likely irrelevant. More significant elevations and the presence of risk factors or evidence of liver failure should prompt further investigation. In a retrospective analysis of patients with cirrhosis undergoing cardiothoracic surgery, those with Child-Pugh score <8 had no significant increase in mortality or morbidity. In another review of over 700 cirrhotic patients undergoing major gastrointestinal, cardiothoracic, and orthopedic surgery, MELD score, age, and ASA physical status predicted perioperative mortality. MELD score correlated linearly with mortality, with 30-day mortality ranging from 6% (MELD score <8) to >50% (MELD score >20).

E. Intraoperative Management

Hemodynamic monitoring for patients with end-stage liver disease should include an arterial catheter and other invasive monitoring, depending on the extent of the surgery and the patient's comorbidities. Transesophageal echocardiography is a relative contraindication because of the risk of bleeding from

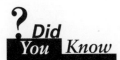

? Did You Know

Although many drugs are metabolized in the liver, the duration of action following a single dose is frequently quite short. This is because cardiac output is high in advanced liver disease and drug action is terminated primarily by redistribution.

esophageal varices, although the data from published case series suggest the risk is low.

Ascites and variceal bleeding can increase the risk of aspiration during anesthetic induction. Induction doses of intravenous induction agents are **short acting** despite liver disease, because the action is terminated by redistribution. However, with repeat doses or infusions, a prolonged duration of action can be expected. Isoflurane and sevoflurane preserve hepatic blood flow and oxygen delivery. The action of opioid agents is often prolonged. In addition, patients with liver disease often have an enhanced response to sedatives. Cisatracurium is the neuromuscular blocker of choice.

Maintenance of circulating volume and renal perfusion is important. Cirrhotic patients may require albumin for replacement after large-volume paracentesis in the presence of spontaneous bacterial peritonitis or hepatorenal syndrome. Patients often exhibit a reduced response to endogenous and exogenous vasoconstrictors. Hypotension, high mean airway pressures during mechanical ventilation, and sympathetic stimulation should be avoided to the extent possible.

F. Specific Procedures

Transjugular Intrahepatic Portosystemic Shunt Procedure

TIPS is indicated for decompression of portal hypertension in the setting of esophageal varices or intractable ascites. A shunt is placed transvenously, connecting the portal circulation to a hepatic vein (Fig. 28-4). Monitored anesthesia care or general anesthesia may be used. Acute volume overload due to influx of portal blood into the systemic circulation is a frequent complication. Because the shunted blood bypasses the liver, new or worsening hepatic encephalopathy is seen in up to 30% to 35% patients after the procedure, occurring soon after TIPS insertion.

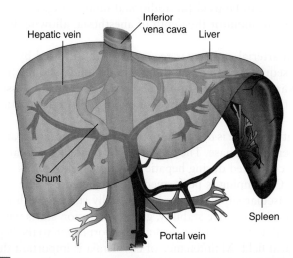

Figure 28-4 Transjugular intrahepatic portosystemic shunt (TIPS) procedure. A stent (or stents) is passed through the internal jugular vein over a wire into the hepatic vein. The wire and stent or stents are then advanced into the portal vein, after which blood can pass through the portal vein into the hepatic vein and bypass and decompress dilated esophageal veins. (From Steadman RH, Braunfeld MY. The liver: surgery and anesthesia. In: Barash PG, Cullen BF, Stoelting RK, et al. *Clinical Anesthesia*, 7th ed. Philadelphia: Lippincott Williams & Wilkins, 2013:1319.)

Hepatic Resection

Hepatic resections are most commonly performed for malignancy (primary hepatobiliary or metastatic) and carry a high perioperative mortality rate. Adequate vascular access and cross-matched blood should be available to combat massive hemorrhage. Prevention of hypothermia is essential to allow normal hemostasis. In the initial stages of the surgery, drainage of ascites can lead to significant fluid shifts, and placement of retractors for exposure can cause respiratory and hemodynamic compromise. Compression of the inferior vena cava (IVC) during exposure and control of vascular supply leads to diminished preload. Liver blood flow can be manipulated with vascular clamping below and above the liver, causing hemodynamic fluctuations. Maintaining a low central venous pressure (<5 cm H_2O) helps decrease blood loss and transfusion. Laboratory testing–guided administration of procoagulants is necessary to improve clotting without unwanted thrombotic complications. An abrupt *drop in end-tidal* CO_2, with rising pulmonary artery pressures, should raise suspicion of a significant air embolism.

G. Hepatic Transplantation

Alcohol- or hepatitis-induced chronic, severe hepatocellular disease is the most common indication for liver transplantation. The MELD scoring system allows for prioritization of organ allocation, with score adjustments for patients with hepatocellular carcinoma and hepatopulmonary syndrome. Fulminant hepatic failure puts patients on the top of the waiting list.

Patients presenting for liver transplantation have usually had an extensive diagnostic workup. Immediate preoperative assessment should include evaluation for a change in functional status since the last assessment, recent oral intake, options for vascular access, and neurologic and renal function.

Multiple, large bore *venous access* is necessary for rapid volume administration, often through a rapid infusion device. Arterial and central venous catheterization is necessary, and a pulmonary artery catheter or transesophageal echocardiogram can be used for additional monitoring. Electroencephalogram can be used to monitor the depth of anesthesia, allowing for titration of anesthetic agents.

A preinduction arterial catheter is recommended, followed by preoxygenation and rapid-sequence induction. Intravenous fluids should be warmed and forced-air warming devices should be used. Immunosuppressive drugs, their doses, and timing should be discussed with the surgical team prior to surgery.

The intraoperative course is divided into the preanhepatic, anhepatic, and the neohepatic or reperfusion phase. The *preanhepatic* phase has similar anesthetic implications as encountered during hepatic resection. Venovenous bypass may be necessary if IVC clamping is performed. The *anhepatic* phase begins with clamping of the vascular supply to the liver, usually starting with the hepatic artery. After a period of relative stability, graft reperfusion starts with flushing of the preservative fluid by perfusion through the portal vein to the hepatic vein and into the surgical field. Maintenance of euvolemia is important during this phase of controlled bleeding. With reanastomosis of the hepatic vein, acidemia and embolism can cause pulmonary hypertension with severe cardiopulmonary instability. Vasopressors, inotropes, and pulmonary vasodilators are often necessary to support blood pressure. The anesthesiologist also needs to monitor the serum electrolyte, glucose, and acid-base status. Patients are at particular risk of hypocalcemia, due to high volume infusion of citrated blood products,

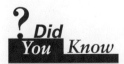

? Did You Know

Massive transfusion is associated with hypocalcemia (due to citrate in bank blood) and hyperkalemia (due to K+ leaking out of stored red blood cells).

and hyperkalemia, because of underlying renal function, potassium-sparing diuretic use, blood transfusion, splanchnic ischemia, and acidosis.

Early in the *neohepatic* phase, patients develop a hypocoagulable, fibrinolytic state. Maintenance of hemostasis is accomplished with guidance from conventional coagulation tests and thromboelastography. Postoperatively, patients can develop fluid overload, transfusion-related acute lung injury, and intra-abdominal hypertension related to massive transfusion. Anastomotic leaks or stenosis or thrombosis of a vascular anastomosis may require urgent re-exploration.

III. Anesthetic Management for Gastrointestinal Surgery

The care of patients undergoing gastrointestinal surgery forms a major part of anesthesia practice in most hospitals.

A. Pharmacology

Nitrous oxide (N_2O) will diffuse into bowel, particularly if it is already distended with bowel gas. This can result in bowel distension and increased intraluminal pressure, which can lead to difficulty with abdominal closure and, in extreme situations, bowel ischemia. N_2O should be used rarely, if at all.

Opioids decrease *lower esophageal sphincter (LES)* tone and reduce gastric and bowel motility, often causing ileus and constipation in intensive care patients sedated with opioids. Opioids, particularly morphine, cause contraction of the *common bile duct sphincter*, which can be problematic if intraoperative cholangiograms are taken. Cholinesterase inhibitors and high neuraxial blocks can cause hyperperistaltic activity because of parasympathetic action and inhibition of sympathetic action, respectively. This may be detrimental in patients with bowel obstruction.

B. Pulmonary Function

Patients undergoing upper abdominal surgery are at increased risk for postoperative pulmonary complications, likely related to atelectasis, reduced cough (pain, edema, ileus), and the risk of perioperative aspiration. Intraoperatively, supine or head-down positioning and abdominal retractors can impair diaphragmatic movement and induce atelectasis and hypoxia. Strategies to prevent pulmonary complications include preoperative cessation of smoking and optimization of pre-existing pulmonary disease, intraoperative avoidance of long-acting neuromuscular blockers, and postoperative pain control and nasogastric drainage in selected patients. The evidence to favor the use of spinal and epidural techniques to reduce postoperative pulmonary complications is suggestive but not conclusive. The impact of laparoscopic surgery on the respiratory system is discussed elsewhere in this book.

C. Mechanical Obstruction and Paralytic Ileus

Patients may present with impaired gastrointestinal motility. Postoperative ileus is common, usually related to physical manipulation of the abdominal viscera. Small bowel motility recovers within a few hours after surgery, gastric peristalsis returns after 24 to 48 hours, and colonic activity returns after 48 hours. Passage of flatus, cramping, and return of appetite signify the return of peristaltic activity. Paralytic ileus can also develop after blunt abdominal trauma, bowel perforation, bilious peritonitis and intra-abdominal sepsis, and after extra-abdominal pathologies like severe pneumonia, trauma, sepsis and myocardial infarction, and electrolyte abnormalities.

Mechanical obstruction of the bowel usually requires surgical management. Patients present with pain, distension, vomiting, and obstipation. Up to 7 to 9 L of fluid may be secreted daily into the gut in an adult (approximately 1 L of saliva, 2 L of gastric juice, 1 L of bile, 2 L of pancreatic juice, and 1 L of succus entericus), and patients can present with severe dehydration and electrolyte abnormalities. Perioperative management concerns for the anesthesiologist include the management of aspiration risk, fluid resuscitation, and management of postoperative analgesia.

D. Bowel Perforation and Peritonitis
Perforation of the gastrointestinal tract into the peritoneal cavity leads to peritonitis and sepsis. Treatment usually involves surgical repair. Advanced age, delayed presentation (>24 hours), organ failure on presentation, diffuse generalized peritonitis, and fecal contamination of the peritoneum are associated with increased hospital stay and increased mortality.

Patients with severe peritonitis are often severely *hypovolemic*. Preoperative and intraoperative restoration of hemodynamics and early institution of appropriate antibiotic therapy are essential. Postoperatively, these patients require admission to an intensive care unit.

IV. Aspiration of Gastric Contents

Irrespective of the surgical procedure, an understanding of gastric emptying and the risk of aspiration is vital to safe anesthesia. The incidence of clinically significant pulmonary aspiration is highest for emergency procedures (~1 in 600 to 800) and relatively rare during elective procedures (~1 in 2,100 to 3,500). The mortality rate associated with aspiration is 1 in 45,000 to 70,000 across a large variety of patient populations. The incidence of aspiration is higher in the presence of ileus, obstetric emergencies, and light planes of anesthesia. Factors predisposing to an increased risk of aspiration are listed in Table 28-5. Regurgitation and aspiration are most common during induction of anesthesia and laryngoscopy.

Table 28-5 Predisposing Factors for Aspiration

Emergency surgery

Inadequate anesthesia

Abdominal pathology

Obesity

Opioid medication

Neurologic deficit

Lithotomy

Difficult intubation/airway

Reflux

Hiatal hernia

Adapted from Kluger MT, Short TG. Aspiration during anesthesia: A review of 133 cases from the Australian Anaesthetic Incident Monitoring Study (AIMS). *Anaesthesia.* 1999;54:19–26.

A. Gastric Emptying

Patients presenting for surgery are routinely asked to fast. The goal of a gastric volume <25 to 30 mL has been extrapolated from animal studies. Clear fluids (water, fat-free and protein-free liquids, pulp-free fruit juice, carbonated drinks, black tea, and black coffee) are emptied within 2 hours of ingestion. Breast milk requires 2 to 4 hours to empty from the stomach, while nonhuman milk takes up to 6 hours. Although light, nonfatty meals (e.g., toast and clear liquids) may be emptied from the stomach in 6 hours, larger meals with fatty food or meat take 8 hours or more to empty from the stomach. Nasogastric drainage can reduce gastric volume but *does not guarantee* an empty stomach.

Several patient conditions prolong gastric emptying time. Diabetic patients commonly develop gastroparesis in correlation with the degree of autonomic neuropathy but not peripheral neuropathy. Patients with renal failure, irrespective of mode of dialysis, also have delayed gastric emptying. Pregnancy causes physical impairment of gastric emptying. Patients with ileus or bowel obstruction have increased gastric volumes. Opioids, antimuscarinics (atropine and glycopyrrolate), and trauma can delay gastric emptying as well.

B. Regurgitation Risk

Passive reflux and regurgitation of gastric contents is normally prevented by the LES. Diseases that affect LES tone (hiatal hernia, gastroesophageal reflux disease) increase the risk. Elevated intra-abdominal pressures (e.g., laparoscopy, abdominal compartment syndrome) can raise the intragastric pressure, overwhelm the LES, and provoke reflux. The presence of a nasogastric tube decreases LES pressure and increases episodes of reflux.

Opioids and antimuscarinics reduce LES tone, as do hormonal changes in pregnancy. An impaired level of consciousness interferes with upper airway reflexes and is also associated with reduced LES tone and delayed gastric emptying.

Metoclopramide is a dopamine antagonist that stimulates upper gastrointestinal motility, increases LES tone, and relaxes the pylorus and duodenum, thus reducing gastric volume. A parenteral dose of 5 to 10 mg administered over 3 to 5 minutes can be given 15 to 30 minutes before induction. Low-dose erythromycin (200 mg orally, given 1 hour before induction of anesthesia) also reduces gastric volume. The actual impact of this on the incidence of aspiration is unknown, and prokinetics are not recommended for patients with bowel obstruction.

Cricoid pressure is the term given to placement of pressure on the trachea to compress the esophagus against the body of the sixth cervical vertebra, thus decreasing regurgitation of stomach contents through the upper esophageal sphincter. Although it is widely used, there is little evidence to prove that cricoid pressure decreases the incidence of aspiration. On the other hand, cricoid pressure can make visualization of the vocal cords during laryngoscopy more difficult.

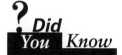

? *Did* **You** *Know*

Application of cricoid pressure is a standard practice to prevent reflux of gastric contents during induction of anesthesia, but its efficacy has never been proven.

C. Pulmonary Injury due to Aspiration

Aspiration of gastric contents can lead to acute lung injury due to acid aspiration, bacterial pneumonia, or obstructive symptoms related to particulate matter. Radiologic findings may be visible within a few hours, and the clinical course can vary depending on the volume, acidity, and particulate makeup of the gastric contents aspirated.

Histamine-2 receptor antagonists (cimetidine, ranitidine, and famotidine) reduce gastric volume and acidity by decreasing acid secretion. Proton-pump inhibitors (omeprazole and pantoprazole) also decrease gastric acid secretion and can last for as long as 24 hours. Antacids neutralize the acid in gastric contents, but use of particulate antacids is not recommended. A single dose of nonparticulate sodium citrate is commonly given before induction of anesthesia to increase gastric fluid pH prior to emergency operations.

D. Fasting Guidelines

In 2011, the ASA published its practice guidelines for preoperative fasting and pharmacologic intervention for the prevention of perioperative aspiration in healthy patients (i.e., without disorders that affect gastric emptying) undergoing elective surgery. The guidelines recommend a minimum fasting period of 2 hours after ingestion of clear liquids, 4 hours after breast milk, and 6 hours after infant formula, nonhuman milk, and light meals. Drugs that reduce gastric acidity or promote gastric motility may be used in patients at risk for pulmonary aspiration, although their routine use is not recommended.

Suggested Readings

Chau EHL, Lam D, Wong J, et al. Obesity hypoventilation syndrome. A review of epidemiology, pathophysiology, and perioperative considerations. *Anesthesiology.* 2012; 117:188–205.

Dellinger RP, Levy MM, Rhodes A, et al. Surviving sepsis campaign: International guidelines for management of severe sepsis and septic shock. *Crit Care Med.* 2013;41(2):580–637.

Giannini EG, Testa R, Savarino V. Liver enzyme alteration: a guide for clinicians. *CMAJ.* 2005;172:367–379.

Ingrande J, Lemmens HJM. Dose adjustment of anaesthetics in the morbidly obese. *BJA.* 2010;105(S1):i16–i23.

King DR, Velmahos GC. Difficulties in managing the surgical patient who is morbidly obese. *Crit Care Med.* 2010;38(Suppl):S478–S482.

Kluger MT, Short TG. Aspiration during anaesthesia: Review of 133 cases from the Australian Anaesthetic Incidence Monitoring Study (AIMS). *Anaesthesia.* 1999;54:19–26.

Practice guidelines for preoperative fasting and the use of pharmacologic agents to reduce the risk of pulmonary aspiration: Application to healthy patients undergoing elective procedures. An updated report by the American Society of Anesthesiologists Committee on standards and practice parameters. *Anesthesiology.* 2011;114:495–511.

Practice guidelines for the perioperative management of patients with obstructive sleep apnea. A Report by the American Society of Anesthesiologists Task Force on Perioperative Management of Patients with Obstructive Sleep Apnea. *Anesthesiology.* 2006;104: 1081–1093.

Questions

1. Which of the following patients meets the criteria for morbid obesity?
   A. 5′ 4″ and 230 lb
   B. 5′ 0″ and 200 lb
   C. 4′ 8″ and 180 lb
   D. 4′ 4″ and 150 lb

2. In an obese patient, the lean body weight should be used when calculating the initial dose for all of the following drugs EXCEPT:
   A. Succinylcholine
   B. Fentanyl
   C. Etomidate
   D. Propofol

3. In the obese patient, which of the following positions is associated with the greatest negative impact on ventilation and oxygenation?
   A. Supine
   B. Lateral
   C. Sitting
   D. Head down

4. In the obese patient, all of the following statements regarding blood pressure measurement with a standard automated cuff are true EXCEPT:
   A. The time required to make a blood pressure measurement can be prolonged
   B. The blood pressure cuff should be longer and more narrow
   C. The forearm is an appropriate site for cuff placement
   D. The conical shape of the upper arm may cause errors

5. Laryngoscopy and tracheal intubation is more likely to be successful when an obese patient is placed in which of the following positions?
   A. Supine with the head in a neutral position on a small pillow
   B. Supine with the head extended over the edge of the table
   C. Semisitting with the head in a neutral position on a small pillow
   D. Semisitting on a ramp with the head extended

6. A patient with a BMI of 46 kg/m², hypertension, and diabetes mellitus has just undergone an unremarkable 3-hour bariatric surgical procedure. Which of the following would be LEAST advantageous in the first 24 hours postoperative?
   A. Thoracic epidural administration of dilute local anesthetic
   B. Continued tracheal intubation with assisted ventilation
   C. Administration of antiemetic(s)
   D. Positioning the patient in the semisitting position

7. Regarding use of propofol in a patient with advanced hepatic cirrhosis, which of the following is TRUE?
   A. The duration of action of a single induction dose will be shorter than normal.
   B. The duration of action of a second, single dose, given 5 minutes after induction will be prolonged.
   C. The duration of action of a continuous infusion will be shorter than normal.
   D. None of the above.

8. For patients undergoing hepatic transplantation, the period of greatest hemodynamic instability is typically during:
   A. Anesthetic induction
   B. The preanhepatic phase
   C. The anhepatic phase
   D. The neohepatic or reperfusion phase

9. A patient is to undergo laparotomy for a bowel obstruction with associated significant bowel distension. Which of the following agents is relatively contraindicated?
   A. Nitrous oxide
   B. Sevoflurane
   C. Isoflurane
   D. Fentanyl

10. A healthy patient about to undergo elective outpatient inguinal hernia repair had a 6-oz glass of clear (pulp free) apple juice and a cup of black coffee on the morning of surgery. According to ASA guidelines, it would be acceptable to induce general anesthesia after waiting a minimum of how many hours:
    A. 8
    B. 6
    C. 4
    D. 2

29 Anesthesia for Otolaryngologic and Ophthalmic Surgery

R. Mauricio Gonzalez
Joseph Louca
Sofia Maldonado-Villalba

I. General Considerations

The anesthetic management of otolaryngologic (ORL) surgery is complex. Many variables must be considered, including understanding the surgical indications and procedures. Depending on the operation, the anesthesiologist may jointly manage the airway with the surgeon. Additionally, airway anatomy may be distorted by tumor, infection, trauma, congenital abnormalities, radiation exposure, or prior surgery. Age-specific differences in anatomy and physiology, along with existing comorbidities, must also be considered.

Assessing the airway extends beyond the physical examination. Familiarity with airway imaging, particularly computed tomography and magnetic resonance imaging, is critical. Review the digital videos of airway fiberoptic examinations if they are available. If they are not available, the anesthesiologist may consider performing a fiberoptic examination of the airway under topical anesthesia prior to induction.

The selection and dosage of anesthetics and adjuvant medications should be tailored to the procedure being performed. Patients undergoing ORL procedures must also be carefully monitored for blood loss, which can be underestimated due to spillage onto the surgical field, swallowing, and distance of the surgical field from the anesthesiologist.

Topical α-agonists for vasoconstriction can cause hypertension and increased blood flow to the pulmonary circulation. This can be associated with pulmonary edema and death, especially if patients are subsequently treated with β-blockers because of their negative inotropic effects. Given the short duration of action of topical vasoconstrictors, moderate hypertension can be allowed to self-resolve or it can be treated by increasing the depth of anesthesia. Direct vasodilators are the proper treatment for a severe hypertensive response to topical vasoconstrictors.

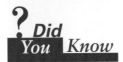

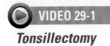
II. Anesthetic Considerations in the Pediatric Population

A. Anatomy and Physiology

Diseases of the ear in children can be better understood by reviewing the anatomy and physiology of the middle ear and adjacent structures. The eardrum is a thin, well-innervated membrane sitting at the deepest part of the external auditory canal. It borders the middle ear laterally. The middle ear drains into the nasopharynx via the eustachian tube. During infancy, it drains poorly because of its small cross-sectional area, floppy cartilaginous walls, and the low angle it travels toward the nasopharynx. Additionally, its short length increases exposure of the middle ear to the mucous and bacteria of the nasopharynx. These factors increase the risk of otitis media, whose peak incidence occurs at 1 year of age. By age 7, the risk of otitis media is roughly that of adults.

B. Myringotomy and Tube Insertion

Myringotomy and ear tube placement requires general anesthesia (GA) to provide the surgeon with the stillness required for work under a microscope. The short length of the procedure and its noninvasive nature allow use of inhaled anesthetics alone. These procedures are often performed without intravenous (IV) access or securing the airway. Induction using a face mask with a mixture of oxygen, nitrous oxide (N_2O), and sevoflurane can be followed by maintenance with sevoflurane. Positioning the head with 30 to 45 degrees of axial rotation allows adequate surgical access.

C. Tonsillectomy and Adenoidectomy

Tonsillar hypertrophy may be asymptomatic or lead to obstructive sleep apnea (OSA) and recurrent tonsillitis, which are frequent indications for removal of tonsils or adenoids. The *tonsils* grow rapidly between the ages of 1 and 3 and are often the largest between ages 3 and 7. Thus, this is the most common age range for this procedure.

The assessment of a child undergoing a tonsillectomy should include evaluating the overall respiratory function. Severe cases of OSA may warrant postoperative intensive care. The worst cases of OSA may also be complicated by pulmonary hypertension with cor pulmonale and may require pharmacologic cardiovascular support prior to induction.

In the setting of a mild or improving upper respiratory infection (URI), proceeding with the operation may increase the risk of respiratory complications. However, a delay often results in the patient returning to the physician until their next URI. Therefore, it may be sensible to proceed in the presence of a mild URI because complete optimization is rarely possible (1).

A variety of regimens exist for postoperative analgesia:

1. Given prior incision, acetaminophen (10 to 40 mg/kg rectally) for analgesia and dexamethasone (0.5 mg IV) for edema, postoperative nausea and vomiting (PONV), may reduce or eliminate the need for IV opioids.
2. If opioids are required, IV fentanyl (0.25 to 1.0 µg/kg) can provide effective relief while reducing the incidence or severity of emergence agitation.
3. Ibuprofen orally, given either pre- or postoperatively, is a safe and effective analgesic, although some surgeons are concerned with postoperative bleeding after its use (2).

D. Posttonsillectomy Hemorrhage

Although rare (<1% to 2% of patients), *posttonsillectomy hemorrhage* can be life-threatening. Risk factors include chronic tonsillitis, older age (>11 years old), intraoperative blood loss >50 cc, and hypertension. Primary hemorrhage occurs within 24 hours of the surgery. Secondary hemorrhage typically occurs within 5 to 10 days of the surgery, the time period when a fibrin clot sloughs off.

The management of posttonsillectomy hemorrhage includes addressing the airway, circulation, and breathing. Assess cardiovascular stability and obtain IV access. Examine the airway, look for active bleeding or a clot, and obtain the history of any bleeding expeditiously. Keep the patient leaning forward and face down to drain blood away from the laryngopharynx. When minor or recurrent bleeding is present, there is a significant risk (perhaps >40%) for severe hemorrhage due to relaxation of vasospasm or the displacement or lysis of a clot. One must notify the blood bank and prepare for surgery.

In the operating room (OR), a gauze soaked in 1:10,000 epinephrine should be available. Direct pressure can be applied to tonsillar fossae using a *Magill forceps* wrapped with gauze. Suction and airway equipment should also be available before the patient is placed supine. Children may not tolerate efforts at hemostasis while awake and may need sedation or GA before attempts are made. Ketamine may be an excellent choice. It has a low risk of respiratory compromise and hypotension in hypovolemic patients (3).

E. Emergencies or Stridor

Stridor, a high-pitched or musical breathing caused by obstruction of the larynx, is a medical emergency that must be considered life-threatening. Common causes include foreign body aspiration (FBA), epiglottitis, and croup (Table 29-1).

FBA is a common problem in children, particularly ages 1 to 5, that can be difficult to diagnose unless the event is witnessed and reported. FBA may present with wheezing and coughing, decreased breath sounds, and stridor. It may also mimic common allergies, asthma, OSA, gastroesophageal reflux disease, bronchiolitis, or airway obstruction due to abscess or congenital anomaly. Although radiography may detect atelectasis and hyperinflation, it cannot rule out FBA when the aspirated body is radiolucent. If there is a high index of suspicion for FBA, rigid bronchoscopy may be the necessary next step (Fig. 29-1).

? Did You Know

Stridor, a high-pitched or musical breathing caused by obstruction of the larynx, is a medical emergency and must be considered life-threatening.

Table 29-1 Causes of Stridor

Supraglottic Airway	Larynx	Subglottic Airway
Laryngomalacia	Laryngocele	Tracheomalacia
Vocal cord paralysis	Infection (tonsillitis, peritonsillar abscess)	Vascular ring
Subglottic stenosis	Foreign body	Foreign body
Hemangiomas	Choanal atresia	Infection (croup, epiglottitis)
Cysts	Cysts Mass Large tonsils Large adenoids Craniofacial abnormalities	

From: Ferrari LR, Nargozian C. Anesthesia for otolaryngologic surgery. In: Barash PG, Cullen BF, Stoelting RK, et al. *Clinical Anesthesia*, 7th ed. Philadelphia: Lippincott Williams & Wilkins, 2013:1363.)

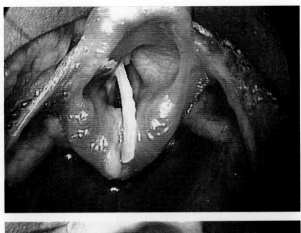

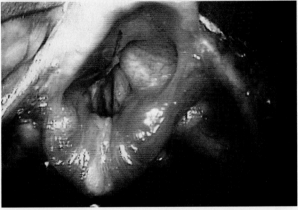

Figure 29-1 A radiolucent plastic strip is visible in the glottic inlet (just above the vocal cords) in a child who presented with inspiratory and expiratory stridor. Following foreign body removal, a small endothelial laceration is visible on the posterior surface of the epiglottis.

? Did You Know

A chest x-ray may detect atelectasis and hyperinflation but it cannot rule out FBA if the aspirated body is radiolucent. When there is a high index of suspicion for FBA, rigid bronchoscopy may be necessary to establish a diagnosis.

Epiglottitis, a life-threatening condition typically caused by a bacterial infection, often affects the epiglottis, aryepiglottic folds, arytenoids, and uvula. Its incidence has declined in the pediatric population due to widespread vaccination against *Haemophilus influenzae B* (Hib). Other bacteria, however, including *Streptococcus pneumoniae*, may also cause epiglottitis.

Epiglottitis presents with stridor, drooling, odynophagia, outright avoidance of food and drink, dysphagia, or high fever. Other signs include malaise and agitation or a history of rapid symptom onset (within hours). An absence of Hib vaccination is of obvious concern. A child growing tired or lethargic suggests imminent respiratory collapse requiring securing the airway. Hypotension, hypoxemia, and bradycardia are also indications for rapid intervention.

Manage patients with suspected epiglottitis swiftly by obtaining radiologic images, monitoring with pulse oximetry, and administering supplemental oxygen. Do not agitate the patient prior to a procedure as it may lead to laryngospasm.

Keep the child upright during transport and proceed directly to the OR for an inhaled anesthetic induction with continuous positive airway pressure ventilation. After induction and IV line placement, weigh the benefit of preventing laryngospasm with a neuromuscular blocking agent against the risk of abolishing spontaneous respiration should tracheal intubation fail. For direct laryngoscopy, a curved Macintosh blade placed gently into the vallecula is likely the best approach. Prevent contact with the epiglottis as this may induce bleeding or swelling. An endotracheal tube 0.5 cm smaller in diameter than would normally be age appropriate should be placed due to the likelihood that edema has reduced patency of the airway. Smaller tubes should also be available.

Have atropine and succinylcholine ready for intramuscular administration to treat cardiac depression or laryngospasm. Alternative airway management plans are essential, and they include having immediate access to rigid bronchoscopy, emergency tracheostomy, or cricothyroidotomy.

Postoperative sedation and mechanical ventilation allow time for airway inflammation to subside. The infection must also be cultured and treated. Extubation should only occur after inspection reveals that the swelling and friability of airway tissues has decreased. A leak test may be helpful in determining readiness.

Laryngotracheobronchitis, or croup, is another cause of stridor, although it tends to have a milder course than epiglottitis. Croup presents with a barking, high-pitched cough and less severe systemic involvement. Consider croup in a vigorously coughing, alert toddler with a hoarse voice. For croup in an otherwise healthy child, it is unlikely that intubation and mechanical ventilation will be necessary.

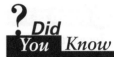

? Did You Know

Laryngotracheobronchitis, also known as croup, may cause stridor; however, it tends to have a milder course than epiglottitis.

III. Anesthesia for Adult Otolaryngologic Surgery

A. Middle Ear and Mastoid

Common procedures for adult middle ear and mastoid issues include stapedectomy, tympanoplasty, mastoidectomy, and myringotomy. Intraoperative considerations for middle ear and mastoid surgery include preservation of the facial nerve, prevention of brachial plexus or cervical injuries, and management of the adverse effects of N_2O.

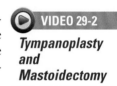

▶ VIDEO 29-2

Tympanoplasty and Mastoidectomy

Facial nerve integrity can be monitored and maintained with intraoperative electromyography and avoidance of neuromuscular blocking agents. Preoperative evaluation of cervical spine range of motion is essential to prevent injuries to the brachial plexus and cervical spine. Avoid extreme neck extension or rotation during surgery.

N_2O can result in increased middle ear pressure if the eustachian tube is not patent. Sudden discontinuation of this gas leads to rapid absorption of N_2O, creating negative pressure that may result in changes to middle ear anatomy, rupture of tympanic membrane, disruption of grafts, and PONV.

B. Nasal and Sinus Surgery

Nasal and sinus surgeries can be performed under local anesthesia with sedation or under GA when there is concern regarding arterial damage or advancing into the intracranial space, the latter being a concern during *endoscopic sinus surgery*.

Minimize intraoperative bleeding with intranasal vasoconstriction, elevation of the head to facilitate venous drainage, and induced mild hypotension.

C. Maxillofacial Trauma and Orthognathic Surgery

High-speed impact trauma, with or without external evidence of injury, is frequently associated with life-threatening injuries. The anesthetic plan must consider the possibility of cervical spine injuries and skull fractures. Cervical spine stabilization prior to intubation and oral versus nasal intubation (contraindicated in *LeFort III fracture*) are important considerations. Orthognathic surgery for reconstruction of facial skeletal malformations is often achieved by performing LeFort or mandibular osteotomies, so understanding of these procedures is beneficial.

D. Craniofacial Bone Structure

Knowledge of basic craniofacial bone structure is important. The facial skeleton comprises three parts. The lower third is the mandible. The middle portion includes the zygomatic arch of the temporal bone, zygomaticomaxillary complex, maxilla, nasal bones, and orbits. Lastly, the superior portion comprises the frontal bone.

E. Temporomandibular Joint Arthroscopy

▶ **VIDEO 29-3**

Temporomadibular Joint Assessment

Temporomandibular joint arthroscopy is indicated when there is displacement of the temporomandibular joint cartilage, causing clicking, trismus, fibrosis, or osteoarthritis. Intubation may be oral (if immobility is achieved with GA) or with nasal fiberoptic assistance if the patient is in trismus. Swelling around the surgical site due to irrigation may result in partial or complete airway obstruction.

F. Surgery of the Airway

Suspension Laryngoscopy and Microlaryngoscopy

Suspension laryngoscopy and microlaryngoscopy provide direct access and visualization of the airway, while protecting the trachea and maintaining ventilation and oxygenation.

Jet ventilation provides an airway without the use of endotracheal intubation. Short cases (<30 minutes) may require succinylcholine infusion to achieve an immobile field. Lower pressure (30 to 50 pounds per square inch) jet ventilation is used to reduce the risk of barotrauma, which is more likely to occur in children, those with chronic pulmonary disease, and the obese. Stimulation of the larynx may trigger arrhythmias, tachycardia, or hypertension. To block a severe sympathetic response due to stimulation of the larynx, lidocaine (IV or topical), opiates (e.g., remifentanil infusion for faster recovery), or β-blockers can be administered (Fig. 29-2).

Laser surgery of the airway can be used for microsurgery of the upper airway or trachea. Benefits include coagulation of small vessels, reduced tissue inflammation, and better precision. A serious complication is airway fire. Usage of fire-resistant, impregnated, or shielded endotracheal tubes, a low fraction of inspired oxygen, and avoidance of N_2O are prudent precautions (4).

Bronchoscopy

Bronchoscopy can be flexible or rigid. Flexible bronchoscopy is used to examine the smaller airways. Rigid bronchoscopy is used when there is bleeding of

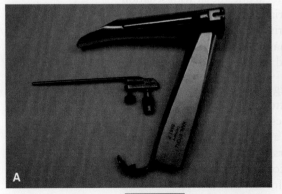
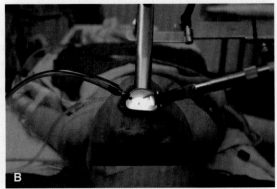

Figure 29-2 The surgical laryngoscope and the jet ventilator needle (**A**). The surgical view of the laryngoscope positioned in the patient's pharynx and connected to a continuous flow of oxygen through the jet ventilator needle (**B**).

the airway or to perform large airway biopsies, dilate the airway, or remove foreign bodies.

Rigid bronchoscopy is performed under GA to prevent airway injury due to coughing, bucking, or straining. Ventilation is administered through a side port of the rigid bronchoscope. Emergence may proceed with mask-assisted ventilation, laryngeal mask airway, or endotracheal intubation. Endotracheal intubation may be needed if the patient has received neuromuscular blocking agents or if the protective airway reflexes are compromised.

Tracheostomy

Tracheostomy is indicated when there is severe upper airway obstruction, loss of protective reflexes, or vocal cord paralysis. In conscious patients with respiratory distress, it is important to perform a physical examination and determine if a tracheostomy should be done with the patient awake or under GA.

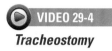

VIDEO 29-4

Tracheostomy

G. Infection

Infections of the ear, nose, and throat are mainly by gram-negative bacteria. These may be associated with fever, chills, drooling, and difficulty swallowing and speaking.

Peritonsillar or Retropharyngeal Abscess and Ludwig's Angina

Occasionally, an abscess must be decompressed under local anesthesia prior to induction. This decreases airway obstruction and the risk of abscess rupture while placing the endotracheal tube. Difficult intubation due to distorted anatomy or trismus may require awake intubation, mask induction with spontaneous breathing, or tracheostomy (Fig. 29-3).

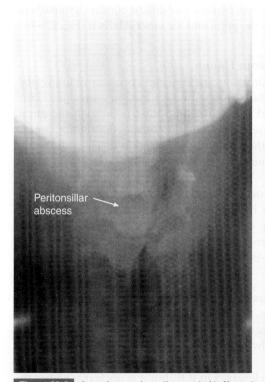
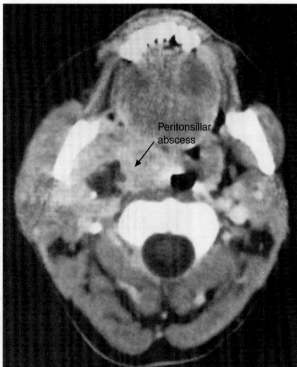

Peritonsillar abscess

Peritonsillar abscess

Figure 29-3 Anterior neck radiograph (*left*) and computed tomography scan (*right*) of a patient with a right peritonsillar abscess. Note displacement of the airway to the left and external compression of the supraglottic airway. (From Ferrari LR, Nargozian C. Anesthesia for otolaryngologic surgery. In: Barash PG, Cullen BF, Stoelting RK, et al. *Clinical Anesthesia*, 7th ed. Philadelphia: Lippincott Williams & Wilkins, 2013:1360–1361.)

Ludwig's angina is a cellulitis of the submandibular region that displaces the tongue upward and obstructs the airway.

H. Neck Dissections and Free Flaps

Patients with head or neck cancer often have a history of heavy smoking and alcohol use with underlying malnutrition and pulmonary and cardiovascular disease. Preparations for difficult intubation must be taken.

A free flap is a transfer of cutaneous and subcutaneous tissue from one part of the body to another. The vascular supply is disconnected during the transfer and reconnected microsurgically. Vasopressors may compromise flap viability and should be avoided.

IV. Extubation

It is necessary to engage in *closed-loop communication* with the entire surgical team and to have a systematic step-wise approach to tracheal extubation. All decisions must be individualized for each patient and take into account multiple factors (5).

V. Anesthesia for Ophthalmic Surgery

A. Ocular Anatomy

The eye is formed by the orbit, globe, extraocular muscles, eyelid, and lacrimal system. The outer fibrous layer forms the sclera, cornea, and corneoscleral junction. The middle layer is formed by the choroid, ciliary body, ciliary processes, and the iris. The choroid contains a dense vascular bed, while the ciliary body controls lens thickness. The pupil is an aperture, the diameter of which is controlled by the sphincter pupillae (parasympathetic innervation) and dilator pupillae (sympathetic innervation). The former constricts the pupil and the latter dilates it (Fig. 29-4).

B. Ocular Physiology

Formation and Drainage of Aqueous Humor

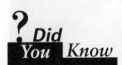

Aqueous humor production and drainage are vital aspects of maintaining normal intraocular pressure (IOP) and vision. Aqueous humor is produced continuously by the *ciliary body* and secreted behind the iris through the pupil. Stimulation of β_2 receptors increases the production of aqueous humor. Stimulation of α_2 receptors decreases the production. Secretion of chloride by the ciliary epithelium leads to an osmotic influx of fluid, a secondary mechanism mediated by carbonic anhydrase.

Drainage of aqueous humor occurs primarily through the canal of Schlemm. Aqueous humor can also be reabsorbed via the ciliary muscle. This uveoscleral flow is increased by ciliary muscle relaxation and is typically mediated by prostaglandins. Therefore, topical prostaglandin analogues can be used to relieve IOP. Topical β-blockers can also decrease IOP by reducing aqueous humor production.

Maintenance of Intraocular Pressure

Volatile anesthetics and sedatives or hypnotics (with the exception of ketamine) reduce IOP. Opioids have no direct effect on IOP. Nondepolarizing paralytics indirectly reduce IOP by attenuating mechanical reflexes that raise IOP, such as coughing.

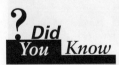

Succinylcholine may cause an elevation in IOP, but it is unclear whether the effect is of clinical significance. Because it is the drug of choice for rapid-onset paralysis, the risks of elevated IOP must be weighed against the risk of not obtaining ideal intubation conditions (6).

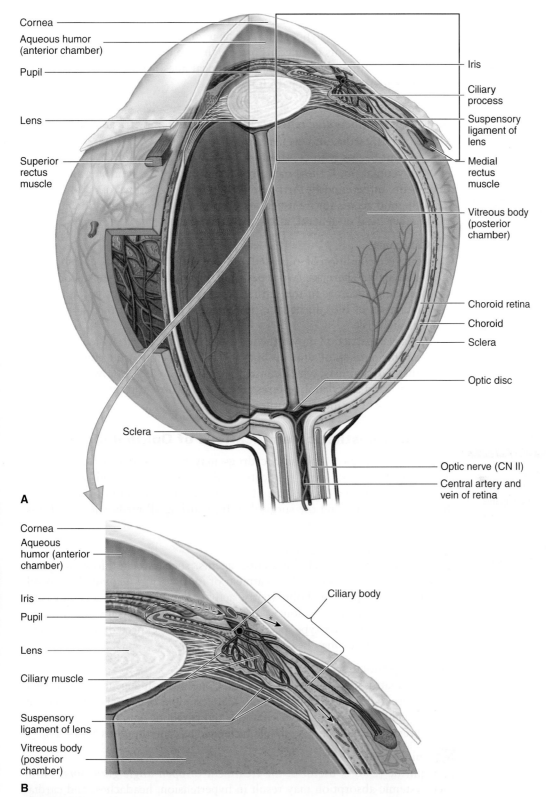

Cornea

Aqueous humor
(anterior chamber)

Pupil

Lens

Superior
rectus
muscle

Iris

Ciliary
process

Suspensory
ligament of
lens

Medial
rectus
muscle

Vitreous body
(posterior
chamber)

Choroid retina

Choroid

Sclera

Optic disc

Sclera

Optic nerve (CN II)

Central artery and
vein of retina

A

Cornea

Aqueous
humor (anterior
chamber)

Iris

Pupil

Lens

Ciliary muscle

Suspensory
ligament of lens

Vitreous body
(posterior
chamber)

Ciliary body

B

Figure 29-4 Diagram of ocular anatomy. (Adapted from Moore KL, Agur AMR, Dalley AF. *Clinically Oriented Anatomy*. 7th ed. Philadelphia: Wolters Kluwer; 2013, with permission).

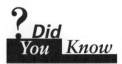

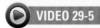

Oculocardiac Reflex

To relieve IOP acutely, raise the head and prevent other causes of venous congestion. Under GA, hypocapnia can be used. Additional tactics include the use of muscle relaxants during intubation, the use of a laryngeal mask airway in lieu of intubation, deep extubation, or local anesthetization of the airway. IV agents can also rapidly relieve IOP.

Oculocardiac Reflex
Through the *oculocardiac reflex*, ocular stimulation may trigger hypotension, syncope, bradycardia, and even asystole.

Treatment begins with cessation of any stimuli and ensuring adequate airway and ventilation. If these measures do not succeed, administer antimuscarinic agents intravenously. Atropine (20 µg/kg) or glycopyrrolate (15 µg/kg) are both good agents for treatment or prophylaxis. Deepening of the anesthesia, whether local or general, also blunts the reflex.

C. Glaucoma
Glaucoma is a condition of increased pressure within the eyeball, causing gradual loss of sight. There are two types of glaucoma: open-angle glaucoma and closed-angle glaucoma. In the setting of either type of glaucoma, additional acute increases in IOP during the perioperative period can put the patient's vision at high risk.

Pupillary constriction moves the iris away from the canal, which lowers the resistance for outflow of aqueous humor. Therefore, muscarinic antagonists or sympathetic α_1 agonists, which cause mydriasis, decrease outflow. Conversely, cholinergics and acetylcholinesterase inhibitors, whose topical forms are indicated for glaucoma, increase outflow (7).

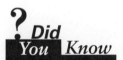

VI. Anesthetic Ramifications of Ophthalmic Drugs
Absorption of topical ophthalmic drugs may be enough to cause systemic effects. Additionally, some medications that are administered systemically may have significant ophthalmic effects. Constant communication between the anesthesia team and the surgical staff regarding all medications and dosages administered is required.

A. Anticholinesterase Agents
Long-acting topical anticholinesterase agents, such as echothiophate (phospholine iodide), are used in the treatment of *refractory glaucoma*. They result in a reduction of pseudo-cholinesterase activity that can last for several weeks. In the setting of their use, a longer duration of action for succinylcholine (prolonged apnea) and ester-type local anesthetics can be expected; lower dosages of these medications may be required.

B. Cyclopentolate
Cyclopentolate is used as a mydriatic agent. Concentration-dependent central nervous system toxicity occurs with its use. Manifestations of central nervous system toxicity include dysarthria, disorientation, and psychotic episodes. Seizures have been observed in children. Use should be limited to concentrations below 1%.

C. Epinephrine
Epinephrine (2%) is useful in the treatment of *open-angle glaucoma*. However, systemic absorption may result in hypertension, headaches, and cardiac dysrhythmias (especially in the presence of halothane). Dipivefrin is a prodrug of epinephrine that reduces the production of aqueous humor, increases its outflow, and has fewer side effects than epinephrine.

D. Phenylephrine

Phenylephrine decreases capillary congestion and causes mydriasis. Systemic absorption may result in hypertension, headaches, tremors, and bradycardia. In patients with coronary artery disease, it could trigger myocardial ischemia. A solution of 2.5% phenylephrine should be used instead of the usual 10% in small children and the elderly. To minimize absorption, its use should be limited to the time before incision.

E. Topical β-blockers

Timolol is a nonselective β-blocker that decreases aqueous humor production. Systemic absorption may cause bradycardia, bronchospasm, congestive heart failure, exacerbation of myasthenia gravis, and postoperative apnea in neonates. Exercise caution when prescribing to patients with pre-existing reactive airway diseases, congestive heart failure (CHF), and conduction abnormalities greater than first-degree heart block.

Betaxolol is a newer antiglaucoma β-blocker that is more oculoselective than timolol and has minimal systemic effects. Nonetheless, it may potentiate the effects of systemic β-blockers and is contraindicated in patients with sinus bradycardia, first-degree or higher heart block, CHF, and cardiogenic shock.

F. Intraocular Sulfur Hexafluoride

Intraocular sulfur hexafluoride (SF6) and other gases are used in retinal detachment repair to replace the volume of vitreous humor lost during surgery. The low water solubility of SF6 ensures persistence of the intraocular bubble for several days to weeks.

N_2O is 34 times more soluble than nitrogen so it can enter the bubble quicker than nitrogen can exit. This "entrapment" of N_2O causes expansion of the gas bubble, increasing the IOP and potentially compromising the retinal blood flow, especially in the presence of systemic hypotension. N_2O should be discontinued 15 minutes prior to injecting SF6 or any other gas. Abrupt discontinuation of N_2O after injection of SF6 will result in a sharp decrease in the volume of the bubble with a corresponding drop in IOP to below awake levels, possibly jeopardizing the surgical repair. N_2O must be avoided up to 5 days after injection of air, 10 days after the injection of SF6, and 70 days after injection of *perfluorocarbons*. A Medic Alert bracelet should be considered after use of perfluorocarbons.

G. Systemic Drugs
Oral Glycerol
Oral glycerol is used to lower the IOP during the treatment of acute glaucoma attacks. Its side effects include hyperglycemia, glycosuria, disorientation, and seizures.

Mannitol
Mannitol is used to decrease IOP to enhance surgical exposure (achieve a "soft eye") and occasionally to treat glaucoma. Rapid administration of large doses of mannitol has been associated with renal failure, CHF, fluid overload, electrolyte imbalance, hypertension due to rapid increase in intravascular oncotic pressure, hypotension from the subsequent diuresis, and myocardial ischemia. Allergic reactions have been described as well.

Acetazolamide
Acetazolamide, a carbonic anhydrase inhibitor, is used to decrease IOP. Because of its renal tubular effects, acetazolamide can result in loss of sodium bicarbonate and potassium. Metabolic acidosis and cardiac arrhythmias have

been described as well. Acetazolamide should not be used in patients with severe liver or renal dysfunction.

VII. Preoperative Evaluation

All patients undergoing ophthalmologic surgery should receive a thorough preoperative (preanesthesia) evaluation by an anesthesiologist. Timing for the preanesthesia evaluation is based on the invasiveness of the procedure and the general medical condition of the patient.

The components of the preanesthesia evaluation are a full patient history, including allergies, medications, and anesthetic history (personal and familial), and an anesthesia-focused physical examination. A complete account of the use of all topical and systemic medications is necessary. This includes over-the-counter medications and alternative therapies. Give clear instructions to the patient regarding which medications to take and which to avoid prior to surgery. Special attention should be paid to anticoagulants and antiplatelet medications. Continue warfarin (at least for cataract surgery) because of a lack of evidence for a clinically significant increase in the risk of hemorrhage. Dual antiplatelet therapy should be continued in patients with cardiac stents during the perioperative period. Consultation with the patient's cardiologist, primary care physician, and ophthalmologist regarding management of anticoagulants and antiplatelet medications is necessary. The physical examination must include, at a minimum, general condition and vital signs, airway examination (including range of motion of the cervical spine), and dental, cardiac, and lung examinations.

VIII. Anesthetic Techniques

Several types of blocks may be used for intraocular surgery.

A. Retrobulbar, Peribulbar, and Subtenon Blocks

For the *retrobulbar block*, the patient is placed supine with the eye in a neutral position. A 23- to 25-gauge needle is inserted through the lower lid or conjunctiva at the level of the inferior orbital rim in the inferotemporal quadrant. The needle is advanced toward the apex of the orbit until loss of resistance is felt (a "pop"). Then 4 to 6 mL of local anesthetic is injected within the muscle cone (four recti muscles and two oblique muscles), obtaining fast and reliable anesthesia and akinesia (Fig. 29-5).

For the *peribulbar block*, the needle is advanced along the inferior orbital floor parallel to the globe, and local anesthetics are injected in the extraconal space, diffusing to adjacent tissue. Greater amounts of local anesthetics are needed in comparison with a retrobulbar block, raising the concern of an increase in IOP, perforation of the globe, and myotoxicity.

Aspiration before injection is required for both blocks, followed by gentle massage or orbital compression to promote spread of the anesthetic. For the episcleral (subtenon) block, local anesthetic is injected into the episcleral space (posterior subtenon space) using a cannula. Needle entry is into the fornix at the angle tangential to the globe, between the conjunctival semilunaris fold and globe. Upon entry into the conjunctiva, the needle is shifted medially and advanced posteriorly until a click is felt (8).

Complications of regional eye blocks include optic nerve trauma, brainstem anesthesia (amaurosis, gaze palsy, apnea, dilatation of the contralateral pupil, cardiac arrest), retrobulbar hemorrhage (proptosis of the eye), globe perforation, oculocardiac reflex, seizures, and myocardial depression.

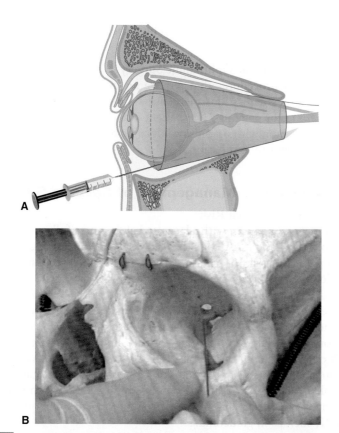

Figure 29-5 Schematic illustration **(A)** and skeletal demonstration **(B)** of proper needle placement for the retrobulbar block. (From McGoldrick KE, Gayer SI. Anesthesia for ophthalmologic surgery. In: Barash PG, Cullen BF, Stoelting RK, et al. *Clinical Anesthesia*, 7th ed. Philadelphia: Lippincott Williams & Wilkins, 2013:1384.)

B. Topical Anesthesia
Topical anesthesia includes drops or gels. Local anesthetics include proparacaine (least irritating), lidocaine, bupivacaine, and tetracaine. Benefits of topical anesthesia include no risk of hemorrhage, brainstem anesthesia, optic nerve damage, or perforation of the globe. Disadvantages include lack of akinesia and limited use for cataract surgery.

C. Choice of Local Anesthetic, Block Adjuvants, and Adjuncts
The anesthetic approach for ophthalmologic surgery is based on the procedure length and type. Topical anesthesia combines local anesthetics and vasoconstrictors. Vasoconstrictors delay the washout of local anesthetics, prolonging their action.

Adjuvants like clonidine, sodium bicarbonate, morphine sulfate, vecuronium, and hyaluronidase (increased tissue permeability) may also be used to prolong the duration of the blocks.

Increased IOP after administration of local anesthetics can be reduced with the aid of IV osmotic agents or mechanical devices to compress the globe. Mechanical devices may compromise blood flow and result in ischemic optic neuropathy or central retinal artery occlusion.

D. Monitored Anesthesia Care
The goals of this type of sedation are to provide deep sedation during the administration of regional anesthesia and to keep the patient comfortable

during the procedure. The patient should be responsive, cooperative, and able to protect the airway.

E. General Anesthesia for Ophthalmic Surgery

GA is indicated in procedures that require an immobile surgical field or in patients unable to remain still. Emergence should be smooth, with minimal coughing, bucking, or gagging. The patient should be spontaneously breathing, and premedication with opioids or lidocaine to blunt the cough reflex may be administered prior to extubation.

IX. Anesthetic Management of Specific Situations

A. Open Eye, Full Stomach Risk

The management of a patient with a lacerated globe and a full stomach requires awareness of risks. The most controversial issue is how to quickly secure an airway in a patient at risk for aspiration without causing a significant increase in IOP, which could extrude eye contents and cause blindness.

A large dose of an induction agent such as propofol (2 mg/kg) addresses both problems by facilitating conditions for endotracheal intubation while reducing the risk of straining or coughing. Although succinylcholine is the most appropriate paralytic for rapid sequence induction in a patient at risk for aspiration, it is known to increase IOP 10 to 20 mm Hg, which peaks at 2 to 4 minutes and lasts 7 to 10 minutes. There is also anecdotal evidence of succinylcholine causing extrusion of vitreous humor in an open globe. There is no evidence that succinylcholine causes damage to an intact globe that has elevated IOP, such as in glaucoma.

Alternatively, a high dose of a nondepolarizing agent (e.g., rocuronium 2 mg/kg) has been shown to provide paralysis within 60 seconds 90% of the time. The major drawback is the prolonged paralysis, which carries a risk of preventing the patient from recovering his or her own respiratory effort in the event of difficult intubation.

If GA is contraindicated, local anesthesia should be considered. With an open globe, penetrating nerve blocks are contraindicated because the pain of injection and the fluid injected may raise IOP. Topical agents are a safer alternative in such situations.

Important measures to take, regardless of the anesthetic type used, include eliminating any sharp increases in IOP, keeping the head elevated, not impinging venous drainage at the neck through the application of cricoid pressure or palpation of the carotid artery, avoiding direct pressure on the globe (e.g., face mask), and avoiding painful or intense stimuli of the eye prior to the full onset of the chosen anesthetic.

B. Strabismus Surgery

Strabismus is a persistent misalignment of the visual fields, typically correctable by surgery to counteract the deviation. Surgical repair provides the most benefit when performed before the age of 5, at which time the neural pathways involved in vision have neared maturation (6).

Typically, these repairs are performed under GA due to the stillness required for the work and the pain of the skin and muscle incisions. Endotracheal intubation is preferred to secure the airway due to its proximity to the surgical field and the risk of inadvertent contact.

Acetaminophen may combat the eye irritation felt postoperatively. Fentanyl IV is also an appropriate adjunct.

? Did You Know

With an open globe, penetrating nerve blocks are contraindicated because the pain of injection and the fluid injected may raise IOP.

Strabismus repair has one of the highest rates of PONV of any commonly performed operation, with some studies showing up to 80% in patients who receive no prophylaxis.

Dexamethasone (0.5 mg/kg IV up to 4 mg), ondansetron (0.15 mg/kg IV up to 4 mg), and full replacement of fluid deficits with crystalloids have been shown to reduce the incidence of PONV. Consider gastric emptying with oronasogastric tube while the patient is still deeply anesthetized, in the absence of any contraindications.

C. Intraocular Surgery

The majority of intraocular surgery is performed under local anesthesia rather than GA, the latter having a higher morbidity, higher resource consumption, and longer hospital stay. Various nerve blocks are used to provide surgical analgesia, but are also critical for blunting the oculocardiac reflex. Contraindications to using regional anesthesia for eye surgery include, but are not limited to, inability to lie supine, procedure lasting >2 hours, local anesthetic allergy, and inability to lie still and remain awake throughout the surgery. Some surgeons may tolerate a sleeping patient, although it carries the risk of sudden movement upon awakening.

D. Retinal Detachment Surgery

As with other ophthalmic surgeries, the primary concern is choosing GA versus nerve block. For vitreoretinal surgery, a gas bubble is often placed by the surgeon to provide steady pressure that will aid reattachment of the retina to the pigment epithelium. N_2O should be avoided during surgery and, depending on the type of gas installed in the eye, for the next 2 to 12 weeks (9).

X. Perioperative Ocular Complications

A. Corneal Abrasion

Corneal abrasions are the most common ophthalmic complications after anesthesia. Decreased tear production and incomplete eyelid closure increase the susceptibility of the cornea to mechanical trauma. Chemical trauma and laser injuries may also occur.

Several risk factors have been correlated to corneal abrasion, including advanced age, high blood loss, Trendelenburg position, prolonged length of stay in the postanesthesia care unit, and oxygen supplementation during recovery. Patients with corneal abrasion report a foreign body sensation, photophobia, tearing, blurry vision, and pain that tends to increase with blinking. Corneal abrasions heal within 24 to 48 hours and rarely result in long-term sequelae.

Anesthesiologists must evaluate patients who complain of symptoms suggestive of a corneal abrasion. An eye examination usually reveals conjunctival injection with normally reactive pupils. One recommendation is to start ophthalmic antibiotic ointment immediately and continue four times daily for 48 hours. Erythromycin is first-line therapy, while bacitracin may be used for patients with a contraindication to erythromycin. Patients need to be evaluated by ophthalmology while in the hospital or shortly after discharge, depending on symptom severity. Topical nonsteroidal anti-inflammatory drug can mask unresolved damage and should not be used because unresolved pain is an important reason for patients to follow up. Do not occlude the affected eye because it has not been shown to improve symptoms and the loss of binocular vision may place the patient at risk for falls or other accidents.

Precautions in the OR need to be considered on a case-by-case basis. Taping is the preferred method of eye protection. Aggressive application and removal of tape have been associated with corneal abrasion and periocular soft tissue damage. Ointments must be used with care. Both petroleum-based and methylcellulose ointments can result in irritation or allergic reactions, and may induce the patient to rub their eyes.

B. Perioperative Visual Loss

Perioperative visual loss (POVL) is a rare but devastating complication with a prevalence of <0.1%. Cardiac surgery and major spine surgery have the highest frequency of POVL. There are two major types of POVL: retinal artery occlusion (central and branch) and ischemic optic neuropathy.

Retinal Artery Occlusion

Central retinal artery occlusion (RAO) affects the entire retina and is associated with improper positioning and direct external pressure to the eye. Branch RAO has a segmental deficit distribution and is likely the result of microemboli or vasospasm. Branch RAO is associated with visual loss after cardiac surgery. Retrobulbar hemorrhage may result in ischemic ocular compartment syndrome.

All types of RAO have poor prognoses and no effective treatment. Therefore, prevention is critical. Prone patients must be positioned using modern foam headrests with cutouts and goggles must not be used. Positioning and eyes must be checked every 20 minutes. Horseshoe head rests should not be used.

Ischemic Optic Neuropathy

The causative factors of ischemic optic neuropathy (ION) are poorly understood, but it is known that ION results from disruption of the blood supply to the optic nerve. Anterior ION is associated with cardiac surgery. Posterior ION is associated with lengthy spine surgery (~6.5 hours) when performed in the prone position with elevated blood losses. There are also case reports of ION being associated with the steep Trendelenburg position during laparoscopic robotic radical prostatectomies.

As with RAO, there is no effective treatment for ION, so prevention is paramount. The Postoperative Visual Loss Study Group recently identified the use of a Wilson frame as an independent significant risk factor. It is the only significant risk factor that is easily controllable. The American Society of Anesthesiologists recommends positioning the head at or higher than the level of the heart and in a neutral position to prevent venous congestion (10).

Patients deemed to be at high risk for POLV after spinal surgery must be immediately evaluated postoperatively. In the event of positive findings or concerns, obtain an immediate ophthalmology consult. Without delay, optimize hemoglobin or hematocrit, hemodynamics, and oxygenation. Consider magnetic resonance imaging to rule out an intracranial cause.

References

1. Isaacson G. Tonsillectomy care for the pediatrician. *Pediatrics*. 2012;130(2):324–334.
2. Jeyakumar A, Brickman TM, Williamson ME, et al. Nonsteroidal anti-inflammatory drugs and postoperative bleeding following adenotonsillectomy in pediatric patients. *Arch Otolaryngol Head Neck Surg*. 2008;134(1):24–27.
3. Malone E, Meakin GH. Acute stridor in children. *Contin Educ Anaesth Crit Care Pain*. 2007;7(6):183–186.

4. Mariano ER. Anesthesia for otorhinolaryngology surgery. In: Butterworth JF, Mackey DC, Wasnick J, eds. *Morgan & Mikhail's Clinical Anesthesiology.* 5th ed. New York: McGraw-Hill; 2013:773–787.
5. Popat M, Mitchell V, Dravid R, et al. Difficult airway society guidelines for the management of tracheal extubations. *Anaesthesia.* 2012;67:318–340.
6. Coté CJ, Lerman J, Anderson BJ, eds. *A Practice of Anesthesia for Infants and Children.* Philadelphia: Elsevier Saunders; 2013.
7. Raw D, Mostafa SM. Drugs and the eye. *Br J Anaesth CEPD Rev.* 2001;1:161–165.
8. Canavan KS, Dark A, Garrioch MA. Sub-Tenon's administration of local anaesthetic: A review of the technique. *BJA.* 2003;90:787–793.
9. Hunnigher A. Anesthesia for retinal detachment. *BMJ.* 2008;336(7657):1325–1326.
10. An updated report by the American Society of Anesthesiologists Task Force on Perioperative Visual Loss. Practice advisory for perioperative visual loss associated with spine surgery. *Anesthesiology.* 2012;116:275–285.

Questions

1. Which of the following factors increase the risk of otitis media in children?
   A. During infancy, the eustachian tube has a large cross-sectional area.
   B. During infancy, the eustachian tube is relatively short.
   C. Children have a poorly developed immune system.
   D. During infancy, the eustachian tube has more rigid walls.

2. Myringotomy and ear tube placement is most frequently performed with which of the following anesthetic techniques?
   A. Intravenous induction of general anesthesia
   B. Local anesthesia with moderate sedation
   C. General anesthesia with endotracheal intubation
   D. Inhalation induction with a face mask

3. A child presents to the emergency room with stridor, drooling, odynophagia, outright dysphagia, and high fever. The most likely diagnosis is:
   A. Allergic reaction
   B. Foreign body aspiration
   C. Croup
   D. Epiglottitis

4. A patient is undergoing surgery to correct strabismus. Suddenly, the heart rate decreases to 20 beats per minute. The next step should be:
   A. Administration of intravenous epinephrine
   B. Removing any stimulation
   C. Administration of intravenous atropine
   D. Decreasing the anesthetic depth

5. Which of the following drugs should be avoided in patients who have received intraocular sulfur hexafluoride?
   A. Desflurane
   B. Nitrous oxide
   C. Timolol
   D. Phenylephrine

30 Anesthesia for Neurosurgery

John F. Bebawy
Antoun Koht

Neuroanesthesia is the practice of anesthesia related to the treatment of real or impending neurologic injury to the ***central nervous system (CNS)*** or peripheral nervous system (PNS). The CNS encompasses the brain and spinal cord, while the PNS includes all of the peripheral nerves of the body emanating from the spinal cord. As such, neuroanesthesia is the provision of anesthesia and analgesia for a multitude of procedures, including invasive, minimally invasive, and neurointerventional procedures, involving the brain, spinal cord, and peripheral nerves.

I. Neuroanatomy

The adult brain accounts for only 2% of total body weight but 20% of total body oxygen consumption. The different regions of the brain and spinal cord are responsible for distinct functions (Table 30-1). Blood flow to the brain is accomplished by two carotid arteries anteriorly (70%) and two vertebral arteries posteriorly (forming the basilar artery) (30%), which subsequently converge to form an anastomotic ring at the base of the skull known as the circle of Willis (Fig. 30-1). The spinal column is composed of 33 vertebrae (7 cervical, 12 thoracic, 5 lumbar, and 9 fused sacral and coccygeal), with nerve roots leaving the enclosed spinal cord and exiting through corresponding intervertebral foramina. The blood supply to the spinal cord entails one anterior spinal artery and two posterior spinal arteries. The anterior spinal artery originates from radicular arteries branching off the aorta, with the largest one being the artery of Adamkiewicz (usually at L1 or L2). The posterior spinal arteries originate from the posterior cerebral circulation (Fig. 30-2). The spinal cord itself terminates at L1 or L2 in adults, ending in structures known as the conus medullaris terminus and filum terminale.

II. Neurophysiology

The *cerebral metabolic rate of oxygen consumption (CMRO$_2$)* is normally 3 to 3.8 mL/100 g/min in adults. Normal *cerebral blood flow (CBF)*

Table 30-1   Functionality of Central Nervous System Structures

Anatomic Location	Structure	Function
Postcentral gyrus	Primary somatosensory cortex	Sensation
Precentral gyrus	Primary motor cortex	Movement
Occipital lobe	Primary visual cortex	Vision
Temporal lobe	Primary auditory cortex	Hearing
Wernicke's area (angular gyrus of dominant hemisphere)	Primary language association cortex	Language
Frontal lobe	Primary personality cortex	Personality/intellect
Medial brain	Limbic cortex	Emotion
Medial brain	Hippocampus	Memory
Medial brain	Hypothalamus	Vegetative regulation
Brainstem	Reticular activating system	Consciousness
Brainstem	Vasomotor center	Circulatory/respiratory control
Spinal cord	Dorsal horn (sensory)/ventral horn (motor)	Movement/sensation/reflexes

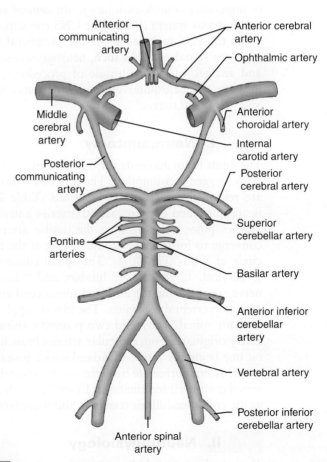

Figure 30-1 The circle of Willis, demonstrating the anterior and posterior blood supply to the brain.

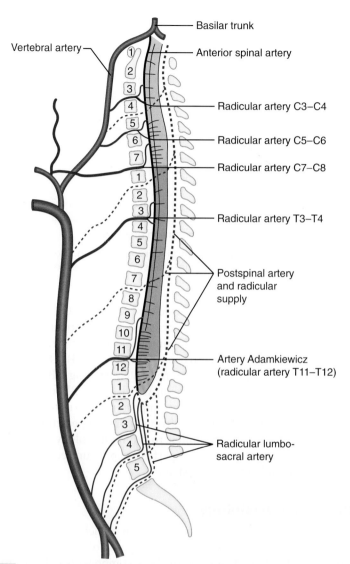

Basilar trunk

Vertebral artery

Anterior spinal artery

① ② ③ ④ ⑤ ⑥ ⑦

Radicular artery C3–C4

Radicular artery C5–C6

Radicular artery C7–C8

① ② ③ ④ ⑤ ⑥ ⑦ ⑧ ⑨ ⑩ ⑪ ⑫

Radicular artery T3–T4

Postspinal artery and radicular supply

Artery Adamkiewicz (radicular artery T11–T12)

① ② ③ ④ ⑤

Radicular lumbo-sacral artery

Figure 30-2 The spinal blood supply. Note that the cervical spine is served by the posterior circulation emanating from the circle of Willis.

is 50 mL/100 g/min at rest, while glucose consumption is approximately 5 mg/100 g/min. The brain is dependent on a continuous supply of oxygen and glucose, with starvation and hypoxic damage resulting after roughly 5 minutes of global ischemia. The results of focal ischemia are less certain.

Cerebral perfusion pressure (CPP) is the difference between mean arterial pressure (MAP) and either *intracranial pressure (ICP)* or central venous pressure (CVP), depending on which is higher. Fortunately, even wide swings in MAP will yield a consistent CBF of 50 mL/100 g/min, thanks to *autoregulation*, which remains intact between a MAP of approximately 60 to 160 mm Hg (Fig. 30-3). The autoregulatory curve is shifted rightward in cases of chronic hypertension. Above and below these limits, CBF becomes pressure dependent as cerebral vessels are either maximally vasodilated (lower limit of autoregulation) or vasoconstricted (upper limit of autoregulation).

Besides MAP, other physiologic parameters play an important role in controlling CBF. Arterial carbon dioxide tension ($PaCO_2$) is the most important

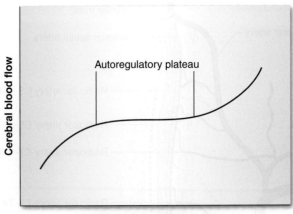

Figure 30-3 Autoregulation in the central nervous system. Cerebral blood flow remains constant between mean arterial pressures (denoted here as cerebral perfusion pressure) of 60 to 160 mm Hg.

of these variables. CBF is linearly associated with $PaCO_2$ between 20 and 80 mm Hg. Hence, hyper- and hypoventilation (both patient determined and iatrogenic) play critical roles in maintaining, decreasing (with hyperventilation), or increasing (with hypoventilation) CBF (Fig. 30-4). Oxygen tension in the arterial blood (PaO_2) plays less of a role in controlling CBF unless marked hypoxemia (PaO_2 <50 mm Hg) occurs, in which case CBF increases dramatically (Fig. 30-5). Temperature is also an important determinant of CBF, with a 6% to 7% decrease in CBF per 1°C drop in core temperature.

Spinal cord physiology is very similar to brain physiology in that autoregulation is maintained and spinal cord perfusion pressure equals MAP minus ICP (pressure in the subarachnoid space).

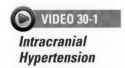

VIDEO 30-1

Intracranial Hypertension

III. Pathophysiology

Intracranial hypertension is any condition in which ICP is raised above 15 mm Hg. The cranium is a closed vault, composed of brain tissue, blood, and cerebrospinal fluid (CSF). When one of these components enlarges to occupy

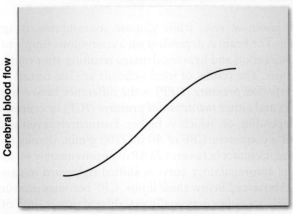

Figure 30-4 Autoregulation in the central nervous system. Cerebral blood flow varies linearly between arterial carbon dioxide partial pressures of 20 to 80 mm Hg.

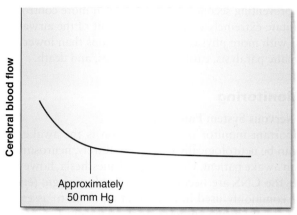

Figure 30-5 Autoregulation in the central nervous system. Cerebral blood flow remains constant above an arterial oxygen partial pressure of 50 mm Hg.

more space (e.g., brain tumor, bleeding), compensation occurs, usually by vasoconstriction and CSF drainage out of the cranium and into the spinal column. *Intracranial elastance* (as this is called), however, becomes very limited as ICP reaches a critical point, where sudden, even very small increases in volume can lead to dramatic increases in pressure within the cranium (Fig. 30-6). The results can be neurologically devastating, with herniation of the brain into the foramen magnum and subsequent irreversible damage or even death. Hence, meticulous care in those patients in whom elevated ICP is suspected (e.g., avoiding hypoventilation, emergent surgical decompression, or CSF diversion) is critical.

As for the spinal cord, damage can be acute (leading to weakness, loss of sensation, or paralysis) or chronic (causing pain and deformity). *Acute spinal cord compression*, due to trauma or tumor, is usually a surgical emergency, as time to decompression is correlated with functional outcome. Patients may be flaccid initially and severely hypotensive, due to a relative sympathectomy. Resuscitation and hemodynamic support are mainstays of treatment at this time. The role

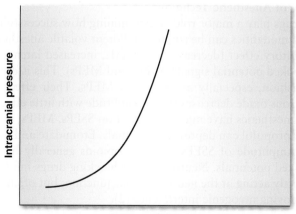

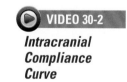

VIDEO 30-2

Intracranial Compliance Curve

Figure 30-6 The intracranial elastance curve is composed of three sections. (**1**) Intracranial pressure remains low and relatively constant at low volumes until the "elbow" of the curve is reached. (**2**) At this point, small changes in volume lead to moderate changes in pressure. (**3**) When a critical intracranial volume is reached, the pressure increases precipitously.

of steroids in preventing secondary injury is much more controversial. Cervical injuries necessitate extremely careful management of the airway. These injuries are associated with more physiologic perturbations than lower injuries, including diaphragmatic paralysis, cardiac disturbances, and death.

IV. Monitoring

A. Central Nervous System Function

The most important monitor of CNS function is the awake and responsive patient who can be neurologically examined. Rarely, neurosurgery can be performed with an awake patient. Under general anesthesia, however, other modes of monitoring the CNS are necessary. *Electrophysiologic (evoked potential) monitoring* is commonly used in the operating room to assess the functional integrity of the CNS during surgeries that might put CNS structures at risk (1). The most commonly used modalities of evoked potential monitoring are *somatosensory-evoked potentials (SSEPs), motor-evoked potentials (MEPs), and electromyography (EMG),* with brainstem auditory-evoked potentials and visual-evoked potentials being less commonly used.

SSEPs are elicited from a peripheral nerve (e.g., median, ulnar, posterior tibial) and usually measured at the level of the subcortex and cortex. This modality is especially useful for monitoring the integrity of the dorsal columns of the spinal cord and the sensory cortex of the brain, where sensory fibers travel. MEPs are produced at the level of the cortex by direct or indirect stimulation and measured as compound muscle action potentials at the muscular level. MEPs are useful for assessing the motor cortex and the anterior spinal cord (corticospinal tracts) during surgeries that may put these structures at risk. EMG is a monitor that continuously assesses distinct nerve or nerve root integrity, either spontaneously or through elicited current, and is sensitive to mechanical and thermal damage to these structures.

Other monitoring modalities used to monitor the CNS (many referenced below) include transcranial Doppler ultrasonography, raw and processed electroencephalography (EEG), cerebral oximetry, and functional magnetic resonance imaging, among others.

B. Influence of Anesthetic Technique

Anesthetic drugs play a major role in determining how successfully these neuromonitoring modalities can be employed. Potent volatile anesthetics have the greatest inhibitory effect (decreased amplitude, increased latency) on obtaining robust evoked potential signals (SSEPs and MEPs). This is done in a dose-dependent fashion, especially as related to MEPs. Their effect on EMG is minimal. Nitrous oxide decreases signal amplitude with little effect on latency. Intravenous anesthetics have much less effect on SSEPs, MEPs, and EMG, but high doses of propofol can depress these signals. Etomidate and ketamine may increase the amplitude of SSEPs, whereas opioids generally have very little effect on evoked potentials. Neuromuscular blocking drugs inhibit MEPs and EMG by directly acting at the neuromuscular junction, but often will improve SSEPs by removing myogenic interference (2).

V. Cerebral Perfusion

A. Laser Doppler Flowmetry

Laser Doppler flowmetry (LDF) is a relatively new technique used in the study of hemodynamics to quantify blood flow in human tissue such as the brain. LDF employs a very small laser that can be implanted into the brain and measures the "scatter," or Doppler shift, caused by passing red blood cells into microscopic vessels. Such measurements are useful in detecting the effects of various physiologic changes (e.g., anemia, hyperventilation) on CBF. Recent studies have shown LDF to yield measurements of CBF similar to xenon (^{133}Xe), which is an isotope whose decay is measured in the brain as a marker of CBF. It is considered the gold standard of experimental CBF measurement (3).

B. Transcranial Doppler Ultrasonography

Transcranial Doppler ultrasonography (TCD) is a tool used in neurosurgery and neurocritical care by which an ultrasound probe is placed over a "window" (usually the temporal bone) to measure flow velocities of major cerebral vessels (usually the middle cerebral artery). Blood flow velocity is recorded by the ultrasound probe, which emits a high-pitched sound wave. That sound wave bounces off red blood cells and returns to the probe. The speed of the blood in relation to the probe causes a phase shift, with a higher or lower frequency directly correlated to a higher or lower velocity, respectively. Changes in these flow velocities (higher velocities) can indicate narrowing, emboli, or vasospasm of these vessels. Notably, TCD is unable to determine actual CBF; rather, it is primarily a technique for measuring relative changes in CBF over time (4).

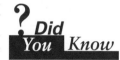

Transcranial Doppler ultrasonography can noninvasively assess changes in cerebral blood flow.

C. Intracranial Pressure Monitoring

ICP monitoring is a useful tool for patients suffering from any cause of dangerously elevated ICP (e.g., brain trauma, bleeding, mass). Normal ICP is 5 to 15 mm Hg, and monitoring or treatment is generally initiated when ICP is >20 mm Hg. Waveforms of ICP can be transduced (A, B, and C waves) and may be useful diagnostically over time. ICP monitoring can be accomplished using a variety of devices, all of which currently are invasive. The most commonly used device is an *external ventricular drain*, which measures ICP by way of a transducer connected via tubing to the ventricle. It is also capable of removing CSF to relieve ICP. Other methods of monitoring ICP include the use of a *subdural screw* (usually performed urgently) placed through the skull and dura mater, an epidural sensor placed between the skull and the dura mater, or a tissue sensor placed directly in the brain parenchyma. These methods are incapable of diverting CSF.

D. Cerebral Oxygenation and Metabolism Monitors

Other devices used to monitor the homeostasis of the brain, including its oxygenation and metabolism, are available (often experimental) but may not be commonly used in the clinical setting. Jugular bulb venous oximetry is the most common of these techniques, which involves a fiberoptic catheter placed in a retrograde fashion into the jugular vein. This catheter is capable of measuring the mixed cerebral venous oxygen tension, which is indicative of the brain's oxygen consumption or extraction. Other monitors used to measure *cerebral metabolism* include microdialysis catheters, which are multiparameter catheters that can detect focal brain tissue oxygen tension, glucose, pyruvate, lactate, glutamate, and glycerol levels by way of obtaining local perfusate from the brain. These catheters are becoming more popular in neurocritical care units but remain highly experimental (5). Lastly, cerebral oximetry has become more prevalent in the clinical setting recently, which involves a noninvasive measurement of regional cerebral blood oxygenation over the frontal

? Did
You Know

The brain is particularly susceptible to rapid ischemic injury because of its high oxygen and glucose consumption, inability to store substrate, and inability to dispose of toxic metabolites.

cortices bilaterally. Oxygenation is given as a percentage, reflecting the contribution of both arterial (25%) and venous (75%) blood (6).

VI. Cerebral Protection

A. Ischemic and Reperfusion

Because of its high oxygen and glucose consumption, inability to store substrate, and inability to dispose of toxic metabolites, the brain is especially susceptible to rapid ischemic injury. With the accumulation of intracellular calcium under these ischemic conditions, neuronal damage quickly occurs and is compounded by the accumulation of lactic acid. Global ischemia, as is seen in conditions such as cardiac arrest, is responsive to interventions that restore total cerebral perfusion and oxygen-carrying capacity, such as cardiopulmonary resuscitation or red blood cell transfusion. Focal ischemia, on the other hand, is usually due to a regional insult, such as an embolus or intentional or unintentional arterial disruption. Treatment must be focused on restoring perfusion to the region in question. In cases of focal ischemia, a penumbra of salvageable tissue (watershed) usually surrounds the area that is damaged. Efforts must also be directed at "saving" this tissue, which is being supplied by some degree to collateral circulation. Much of the research being performed in *cerebral protection* today deals with this concept of "saving the penumbra." Practical methods include augmentation of CPP and reducing brain edema in the acute setting (see below). Another area under heavy study is that of reperfusion and "reperfusion injury," in which reperfusion of previously ischemic brain tissue can actually worsen neurologic outcomes largely due to the production of free radicals derived from oxygen and mediators of inflammation.

B. Hypothermia

Research into the cerebroprotective effects of *hypothermia* in humans has been largely disappointing, despite some encouraging animal studies. Theoretically, hypothermia should be extremely protective to the brain and spinal cord, as it lowers the $CMRO_2$ for the CNS to a much greater extent than anesthetics would. Although anesthetics can cause an isoelectric EEG (electrical silence), reducing the brain's metabolic activity by up to 60%, hypothermia can do far more by reducing even the brain's homeostatic (e.g., mitochondrial) need for oxygen, which is required for basic neuronal survival. Despite this, mild to moderate reductions in core temperature in the face of cerebral ischemia have not yielded protective results in human studies and have been associated with worsened immunologic and clotting function (7).

C. Medical Therapy for Cerebral Protection

Similar to hypothermia, medical therapy for *cerebral protection* in its application to humans has been difficult to ascertain. Anesthetics, especially barbiturates, have been widely used in an attempt to lessen the burden of ischemia on neurons. Nearly all anesthetics (notable exceptions being ketamine and etomidate in low doses) can lower $CMRO_2$ and theoretically protect the brain. But only barbiturates have been shown in humans to provide some protection from focal (not global) ischemia. No agents have been definitively shown to provide protection from global ischemia. Nimodipine, a calcium channel blocker, is frequently used in the setting of subarachnoid hemorrhage. It may have the benefit in neurologic protection during brain ischemia, although its protective mechanism remains elusive. Within 8 hours of acute spinal cord injury, methylprednisolone (a steroid) has been used to limit the degree of secondary injury due to edema, although controversy still surrounds this technique. Other more experimental agents, such as lidocaine, tirilazad (steroid), magnesium, dexmedetomidine (α_2 agonist), and vitamin E (antioxidant) have been used in various ischemic settings, all with mixed results on neurologic protection and outcomes.

D. Glucose and Cerebral Ischemia

As mentioned previously, ischemia is rapidly detrimental to the nervous system not only because of oxygen starvation, but also because glucose is the only substrate that can be aerobically metabolized by the brain under normal conditions. Glucose is not stored in the nervous system, so when glucose is absent due to limited or absent cerebral circulation, adenosine triphosphate is no longer available to neurons and cellular injury quickly ensues. Cerebral glucose consumption (5 mg/100 g/min), on a time scale, mimics $CMRO_2$, so hypoxemia and hypoglycemia are roughly equally detrimental to the brain. With cerebral ischemia and hypoglycemia, lactate is metabolized to some extent in the brain, but with much less efficacy than glucose. Hyperglycemia (serum blood glucose >180 mg/dL) in the setting of cerebral ischemia has also been shown to worsen neurologic outcomes, presumably by worsening cerebral acidosis in an anaerobic setting in which glucose is converted to lactic acid (8).

E. A Practical Approach

"True" cerebral protection is hard to achieve or to prove, but practically speaking, certain techniques are commonly used for their possible benefit. Inhaled and intravenous anesthetics are generally "protective," based on their known effect on $CMRO_2$. For operations in which there is planned regional ischemia (e.g., temporary clipping of cerebral vessels during aneurysm surgery), propofol given in a large bolus (1 to 2 mg/kg) followed by a high-dose infusion (150 µg/kg/min) is often used and titrated to induce burst suppression on the EEG *prior* to the planned ischemia (ischemic preconditioning). In cardiac or neurologic surgeries in which circulatory arrest is planned (e.g., aortic arch repair, giant basilar aneurysm clipping), deep hypothermia (12 to 18°C) has been instituted to "protect" the nervous system with seemingly great success. Another example of practical neurologic protection involves the placement of a lumbar CSF drain prior to thoracoabdominal aortic repair, used to lower CSF pressure and ostensibly maintain spinal cord perfusion when radicular arteries originating from the aorta are at surgical risk.

VII. Anesthetic Management

A. Preoperative Evaluation

The preoperative evaluation of the neurosurgical patient is of paramount importance in ensuring a safe and successful anesthetic. For patients with intracranial mass lesions, the most important fact to ascertain is the presence and extent of intracranial hypertension, or elevated ICP, and this should be assumed until information proves otherwise. This information can be obtained most readily from the history and physical examination, computed tomography (CT) and magnetic resonance imaging (MRI) scans, and ICP measurements (if available). Patients with elevated ICP may complain of headaches, dizziness, visual or gait disturbances, nausea or vomiting, and seizures. On physical examination, such patients may exhibit abnormalities such as papilledema, loss of strength or sensation, and cranial nerve dysfunction. CT or MRI of the brain are generally most helpful in quantifying the degree of

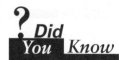

Glucose is the only substrate that can be aerobically metabolized by the brain under normal conditions.

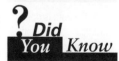

The reason cellular injury ensues more quickly in the nervous tissue is because glucose is not stored in the nervous system, so when glucose is absent due to limited or absent cerebral circulation, adenosine triphosphate is no longer available to neurons and cellular injury quickly ensues.

? Did You Know

Hyperglycemia (serum blood glucose >180 mg/dL) in the setting of cerebral ischemia has also been shown to worsen neurologic outcomes, presumably by worsening cerebral acidosis in an anaerobic setting in which glucose is converted to lactic acid.

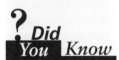

ICP derangement, with slit ventricles and a midline shift >5 mm indicating advanced pathology. Lastly, a careful evaluation of laboratory values may demonstrate electrolyte disturbances, which can be due to pituitary pathology (e.g., *syndrome of inappropriate antidiuretic hormone [SIADH] secretion*), diuretics, or anticonvulsants being taken by the patient.

In patients with elevated ICP, sedative or anxiolytic premedication must be carefully titrated or avoided completely. Benzodiazepines and opioids, even in small doses, can depress respiration, leading to elevated $PaCO_2$ and subsequent brain herniation. On the other hand, steroids (e.g., dexamethasone) and anticonvulsants should be continued preoperatively.

Preoperative evaluation of patients presenting for spine surgery, especially in the acute setting, should focus on (a) the level of injury, (b) the degree of neurologic impairment (complete vs. incomplete), (c) the timing of injury (less or more than 8 hours), (d) the complete neurologic examination, (e) current hemodynamic conditions, and (f) the airway examination. Carefully planning endotracheal intubation and subsequent hemodynamic management of these patients is vital. Advanced airway techniques (e.g., awake fiberoptic intubation) and critical blood or fluid management with concomitant vasopressor use (e.g., during spinal shock) may be required.

B. Induction of Anesthesia and Airway Management

Proper induction of anesthesia and airway management are critically important in neuroanesthesia, especially in those patients who have elevated ICP and unsecured aneurysm or cervical spinal cord injury. Elevated ICP demands constant attention during induction and intubation; ICP must be controlled, while CPP must be maintained. To that end, the induction of patients with elevated ICP should be slow and controlled, with constant attention to the blood pressure throughout the process. In many cases, preinduction arterial catheterization, osmotic diuresis, and CSF drainage are helpful. Patients with elevated ICP should receive a generous dose of opioid and intravenous lidocaine (1.5 mg/kg) prior to the induction drug to blunt the sympathetic response to laryngoscopy, at the same time maintaining normo- to hyperventilation to ensure eucapnia. Following induction and muscle relaxation, hyperventilation by mask should be performed in anticipation of the period of apnea that will accompany the intubation attempt. During intubation, strict control of blood pressure is important, as a rapid increase in arterial blood pressure will worsen ICP, while hypotension and decreased CPP would also be detrimental. In the case of a cervical spinal cord injury, maintenance of MAP is important during induction, while the actual performance of intubation may require more complex techniques (e.g., awake fiberoptic intubation, midline stabilization, etc.) to ensure that the spinal cord is not further compromised.

C. Maintenance of Anesthesia

The maintenance of anesthesia in neurosurgical patients requires regimens that vary depending on the hemodynamic and monitoring goals for that procedure. Generally speaking, for intracranial surgeries, ICP control is paramount until the dura is opened. To this end, once Mayfield fixation of the head and positioning are safely completed, mannitol (0.5 to 1.5 g/kg) is administered, as are steroids (e.g., dexamethasone 10 to 20 mg) and, in some cases, a prophylactic anticonvulsant. Anesthetic regimen depends on the ICP and whether neuromonitoring is being employed. For patients with elevated ICP, volatile anesthetics are often limited to 0.5 minimum alveolar concentration (MAC) to minimize the degree of cerebral vasodilation and inhibition of autoregulation that they cause. This is supplemented with intravenous agents such as propofol or opioid by infusion. This regimen works well in neuromonitoring cases as well, where >0.5 MAC of volatile agent may interfere with SSEP and MEP monitoring (MEP is more sensitive than SSEP). Muscle relaxants are generally used, unless they are limited by the MEP monitoring. Nitrous oxide is generally avoided because of its mild vasodilating effects, potential for expanding pneumocephalus, and unfavorable effects on neuromonitoring. Throughout the procedure, CPP must be maintained (often requiring a vasopressor). If autoregulation is greatly inhibited due to the disease process or the anesthetic, CBF will be directly dependent on MAP (or CPP). In cases of acute spinal cord injury, many of the same principles apply regarding maintenance of anesthesia, as spinal cord perfusion (especially in cervical spine surgery) and the ability to perform neuromonitoring are of great concern.

D. Ventilation Management

Ventilatory management of patients undergoing neurosurgery is also a key consideration. For patients undergoing an intracranial procedure, tidal volume should be maintained at 6 to 8 mL/kg (i.e., lung-protective strategy) to minimize potential inflammatory injury to the lungs, with peak pressures kept at <40 cm H_2O. These principles hold especially true for patients with subarachnoid hemorrhage, who may already exhibit acute lung injury or adult respiratory distress syndrome. Positive end-expiratory pressure (PEEP) should be avoided unless needed to improve oxygenation, as it increases intrathoracic pressure and may impede cerebral venous drainage. Positive pressure ventilation is generally used for neurosurgical procedures, as it allows direct control of $PaCO_2$. It is especially beneficial during sitting craniotomies, where negative intrathoracic pressure that would occur during a spontaneous breath may contribute to the development of venous air embolism.

E. Fluids and Electrolytes

For many years, the teaching of fluid maintenance during craniotomy was to keep the patient "dry," so as to minimize the amount of reactive cerebral edema both during the surgery and postoperatively. This is generally not considered optimal, as it is now known that the primary goal of fluid management in these cases should be to maintain cerebral perfusion, which is a more important consideration and will actually lessen cerebral edema. Hence, the goal of fluid management should be to keep the patient euvolemic at all times. Isotonic solutions should always be used (e.g., 0.9% normal saline), as hypotonic solutions (e.g., 0.45% half normal saline) in greater amounts can contribute to cerebral edema. Glucose-containing solutions are avoided, as hyperglycemia is detrimental to cerebral metabolism (see above), and because glucose is quickly metabolized and not osmotically active, leaving hypotonic free water, which can worsen edema.

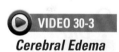

VIDEO 30-3
Cerebral Edema

Depending on patient comorbidities and length of the surgery, electrolyte derangements may be common and require close monitoring. Certainly, patients with pre- or intraoperative SIADH or *diabetes insipidus (DI)* will require careful monitoring of electrolytes. Hypertonic saline (3%) supplementation (given slowly to prevent central pontine myelinolysis) may also be needed. *Mannitol*, especially at large doses, can cause mild electrolyte derangements, which are generally short lived (e.g., hyponatremia, hyperkalemia). These should be monitored as well. Given in large amounts, 0.9% normal saline can cause hyperchloremic metabolic acidosis, and care should be taken to avoid this.

F. Transfusion Therapy

The transfusion of blood and blood products is often needed during neurosurgical procedures. Preoperatively, coagulation studies should be noted. Anticoagulants should be discontinued in consultation with the physician prescribing anticoagulation. Neurosurgical patients having nonemergency surgery should have a platelet count >100,000 mm^3. Red blood cells that have been typed and crossed should be available for most craniotomies, especially for neurovascular procedures (e.g., aneurysm clipping, arteriovenous malformation [AVM] resection) or for resection of tumors that invade the cranial sinuses. Coagulopathies may develop with the release of brain tissue thromboplastin. These should be treated with fresh frozen plasma, platelets, or cryoprecipitate as needed. Complex spine surgery (especially with planned osteotomies or due to tumor) is usually associated with more profound blood loss and transfusion therapy. In these cases, multiple units of blood products should be immediately available and close, repetitive monitoring of the hemoglobin level and coagulation studies should be performed.

G. Glucose Management

As discussed previously, glucose management is very important in neurosurgical cases, with the desire to avoid both hypo- and hyperglycemia. Some have advocated for "tight glucose control," in which the range of acceptable serum glucose perioperatively is very narrow (e.g., 90 to 120 mg/dL) and tightly controlled with insulin. Others disagree with such intensive glucose control, arguing that the incidence of hypoglycemia is increased with such a strategy. In any case, most neuroanesthesiologists agree that serum glucose during neurosurgical procedures should be maintained in the 90 to 180 mg/dL range. For hyperglycemia exceeding this range, regular insulin should be readily available and can be given intravenously as a bolus with or without an infusion. In these cases, monitoring of serum glucose must be frequent enough to capture episodes of hypoglycemia. In cases of hypoglycemia, dextrose (e.g., dextrose 50% in water) should be administered in 20 to 50 mL doses depending on the degree of hypoglycemia.

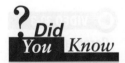

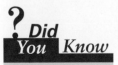

H. Emergence

Emergence from anesthesia after neurosurgical procedures requires meticulous attention to maintaining stable hemodynamic and ventilatory parameters, yet ensuring a patient is sufficiently responsive as to allow neurologic examination immediately after the operation. Postcraniotomy hypertension is a well-described, albeit poorly understood, phenomenon, but can certainly be detrimental as it may increase cerebral bleeding from the resection bed and worsen cerebral edema. Careful analgesia (so as not to obtund the patient postoperatively) is helpful in controlling this hypertension, but usually antihypertensive medications are required as well (e.g., labetalol, nicardipine). Patients emerging from cerebral AVM resection are particularly vulnerable because the resection bed is more likely to bleed. Patients having undergone posterior fossa surgery, who may also have brainstem compromise, may emerge more slowly and the time to safe extubation may be prolonged. Coughing on emergence should be avoided for all patients because it increases the risk of bleeding and elevation in ICP. A low-dose opioid infusion or intravenous lidocaine may be helpful in this regard. Likewise, postoperative nausea and vomiting should be prophylactically treated in these cases for the same reasons.

VIII. Common Surgical Procedures

A. Surgery for Tumors

Neurosurgery is commonly performed to remove tumors, both benign and malignant, that emanate from or spread to the CNS or PNS. Common primary tumors include meningiomas, astrocytomas, glioblastomas, schwannomas, and oligodendrogliomas, whereas metastatic tumors may arise from various primary sites (e.g., lung, breast, skin). Independent of their histology, the morbidity of brain tumors is associated with their size, rate of growth, and proximity to or invasion of nearby structures. Patients with dangerously elevated ICP preoperatively may requiring preoperative CSF drainage and intravenous glucocorticoids. Generally speaking, surgery for intracranial tumors can be safely accomplished with the induction and maintenance regimen mentioned above, as well as normo- or hyperventilation and adequate vascular access (usually two peripheral intravenous catheters and an arterial catheter). ICP and CPP are of great concern for these cases. An arterial catheter is very helpful in monitoring CPP closely while also allowing the titration of $PaCO_2$ (by revealing its gradient with end-tidal carbon dioxide via arterial blood gas measurement). Usually, patients are extubated in the operating room at the conclusion of the case.

B. Pituitary Surgery

Although elevated ICP is of great importance for supratentorial and infratentorial masses, it is not usually a grave concern in pituitary surgery, as the sellar space usually has room to accommodate most tumors. Pituitary surgery is usually performed endoscopically and transnasally. Anesthetic concerns for pituitary surgery include optic chiasm compression (leading to cranial nerve III compression and classically a bitemporal hemianopsia), acromegaly, electrolyte and fluid disturbances caused by SIADH or DI, and inadvertent surgical trespass into the cavernous sinus or internal carotid artery. Patients with a sellar mass (usually a pituitary adenoma or a craniopharyngioma) may exhibit visual field defects. It is important to differentiate between organic and anesthetic causes of visual problems after surgery. Growth hormone–secreting tumors can commonly cause acromegaly, which is vitally important to the anesthesiologist as airway and hemodynamic management can be much more difficult. Despite an adequate oral opening, acromegalic patients tend to have an abundance of pharyngeal soft tissue and a small glottic opening, which may make mask ventilation and intubation challenging and may require a smaller-sized endotracheal tube and awake fiberoptic intubation. Furthermore, long-standing acromegalics are prone to cardiac rhythm disturbances and cardiomyopathies, and caution with cardiac depressant medications is warranted.

SIADH is common with sellar tumors due to compression of the posterior pituitary and an oversecretion of antidiuretic hormone (ADH), which may lead to intravascular volume overload and hyponatremia. Extracellular body water is usually normal, and edema or hypertension are usually not seen. Treatment of perioperative SIADH involves judicious water restriction, removing the underlying cause (the tumor), and demeclocycline (which is a long-acting inhibitor of ADH, but less helpful in the acute setting). Perioperatively, central DI is also occasionally seen (due to a lack of ADH secretion), the hallmark being a large, dilute urine output. Postoperative DI is usually short lived and can be treated with fluid restriction. Rarely is exogenous desmopressin needed.

Because accidental surgical entry into the cavernous sinus or internal carotid artery is a potential, albeit infrequent, complication of pituitary surgery, two intravenous catheters and an arterial catheter are recommended. Intraoperative hyperventilation is generally not used in pituitary surgery and may make the sellar structures more difficult to access endoscopically. Similarly, a lumbar subarachnoid catheter is sometimes placed before or after pituitary surgery, both to inject small amounts of sterile saline to facilitate surgical exposure and to drain CSF postoperatively to decrease CSF pressure where a dural sealant or fat graft has been used.

C. Cerebral Aneurysm Surgery and Endovascular Treatment

Anesthesia for *cerebral aneurysm* clipping requires stable blood pressure so as not to rupture the aneurysm prior to exposure, to maintain CPP, and to have a plan in place in the event of intraoperative rupture. The maintenance regimen should allow neuromonitoring that is used to detect regional ischemia. During exposure of the aneurysm, burst suppression on the EEG is often sought (Fig. 30-7) to decrease the impending ischemic burden on the brain from temporary occlusion of large cerebral vessels. Additional vasopressor may be required during this time. Prior to direct clipping of the aneurysmal neck, the surgeon may place temporary clips to "soften" the neck and make it more amenable to direct clipping while minimizing the chances of rupture. Alternatively, when temporary clips are anatomically difficult to place, adenosine 0.3 to 0.4 mg/kg may be safely given as a bolus to cause transient circulatory arrest and profound hypotension, allowing safe permanent clip application (9).

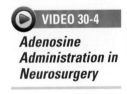

VIDEO 30-4

Adenosine Administration in Neurosurgery

Inadvertent rupture is possible during dissection around the aneurysm. The plan for this must include the availability of blood products and adenosine for rescue. Thus, large bore intravenous access is required for these cases and central venous access is recommended. Arterial catheters are routinely used for aneurysm surgery.

The endovascular treatment of aneurysms involves femoral arterial access and coils deployed to the aneurysmal sac to cause thrombosis and eventual obliteration of the aneurysm. General anesthesia is used and movement should be prevented. An arterial catheter is needed to monitor the blood pressure closely and to obtain blood samples for coagulation measurements at repeated intervals, as heparin is given periodically. The anesthesiologist should

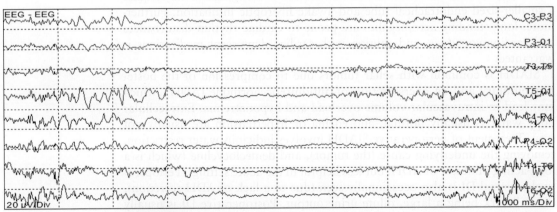

Figure 30-7   Burst-suppression electroencephalogram. Note the "burst" of electrical activity, followed by a period of "suppression," followed again by a "burst."

communicate very closely with the interventionalist throughout the procedure, as any extravasation of dye into the brain parenchyma may be indicative vascular rupture. Coils may embolize to other parts of the brain. Thus, prompt neurologic examination at the procedure's conclusion is important.

D. Arteriovenous Malformations

Cerebral AVMs are congenital abnormalities in which a plexus of arteries and "arterialized" veins are bunched together and may lead to cerebral hemorrhage, headaches, or seizures, usually between the ages of 10 and 40 years. These lesions may be embolized in the interventional radiology suite (preoperatively or curatively), radiated, or surgically removed. More than in any other intracranial neurosurgical procedure, vascular access is of great importance and a central venous catheter is highly recommended. The greatest risk of AVM resection is bleeding, both intraoperatively and postoperatively, and strict control of blood pressure is required to maintain CPP without worsening blood loss from the resection bed. Blood products should be immediately available, and vasodilators are very often needed, especially at emergence. The phenomenon of normal perfusion pressure breakthrough is a type of autoregulatory inhibition caused by the AVM and affecting the surrounding "normal" brain, in which previously normal cerebral vessels are maximally vasodilated due to long-standing "steal" caused by the AVM. After the AVM has been resected, these "vasoparalyzed" vessels are unable to constrict, leading to cerebral hyperemia, cerebral congestion, headache, and possibly worsened postoperative bleeding. Neuromonitoring is increasingly being used for cerebral AVM resections. Arterial catheterization and careful induction and intubation, as described with cerebral aneurysms, are standard.

 VIDEO 30-5
Indocyanine Green in Neurosurgery

E. Carotid Surgery

Carotid endarterectomy to remove carotid plaque that is ≥70% occlusive is performed either awake (regional technique) or asleep (general anesthesia), with neither technique proven to be superior in terms of neurologic outcome. Awake carotid surgery usually involves a superficial and sometimes deep cervical plexus block, along with low-dose analgesia and sedation (e.g., remifentanil, propofol), while ensuring that the patient is responsive to commands and able to perform manual tasks on the contralateral side. Asleep carotid surgery employs general endotracheal anesthesia. Frequently some form of neuromonitoring is used (e.g., EEG, SSEPs, cerebral oximetry), or the measurement of carotid stump pressure is performed (>50 mm Hg is desirable) to ensure adequate CBF during cross-clamping. In either case, arterial blood pressure monitoring is preferred, as operative morbidity is generally due to neurologic complications, while mortality is usually due to cardiac complications, and blood pressure control is critical. During manipulation of the carotid baroreceptor, bradycardia is not uncommon, and the surgeon may infiltrate the carotid sinus with lidocaine to prevent this response. Surgical denervation of the carotid baroreceptor causes hypertension and tachycardia upon emergence, which must be tightly controlled. Because cerebral vessels distal to the carotid have been maximally vasodilated for a long period of time, autoregulation is not intact and a "steal" phenomenon can occur in which cerebral hyperemia and bleeding can potentially occur. Beta-blockers are helpful in this regard. Lastly, the anesthesiologist must be keenly aware of the potential for a postoperative neck hematoma, which may quickly compromise the airway. Immediate intubation, which may be more difficult, and surgical exploration of the wound is required.

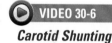 **VIDEO 30-6**
Carotid Shunting

VIDEO 30-7
Carotid Sinus Stimulation

F. Epilepsy Surgery and Awake Craniotomy

Surgery for intractable epilepsy that is not responsive to medical management requires a keen understanding of the pharmacologic effects of both anesthetics and anticonvulsants. Anticonvulsants taken by the patient can induce liver enzymes to a great extent and generally cause a very high metabolism of muscle relaxants and opioids. This leads to a "resistance" to the effects of these drugs and the need for higher dosages. On the other hand, anesthetics have very mixed and variable excitatory and inhibitory effects on seizure activity, and if used improperly can be detrimental to seizure focus mapping. Generally speaking, benzodiazepines should be avoided when electrocorticography (ECoG) is planned. Induction of anesthesia with propofol, muscle relaxant, and opioid is acceptable. During maintenance of anesthesia and prior to ECoG, any anesthetic regimen that allows craniotomy is used, but 30 minutes prior to ECoG initiation, propofol infusion should be stopped and potent volatile anesthetic held to a minimum or stopped as well. To prevent awareness, scopolamine, nitrous oxide, and high-dose opioid infusion can be used with very little adverse effect on ECoG. In any case, the patient should be counseled about the possibility of intraoperative awareness. In some cases, methohexital or etomidate can be used to elicit seizure activity. Once ECoG is complete, a "routine" general anesthetic can be resumed during the resection.

Awake craniotomy has gained popularity in some institutions and is used in cases in which a cranial lesion lies adjacent to either "eloquent," motor, or sensory cortex. The advantage of awake craniotomy lies in its ability to allow speech, motor, or sensory mapping in real time, hence facilitating a subtotal resection of the tumor and avoiding the loss of these functions. The anesthesiologist must be attentive to the patient's analgesic, ventilatory, and emotional needs. Thus, constant communication with the patient is of paramount importance. Generally, an arterial catheter is placed and very light sedation or analgesia (e.g., propofol, remifentanil, dexmedetomidine) is used. A selective scalp nerve block may be performed preoperatively, either unilaterally or bilaterally, blocking the six nerves on each side that innervate the scalp and dura mater. The brain itself has no pain or sensory receptors, so only the scalp and dura require anesthesia.

IX. Anesthesia and Traumatic Brain Injury

A. Overview of Traumatic Brain Injury

Traumatic brain injury is often associated with other trauma (e.g., thoracic, abdominal, and orthopedic injuries) and is a common cause of death and disability in young people. Death following traumatic brain injury is often associated with secondary insults, which emergency and anesthetic management are designed to minimize. Patients presenting with traumatic brain injury are graded according to the *Glasgow coma scale (GCS)* on presentation (score of 3 to 15) and are intubated when GCS is 8 or less, as this corresponds to 35% mortality (Table 30-2). Noncontrast CT scan that shows midline shift >5 mm or absent ventricles should also lead to immediate intubation, as ICP is very high in these cases and ventilation must be controlled. ICP monitoring is frequently used in these cases and can be instituted in the emergency department by an external ventricular drain, where mannitol, hyperventilation, and propofol are used to control elevated ICP. Operative management is normally indicated for depressed skull fractures and expanding brain bleeding, including subdural and epidural hematomas.

Table 30-2	Glasgow Coma Scale					
	1	**2**	**3**	**4**	**5**	**6**
Eye	Does not open	Opens to painful stimulus	Opens to voice	Opens spontaneously	NA	NA
Verbal	Makes no sound	Incomprehensible sound	Inappropriate words	Disoriented, confused	Normal speech	NA
Motor	Makes no movement	Extension to painful stimulus (decerebrate movement)	Flexion to painful stimulus (decorticate movement)	Withdrawal to painful stimulus	Localizes to painful stimulus	Follows commands

NA, not applicable.
Note that the lowest attainable score is 3 and the highest is 15.

B. Anesthetic Management

Patients presenting with traumatic brain injury are assumed to have concomitant cervical spine injury, and the plan for intubation must take this into account. Hypoxemia is common, which may be further exacerbated by pulmonary injury. Induction doses of anesthetics must be tailored so as to avoid worsening systemic hypotension. Succinylcholine is controversial in the face of a closed head injury, as it may raise ICP transiently. But most anesthesiologists would use it to facilitate securing the airway in a rapid and predictable fashion. Nasal intubation is contraindicated if a basilar skull fracture is present or suspected. Once the airway is secured, attention must be paid to hemodynamics, as systolic blood pressure <80 mm Hg is associated with a worse neurologic outcome. Fluid resuscitation and vasopressors are needed to ensure an adequate systemic and cerebral perfusion pressure. Intravascular access should include an arterial catheter and large-bore intravenous cannulae, if not a central venous line. Anesthetic maintenance hinges on a good understanding of ICP management (see above), with intravenous agents and inhalational agents used in balance to avoid excessive cerebral vasodilation. Additional mannitol may be given, but hyperventilation should not continue beyond 2 to 6 hours, as normalization of the pH in the CSF begins to occur and its effect is only to decrease cerebral perfusion. Of note, the release of brain tissue thromboplastin may lead to disseminated intravascular coagulation, and coagulopathy must be aggressively sought and treated. Likewise, neurogenic pulmonary edema may be present, and a "lung-protective strategy" using PEEP and low tidal volumes may be needed to maintain oxygenation. Extubation at the conclusion of surgery depends on the degree of ICP elevation and the severity of injury, with most of these patients being admitted to the neurointensive care unit intubated and sedated.

X. Anesthesia for Spine Trauma and Complex Spine Surgery

A. Spinal Cord Injury

Acute spinal cord injury often necessitates emergency surgery to stabilize the spinal column and prevent secondary injury. Spinal cord injuries, like traumatic brain injuries, often involve young people, and may be due to motor vehicle accidents, falls, violence, or sports-related accidents. Cervical spine injuries are most common, as this is the most mobile part of the spine, followed by thoracic and lumbar injuries. Incomplete tetraplegia (C3-5) is the most common neurologic outcome, followed by complete paraplegia (T1 and below), complete tetraplegia, and incomplete paraplegia. Cervical injuries are the most devastating from a neurologic perspective, as high cervical injuries may impair vital respiratory function (C3-5) and cardiac accelerator function (T1-5), necessitating permanent tracheotomy and ventilator support. Following acute spinal cord injury, spinal cord autoregulation is impaired and "spinal shock" may be seen, characterized by flaccid paralysis and decreased spinal cord perfusion, lasting 24 hours. During this time, it is critical to prevent secondary injury by providing aggressive hemodynamic support.

B. Comorbid Injuries

Up to 42% of patients presenting with acute spinal cord injury may also have a concomitant injury. Life-threatening injuries must be addressed, while ensuring that spinal alignment is maintained to avoid adding secondary injury to the spinal cord.

C. Initial Management

Patients presenting with acute spinal cord injury must be immediately evaluated for compromised ventilatory and hemodynamic function. Airway management in cervical spinal injury focuses on maintaining in-line stabilization throughout the intubation process, and may require the use of fiberoptic intubation. In a stable patient, radiographic studies are helpful in assessing the degree of cervical injury and options for intubation. Succinylcholine is safe in the initial 24 hours following spinal cord injury. Extrajunctional nicotinic receptors, which may cause a hyperkalemic response, have not yet fully developed. Fluid or blood product resuscitation and vasopressors or inotropes are often needed to support the blood pressure, which is important both from a systemic standpoint and to prevent secondary injury in the spinal cord due to ischemia and worsening edema due to cellular dysfunction. Arterial blood pressure monitoring and large-bore intravenous access (preferably central venous access) are required. Other strategies to protect the spinal cord, such as corticosteroids, naloxone, or hypothermia, may be instituted at this time, but convincing data for these therapies are lacking. Most anesthesiologists will, however, maintain the mean arterial pressure above 85 mm Hg to ensure adequate spinal cord perfusion (recommended for at least 7 days from the date of injury).

D. Intraoperative Management

Anesthetic choice during maintenance of anesthesia for spinal cord injury should focus on two key considerations: maintaining blood pressure (mean >85 mm Hg) and allowing for intraoperative neuromonitoring (SSEPs, MEPs, EMG). Complex spine surgery, which often involves multiple level fusions and osteotomies, should also take into account the real possibility of significant (sometimes multiple blood volumes) surgical bleeding and the need for postoperative mechanical ventilation in light of massive transfusion. Adequate intravascular access is vitally important. Measurements of arterial blood gas, coagulation parameters, and hemoglobin levels should be performed frequently. Close communication with the surgeon is important. In noninfectious, nontumor cases, intraoperative cell salvage can be quite helpful in reducing the total amount of allogeneic blood transfused. Other blood-sparing techniques, such as acute normovolemic hemodilution and deliberate hypotension, have largely fallen out of favor, due to the known harmful effects of anemia and hypotension on the neurologic and cardiovascular systems.

E. Complications of Anesthesia for Spine Surgery

Fortunately, complications specifically related to anesthesia for spine surgery are rare, but they are often devastating when they occur. *Postoperative visual loss (POVL)* is one such complication, with an incidence of 0.3% after spine surgery (10). Most cases of POVL are thought to be due to posterior ischemic optic neuropathy, with central retinal artery occlusion and cortical blindness being much less common. Risk factors for POVL (associated but not necessarily causative) include hypotension, anemia, blood loss >1,000 mL, surgical duration >6 hours, and the prone position itself (leading to increased intraocular pressure). Ophthalmologic consultation should be immediately undertaken if this complication is suspected. Another complication of spine surgery in which anesthetic technique may be implicated is anterior spinal artery syndrome, which is caused by a sustained hypoperfusion of the anterior spinal artery and leads to motor weakness. Finally, deliberate hypotension, hypothermia, and hypovolemia may predispose spine surgery patients to the formation of deep venous thromboses (DVT) and subsequent pulmonary emboli (PE). Lumbar fusion is associated with an incidence of symptomatic DVT of up to 4%, with a 2% incidence of PE. Because prophylaxis with an anticoagulant is often impossible prior to spine surgery (for fear of worsening blood loss and formation of epidural hematoma), an inferior vena cava filter is often placed prior to these surgeries to minimize the chance of developing a significant PE.

References

1. Isley MR, Edmonds HL Jr, Stecker M. American Society of Neurophysiological Monitoring. Guidelines for intraoperative neuromonitoring using raw (analog or digital waveforms) and quantitative electroencephalography: A position statement by the American Society of Neurophysiological Monitoring. *J Clin Monit Comput.* 2009;23(6):369–390.
2. Sloan TB, Heyer EJ. Anesthesia for intraoperative neurophysiologic monitoring of the spinal cord. *J Clin Neurophysiol.* 2002;19(5):430–443.
3. Sutherland BA, Rabie T, Buchan AM. Laser Doppler flowmetry to measure changes in cerebral blood flow. *Methods Mol Biol.* 2014;1135:237–248.
4. Kalanuria A, Nyquist PA, Armonda RA, et al. Use of transcranial Doppler (TCD) ultrasound in the neurocritical care unit. *Neurosurg Clin North Am.* 2013;24(3):441–456.
5. Kitagawa R, Yokobori S, Mazzeo AT, et al. Microdialysis in the neurocritical care unit. *Neurosurg Clin North Am.* 2013;24(3):417–426.
6. Ghosh A, Elwell C, Smith M. Cerebral near-infrared spectroscopy in adults: A work in progress. *Anesth Analg.* 2012;115(6):1373–1383.
7. Todd MM, Hindman BJ, Clarke WR, et al. Intraoperative Hypothermia for Aneurysm Surgery Trial (IHAST) Investigators. Mild intraoperative hypothermia during surgery for intracranial aneurysm. *N Engl J Med.* 2005;352(2):135–145.
8. Pasternak JJ, McGregor DG, Schroeder DR, et al. IHAST Investigators. Hyperglycemia in patients undergoing cerebral aneurysm surgery: Its association with long-term gross neurologic and neuropsychological function. *Mayo Clin Proc.* 2008;83(4):406–417.
9. Bebawy JF, Gupta DK, Bendok BR, et al. Adenosine-induced flow arrest to facilitate intracranial aneurysm clip ligation: Dose-response data and safety profile. *Anesth Analg.* 2010;110(5):1406–1411.
10. American Society of Anesthesiologists Task Force on Perioperative Visual Loss. Practice advisory for perioperative visual loss associated with spine surgery: An updated report by the American Society of Anesthesiologists Task Force on Perioperative Visual Loss. *Anesthesiology.* 2012;116(2):274–285.

Questions

1. The blood supply to the cervical spinal cord originates from:
   A. The internal carotid arteries bilaterally
   B. The aortic arch
   C. The posterior Circle of Willis
   D. The artery of Adamkiewicz
   E. The external carotid arteries bilaterally

2. Cerebral perfusion pressure is calculated as the difference between:
   A. Cerebral blood flow and cerebral vascular resistance
   B. Mean arterial pressure and intracranial pressure
   C. Central venous pressure and intracranial pressure
   D. Systolic blood pressure and diastolic blood pressure
   E. Diastolic blood pressure and intracranial pressure

3. Autoregulation in the brain between a range of blood pressures is responsible for maintaining:
   A. Intracranial pressure
   B. Cerebral perfusion pressure
   C. Cerebrovascular resistance
   D. Cerebral blood flow
   E. Jugular venous pressure

4. Cerebral blood flow is directly controlled by all of the following physiologic parameters EXCEPT:
   A. pH
   B. $PaCO_2$
   C. PaO_2
   D. MAP
   E. $CMRO_2$

5. All of the following techniques are known to mitigate the effects of intracranial hypertension EXCEPT:
   A. Administration of mannitol
   B. Administration of hyperventilation
   C. Total intravenous anesthesia
   D. Administration of opioids
   E. Elevation of the head of the bed

6. Neuromuscular blocking agents may limit the success of which of the following neuromonitoring modalities?
   A. Somatosensory evoked potentials (SSEPs)
   B. Electroencephalography (EEG)
   C. Brainstem auditory evoked potentials (BAEPs)
   D. Visual evoked potentials (VEPs)
   E. Electromyography (EMG)

7. Cerebral protection for global ischemia in humans is known to occur with which of the following?
   A. Steroids
   B. Mild hypothermia
   C. Barbiturates
   D. Hyperglycemia
   E. None of the above

8. All of the following are important considerations for reducing morbidity and mortality after a traumatic brain injury EXCEPT:
   A. Maintaining a systolic blood pressure > 80 mm Hg
   B. Administering hyperventilation for 48 hours
   C. Ensuring adequate oxygenation
   D. Emergent intubation with a Glasgow coma scale (GCS) score < 8
   E. Administering mannitol for 24 hours

9. Acute cervical spine injury may cause all of the following EXCEPT:
   A. Hyperthermia
   B. Bradycardia
   C. Respiratory impairment
   D. Hypotension
   E. Flaccid paralysis

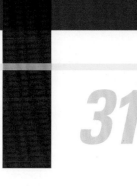

31

Obstetric Anesthesia

Melissa L. Pant
Barbara M. Scavone

I. Physiologic Changes of Pregnancy

Pregnancy induces many *physiologic changes*, most of which are adaptations to support blood flow and oxygen delivery to the fetus.

A. Hematologic Changes

Blood volume increases by 40% to approximately 100 mL/kg; plasma volume increases by 30% to 50% and red blood cell volume by 20% to 30%, causing a physiologic *anemia of pregnancy* (Table 31-1). Blood viscosity is decreased, allowing easier flow to the fetus. Normal hemoglobin range during pregnancy is 10.5 to 14 g/dL and is lowest in the second trimester (Table 31-2).

Pregnancy is a prothrombotic state, and pregnant patients carry a greater risk of venous thromboembolism. Production of all clotting factors, except factors XI and XIII, increase. Fibrinogen levels significantly increase and are normally >400 mg/dL in the third trimester. A secondary fibrinolysis occurs later in pregnancy, and coagulation changes resemble a state of compensated disseminated intravascular coagulation (DIC). Platelet count may decrease during pregnancy due to dilution as well as increased consumption. Gestational thrombocytopenia is common, occurring in 8% of pregnancies, and is not associated with an increased risk of neuraxial hematoma.

Mild leukocytosis is normal during pregnancy. However, pregnancy is an immunosuppressed state, and pregnant patients do not tolerate the physiologic effects of systemic infection well, and mortality from sepsis is increased. In general, autoimmune diseases improve during pregnancy due to relative immunosuppression.

B. Cardiovascular Changes

Due to increased blood volume, stroke volume, and heart rate, cardiac output increases up to 45% by the end of the first trimester. During labor, cardiac output increases by another 50%, up to 80% over prelabor values immediately postpartum. Cardiovascular changes resolve several days postpartum. Systemic vascular resistance decreases, sometimes causing a mild decrease in blood pressure. Pregnant patients are less responsive to vasopressors

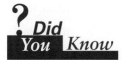

Did You Know

The anemia of pregnancy is caused by a disproportionate increase in plasma volume relative to red cell volume.

Table 31-1	Summary of Physiologic Changes of Pregnancy at Term	
Variable	Change	Amount
Plasma volume	↑	40–50%
Total blood volume	↑	25–40%
Hemoglobin	↓	11–12 g/dL
Fibrinogen	↑	100%
Serum cholinesterase activity	↓	20–30%
Systemic vascular resistance	↓	50%
Cardiac output	↑	30–50%
Systemic blood pressure	↓	Slight
Functional residual capacity	↓	20–30%
Minute ventilation	↑	50%
Alveolar ventilation	↑	70%
Functional residual capacity	↓	20%
Oxygen consumption	↑	20%
Carbon dioxide production	↑	35%
Arterial carbon dioxide tension	↓	10 mm Hg
Arterial oxygen tension	↑	10 mm Hg
Minimum alveolar concentration	↓	32–40%

Reprinted from Braveman FR, Scavone BM, Blessing ME, et al. Obstetrical anesthesia. In: Barash PG, Cullen BF, Stoelting RK, et al., eds. *Clinical Anesthesia*. 7th ed. Philadelphia: Wolters Kluwer Health; 2013:1144–1177, with permission.

Table 31-2	Normal Lab Values in Pregnant Patients			
Laboratory Value	Nonpregnant Female	First Trimester	Second Trimester	Third Trimester
Hemoglobin (g/dL)	12–16	11.5–14	9.7–15	9.5–15
Platelets ($\times 10^9$/L)	160–420	180–400	155–420	145–420
WBC ($\times 10^3$/mm^3)	3.5–9	6–14	5.5–15	6–17
Creatinine (mg/dL)	0.5–0.9	0.4–0.7	0.4–0.8	0.4–0.9
Fibrinogen (mg/dL)	230–490	245–500	290–540	370–620
pH	7.38–7.42			7.39–7.45
PCO$_2$ (mm Hg)[a]	38–42			25–33
Bicarbonate (mEq/L)	22–26			16–22
PO$_2$ (mm Hg)[a]	90–100			92–107

[a]Blood gas values are arterial.

and more sensitive to decreases in preload. After 20 weeks gestation, pregnant patients may experience *supine hypotension syndrome* when lying flat, because the gravid uterus can compress the IVC and decrease venous return. Therefore, LUD is the preferred position for pregnant patients over 20 weeks' gestation.

C. Respiratory Changes

Oxygen consumption increases by 20% to 50% and minute ventilation by 50% at term. Minute ventilation increases mainly due to an increase in tidal volume and to a lesser extent respiratory rate. This physiologic hyperventilation decreases arterial partial pressure of carbon dioxide ($PaCO_2$) levels to 28 to 32 mm Hg and may cause a slight increase in arterial partial pressure of oxygen (PaO_2) levels. Compensatory metabolic acidosis occurs, bicarbonate levels are normally 18 to 22 mEq/L, and pH only slightly increases (7.45). Vital capacity and closing volume remain the same, but expiratory reserve volume and functional residual capacity decrease, making the pregnant patient quick to desaturate during periods of apnea, in particular in the supine position. A rightward shift in the hemoglobin–oxygen dissociation curve occurs, facilitating oxygen transfer to the fetus.

D. Airway Changes

Mucosal edema and capillary engorgement occur as pregnancy progresses, and Mallampati class increases at term. The incidence of difficult mask ventilation and laryngoscopy also increases, with difficult or failed intubation occurring in one of 224 pregnant patients versus one of 2,500 in the general surgical population (1). A longer second stage of labor and preeclampsia are both associated with increased *airway edema*. Proper positioning and preoxygenation assume additional importance during induction of general anesthesia and intubation of pregnant versus nonpregnant patients (Fig. 31-1).

E. Gastrointestinal Changes

The gravid uterus causes *mechanical gastroesophageal sphincter dysfunction*. Progesterone decreases lower esophageal sphincter tone, predisposing pregnant patients to reflux of stomach contents into the oropharynx. In addition, the gravid uterus increases abdominal pressure and, thus, intragastric pressure, furthering reflux of stomach contents. Gastrin secretion by the placenta causes greater acidity of stomach contents. Finally, progesterone slows gastric emptying and gastrointestinal mobility. Pregnant women often have a gastric volume of over 25 mL with pH <2.5, both of which are associated with aspiration pneumonitis syndrome. Administration of a nonparticulate antacid is the only reliable way to change gastric content pH and possibly reduce the chance of aspiration pneumonitis syndrome should aspiration occur.

F. Neurologic and Musculoskeletal Changes

Minimum alveolar concentration (MAC) decreases by 40% during pregnancy, possibly due to elevated progesterone levels, and returns to baseline by 1 week postpartum. Pregnant women are also more sensitive to neuraxial local anesthetics and require lower doses than nonpregnant patients. Epidural space volume is decreased due to epidural vein engorgement, and cerebrospinal fluid (CSF) pH is decreased. Ligamentous relaxation occurs, and lumbar lordosis is accentuated, raising the intercristal line from L4-5 in nonpregnant patients to L3-4 in pregnant patients.

VIDEO 31-1

Left Uterine Displacement

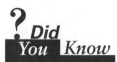
? *Did* You *Know*

Left uterine displacement should be used for pregnant patients over 20 weeks' gestation to prevent compression of the inferior vena cava by the gravid uterus.

? *Did* You *Know*

The normal arterial partial pressure of carbon dioxide during pregnancy is 28 to 32 mm Hg.

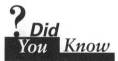
? *Did* You *Know*

The incidence of difficult mask ventilation and laryngoscopy is greater in pregnant patients than in the general surgical population.

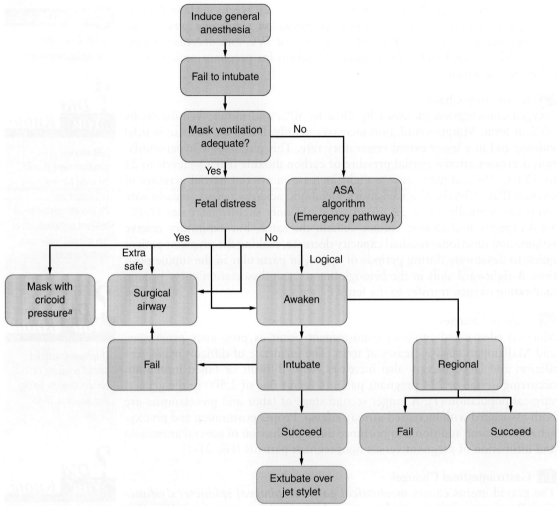

Figure 31-1 Management of the difficult airway in pregnancy with special reference to the presence or absence of fetal distress. When mask ventilation is not possible, the clinician is referred to the American Society of Anesthesiologists algorithm for the emergency airway management. [a]Conventional face mask or laryngeal mask airway. (From Braveman FR, Scavone BM, Blessing ME, et al. Obstetrical anesthesia. In: Barash PG, Cullen BF, Stoelting RK, et al., eds. *Clinical Anesthesia*. 7th ed. Philadelphia: Wolters Kluwer Health; 2013:1144–1177, with permission.)

G. Endocrine Changes
Glucose Control
Pregnancy is a diabetogenic state, due to human placental lactogen's anti-insulin effects. Routine screening for gestational diabetes is done via a carbohydrate load between 24 to 26 weeks. Women with gestational or pregestational diabetes are at greater risk for fetal macrosomia and pregnancy complications. Tight glucose control during labor is the standard of care for diabetic women, with goal blood sugar range between 80 to 110 mg/dL in order to avoid neonatal hypoglycemia.

Thyroid
Human chorionic gonadotropin is similar in structure to thyroid-stimulating hormone and causes thyroid hormone levels to increase during pregnancy.

Estrogen stimulates production of thyroid-binding globulin, allowing more thyroid hormone to circulate.

H. Renal and Hepatic Changes

Blood flow to the kidneys and renal autoregulation remains unchanged during pregnancy as long as blood pressure remains stable. Increased glomerular filtration rate and decreased creatinine occur due to increases in cardiac output, and serum creatinine over 0.8 is abnormal. Proteinuria is common, as is asymptomatic bacteriuria. Ureteral tone decreases and asymptomatic bacteriuria can lead to pyelonephritis. Therefore, urine is screened for infection during routine prenatal visits.

Hepatic blood flow is not altered during pregnancy. Elevated alkaline phosphatase levels are seen due to secretion by the placenta. Liver transaminase levels are unchanged. Plasma osmolality is lower, leading to tissue edema. Pseudocholinesterase levels decrease, without much clinical significance. Clotting factor production increases. Cholestasis of pregnancy can occur due to the effects of estrogen, and causes pruritus and an increased risk of stillbirth.

II. Uteroplacental and Fetal Circulation

The uterus receives 15% of the cardiac output at term; normal uterine blood flow is 700 to 900 mL/min. Uterine blood flow is derived from the uterine arteries and additionally via collaterals from the ovarian and cervical arteries. Uterine (and therefore placental and fetal) blood flow is directly proportional to uterine perfusion pressure (defined as the difference between uterine arterial pressure vs. uterine venous pressure), and inversely proportional to uterine artery vascular tone. The uterine vasculature is maximally vasodilated during pregnancy. A lack of uterine autoregulation makes blood flow proportional to perfusion pressure. Uterine vasculature maintains responsiveness to vasoconstrictors. Increases in uterine smooth muscle tone constrict uterine vessels, decreasing flow.

The fetus exchanges gases and nutrients with its mother via the placenta. Fetal placental villi containing fetal capillaries are bathed in maternal blood supplied by the spiral arteries, which are branches of the uterine arteries. A normal umbilical cord has three vessels: one vein containing oxygenated blood from the placenta and two arteries carrying deoxygenated blood and waste back to the placenta. A number of mechanisms of transport from mother to fetus and back exist, including simple diffusion (most common, due to fetal or maternal concentration gradient), transcellular transfer, and endocytosis and exocytosis. Oxygen and carbon dioxide exchange occurs via simple diffusion; higher maternal PaO_2 favors diffusion to the fetus, and fetal CO_2 is higher than maternal CO_2, favoring diffusion back to the mother.

Fetal hemoglobin has greater O_2 carrying capacity. The Bohr effect is more profound in the fetus because fetal hemoglobin encounters more hydrogen ions (H^+) in the fetus, which is relatively more acidotic than in the mother, and is more likely to release O_2 it is carrying to fetal tissues. *Fetal circulation* differs from adult circulation in that it bypasses the lungs (Fig. 31-2).

The majority of maternally administered drugs will be delivered to the fetus via the placenta. The fetal/maternal ratio describes the concentration of drug in the fetal umbilical vein versus maternal serum concentration. Nonionized, nonprotein bound, lipid-soluble drugs with molecular weights below 600 Da easily cross the placenta. Large, ionized, hydrophilic drugs are less likely to

? Did You Know

Oxygen and carbon dioxide exchange occurs via simple diffusion; higher maternal PaO_2 favors diffusion to the fetus, and fetal carbon dioxide is higher than maternal carbon dioxide, favoring diffusion back to the mother.

? Did You Know

Most anesthetic drugs cross the placenta, with the exception of paralyzing agents and glycopyrrolate. Heparin and insulin also do not cross the placenta.

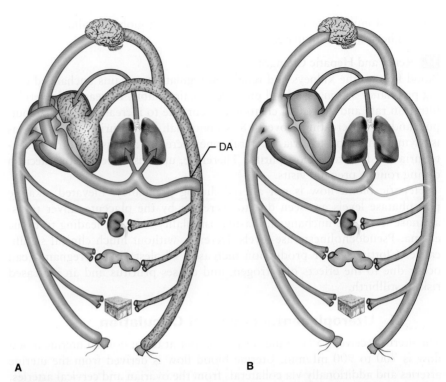

Figure 31-2 **A:** Schematic representation of the fetal circulation. Oxygenated blood leaves the placenta in the umbilical vein (*vessel without stippling*). Umbilical blood joins blood from the viscera (represented here by the kidney, gut, and skin) in the inferior vena cava. Approximately half of the inferior vena cava flow passes through the foramen ovale to the left atrium, where it mixes with a small amount of pulmonary venous blood. This relatively well-oxygenated blood (*light stippling*) supplies the heart and brain by way of the ascending aorta. The other half of the inferior vena cava stream mixes with superior vena cava blood and enters the right ventricle (blood in the right atrium and ventricle has little oxygen, which is denoted by *heavy stippling*). Because the pulmonary arterioles are constricted, most of the blood in the main pulmonary artery flows through the ductus arteriosus (DA) so the descending aorta's blood has less oxygen (*heavy stippling*) than does blood in the ascending aorta (*light stippling*). **B:** Schematic representation of the circulation in the normal newborn. After expansion of the lungs and ligation of the umbilical cord, pulmonary blood flow and left atrial and systemic arterial pressures increase. When left atrial pressure exceeds right atrial pressure, the foramen ovale closes so all inferior and superior vena cava blood leaves the right atrium, enters the right ventricle, and is pumped through the pulmonary artery toward the lung. With the increase in systemic arterial pressure and decrease in pulmonary artery pressure, flow through the ductus arteriosus becomes left to right, and the ductus constricts and closes. The course of circulation is the same as in the adult. (From Hall SC, Suresh S. Neonatal anesthesia. In: Barash PG, Cullen BF, Stoelting RK, et al., eds. *Clinical Anesthesia.* 7th ed. Philadelphia: Wolters Kluwer Health; 2013:1179, with permission.)

transfer. Most anesthetic drugs cross the placenta, with the exception of paralyzing agents and glycopyrrolate. Heparin and insulin also do not cross the placenta. Transient fetal or neonatal depression can be seen after administration of induction agents, anesthetic gases, opioids, and benzodiazepines. The long-term effects of general anesthetic agents on neonatal outcome are unknown. Theoretically, nitrous oxide can interfere with DNA synthesis via oxidation of vitamin B_{12}. However, in animal studies only prolonged (>24 hours) exposure to high-concentration nitrous oxide produces fetal loss.

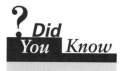

III. Pain Pathways in Labor, Anatomy of the Spine, and Neuraxial Analgesia and Anesthesia

Pain is transmitted via different means in different stages of labor. Pain during the first stage of labor, which commences with the beginning of regular contractions and cervical dilation and ends at complete cervical dilation, is transmitted via visceral afferent fibers entering the spinal cord from T10-L1. During the second stage, which begins with complete cervical dilation and ends with delivery of the fetus, additional pain is caused by stretching of vaginal and perineal tissues and is transmitted via sacral somatic fibers. The third stage of labor begins after delivery of the fetus and ends with delivery of the placenta, and pain during this stage is also transmitted via sacral somatic fibers.

The *spine* has 33 levels: 7 cervical, 12 thoracic, 5 lumbar, 5 sacral, and 4 coccygeal. Skin dermatomal levels correspond to the vertebral level at which their nerve roots enter (Fig. 31-3). The spinal cord is protected by the bony spine, ligaments, and layers of connective tissue and is bathed in CSF. The spinal cord is covered by three membranes, called the spinal meninges. The outermost layer is the dura mater, deep to the dura is the arachnoid, under the arachnoid layer lies CSF, and the pia mater is adherent to the spinal cord. The spinal cord extends from its inception off the brainstem through the foramen magnum and continues to L1 in most adults. About 10% of adults have

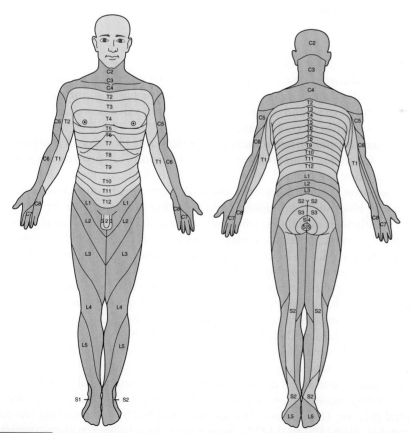

Figure 31-3 Human sensory dermatomes. (From Bernards CM, Hostetter LS. Epidural and spinal anesthesia. In: Barash PG, Cullen BF, Stoelting RK, et al., eds. *Clinical Anesthesia*. 7th ed. Philadelphia: Wolters Kluwer Health; 2013:905–933, with permission.)

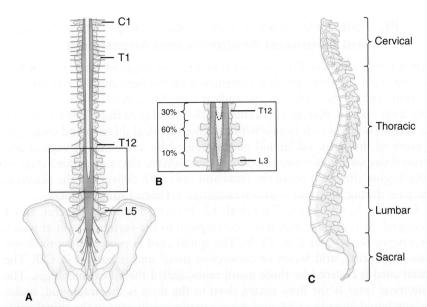

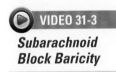

VIDEO 31-3

Subarachnoid Block Baricity

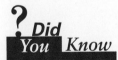

? Did You Know

The goal of avoiding excessive motor blockade, while still providing adequate analgesia, is commonly accomplished by administering low-concentration (0.0625% to 0.125% bupivacaine), high-volume, patient-controlled epidural anesthesia, with small amounts of opioid in the solutions.

spinal cords that terminate lower, at L3. It is therefore prudent to perform neuraxial procedures below this level.

The spinal cord terminates as the cauda equina and the dural sac extends to S2. The epidural space spans from the foramen magnum to the sacral hiatus. It is a potential space and contains nerve roots, fat, valveless veins, lymphatics, and spinal arteries (Figs. 31-4 and 31-5).

Neuraxially administered local anesthetics cause blockade of sympathetic, sensory, and motor input and, depending on the dose, can provide analgesia or complete anesthesia. Small, myelinated, rapidly firing, active nerve fibers are more sensitive to local anesthetic blockade than larger, unmyelinated fibers. Degree of blockade from highest to lowest after administration of neuraxial local anesthetic is as follows: temperature sensation, vasomotor tone, sensory, and finally motor. Spinal anesthesia occurs via direct action of local anesthetic on the spinal cord, and block level depends on several factors, of which baricity and dose are the most significant.

Epidural anesthesia occurs via local anesthetic action on nerve roots and, to a lesser extent, has a direct effect on the spinal cord, via diffusion of local anesthetic into the intrathecal space. Usually 1 to 2 mL of epidural local anesthetic is required per lumbar dermatomal level requiring blockade.

Neuraxial labor analgesia provides excellent pain relief without effects on fetal or labor outcomes, with the exception of slightly increasing the length of the first and second stages of labor and the risk of instrumented vaginal delivery (2). Avoiding excessive motor blockade, while still providing adequate analgesia, is ideal in labor. This goal is commonly accomplished by administering low concentration (0.0625% to 0.125% bupivacaine) high-volume, patient-controlled epidural anesthesia (PCEA), with small amounts of opioid in the solutions.

After history, physical examination, and determination that the patient is a candidate for neuraxial anesthesia (Table 31-3), preparation for placement of

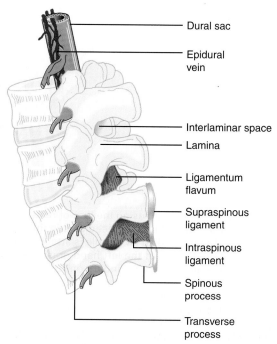

Figure 31-5 Detail of the lumbar spinal column and epidural space. Note that the epidural veins are largely restricted to the anterior and lateral epidural space. (From Bernards CM, Hostetter LS. Epidural and spinal anesthesia. In: Barash PG, Cullen BF, Stoelting RK, et al., eds. *Clinical Anesthesia*. 7th ed. Philadelphia: Wolters Kluwer Health; 2013:905–933, with permission.)

a neuraxial block begins. A functioning intravenous line, resuscitation equipment, and blood pressure and heart rate monitoring are required, as are sterile precautions including hat, mask, hand hygiene, and sterile gloves. The patient is placed in either the sitting or lateral decubitus position, and the desired lumbar level is identified by palpation of the iliac crests and spinous processes. Most neuraxial catheters for labor are placed between L2-3 to L5-S1. After sterilizing the back with an antiseptic and placing a sterile drape, the anesthesiologist places a skin wheal of local anesthesia at the intended needle placement site. Either a midline or paramedian approach to the epidural space is possible. Midline is more common and easier to perform for beginners. Layers traversed by the epidural needle during placement of epidural block include, from superficial to deep, skin, subcutaneous tissue, supraspinous ligament, interspinous

Table 31-3	**Contraindications to Neuraxial Block**
Patient refusal	
Severe hypovolemia or shock	
Coagulopathy	
Condition in which hypotension is physiologically very undesirable (i.e., right heart failure, severe aortic stenosis)	
Elevated intracranial pressure	
Infection at the block site	

Labels on figure:
- Dural sac
- Epidural vein
- Interlaminar space
- Lamina
- Ligamentum flavum
- Supraspinous ligament
- Intraspinous ligament
- Spinous process
- Transverse process

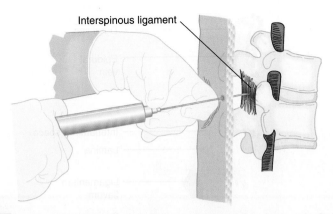

Interspinous ligament

Figure 31-6 Proper hand position when using the loss-of-resistance technique to locate the epidural space. After embedding the needle tip in the ligamentum flavum, a syringe with 2 to 3 mL of saline and an air bubble is attached. The left hand rests securely on the back and the fingers of the left hand grasp the needle firmly. The left hand advances the needle slowly and under control by rotating at the wrist. The fingers of the right hand maintain constant pressure on the syringe plunger but do not aid in advancing the needle. If the needle tip is properly engaged in the ligamentum flavum, it should be possible to compress the air bubble without injecting the saline. As the needle tip enters the epidural space, there will be a sudden loss of resistance and the saline will be suddenly injected. (From Bernards CM, Hostetter LS. Epidural and spinal anesthesia. In: Barash PG, Cullen BF, Stoelting RK, et al., eds. *Clinical Anesthesia.* 7th ed. Philadelphia: Wolters Kluwer Health; 2013:905–933, with permission.)

ligament, and ligamentum flavum. The epidural space is a potential space lying deep to the ligamentum flavum. The hollow, large-bore epidural needle with stylet is placed into the superficial ligaments, the stylet is removed, and an air- or saline-filled syringe is attached. The syringe will give tactile resistance when pushed until the ligamentum flavum is traversed, and the epidural space is entered, at which time tactile resistance disappears. Both the thickness of the ligamentum flavum and depth of the epidural space are usually 3 to 5 mm. Once the space is entered, saline may be injected to confirm loss of resistance, and the depth at which the epidural space was entered is noted (most epidural needles have centimeter markings on them). A soft catheter is then threaded into the space 3 to 5 cm. A test dose of lidocaine mixed with 15 μg of epinephrine is commonly administered via the catheter to ensure that it is not intravascular or intrathecal. Criteria for a positive intravascular test dose include an increase in heart rate by 20 beats per minute or an increase in systolic blood pressure by 15 mm Hg within 45 seconds of administration. The catheter must be removed and replaced at the same or a different interspace if a positive intravascular test occurs. A profound sensory and motor block within 5 minutes after administration of test dose confirms a positive intrathecal. If an intrathecal catheter is accidentally placed, it may be used for labor analgesia with appropriate dosing or it may be removed and replaced at a *different* level (Fig. 31-6).

Epidural activation begins with an initial bolus of dilute local anesthetic mixed with lipid soluble opioid, such as 0.125% bupivacaine mixed with fentanyl 50 to 100 μg, given in 5-mL increments, for a total of 10 to 20 mL. Time to analgesia is typically 10 to 20 minutes.

Alternatively, combined spinal epidural (CSE) has gained popularity because time to initial analgesia is shorter (3). Placement resembles an epidural procedure, expect that once the epidural space has been located, a long, small-gauge, noncutting spinal needle is inserted through the epidural needle. Then an intrathecal dose of lipid soluble opioid, such as fentanyl or sufentanil, with or without a low dose of local anesthetic, is administered. The clinician commonly administers a test dose, but no epidural bolus is necessary, and time to analgesia is typically <5 minutes. Postdural puncture headache risk is not increased, and the risk of epidural failure may be *lower* with CSE, although data yield conflicting results (3,4).

If an intrathecal catheter is placed, the dose is about one-tenth the volume of a typical epidural dose, administered either as a continuous infusion or via intermittent *provider-administered* bolus every 1 to 2 hours. The patient's nurse and any subsequent providers must be notified that the catheter is intrathecal, and both the catheter and pump must be clearly labeled so that accidental overdose does not occur.

The use of ultrasound guidance for placement of neuraxial catheters is becoming more common and can be useful in obese patients or for patients with spinal abnormalities. Location of midline, accurate assessment of lumbar level, and measurement of depth of the epidural and intrathecal spaces are all possible via ultrasound.

IV. Anesthesia for Cesarean Delivery

In the United States, 32% of babies are born via cesarean delivery (5), and vaginal birth after cesarean delivery is losing popularity due to perceived risks by both patients and providers. Most cesarean deliveries are performed under neuraxial anesthesia, either spinal, epidural, or CSE.

Elective cesarean deliveries are performed at term (≥39 weeks), under *neuraxial* anesthesia unless there is a contraindication, because the risk to both mother and fetus is lower with neuraxial versus general anesthesia. In preparation for surgery, patients are instructed not to eat solids for 8 hours prior to surgery and not to drink clear fluids for 2 hours prior to surgery. Preoperative labs may include a complete blood count and type and screen. An 18-gauge or larger peripheral intravenous line is placed and balanced salt solution is administered.

Pfannenstiel skin incision with low transverse uterine incision is the most common type of operative approach. To provide adequate anesthesia for cesarean delivery, blockade must include both incisional or somatic and peritoneal pain fibers up to the celiac plexus. Therefore, a dermatomal block from at least T6 to sacrum is required. Anesthesia care providers commonly employ either spinal or epidural anesthesia to achieve this level.

Spinal bupivacaine (dose 10 to 12 mg) or lidocaine (dose 60 to 100 mg) represents a viable option for cesarean delivery anesthesia. Intrathecal lidocaine spinal has become less popular due to concern about transient neurologic symptoms (TNS). The anesthesiologist commonly administers short-acting and long-acting intrathecal opioids along with the local anesthetic. Typically fentanyl (10 to 20 µg) or sufentanil (2.5 to 5 µg) is given. The duration of either is 2 hours, and intraoperative pain, nausea, and vomiting occur less frequently when they are used. Long-acting hydrophilic morphine provides postoperative analgesia.

Hypotension commonly accompanies initiation of spinal anesthesia for cesarean delivery and can be prevented or lessened by placing the patient in left uterine displacement and administering a coload of crystalloid 10 to 20 mL/kg or colloid 5 mL/kg. Prophylactic phenylephrine infusion decreases

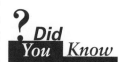

? *Did*
You *Know*

Nausea is common after initiation of spinal anesthesia and may be related to hypotension or to increased vagal tone from sympathectomy.

the incidence of spinal-related hypotension, nausea, and vomiting (6). Nausea is common after initiation of spinal anesthesia and may be related to hypotension or to increased vagal tone from sympathectomy.

Epidural anesthesia for cesarean delivery is achieved via 2% lidocaine or 3% chloroprocaine, 15 to 25 mL, incrementally dosed in nonemergent situations. In emergent situations, 3% 2-chloroprocaine 20 mL is preferred because it has the shortest onset time (3 to 4 minutes) and desirable maternal and fetal safety profiles. Of note, chloroprocaine may decrease the efficacy of opioids and local anesthetics administered subsequently. The addition of sodium bicarbonate will decrease time to blockade by converting more of the local anesthetic to its nonionized form. The dose is typically 1 mEq/10 mL local anesthetic volume. Epinephrine (5 μg/mL) can be added to increase the density and extend the duration of block and to test dose a labor epidural catheter that will be used for cesarean delivery anesthesia. Preservative-free morphine can be given via the epidural catheter for postoperative analgesia, typically after umbilical cord clamping.

General anesthesia for cesarean delivery is generally reserved for emergency cases or when contraindications to neuraxial anesthesia exist. Standard of care requires American Society of Anesthesiologists' (ASA) standard monitors and preoxygenation. Proper positioning and preoxygenation help mitigate the desaturation that occurs, and they assume special importance in pregnant patients who are particularly prone to desaturation after a period of apnea. Administration of a nonparticulate antacid and rapid sequence induction and intubation, with an assistant providing cricoid pressure, are also standard, due to the increased risk of aspiration. The surgeon prepares and drapes the patient's abdomen prior to induction to be ready to perform surgery immediately after endotracheal tube placement is confirmed. Induction was historically with thiopental; however, propofol has replaced thiopental as the induction agent of choice, mainly because of its availability. Succinylcholine (1 mg/kg) given with induction provides muscle relaxation. Once the trachea is intubated, the anesthesiologist notifies the obstetrician and surgery begins.

Temperature monitoring and stomach decompression with an OG tube are generally recommended. Oxygen and inhaled anesthetic are administered until delivery of the fetus. Inhaled anesthetic over 1 MAC may decrease uterine tone, so after delivery of the fetus, a nitrous oxygen mixture is started, along with low concentration inhaled anesthetic. An analgesic, amnestic, and sometimes additional muscle relaxant are given. After delivery of the placenta, an oxytocin infusion is started, and additional uterotonics are given as needed.

A. Postoperative Analgesia

Intrathecal or epidural morphine provides long lasting analgesia and appears to have a ceiling effect around 150 μg (intrathecal) and 3 to 4 mg (epidural) (7,8). Higher doses do not increase analgesia and cause more nausea, respiratory depression, and pruritus. Peak morphine effects occur about 6 hours postadministration and cease by 12 to 18 hours postadministration. Published ASA recommendations call for monitoring of sedation and respiratory rate every hour during the first 12 hours and every 2 hours for the next 12 hours after dosing (9). Medications to treat side effects include naloxone to treat respiratory depression or sedation, a mixed opiate agonist or antagonist to treat pruritus, and an intravenous antiemetic. Oral analgesics should be ordered, such as acetaminophen and nonsteroidal anti-inflammatory drugs. Additional opiates may be administered if needed, as long as vigilant monitoring takes place. Prophylaxis with an intraoperative dose of antiemetic decreases the incidence of nausea and vomiting associated with neuraxial morphine. Alternatively, the anesthesiologist may leave the epidural catheter in place and administer PCEA with low concentration local anesthetic and lipid soluble opioid, typically for 24 hours postdelivery.

For patients who do not receive neuraxial morphine or PCEA, transversus abdominis plane (TAP) blocks improve analgesia by decreasing incisional pain. TAP blocks may be performed immediately postoperatively with ultrasound guidance, typically with 10- to 15-mL long-acting local anesthetic per side.

V. Fetal Assessment and Neonatal Resuscitation

Fetal heart rate (FHR) monitoring during labor attempts to identify fetal hypoxemia or acidosis and avoid resultant fetal neurologic damage or death. FHR monitoring can be intermittent, via auscultation or Doppler, or continuous, via external Doppler or fetal electrocardiogram (ECG). Fetal ECG requires internal monitor placement on the fetal scalp. The mother must be dilated and ruptured for this to occur. Continuous FHR monitoring is recommended by major obstetric organizations and accompanies almost 90% of US deliveries (10). Despite the emphasis on FHR patterns and neonatal neurologic outcome, cerebral palsy is most often due to an antepartum, not intrapartum, event. Continuous FHR monitoring is associated retrospectively with lower rates of cerebral palsy and death. However, no randomized prospective data are available due to ethical issues. Intermittent versus continuous fetal monitoring has been compared prospectively, and the only difference in outcome is a higher rate of cesarean delivery *without benefit to the neonate*, and in general a lower risk of neonatal seizures (11).

FHR tracing interpretation is very sensitive but not very specific. Therefore, a normal FHR and variability without decelerations almost always indicates a nonacidotic fetus, but a healthy fetus may have FHR abnormalities not caused by acidosis or distress. Fetal tachycardia may be due to hypoxemia, but it may also result from maternal fever or infection or maternally administered drugs (β agonists in particular). Many maternally administered drugs, including magnesium and opioids, may decrease FHR variability (Fig. 31-7).

The American Congress of Obstetrics and Gynecology (ACOG) classifies FHR tracings into three categories (10). A Category I tracing is highly predictive of a healthy nonacidotic fetus and must have the following characteristics: normal baseline heart rate, normal variability, and no decelerations other than early. A Category III designation is associated with fetal acidosis and has the following characteristics: absent variability *accompanied by* late or variable decelerations occurring with >50% of contractions or sinusoidal pattern. Category II includes any tracing not meeting the qualifiers of Category I or III (Fig. 31-8).

A. Intrauterine Resuscitation

Fetuses with Category III tracings or with prolonged bradycardia require rapid treatment. Treatment of maternal hypotension with lateral positioning, fluid bolus, and vasopressors, administration of high-flow oxygen via face mask, and cessation of uterine contractions with nitroglycerin or terbutaline are primary therapy. If no improvement is seen, immediate delivery is indicated.

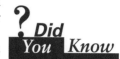

Continuous fetal heart rate monitoring is recommended by major obstetric organizations and accompanies almost 90% of US deliveries.

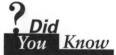

Fetal heart rate tracing interpretation is very sensitive, but not very specific. Thus, a normal fetal heart rate and variability without decelerations almost always indicates a nonacidotic fetus, but a healthy fetus may have fetal heart rate abnormalities not due to acidosis or distress.

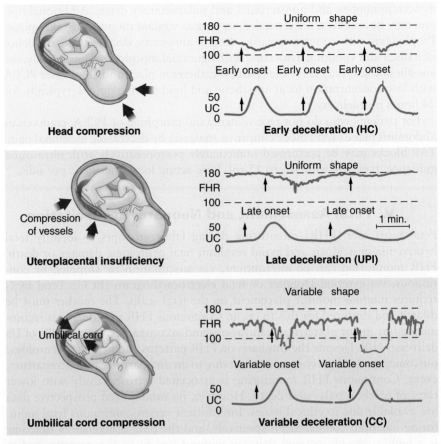

Uniform shape
FHR
180
100
Early onset   Early onset   Early onset
50
UC
0
Head compression   **Early deceleration (HC)**

Uniform shape
180
FHR
100
Late onset   Late onset   1 min.
50
UC
0
Compression of vessels
Uteroplacental insufficiency   **Late deceleration (UPI)**

Variable shape
180
FHR
100
Umbilical cord
Variable onset   Variable onset
50
UC
0
Umbilical cord compression   **Variable deceleration (CC)**

Figure 31-7 Classification and mechanism of fetal heart rate patterns. HC, head compression; UPI, uteroplacental insufficiency; CC, cord compression. (From Braveman FR, Scavone BM, Blessing ME, et al. Obstetrical anesthesia. In: Barash PG, Cullen BF, Stoelting RK, et al., eds. *Clinical Anesthesia*. 7th ed. Philadelphia: Wolters Kluwer Health; 2013:1144–1177, with permission.)

Prolonged *fetal bradycardia* will lead to emergency cesarean delivery if intrauterine resuscitation measures are ineffective. An existing epidural catheter can be dosed with 20 mL of 3% chloroprocaine, which should provide a surgical level within 3 to 4 minutes. General anesthesia is usually chosen if fetal bradycardia persists in the operating room and no neuraxial catheter is present.

B. Ancillary Fetal Testing

High-risk fetuses or pregnancies sometimes require closer monitoring or additional testing to assess fetal status. A nonstress test (NST) consists of 30 minutes of continuous external fetal heart rate monitoring, during which time at least two accelerations of at least 15 beats per minute lasting 15 seconds or more must be seen, indicating a healthy fetus. NSTs are done weekly or daily depending on the diagnosis. A biophysical profile further assesses fetal status. It has five components each with a maximum of two points, including an NST, measurement of amniotic fluid index, fetal tone, fetal movement, and fetal breathing attempts. Lower scores are indications for admission and continuous monitoring and sometimes delivery. Umbilical artery Doppler studies are

Three-Tier Fetal Heart Rate Interpretation System

Category I

Category I fetal heart rate (FHR) tracings include <u>all</u> of the following:

- Baseline rate: 110–160 beats per minute (bpm)
- Baseline FHR variability: moderate
- Late or variable decelerations: absent
- Early decelerations: present or absent
- Accelerations: present or absent

Category II

Category II FHR tracings include all FHR tracings not categorized as Category I or Category III. Category II tracings may represent an appreciable fraction of those encountered in clinical care. Examples of Category II FHR tracings include any of the following:

Baseline rate

- Bradycardia not accompanied by absent baseline variability
- Tachycardia

Baseline FHR variability

- Minimal baseline variability
- Absent baseline variability not accompanied by recurrent decelerations
- Marked baseline variability

Accelerations

- Absence of induced accelerations after fetal stimulation

Periodic or episodic decelerations

- Recurrent variable decelerations accompanied by minimal or moderate baseline variability
- Prolonged deceleration ≥2 minutes but <10 minutes
- Recurrent late decelerations with moderate baseline variability
- Variable decelerations with other characteristics, such as slow return to baseline, "overshoots," or "shoulders"

Category III

Category III FHR tracings include either:

- Absent baseline FHR variability and any of the following:
  - Recurrent late decelerations
  - Recurrent variable decelerations
  - Bradycardia
- Sinusoidal pattern

Figure 31-8 Three-tiered fetal heart interpretation system. (From the 2008 National Institute of Child Health and Human Development Workshop on Electronic Fetal Monitoring: Updates on definitions, interpretations, and research guidelines. *Obstet Gynecol.* 2008;112:661, with permission.)

performed in fetuses with growth restriction or in mothers with hypertension or placental abnormalities to monitor for signs of worsening fetal perfusion (indicated by poor flow in diastole or elevation in placental resistance). The ratio of flow in systole versus diastole is measured, and a score over 3 is concerning. The resistance index is also measured, and a score of >0.6 is indicative of elevated placental resistance. Absent end diastolic flow (AEDF) occurs when flow in diastole stops due to increased placental resistance. Reverse end diastolic flow (REDF) occurs when flow in diastole moves from the placenta to the fetus in the umbilical artery, indicating very elevated placental resistance. REDF is always an indication for delivery. AEDF is an indication for

Table 31-4	Apgar Scores		
Sign	**0**	**1**	**2**
Heart rate	Absent	<100 beats/min	>100 beats/min
Respiratory effort	Absent	Slow, irregular	Good, crying
Muscle tone	Limp	Some flexion of extremities	Active motion
Reflex irritability	No response	Grimace	Cough, sneeze, or cry
Color	Pale, blue	Body pink, extremities blue	Completely pink

Reprinted from Braveman FR, Scavone BM, Blessing ME, et al. Obstetrical anesthesia. In: Barash PG, Cullen BF, Stoelting RK, et al., eds. *Clinical Anesthesia*. 7th ed. Philadelphia: Wolters Kluwer Health; 2013:1144–1177, with permission.

delivery depending on gestational age and other factors. Both are associated with increased fetal morbidity and mortality.

The *Apgar score* is a global assessment of neonatal status immediately after birth. The score's intended use is to guide acute intervention, not to provide prognosis. Neonatal breathing, heart rate, reaction to stimulus, tone, and color are each assessed at 1, 5, and sometimes 10 minutes postnatal and given a score of 0 to 2 per category. A score of ≥7 is considered normal. Scores <7 necessitate further intervention (Table 31-4 and Fig. 31-9).

VI. Comorbidities and Obstetric Diseases

A. Pregnancy-induced Hypertensive Disorders

The pregnancy-induced hypertensive disorders include gestational hypertension, preeclampsia or eclampsia, and hemolysis-elevated liver enzymes with low platelets (HELLP) syndrome. Pregnancy normally causes a slight decrease in blood pressure. Elevated blood pressure in pregnancy is pathologic and associated with fetal and maternal morbidity and mortality. Gestational hypertension is defined as elevated blood pressure occurring after 20 weeks' gestation, without accompanying proteinuria. Preeclampsia is defined by elevated blood pressures after 20 weeks' gestation, accompanied by proteinuria or other organ-system effects. Eclampsia is preeclampsia with seizure (12). The HELLP syndrome is a variant of severe preeclampsia associated with liver dysfunction and thrombocytopenia.

Preeclampsia can be further categorized as having severe features if any of the following conditions are met: blood pressure elevated over 160 mm Hg systolic or 110 mm Hg diastolic, or end-organ dysfunction, which can manifest as severe headache, vision or cerebral disturbance, pulmonary edema or cyanosis, oliguria or renal failure, liver dysfunction, or severe epigastric pain. Severe proteinuria and fetal growth restriction are no longer used as indicators of severe features but do frequently occur with the disorder (12).

The etiology of preeclampsia is still being studied, but abnormalities in placental implantation and placental production of thromboxane and prostacyclin may play a role. Poor placental perfusion causes systemic endothelial dysfunction and activation of the renin-angiotensin-aldosterone system,

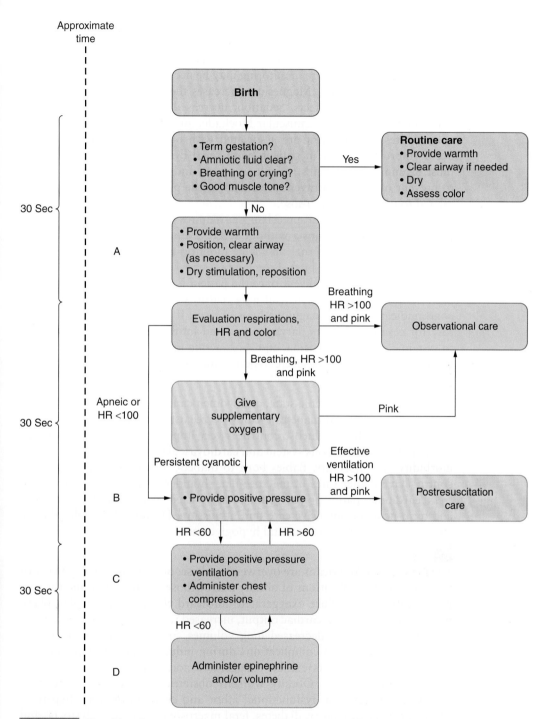

Approximate
time

Birth

• Term gestation?
• Amniotic fluid clear?
• Breathing or crying?
• Good muscle tone?

Yes

Routine care
• Provide warmth
• Clear airway if needed
• Dry
• Assess color

No

30 Sec

A

• Provide warmth
• Position, clear airway
  (as necessary)
• Dry stimulation, reposition

Evaluation respirations,
HR and color

Breathing
HR >100
and pink

Observational care

Apneic or
HR <100

Breathing, HR >100
and pink

30 Sec

Give
supplementary
oxygen

Pink

Persistent cyanotic

Effective
ventilation
HR >100
and pink

B

• Provide positive pressure

Postresuscitation
care

HR <60

HR >60

30 Sec

C

• Provide positive pressure
  ventilation
• Administer chest
  compressions

HR <60

D

Administer epinephrine
and/or volume

Figure 31-9 Algorithm for neonatal resuscitation. HR, heart rate. (From Kattwinkel J, Perlman JM, Aziz K, et al. Special report–Neonatal resuscitation; 2010. American Heart Association guidelines for cardiopulmonary resuscitation and emergency cardiovascular care. *Circulation.* 2010;122:S9, with permission.)

resulting in arteriolar hypertension and edema. Platelet aggregation occurs at sites of endothelial injury, resulting in coagulopathy.

Severe hypertension can cause focal cerebral ischemia, cerebral edema, or hemorrhage, leading to eclampsia or seizures and death or major disability. A recent ACOG Executive Summary recommends immediate control of blood pressure with intravenous antihypertensives to prevent morbidity and mortality (12). Intravenous labetalol and hydralazine are most commonly used, and direct arterial pressure monitoring may be necessary. Magnesium infusion prevents eclampsia (13). Magnesium increases the seizure threshold and has many unwanted side effects. Sedation, decreased reflexes, muscle weakness and potentiation of neuromuscular blockade, and respiratory and cardiovascular depression or arrest are associated with magnesium overdose, which occurs more frequently in patients with renal dysfunction. The practitioner must examine the patient's neurologic status and monitor magnesium levels to prevent overdose. Intravenous calcium is the primary treatment for arrest related to magnesium overdose.

Ultimately, treatment of preeclampsia requires delivery and removal of the placenta. Early preeclampsia without severe features can be managed expectantly with careful maternal and fetal monitoring and antihypertensives in order to prevent preterm birth. Preeclampsia with severe features usually represents an indication for delivery once the patient is stabilized and steroids have been administered to hasten fetal lung maturity. Neuraxial anesthesia is not contraindicated unless coagulopathy is present. If general anesthesia is necessary for cesarean delivery, laryngoscopy and intubation may be difficult due to systemic and airway edema, and short-acting intravenous antihypertensives should be used to prevent severe hypertension during airway management.

B. Diabetes Mellitus

Pregnancy is a diabetogenic state, and women can develop diabetes related to pregnancy (gestational diabetes mellitus). Preexisting diabetes often requires insulin therapy. Blood glucose control is very important during pregnancy to avoid fetal central nervous system and cardiovascular malformations and fetal morbidity and mortality. Babies born to diabetic women with poor glucose control have higher rates of macrosomia, shoulder dystocia, respiratory distress, cardiomyopathy, polycythemia and persistent pulmonary hypertension, and term neonatal intensive care unit admission. During labor, tight glucose control will help prevent neonatal hypoglycemia.

C. Obesity

The majority of Americans are overweight, obese, or morbidly obese. Many of the physiologic implications of obesity mirror those of pregnancy and the two may combine to produce exaggerated untoward effects. In particular, obese patients have increased cardiac output, increased work of breathing, increased oxygen consumption, decreased lung volumes, and more redundant tissue, making them prone to complications during induction and airway management. Obese parturients exhibit exaggerated aortocaval compression when in the supine position. Obesity worsens obstetric and neonatal outcomes, increasing the rates of dysfunctional labor and cesarean delivery, hypertensive diseases of pregnancy, diabetes, fetal macrosomia, shoulder dystocia, and intrauterine fetal demise. Postoperatively these patients demonstrate increased rates of infection, wound disruption, and thromboembolic disease.

Neuraxial anesthetic techniques are fraught with difficulty, and ultrasound guidance may facilitate block placement. Airway management during administration of general anesthesia should cause concern for failure to ventilate, failure to intubate, and aspiration of gastric contents. The clinician should have a low threshold for awake fiberoptic intubation. Obese parturients should be evaluated soon after admission to the labor and delivery unit and early neuraxial analgesia is encouraged to decrease the risk of general anesthesia being required should an emergency cesarean delivery become necessary.

D. Fever and Infection

Pregnancy is an immunosuppressed state, and systemic infection is poorly tolerated. Chorioamnionitis is a common severe infection in pregnant patients that can lead to preterm labor, atony, hemorrhage, and sepsis. Urinary tract infections are also frequent and can lead to ascending infection and pyelonephritis due to poor ureteral valve function in pregnancy. Systemic inflammatory response syndrome and sepsis are treated in the same manner as for nonpregnant patients, but mortality rates are higher in pregnant patients.

Genital *herpes simplex virus* (HSV) is a common sexually transmitted disease and is an indication for cesarean delivery if active genital or cervical lesions are present because of the risk of neonatal HSV infection. Primary herpes infection is associated with flu-like symptoms and genital lesions. Neuraxial anesthesia is controversial during primary infection because of the potential risk of seeding the central nervous system with HSV. Many anesthesia practitioners will not administer neuraxial anesthesia until the lesions associated with primary HSV have begun healing and no signs or symptoms of systemic infection are present. Secondary infections are not considered a contraindication to neuraxial techniques. *Oral HSV* more commonly recurs in patients who receive neuraxial morphine. The etiology of the recrudescence is unclear and may be related to immunomodulation or to facial pruritus and scratching.

Pregnant patients with human immunodeficiency virus (HIV) are treated with highly active antiretroviral therapy, with the goal viral load being <1,000 copies/mL. Vaginal delivery is allowed if viral load is <1,000 copies/mL. If viral load is >1,000 copies/mL, cesarean delivery helps prevent vertical transmission to the infant. During labor and delivery, the administration of intravenous zidovudine decreases the rate of vertical HIV transmission. Breastfeeding is contraindicated. Neuraxial analgesia and anesthesia are not contraindicated.

E. Epidural Fever

Temperature rises about 0.4 degrees per hour in women with epidural labor analgesia versus those without, even when controlling for other factors such as pain medication and infection (14). The etiology of this temperature rise is unclear, and the actual temperature difference's clinical significance is also unclear. Women with epidural-related fever during labor may be incorrectly diagnosed with chorioamnionitis.

F. Bleeding Disorders

Von Willebrand disease represents the most common inherited coagulopathy in pregnant women. Von Willebrand factor (vWF) is important for normal hemostasis, as it causes adhesion of platelets to injured tissue and serves as a cofactor to factor VIII. Three subtypes of vWF deficiency exist, with deficiencies in either quantitative amount of or qualitative function of vWF. The most common subtype, vWF deficiency type 1, is a result of a decrease in circulating vWF levels. Pregnancy increases circulating levels of vWF and may decrease symptoms or need for treatment. If required, initial therapy for type 1 is with desmopressin (DDAVP), which increases vWF release, doubling to quadrupling the circulating concentrations. Intravenous or intranasal DDAVP begins working in 30 to 60 minutes and lasts for 6 hours. Type 2 has four subcategories and is a result of qualitative abnormalities in vWF causing abnormal function. Subtype 2b is associated with thrombocytopenia and thrombosis if DDAVP is given. Therefore, therapy must include factor VIII concentrate containing vWF (Humate). Fresh frozen plasma (FFP) and cryoprecipitate also contain vWF. However, factor VIII concentrate is recommended if available because of a lower risk of viral disease transmission. Type 3 is a severe, recessive disorder with very low circulating vWF levels and severe bleeding. A hematology consult may guide the therapy.

Acquired coagulopathies commonly occur associated with hemorrhage and are due to dilution or DIC. Dilutional coagulopathy occurs after massive hemorrhage, when resuscitation consists primarily of packed red blood cells (pRBC) without plasma or platelets. Additionally, DIC is associated with placental abruption and amniotic fluid embolism. Therapy for acquired coagulopathy is supportive and includes transfusion of plasma, cryoprecipitate, and platelets.

VII. Emergencies

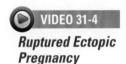
VIDEO 31-4
Ruptured Ectopic Pregnancy

Antepartum hemorrhage occurs due to either acute abnormalities associated with the uterus or placenta (placental abruption or uterine rupture) or abnormal implantation of the placenta (previa).

Placental abruption occurs when a portion of the placenta prematurely separates off its implant site on the uterus. Large abruptions can cause significant blood loss, DIC, and maternal instability, in addition to fetal distress or demise. Risk factors for abruption include advanced age, hypertension, diabetes, smoking, trauma, and cocaine use. Treatment is delivery and fluid and blood product administration. Coagulation should be monitored, including fibrinogen level.

Uterine rupture occurs most often in women with a history of previous cesarean delivery, in particular with a "classical" vertical uterine scar. Uterine rupture is a surgical emergency and can be associated with severe bleeding. Uterine rupture is less common if a low transverse uterine scar is present, and a vaginal trial of labor (VTOL) may be offered to appropriate patients. A team must be immediately available to provide cesarean delivery for patients undergoing a VTOL.

Placenta previa occurs when the placenta implants either very close to or completely over the cervical os. Vaginal delivery is not possible without maternal and fetal consequences. Placenta previa is associated with maternal hemorrhage and with other abnormalities of placentation such as placenta accreta. When placenta previa occurs in the setting of five or more cesarean deliveries, the risk of invasive placentation or accreta is at least 75%. Continued bleeding from placenta previa is an indication for emergency cesarean delivery.

Vasa previa occurs when unprotected fetal vessels lie over the cervical os. Any vaginal bleeding may be fetal, and therefore represents an obstetric emergency requiring immediate delivery. Fetal mortality (in an otherwise normal fetus) is higher from vasa previa than any other condition. Therefore, mothers are admitted and fetuses are continuously monitored until planned early cesarean delivery.

Patients with placenta or vasa previa are more likely to experience postpartum hemorrhage, so blood should be cross matched and adequate access placed prior to cesarean delivery.

Postpartum hemorrhage (PPH) is the primary cause of maternal death worldwide and a leading contributor to maternal mortality and severe morbidity in the United States. PPH complicates 3% of deliveries (16) and is classically defined as estimated blood loss greater than 500 mL for a vaginal delivery or 1,000 mL for a cesarean delivery. However, in clinical practice, these values

Table 31-5	Uterotonic Therapy	
Drug	**Dose**	**Side Effects**
Oxytocin	20–40 U in 1,000 mL LR by continuous IV infusion	Hypotension, tachycardia
Ergot alkaloids (Methergine)	0.2 mg IM q2–4h prn	Hypertension, vasoconstriction Coronary vasospasm V/Q mismatch (ventilation perfusion mismatch), elevated pulmonary vascular resistance, and nausea and vomiting
Carboprost (prostaglandin F 2 alpha/ Hemabate)	0.25 mg q15 min × 8 doses, maximum 2 mg	↑ pulmonary vascular resistance Bronchospasm Diarrhea/nausea Fever
Misoprostol	800–1,000 mg PR/PV/PO q2h	Fever Nausea
Dinoprostone	20 mg PO q2h	Hypotension Nausea

LR, Lactated ringers; IV, intravenous; IM, intramuscular; prn, as needed; PR/PV/PO, per rectum/per vaginum/per os.
Reprinted from Braveman FR, Scavone BM, Blessing ME, et al. Obstetrical anesthesia. In: Barash PG, Cullen BF, Stoelting RK, et al., eds. *Clinical Anesthesia*. 7th ed. Philadelphia: Wolters Kluwer Health; 2013:1144–1177, with permission.

approximate average blood loss totals. A better way to define PPH may be heavy bleeding associated with symptoms or requiring fluid resuscitation or blood transfusion. The uterine blood flow at term is 700 to 900 mL/min. The uterus normally contracts postpartum, causing mechanical obstruction of bleeding vessels to prevent major maternal hemorrhage. The lack of uterine contraction postdelivery is called *atony* and 80% of PPH is due to uterine atony (16). Risk factors for atony include a history of atony with previous pregnancy, retained placenta, chorioamnionitis, augmented or prolonged labor, uterine relaxants, and an overdistended uterus (macrosomic fetus, polyhydramnios, multiple gestation). Treatment of atony includes bimanual uterine massage, uterotonic drugs, discontinuation of drugs that may impair uterine contraction (inhaled anesthetics), or internal (Bakri balloon) or external (B-Lynch suture) compression of the uterus. Hysterectomy is indicated for severe unresponsive atony.

Medications commonly used for atony include oxytocin, prostaglandins, and methylergonovine (Table 31-5).

Abnormalities of placentation represent a major source of massive obstetric hemorrhage. Placenta accreta, increta, and percreta occur when the placenta abnormally adheres to (accreta) or invades (increta) the uterine myometrium or serosa (percreta). Previous cesarean deliveries or uterine surgery are associated with placental implantation abnormalities. Accreta can be diagnosed via ultrasound or magnetic resonance imaging (MRI), although both remain imperfectly sensitive or specific. Planning for cesarean delivery and the possibility of large blood loss is crucial, and adequate large bore intravenous access and type and cross-matched blood products are needed. Safe surgical management of hysterectomy in patients with placenta percreta requires the involvement of subspecialties, including interventional radiology, gynecologic oncology, and general surgery.

Massive blood loss and transfusion can occur in obstetrical patients. Many hospitals are creating massive transfusion protocols to facilitate the timely delivery of blood products when needed. High ratios of FFP to pRBC are recommended in the setting of ongoing loss and transfusion. Although the optimal ratio remains controversial, most experts endorse administration of 1:1 or 1:2 FFP to pRBC. One pooled unit of cryoprecipitate and one pooled unit of platelets should be given for every six pRBC transfused or based on laboratory values. Experts recommend early identification and aggressive treatment of coagulopathy, and frequent laboratory monitoring can help guide therapy (e.g., complete blood cell count, prothrombin time and international normalized ratio, partial thromboplastin time, fibrinogen, or thromboelastogram). Cell saver can be used during massive hemorrhage or for patients who refuse blood transfusion.

Amniotic fluid embolism (AFE) occurs when amniotic fluid enters the mother's circulation and causes a severe inflammatory response. AFE often occurs immediately surrounding delivery, and the intact survival rate remains poor. Bronchospasm, acute pulmonary hypertension, circulatory shock, and DIC can all occur with AFE. Treatment is supportive and can include massive transfusion for DIC and resultant hemorrhage.

A. Cardiopulmonary Arrest

The incidence of peripartum maternal arrest is 1 in 30,000 deliveries (17). Maternal arrest has many etiologies, including pulmonary or amniotic fluid embolism, drug errors, maternal comorbidities such as preeclampsia, coronary artery disease or severe valvular disease, or complications of general or neuraxial anesthesia. Initial treatment is cardiopulmonary resuscitation (CPR) modified for the pregnant patient, using either manual left uterine displacement or a Cardiff wedge or a "human wedge" on the knees of a provider. Other CPR modifications due to the pregnant state include a slightly higher sternal placement of hands for chest compressions, use of cricoid pressure during bag mask ventilation until the trachea is intubated, and a high index of suspicion for drug errors, in particular magnesium overdose. Use of defibrillation, vasopressors, and inotropes all remain unchanged from adult advanced cardiac life support guidelines. Maternal CPR is almost always suboptimal due to the gravid uterus. If the source of the arrest is unknown or not immediately reversible, cesarean delivery should be performed *in the labor and delivery room within 5 minutes of arrest*. To achieve this goal, the team must make the decision to perform a cesarean delivery and make the incision within 4 minutes of arrest. With delivery of the fetus, adequate CPR can be delivered to the mother. Longer arrest-to-delivery intervals are associated with worse neonatal and maternal outcomes.

B. Maternal Mortality

The maternal mortality ratio refers to the number of maternal deaths during a given time period per 100,000 live births. In the United States and other developed countries, the maternal mortality ratio is 14.5 in 100,000 (18). The leading contributors to mortality in the United States are hemorrhage, venous thromboembolism, infection, hypertensive diseases, cardiomyopathy, cardiovascular comorbidities, and noncardiovascular comorbidities. Globally, the maternal mortality ratio is 260 per 100,000 live births (19). Hemorrhage, sepsis, and pregnancy-induced hypertension are the leading causes of maternal death in undeveloped countries. The anesthesia-related maternal mortality ratio is 1.2 in 1 million; anesthesia is the cause of about 1.5% of maternal deaths in the United States (20).

VIII. Complications of Neuraxial Anesthesia

A. Postdural Puncture Headache or Epidural Blood Patch

Postdural puncture headache (PDPH) occurs after puncture of the dura, with resultant leakage of CSF. The associated headache is theorized to occur because CSF loss is greater than production, resulting in low CSF volume and pressure. Reflexive cerebral vasodilation then occurs, causing headache. The headache is classically frontal or occipital, may be associated with neck stiffness or pain, increases in severity with sitting position, and is relieved by supine position. It may be accompanied by cranial nerve palsies (abducens palsy is most common), nausea and vomiting, or tinnitus. The majority of PDPHs resolve within 1 week, but some may persist longer. Development of PDPH after dural puncture is higher in young, thin, women with histories of headaches and when larger gauge, cutting needles are used. The risk of headache development in pregnant women after dural puncture with an epidural needle (17 to 18 gauge) is over 50% (21).

Treatment of PDPH is either conservative (intravenous fluid and oral caffeine and analgesics) or with epidural blood patch (EBP). During an EBP, the anesthesiologist draws the patient's blood sterilely drawn and injects it into the epidural space, "patching" the dural hole with clot and stopping the CSF leakage. Usually, 15 to 20 mL of blood is given. Sometimes development of back or neck pain with injection limits the volume of blood administered. EBP typically relieves pain immediately, but may need to be repeated if headache recurs as the clot is resorbed. When PDPH does not respond to EBP or is associated with fever or other neurologic abnormalities, further diagnostic testing is indicated to rule out meningitis or intracranial hemorrhage or thrombosis.

B. Local Anesthetic Overdose

Epidural catheters can unintentionally become intravascular during either initial placement or from migration later. If a large dose of intravenous local anesthetic is accidentally given, systemic toxicity can occur. Neurotoxicity typically manifests before cardiotoxicity and includes changes in mental status, seizures, and obtundation. Cardiovascular effects first become evident as widening of the QRS complex and progress to ventricular tachycardia or ventricular fibrillation and arrest. At the first signs of overdose, local anesthetic should be discontinued and oxygen and lipid emulsion administered. Lipid emulsion binds free local anesthetic to prevent further blockage of cardiac sodium channels. However, channels that are already affected will not be altered. Therefore, circulatory support, CPR, and even cardiopulmonary bypass may be necessary to rescue, particularly in the case of bupivacaine overdose (Fig. 31-10).

C. Nerve Damage

Nerve injuries may arise independently of obstetric or anesthetic interventions. They occur at a rate of 0.8% and are thought to be due to fetal head compression of nerves during passage through the pelvis or nerve stretch or compression from patient positioning during labor and delivery. Mean duration of injury is 2 to 3 months. The lateral femoral cutaneous nerve is most often affected and presents with numbness over the lateral thigh. The femoral nerve is the second most common site of injury, and palsies of this nerve can be

AMERICAN SOCIETY OF
REGIONAL ANESTHESIA AND PAIN MEDICINE

Checklist for Treatment
of Local Anesthetic Systemic Toxicity

**The Pharmacologic Treatment of Local Anesthetic Systemic Toxicity (LAST)
is Different from Other Cardiac Arrest Scenarios**

❑ **Get Help**
❑ **Initial Focus**
  ❑ **Airway management:** ventilate with 100% oxygen
  ❑ **Seizure supperssion: benzodiazepines are preferred; AVOID propofol**
    in patients having signs of cardiovascular instability
  ❑ **Alert** the nearest facility having **cardiopulmonary bypass** capability
❑ **Management of Cardiac Arrhythmias**
  ❑ **Basic and Advanced Cardiac Life Support (ACLS)** will require
    adjustment of medications and perhaps prolonged effort
  ❑ **AVOID vasopressin, calcium channel blockers, beta blockers, or local anesthetic**
  ❑ **REDUCE individual epinephrine doses to <1 mcg/kg**
❑ **Lipid Emulsion (20%) Therapy** (values in parenthesis are for 70 kg patient)
  ❑ **Bolus 1.5 mL/kg** (lean body mass) intravenously over 1 minute (~100 mL)
  ❑ **Continuous infusion 0.25 mL/kg/min** (~18 mL/min; adjust by roller clamp)
  ❑ Repeat bolus once or twice for persistent cardiovascular collapse
  ❑ Double the infusion rate to 0.5 mL/kg/min if blood pressure remains low
  ❑ **Continue infusion** for at least 10 minutes after attaining circulatory stability
  ❑ Recommended upper limit: Approximately 10 mL/kg lipid emulsion
    over the first 30 minutes
❑ **Post LAST events at** www.lipidrescue.org and report use of lipid to www.lipidregistry.org

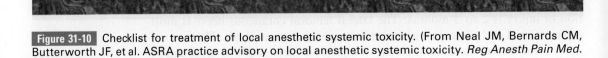

Figure 31-10 Checklist for treatment of local anesthetic systemic toxicity. (From Neal JM, Bernards CM, Butterworth JF, et al. ASRA practice advisory on local anesthetic systemic toxicity. *Reg Anesth Pain Med.* 2010;35:152–161, with permission.)

BE PREPARED

- We strongly advise that those using local anesthetics (LA) in doses sufficient to produce local anesthetic systemic toxicity (LAST) establish a plan for managing this complication. Making a *Local Anesthetic Toxicity Kit* and posting instructions for its use are encouraged.

RISK REDUCTION (*BE SENSIBLE*)

- Use the least dose of LA necessary to achieve the desired extent and duration of block.
- Local anesthetic blood levels are influenced by site of injection and dose. Factors that can increase the likelihood of LAST include: advanced age, heart failure, ischemic heart disease, conduction abnormalities, metabolic (e.g., mitochondrial) disease, liver disease, low plasma protein concentration, metabolic or respiratory acidosis, medications that inhibit sodium channels. Patients with severe cardiac dysfunction, particularly very low ejection fraction, are more sensitive to LAST and also more prone to 'stacked' injections (with resulting elevated LA tissue concentrations) due to slowed circulation time.
- Consider using a pharmacologic marker and/or test dose, e.g. epinephrine 5 mcg/mL of LA. Know the expected response, onset, duration, and limitations of "test dose" in identifying intravascular injection.
- Aspirate the syringe prior to *each* injection while observing for blood.
- Inject incrementally, while observing for signs and querying for symptoms of toxicity between each injection.

DETECTION (*BE VIGILANT*)

- Use standard American Society of Anesthesiologists (ASA) monitors.
- Monitor the patient during and after completing injection as clinical toxicity can be delayed up to 30 minutes.
- Communicate frequently with the patient to query for symptoms of toxicity.
- Consider LAST in any patient with altered mental status, neurological symptoms or cardiovascular instability after a regional anesthetic.
- Central nervous system signs (may be subtle or absent)
  - *Excitation* (agitation, confusion, muscle twitching, seizure)
  - *Depression* (drowsiness, obtundation, coma or apnea)
  - *Non-specific* (metallic taste, circumoral numbness, diplopia, tinnitus, dizziness)

- Cardiovascular signs (often the only manifestation of severe LAST)
  - *Initially may be hyperdynamic* (hypertension, tachycardia, ventricular arrhythmias), then
  - *Progressive hypotension*
  - *Conduction block, bradycardia or asystole*
  - *Ventricular arrhythmia* (ventricular tachycardia, Torsades de Pointes, ventricular fibrillation)
- Sedative hypnotic drugs reduce seizure risk but even light sedation may abolish the patient's ability to recognize or report symptoms of rising LA concentrations.

TREATMENT

- Timing of lipid infusion in LAST is controversial. The most conservative approach, waiting until after ACLS has proven unsuccessful, is unreasonable because early treatment can prevent cardiovascular collapse. Infusing lipid at the earliest sign of LAST can result in unnecessary treatment since only a fraction of patients will progress to severe toxicity. The most reasonable approach is to implement lipid therapy on the basis of clinical severity and rate of progression of LAST.
- There is laboratory evidence that epinephrine can impair resuscitation from LAST and reduce the efficacy of lipid rescue. Therefore it is recommended to avoid high doses of epinephrine and use smaller doses, e.g., <1mcg/kg, for treating hypotension.
- Propofol *should not be used* when there are signs of cardiovascular instability. Propofol is a cardiovascular depressant with lipid content too low to provide benefit. Its use is discouraged when there is a risk of progression to cardiovascular collapse.
- Prolonged monitoring (> 12 hours) is recommended after any signs of systemic LA toxicity, since cardiovascular depression due to local anesthetics can persist or recur after treatment.

Neal JM, Bernards CM, Butterworth JF, Di Gregorio G, Drasner K, Hejtmanck MR, Mulroy MF, Rosenquist RW, Weinberg GL. ASRA practice advisory on local anesthetic systemic toxicity. *Reg Anesth Pain Med* 2010;35:152-161.

Figure 31-10 (*Continued*)

sensory, motor, or mixed and occasionally occur bilaterally. Nulliparity, fetal macrosomia, prolonged second stage of labor, and prolonged duration of hip hyperflexion are associated with increased rates of injury. Regional labor analgesia was not associated with nerve injury in a large prospective study (22). Occasionally, root injuries or radiculopathy may present postpartum due to exacerbation of underlying pathologies such as disk herniation. During neuraxial block, a needle or catheter may directly traumatize nerves, resulting in injury. Such an injury is usually preceded by paresthesias during block placement. Persistence of paresthesias or severe pain during a neuraxial technique should prompt withdrawal of the needle or catheter.

Documentation of neurologic examination and pre-existing deficits prior to neuraxial procedures is important, and intrinsic nerve injuries due to labor and delivery must be distinguished from those resulting from neuraxial anesthesia. Electromyogram may be helpful in determining the amount of time a deficit has been present.

D. Neuraxial Hematoma or Abscess

Epidural bleeding or abscess can be catastrophic because of pressure exerted on the spinal cord or cauda equina. Neuraxial hematoma is a rare event, but traumatic or difficult placement and coagulopathy or anticoagulant use increase the likelihood of occurrence. The American Society of Regional Anesthesia recommendations for use of anticoagulants and placement of neuraxial anesthesia can be viewed at their website. Motor weakness that persists or worsens despite discontinuation of local anesthetic is the most common presentation for a neuraxial hematoma. Back pain sometimes accompanies the weakness. Time is important in cases of neuraxial hematoma because neurologic outcomes are worse the longer treatment is delayed. MRI represents the best imaging modality for diagnosis. Neuraxial hematoma necessitates immediate neurosurgical consultation for possible emergent decompression of the clot.

Neuraxial infection may manifest as either meningitis or abscess; both are very uncommon events. Contaminants causing meningitis tend to arise from the nasopharynx of the provider who placed the block. Abscess may be due to the patient's skin flora. Sterile preparation, draping, and use of a surgical mask are standard during placement of neuraxial blocks to prevent iatrogenic infection.

IX. Anesthesia for Nonobstetric Surgery during Pregnancy

Nonobstetric elective surgery during a desired pregnancy is not recommended. Occasionally emergency conditions warrant surgery during pregnancy, the most common of which are appendicitis or trauma. The safest time to perform surgery during pregnancy is the second trimester because surgery during the first trimester is associated with spontaneous abortion and during the third trimester with preterm labor. Organogenesis occurs early in the first trimester, and it is still unclear what effects anesthetic agents may have on the developing fetus.

Confirmation of fetal heart tones both pre- and postoperatively is recommended. In certain cases, continuous fetal monitoring may be indicated, specifically if the fetus is viable and if staff qualified to perform emergency cesarean delivery are available. Most abdominal surgeries preclude the use of continuous fetal monitoring. Observation postoperatively is generally recommended due to the increased risk of preterm labor.

Regional anesthesia is preferred whenever possible, including for short, uncomplicated open abdominal surgery, such as appendectomy. If not possible (e.g., for laparoscopic surgery), general anesthesia should be induced via rapid sequence induction and intubation with cricoid pressure. Patients over 14 weeks' gestation should be positioned in left uterine displacement if feasible. Normotension, maintenance of eucarbia, and adequate oxygenation will provide the fetus and mother with adequate perfusion and oxygenation. Most anesthetic agents, other than the neuromuscular blocking agents, cross the placenta with unknown fetal effects. Neuromuscular blockade reversal agents do cross the placenta, but glycopyrrolate does not. Therefore, the anesthesiologist should reverse blockade with atropine to avoid fetal effects of reversal, including bradycardia.

In summary, providing optimal anesthetic care to pregnant patients requires consideration of the many maternal physiologic changes pregnancy induces, as well as recognition of the effects of anesthesia on both the mother and the fetus. The anesthesiologist is responsible for providing analgesia for labor, but also for guiding the response to complex medical and emergency clinical situations. A thorough knowledge of the medical histories of patients who are admitted to labor and delivery, as well as coordinated multidisciplinary care, is of the utmost importance to ensure optimal outcomes for both mothers and babies.

References

1. Quinn A, Milne D, Columb M, et al. Failed tracheal intubation in obstetric anaesthesia: 2 yr national case–control study in the UK. *Brit J Anaesth*. 2013;110(1):74–80.
2. Sharma S, Alexander J, Messick G, et al. Cesarean delivery: A randomized trial of epidural analgesia versus intravenous meperidine analgesia during labor in nulliparous women. *Anesthesiology*. 2002;96:546–551.
3. Gambling D, Berkowitz J, Farrell T, et al. Randomized controlled comparison of epidural analgesia and combined spinal-epidural analgesia in a private practice setting: Pain scores during first and second stages of labor and at delivery. *Anesth Analg*. 2013; 116(3):636–643.
4. Pan P, Bogard T, Owen M. Incidence and characteristics of failures in obstetric neuraxial analgesia and anesthesia: A retrospective analysis of 19,259 deliveries. *Int J Obstet Anesth*. 2004;13:227–233.
5. Hamilton B, Martin J, Ventura S. Births: Preliminary data for 2011. *Natl Vital Stat Rep*. 2012;61(5):1–20.
6. Siddik-Sayyid S, Taha S, Kanazi G, et al. A randomized controlled trial of variable rate phenylephrine infusion with rescue phenylephrine boluses versus rescue boluses alone on physician interventions during spinal anesthesia for elective cesarean delivery. *Anesth Analg*. 2014;118:611–618.
7. Palmer C, Emerson S, Volgoropolous D, et al. Dose-response relationship of intrathecal morphine for postcesarean analgesia. *Anesthesiology*. 1999;90:437–444.
8. Palmer C, Nogami W, Van Maren G, et al. Postcesarean epidural morphine: A dose-response study. *Anesth Analg*. 2000;90:887–891.
9. Horlocker T, Burton A, Connis R, et al. Practice guidelines for the prevention, detection, and management of respiratory depression associated with neuraxial opioid administration: An updated report by the American Society of Anesthesiologists Task Force on Neuraxial Opioids. *Anesthesiology*. 2009;110:218–230.
10. ACOG Practice Bulletin. Intrapartum fetal heart rate monitoring: Nomenclature, interpretation, and general management principles. *Obstet Gynecol*. 2009;114(1):192–202.
11. Alfirevic Z, Devane D, Gyte GM. Continuous cardiotocography (CTG) as a form of electronic fetal monitoring (EFM) for fetal assessment during labour. *Cochrane Database Syst Rev*. 2006;3:CD006066.
12. ACOG Task Force on Hypertension in Pregnancy. Hypertension in pregnancy: Report of the American College of Obstetricians and Gynecologists' Task Force on Hypertension in Pregnancy. *Obstet Gynecol*. 2013;122:1122.

13. The Eclampsia Trial Collaborative Group. Which anticonvulsant for women with eclampsia? Evidence from the Collaborative Eclampsia Trial. *Lancet.* 1995;345:1455–1463.
14. Segal S. Labor epidural analgesia and maternal fever. *Anesth Analg.* 2010;111:1467–1475.
15. American College of Obstetricians and Gynecologists. ACOG practice bulletin no. 115: Vaginal birth after previous cesarean delivery. *Obstet Gynecol.* 2010;116(1 Pt 1):450–463.
16. Bateman B, Berman M, Riley L, et al. The epidemiology of postpartum hemorrhage in a large, nationwide sample of deliveries. *Anesth Analg.* 2010;110:1368–1373.
17. Morris S, Stacey M. Resuscitation in pregnancy. *BMJ.* 2003;327:1277–1279.
18. Berg C, Callaghan W, Syverson C, et al. Pregnancy-related mortality in the United States, 1998 to 2005. *Obstet Gynecol.* 2010;116:1302–1309.
19. World Health Organization: Trends in Maternal Mortality: 1990 to 2010. Geneva: World Health Organization; 2012;1–59.
20. Hawkins J, Chang J, Palmer S, et al. Anesthesia-related maternal mortality in the United States: 1979–2002. *Obstet Gynecol.* 2011;117:69–74.
21. Choi P, Galinski S, Takeuchi L, et al. PDPH is a common complication of neuraxial blockade in parturients: A meta-analysis of obstetrical studies. *Can J Anesth.* 2003; 50(5):460–469.
22. Wong C, Scavone B, Dugan S, et al. Incidence of postpartum lumbosacral spine and lower extremity nerve injuries. *Obstet Gynecol.* 2003;101:279–288.

Questions

1. The physiologic anemia of pregnancy is most frequently caused by:
   A. Decreased hematopoiesis and decreased red cell production
   B. Disproportionate increase in plasma volume relative to red cell volume
   C. Shorter red blood cell circulating life
   D. Iron deficiency in pregnant women

2. The most common reason for difficult mask ventilation and laryngoscopy in the pregnant patient is because:
   A. Pregnant women have less neck mobility, making the head-tilt required difficult
   B. Pregnant women tend to have higher Mallampati scores
   C. Pregnant women have a difficult time breathing in the supine position
   D. Pregnant women develop mucosal edema and capillary engorgement, creating mechanical obstruction to the instruments used

3. By what mechanism do oxygen and carbon dioxide move from the maternal placental circulation to the fetal circulation?
   A. By diffusion
   B. By transcellular transfer
   C. By endocytosis
   D. By exocytosis

4. Which commonly used anesthetic drugs do not cross the placenta and do not affect the fetus?
   A. Propofol
   B. Sevoflurane
   C. Succinyl choline
   D. Fentanyl

5. What level spinal fibers should be targeted to receive local anesthetic drugs when an epidural catheter will be used for analgesia for the first stage of labor?
   A. T1-10
   B. T10-L1
   C. L1-5
   D. T6-S5

6. What is the best strategy for providing adequate labor analgesia while avoiding excessive motor blockade?
   A. Epidural administration of low concentration local anesthetics
   B. Encouraging the parturient to ambulate
   C. Adding epinephrine to the epidural local anesthetic
   D. Administering subsequent doses of epidural local anesthetic only after evaluation by a provider from the labor and delivery care team

7. When a healthy fetus exhibits changes in fetal heart rate or variability, one can conclude that:
   A. The fetus is almost certainly acidotic or in distress
   B. A cesarean delivery is imminent
   C. There are maternal factors that could be causing these changes
   D. The magnesium infusion to the mother should be discontinued

32 Trauma and Burn Anesthesia

Joshua M. Tobin
Andreas Grabinsky

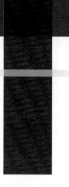
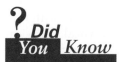
I. Initial Trauma Evaluation and Resuscitation

The treatment of seriously injured patients is time-sensitive and requires a coordinated and systematic approach from all medical providers. This should include those with anesthesiology training who are providing acute resuscitative care in the emergency medical setting or perioperative care in the operating room and intensive care unit (1). Rapid assessment of injuries and institution of life-saving therapies is guided by tenets of the American College of Surgeons' *Advanced Trauma Life Support (ATLS)* program. ATLS management of injured patients consists of the *primary survey* (identification of life-threatening injuries), *resuscitation* (immediate treatment of such injuries as they are identified), the *secondary survey* (comprehensive assessment of all other injuries and associated conditions), and *definitive care* (medical, surgical, or critical care).

A. Airway Evaluation and Management

Assessing and securing the airway of the trauma patient is the first step of the primary survey and associated resuscitation. Chapter 20 provides comprehensive details of airway management in elective and emergent settings, including application of the American Society of Anesthesiologists (ASA) difficult airway algorithm (see Appendix F).

Airway assessment (Tables 20-4, 20-5, 20-6) can be limited in the trauma setting by lack of patient cooperation and preclude use of the *Mallampati classification* (Fig. 20-3). Thus, trauma airway assessment largely relies on visual inspection of the patient's face, head, and neck. A short, fat neck with fewer than three finger-breadths from the thyroid notch to the jaw tip (i.e., thyromental distance) is concerning for a difficult airway. Obvious facial asymmetry further suggests an underlying anatomic abnormality, be it traumatic, congenital, or neoplastic. Limited neck range of motion further suggests a more challenging airway, although cervical motion should not be assessed in patients with suspected cervical spine injuries.

Mask ventilation and tracheal intubation can both be challenging in trauma patients due to head and neck injuries, recent oral intake that increases aspiration risk, and possible lung injury that can negatively impact both oxygenation and ventilation. Adherence to the ASA difficult airway algorithm is essential, including planning and preparation of multiple backup airway management techniques.

To assist the laryngoscopist with visualization of the vocal cords, cricoid pressure is typically applied in a backward, upward, rightward fashion (i.e., BURP). Although this is common practice, the literature supporting cricoid pressure is controversial, and the technique may in some cases interfere with vocal cord viewing or tracheal tube placement. Cricoid pressure is not intended to prevent aspiration in a vomiting patient, but rather to prevent passive reflux of gastric contents into the posterior pharynx and facilitate laryngeal viewing. In fact, if a patient begins to vomit, one must release cricoid pressure, turn the patient on his or her side (if possible), and suction the emesis. Maintenance of cricoid pressure during active vomiting risks esophageal injury.

Manual in-line stabilization (MILS) of the cervical spine is routinely used in emergency airway management of trauma patients in whom a spinal cord injury is suspected. Patients with documented spinal cord injuries rarely have worsening of their neurologic injury with proper MILS during direct laryngoscopy and tracheal intubation. Cadaveric studies have shown that MILS does not ensure spine immobility, however. Persisting with rigid adherence to MILS in the context of a poor view of the vocal cords can increase the difficulty and duration of tracheal intubation; therefore, application and possible relaxation of MILS must be considered in the context of the overall clinical picture.

B. Breathing Evaluation and Management

Respiratory assessment is a critical component of the primary survey and resuscitation phases. Indications for tracheal intubation include obvious respiratory distress, inability to speak in complete sentences, an elevated respiratory rate, poor oxygenation, poor ventilation, or significant traumatic brain injury.

Patients who arrive with an airway device placed prior to hospital arrival must be immediately evaluated to ensure proper position and function of the device. End-tidal carbon dioxide and the presence of bilateral breath sounds should be evaluated and documented to confirm satisfactory ventilation. Alternative airway devices such as the King LT (King System, Noblesville, IN) airway, Combitube (Moore Medical, Farmington, CT), or laryngeal masks do not protect the airway from aspiration of stomach contents, blood, saliva, or tooth fragments. They should be replaced with a cuffed endotracheal tube as soon as possible. A gastric tube should also be placed soon after tracheal intubation to further mitigate the risk of aspiration.

C. Circulation Evaluation and Shock Management

Shock is defined as inadequate tissue perfusion. Delayed capillary refill, cold and "clammy" skin, impaired mentation, and oliguria are classic signs in trauma patients that most often suggest *hypovolemic shock* due to massive hemorrhage. Blood pressure and heart rate can help provide more quantifiable assessment of systemic perfusion and shock. For example, low blood pressure is typically compensated for with an elevated heart rate (see Chapter 3). The assessment of blood consumption score (Table 32-1) is a tool that uses four simple clinical assessments to determine the likelihood

Table 32-1 Assessment of Blood Consumption	
Penetrating injury mechanism?	YES / NO
Systolic blood pressure <90 mm Hg?	YES / NO
Heart rate >120 beats per minute?	YES / NO
Positive FAST examination?	YES / NO
If 2 or more YES answers, then activate massive transfusion protocol.	

FAST, focused assessment with sonography in trauma.

of hemorrhagic shock and the associated need for early massive blood transfusion.

The immediate treatment goals for hemorrhagic shock are to stop ongoing bleeding and restore tissue perfusion by replacing intravascular volume (see Chapter 23). The use of tourniquets for massive bleeding from extremities is supported by recent military experience with blast injuries. Ultimately, any patient in extremis must have his or her blood volume restored and be rapidly transported to the operating room for definitive control of internal or external bleeding.

D. Neurologic Evaluation and Management

A prompt neurologic evaluation during the primary survey is important for establishing a baseline examination for future treatments. Given that the anesthesiologist is often the last person to speak to a conscious patient prior to induction of anesthesia or tracheal intubation, an understanding of the *Glasgow coma scale* (Table 32-2) is critical to rapidly evaluate the mental

Table 32-2   Glasgow Coma Scale
Motor
6 = Obeys Commands
5 = Localizes Pain
4 = Withdraws from Pain
3 = Decorticate Flexion
2 = Decerebrate Extension
1 = Flaccid
Verbal
5 = Oriented & Appropriate
4 = Disoriented
3 = Inappropriate Words
2 = Incomprehensible Sounds
1 = None
Eyes
4 = Open Spontaneously
3 = Open to Verbal Stimulus
2 = Open to Pain
1 = None
If GCS <8, then tracheal intubation should be performed.

status and motor function of trauma patients. It also guides the need for tracheal intubation in patients with *traumatic brain injury (TBI)*. Of note, the iris contains no nicotinic acetylcholine receptors; therefore, neuromuscular blocking agents do not affect pupil size.

TBI is the leading cause of death in trauma. Any suspicion of TBI should be evaluated with a head computed tomography (CT) scan to identify primary injuries (e.g., intracranial hematoma) that require immediate surgery or specialized critical care. Throughout the initial evaluation and treatment period, however, priority is given to maintaining adequate blood pressure and oxygenation to avoid *secondary brain injury* due to neuronal ischemia. Guidelines from the Brain Trauma Foundation recommend that systolic blood pressure be >90 mm Hg and oxygen saturation be >90% at all times. Even transient reductions in blood pressure or oxygen saturation can profoundly affect the mortality of these patients (2). Perioperative anesthetic management of TBI is discussed in detail in Chapter 30.

In patients who have sustained a *spinal cord injury (SCI)*, it is important to assess the anatomic level of the neurologic deficit as soon after the event as possible. Sensory level is determined by dermatome level of touch or pain. Motor function is assessed using the American Spinal Injury Association score (Table 32-3). Assessment of anal sphincter tone is also an important component of the motor examination.

In the past, patients with SCI were treated with methylprednisolone infusions to decrease spinal cord swelling and enhance recovery of function. Recent literature, however, has not demonstrated a significant benefit of such therapy and instead showed an increased risk of infection. Thus, steroid administration is not currently recommended in SCI.

Initial management of suspected cervical spine injuries includes placement of a rigid cervical collar to minimize cervical motion. Because it is often challenging to rule out SCI in intoxicated or head-injured patients, these patients should remain in a cervical collar until definitive imaging can be performed. Recent data support removal of a cervical collar in adult patients with normal cervical spine CT scans who spontaneously move all four extremities.

E. Other Major Vascular Injuries

Initial evaluation of major vascular injuries includes assessment of the affected extremity for presence and character of pulse as well as skin color and

Table 32-3 American Spinal Injury Association (ASIA) Spinal Cord Injury Classification

Grade	Type of Injury	Description
A	Complete	No motor or no sensory function in S4-5
B	Incomplete	No motor or sensory function preserved below the level of injury including S4-5
C	Incomplete	Motor and sensory function is preserved below the level of injury (motor strength <3/5 in half of the major muscles)
D	Incomplete	Motor and sensory function is preserved below the level of injury (motor strength ≥3/5 in half of the major muscles)
E	Normal	Motor and sensory functions are intact

temperature. A cool and poorly perfused limb must be immediately evaluated for possible arterial injury and revascularization. Similarly, obvious vascular injury with external hemorrhage must be immediately addressed with hemorrhage control and fluid resuscitation. Placement of temporary tourniquets on a limb with life-threatening bleeding is a simple and effective hemostasis measure. In cases of significant pelvic trauma and retroperitoneal bleeding, placement of a *pelvic binder* can reapproximate pelvic fractures to a degree sufficient to temporarily limit blood loss. Interventional, endovascular radiology techniques are frequently used to control pelvic and liver bleeding, thereby avoiding complications associated with open surgical repairs. Aortic injuries are evaluated with a contrast CT scan of the chest and abdomen. Transesophageal echocardiography can be used to evaluate the ascending aorta, aortic arch, and descending aorta for potential disruption.

F. Interdisciplinary, Team-Based Management
Crew resource management is a concept developed by the aviation industry in which each member of the multidisciplinary team has equal responsibility for passenger safety. For example, any member of a flight crew can alert the pilot in command of a potential hazard. This concept is particularly relevant to trauma, when care is necessarily multidisciplinary and critical events must occur in a timely fashion. Central to the concept of crew resource management is clear and free communication between all parties, regardless of hierarchy. When several events and therapies must occur simultaneously, it can be valuable to use a checklist to ensure that no critical steps are overlooked (3). The recommended checklist for trauma and emergency anesthesia is shown in Figure 32-1. Assigning predetermined positions to members of the anesthetic resuscitation team is also an effective way to maintain organization in the trauma operating room (Fig. 32-2).

II. Operative Management: General Considerations
A. Monitoring
Standard ASA monitors are described in Chapter 15. In emergencies, the oxygen saturation monitor can provide reasonably accurate heart rate and numeric oxygen saturation information. It also is an indirect indicator of peripheral perfusion, as a poor quality waveform suggests poor peripheral perfusion. An arterial line can provide accurate beat-to-beat measurement of blood pressure and facilitate frequent blood sampling. It can also use emerging technologies for arterial waveform analysis (see Chapter 23) to estimate cardiac output and intravascular volume status. Placement of an arterial line, however, should never delay the start of an emergent surgical case.

B. Anesthetic and Adjunct Drugs
Severely injured patients with hypovolemia are very susceptible to the negative inotropic and vasodilatory effects of anesthetics, especially volatile anesthetics. Thus, all anesthetic drugs should be slowly and carefully titrated to avoid cardiovascular collapse in such patients. A partial list of commonly used perioperative anesthetic and adjunct drugs, along with specific cautions for use in trauma patients, is provided in Table 32-4.

C. Induction and Airway Management
Rapid sequence induction (RSI) is the process by which an endotracheal tube is rapidly placed by direct laryngoscopy during emergency airway management

BEFORE PATIENT ARRIVAL
☐ Room temperature 25°C or higher
☐ Warm IV line
☐ Machine check
☐ Airway equipment
☐ Emergency medications
☐ **BLOOD BANK: "6U O Neg PRBC, 6U AB FFP, 5–6 units of random donor platelets (1 standard adult dose) available"**

PATIENT ARRIVAL
☐ Patient identified for trauma/emergency surgery?
☐ **BLOOD BANK: "Send blood for T&C and initiate MTP now!"**
☐ IV access
☐ Monitors (SaO_2, BP, ECG)
☐ **SURGEON: "PREP & DRAPE!"**
☐ Pre-oxygenation

INDUCTION
☐ Sedative hypnotic (ketamine v. propofol v. etomidate)
☐ Neuromuscular blockade (succinylcholine v. rocuronium)

INTUBATION
☐ (+) $ETCO_2$ → SURGEON : "GO!"
☐ Place orogastric tube

ANESTHETIC
☐ (Volatile anesthetic and/or benzodiazepine) + narcotic
☐ Consider TIVA
☐ Insert additional IV access if needed and an arterial line

RESUSCITATION
☐ Send baseline labs
☐ Follow MAP trend
☐ Goal FFP: PRBC controversial, but consider early FFP
☐ Goal urine output 0.5–1 mL/kg/hr
☐ Consider tranexamic acid if <3 hr after injury; 1 gm over 10 min ×1, then 1 gm over 8 hrs
☐ Consider calcium chloride 1 gm
☐ Consider hydrocortisone 100 mg
☐ Consider vasopressin 5–10 IU
☐ Administer appropriate antibiotics
☐ Special considerations for TBI (SBP > 90–100 mm Hg, SaO_2 > 90%, pCO2 35–45 mm Hg)

CLOSING/POST-OP
☐ **ICU: "Do you have a bed?"**
☐ Initiate low lung volume ventilation (TV = 6 mL/kg ideal body weight)

? *Did You Know*

Whereas rapid sequence induction and intubation is generally a two-person procedure, a minimum of three providers are required when performing the procedure in a patient with possible cervical spin injury: one to hold manual in-line neck stabilization, one to provide cricoid pressure, and one to perform tracheal intubation.

Figure 32-1 Emergency and trauma anesthesia checklist. Critical preparation and treatment strategies are shown for each successive step in the emergent, perioperative care of the major trauma victim. PRBC, packed red blood cells; AB FFP, type AB fresh frozen plasma; T&C, type and cross; MTP, massive transfusion protocol; SaO_2, oxygen saturation; BP, blood pressure; ECG, electrocardiogram; $ETCO_2$, end-tidal carbon dioxide; TIVA, total intravenous anesthesia; MAP, mean arterial blood pressure; TBI, traumatic brain injury; SBP, systolic blood pressure.

(see Chapter 20). RSI is commonly employed in trauma patients. When it is combined with MILS in patients at risk for cervical spinal cord injury, it is a safe, effective method to secure the airway. When a hard cervical collar is in place, the front portion of the collar can be removed (with MILS applied) immediately after induction to facilitate mandible subluxation and laryngeal viewing.

Video laryngoscopy (e.g., Glidescope, Verathon Inc., Bothell, WA) is increasingly used in emergency settings. Although video laryngoscopy can improve visualization of the vocal cords, it does not decrease time to intubation or improve successful first attempt intubation (4). The benefit of video

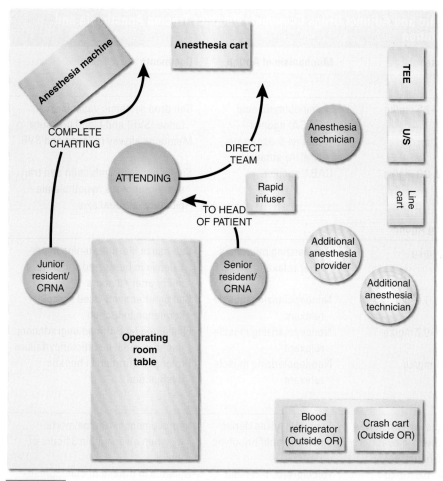

Figure 32-2 Trauma anesthesia team work flow diagram. The ideal floor plan setup for anesthetic care of the major trauma patient includes assigned spaces for various anesthesia providers, the anesthesia workstation, and critical equipment.

laryngoscopy may be confined to patients with difficult airway anatomy (e.g., limited mouth opening or neck mobility) or to novices or those who do not perform direct laryngoscopy regularly (5). Supraglottic airways (e.g., laryngeal mask) provide a blind insertion alternative to tracheal intubation. In the prehospital environment, such devices may be easier to place by providers with limited tracheal intubation experience. In the hospital setting, they serve as effective rescue devices in "can't intubate, can't ventilate" scenarios.

D. Hypotension

As noted previously, ongoing blood loss frequently leads to hypovolemic shock in patients with major or multiple injuries. Aggressive resuscitation in the presence of untreated injuries can actually worsen blood loss by increasing intravascular pressure in injured vessels. The concept of *"hypotensive resuscitation"* aims to mitigate blood loss in these cases by targeting a lower-than-normal blood pressure—yet still provide vital organ perfusion—until source control of hemorrhage is achieved. Although animal models have offered encouraging results with hypotensive resuscitation, human data have been less

Table 32-4   Anesthetic and Adjunct Drugs Commonly Used for Trauma Anesthesia and Resuscitation

Medication	Dose	Mechanism of Action	Comments
Sedative/Hypnotics			
Propofol	1.5–2.5 mg/kg	γ-aminobutyric acid (GABA) agonist	Can drop systemic vascular resistance (SVR) and blood pressure
Ketamine	1–2 mg/kg	N-methyl-D-aspartate (NMDA) antagonist	Maintains airway reflexes and SVR
Etomidate	0.2–0.3 mg/kg	GABA agonist	Single doses for induction can transiently suppress hypothalamic–pituitary–adrenal axis
Neuromuscular Blocking Agents			
Succinylcholine	1 mg/kg	Depolarizing neuromuscular relaxant	Can cause life-threatening hyperkalemia in burns and spinal cord injury after 48 hours
Rocuronium	0.6–1.0 mg/kg	Nondepolarizing muscle relaxant	Can be effectively used in rapid sequence induction
Cisatracurium	0.1–0.2 mg/kg	Nondepolarizing muscle relaxant	Eliminated by Hoffman degradation; useful in renal insufficiency/failure
Vecuronium	0.1 mg/kg	Nondepolarizing muscle relaxant	Prolonged duration in hepatic dysfunction
Adjuncts			
Tranexamic acid	1 g over 10 minutes, then 1 g over 8 hours	Synthetic lysine derivative and antifibrinolytic	Improvement in trauma mortality when given within 3 hours of injury
Recombinant factor VII	20–100 µg/kg	Accelerates thrombin formation at site of endothelial injury	Benefits in trauma unclear; potential risk of thrombosis; expensive
Vasopressin	5–20 IU	Potent vasoconstrictor	Shunts blood to cerebral, cardiac and pulmonary vascular beds
Calcium chloride	1 g	Facilitates smooth muscle contraction	Used to restore low calcium levels and inotropy during massive transfusion
Hydrocortisone	100 mg	Potent mineralocorticoid	Treats adrenal suppression seen in critical illness

encouraging, and documented benefit appears limited to victims of penetrating injury.

Although it is difficult to quantify the ideal blood pressure goal during resuscitation, mean arterial pressure trends often provide a better assessment of resuscitation progress than reliance on discrete systolic blood pressure values. Recent literature suggests that the risk of acute kidney or myocardial injury is increased with mean arterial pressures below 55 mm Hg (6), thus supporting this value as a lower target limit during resuscitation.

Resuscitation is often initiated with isotonic crystalloid, such as Plasma-Lyte or lactated Ringer's. Sodium chloride 0.9% should be avoided because of its associated risk of acute kidney injury (see Chapter 23). Volume resuscitation should be converted to blood products as quickly as possible. Early use of packed red blood cells and empiric administration of fresh frozen plasma before a documented coagulopathy develops has improved survival of severely injured trauma patients in both the combat environment (7) and the civilian population (8). A ratio of packed red blood cells to fresh frozen plasma to platelets approaching 1:1:1 is the general goal of such trauma resuscitation, although the exact relative ratios remain to be determined.

Tranexamic acid is a synthetic lysine derivative that inhibits fibrinolysis and can decrease blood loss in some high-risk surgical procedures (e.g., liver transplantation, major spine surgery). Its early administration has also been shown to reduce mortality in major trauma patients (9) and is increasingly used in this setting.

The use of vasopressors (with the possible exception of vasopressin) is associated with increased mortality in trauma resuscitation, and their use should be avoided (10). Because shock in the trauma setting is generally due to hypovolemia, therapeutic efforts must be aimed at controlling hemorrhage and replacing lost intravascular volume.

E. Hypothermia

The *"lethal triad" of trauma resuscitation* consists of hypothermia, coagulopathy, and acidosis. To avoid hypothermia in perioperative trauma care, the operating room should be heated as warm as possible (even to the point of discomfort for the operating team), intravenous fluids warmed, and convective warming devices used to maintain a core temperature as close to normal as possible.

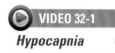

VIDEO 32-1

Hypocapnia

Therapeutic hypothermia has demonstrated improved neurologic recovery in patients who have suffered out-of-hospital cardiac arrest, and animal models have suggested potential benefit in the setting of hypovolemic shock. However, at this time there are no clinical data to support this practice in trauma.

F. Coagulation Abnormalities

Although empiric administration of fresh frozen plasma before documented coagulopathy improves survival, as noted previously, accurate assessment of coagulation status remains an important component of trauma resuscitation. Traditionally, blood samples are sent for cross-matching, as well as prothrombin time (PT)/international normalized ratio (INR), partial thromboplastin time (PTT), hemoglobin/hematocrit, platelet count, and fibrinogen. Low platelet counts, hemoglobin/hematocrit, and fibrinogen are treated with platelets, packed red blood cells, and cryoprecipitate, respectively. Elevated PT/INR and PTT are treated with fresh frozen plasma.

More recently, *thromboelastography* has been used to evaluate various functional aspects of coagulation (Figs. 32-3 and 32-4). The reaction time (R) and clot kinetic time (K) are measures of the enzymatic process of clot formation. Prolongations of either are treated with fresh frozen plasma. The maximum amplitude (MA) and the α angle are measures of clot kinetics and cross-linking. A shallow α angle and decreased MA are treated with platelet infusions. Clot lysis is measured at specific intervals throughout the process and indicates the status of fibrinolysis. Abnormally narrowed waveforms can be treated with antifibrinolytics such as tranexamic acid.

G. Electrolyte and Acid–Base Disturbances

During massive transfusion, the citrate preservative in packed red blood cells can chelate calcium, decreasing the serum calcium level and contributing to

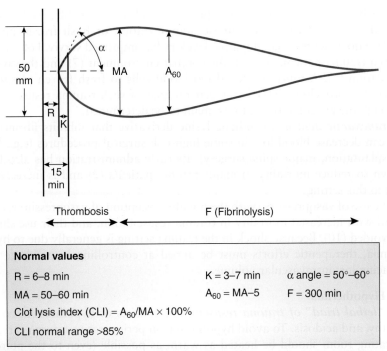

Normal values

R = 6–8 min   K = 3–7 min α angle = 50°–60°

MA = 50–60 min A_{60} = MA–5   F = 300 min

Clot lysis index (CLI) = $A_{60}/MA \times 100\%$

CLI normal range >85%

Figure 32-3 A normal thromboelastogram's associated values are shown (see text for details). R, interval from blood deposition in the cuvette to an amplitude of 1 mm on the thromboelastogram; K, time between the end of R and a point with an amplitude of 20 mm on the thromboelastogram; α angle, slope of the external divergence of the tracing from the R value point; MA, maximum amplitude of thromboelastogram; A60, amplitude of thromboelastogram 60 minutes after maximum amplitude; F, time from MA to return to 0 amplitude (normal, >300 minutes). (From Capon LM, Miller SM, Gingrich KJ. Trauma and burns. In: Barash PG, Cullen BF, Stoelting RK, et al. *Clinical Anesthesia.* 7th ed. Philadelphia: Lippincott Williams & Wilkins; 2013: 1490–1534, with permission.)

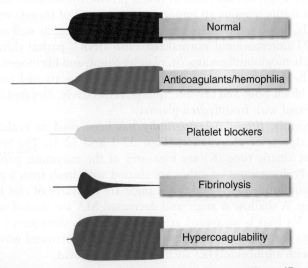

Figure 32-4 Examples of abnormal thromboelastogram tracings. (From da Luz LT, Nascimento B, Rizoli S. Thrombelastography (TEG®): Practical considerations on its clinical use in trauma resuscitation. *Scand J Trauma Resusc Emerg Med.* 2013;21:29, with permission.)

hypotension. Calcium is highly protein bound; therefore, the biochemical assay for ionized calcium provides a more accurate estimate of total calcium level. *Hypocalcemia* is associated with increased mortality, and ionized calcium levels below 1 mmol/L should be promptly treated with calcium chloride.

Lysis of red blood cells during blood transfusion can result in *hyperkalemia*. This is particularly true when older blood products are used and in small children. Hyperkalemia is characterized by peaked T waves on the electrocardiogram. Potassium levels >5 mEq/L should be treated with calcium chloride to stabilize cardiac membrane potentials. Insulin can also be administered to drive potassium into the cell, lowering the serum potassium level. Care must be taken to avoid hypoglycemia; thus, blood glucose must be frequently checked and dextrose readily available.

The *base deficit* is the quantity of base required to normalize a blood sample at 37°C to a pH of 7.4 with an assumed carbon dioxide tension of 40 mm Hg. By eliminating the respiratory component of the acid–base assessment, a more specific measurement of the metabolic component is possible. Base deficit is quickly available and more rapidly responsive to therapeutic interventions than other biochemical assays (e.g., serum lactate).

III. Anesthetic Management of Specific Injuries

A. Traumatic Brain Injuries or Head Injury

The most important consideration in the anesthetic management of patients with TBI is the prevention of secondary neurologic injury. As noted previously, drops in blood pressure or oxygenation contribute significantly to mortality and must be avoided in head-injured patients. Perioperative anesthetic management of TBI is discussed in detail in Chapter 30.

B. Spine and Spinal Cord Injury

As noted previously, steroids are not indicated in SCI and may worsen outcome by increasing the risk of infection. As with TBI, avoidance of secondary neurologic injury is critical. Improved neurologic recovery with intentional hypothermia is an exciting avenue of research, but it is not currently supported in the literature. Perioperative anesthetic management of SCI and spine surgery is discussed in detail in Chapter 26.

C. Soft Tissue Neck Injury

The neck is divided into three anatomic zones: zone 1 extends from the clavicle to the cricoid cartilage, zone 2 from the cricoid cartilage to the angle of the mandible, and zone 3 from the angle of the mandible to the mastoid. Injuries in zones 1 and 3 are generally treated with watchful waiting or interventional radiology due to challenging surgical exposure. Zone 2 injuries that penetrate the platysma are typically explored in the operating room. The primary anesthetic consideration with these injures is airway management, as the trachea may be involved. Large hematomas outside the airway can cause a midline shift of the trachea. Direct injury to the trachea can create a false passage for the endotracheal tube, even after it is visualized passing through the vocal cords. Signs of tracheal or laryngeal injury in the trauma patient with neck injury include difficulty with or altered phonation, hoarseness, stridor, and subcutaneous emphysema. As in the management of any traumatized airway, careful preoxygenation, RSI, and direct laryngoscopy are generally safe. However, if there is significant concern for airway involvement, awake fiberoptic intubation is indicated.

D. Chest Injury

Chest injuries can involve the heart, lungs, great vessels, and aerodigestive tract. Primary survey evaluation includes assessment of breath sounds and heart tones. Absent or asymmetric breath sounds suggest *pneumothorax* or *hemothorax*, while distant heart tones, especially when accompanied by distended jugular veins, suggest *cardiac tamponade*. A portable chest x-ray can confirm pneumothorax or hemothorax but should not delay immediate decompression of a *tension pneumothorax* if cardiovascular instability is present. Hemothorax and pneumothorax are both treated by placement of a chest tube. If >2 L of blood drains upon placement of the chest tube, or if >150 mL of blood drains from the chest tube per hour, then an exploratory thoracotomy is indicated. The surgeon will often require one-lung ventilation in these cases, necessitating placement of a double-lumen endotracheal tube or bronchial blocker (see Chapter 34). In an emergency, a simple endotracheal tube can be blindly advanced into the right main-stem bronchus to isolate the left lung.

Cardiac tamponade in trauma is a life-threatening condition in which blood fills the pericardium and restricts both venous return and cardiac output. Right and left heart pressures equalize and forward flow stops, resulting in cardiac arrest. Transthoracic ultrasound is used to quickly assess cardiac function and evaluate for the presence of fluid around the heart. Cardiac tamponade can be relieved by *pericardiocentesis* or in the operating room by a *pericardial window*. While the surgical team is preparing for this procedure, care must be taken to minimize positive intrathoracic pressure (facilitating venous return) and maintain systemic vascular resistance (e.g., phenylephrine) to ensure adequate coronary perfusion.

E. Abdominal and Pelvic Injuries

The *focused assessment with sonography in trauma (FAST)* examination evaluates the pericardium, hepatorenal recess (Morison's pouch), splenorenal region, and pelvic floor. Hypoechoic (dark) signals represent free fluid (blood) and suggest the need for exploratory surgery in victims of blunt abdominal trauma. In hemodynamically stable patients, an abdominal CT scan identifies intra-abdominal and pelvic injuries with more anatomic specificity than the FAST examination. Unstable patients, however, should be taken immediately to the operating room without CT imaging. Major abdominal trauma can include devastating solid organ injury, major vascular injury, and hollow organ contamination. To facilitate surgical exposure of the entire peritoneal cavity, abdominal wall relaxation must be maintained for the duration of the surgery. In cases of hepatic injury, splenic injury, or major vascular injury, a massive transfusion must be anticipated. In such cases, one must also be alert that manual pressure on the inferior vena cava by the operating surgeon can intermittently obstruct venous return and be an occult cause of hypotension. When nonarterial bleeding cannot be easily controlled, surgeons may elect to perform *"damage control" surgery*, with the limited goals of packing sites of major hemorrhage and temporary abdominal closure. This is followed with plans to return to the operating room several hours later for definitive surgical repairs after resuscitation, hypothermia, coagulopathy, and acidosis have been corrected. Broad-spectrum antibiotics may be given empirically to patients with widespread peritoneal contamination resulting from intestinal injury to prevent the development of septic shock.

Pelvic vascular injuries are increasingly being treated in the *interventional radiology* setting, as noted previously. Therefore, these facilities will require

VIDEO 32-2
Tension Pneumothorax

VIDEO 32-3
Chest Tube Insertion

? Did You Know

"Damage control surgery" refers to emergent surgical procedures or emergency interventional radiology procedures with the specific limited goals of rapidly identifying and treating life-threatening blood loss or other conditions, but transiently postponing definitive surgical repair until the patient can be medically stabilized.

Table 32-5	Estimated Internal (Occult) Blood Loss for Closed Fractures in Adults	
Pelvic fracture	2–3 L
Femur fracture	1–2 L
Proximal tibia fracture	0.5–1 L
Humerus fracture	~0.5 L

the same level of anesthesia equipment and staffing as a standard operating room to ensure appropriate care can be provided in such nontraditional locations for anesthetic resuscitation.

F. Extremity Injuries
Extremity injuries can run the spectrum from isolated closed fractures and simple lacerations to traumatic amputation secondary to blast injury. Blood loss from extremity injury can be surprisingly high (Table 32-5) and must be anticipated. Pain control is an important goal during all phases of trauma care. Not only is appropriate analgesia humane, but it also decreases inflammatory markers and the stress response, with theoretical benefit on wound healing. Obvious bleeding from an extremity should be promptly controlled initially with direct pressure and elevation of the extremity. Tourniquets should be considered early in cases of uncontrolled hemorrhage and can be left in situ for 2 to 3 hours and be released only when the team is fully prepared for surgical intervention.

G. Major Vascular Injuries
Truncal hemorrhage (e.g., iliac arteries, aorta) presents a unique challenge in that tourniquets are not an option and direct pressure with pelvic or abdominal binders is of limited utility. Bleeding from major retroperitoneal vascular injuries may be transiently self-limited by the tamponade effect of adjacent anatomic structures or the peritoneum. Surgical incision to expose the injury will release that tamponade effect, however, and incur the need for potential massive intraoperative transfusion. Open repair of thoracic aortic and aortic arch injuries may require median sternotomy, although such injuries are increasingly repaired with closed endovascular techniques.

After certain arterial vascular repairs, the surgeon may request heparinization to maintain vessel patency and minimize thrombotic occlusion. The benefit of heparinization to the vascular repair must be weighed, however, against the risk of potential catastrophic bleeding from other traumatized sites in the multiply injured patient. A collegial, multidisciplinary discussion is necessary to prioritize the various risks and benefits and resolve any discrepancies.

H. Open Globe Injuries
Ocular injuries can occur from both blunt and penetrating trauma. Care must be taken during the initial evaluation and any operative treatment to avoid increases in the *intraocular pressure* that could lead to extruded vitreous and loss of vision. For these reasons, succinylcholine should be avoided during induction, and rocuronium is used as an alternative neuromuscular blocker for RSI. Similarly, increases in intraocular pressure associated with coughing or vomiting in the postoperative period should be minimized with regular use of antiemetics (e.g., ondansetron) prior to emergence.

IV. Burn Injuries

A. Burn Size and Depth

Burns have classically been characterized as first degree (painful redness), second degree (blisters in addition to painful redness), and third degree (painless eschar). More recently, burns are characterized as either *partial thickness* or *full thickness*. Full-thickness burns penetrate all layers of the skin down to the dermis and require surgical debridement. A general rule of thumb is that the area covered by the patient's handprint is equivalent to 1% of the total body surface area (TBSA). There are a number of methods for estimating the TBSA of a larger burn, the most common being the "Rule of Nines" (Fig. 32-5). However, the Rule of Nines frequently overestimates the estimated TBSA, especially in obese patients.

> **VIDEO 32-4**
>
> *Body Surface Area Rule of Nines*

B. Initial Evaluation and Management of Burn Injuries

Burn-injured patients merit special consideration in the primary trauma survey, given the possibility for airway involvement with thermal injury or smoke inhalation. Airway edema can quickly decrease both upper and lower airway patency, making laryngoscopy and tracheal intubation nearly impossible if delayed. If the patient was injured in an enclosed space (e.g., house fire), has

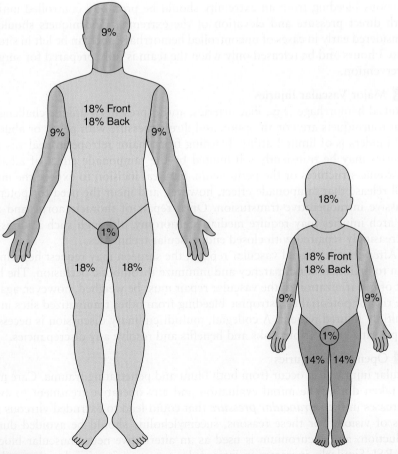

Figure 32-5 Rule of Nines burn man/child diagram. The percentage of total body surface area (TBSA) for burn injuries can be estimated from age-specific figures of percentage surface areas for different anatomic regions.

carbonaceous sputum, singed nasal hairs, or other signs suggesting *inhalation injury*, it is prudent to perform tracheal intubation immediately. Delaying tracheal intubation can allow airway edema to form—particularly during initial burn fluid resuscitation—and make later airway management extremely difficult. As noted in Table 32-4, succinylcholine can precipitate life-threatening hyperkalemia in burn-injured patients, but not in the first 48 hours following injury when neuromuscular acetylcholine receptors are yet to be upregulated. Thus, either succinylcholine or rocuronium can be used for RSI in the immediate postinjury setting.

Carbon monoxide (CO) has an affinity for the heme moiety in hemoglobin several hundred times higher than that of oxygen. CO poisoning can result from inhalation of the products of combustion. Patients rarely present with the classic cherry red complexion, and oxygen saturation by pulse oximetry will erroneously appear normal. In contrast, co-oximetry of arterial blood in this setting will yield accurate values for both elevated *carboxyhemoglobin* and reduced hemoglobin oxygen saturation. CO poisoning interferes with oxygen delivery to peripheral tissues and with cellular respiration, leading to severe metabolic acidosis. It is also associated with *central demyelination* and long-term neurologic sequelae. In cases of suspected CO poisoning, high-flow oxygen should be initiated immediately and the carboxyhemoglobin level determined. High-flow oxygen establishes an oxygen gradient that will favor rapid displacement of CO from heme and replacement with oxygen. Hyperbaric oxygen therapy can be used to deliver oxygen concentrations >100%, although such facilities are rarely available and pose logistic issues for other important intensive and burn care issues.

Cyanide toxicity can result from inhalation of combustion products, as well as prolonged use of sodium nitroprusside, leading to impaired cellular respiration and metabolic acidosis. When sodium nitroprusside releases nitric oxide, cyanide is also created and can reach toxic levels in patients receiving prolonged, high-dose infusions. Cyanide toxicity is treated with *hydroxocobalamin*; it combines with cyanide to form cyanocobalamin, which is eliminated in the urine. *Sodium thiosulfate* can also be administered to form thiocyanate, which is eliminated via the kidneys. Cyanide antidote kits also contain *amyl nitrite*, which can clear cyanide through formation of *methemoglobin*. Amyl nitrite is a temporizing measure that should be used only if intravenous access or hydroxocobalamin are unavailable.

Burn-injured patients develop a capillary leak syndrome at both the burn site and distal anatomic locations, resulting in intravascular fluid loss and hypovolemic shock. Aggressive fluid resuscitation is required in the first 24 hours and is guided by various crystalloid and colloid algorithms (Table 32-6), with the goal of maintaining adequate tissue perfusion. Overresuscitation can lead to serious complications (e.g., acute lung injury, abdominal compartment syndromes); thus, fluid resuscitation should be carefully titrated up or down to maintain urine output at ~1 mL/kg/hr and avoid overresuscitation.

C. Perioperative Management of Burn-Injured Patients

Burn-injured patients require specialized perioperative care for several injury-specific risks (11). These patients are at increased risk for hypothermia (because of poor skin integrity and aggressive intravenous fluid therapy). They require special efforts to maintain their body temperature, including elevated operating room temperature, convective warming devices, and warmed intravenous fluids. Patients with severe inhalation injury may

? Did You Know

Even if respiratory distress is not present upon hospital arrival, patients with significant facial burns or inhalation injury should undergo early tracheal intubation when the procedure is easier to perform, rather than delay until fluid resuscitation and inflammation create a difficult airway due to massive soft tissue edema.

Table 32-6	Guidelines for Initial Fluid Resuscitation after Burn Injury
Adults and Children >20 kg	
Parkland formula[a]	
4.0 mL crystalloid/kg/% burn/first 24 hr	
Modified Brooke Formula[a]	
2.0 mL lactated Ringer's/kg per % burn per first 24 hr	
Children <20 kg	
Crystalloid 2–3 mL/kg per % burn per 24 hr[a]	
Crystalloid with 5% dextrose at maintenance rate	
100 mL/kg for the first 10 kg and 50 mL/kg for the next 10 kg for 24 hr	
Clinical End Points of Burn Resuscitation	
Urine output: 0.5–1 mL	
Pulse: 80–140 per min (age dependent)	
Systolic BP: 60 mm Hg (infants); children 70–90 plus 2 × age in years mm Hg; adults MAP >60 mm Hg	
Base deficit: <2	

BP, blood pressure; MAP, mean arterial pressure.
[a]50% of calculated volume is given during the first 8 hr, 25% is given during the second 8 hr, and the remaining 25% is given during the third 8 hr.
From Capon LM, Miller SM, Gingrich KJ. Trauma and burns. In: Barash PG, Cullen BF, Stoelting RK, et al. *Clinical Anesthesia*. 7th ed. Philadelphia: Lippincott Williams & Wilkins; 2013:1490–1534, with permission.

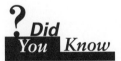

Did You Know

Burn excision and skin grafting procedures are associated with potentially significant blood loss, hypothermia, cardiovascular instability, as well as significant postoperative pain at both the injury and skin donor sites, all of which require comprehensive perioperative planning.

require special ventilation strategies (e.g., high-frequency percussive ventilation) and necessitate use of the intensive care unit ventilator in the operating room. Such cases will require total intravenous anesthesia to provide hypnosis and analgesia. If neuromuscular blockade is required, succinylcholine should be avoided after the first 48 hours, as noted previously. Nondepolarizing muscle relaxants are safe but will have shortened durations of action in burn patients because of the quantitative and qualitative changes in neuromuscular acetylcholine receptors that occur in the early days following injury. Postoperative pain control is a major priority for the burn patient, and multimodal therapy should be considered wherever possible. Patient-controlled analgesia, regional anesthesia, opioids, gabapentin, acetaminophen, and ketamine are all options in the burn patient, and consultation with a pain specialist is often helpful.

D. Sedation and Analgesia for Nonoperating-Room Burn Care
Burn dressing changes and other wound care procedures are often undertaken in special procedure rooms outside the operating room with full ASA monitoring and resuscitation capabilities. This procedure room is particularly important to pediatric patients who should feel a sense of safety and comfort in their own hospital rooms. Propofol, generous opioid dosing, benzodiazepines, and ketamine are commonly used sedative hypnotic medications for moderate or deep sedation in this setting. Nonpharmacologic analgesic therapies (e.g., meditation, video games, virtual reality) are also frequently used as adjuncts in the multimodal approach to burn pain control.

V. Disaster Preparedness

A. Mass Casualties

Any event that overwhelms the medical capacity of a given facility is defined as a *mass casualty incident*. These events run the spectrum from natural disasters to public transit accidents to warfare. The concept of *triage* is used to sort patients who are mostly likely to benefit from the limited medical resources that are available. Patients who are conscious, able to maintain their airway, and are ambulatory are considered "walking wounded" and are labeled low priority. Patients in cardiac arrest are considered nonsalvageable and are managed expectantly. Conscious or unconscious patients who are in need of emergent surgery to save life, limb, or eyesight are given the highest priority. Less critically ill patients, including those who will survive for at least several hours without surgery, are given medium priority.

Anesthesia departments should have an established *disaster plan* to structure procedures and staffing in mass casualties events. This plan should include anesthesia staffing in the triage area or emergency department to coordinate the flow of patients to the operating room and to coordinate anesthesia resources. In the operating room, all cases already undergoing surgery should be finished, while new elective cases should be postponed. The departmental disaster plan should also include a process for mass casualty deactivation and return to the usual activity.

B. Biologic, Chemical, and Nuclear Warfare

The role of the anesthesiologist in a biologic, chemical, or nuclear attack is limited. Any therapy that is undertaken will be of a basic nature. Proper training with chemical or biologic protective gear is necessary to manage patients at any level of care. Proper decontamination is mandatory before patients enter a "clean" environment (e.g., the hospital).

In biologic attacks, a healthy immune system and appropriate vaccinations are the main line of defense for care providers. Prompt identification of the involved organism can guide antimicrobial therapy. In chemical attacks, agents are typically dispersed quickly, and protective gear is needed to survive the initial phases of the attack. Similarly, identification of the chemical is mandatory to guide therapy with appropriate antidotes. In nuclear attack, the initial and secondary blasts do the most damage. Nuclear fallout presents a risk of radiation exposure. The only protection against this sort of attack is reinforced shelter and distance from the event. The long-term risk of cancer from radioactive fallout is unclear and often overestimated. Interestingly, the citizens of Hiroshima and Nagasaki experienced lower-than-expected rates of cancer following the nuclear attacks there in 1945. Some groups advocate iodine supplementation in the event of nuclear disasters (i.e., nuclear power plant meltdown). However, any protection from radiation exposure that is provided by iodine is limited to the thyroid gland and is not a widely recommended practice.

References

1. Capon LM, Miller SM, Gingrich KJ. Trauma and burns. In: Barash PG, Cullen BF, Stoelting RK, et al. *Clinical Anesthesia*. 7th ed. Philadelphia: Lippincott Williams & Wilkins; 2013:1490–1534.
2. Chesnut RM, Marshall LF, Klauber MR, et al. The role of secondary brain injury in determining outcome from severe head injury. *J Trauma*. 1993;34(2):216–222.
3. Tobin JM, Grabinsky A, McCunn M, et al. A checklist for trauma and emergency anesthesia. *Anesth Analg*. 2013;117(5):1178–1184.

4. Griesdale DE, Liu D, McKinney J, et al. [Glidescope® video-laryngoscopy versus direct laryngoscopy for endotracheal intubation: A systematic review and meta-analysis.] *Can J Anaesth*. 2012;59(1):41–52.

5. Nouruzi-Sedeh P, Schumann M, Groeben H. Laryngoscopy via Macintosh blade versus GlideScope: Success rate and time for endotracheal intubation in untrained medical personnel. *Anesthesiology*. 2009;110(1):32–37.

6. Walsh M, Devereaux PJ, Garg AX, et al. Relationship between intraoperative mean arterial pressure and clinical outcomes after noncardiac surgery: Toward an empirical definition of hypotension. *Anesthesiology*. 2013;119(3):507–515.

7. Borgman MA, Spinella PC, Perkins JG, et al. The ratio of blood products transfused affects mortality in patients receiving massive transfusions at a combat support hospital. *J Trauma*. 2007;63(4):805–813.

8. Holcomb JB, Wade CE, Michalek JE, et al. Increased plasma and platelet to red blood cell ratios improves outcome in 466 massively transfused civilian trauma patients. *Ann Surg*. 2008;248(3):447–458.

9. Shakur H, Roberts I, Bautista R, et al. Effects of tranexamic acid on death, vascular occlusive events, and blood transfusion in trauma patients with significant haemorrhage (CRASH-2): A randomised, placebo-controlled trial. *Lancet*. 2010;376(9734):23–32.

10. Plurad DS, Talving P, Lam L, et al. Early vasopressor use in critical injury is associated with mortality independent from volume status. *J Trauma*. 2011;71(3):565–572.

11. Kaiser HE, Kim CM, Sharar SR, et al. Advances in perioperative and critical care of the burn patient: anesthesia management of major thermal burn injuries in adults. *Adv Anesth*. 2013;31:137–161.

Questions

1. All of the following statements regarding manual in-line stabilization (MILS) during laryngoscopy and tracheal intubation are true, EXCEPT:
   A. MILS must be performed whenever the rigid cervical collar is removed from any trauma patient with potential cervical spine or spinal cord injury.
   B. MILS facilitates direct laryngoscopy and tracheal intubation by improving the laryngoscopist's view of the vocal cords.
   C. During rapid sequence induction, MILS should be the sole responsibility of one properly trained provider.
   D. Patients with cervical spinal cord injury rarely have worsening of their neurologic function when laryngoscopy and tracheal intubation are performed with MILS.

2. A 32-year-old unhelmeted female bicyclist is struck by a car at an urban intersection, evaluated at the scene by prehospital emergency medical providers, and transported to the hospital on a backboard with a rigid cervical collar. In the emergency department, her airway, breathing, and vital signs are within normal range, and she has a grossly deformed right ankle that appears to be dislocated. On neurologic examination, she speaks no words or sentences, and can only grunt and moan. She withdraws each extremity to pinprick; her eyes are closed and only open when her right leg is moved. Her Glasgow coma scale (GCS) score is:
   A. 6
   B. 8
   C. 10
   D. 12

3. You are asleep in the on-call room at 3:00 a.m. when you receive a call from the operating room notifying you that a 37-year-old woman with a single, high-caliber gunshot wound to the epigastrium just arrived in the emergency room. Because of her unstable vital signs (blood pressure 72/38, heart rate 132, respiration rate 36), the patient will be transported to the operating room within the next 10 minutes for an exploratory laparotomy. The "Emergency and Trauma Anesthesia Checklist" can guide your rapid preparation for this procedure in which of the following areas?
   A. Drugs for general anesthesia induction and tracheal intubation
   B. Drugs and equipment for intraoperative resuscitation
   C. Preparation of operating room equipment and anesthesia workstation
   D. All of the above

4. Which of the following statements regarding "hypotensive resuscitation" of the hemodynamically unstable trauma victim is TRUE?
   A. The hemodynamic goal of the resuscitation is a lower-than-normal blood pressure that still provides sufficient perfusion to vital organs until hemostasis is achieved, after which the blood pressure is normalized.
   B. Hypotensive resuscitation is of potential value in patients with traumatic brain injury (TBI).
   C. The hemodynamic goal of the resuscitation is normal, age-appropriate blood pressure until hemostasis is achieved, after which the blood pressure is pharmacologically reduced to lower-than-normal levels that still provide vital organ perfusion.
   D. Hypotensive resuscitation is of greater value in patients with blunt abdominal trauma than those with penetrating trauma.

5. The concept of "1:1:1 volume resuscitation" in hypovolemic, hypotensive trauma victims refers to administering equivalent numbers of units of packed red blood cells, fresh frozen plasma, and platelet. TRUE or FALSE?
   A. True
   B. False

6. When caring for trauma and burn patients, unintended hyperkalemia can result in all of the following clinical settings EXCEPT:
   A. Administration of six units of 23-day-old packed red blood cells to a 3-year-old girl with a traumatic leg amputation from a lawn mower accident
   B. Rapid administration of 12 units of 2-day-old packed red blood cells containing citrate preservative to a 53-year-old woman undergoing emergent splenectomy for blunt abdominal trauma
   C. Hemolytic transfusion reaction in a 23-year-old woman who received improperly cross-matched packed fresh frozen plasma following traumatic brain injury
   D. Succinylcholine administration to a 44-year-old man with 43% total body surface area flame burn on day 5 of hospitalization

7. A 35-year-old male competitive bicycle racer sustains an isolated closed pelvic fracture (iliac wing and pubic ramus) in a bicycle crash. Assuming that his preinjury hematocrit was 45% and that during the first 24 hours of his hospitalization he maintained normal vital signs while being resuscitated to euvolemia with isotonic crystalloid only, what is his predicted hematocrit on day 2 of hospitalization?
   A. 45%
   B. 35%
   C. 25%
   D. 15%

8. A 3-year-old, 21-kg girl sustains a 29% total body surface area burn after pulling a pot of boiling water off the stove. Using the Parkland formula for postburn fluid resuscitation, what volume of isotonic crystalloid should she receive in the first 8 hours of hospitalization?
   A. ~400 mL
   B. ~800 mL
   C. ~1,200 mL
   D. ~2,400 mL

9. A 75-year-old otherwise healthy woman is rescued from a house fire and arrives shortly thereafter at the hospital receiving supplemental face-mask oxygen at 10 L/min. She has no apparent burn injuries, but is lethargic and coughing up carbonaceous sputum. Which of the following laboratory assessments would you NOT EXPECT to observe?
   A. Pulse oximetry reading of 95%
   B. Carboxyhemoglobin level of 26%
   C. Arterial blood gas with partial pressure of oxygen (PO_2) of 57 mm Hg
   D. Co-oximeter measured arterial oxyhemoglobin saturation of 72%

10. In a mass casualty incident, patients are triaged based on the severity of their injuries. In general, those with the most severe, multiple injuries and near death receive the highest priority for care. TRUE or FALSE?
    A. True
    B. False

33 Neonatal and Pediatric Anesthesia

Jorge A. Gálvez
Paul A. Stricker
Alan Jay Schwartz

I. Physiology

A. Cardiovascular System

Normal Fetal to Pediatric Cardiovascular Transition

Development of *normal cardiovascular physiology* in the pediatric patient depends on the transition from fetal circulation to an adult flow pattern (1,2). The fetus uses the low vascular resistance placenta as the organ of respiration and therefore does not require pulmonary blood flow. Placental venous blood streams past the liver through the ductus venosus to provide venous inflow to the right atrium and is shunted across the foramen ovale and ductus arteriosus into the left heart and aorta bypassing the right heart flow and the pulmonary circuit (Fig. 33-1).

During the birthing process, elimination of the low resistance placental circulatory bed results in a rise in the neonate's *systemic vascular resistance*. This is coupled with the decrease in neonatal pulmonary vascular resistance. This reduces and eventually eliminates the blood flow that had been directed away from the lungs through the foramen ovale and ductus arteriosus. The rise in arterial oxygen level when the neonate initiates breathing is essential to maintain blood flow through the alveolar vascular bed.

Although the pulmonary vascular resistance declines at birth, it is not at the normal adult level until the end of the neonatal period. Any factor that can cause a rise in the *pulmonary vascular resistance* (e.g., hypoxia, hypothermia, respiratory or metabolic acidosis) can precipitate a reversion to a fetal circulatory pattern, with reopening of the foramen ovale and ductus arteriosus shunting blood away from the neonate's lungs. There are other differences in cardiac function that distinguish the pediatric heart from the adult heart. Most notable is the fact that the young child has a relatively noncompliant heart that depends on rate rather than contractility to boost cardiac output.

Common Congenital Cardiac Malformations

Malformations of the cardiac anatomy include many variations in which the ventricular and atrial chambers and the cardiac valves are deformed, causing

Fetal circulation

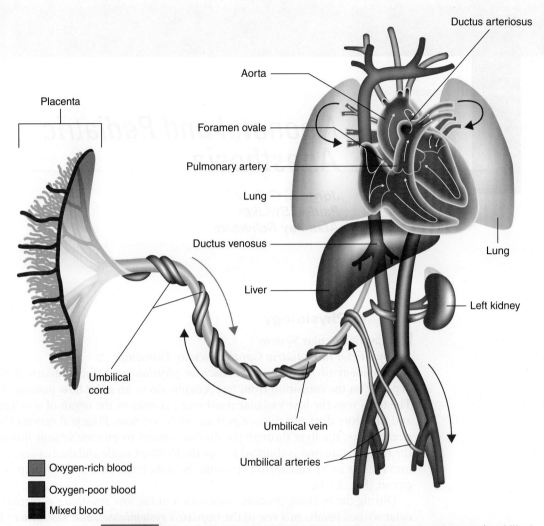

Placenta

Aorta

Ductus arteriosus

Foramen ovale

Pulmonary artery

Lung

Lung

Ductus venosus

Liver

Left kidney

Umbilical
cord

Umbilical vein

Umbilical arteries

Oxygen-rich blood

Oxygen-poor blood

Mixed blood

Figure 33-1 Fetal circulation showing direction of blood from the placenta (umbilical artery) that allows blood to bypass the fetal lungs via the foramen ovale, ductus arteriosus, and ductus venosus.

abnormal blood flow patterns. It is quite difficult to remember all of the possible anatomic variations that comprise congenital heart disease. Viewing congenital heart disease as a physiologic assessment enables the clinician to group the various lesions into three general categories: lesions that cause obstruction to blood flow without shunting, lesions that result in an increase in pulmonary blood flow through a shunt pathway, and lesions that result in a decrease in pulmonary blood flow through a shunt pathway.

Congenital aortic stenosis and *coarctation of the aorta* represent examples of nonshunt-obstructing congenital cardiac defects (Fig. 33-2A,B). The major physiologic impairment is an increase in myocardial workload. Congenital aortic stenosis can be associated with rapid cardiac arrest when the stenotic valve is so narrow that the left ventricle fails to generate sufficient forward cardiac output to supply oxygen to the coronary circulation. A critical difference from adult aortic stenosis is that the pediatric heart does not have

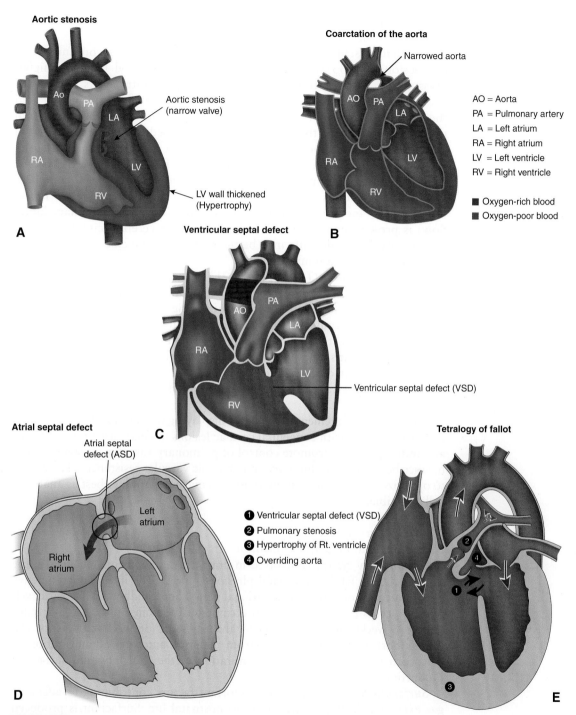

Aortic stenosis

Ao
PA
LA
RA
LV
RV

Aortic stenosis
(narrow valve)

LV wall thickened
(Hypertrophy)

A

Coarctation of the aorta

Narrowed aorta

AO
PA
LA
RA
LV
RV

AO = Aorta
PA = Pulmonary artery
LA = Left atrium
RA = Right atrium
LV = Left ventricle
RV = Right ventricle

■ Oxygen-rich blood
■ Oxygen-poor blood

B

Ventricular septal defect

AO
PA
LA
RA
LV
RV

Ventricular septal defect (VSD)

C

Atrial septal defect

Atrial septal
defect (ASD)

Left
atrium

Right
atrium

D

❶ Ventricular septal defect (VSD)
❷ Pulmonary stenosis
❸ Hypertrophy of Rt. ventricle
❹ Overriding aorta

Tetralogy of fallot

❷
❹
❶
❸

E

Figure 33-2 **A:** Aortic stenosis. **B:** Coarctation of the aorta also can lead to intracardiac shunting. Depending on the location of coarctation in relation to a patent ductus arteriosus, intracardiac shunting can be either right to left (preductal) or left to right (postductal). **C:** Ventricular septal defect leads to intracardiac shunting. Direction (right to left or left to right) depends on associated cardiac anatomy. **D:** Atrial septal defect leads to intracardiac shunting. Direction (right to left or left to right) depends on associated cardiac anatomy. **E:** Tetralogy of Fallot (TOF) consists of four anatomical abnormalities: (1) ventricular septal defect, (2) right ventricular outflow tract obstruction, (3) overriding aorta, and (4) left ventricular hypertrophy. (If an atrioventricular defect is present, the malformation is termed a pentalogy of Fallot.) TOF lesion leads to a right to left intracardiac shunt. ASD, atrial septal defect; VSD, ventriculoseptal defect; RA, right atrium; RV, right ventricle; PA, pulmonary artery; LA, left atrium; LV, left ventricle; Ao, aorta.

sufficient time to adapt and hypertrophy to compensate and overcome the valvular obstruction.

Ventricular septal defect (VSD) is the most common congenital cardiac lesion (Fig. 33-2C). It results in shunting of blood from the higher pressure left ventricle to the lower pressure right ventricle. As long as the shunt communication is sufficiently large to allow flow through it and the pulmonary vascular resistance is sufficiently low to allow flow from the right ventricle to the pulmonary vascular bed, lesions like VSD will increase pulmonary blood flow. The overall shunt is from left to right. However, at any time during the cardiac cycle, the flow may cease or become right to left, highlighting the distinct possibility for paradoxical embolization from the venous to arterial circulation. When an *atrial septal defect* (Fig. 33-2D) (another example of a lesion that increases pulmonary blood flow) is present, paradoxical embolization to the cerebral circulation that causes a stroke in adult life may be the first diagnostic clue of the presence of the intracardiac communication.

Tetralogy of Fallot (TOF) (Fig. 33-2E) is an example of those congenital cardiac abnormalities that result in a decrease in pulmonary blood flow. The obstruction to normal blood flow out of the right ventricle into the pulmonary outflow tract causes shunting from the right to left circulations through the VSD that is part of TOF (right to left shunt [cyanotic]). All congenital cardiac lesions that shunt blood flow away from the lungs have some obstruction to right heart outflow into the pulmonary circuit. Understanding this principle makes it easier to understand the physiology and anatomy of the congenital lesions.

Anesthetic management of neonates displaying transitional circulation and pediatric patients with congenital cardiac lesions mandate use of medications and techniques that promote control of pulmonary vascular resistance and a balance between the pulmonary and systemic vascular resistances. The goal is to optimize the ratio of pulmonary to systemic circulation as best as anatomically possible.

B. Pulmonary System
Normal Fetal to Pediatric Transition
The *pulmonary system* is involved in dramatic developmental changes in the transition from fetal to postnatal physiology (1,2). The lungs undergo active development throughout the gestational period and childhood. Alveolar development occurs primarily in the third trimester beginning in the saccular stage (24 to 38 weeks) and peaking in the alveolar stage (36 weeks to 8 years) (1). Infants born prematurely benefit from maternal antenatal administration of glucocorticoids, which promote maturation of the fetal lung and surfactant production.

Surfactant is one of the most important factors contributing to adequate gas exchange during the transition to postnatal life. Surfactant is produced by type II endothelial cells, which proliferate during the alveolar stage. It is a mixture of neutral lipids, phospholipids, and specific proteins with an amphipathic nature, which leads to a decrease in surface tension that stabilizes alveoli and provides alveolar inflation while reducing hydrostatic forces that cause pulmonary edema.

During the transition to extrauterine life, the first breaths lead to an increase in pulmonary arterial oxygen (PO_2) and a decrease in partial pressure of carbon dioxide (PCO_2), which stimulates pulmonary vascular dilation,

Table 33-1   Normal Arterial Blood Gas Values in Neonate

Subject	Age	PO$_2$ (mm Hg)	PCO$_2$ (mm Hg)	pH (u)
Fetus	Before labor	25	40	7.37
Fetus	End of labor	10–20	55	7.25
Newborn (term)	10 min	50	48	7.20
Newborn (term)	1 hour	70	35	7.35
Newborn (term)	1 week	75	35	7.40
Newborn (preterm, 1,500 g)	1 week	60	38	7.37

PO$_2$, pulmonary arterial oxygen; PCO$_2$, partial pressure of carbon dioxide.
From Hall SC, Suresh S. Neonatal anesthesia. In: Barash PG, Cullen B, Stoelting RK, et al., eds. *Clinical Anesthesia*. 7th ed. Philadelphia: Wolters Kluwer/Lippincott Williams & Wilkins; 2013:1178–1215, with permission.

decreased *pulmonary vascular resistance*, and constriction of the ductus arteriosus (Table 33-1).

Respiratory Function
Respiratory function differs significantly in infants and children. Oxygen consumption is dramatically higher than adult levels, at approximately 7 to 9 mL/kg/min (Table 33-2). The demand for oxygen is met with increased minute ventilation and with an increased ratio of minute ventilation to functional residual capacity (FRC) ratio. However, the FRC is relatively low compared with the minute ventilation. The oxygen consumption is higher, thus infants and children have a lower oxygen reserve and can rapidly develop hypoxemia.

Chest wall compliance is higher than that in adults, because the ribs and intercostal muscles are not fully developed, which can lead to significant retractions that do not provide efficient effort for gas exchange. The primary mechanism driving respiratory effort in neonates is the diaphragm, which is easily fatigued when the work of breathing is increased due to increased resistance to ventilation or hyperventilation.

? Did You Know

Inhalation induction as well as emergence of anesthesia are faster in infants and children as a result of increased minute ventilation relative to adults.

Table 33-2   Normal Respiratory Function Values in Infants and Adults

Parameter	Infant	Adult
Respiratory frequency	30–50	12–36
Tidal volume (mL/kg)	7	7
Dead space (mL/kg)	2–2.5	2.2
Alveolar ventilation (mL/kg/min)	100–150	60
Functional residual capacity (mL/kg)	27–30	30
Oxygen consumption (mL/kg/min)	7–9	3

From Hall SC, Suresh S. Neonatal anesthesia. In: Barash PG, Cullen B, Stoelting RK, et al., eds. *Clinical Anesthesia*. 7th ed. Philadelphia: Wolters Kluwer/Lippincott Williams & Wilkins; 2013:1178–1215, with permission.

Table 33-3   Factors that Impair Vasodilation of the Pulmonary Vascular Tree

Anatomic	Physiologic
Congenital heart syndromes (i.e., pulmonary artery hypoplasia)	Hypoxemia
Prematurity with lack of surfactant and broncho-alveolar development	Hypercarbia
Congenital diaphragmatic hernia	Hypothermia
Maternal diabetes	Meconium aspiration
Maternal asthma	Birth asphyxia Polycythemia Sepsis Chronic aspiration (postnatal)

? Did You Know

During resuscitation of a newborn with a very low Apgar score, suctioning may delay other very important therapeutic interventions such as stimulation, assisted ventilation, and chest compressions.

Meconium Aspiration

Fetal hypoxemia may result in intrauterine passage of meconium that mixes with amniotic fluid. The fetal breath movements will then result in pulmonary exposure to meconium prenatally. During birth, infants may also aspirate meconium produced during labor. The latter scenario is consistent with thick meconium that can cause a mechanical airway obstruction. Current Pediatric Advanced Life Support recommendations do not support routine suctioning for infants born with meconium-stained amniotic fluid. Meconium aspiration may result in alveolar damage, which results in impaired oxygenation as well as increased pulmonary vascular resistance.

Persistent Pulmonary Hypertension of the Newborn

The pulmonary circulation is highly sensitive to pH and oxygen levels, as well as other mediators such as nitric oxide, adenosine, prostaglandins, and lung inflation (3). During the newborn period, certain factors can impair vasodilation of the pulmonary vascular tree (Table 33-3) and result in elevated pulmonary vascular resistance. Systemic hypotension and cardiac arrhythmias may result, particularly if the right ventricle is not able to compensate and right atrial dilation ensues.

C. Renal System

The kidneys begin to receive increased blood flow after the transition to postnatal circulation. However, the *glomerular filtration rate (GFR)* remains lower than adult levels for the first two years of life. As a result, infants have impaired ability to retain free water. Therefore, infants are less likely to tolerate prolonged fasting periods, particularly during the first few weeks of life. Their inability to regulate GFR to excrete large amounts of water also leads to an inability to tolerate fluid overload without resulting electrolyte abnormalities. Urine output is initially low, but increases to 1 to 2 mL/kg/hour after the first day of life.

D. Hepatic System

The synthetic and metabolic functions of the *liver* remain immature in term newborns. The enzymes required for metabolism and drug elimination are present but have not been induced yet (4). The results are variable, depending on the medication and elimination pathways. Morphine relies on hepatic biotransformation for elimination; therefore, it has a prolonged half-life in neonates. Alternatively, lidocaine does not demonstrate prolonged elimination. Synthetic function is also limited, as exhibited by decreased albumin and vitamin K production, which is one of the medications routinely administered at birth to prevent postpartum hemorrhagic complications such as intraventricular hemorrhage.

E. Central Nervous System

The central nervous system has recently come under close scrutiny in pediatric anesthesia. Specifically, there has been evidence of anesthetic-induced *neuro-apoptosis* in animal models that is being closely studied for implications in humans (5). Data in humans are limited to retrospective studies that suggest an association between administration of general anesthesia under the age of 3 years and an increased incidence of learning deficits (5). The U.S. Food and Drug Administration provided comments on the issue and recommends that medications to provide general anesthesia should be used except for the rare scenario of an infant or child undergoing a purely elective procedure before the age of 3 years (5). In this case, a thorough conversation between the parents, the surgeon, and the anesthesiologist detailing the risks and benefits of the proposed surgical procedure and anesthetic should be undertaken. Most surgical procedures in children are not truly elective, as delaying surgical care can have effects on growth and development at later stages. Furthermore, untreated pain can have detrimental effects on behavioral and neurologic development and should be treated (5).

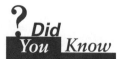

? Did You Know

Neonatal glycogen stores are decreased, especially in preterm infants, thus increasing the risk of hypoglycemia.

II. Pharmacology

Administration of appropriate doses of anesthetic agents, analgesics, and all medications in the pediatric setting requires consideration of *pharmacologic differences* between children and adults (4). Several variables in pediatric patients affect pharmacokinetics. For nearly all parameters, developmental differences are greatest in neonates and premature infants. For example, total body water comprises 70% to 83% of weight in premature babies and term neonates, whereas it is approximately 60% of weight in infants 6 months through adulthood. Increased total body water translates to larger volumes of distribution of hydrophilic medications, which (assuming similar pharmacodynamics) translates to increased dosing requirements per kilogram of body weight. A selection of pharmacokinetic variables and their influence on drug metabolism are presented in Table 33-4. Volatile anesthetic MAC requirements are greatest at approximately 1 month of age.

III. Equipment

The three factors that affect design and choice of *pediatric breathing circuits* are excessive resistance to flow, excessive dead space, and decreased heat and humidification. It is for these reasons that a variety of valveless breathing systems have been devised (Fig. 33-3) (1,2).

Ayre's T-piece has no unidirectional gas flow valve and is effective for the spontaneously breathing patient. It is compact, can provide supplemental oxygen, and is not associated with rebreathing of carbon dioxide. Once neuromuscular relaxants were introduced into anesthesia practice, however, Ayre's T-piece became ineffective, as it was difficult to provide the required

Table 33-4   Pharmacokinetic Variables and Their Clinical Influence in Infants and Children

Pharmacokinetic Variable	Physiology	Effect	Clinical Example
Hepatic metabolism	Immature phase 1/phase 2 metabolic pathways in neonates and infants	Decreased metabolism, longer drug half-lives	Phase 1: Amide local anesthetic accumulation with infusion Phase 2: Immature morphine glucuronidation in neonates and early infancy
Renal clearance	Adult glomerular filtration rate not achieved until 6–12 months	Renally excreted drugs prolonged half-life in infants under 6 months	Prolonged effect of pancuronium, reduced infusion requirements of other renally excreted drugs (e.g., aminocaproic acid)
Total body water	Increased in neonates and infants	Increased volume of distribution for hydrophilic drugs	Increased succinylcholine dose requirement in neonates and infants
Plasma protein content and composition	Reduced α_1-acid glycoprotein and albumin, fetal albumin in neonates	Increased free (unbound) fraction both for acidic and basic drugs	Potentially increased pharmacodynamic effects for a wide variety of drugs

positive pressure breathing with this device. The Jackson Rees modification of the Ayre's T-piece solved this problem while maintaining the valveless system by adding a reservoir bag with a variable occlusion pop-off (a variably occluded pigtail on the bag). Although the Jackson Rees modification of the Ayre's T-piece solved the need to be able to provide positive pressure breathing, it became apparent that another technical issue had to be solved—the potential for rebreathing carbon dioxide.

Mapleson introduced variations on the Jackson Rees system to address the potential for rebreathing. Mapleson recognized that while rebreathing could

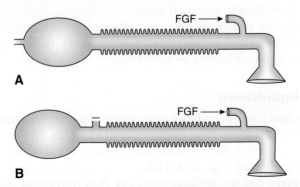

Figure 33-3 Anesthesia breathing circuits. **A:** Jackson-Rees modification of Ayre's T-piece. **B:** Mapleson D circuit. FGF, fresh gas flow. (From Ruitort KT, Eisenkraft JB. The anesthesia work station and delivery systems for inhaled anesthetics. In: Barash PG, Cullen B, Stoelting RK, et al., eds. *Clinical Anesthesia*. 7th ed. Philadelphia: Wolters Kluwer/Lippincott Williams & Wilkins; 2013:1178–1215, with permission.)

occur because this system did not contain unidirectional gas flow valves, the sequential placement of the fresh gas inlet, the pop-off, the reservoir bag, and the connection to the patient can be varied. Depending on whether the patient was breathing spontaneously or was controlled with positive pressure, if the fresh gas flow was sufficient, carbon dioxide rebreathing could be minimized. There are six variations of the Mapleson system, the Mapleson D being commonly used in pediatric patient care. *The Mapleson D system* places the fresh gas inlet close to the connection to the patient's airway. The pop-off is farther away from the patient and fresh gas inflow, and the bag is distal to the pop-off. The popularity of the Mapleson D system results from its ability to minimize carbon dioxide rebreathing when controlled ventilation is the ventilatory mode. Rebreathing is also eliminated during spontaneous ventilation when the fresh gas flow is two to three times the patient's minute ventilation.

Modern-day pediatric anesthesia patient care effectively employs the *circle breathing system*, without undue resistance to the patient when opening the valves. It has the added benefit of conservation of the patient's heat and airway humidity. If concern exists that airway heat and humidity will be lost during ventilation with the anesthesia machine, a heater and humidifier can be incorporated into the circle system.

Recent reports demonstrate that by using the proper-sized *cuffed endotracheal tube*, the ability to provide positive pressure ventilation was enhanced. There was also less operating room anesthetic gas contamination, better isolation of the airway from gastric contents, and less need for additional laryngoscopies in attempts to select the proper size tube.

IV. Perioperative Management

A. Preoperative Assessment

Children should be evaluated for common coexisting conditions (1,2). One of the most common questions relates to children with ongoing *upper respiratory infections*. A large prospective trial evaluated healthy children scheduled for elective surgery. It assessed their respiratory symptoms for nasal drainage (clear or discolored yellow/green) as well as cough (dry or productive and color of sputum), lethargy, and fever for correlation with respiratory complications, including bronchospasm and laryngospasm (6). The relative risk for respiratory complications was >1.5 if the child had active symptoms, including clear runny nose, green runny nose, moist cough, and fever. A general discussion between the parents, child, surgeon, and anesthesiologist should take place to determine the risk–benefit ratio for every scenario. A thorough preanesthetic discussion with the parents or responsible guardians should include the possibility of admission to the hospital for postoperative management.

The first observation of a child's behavior offers great insight into the developmental stage, as the *developmental stages* may not always correlate with a child's age. Children will naturally express anxiety around strangers and may not tolerate a thorough physical examination. *Neurologic examination* should focus on the child's activity level and note any anomalies such as contractures, weakness of extremities, or abnormal appearance. The *cardiovascular examination* focuses on auscultation of the heart sounds, noting that heart murmurs are common in newborns (patent ductus arteriosus continuous murmur, patent foramen ovale, atrial septal defect, and ventricular septal defect). The presence of a murmur should warrant further exploration of signs or symptoms of cardiac disease, particularly fainting, discoloration such as blue lips, or failure to thrive. Furthermore, the *abdominal examination* may reveal a large or very small liver, which correlates with volume status as well as the ability for the heart to handle preload.

Pulmonary examination focuses on determining the presence of abnormal air movement, including absent breath sounds, wheezing, or coarse breath sounds. It can often be challenging to differentiate coarse lung sounds from transmitted upper airway sounds in the presence of nasal congestion. The abdominal examination evaluates for signs of trauma, distention, or discomfort. Furthermore, umbilical hernias may be appreciated. The extremities should be assessed for range of motion, contractures, or deformities as well as possible sites for intravenous access. There should be a discussion with the patient and guardians regarding the risks and benefits of delivering general versus regional anesthesia to the child. The risks of anesthesia that are specific to pediatrics include, in particular, respiratory depression, particularly in ex-premature infants, respiratory complications, such as bronchospasm and laryngospasm, hypoxia, and aspiration pneumonia.

B. Fasting Guidelines

Children are particularly sensitive to dehydration during *preoperative fasting*. It is important to emphasize the most recent recommended guidelines by the American Society of Anesthesiologists' taskforce (7). In general, there is consensus that:

1. Clear liquids should be allowed up to 2 hours before the procedure;
2. Breast milk 4 hours before the procedure;
3. Formula 6 hours before the procedure;
4. Solids about 8 hours or longer (i.e., midnight the night before) before the procedure.

C. Premedication

Oral premedication with a benzodiazepine (e.g., midazolam 0.5 mg/kg up to 10 mg) is an effective method (8). Oral midazolam has a rapid onset (5 to 15 minutes to peak effect) and short duration of action, which makes it well suited for ambulatory surgical procedures.

D. Parental Presence

Another approach to mitigating the stress of separation from parents is to allow a parent or caregiver to be present during induction. This approach is most effective when parents are calm and is not effective for all parents or children (8). In addition to selecting the appropriate parents or children for which to use this approach, to be successful the parent or guardian should be adequately prepared in terms of what to expect during the course of induction. Parents should be coached regarding how they can be most helpful to their child.

E. Induction of Anesthesia

Induction of anesthesia represents a stressful event for children (and parents!). Beyond the mandatory goals of maintaining a patent airway and stable hemodynamics, the goals of a pediatric induction also include a smooth separation from the parent (if a parent is not present for induction) and a cooperative child during the process of induction, while establishing and meeting parental expectations during the process. Two of the most commonly used approaches for minimizing the stress of induction (which may be used alone or in combination) are discussed in the sections that follow (1,2).

Inhalation Induction of Anesthesia

In the absence of contraindications, an *inhaled induction* of anesthesia has a number of advantages in children. It is painless and it is successful on the first attempt (whereas intravenous cannulation has an inherent failure rate). In the United States, inhalation inductions are performed almost exclusively with sevoflurane, as the availability of halothane is severely limited. In cooperative patients, 70% nitrous oxide in oxygen may be delivered first (which is odorless), with 8% sevoflurane added after a minute or two. This may allow the child to both tolerate and not remember the less pleasant volatile agent. Because inhaled inductions are performed in children prior to securing vascular access and there is the potential for laryngospasm and bradycardia, succinylcholine (4 mg/kg) and atropine (0.02 mg/kg) should be immediately available for intramuscular administration.

Intravenous Induction

Intravenous induction is typically preferred in children who have established venous access. For children coming for elective surgery, some centers routinely place an intravenous line for induction of anesthesia. Premedication with a benzodiazepine and application of topical local anesthetic cream can minimize the stress of intravenous line placement.

Intramuscular Induction

Occasionally a patient may not be able to cooperate with any element of preoperative preparation (e.g., autistic children) or induction of anesthesia (including taking oral premedication). *Intramuscular injection* of ketamine (3 to 5 mg/kg) may be the best option in these circumstances, but this requires a careful team approach and family preparation to be safe and successful.

F. Pediatric Airway Management

Understanding the anatomical and physiologic differences between adults, infants, and children is necessary to provide safe and successful airway management tailored to the infant or child. In general, these differences and their impact on *airway management* are greatest in the neonatal and infant period.

Anatomically, an infant has a larger occiput, a larger tongue size relative to the size of the oropharynx, and a more cephalad larynx (Table 33-5). The larger occiput may promote airway obstruction and interfere with laryngoscopy when a head pillow is used to achieve the classic sniffing position. Instead, a shoulder roll is often more useful both for promoting a patent airway and for facilitating direct laryngoscopy. Although it was originally postulated that the narrowest portion of the pediatric airway is at the level of the cricoid ring, newer magnetic resonance imaging–based research suggests the glottic opening and the immediate subvocal cord level are the narrowest. Furthermore, the shape of the larynx is cylindrical, as in the adult, so it is important to remember clinically because the endotracheal tube fit (resistance to endotracheal tube passage) must be assessed after it has passed through the vocal cords. Tightly fitting tubes may cause *postextubation stridor* and postextubation croup. A leak pressure of less than 20 to 25 cm H_2O should be targeted to minimize this risk.

Normal healthy infants have overlap with tidal breathing and closing volumes, and their oxygen consumption rates are nearly three times that of an adult, so under anesthetized conditions, their functional residual capacity is reduced (Table 33-2). The clinical impact of this is rapid oxyhemoglobin desaturation following brief periods of apnea, resulting in shorter times to perform apneic intubation techniques. Additionally, oxyhemoglobin desaturation

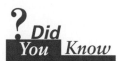
? Did You Know

Infants and young children have a relatively large tongue and a more cephalad larynx effectively shortening the distance in which the oral, pharyngeal, and tracheal axes must be aligned to achieve laryngeal exposure during direct laryngoscopy.

Table 33-5	Anatomic Differences between Infant and Adult Airways	
Anatomic Relationship	**Pediatric**	**Adult**
Occiput	Large	Normal
Tongue	Large	Normal
Epiglottis	Relatively longer, narrower, and stiffer	Firm
Epiglottis shape	Omega shaped	Flat, broad
Relative larynx location	Cephalad	Caudal
Larynx size/shape	Proportionately smaller/ cylindrical	Cylindrical
Glottic level	C3–C4	C5–C6
Narrowest point	Vocal cords	Vocal cords
Vocal cords	Inclined posterior to anterior	Perpendicular to larynx
Mucosa	More vulnerable to trauma	Less vulnerable to trauma

Data from Lerman J. Pediatric anesthesia. In: Barash PG, Cullen B, Stoelting RK, et al., eds. *Clinical Anesthesia.* 7th ed. Philadelphia: Wolters Kluwer/Lippincott Williams & Wilkins; 2013:1216–1256. Litman RS, Weissend EE, Shibata D, et al. Developmental changes of laryngeal dimensions in unparalyzed, sedated children. *Anesthesiology.* 2003;98:41–45, with permission.

will rapidly occur when ventilation is compromised (e.g., coughing, airway obstruction). *Difficult airway management* in pediatric patients often requires deep sedation or general anesthesia.

Anesthetic Conditions for Laryngoscopy and Endotracheal Intubation
Traditionally, intubation of the trachea in children is performed following induction of anesthesia and administration of a nondepolarizing neuromuscular blocker. It has become common practice to perform *laryngoscopy* and *endotracheal intubation* under deep anesthesia without neuromuscular blockade. This can be done with deep sevoflurane anesthesia alone, but it is also often performed with a propofol bolus (e.g., 2 mg/kg) or a fast-acting opioid (e.g., remifentanil or fentanyl 2 µg/kg) following inhalational induction of anesthesia with sevoflurane. Insufficient depth of anesthesia without neuromuscular blockade may result in coughing, laryngospasm, oxyhemoglobin desaturation, and regurgitation.

Succinylcholine
In the early 1990s, the U.S. Food and Drug Administration applied a black box warning for succinylcholine contraindicating its use for routine airway management. However, in the absence of absolute contraindications to succinylcholine (malignant hyperthermia susceptibility, history of burns, etc.) is acceptable in scenarios such as laryngospasm and rapid sequence induction and intubation and may be the preferred agent.

Direct Laryngoscopy
Traditionally the *straight blade (Miller)* has been used in children, although there is little or no comparative evidence to show that this blade performs better than

the *curved blade (Macintosh)* (see Chapter 20, Fig. 20-5). After sweeping the tongue, the blade tip is advanced beyond the vallecula and the epiglottis is directly lifted. Alternatively, the straight blade can be used in the manner of the Macintosh and the epiglottis lifted indirectly with the blade tip in the vallecula.

Laryngeal Masks and Supraglottic Airways

Laryngeal mask airways are frequently used in pediatric anesthesia. In general, the indications and contraindications are similar to adults. Laryngeal masks with gastric drain channels as well as laryngeal masks designed to facilitate intubation are available in pediatric sizes.

Endotracheal Tube Selection

Historically, *uncuffed endotracheal tubes* were recommended in children; however, in the current era, cuffed tubes are in most circumstances superior. The incidence of postintubation stridor is less when properly sized cuffed tubes are used, possibly from the decreased need or frequency of repeated laryngoscopy for tube change when too small a tube is placed initially. *Cuffed endotracheal tubes* also offer advantages of improved sealing of the trachea, which decreases operating room pollution, allows for lower fresh gas flows, improves ventilator performance, and may offer greater protection from macroaspiration. Although cuffed tubes can be safely used and often preferred for surgical procedures in neonates and preterm infants, uncuffed tubes are commonly used for long-term ventilation in the neonatal intensive care unit (NICU). When tracheal intubation is performed, the correct tracheal tube size must be chosen. Most commonly, the modified *Cole's formula* is used for uncuffed endotracheal tubes, where the predicted tube size is 4 plus the age divided by 4. In infants and smaller children, a half-size smaller should be selected when a cuffed tube is used. For example, for a 4-year-old child, one would select a (4 + 4/4 = 5) 5.0 uncuffed endotracheal tube, or a (4 + 4/4 − 0.5 = 4.5) 4.5 cuffed endotracheal tube.

Tracheal Intubation and Positioning of the Endotracheal Tube

Indications for tracheal intubation in children are largely similar to those for adults. In addition, many anesthesiologists intubate the trachea and control ventilation in neonates and preterm infants in the absence of other traditional indications. Careful attention must be paid to positioning the tracheal tube tip in the midtrachea. Small tube movements may result in endobronchial intubation or inadvertent extubation in infants. Assessing the adequate depth of the endotracheal tube can be performed by deliberately advancing the endotracheal tube into the main-stem bronchus while simultaneously auscultating and providing breaths with hand-bag ventilation. When the endotracheal tube enters the right or left mainstem bronchus, breath sounds will be absent in the opposite side respectively. The tube is then withdrawn by 1 cm in infants and 2 cm above the carina and breath sounds should be used to confirm both lungs are being ventilated. When a cuffed tube is used, it may be easier and more reliable to position the tube so that the cuff can be palpated by ballottement in the suprasternal notch. This translates to the tip of the tube being in an intrathoracic and midtracheal location.

Rapid Sequence Induction and Intubation in Pediatrics

One of the clinical manifestations of the high oxygen consumption rate and reduced FRC of an infant under anesthesia is rapid oxyhemoglobin desaturation following apnea. If a "traditional" *rapid sequence induction* is performed, nearly all infants will have an oxyhemoglobin saturation below 90% after 1 minute of apnea. Therefore, many pediatric anesthesiologists perform a modified rapid sequence induction with gentle positive pressure ventilation in addition to cricoid pressure prior to intubation, because oxygen delivery is prioritized over aspiration risk from a risk–benefit standpoint (9).

V. Temperature Management

Children are at increased risk of *hypothermia* under anesthesia; infants and in particular premature infants and neonates are at greatest risk. Similar to adults, the primary modes of heat loss are:

1. Radiation
2. Evaporation
3. Convection
4. Conduction

Neonates under anesthesia behave as poikilotherms; their temperature approaches that of their surroundings. Hypothermia can be prevented and normothermia maintained using a combination of strategies tailored to the individual patient. Warming the operating room prior to arrival (convection or radiation), forced air warming (convection), use of a circulating warm water mattress (conduction), heated humidified gases or humidified moisture exchanger (evaporation), and overhead infrared warming lights (radiation) are among the available methods.

VI. Fluid and Blood Management

A. Intravenous Fluid Requirements

Intravenous fluid requirements in fasting children are usually determined using the *4-2-1 rule*. The hourly infusion rate is calculated as 4 mL/kg for the first 10 kg, plus 2 mL/kg for the second 10 kg, and 1 mL/kg for each additional kilogram. Fasting fluid deficits are calculated based on this formula and the duration the child has been non per os. These are replaced intraoperatively in a manner similar to adults. The generally accepted guideline is 50% of the deficit replaced in the first hour, followed by 25% of the deficit replaced in hour 2, and hour 3 to complete the entire deficit.

Infants under 6 months of age, and neonates in particular, are at increased risk of hypoglycemia with fasting durations commonly seen in anesthetic practice. Liberalized fasting guidelines (e.g., clear liquids until 2 hours prior to surgery) may help prevent hypoglycemia and improve patient comfort.

B. Blood Loss Replacement and Transfusion

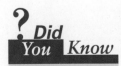

Did You Know

Hypovolemia associated with hemorrhage is the most common cardiovascular cause of perioperative cardiac arrest in children.

Underestimation of blood loss, inadequate preparation (vascular access, blood preparation), and massive hemorrhage are identified as contributors to *cardiac arrest* in the pediatric patient (10–12). Blood loss is replaced with crystalloids (without glucose). Although *transfusion thresholds* are ultimately tailored to the individual patient and clinical scenario, in most scenarios red blood cell transfusion is indicated when the hemoglobin is below 7 g/dL (13,14) and is often indicated sooner depending on the age of the patient and clinical scenario (10,11). Packed red blood cells (5 mL/kg) can be expected to raise the hemoglobin approximately 1 g/dL. Indications for hemostatic blood component therapy are similar to those for adults. Suggested dosing for blood components are presented in Table 33-6.

Table 33-6	Pediatric Blood Component Administration	
Component	**Dosing Guideline**	**Comments**
PRBCs	5–10 mL/kg	Expected hemoglobin increase of 1–1.5 g/dL for every 5 mL/kg. Infants/small children at risk of hyperkalemia with rapid infusion of PRBCs with prolonged storage during hypovolemia. Consider fresh/washed PRBCs when anticipated.
FFP	10–15 mL/kg	During massive hemorrhage dilutional coagulopathy of soluble clotting factors develops after >1 blood volume of loss; FFP treatment recommended.
Platelets	10–15 mL/kg	Usually indicated for platelet counts <50,000/μL; higher thresholds may be used for certain procedures (e.g., neurosurgery).
Cryoprecipitate	0.1 units/kg	Indicated for fibrinogen levels <80–100 mg/dL.

PRBC, packed red blood cells; FFP, fresh frozen plasma.

VII. Surgical Procedure Considerations

A. Myelomeningocele

Spina bifida refers to a range of congenital anomalies of the central nervous system. The most common is a myelomeningocele, which involves bulging of the spinal cord into a sac filled with cerebrospinal fluid (Fig. 33-4). The incidence of myelomeningocele remains at 3.4 per 10,000 live births. Long-term survivors with myelomeningocele have neurologic deficits, including bladder and bowel incontinence as well as sensory and motor deficits related to the level of spinal cord involved in the defect. Early surgical treatment may not be entirely protective. Long-term care involves frequent bladder catheterization and potential risk of developing sensitivity to latex products. Latex precautions should be exercised regardless of any history of allergic sensitivity to latex products.

B. Ventriculoperitoneal Shunts

Children may present with *elevated intracranial pressure* as a result of various lesions, including anatomic obstruction of cerebrospinal fluid (CSF) flow

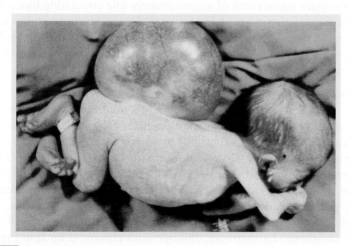

Figure 33-4   Neonate with spina bifida cystica.

such as Chiari malformations or tumors. In order to relieve the obstruction of CSF flow, an intraventricular shunt may be placed to redirect flow to a body cavity such as the peritoneal cavity, the pleura, or less commonly an intravascular location such as the right atrium. Patients with existing shunts may present with shunt malfunction or infection and may require emergency surgery to alleviate the shunt malfunction. Preanesthetic evaluation should focus on assessing signs of *increased intracranial pressure*, such as depressed consciousness, nausea, vomiting, bradycardia, and hypertension. Induction of anesthesia should weigh the potential risk of aspiration with the risk of brain herniation in the setting of elevated intracranial pressure. Surgical approach typically requires access to the head, neck, thorax, and abdomen. Infants and children are particularly prone to hypothermia due to exposure to surgical preparation solution as well as an inability to provide adequate heat source during the procedure. Patient positioning may also result in endobronchial intubation, particularly in small children. Although the risk of hemorrhage is small, it is significant particularly in young children as well as shunt revisions that may involve a vascular component. Patients should be considered for an awake examination after surgery unless the patient's baseline condition is not suitable for extubation and emergence.

C. Craniofacial Surgery

Craniofacial reconstruction is performed for children with premature fusion of cranial sutures during development (11). Surgical correction is performed to improve appearance as well as to reduce the risk of increased pressure on areas of the developing brain and potential long-term effects on development resulting from inhibited brain growth. Depending on the type and severity of the deformity, it may be corrected in one or more stages typically during the first years of life. Each surgical procedure is associated with variable scalp dissection and cranial osteotomies. Children should be evaluated for associated syndromes (i.e., *Crouzon* and *Saethre-Chotzen*), which can be associated with difficult airway as well as difficult intravascular access (15). Intraoperative management typically includes continuous arterial blood pressure monitoring. To detect *air embolism*, use of a Doppler monitor is suggested. Central venous access should be considered to assist management in complex procedures, particularly if peripheral vascular access is not adequate (at least two large-bore intravenous lines). Despite surgical efforts to minimize hemorrhage, patients typically require transfusion of approximately one circulating blood volume. Pre-emptive administration of fresh-frozen plasma during surgery has been demonstrated to reduce the incidence of postoperative coagulopathy. Surgical complications may include tearing of dural sinuses as well as tearing of the dura during osteotomies.

D. Tonsillectomy

Children presenting for tonsillectomy or adenoidectomy comprise a large amount of all pediatric anesthesiology practices. The indications for the procedures range from recurrent tonsillitis to *obstructive sleep apnea* with various levels of symptomatology (16). Children with Down syndrome, craniofacial anomalies, neuromuscular disorders, sickle cell disease, or mucopolysaccharidoses are at increased risk for postoperative complications from adenotonsillectomy, particularly in terms of postoperative airway obstruction. Airway obstruction can increase the duration of inhalation induction as well as emergence of anesthesia. Furthermore, children with chronic sleep apnea may have increased sensitivity to the respiratory depressant effects of opioids. Airway management is typically performed with an oral RAE (Ring-Adair-Elwyn) endotracheal tube that allows surgical access to the airway for the procedure. During emergence, anesthesiologists should take care to avoid contact with the tonsillar beds by oral airways or suctioning equipment to minimize the risk of hemorrhage (16). Postsurgical hemorrhage is associated with morbidity and mortality, particularly if there is active hemorrhage during airway management phases such as induction or emergence of anesthesia. Postoperative care ranges from ambulatory surgical care to monitoring in an intensive care unit and is based on the individual comorbidities as well as the postoperative course exhibited by an individual patient. Postoperative nausea and vomiting is a significant risk and should be treated prophylactically with dexamethasone and ondansetron unless otherwise contraindicated (i.e., dexamethasone is contraindicated for patients with leukemia patients due to possibility of tumor lysis syndrome and interference with chemotherapy protocols). Children scheduled for ambulatory tonsillectomy or adenoidectomy should be carefully observed for adequate analgesia and any signs of airway obstruction prior to discharge from the facility.

E. Cleft Lip and Palate

Cleft lip and palate make up the ***most common congenital deformity*** of the head and neck, affecting between 0.5 to 1 child per 1,000 births with variation across ethnic groups worldwide (Fig. 33-5) (17). Maternal exposure to phenytoin has been shown to increase the risk of cleft lip, and tobacco use nearly doubles the risk of cleft lip. Various syndromes and genetic disorders may be associated with cleft lip or palate as well and may be a predisposing factor for perioperative airway complications. The anesthetic management plan should recognize these comorbidities. Surgical correction varies based on the type of defect as well as the age of the child and may be performed in one or more stages. Anesthetic management may be highlighted by difficulty with laryngoscopy if either the laryngoscope blade or endotracheal tube is caught in the cleft. Furthermore, positioning of the child during surgery may result in dislodgement of the endotracheal tube or endobronchial intubation. Typically, an oral RAE endotracheal tube is preferred to facilitate surgical access to the airway. Children undergoing repair may be as young as 10 weeks, thus choosing an appropriately sized endotracheal tube is critical. Cuffed oral RAE tubes

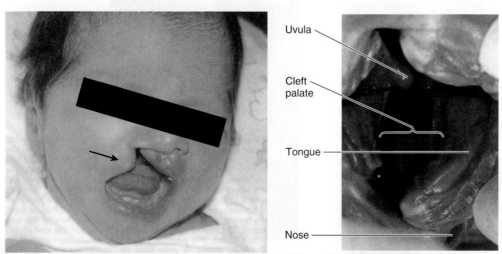

Figure 33-5 **A:** Unilateral cleft lip (*arrow*). **B:** Bilateral cleft palate (laryngoscopic view).

may not be universally available. As a result, uncuffed endotracheal tubes may result in a large leak or inappropriate depth. When uncuffed tubes are used, large leaks may be managed by inserting a throat pack. Following the repair, children are prone to airway obstruction upon extubation. It is critical that nasopharyngeal airways are avoided unless they are placed by the surgeon at the time of the repair. Postoperative care should focus on maintaining adequate respiration while managing analgesia and hydration.

F. Diaphragmatic Hernia

Diaphragmatic hernias occur as a result of a defect in the diaphragm that results in *herniation of abdominal contents* into the thoracic cavity (Fig. 33-6). There are anatomic variants, including Bochdalek (70% to 90%), Morgagni (20% to 30%), and central (1% to 2%) diaphragmatic hernias (18). This condition usually begins to develop in early gestation during the first trimester. As a result, the affected lung is compressed and not able to develop due to the presence of abdominal organs in the hemithorax. The diagnosis can be made by prenatal diagnostic tests such as ultrasound and magnetic resonance imaging.

Because one lung will be underdeveloped, the patient will have elevated pulmonary vascular resistance as well as limited capacity for gas exchange, which can be life-threatening. The prevalence ranges from 1 in 2,500 to 4,000 and has a 30% to 60% mortality rate. Even after surgical correction, children may develop chronic lung disease as well as pulmonary hypertension. Furthermore, the herniated organs can become distended (i.e., stomach distention during mask ventilation or crying), which could result in further impairment of lung mechanics for both lungs. Depending on the severity of the condition, the child may not be able to sustain oxygenation and circulation without assistance. In some cases, the patient may be placed on *extracorporeal membrane oxygenation (ECMO)* as a bridge prior to surgical repair.

Considerations for anesthetic management depend on the severity of the case and whether the child can be safely transported from the NICU to the

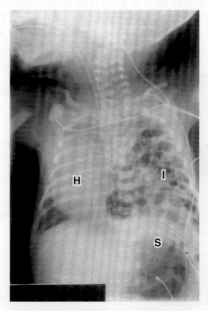

Figure 33-6 Diaphragmatic hernia showing intestine (I) in left thorax. Note position of stomach bubble (S) and shift of heart (H) into right thorax.

operating room. In some cases, the procedure may be done at the NICU bedside with ECMO. If a patient is not intubated or on ECMO, the anesthesiologist must take care to avoid airway obstruction and ensure ventilation takes place without excessive pressure to avoid overdistention of the stomach and intestines. Distended organs may lead to increased difficulty with ventilation as well as increased difficulty of the surgical procedure. Adequate intravenous access should be ensured with at least two peripheral intravenous lines. The surgical approach may be by laparotomy or thoracotomy. Laparotomy precludes the use of umbilical lines for vascular access. Continuous arterial monitoring is warranted to allow for blood gas monitoring for oxygenation and ventilation as well as for monitoring hemoglobin during the procedure.

G. Anterior Mediastinal Mass

Anterior mediastinal masses range from benign to malignant but may become life-threatening due to *compression of vital structures* such as the trachea, great vessels, or the heart (see Chapter 34) (19). The etiology includes lymphoma, thymoma, germ cell tumors, metastatic lesions, bronchogenic masses, or thyroid masses. Preoperative assessment is critical to determine the extent of symptomatology, particularly if there is dyspnea, stridor, or syncope and any postural component. History and examination should focus on identifying any position that exacerbates the symptom to assist in perioperative care. Diagnostic imaging may include plain radiographs, computed tomography scan, and echocardiogram to characterize the mass as well as signs of cardiovascular compromise. Initial management typically involves obtaining a tissue sample to establish a diagnosis prior to initiating treatment such as chemotherapy or radiation to reduce the size of the mass. Induction of general anesthesia may be catastrophic if the mass shifts in position and compresses the airway or cardiovascular structures in the chest, resulting in an inability to ventilate and marked reduction in cardiac output. In high-risk scenarios, the priorities should always be to maintain spontaneous ventilation and to avoid neuromuscular blockade and positive pressure ventilation. In the event that cardiovascular collapse or difficulty with ventilation is encountered, the patient should be placed in a rescue position, which consists of the positions that improved the symptoms based on preoperative history. This may involve the upright sitting, lateral decubitus, or prone position. Furthermore, cardiopulmonary bypass may be required for a patient with a critical mediastinal mass.

H. Tracheoesophageal Fistula or Esophageal Atresia

Tracheoesophageal fistula results when an abnormal connection from the esophagus to the trachea is present due to failed fusion of tracheoesophageal ridges in early embryonal development (20). This can occur in 1 of 3,500 live births and is usually a postnatal diagnosis. Children may present with inability to eat or recurrent aspiration with oxygen requirement. In most cases, a nasogastric or orogastric tube is advanced and is unable to pass to the stomach. The specific diagnosis is usually confirmed by bronchoscopy prior to surgical repair. There are five types of tracheoesophageal fistula (Fig. 33-7). The most common is a proximal blind esophageal pouch and a distal esophageal segment that communicates with the trachea (approximately 90% of cases), with the other types being less common.

There can be associated conditions, most notably the VATER or VACTERL syndromes (Vertebral anomalies, Anal atresia, Cardiac defects, Tracheoesophageal fistula and/or Esophageal atresia, Renal and radial anomalies and Limb

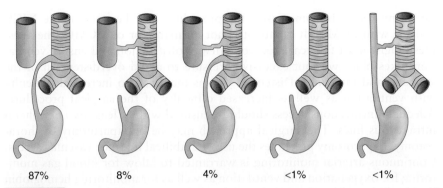

87%   8%   4%   <1%   <1%

Figure 33-7 Relative frequencies of anatomic variations of esophageal atresia and tracheoesophageal atresia.

defects). Although surgical correction is paramount to allow the child to eat and grow, a complete workup including echocardiogram should be performed to rule out any associated cardiac anomalies.

Prior to surgical correction, a Replogle tube is typically placed in the esophagus to empty any secretions. The child is not fed and efforts should be made to soothe the child, as crying may lead to stomach distention, resulting in abdominal compression and respiratory distress. The initial approach typically requires flexible or rigid bronchoscopy to establish the anatomic location of the defect. The surgical approach will be dictated by the location of the defect, ranging from a thoracotomy or laparotomy, and may be completed over multiple stages. Induction of general anesthesia should focus on limiting stomach distention as well as adequate positioning of the endotracheal tube in relation to the fistula. In some cases, the fistula can be large enough to fit the endotracheal tube, and changing the patient's position throughout the procedure may result in "intubation" of the fistula.

I. Pyloric Stenosis

Pyloric stenosis is one of the most common conditions requiring surgical intervention in infants, with an incidence of 2 to 9 per 1,000 live births (1). Infants typically present with an inability to tolerate oral feeding and classic projectile vomiting in the first three months of life, resulting in *hypochloremic, hypokalemic metabolic alkalosis.* If untreated, the condition can be fatal. Initial management consists of adequate resuscitation with intravenous fluids to restore normal circulating blood volume and electrolyte anomalies. The diagnosis may be confirmed with palpation of the thickened pylorus or by ultrasound studies. Anesthetic management should focus on minimizing aspiration of gastric contents.

J. Necrotizing Enterocolitis

Necrotizing enterocolitis (NEC) remains a devastating problem affecting preterm infants during the first weeks to months of life (1). Despite advances in perinatal and neonatal care, the incidence of NEC has not decreased, and its *morbidity and mortality remain high*. Infants may present with abdominal distention resulting in hemodynamic instability and respiratory failure. Breast milk has been found to offer protection against developing NEC, despite advances in neonatal formula mixtures over the years. Though management strategies have evolved, the common therapies include cessation of gastric feeding, mechanical ventilation, and antibiotic therapy. Infants

? Did You Know

Suctioning the infant's stomach immediately prior to the induction of anesthesia until little or no gastric fluid is retrieved has been successfully applied to reduce the risk of gastric content reflux during induction of anesthesia.

requiring surgical management are at the highest risk for morbidity and mortality and may not be stable enough to be transported out of the NICU. In such extreme cases, the surgical procedure may be performed at the NICU bedside. Surgical procedures may be complicated by hemorrhage as well as large fluid shifts. Infants may require transfusions in excess of 100 mL/kg and are at risk of transfusion-related complications such as coagulopathy and hyperkalemia.

K. Omphalocele and Gastroschisis

Omphalocele and *gastroschisis* are rare abdominal wall defects affecting 2 in 10,000 live births and 3 in 10,000 live births, respectively (1). Gastroschisis is not associated with an overlying sac and results in exposed intra-abdominal organs. Gastroschisis is not usually associated with other congenital defects. Omphalocele is characterized by herniation of abdominal contents through a defect, although they are protected from the environment by a membrane. Omphalocele is associated with other anomalies including pentalogy of Cantrell, bladder or cloacal exstrophy, trisomy 21 (Down syndrome), or Beckwith-Wiedemann syndrome (15). Both gastroschisis and omphaloceles require surgical management, which typically involves gradual reduction of the externalized abdominal contents via a mesh or silo. The process can be performed through various procedures to allow for gradual expansion of the abdominal cavity. It can be complicated by abdominal competition and difficulty with ventilation due to increased intrathoracic pressures from a bulging diaphragm.

L. Scoliosis

Children may present for surgical correction of *scoliosis* that results from neuromuscular defects with misalignment of the vertebral column or simply as "idiopathic" scoliosis (2). In severe cases, gross deformities of the chest and abdomen may result in thoracic insufficiency and impair lung development. Furthermore, some patients may suffer neurologic sequelae such as nerve compression, which manifests as weakness, and sensory defects depending on the affected area. Surgical correction of scoliosis in a growing child remains controversial and treatment alternatives vary by surgeon, patient age, and coexisting disease. Surgical options include posterior spine fusion and vertical expandable prosthetic titanium rib. Anesthetic management should be tailored to meet the monitoring needs, as neurophysiologic monitoring may be used to assist and provide safety in the surgical approach. Agents that may affect the quality of motor and somatosensory-evoked potentials should be avoided, including volatile anesthetics, nitrous oxide, and neuromuscular blockade. Total intravenous anesthesia with propofol infusion and opioid infusions such as fentanyl or remifentanil are commonly used. The surgical procedures may be associated with significant hemodynamic derangements, including massive hemorrhage, spinal shock, coagulopathy, and hypothermia. Furthermore, positioning the patient should be done carefully to avoid pressure on the eyes, shoulders, and genitals to minimize position-related complications. Postoperative visual loss is uncommon but devastating and may occur as a result of ischemic optic neuropathy associated with the long duration of surgery. Intraoperative management should place specific emphasis on adequate intravascular access, with consideration for continuous arterial blood pressure monitoring as well as central venous access on a case-by-case basis. Blood conservation strategies such as antifibrinolytic agents, blood salvage techniques, and autologous blood donation may be used based on the resources available. Postoperative pain management may require support from a dedicated team.

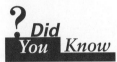

VIII. Common Pediatric Perioperative Complications

A. Postoperative Apnea

Infants and neonates born preterm are at increased risk for postoperative apnea following administration of anesthetic and sedative agents (21). In addition to prematurity, a history of apnea and anemia are risk factors for postoperative apnea. Intravenous caffeine may be administered and is effective in reducing the incidence of apnea, although postoperative admission is still warranted based on postconception age. Based on the available data, many institutions admit all former preterm infants until they reach an age of *60 weeks postconception age*. Children with obstructive sleep apnea may be especially sensitive to respiratory depression associated with narcotics and general anesthesia.

B. Laryngospasm

Incidence of *laryngospasm* is more common in children than adults. The estimated incidence rate ranges from 1 to 17.4 per 1,000 anesthetics (22). When properly managed, laryngospasm typically results in no significant sequelae. However, it is a significant concern and continues to be a cause of cardiac arrest in children (12). Treatment is with 100% oxygen, positive pressure, and maneuvers to ensure that upper airway obstruction is not present. Laryngospasm not relieved by these maneuvers should be treated with succinylcholine (22). If there are contraindications to succinylcholine, such as malignant hyperthermia or extensive burn injuries, a nondepolarizing neuromuscular blocking agent may be appropriate. Deepening the anesthetic (e.g., with 1 to 2 mg/kg of propofol) is an option in the early management of laryngospasm. Once desaturation has occurred, rapid neuromuscular blockade (succinylcholine) without delay is the treatment of choice. Secondary complications such as gastric insufflation, regurgitation, and aspiration can occur as a result of the sustained positive upper airway pressure that comprises appropriate management of laryngospasm.

C. Postextubation Stridor

Smaller children and infants are at increased risk for *postextubation stridor* due to their smaller diameter tracheas. Symptoms include a barky sounding cough (similar to infectious croup). More severe symptoms include respiratory compromise with retractions and dyspnea. Treatment for mild symptoms includes humidified air or mist. Dexamethasone 0.5 mg/kg up to 10 mg may be administered intravenously. More severe cases are treated with nebulized racemic epinephrine in addition to dexamethasone. Following treatment with racemic epinephrine, patients with improved symptoms should be observed for at least 4 hours to ensure rebound edema does not occur. Recrudescence of symptoms necessitates admission.

D. Emergence Agitation or Delirium

Emergence delirium is characterized by a state of delirium (confusion, lack of orientation to surroundings, agitation) in the immediate postoperative period following emergence from anesthesia (23). Since the introduction of sevoflurane into clinical practice, the incidence of emergence agitation has surged. Risk factors include young age (2 to 7 years), sevoflurane use, poor adaptability, and procedures near the face (ear, nose, throat, or ophthalmology). Emergence agitation is a significant concern because agitated children can injure themselves, injure staff, or pull out catheters or drains and require additional staff to safely restrain and protect them. Emergence agitation also upsets parents and creates dissatisfaction. Most strategies have focused on prevention, and a variety of regimens are effective, including maintenance of anesthesia with propofol or intraoperative administration of dexmedetomidine, clonidine, and opioids. Initial management is typically observation and protection of the child from harm. More severe cases or prolonged cases may be managed with benzodiazepines, opioids, or subhypnotic doses of other sedatives.

IX. Outpatient Procedures or Ambulatory Surgery

A. Indications and Contraindications

In general, children presenting for outpatient procedures require being in optimal health and having no ongoing cardiorespiratory processes such as upper respiratory infections (1,2,5). Furthermore, the procedure must be amenable to pain control with medications administered by mouth. Although it is not necessary to demonstrate that a child is able to eat prior to discharge, the child should be willing and able to drink fluids and ensure he or she can take the necessary medications as indicated. Additional elements to consider for eligibility for outpatient surgery include the care environment at home as well as the distance to travel home. For example, it may not be prudent to discharge a child from the hospital in the evening if the family has to drive several hours to get home.

There is a clear contraindication to ambulatory surgery in ex-premature infants during the first months of life due to the risk of postoperative apnea. The recommendation applies to premature infants defined as postgestational age of 37 weeks and 5 days or less. There is an absolute cutoff at 52 weeks of postconceptual age where children must be admitted for overnight observation. Premature infants between 52 and 60 weeks postconceptual age may be observed in the postanesthesia care unit, and the decision to discharge the child can be left to the discretion of the providers caring for the child.

B. Premedication

Children as young as 10 months of age may begin to experience anxiety when transferring to the operating room. Although all children can experience anxiety, the highest risk population is the toddler or preschool range (ages 1 to 7). Strategies to mitigate the anxiety range from *premedication* with short-acting benzodiazepines such as midazolam to induction with parental presence (8). Options for medication administration are typically limited, as most children may not have intravenous access until after induction of general anesthesia.

Some institutions have an induction room specially designed to minimize the child's anxiety and allow the child to enter with their parent(s). There are many strategies available to mitigate anxiety, including imaginative play (the anesthesia machine game), singing, and even providing flavored air through the anesthesia mask (flavored lip balm or oils). It is particularly important to address anxiety, as children who require multiple procedures can develop stress reactions ranging from defiant, aggressive reactions in the short term to regression of certain behaviors or depression in the long term.

C. Regional Anesthesia

There are many useful applications for *regional anesthetic* techniques in pediatrics (24,25). Caudal injections are among the most common procedures performed in pediatric anesthesia. Conversely, rare scenarios may require spinal anesthesia in infants, such as the evaluation of a child for a congenital myopathy that may be associated with malignant hyperthermia. In such cases, a spinal anesthetic would provide adequate conditions for a muscle biopsy of the thigh. Epidural catheters may be threaded to various levels via a caudal approach. Furthermore, peripheral nerve blocks may be helpful for a variety of orthopedic procedures, ranging from osteotomies to arthroscopic procedures for tendon repairs. Ultrasound imaging provides visualization of nerves, anatomic landmarks, and the needle and spread of local anesthetic, which allows for safe and effective administration of regional anesthesia. Other chapters of this book discuss epidural or regional anesthesia blocks.

Prior to administration of caudal anesthesia, informed consent should be obtained from the patient's parent or legal guardian. Physical examination should note the presence of any sacral dimples, which may be associated with occult spina bifida or tethered cord, thus increasing the risk of neurologic complications from the administration of local anesthetics via the caudal approach. The surface landmarks that should be palpated include the sacral cornua as well as the coccyx. The sacral hiatus and sacrococcygeal ligament are located inferior to the cornua. The block can be safely performed with either bupivacaine 0.25% with epinephrine (limit 1 mL/kg) or ropivacaine 0.2% (limit 1 mL/kg) (25). A test dose should consist of epinephrine 5 µg/kg. Criteria for intravascular injection should consider an increase in 10 beats per minute in heart rate as positive, as well as the fact that the heart rate changes can be delayed by as much as a minute after medication administration.

References

1. Hall SC, Suresh S. Neonatal anesthesia. In: Barash PG, Cullen B, Stoelting RK, et al., eds. *Clinical Anesthesia.* 7th ed. Philadelphia: Wolters Kluwer/Lippincott Williams & Wilkins; 2013:1178–1215.
2. Lerman J. Pediatric anesthesia. In: Barash PG, Cullen B, Stoelting RK, et al., eds. *Clinical Anesthesia.* 7th ed. Philadelphia: Wolters Kluwer/Lippincott Williams & Wilkins; 2013:1216–1256.
3. Healy F, Hanna BD, Zinman R. Clinical practice. The impact of lung disease on the heart and cardiac disease on the lungs. *Eur J Pediatr.* 2010;169(1):1–6.
4. Alcorn J, McNamara PJ. Pharmacokinetics in the newborn. *Adv Drug Deliv Rev.* 2003;55(5):667–686.
5. FDA Advisory Committee background document to the Anesthetic and Life Support Drugs Advisory Committee (ALSDAC). March 10, 2011. Available at: www.fda.gov/downloads/AdvisoryCommittees/CommitteesMeetingMaterials/Drugs/AnestheticAndLifeSupportDrugsAdvisoryCommittee/UCM245769.pdf.
6. Ungern-Sternberg von BS, Boda K, Chambers NA, et al. Risk assessment for respiratory complications in paediatric anaesthesia: A prospective cohort study. *Lancet.* 2010;376(9743):773–783.
7. Apfelbaum J, Caplan RA, Connis RT, et al. Practice guidelines for preoperative fasting and the use of pharmacologic agents to reduce the risk of pulmonary aspiration: Application to healthy patients undergoing elective procedures. *Anesthesiology.* 2011;114:495–511.
8. Kain ZN, Mayes LC, Wang SM, et al. Parental presence during induction of anesthesia versus sedative premedication: Which intervention is more effective? *Anesthesiology.* 1998;89:1147–1156.
9. Weiss M, Gerber AC. Rapid sequence induction in children—it's not a matter of time! *Paediatr Anaesth.* 2008;18(2):97–99.
10. Practice guidelines for perioperative blood management: An updated report by the American Society of Anesthesiologists Task Force on Perioperative Blood Management. *Anesthesiology.* 2015;122:241–275.
11. Stricker PA, Shaw TL, Desouza DG, et al. Blood loss, replacement, and associated morbidity in infants and children undergoing craniofacial surgery. *Pediatr Anesth.* 2010;20:150–159.

12. Bhananker SM, Ramamoorthy C, Geiduschek JM, et al. Anesthesia-related cardiac arrest in children: Update from the Pediatric Perioperative Cardiac Arrest Registry. *Anesth Analg.* 2007;105:344–350.

13. Lacroix J, Hebert PC, Hutchison JS, et al. Transfusion strategies for patients in pediatric intensive care units. *N Engl J Med.* 2007;356:1609–1619.

14. Rouette J, Trottier H, Ducruet T, et al. Red blood cell transfusion threshold in postsurgical pediatric intensive care patients: a randomized clinical trial. *Ann Surg.* 2010;251: 421–427.

15. OMIM. Available at: www.ncbi.nlm.nih.gov/omim.

16. Roland PS, Rosenfeld RM, Brooks LJ, American Academy of Otolaryngology—Head and Neck Surgery Foundation. Clinical practice guideline: Polysomnography for sleep-disordered breathing prior to tonsillectomy in children. *Otolaryngol Head Neck Surg.* 2011;145(1 Suppl):S1–15.

17. Jackson O, Basta M, Sonnad S, et al. Perioperative risk factors for adverse airway events in patients undergoing cleft palate repair. *Cleft Palate Craniofac J.* 2013;50:330–336.

18. Bösenberg AT, Brown RA. Management of congenital diaphragmatic hernia. *Curr Opin Anaesthesiol.* 2008;21:323–331.

19. Blank RS, de Souza DG. Anesthetic management of patients with an anterior mediastinal mass: Continuing professional development. *Can J Anaesth.* 2011;58:853–859, 860–867.

20. Pinheiro PF, Simões e Silva AC, Pereira RM. Current knowledge on esophageal atresia. *World J Gastroenterol.* 2012;18:3662–3672.

21. Coté CJ, Zaslavsky A, Downes JJ, et al. Postoperative apnea in former preterm infants after inguinal herniorrhaphy. A combined analysis. *Anesthesiology.* 1995;82:809–822.

22. Burgoyne LL, Anghelescu DL. Intervention steps for treating laryngospasm in pediatric patients. *Paediatr Anaesth.* 2008;18:297–302.

23. Voepel-Lewis T, Malviya S, Tait AR. A prospective cohort study of emergence agitation in the pediatric postanesthesia care unit. *Anesth Analg.* 2003:1625–1630.

24. Gurnaney H, Kraemer FW, Maxwell L, et al. Ambulatory continuous peripheral nerve blocks in children and adolescents. *Anesth Analg.* 2014;118:621–627.

25. Suresh S, Long J, Birmingham PK, et al. Are caudal blocks for pain control safe in children? An analysis of 18,650 caudal blocks from the Pediatric Regional Anesthesia Network (PRAN) database. *Anesth Analg.* 2015;120:151–156.

Questions

1. A 2-month-old is scheduled for an elective bilateral Achilles' tenotomy under general anesthesia. He can be given formula:
   A. Up to 2 hours prior to operation
   B. Up to 4 hours prior to operation
   C. Up to 6 hours prior to operation
   D. Up to 8 hours prior to operation

2. A 2-year-old girl is scheduled for emergency exploratory laparotomy for intestinal obstruction. You plan a rapid sequence induction. According to the package insert black box warning:
   A. Succinylcholine is contraindicated in this age group.
   B. Succinylcholine may be used if preceded by a nondepolarizing neuromuscular blocker.
   C. Succinylcholine may be administered.
   D. Rocuronium is not appropriate due to its slower onset.

3. A 1-year-old 10-kg patient is scheduled for strabismus surgery at 7:30 a.m. She had clear liquids at 5:30 a.m. How much fluid (approximately) should she receive during her first hour of surgery?
   A. 40 mL
   B. 60 mL
   C. 80 mL
   D. 120 mL

4. As the pediatric postanesthesia care unit resident, which of these patients has the greatest risk of postoperative apnea?
   A. A 2-year-old undergoing an ophthalmologic examination under anesthesia
   B. A 2-month-old born at 32 weeks following repair of inguinal hernia
   C. A 1-year-old delivered at 40 weeks following inguinal hernia repair
   D. A 2-year-old following elective setting of an arm fracture 2 weeks after an upper respiratory infection

5. Which of the following will cause the greatest difficulty in successfully passing a nasotracheal tube in a 1-month-old child?
   A. Tongue
   B. Cylindrical laryngeal shape of larynx
   C. Cricoid cartilage
   D. Orientation of the vocal chords within the larynx

6. As compared to a normal adult, the oxygen consumption (cc/kg basis) of the neonate is:
   A. The same
   B. Greater than the adult
   C. Three times greater in the neonate
   D. Three times greater in the adult

7. Which of the following best reflects electrolyte and acid-base abnormalities seen in the neonate with pyloric stenosis?

	Sodium	Potassium	Chloride	Acid Base Diagnosis
A.	↓	↓	↓	Metabolic alkalosis
B.	↓	↓	↓	Metabolic acidosis
C.	↑	↑	↑	Metabolic acidosis
D.	↓	↑	↑	Respiratory alkalosis

8. Which of the following represents the normal blood gas values for a full-term neonate at 10 minutes postdelivery?

	PO$_2$ (mm Hg)	PCO$_2$ (mm Hg)	pH (u)
A.	10–20	55	7.25
B.	50	48	7.20
C.	70	35	7.35
D.	60	38	7.37

9. The factor that does not affect design of pediatric breathing circuits is:
   A. Resistance to fresh gas flow
   B. Temperature maintenance
   C. Dead space volume
   D. Facemask fit

10. Which of the following respiratory function variables significantly differ (mL/kg or mL/kg/min) between infant and adult?
    A. Tidal volume
    B. Dead space
    C. Functional residual capacity
    D. Oxygen consumption

34 Anesthesia for Thoracic Surgery

Katherine Marseu
Peter Slinger

The most common indication for thoracic surgery is malignancy (1,2,3). Despite this, a wide variety of pathologies and procedures are commonly encountered when providing anesthetics for patients undergoing thoracic surgery. As a result, there are a number of important preoperative, intraoperative, and postoperative anesthetic considerations for thoracic surgery.

I. Preoperative Assessment

Respiratory and *cardiac complications* are the major cause of perioperative morbidity and mortality in the thoracic surgical population. Thus, the preoperative evaluation of these patients focuses on an assessment of respiratory function and the cardiopulmonary interaction. All pulmonary resection patients should have preoperative spirometry to determine postoperative preservation of respiratory function, which has been shown to be proportional to the remaining number of lung subsegments (right upper, middle, and lower lobes = 6,4,12 subsegments, respectively; left upper and lower lobes = 10 subsegments each, for a total of 42 subsegments). The principles discussed in the sections that follow also apply to thoracic surgical patients who are not having lung resections (1,2).

A. Lung Mechanical Function

A valid single test for postthoracotomy respiratory complications is the *predicted postoperative (ppo) forced expiratory volume* in 1 second (ppoFEV$_1$%), which is calculated as:

$$\text{ppoFEV}_1\% = \text{preoperative FEV}_1\% \times (1 - \text{fraction lung tissue removed}).$$

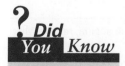

For example, a patient with a preoperative FEV$_1$ of 60% having a right upper lobectomy (6 of 42 lung subsegments) would be expected to have a ppoFEV$_1$% = 60% × [1 − (6/42)] = 51%. Patients with a ppoFEV$_1$ >40% are at low risk for postresection respiratory complications, <40% at moderate risk, and <30% are at high risk (1,2).

Table 34-1   Summary of Important Values in the Preoperative Respiratory Assessment

Parameter	Value	Risk of Respiratory Complications
ppoFEV$_1$%	>40%	Low
	<40%	Moderate
	<30%	High
ppoDLCO	<40%	Increased
	<30%	Very high
$\dot{V}O_2$max	≤15 mL/kg/min	Increased
	≤10 mL/kg/min	Very high

ppoFEV$_1$, predicted postoperative forced expiratory volume in 1 second; DLCO, diffusing capacity of the lung for carbon monoxide; $\dot{V}O_2$max, maximal oxygen consumption.

B. Lung Parenchymal Function

The most useful test of gas exchange is the *diffusing capacity* of the lung for carbon monoxide (DLCO). The preoperative DLCO can be used to calculate a ppo value using the same calculation as for the FEV$_1$, with similar risk categories: increased risk <40% and high risk <30% (1,2,3).

C. Cardiopulmonary Interaction

The most important assessment of respiratory function is an assessment of the *cardiopulmonary reserve*, and the maximal oxygen consumption ($\dot{V}O_2$max) is the most useful predictor of outcome. The risk of morbidity and mortality is increased if the preoperative $\dot{V}O_2$max is ≤15 mL/kg/min and very high if it is ≤10 mL/kg/min. In ambulatory patients, the $\dot{V}O_2$max can be estimated from the distance in meters that a patient can walk in 6 minutes (6-minute walk test [6MWT]) divided by 30 (i.e., 6MWT of 450 m:estimated $\dot{V}O_2$max = 450/30 = 15 mL/kg/min). The ability to climb five flights of stairs correlates with a $\dot{V}O_2$max >20 mL/kg/min, and two flights corresponds to a $\dot{V}O_2$max of 12 mL/kg/min (1,2,3) (Table 34-1).

D. Cardiac Investigations

Thoracic surgery is considered *"intermediate risk"* for cardiac complications, such as myocardial infarction and arrhythmias, according to the American College of Cardiology and the American Heart Association (ACC/AHA) guidelines for the preoperative assessment of cardiac patients undergoing non-cardiac surgery. Patients with cardiac conditions or risk factors (Table 34-2)

Table 34-2   Cardiac Conditions and Risk Factors

Active Cardiac Conditions	Predictors of Risk
Unstable ischemia, recent MI	Ischemic heart disease (stable angina, remote MI)
Decompensated CHF	History of CHF
Significant arrhythmias	History of CVD
Severe valvular disease	Renal insufficiency Diabetes

MI, myocardial infarction; CHF, congestive heart failure; CVD, cerebrovascular disease.
Adapted from Fleisher L, Beckman J, Brown K, et al. ACC/AHA 2007 guidelines on perioperative cardiovascular evaluation and care for noncardiac surgery. *Circulation.* 2007;116:418–500.

should be investigated according to the ACC/AHA guidelines: noninvasive stress testing or cardiac catheterization should be performed in these patients if they have poor or unknown functional capacity, three or more clinical risk factors, and, most important, if the results of the testing will change management (1,2,4).

E. Common Pathologies and Comorbidities
Malignancies
The majority of patients presenting for thoracic surgery will have a malignancy, including lung cancers, pleural and mediastinal tumors, and esophageal cancer. These patients should be assessed for the "4-M's" associated with malignancy: *Mass effects* (obstructive pneumonia, superior vena cava [SVC] syndrome, etc.), *Metabolic abnormalities* (hypercalcemia, Lambert-Eaton syndrome, etc.), *Metastases* (brain, bone, liver, and adrenal), and *Medications* (adjuvant chemotherapy and radiation) (1,2).

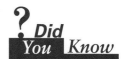

? *Did* **You** *Know*

The "4-M's" associated with malignancy are: Mass effect, Metabolic abnormalities, Metastases, and Medications.

Chronic Obstructive Pulmonary Disease
This is the most common concurrent illness in the thoracic surgical population. Patients should be *free of exacerbation* before elective surgery, and may have fewer postoperative pulmonary complications when intensive chest physiotherapy is initiated preoperatively. Pulmonary complications are also decreased in thoracic surgical patients who cease smoking for more than four weeks before surgery. Patients with chronic obstructive pulmonary disease and limited or unknown exercise tolerance may benefit from an arterial blood gas (ABG) preoperatively, if the results prove helpful in weaning mechanical ventilation at the conclusion of surgery. Other considerations in chronic obstructive pulmonary disease patients include the presence of bullous disease, pulmonary hypertension with right heart dysfunction, and the risk of dynamic hyperinflation due to gas trapping (1,2,3).

II. Intraoperative Management

A. Monitoring
Standard anesthetic monitoring is used in all thoracic surgery cases. An invasive *arterial line* is placed for the majority of surgeries. It is useful to measure baseline preoperative ABGs for intraoperative comparison during *one-lung ventilation (OLV)*, detection of sudden blood pressure changes, and postoperative weaning of mechanical ventilation. A central venous line may be required in some cases for vascular access or for infusion of vasoactive medications. The central venous pressure (CVP) can be a useful intraoperative and postoperative monitor, particularly for cases where fluid management is critical, such as pneumonectomies and esophagectomies. Fluid management for all thoracic procedures should follow either a restricted or a goal-directed protocol. However, recently, concerns about *acute kidney injury* have called into question the strategy of fluid restriction in thoracic surgery (3). No fluids are given for theoretical "third-space" losses. Colloids have not been proven to improve outcome and add considerable expense. Spirometry is particularly useful to monitor breath-by-breath inspired and expired tidal volumes during OLV and may alert the clinician to possible loss of lung isolation, air leaks, and the development of hyperinflation (1,3).

B. Physiology of One-Lung Ventilation
In the majority of thoracic surgery cases, patients transition from being upright, awake, and spontaneously breathing to supine, asleep, and paralyzed.

They are then moved from the supine position to the lateral position. Finally, OLV is initiated and their chest is opened. Changes in ventilation and perfusion accompany each of these circumstances.

First, functional residual capacity (FRC) is the main factor determining oxygen reserve in patients when they become apneic. Patients will experience a decrease in FRC when in the supine position compared with the upright position. This change will be magnified by the induction of anesthesia and administration of muscle relaxants. When upright, the majority of ventilation and perfusion reach the gravity-dependent portions of the lungs (i.e., the bases). With the induction of anesthesia, most of the ventilation now enters the nondependent portions of the lung, increasing ventilation-perfusion ($\dot{V}/\dot{Q}$) mismatch.

Second, in the lateral position, the dependent lung receives more perfusion compared with the nondependent lung. However, the dependent hemidiaphragm is pushed into the thoracic cavity by the abdominal contents, further decreasing FRC and worsening $\dot{V}/\dot{Q}$ mismatch.

Third, when the chest is opened, the compliance of the nondependent lung improves relative to the dependent lung, and it is preferentially ventilated, further increasing the $\dot{V}/\dot{Q}$ mismatch. However, when OLV is initiated in the dependent lung, it receives the majority of both perfusion and ventilation. There will still be some cardiac output shunted through the collapsed, nondependent lung, but $\dot{V}/\dot{Q}$ matching may be improved by hypoxic pulmonary vasoconstriction (HPV) in the nonventilated, nondependent lung (Fig. 34-1). HPV can be inhibited by many factors, such as extremes of pulmonary artery pressures, hypocapnia, vasodilators, and inhalational agents (1,3).

C. Indications for One-Lung Ventilation

High and intermediate priorities for OLV are listed in Table 34-3. The highest priorities include prevention of *contamination* of the healthy lung by infection

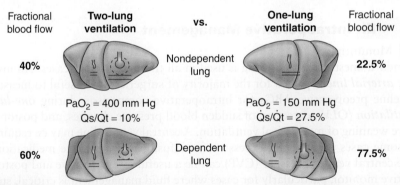

Figure 34-1 Schematic representation of two-lung ventilation versus one-lung ventilation (OLV). Typical values for fractional blood flow to the nondependent and dependent lungs, as well as PaO$_2$ and $\dot{Q}s/\dot{Q}t$ for the two conditions, are shown. The $\dot{Q}s/\dot{Q}t$ during two-lung ventilation is assumed to be distributed equally between the two lungs (5% to each lung). The essential difference between two-lung ventilation and OLV is that, during OLV, the nonventilated lung has some blood flow and therefore an obligatory shunt, which is not present during two-lung ventilation. The 35% of total flow perfusing the nondependent lung, which was not shunt flow, was assumed to be able to reduce its blood flow by 50% by hypoxic pulmonary vasoconstriction. The increase in $\dot{Q}s/\dot{Q}t$ from two-lung to OLV is assumed to be due solely to the increase in blood flow through the nonventilated, nondependent lung during OLV. (From Eisenkraft JB, Cohen E, Neustein SM. Anesthesia for thoracic surgery. In: Barash PG, Cullen BF, Stoelting RK, et al. *Clinical Anesthesia*, 7th ed. Philadelphia: Lippincott Williams & Wilkins, 2013:1041.)

Table 34-3	Indications for Lung Isolation
High Priority	**Intermediate Priority**
Prevention of contamination of healthy lung: • Infection • Hemorrhage	Higher indication for surgical exposure: • Thoracic aortic aneurysm repair • Pneumonectomy • Lung volume reduction • Minimally invasive cardiac surgery • Upper lobectomy
Control of distribution of ventilation: • Bronchopleural fistula • Unilateral bullae • Airway disruption	Lower indication for surgical exposure: • Esophageal surgery • Middle and lower lobectomy • Mediastinal mass resection • Bilateral sympathectomies
Unilateral lung lavage	
Video-assisted thoracoscopic surgery	

or hemorrhage; control of distribution of ventilation in bronchopleural fistula, unilateral bullae, or airway disruption; unilateral lung lavage; and video-assisted thoracoscopic surgery (VATS). Intermediate priorities for OLV include surgical exposure in thoracic aortic aneurysm repair, pneumonectomy, lung volume reduction, minimally invasive cardiac surgery, and upper lobectomy. Lower indications for OLV include surgical exposure in esophageal surgery, middle and lower lobectomy, mediastinal mass resection, and bilateral sympathectomies (1,3).

D. Methods of Lung Isolation

Lung isolation can be achieved with the use of a *double-lumen tube (DLT)*, bronchial blocker, or endobronchial intubation with a regular single-lumen tube (SLT) or specialized endobronchial tube. An SLT is rarely used in an endobronchial fashion in adults except in emergent scenarios, as bronchoscopy, suction, or continuous positive airway pressure (CPAP) cannot be applied to the collapsed lung.

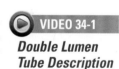

VIDEO 34-1

Double Lumen Tube Description

DLTs are the most commonly used method to achieve lung isolation and OLV (Fig. 34-2). They are available in both left- and right-sided conformations, with the left-sided DLT being the most widely used. Advantages of the DLT include the ability to isolate either lung; apply suction, CPAP, or oxygen insufflation down either lumen; and to perform bronchoscopy down either lumen. The DLT is less likely to dislodge than other methods of lung separation, which makes it the *preferred method* of isolation in cases of infection or hemorrhage. Disadvantages of the DLT include the fact that it is more challenging to place in a difficult airway, and it will usually need to be exchanged for an SLT if a patient is to remain intubated postoperatively.

A *bronchial blocker* placed through an SLT can also be used to achieve lung isolation (Fig. 34-3). A bronchoscope is used to direct the blocker to the lung or lung segment that is to be collapsed. Several advantages of the blocker include the flexibility for use in an oral or nasotracheal fashion and for selective lobar blockade. It is particularly useful in scenarios such as a *difficult airway* or the need for postoperative ventilation. The main disadvantage of a bronchial blocker is that it can be displaced from changes in patient position

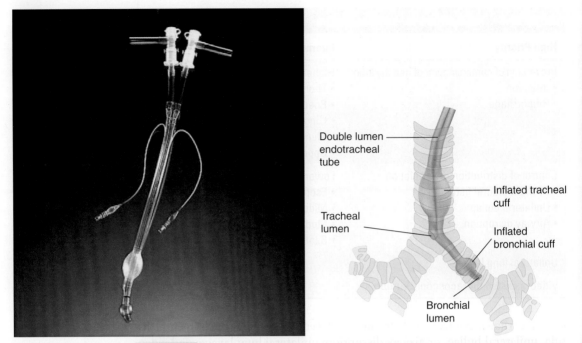

Figure 34-2 A left-sided Robertshaw type double-lumen tube constructed from polyvinyl chloride (*left*). When properly positioned (*right*), the distal "bronchial lumen" is placed in the left mainstem bronchus proximal to the left upper lobe orifice, with the "bronchial cuff" inflated just distal to the carina in the left mainstem bronchus. The proximal "tracheal lumen" is positioned above the carina, with the "tracheal cuff" inflated in the mid-trachea. Proper positioning allows for the options of one-lung ventilation on either side (with contralateral lung deflation), as well as two-lung ventilation. (From Eisenkraft JB, Cohen E, Neustein SM. Anesthesia for thoracic surgery. In: Barash PG, Cullen BF, Stoelting RK, et al. *Clinical Anesthesia*, 7th ed. Philadelphia: Lippincott Williams & Wilkins, 2013:1043.)

or surgical manipulation. This is especially detrimental in a situation where loss of lung separation can lead to contamination from blood or pus (1,3).

E. Management of One-Lung Ventilation

Fraction of Inspired Oxygen
When initiating OLV, a fraction of inspired oxygen (FiO_2) of 1.0 is generally used to prevent hypoxemia. An ABG may be taken to determine arterial partial pressure of O_2. If this is adequate, the FiO_2 may be titrated down (3).

Tidal Volume and Respiratory Rate
The current trend in OLV is to use *lung-protective strategies*. Whether using volume-controlled or pressure-controlled ventilation, tidal volume should be approximately 5 mL/kg. The respiratory rate is then titrated to maintain an acceptable range of end-tidal carbon dioxide (CO_2) or arterial partial pressure of CO_2 (35 to 40 mm Hg). Peak airway pressures should be maintained at <35 cm H_2O, and preferably <25 cm H_2O (1,3). In the presence of bullous disease, even lower airway pressures must be considered.

F. Management of Hypoxemia on One-Lung Ventilation

Hypoxic pulmonary vasoconstriction can take hours to reach full effect. If hypoxemia develops during OLV, the FiO_2 should be increased to 1.0. Bronchoscopy should be performed to confirm tube position. The most effective

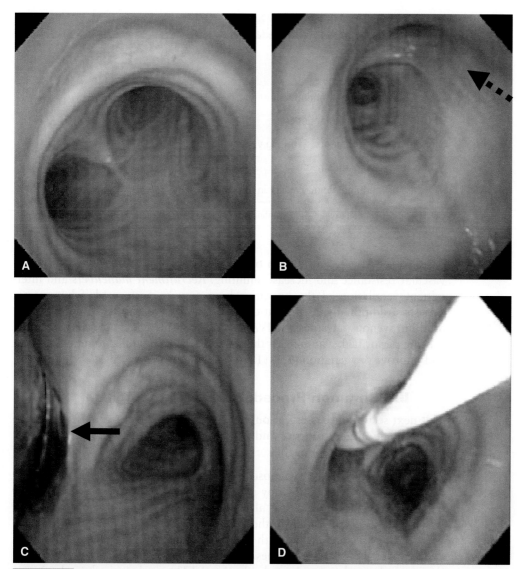

Figure 34-3 **A.** Bronchoscopic view of the carina through the distal opening of a standard endotracheal tube. Note the C-shaped tracheal rings anteriorly orient the viewer to the left and right mainstem bronchi. **B.** Bronchoscopic view of the right upper lobe orifice (*arrow*) only 1.5-2.0 cm distal to the carina. This short distance generally prevents the use of right-sided double-lumen tubes. **C.** Bronchoscopic view of the carina and right mainstem bronchus, demonstrating a properly positioned left-sided double lumen tube with the blue bronchial cuff (*arrow*) inflated just distal to the carina in the left mainstem bronchus. **D.** Bronchoscopic view of a bronchial blocker placed through a single-lumen tube and positioned in the left mainstem bronchus to allow one-lung ventilation on the right. (From Eisenkraft JB, Cohen E, Neustein SM. Anesthesia for thoracic surgery. In: Barash PG, Cullen BF, Stoelting RK, et al. *Clinical Anesthesia*, 7th ed. Philadelphia: Lippincott Williams & Wilkins, 2013:1044–1048.)

treatment of hypoxemia is to apply 5 to 10 cm H_2O of **CPAP** to the non-dependent lung. However, as this is the operative lung, CPAP can interfere with the surgical exposure. Thus, the application of positive end-expiratory pressure (PEEP) to the dependent lung may then be useful to increase FRC and $\dot{V}/\dot{Q}$ matching. This should be limited to approximately 10 cm H_2O in

Table 34-4   Management of Hypoxia on One-Lung Ventilation
FiO_2 1.0
Confirm tube position
CPAP 5–10 cm H_2O to nondependent lung
PEEP 10 cm H_2O to dependent lung
Intermittent recruitments, two-lung ventilation
Total intravenous anesthesia
Clamp ipsilateral pulmonary artery in pneumonectomy

FiO_2, fraction of inspired oxygen; CPAP, continuous positive airway pressure; PEEP, positive end expiratory pressure.

order to prevent overdistension of the alveoli, which can elevate pulmonary vascular resistance and increase shunting. *Recruitment maneuvers* and intermittent ventilation of the operative lung may be performed if hypoxemia persists. Additionally, as inhalational anesthetics are known to inhibit HPV, total intravenous anesthesia (TIVA) may be considered. If a pneumonectomy is being performed, clamping of the pulmonary artery will eliminate the shunt and improve oxygenation (1,3) (Table 34-4).

III. Common Procedures and Pathologies

This next section discusses various procedures that are commonly performed in a thoracic surgery practice and reviews the relevant pathologies and anesthetic considerations for each.

A. Flexible Fiberoptic Bronchoscopy

Flexible fiberoptic bronchoscopy is a diagnostic and therapeutic modality for pathologies of the airways. It is also common to perform bronchoscopy prior to lung resections to reconfirm the diagnosis or determine invasion of the airway. Options include awake with topical anesthesia versus general anesthesia and oral versus nasal approaches. Airway management during general anesthesia can be with an endotracheal tube (ETT) or a laryngeal mask airway. *Intravenous* anesthesia is preferred if this procedure is going to be prolonged, as volatile agents *may* contaminate the operating room (1,3).

B. Rigid Bronchoscopy

Rigid bronchoscopy is the procedure of choice for dilation of *tracheal stenosis* with or without the use of a laser, foreign body removal, and massive hemoptysis. There are four basic methods of ventilation for rigid bronchoscopy: spontaneous ventilation; apneic oxygenation with or without the insufflation of oxygen; positive pressure ventilation (PPV) via the side arm of a ventilating bronchoscope; and jet ventilation with a handheld injector or high-frequency jet ventilator. Rigid bronchoscopy in children is most commonly managed with spontaneous ventilation and a volatile anesthetic. In adults, total intravenous anesthesia (TIVA) and the use of muscle relaxants is more common, with a combination of PPV via the bronchoscope side arm or jet ventilation. Pulse oximetry is vital during rigid bronchoscopy because there is a high risk of desaturation. However, monitoring of end-tidal CO_2 and volatile anesthetics is less useful, because the airway remains essentially open to the

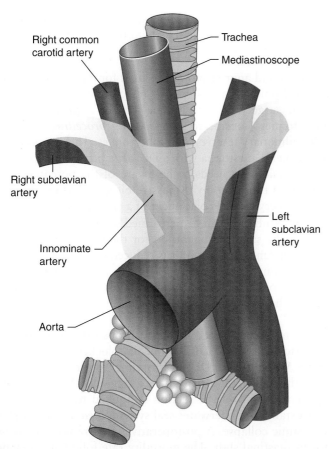

Right common
carotid artery

Trachea

Mediastinoscope

Right subclavian
artery

Left
subclavian
artery

Innominate
artery

Aorta

Figure 34-4 Anatomic relationships during mediastinoscopy. Note the position of the mediastinoscope behind the right innominate artery and aortic arch and anterior to the trachea. (From Eisenkraft JB, Cohen E, Neustein SM. Anesthesia for thoracic surgery. In: Barash PG, Cullen BF, Stoelting RK, et al. *Clinical Anesthesia*, 7th ed. Philadelphia: Lippincott Williams & Wilkins, 2013:1060.)

atmosphere. Unlike during fiberoptic bronchoscopy via an ETT, with rigid bronchoscopy, the airway is never completely secure and there is always the potential for aspiration, especially in patients at increased risk. Complications of rigid bronchoscopy include airway perforation, mucosal damage, hemorrhage, postmanipulation airway edema, and potential airway loss at the end of the procedure (1,3).

C. Mediastinoscopy
Mediastinoscopy is a diagnostic procedure for the evaluation of lymph nodes in the staging of lung cancer and for *anterior mediastinal masses*. The most common mediastinal procedure is a cervical mediastinoscopy, in which the mediastinoscope is inserted through a small incision in the suprasternal notch and advanced toward the carina (Fig. 34-4). The majority of these cases require general anesthesia with placement of an SLT. A pulse oximeter or arterial line can be used to monitor perfusion to the right arm, because compression of the innominate artery by the mediastinoscope may occur. The most severe complication of mediastinoscopy is *major hemorrhage*, which may require emergent sternotomy or thoracotomy. A large-bore intravenous line should be placed in a lower extremity in the event of an SVC tear. Other potential complications

include airway obstruction, pneumothorax, paresis of the recurrent laryngeal, phrenic nerve injury, esophageal injury, chylothorax, and air embolism (1,3,5).

D. Pulmonary Resection

Several techniques and approaches can be used for the resection of pulmonary tissue or tumor. Minimally invasive lung resection can be accomplished with VATS or robotic surgery. Such techniques can be used for wedge resections and segmentectomies (considered *lung-sparing procedures* in patients with limited cardiopulmonary reserve), and lobectomies. These procedures are performed under general anesthesia with a DLT or a bronchial blocker to achieve OLV. The anesthesiologist needs to be aware of the potential for emergent conversion to open thoracotomy if massive bleeding ensues. The majority of thoracoscopic surgery requires placement of a chest tube with underwater seal drainage so that extubation can be performed safely.

Lobectomy is the standard operation for the management of lung cancer because local recurrence of the tumor is reduced compared with that of lesser resections. Lobectomy is commonly performed via *open thoracotomy* or VATS with a DLT or a bronchial blocker. Patients undergoing lobectomy can usually be extubated in the operating room provided preoperative respiratory function is adequate.

? Did You Know

Suction applied to a chest tube placed after pneumonectomy can cause mediastinal shift, resulting in hemodynamic collapse.

Pneumonectomy is performed through an open thoracotomy. Lung isolation can be performed with a DLT, bronchial blocker, or single-lumen endobronchial tube. When using a DLT, it is optimal to use a device that does not interfere with the ipsilateral airway (i.e., a left-sided DLT for a right pneumonectomy). Postoperatively, if suction is applied to a chest drain or it is connected to a standard underwater seal system, *mediastinal shift* may ensue with hemodynamic collapse. A postoperative chest radiograph is mandatory to assess for mediastinal shift. The mortality rate following pneumonectomy exceeds that for lobectomy because of postoperative cardiac complications and acute lung injury. The risk of complications increases fivefold in patients age 65 and older (1,3,6). The complication of cardiac herniation will be discussed in the last section of this chapter.

? Did You Know

Restrictive fluid strategy for patients undergoing pulmonary and esophageal surgery has become controversial because of a concern about its potential to induce acute kidney injury.

E. Esophageal Surgery

General considerations, which apply to almost all esophageal patients, include an increased risk of *aspiration* due to esophageal dysfunction and the possibility of *malnutrition*. Esophagectomy is a potentially curative treatment for esophageal cancer and for some benign obstructive lesions. It is a major surgical procedure and is associated with high morbidity and mortality rates (10% to 15%). There are multiple surgical procedures for esophagectomy that combine three fundamental approaches: transthoracic approach, transhiatal approach, and minimally invasive surgery. Outcomes are improved with early extubation, thoracic epidural analgesia, and vasopressor or inotrope infusions to support blood pressure (1,3,7).

F. Tracheal Resection

Tracheal resection is indicated in patients who have a tracheal obstruction as a result of a tracheal tumor, trauma (most commonly due to postintubation stenosis), congenital anomalies, vascular lesions, or tracheomalacia. The airways of patients with congenital or acquired tracheal stenosis are unlikely to collapse during induction of anesthesia. However, intratracheal masses may lead to *airway obstruction* with induction of anesthesia and should be managed similarly to anterior mediastinal masses (see below). A variety of methods for providing adequate ventilation have been used during tracheal resection, including standard orotracheal intubation; insertion of a sterile SLT into the opened trachea or bronchus distal to the area of resection; high-frequency jet ventilation with a catheter through the stenotic area; high-frequency PPV; and the use of cardiopulmonary bypass (CPB). After the tracheal resection is completed, most patients are kept in a position of neck flexion to reduce tension on the suture line. *Early extubation* in these cases is highly desirable. If a patient requires reintubation, it should be performed with a flexible fiberoptic bronchoscope by advancing an SLT under direct vision over the bronchoscope to avoid damage to the repair (1,3,8).

G. Bronchopleural Fistula

A bronchopleural fistula may be caused by rupture of a lung abscess, bronchus, bulla, cyst, or parenchymal tissue into the pleural space; erosion of a bronchus by carcinoma or chronic inflammatory disease; or stump dehiscence of a bronchial suture line after pulmonary resection. In patients with bullous lung disease, such as emphysema, there is a risk of bulla *hyperinflation* and rupture whenever PPV is used. The complications of bulla rupture can be life-threatening due to *hemodynamic collapse* from *tension pneumothorax* or inadequate ventilation due to a resultant bronchopleural fistula. If bronchial disruption occurs early in postresection patients, it can also be life-threatening. It is possible to redo the thoracotomy and resuture the bronchial stump. Late or chronic postresection disruption is managed with chest tube drainage or with the Clagett procedure, which includes open pleural drainage and the use of a muscle flap to reinforce the bronchial stump.

Concerns for the anesthesiologist in a patient with a bronchopleural fistula include the need for *lung isolation* to protect healthy lung regions, the possibility of tension pneumothorax with PPV, and the possibility of inadequate ventilation due to air leak from the fistula. Placement of a chest drain should be considered prior to induction to avoid the possibility of tension pneumothorax with PPV. A DLT is the optimal choice for airway management, as lung isolation should be performed before initiating PPV or repositioning the patient. This is most commonly performed with a modified rapid sequence induction of anesthesia and immediate fiberoptic positioning of the DLT. However, depending on the context, awake intubation maintenance of spontaneous ventilation may be used (1,3).

H. Bronchiectasis, Lung Abscess, and Empyema

Infectious conditions, including bronchiectasis, lung abscess, and empyema, are indications for thoracic surgery, such as decortication. Anesthetic considerations for these conditions include the need for *lung isolation* to protect uninvolved lung regions from soiling by pus. A DLT facilitates suctioning of debris and copious secretions that are present in the trachea–bronchial tree and is less subject to dislodgement during patient movement or surgical manipulation than would be a bronchial blocker. Due to the inflammation, surgery is technically more difficult, and there is a greater risk of massive hemorrhage, particularly during decortication. Some of these patients may present with sepsis at the time of surgery. If the lung has been chronically collapsed, expansion should be done gradually to avoid the development of pulmonary edema upon re-expansion (1).

I. Mediastinal Masses

Tumors of the anterior mediastinum include thymoma, teratoma, lymphoma, cystic hygroma, bronchogenic cyst, and thyroid tumors. Patients may require anesthesia for biopsy of these masses by mediastinoscopy or VATS or they may require definitive resection via sternotomy or thoracotomy. Mediastinal masses may cause **obstruction** of **major airways** or vascular structures. During induction of general anesthesia, airway obstruction is the most common and feared complication. A history of **supine dyspnea** or cough should alert the anesthesiologist to the possibility of airway obstruction upon induction. General anesthesia and muscle relaxants will exacerbate extrinsic intrathoracic airway compression due to reduced lung volume and tracheobronchial diameters, bronchial smooth muscle relaxation, and loss of the normal transpleural pressure gradient that dilates the airways during spontaneous inspiration and minimizes the effects of extrinsic intrathoracic airway compression. It is important to note that the point of tracheobronchial compression may be in the distal airway, so it may not be bypassed by an ETT. The other major complication is cardiovascular collapse secondary to compression of the heart or major vessels. Symptoms of supine presyncope suggest vascular compression.

Patients who are symptomatic or have evidence of airway or cardiovascular involvement on imaging should have diagnostic procedures performed under local or regional anesthesia whenever possible. When general anesthesia is indicated, awake intubation of the trachea is a possibility in some adult patients, if imaging shows an area of noncompressed distal trachea to which the ETT can be advanced before induction. Alternatively, spontaneous ventilation should be maintained with either an inhalation induction or titration of an agent such as ketamine. If muscle relaxants are required, ventilation should first be gradually taken over manually to ensure that PPV is possible and only then can a short-acting muscle relaxant be administered.

Intraoperative life-threatening **airway compression** may respond to repositioning of the patient (it must be determined before induction if there is a position that causes less symptoms) or rigid bronchoscopy and ventilation distal to the obstruction (this means that an experienced bronchoscopist and equipment must always be immediately available in the operating room for these cases). Institution of femorofemoral CPB before induction of anesthesia is a possibility in some adult patients. The concept of CPB "standby" during attempted induction of anesthesia should not be considered because there is not enough time after a sudden airway collapse to establish CPB before hypoxic cerebral injury occurs (1,3,9).

J. Myasthenia Gravis

Myasthenia gravis is an autoimmune disease of the neuromuscular junction, in which affected patients have weakness due to a decreased number of acetylcholine receptors at the motor endplate. Patients may or may not have an associated thymoma. Thymectomy is frequently performed to induce clinical remission, even in the absence of a thymoma. Thymectomy may be performed via full or partial sternotomy or a minimally invasive approach via a transcervical incision or VATS.

Medical treatments for myasthenia gravis include anticholinesterases, such as pyridostigmine, immunosuppressive drugs, such as steroids, and plasmapheresis. On the day of surgery, patients should continue their usual pyridostigmine dosing. Myasthenic patients are unpredictably **resistant** to **succinylcholine** and extremely **sensitive** to **nondepolarizing blockers**. Ideally, the use of intraoperative neuromuscular relaxation is avoided. Induction of anesthesia with propofol, remifentanil, and topical anesthesia of the airway facilitates intubation without the use of muscle relaxants. Alternatively, inhalational induction with a volatile agent may be performed. Referral for surgery early in the course of the disease, preoperative medical stabilization, and minimally invasive surgical approaches have made the need for postoperative ventilation infrequent (1,3,10).

IV. Postoperative Management

A. Pain Management

Thoracic epidural analgesia (TEA) has been considered the gold standard for postoperative pain control in patients undergoing thoracotomy. When thoracotomy pain is controlled, the risk of pulmonary complications is decreased. In patients with coronary artery disease, thoracic epidural local anesthetics also seem to reduce myocardial oxygen demand. When there is a relative or absolute contraindication to placement of a thoracic epidural, another excellent choice for analgesia is a paravertebral infusion of local anesthetic via a catheter. This may be placed by the anesthesiologist using a landmark or ultrasound-guided technique or directly by the surgeon during an open thoracotomy. A recent systematic review has shown that continuous paravertebral block is as effective as TEA (11). Other options for analgesia include intercostal blocks and the use of patient-controlled opioid analgesia with multimodal analgesia, such as the use of acetaminophen, gabapentin, and nonsteroidal anti-inflammatories. Institutions differ in their practices regarding the use of catheter techniques versus intravenous patient-controlled analgesia for minimally invasive thoracic surgeries (1,3).

B. Complications

As mentioned previously, respiratory and cardiac complications account for the majority of morbidity and mortality following thoracic surgery. There are multiple potential complications that can occur in the immediate postoperative period, such as *torsion* of a remaining lobe after lobectomy, dehiscence of a bronchial stump, hemorrhage from a major vessel, or cardiac ischemia or arrhythmias. Among these possible complications, two will be discussed in more detail: respiratory failure and cardiac herniation.

Respiratory Failure

Patients with decreased respiratory function preoperatively are at increased risk of postoperative respiratory complications. In addition, age, the presence of coronary artery disease, and the extent of lung resection play major roles in predicting postoperative respiratory failure. Decreased pulmonary complications in high-risk patients are associated with the use of TEA during the perioperative period. Chest physiotherapy, incentive spirometry, and early ambulation are also crucial in order to minimize pulmonary complications after lung resection. For an uncomplicated lung resection, *early* extubation is desirable to avoid potential complications that can arise due to *prolonged* intubation and mechanical ventilation. Current therapy to treat acute respiratory failure is aimed at supportive measures that provide better oxygenation, treat infection, and provide vital organ support without further damaging the lungs (1).

Cardiac Herniation

Acute cardiac herniation is an *infrequent complication of pneumonectomy* when the pericardium is incompletely closed or the closure breaks down. It usually occurs immediately or within 24 hours after chest surgery and is associated with >50% mortality. When cardiac herniation occurs after a right pneumonectomy, the impairment of venous return to the heart leads to a sudden increase in CVP, tachycardia, profound hypotension, and shock. An acute SVC syndrome ensues due to the torsion of the heart. In contrast, when the cardiac herniation occurs after a left-sided pneumonectomy, there is less cardiac rotation, but the edge of the pericardium compresses the myocardium. This may lead to myocardial ischemia, the development of arrhythmias, and ventricular outflow tract obstruction.

The differential diagnosis of hemodynamic instability after thoracic surgery should include massive intrathoracic hemorrhage, pulmonary embolism, or mediastinal shift from improper chest drain management. Immediate diagnosis and surgical treatment of cardiac herniation by *relocation of the heart* to its anatomic position is key to patient survival. Maneuvers to minimize the cardiovascular effects include positioning the patient in the full lateral position with the *operated side up*. Vasopressors or inotropes are required to support the circulation while exploration takes place (1).

References

1. Slinger P, Campos J. Anesthesia for thoracic surgery. In: Miller R, ed. *Miller's Anesthesia*. 7e. Philadelphia: Churchill Livingston, 2010:1819–1887.
2. Slinger P, Darling G. Preanesthetic assessment for thoracic surgery. In: Slinger P, ed. *Principles and Practice of Anesthesia for Thoracic Surgery*. New York: Springer; 2011:11–34.
3. Neustein S, Eisenkraft J, Cohen E. Anesthesia for thoracic surgery. In: Barash P, Cullen B, Stoelting R, Cahalan M, Stock M, eds. *Clinical Anesthesia* 6th ed. Philadelphia: Lippincott Williams and Wilkins, 2009:1042–1051.
4. Fleisher LA, Fleischmann KE, Auerbach AD, et al. 2014 ACC/AHA guideline on perioperative cardiovascular evaluation and management of patients undergoing noncardiac surgery: a report of the American College of Cardiology/American Heart Association Task Force on practice guidelines. *Circulation*. 2014;64: e77–e137.
5. Lohser J, Donington JS, Mitchell JD, et al. Anesthetic management of major hemorrhage during mediastinoscopy. *J Cardiothorac Vasc Anesth*. 2005;19:678–683.
6. Powell ES, Pearce AC, Cook D, et al. UK pneumonectomy outcome study. *J Cardiothorac Surg*. 2009;4:41.
7. Buise M, Van Bommel J, Mehra M, et al. Pulmonary morbidity following esophagectomy is decreased after introduction of a multimodal anesthetic regimen. *Acta Anaesth Belg*. 2008;59:257–261.
8. Pinsonneault C, Fortier J, Donati F. Tracheal resection and reconstruction. *Can J Anaesth*. 1999;46:439–455.
9. Takeda S, Miyoshi S, Omori K, et al. Surgical rescue for life-threatening hypoxemia caused by a mediastinal tumor. *Ann Thorac Surg*. 1999;68:2324–2326.
10. White MC, Stoddart PA. Anesthesia for thymectomy in children with myasthenia gravis. *Pediatr Anaesth*. 2004;14:625–635.
11. Joshi G, Bonnet F, Shah R, et al. A systematic review of randomized trials evaluating regional techniques for postthoracotomy analgesia. *Anesth Analg*. 2008;107:1026–1040.

Questions

1. What is the predicted postoperative FEV_1 in a patient with a preoperative FEV_1 of 60% who undergoes a right upper lobectomy?
   A. 50%
   B. 45%
   C. 40%
   D. 35%
   E. None of the above

2. What is the most common concurrent illness identified preoperatively in thoracic surgical patients?
   A. Hypertension
   B. Chronic obstructive pulmonary disease
   C. Coronary artery disease
   D. Diabetes
   E. None of the above

3. Initiation of one-lung ventilation to the dependent lung in a patient in the lateral position decreases ventilation perfusion mismatching because:
   A. It increases functional residual capacity in the dependent lung
   B. It decreases functional residual capacity in the nondependent lung
   C. It increases blood flow in the dependent lung
   D. It increases ventilation in the dependent lung
   E. None of the above

4. If hypoxia occurs during one-lung ventilation, the first step in treatment after confirming administration of 100% oxygen is:
   A. Continuous airway pressure of 5 to 10 cm H_2O to the nondependent lung
   B. Alveolar recruitment maneuvers to the dependent lung
   C. Positive end-expiratory pressure of 5 to 10 cm H_2O to the dependent lung
   D. Bronchoscopy to confirm correct placement of the endotracheal tube
   E. None of the above

5. In a patient requiring lung resection for treatment of right-sided bronchiectasis, the optimal management of the airway would include:
   A. A right-sided endobronchial blocker
   B. A left-sided endobronchial blocker
   C. A left-sided double-lumen endotracheal tube
   D. A right-sided double-lumen endotracheal tube
   E. None of the above

6. During mediastinoscopy, profuse hemorrhage from the operative site is noted. Of the sites listed below, which would be best to provide fluid resuscitation?
   A. Right antecubital vein
   B. Left antecubital vein
   C. Right internal jugular vein
   D. Left femoral vein
   E. None of the above

35

Cardiac Anesthesia

Candice R. Montzingo
Sasha Shillcutt

Patients with heart disease present unique challenges for the anesthesiologist. This chapter provides an overview of those challenges and the associated physiologic changes and anesthetic management strategies needed to safely provide care to patients undergoing cardiac surgical interventions.

I. Coronary Artery Disease

Coronary artery disease (CAD) is one of the most common causes of death in highly developed nations. It results from the buildup of atherosclerotic lesions in the coronary arteries. Myocardial ischemia is a hallmark of CAD. It is caused by an imbalance between myocardial oxygen supply and demand. The anesthesiologist must understand the determinants of this delicate relation and avoid myocardial injury by minimizing myocardial oxygen demand while optimizing myocardial oxygen delivery.

A. Myocardial Oxygen Demand

Systolic wall tension, contractility, and heart rate are the primary determinants of myocardial oxygen demand. *Wall tension* is directly proportional to systolic blood pressure and chamber size (preload) and inversely proportional to wall thickness. Thus, increases in preload increase wall tension exponentially because as chamber size increases, ventricular wall thickness must thin to accommodate the additional volume. Increases in *heart rate* are especially deleterious because increases in heart rate increase oxygen demand directly and decrease oxygen delivery indirectly by shortening diastole. The left ventricle (LV) receives its coronary blood flow only during diastole. Thus, increases in wall tension, *contractility*, and heart rate above normal resting levels must be avoided in patients with CAD.

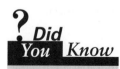

? *Did You Know*

The left ventricle receives its blood flow only during diastole, while the right ventricle is perfused throughout the cardiac cycle.

B. Myocardial Oxygen Supply

The two main factors contributing to myocardial oxygen supply are arterial *oxygen content* and *coronary blood flow*. Recall that arterial oxygen content is represented by the formula:

$$O_2 \text{ content} = (\text{hemoglobin})(1.34)(\% \text{ saturation}) + (0.003)(PO_2).$$

Table 35-1 Treatment of Intraoperative Ischemia	
Clinical Manifestation	
Increased Demand	
↑ HR	Treat usual reasons, beta-blocker
↑ BP	↑ anesthetic depth
↑ PCWP	Nitroglycerin
Decreased Supply	
↓ HR	Atropine, pacing
↓ BP	↓ anesthetic depth, vasoconstrictor
↑ PCWP	Nitroglycerin, inotrope
No Changes	Nitroglycerin, calcium channel blockers, ? heparin

↑, increase; ↓, decrease; HR, heart rate; BP, blood pressure; PCWP, pulmonary capillary wedge pressure. From Skubas NJ, Lichtman AD, Sharma A, et al. Anesthesia for cardiac surgery. In: Barash PG, Cullen BF, Stoelting RK, et al., eds. *Clinical Anesthesia.* 7th ed. Philadelphia: Wolters Kluwer Health/Lippincott Williams & Wilkins; 2013, with permission.

Because hemoglobin levels and blood volume are usually adequately maintained during cardiac surgery, coronary blood flow is the most critical factor in maintaining myocardial oxygen supply. Coronary blood flow is directly related to coronary perfusion pressure and inversely related to coronary vascular resistance and heart rate (time for perfusion in diastole). *Coronary perfusion pressure* is estimated as the difference between systemic (aortic) diastolic pressure and left ventricular diastolic pressure. In normal hearts, coronary blood flow is autoregulated for systolic blood pressures between 50 and 150 mm Hg. In patients with CAD, the area of the heart most at risk for ischemia is the subendocardium of the LV. The right ventricle (RV) is perfused during the entire cardiac cycle due to its low intracavitary pressure. Thus, low left ventricular diastolic pressure, normal systemic diastolic pressure, and low heart rate improve myocardial oxygen supply.

C. Monitoring for Ischemia

Flat or down-sloping *ST segment* depression ≥0.1 mV on the electrocardiogram (ECG) is the most reliable ECG sign of myocardial ischemia. However, transesophageal echocardiography (TEE) has been shown to detect myocardial ischemia earlier and more frequently than the ECG and is very often used in cardiac surgery. Pulmonary artery catheters may reveal acute increases in left atrial pressures associated with ischemia induced stiffening of the LV. However, the pulmonary artery catheters is not a sensitive or specific monitor for myocardial ischemia because so many other things influence left atrial pressure during surgery.

D. Treatment of Ischemia

Myocardial ischemia may occur at any time during coronary bypass surgery. The treatment depends largely on the etiology and can be seen in Table 35-1. Thorough review of the pharmacologic effects of nitrates, peripheral vasoconstrictors, calcium channel blockers and beta-blockers can be found in Chapter 13.

II. Valvular Heart Disease

Growing experience with transesophageal echocardiography has significantly increased the role of anesthesiologists in the intraoperative evaluation and management of valvular heart disease (VHD). VHD can be classified into two primary lesions: *regurgitant* and *stenotic*. *Regurgitant lesions* lead to volume overload, while *stenotic valve disease* leads to pressure overload. Although disease of the tricuspid and pulmonic valves presents unique challenges to the anesthesiologist, this chapter will focus on the much more common left-sided valvular lesions. Additional information is provided in the 2014 AHA/ACC "Guidelines for the Management of Patients with VHD" (1).

A. Aortic Stenosis

The normal adult aortic valve comprises three equally sized cusps and has an area of 2 to 3.5 cm^2. Aortic stenosis (AS) is the *most common* valvular lesion in the heart and can result from congenital or acquired valvular disease. In congenital AS, there is a partial or complete commissural fusion between cusps, resulting in a unicuspid or bicuspid valve. A bicuspid aortic valve is the most commonly occurring congenital heart defect, affecting approximately 1% to 2% of the population. Bicuspid aortic valves are associated with other congenital abnormalities, specifically diseases of the aorta including coarctation and dilatation of the aortic root. Acquired aortic stenosis results from calcific degeneration or, less commonly, rheumatic disease.

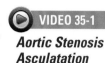

VIDEO 35-1

Aortic Stenosis Asculatation

Progressive narrowing of the aortic valve leads to an increased transvalvular gradient. This in turn increases the work of the LV and over time results in *concentric ventricular hypertrophy*. This compensatory response allows the internal diameter of the LV to remain unchanged and preserves systolic function and stroke volume. However, as the LV thickens, its diastolic function declines, causing an increase in the diastolic filling pressure. Patients often remain asymptomatic until the valve area is <1 to 1.2 cm^2, correlating to a peak transvalvular gradient exceeding 50 mm Hg. The classic triad of symptomatic AS is *angina*, *syncope*, and *congestive heart failure* (dyspnea). The development of any of these is *ominous*, indicating a life expectancy from 2 to 5 years without valve replacement.

The consequence of elevated intraventricular pressure and concentric hypertrophy is increased myocardial oxygen demand. At the same time, diastolic filling pressure is increased, resulting in a lower coronary perfusion pressure. Thus, patients with severe AS may experience myocardial ischemia and angina in the absence CAD, especially if the heart rate increases much beyond resting levels (see prior discussion in the section "Myocardial Oxygen Demand"). Maintenance of *systemic vascular resistance (SVR)* is critical in patients with AS to ensure adequate aortic diastolic pressure and thus coronary perfusion pressure. Vasoconstrictors such as vasopressin or phenylephrine will increase SVR without increasing myocardial oxygen demand because the increase in systemic blood pressure they cause is not "seen" by the LV due to the stenotic aortic valve.

B. Hypertrophic Cardiomyopathy

Although not a disease of a valve, hypertrophic cardiomyopathy (HCM) can cause an obstructive lesion similar to that of AS. HCM is an uncommon autosomal dominant genetic disorder with highly variable penetrance. It leads to ventricular hypertrophy that occurs in varying patterns, not just involving the interventricular septum. Presenting symptoms are often dyspnea on exertion, poor exercise tolerance, syncope, palpitations, and fatigue. Some patients remain asymptomatic much of their lives and unfortunately are diagnosed after sudden cardiac death.

Approximately one-third of patients with HCM will have hypertrophy of the interventricular septum that leads to *dynamic obstruction* of the left ventricular outflow tract. The resulting pressure gradient increases throughout systole, creating obstruction to cardiac output. Any factor decreasing left ventricular size will increase this gradient and further obstruct cardiac output. Examples include increases in heart rate and contractility and decreases in preload and afterload. Therefore, anesthetic management focuses on avoiding tachycardia and maintaining euvolemia and normal systemic vascular resistance. Hypotension in this population is best treated with α-adrenergic agonists and volume. Treatment with inotropic drugs such as *epinephrine is contraindicated* and may worsen the dynamic obstruction and hypotension.

C. Aortic Insufficiency

Aortic insufficiency (AI) can be the result of primary valvular disease or in association with aortic root dilatation (Marfan disease, degenerative aortic dilatation, aortic dissection) despite a normal aortic valve. The natural progression of AI varies depending on the pathophysiology and chronicity of the disease.

Acute AI is often the result of traumatic injury to the aortic root or valvular endocarditis. The consequences of *acute AI* are immediate and profound volume overload to the LV. Frequently, the LV is not able to maintain forward stroke volume despite compensatory mechanisms, including increased sympathetic tone, leading to tachycardia and increased contractility. Rapid deterioration of left ventricular function develops, leading to dyspnea and eventual cardiovascular collapse. Acute AI often requires urgent or emergent surgical intervention.

Chronic AI results in an increased left ventricular end diastolic volume that over time leads to eccentric hypertrophy (cavity dilatation). The course of chronic AI is gradual, limiting the increase in left ventricular diastolic pressure. It is not typical for patients to develop symptoms associated with AI until decades into the disease process when the LV has significantly dilated and myocardial dysfunction occurs. Once symptomatic, life expectancy diminishes dramatically, with expected survival of only 5 to 10 years.

The anesthetic management of AI focuses on *preserving forward stroke volume* and minimizing regurgitant volume by maintaining a relatively rapid heart rate (about 90 beats per minute) and normal to low SVR.

D. Mitral Stenosis

The mitral valve area is typically 4 to 6 cm^2 and is made up of an anterior and posterior leaflet. Mitral stenosis is almost always due to *rheumatic heart disease* and is therefore quite rare in the United States and other highly developed nations. It leads to impaired filling of the LV and a resulting decreased stroke volume. Consequently, the *left atrial pressure* becomes chronically elevated, resulting in left atrial dilatation and increased pulmonary venous pressure. Patients with mitral stenosis are at high risk for developing *atrial fibrillation*, which may be the presenting sign of the disease. Mitral stenosis patients are often asymptomatic for decades until the mitral valve area has decreased to 1 to 1.5 cm^2 and the heart is faced with an increased demand for systemic stroke volume (exercise, pregnancy, infection). Any high cardiac output state or the onset of atrial fibrillation can cause significant increases in the left atrial and pulmonary arterial pressures, leading to acute *congestive heart failure*. Chronically elevated left atrial pressures lead to increases in pulmonary vascular resistance, pulmonary hypertension, restrictive lung disease, and right heart failure.

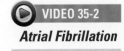

VIDEO 35-2

Atrial Fibrillation

Frequently, patients with mitral stenosis have received diuretics preoperatively to control their pulmonary congestion and are relatively hypovolemic. Induction of anesthesia may unmask the *hypovolemia* and compromise the

Table 35-2   Hemodynamic Goals in Patients with Valvular Heart Disease

	Aortic Stenosis	Hypertrophic Cardiomyopathy	Aortic Insufficiency	Mitral Stenosis	Mitral Regurgitation
Preload	Full	Full	Increase slightly	Maintain; avoid hypo-volemia	Increase slightly
Afterload	Maintain CPP	Increase; treat hypotension aggressively	Decrease to reduce regurgi-tant fraction	Prevent increase	Decrease
Rate	Avoid bradycardia (decrease CO) and tachycardia (ischemia)	Normal	Increase	Low normal	Increase slightly, avoid bradycardia
Rhythm	Sinus	Sinus is critical	Sinus	Sinus or rate controlled atrial fibril-lation	Sinus or rate controlled atrial fibrilla-tion

CO, cardiac output; CPP, coronary perfusion pressure.

transit of blood across the stenotic mitral valve. Thus, adequate fluid administration during anesthesia is crucial, but too much fluid administration can lead to further pulmonary congestion and pulmonary edema. A relatively *slow heart rate* (about 60 to 70 beats per minute) allows ample time for the LV to fill. Tachycardia compromises that filling and may result in severe hypotension. *SVR* should be maintained to ensure adequate coronary perfusion pressure, especially to the RV because it is facing increased pulmonary artery pressures.

E. Mitral Regurgitation

Mitral regurgitation (MR) results from excessive leaflet motion (prolapse or flail) or restricted leaflet motion (ischemic dilatation, rheumatic heart disease). Similar to AI, MR leads to volume overload. In MR, the stroke volume is made up of blood ejected into the systemic circulation and then regurgitated into the left atrium. The regurgitated blood causes left atrial and ventricular dilatation (eccentric ventricular hypertrophy) and increased ventricular compliance. Unless the MR is due to CAD (e.g., ischemic rupture of a papillary muscle), an elevated heart rate (about 90 beats per minute) may be best because it will limit ventricular dilatation. However, the cornerstone in the management of MR is *reduction of the SVR* to promote forward ejection of blood and limit regurgitation. In patients with MR and others undergoing valvular heart surgery, TEE has proven beneficial to assess volume status, ventricular function, and, most important, the adequacy of the surgical procedure. Table 35-2 summarizes the hemodynamic goals in patients with valvular heart disease.

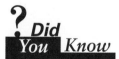

? *Did You Know*

The cornerstone in the management of mitral regurgitation is reduction of the systemic vascular resistance to promote forward ejection of blood and limit regurgitation.

III. Aortic Diseases

The aorta is made up of the aortic root, the ascending aorta, the aortic arch, and the descending thoracic aorta, as seen in Figure 35-1. Diseases of the aorta can be localized to one segment, multiple segments, or involve the entire aorta. Diseases of the aorta may be acquired (traumatic injury, hypertension,

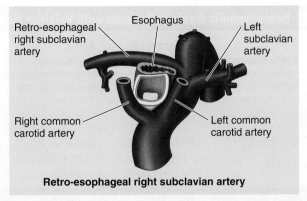

Retro-esophageal right subclavian artery

Figure 35-1 Boundaries of superior mediastinum. The superior mediastinum extends inferiorly from the superior thoracic aperture to the transverse thoracic plane. (From Moore KL, Agur AMR, Dalley AF. *Clinically Oriented Anatomy*. 7th ed. Philadelphia: Wolters Kluwer Health/Lippincott Williams & Wilkins; 2013:160, with permission.)

occlusive disease, inflammation, infection) or congenital (coarctation, patent ductus arteriosus, connective tissue disorders) and can lead to aortic dissection, aortic aneurysm, intramural hematoma, or aortic transection.

A. Aortic Dissection

Aortic dissection occurs due to a tear in the intimal and medial layers of the aorta, which causes separation of the walls and leads to creation of a *false lumen*. Blood travels into the false lumen of the media and can travel the length of the vessel. Intimal tears typically originate from an ulcer due to chronic hypertension or connective tissue disorders, such as Marfan syndrome. As the false lumen propagates, thrombus and dissecting layers can cause disruption in perfusion of vital organs due to decreased blood flow to major arteries such as the carotids, subclavian, spinal, or mesenteric arteries.

Type A aortic dissection, which involves the ascending aorta, is a *surgical emergency* with a mortality that increases exponentially by the hour. It is often associated with cardiac tamponade, myocardial ischemia (due to dissection of coronary arteries), and acute aortic insufficiency. Symptoms may involve syncope, stroke-like sequelae, and chest pain. *Type B dissections* involve the aorta distal to the left subclavian artery and can be *managed medically* unless ongoing symptoms (back pain, abdominal pain, or embolic or ischemic phenomenon) persist or end-organ failure develops. Medical therapy focuses on decreasing aortic wall stress and controlling heart rate and blood pressure with beta-blockers and nondihydropyridine calcium channel blocking agents (2).

Although contrast-enhanced spiral computed tomography scanning is the gold standard for diagnosis, TEE can be used to confirm the diagnosis in unstable patients where immediate surgery is needed. Also, TEE plays an important role in diagnosing concomitant pathology such as aortic insufficiency, tamponade, and left ventricular failure. However, TEE cannot reliably image the distal ascending aorta and proximal aortic arch. Patients with type A dissection require aortic graft placement and may need aortic valve replacement and reattachment of the coronary arteries or arch vessels, depending on the location of the dissection.

Anesthetic management for aortic dissection involves *prevention of hypertension*, adequate intravenous access, including central venous access, invasive

Table 35-3	Acute Aortic Dissection: Hemodynamic Goals
Preload	May be increased if acute AI, increase further in tamponade
Afterload	Decrease with anesthetics, analgesics, arterial dilators (nitroprusside, nicardipine): Keep systolic BP <100–120 mm Hg
Contractility	May be depressed; titrate myocardial depressants carefully
Rate	Decrease to <60–80 bpm: Use beta-blocker; ensure contractility is adequate
Rhythm	If atrial fibrillation present: Control ventricular response
MV̇O₂	Compromised if aortic dissection involves coronary vessels
CPB	Alternate site of inflow (arterial) cannulation, deep hypothermic circulatory arrest possible if cerebral vessels are involved

AI, aortic insufficiency; BP, blood pressure; bpm, beats per minute; MV̇O₂, myocardial oxygen consumption; CPB, cardiopulmonary bypass.
From Skubas NJ, Lichtman AD, Sharma A, et al. Anesthesia for cardiac surgery. In: Barash PG, Cullen BF, Stoelting RK, et al., eds. *Clinical Anesthesia.* 7th ed. Philadelphia: Wolters Kluwer Health/Lippincott Williams & Wilkins; 2013, with permission.

arterial blood pressure monitoring (usually via the right radial artery), and intraoperative TEE. Hemodynamic goals are listed in Table 35-3.

B. Aortic Aneurysm

The aorta is an elastic structure that changes shape with each cardiac contraction. Its normal diameter is 2 to 3 cm. Degenerative diseases, along with age, hypertension, hypercholesterolemia, and atherosclerosis, cause premature loss of its elasticity and are the major cause of aortic aneurysms. Connective tissue diseases such as Marfan syndrome cause cystic medial necrosis, mostly involving the aortic root. Men are more affected than women and the age of presentation is 50 to 70 years (3). The majority of people with aortic aneurysms are asymptomatic when diagnosed, unless there is significant aortic insufficiency or mass effect compressing nearby structures such as the trachea or esophagus (e.g., hoarseness, cough, dysphagia).

Patients with an aortic *diameter of 5.5 cm* or greater should undergo surgical repair. In patients with Marfan syndrome or a bicuspid aortic valve, surgical repair is indicated when the aortic diameter reaches 4.5 cm because in these diseases the rate of aneurysm expansion is faster than in other diseases. Aortic repair with or without coronary implantation and aortic valve replacement may be required in patients with root aneurysms. Involvement of the great vessels may require deep hypothermic circulatory arrest for reconstruction of the aortic arch.

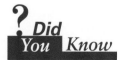

An aortic diameter of >5.5 cm is an indication for surgical repair.

Cerebral protective procedures, such as retrograde or antegrade cerebral perfusion, may also be used to provide hypothermic protective effects on brain tissue, flush toxins, and decrease the cerebral metabolic rate. Cerebral protective effects are controversial and results have been confounding (4). Left heart bypass, from the left atrium to the femoral artery, can provide retrograde aortic perfusion to aortic branches distal to the repair to perfuse the spine and abdomen.

The anesthetic management for patient with aortic aneurysms is similar to that for patients with aortic dissection. The use of *spinal fluid drains* to optimize spinal perfusion pressure during thoracic aortic repair is used in some centers but not others. Intraoperative TEE is recommended to guide hemodynamic management, arterial and venous cannulation, and pre- and postrepair evaluation.

IV. Cardiopulmonary Bypass

The cardiopulmonary bypass machine is made up of four basic parts: venous and arterial cannulae to take blood from and back to the heart, a venous reservoir to collect and transiently store the blood drained from the heart, an oxygenator membrane for exchanging carbon dioxide and oxygen, and a pump to propel blood back to the body. The cannula and oxygenator are primed with approximately 800 to 1,500 mL of solution that approximates normal plasma osmolarity. When cardiopulmonary bypass (CPB) is initiated, this priming volume causes *sudden hemodilution* of the patient's circulating blood volume and transient *hypotension*. Blood is drained from the body via the multiorifice venous cannula that is placed into the right atrium and empties blood from the superior and inferior cavae and right atrium. Venous drainage through this cannula occurs passively by gravity siphon and is dependent on proper cannula position and a drop in height from the heart to the venous reservoir. Once in the venous reservoir, blood travels through a semipermeable membrane oxygenator for carbon dioxide and oxygen exchange. The fraction of inspired oxygen, temperature, the flow rate of the inspired gas, and delivery of volatile agents can all be controlled by the CPB machine. After blood leaves the oxygenator, a roller or centrifugal pump propels the blood via the arterial cannula to the proximal ascending aorta for systemic perfusion. Figure 35-2 illustrates the basic cardiopulmonary bypass circuit.

▶ **VIDEO 35-3**

Extracorporeal Circulation

CPB requires systemic *anticoagulation*, which is usually accomplished by a single intravenous bolus of 300 U/kg of heparin. Anticoagulation is critical to prevent activation of the clotting cascade and clot formation in the CPB machine due to the exposure of blood to CPB circuitry. Activated clotting times (ACT) are checked to confirm adequate anticoagulation (ACT >400 seconds) prior to and during CPB.

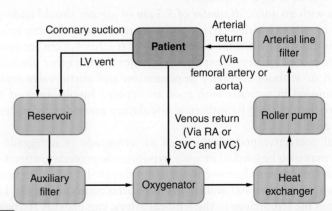

Figure 35-2 The basic circuit for cardiopulmonary bypass. LV, left ventricle; RA, right atrium; SVC, superior vena cava; IVC, inferior vena cava. (From Skubas NJ, Lichtman AD, Sharma A, et al. Anesthesia for cardiac surgery. In: Barash PG, Cullen BF, Stoelting RK, et al., eds. *Clinical Anesthesia*. 7th ed. Philadelphia: Wolters Kluwer Health/Lippincott Williams & Wilkins; 2013:1076, with permission.)

A. Myocardial Protection

Myocardial protection is accomplished through two mechanisms: (a) the delivery of *cardioplegia* solution to arrest, electrically silence, and cool the heart, and (b) removal of blood from the heart to minimize wall tension. Cardioplegia solution is a cold or tepid, high potassium–containing blood solution delivered to the coronaries to decrease myocardial oxygen consumption. It can be delivered antegrade through a cannula placed in the proximal aortic root. However, in the presence of aortic insufficiency, severe coronary stenosis, or valvular surgery, cardioplegia is delivered retrograde by placing a cannula through the right atrium into the coronary sinus. Additional cannulae may be needed to remove any air or blood that collects in the LV from the bronchial circulation or the coronary sinus during CPB. This is critical to prevent dilation of the heart resulting in high wall tension and myocardial ischemia. Surgical blood loss during CPB is returned to the venous reservoir via suction cannulae and a "cardiotomy" reservoir.

V. Preoperative and Intraoperative Management

The preoperative evaluation of the cardiac surgical patient includes the essential elements required for all surgical patients (see Chapter 16). In addition, review of cardiac studies (ECG, echocardiogram, and cardiac catheterization data), laboratory values for hemoglobin, glucose, and renal function, and functional status allow detailed planning of anesthetic management, including the advisability of early extubation after surgery.

A. Current Drug Therapy

In general, *most current medications* should be continued until the time of surgery, including beta-blockers, antihypertensives, antiarrhythmics, calcium channel blockers, nitrates, statins, and aspirin. Insulin administration should be tailored to prevent hyper- or hypoglycemia.

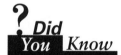

? Did You Know

Most current medications should be continued until the time of cardiac surgery, including beta-blockers, antihypertensives, antiarrhythmics, calcium channel blockers, nitrates, statins, and aspirin.

B. Premedication

Anxiolytics may be administered in hemodynamically stable patients with good underlying left ventricular function and respiratory drive. Caution should be used in patients with heart failure, respiratory failure, pulmonary hypertension, or significant obstructive valvular lesions. Benzodiazepines may produce prolonged sedation in elderly patients and prevent early postoperative extubation.

C. Monitoring

Hemodynamic monitoring is discussed in Chapters 15. This section will address techniques specific to the cardiac surgical patient. *Direct arterial blood pressure monitoring* is essential. During CPB, noninvasive techniques will not work because blood flow is nonpulsatile. Typically, the radial artery of the nondominant hand is cannulated for this purpose except when this artery will be used for coronary artery bypass grafting. Central venous access is required for infusion of vasoactive drugs and monitoring right atrial pressure. The pulmonary artery catheter or TEE can monitor pulmonary pressures, left ventricular filling pressures, and cardiac output. The use of these techniques is dependent on institutional practice and physician preference and varies widely. A recent study on the practice patterns of cardiac anesthesiologists showed that 67% use TEE in coronary artery bypass surgery, with even higher numbers reported for valve surgery (5). TEE provides detailed information, such as new wall motion abnormalities, valvular abnormalities, guidance of cannula placement, detection of intracardiac air, and prosthetic

? Did You Know

Blood flow during CPB is non-pulsatile and therefore blood pressure during CPB cannot be measured with noninvasive techniques.

valve function. Some centers use cerebral oximeters, a noninvasive technique that employs near infrared spectrophotometry to monitor cerebral perfusion.

D. Selection of Anesthetic Drugs

Outcome studies have not demonstrated the optimal anesthetic agent for patients undergoing cardiac surgery. Commonly, a volatile anesthetic agent and low to moderate doses of a narcotic are used in combination. The volatile agent decreases myocardial oxygen demand by lowering blood pressure and decreasing contractility, decreases the likelihood of awareness during surgery, and possibly provides protection from ischemic injury to the heart via a preconditioning mechanism. The narcotic decreases oxygen demand by lowering the heart rate and provides postoperative analgesia. In addition, the narcotic decreases the required dose of the volatile agent, potentially important in patients with depressed ventricular function. This "balanced" anesthetic is optimal if the goal is to extubate the patient's trachea early after surgery (6). Nitrous oxide is often avoided because it can increase pulmonary artery pressure and expand air cavities and air emboli. High-dose narcotic and benzodiazepine techniques are rarely practiced today because *"fast-track"* techniques (extubation within 6 hours after surgery) are safe and cost-effective. Narcotics and benzodiazepines, when used concomitantly for induction of anesthesia, can cause hypotension and bradycardia. These effects can be offset with pancuronium, but may be worsened by administration of vecuronium or cisatracurium. Etomidate, propofol, and barbiturates have been described as adjunct agents along with narcotics and fast-acting benzodiazepines for induction. Selection of one agent over another depends on the patient's underlying ventricular function and vascular tone. Etomidate is often chosen for induction of anesthesia because of its limited effects on hemodynamics. However, in the rare patient with underlying adrenal insufficiency, it may worsen adrenal dysfunction.

E. Intraoperative Management

In addition to the usual operating room preparations, the cardiac operating room requires significant other preparations for intraoperative patient care: fluid warmers; pressure transducers for central venous, arterial and pulmonary artery catheters (if used); inotropes, vasodilators, and vasopressor infusions; and pumps for other medication infusions. *Cross-matched blood* should be immediately available and checked for correct patient identifiers prior to surgical sternotomy. Even in a prepared environment, placing a hemodynamically unstable patient on emergent CPB takes a minimum 15 to 20 minutes. Preparation and checklists, as found in Table 35-4, are key in helping to prevent serious errors.

During the dissection phase of surgery prior to CPB, arrhythmias and hypotension are common, resulting from surgical manipulations near or on the heart, especially in cardiac reoperations. During this time, the anesthesiologist titrates anesthetic depth as needed for the highly variable level of surgical stimulation, performs the baseline TEE examination, and samples arterial blood for determination of blood gas values as well as electrolytes, hemoglobin, and the baseline ACT. *Sternotomy* can cause significant sympathetic stimulation that may be prevented by deepening the anesthetic level with narcotics or the volatile agent. Prior to aortic cannulation and initiation of CPB, heparin is administered and an ACT >400 minutes must be obtained to confirm adequate anticoagulation. During *aortic cannulation* and prior to initiation of cardiopulmonary bypass, the systolic blood pressure should be controlled to no more than 100 mm Hg to minimize the risk of aortic

Table 35-4 Anesthetic Preparation for Cardiac Surgery

Anesthesia machine

Routine check

Airway
Nasal cannula for oxygen
Ventilation/intubation equipment
Suction
Difficult airway anticipated? Special equipment
Inspired gas humidifier

Circulatory access
Catheters for peripheral and central venous and arterial access
Intravenous fluids and infusion tubing and pumps
Fluid warmer

Monitors
Standard ASA: ECG leads, blood pressure cuff, pulse oximeter, neuromuscular
  blockade monitor
Temperature: Various probes (nasal, tympanic, bladder, rectal)
Transducers (arterial, pulmonary, and central venous pressure) zeroed
Cardiac output computer: Proper constant inserted
  Awareness monitor (BIS)
Anticoagulation (ACT) monitor(s)
Recorder

Medications
General anesthetic: Hypnotic/induction, amnestic/benzodiazepine, volatile, opioid,
  muscle relaxant
Heparin (predrawn)
Cardioactive
  In syringes: Nitroglycerin/nicardipine, calcium chloride, phenylephrine/ephedrine,
    epinephrine
  Infusions: Nitroglycerin, inotrope
Antibiotics

Miscellaneous
Pacemaker with battery
  Defibrillator/cardioverter with external paddles and ECG cables
  Ultrasound system for central venous line insertion
Compatible blood in operating room

ASA, American Society of Anesthesiologists; ECG, electrocardiogram; BIS, bispectral index; ACT, activated clotting time.
From Skubas NJ, Lichtman AD, Sharma A, et al. Anesthesia for cardiac surgery. In: Barash PG, Cullen BF, Stoelting RK, et al., eds. *Clinical Anesthesia.* 7th ed. Philadelphia: Wolters Kluwer Health/Lippincott Williams & Wilkins; 2013, with permission.

dissection. Once all cannulae are in place and ***adequate anticoagulation*** confirmed, cardiopulmonary bypass is begun. The patient's head should be examined for any discoloration signaling cannula malposition (plethora may represent venous cannula obstruction or a bright red color may represent aortic cannula malposition), cerebral oximetry monitored (if used), and the surgical field inspected for proper cardiac decompression. Ventilation should stop once cardiopulmonary bypass machine reaches full flow, which is typically 50 to 60 mL/kg/min.

During CPB, volatile or intravenous anesthetic agents are delivered in the cardiopulmonary bypass circuit to maintain anesthesia. Muscle relaxant should be continued and mean arterial pressure controlled to a range of 50 to 75 mm Hg by appropriate use of a volatile agent, vasopressor, or vasodilator. Preoperative vasopressor or inotropic support is discontinued during CPB. Blood glucose should be controlled in the 120 to 200 mg/dL range and hematocrit maintained at >20%.

F. Separation from Cardiopulmonary Bypass
CPB can be discontinued when surgical hemostasis is adequate, the patient rewarmed to at least 36.5°C, sinus rhythm restored at a rate between 70 and 100 beats per minute, mechanical ventilation resumed, and metabolic values optimized including pH >7.35, hematocrit >20%, and serum potassium <6 mEq/L. As the arterial inflow from the CPB machine is decreased, venous drainage from the patient is restricted to allow the heart to generate cardiac output and blood pressure. When these are adequate, CPB is terminated.

Table 35-5   Checklist Before Separation from Cardiopulmonary Bypass

Laboratory values
Hematocrit, ABGs
K+: ? elevated (cardioplegia)
Ionized Ca^{2+}

Anesthetic/machine
Lung compliance: Evaluate (hand ventilation)
Lungs are expanded, no atelectasis, both are ventilated (manual or mechanical)
Vaporizers: Off
Alarms: On

Monitors
Normothermia (37°C nasopharyngeal, 35.5°C bladder, 35°C rectal)
ECG: Rate, rhythm, ST
Transducers rezeroed and leveled
Arterial and filling pressures
Recorder (if available)

Patient/field
LOOK AT THE HEART!
Deaired: Check lead II, TEE
Eyeball contractility, size, rhythm
LV vent clamped/removed, caval snares released
Bleeding: No major sites (grafts, suture lines, LV vent site)
Vascular resistance: CPB flow ∝ MAP ÷ Resistance

Support
As needed

ABGs, arterial blood gases; ECG, electrocardiogram; TEE, transesophageal echocardiography; LV, left ventricle; CPB, cardiopulmonary bypass; MAP, mean arterial pressure.
From Skubas NJ, Lichtman AD, Sharma A, et al. Anesthesia for cardiac surgery. In: Barash PG, Cullen BF, Stoelting RK, et al., eds. *Clinical Anesthesia*. 7th ed. Philadelphia: Wolters Kluwer Health/Lippincott Williams & Wilkins; 2013, with permission.

During this time, blood pressure is monitored closely and TEE is performed to look for intracardiac air, ventricular wall motion abnormalities, and ventricular filling and ejection. Vasoactive and inotropic drugs may be required to obtain adequate hemodynamics and perfusion. Studies have shown risk factors for difficulty in weaning from cardiopulmonary bypass include age >70 years, left ventricular ejection fraction <20%, female sex, reoperation, emergency operation, and recent myocardial infarction (7). A checklist prior to discontinuation of CPB is helpful, as provided in Table 35-5. Electrical pacing of the heart may be required in the setting of AV nodal dysfunction, which is common after CPB.

Once the patient is hemodynamically stable, anticoagulation is reversed by administration of intravenous *protamine*. Protamine is administered first as a small test dose to detect a possible inflammatory reaction, and then if no adverse effect is noted, given slowly over 5 to 10 minutes (typically 1 mg of protamine is administered for every 100 U of heparin). When one-third of the total protamine dose is administered, the perfusionist is alerted and suction of blood from the surgical into the venous reservoir is terminated to prevent clot formation in the CPB machine. After protamine infusion is complete, an ACT is measured to confirm adequate reversal of anticoagulation and arterial blood sampled to confirm maintenance of appropriate blood gas values, electrolytes, and hemoglobin.

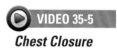

VIDEO 35-4

Protamine Reaction

VIDEO 35-5

Chest Closure

If separation from CPB is difficult, right or left ventricular failure is the likely cause. Ischemia from air embolism, poor myocardial protection, reperfusion injury, and pulmonary hypertension can all cause ventricular dysfunction. Common drug therapy and doses are listed in Table 35-6. Patients who

Table 35-6	Medications Given by Continuous Infusion	
Drugs	**Usual Initial Dose (µg/kg/min)**	**Usual Dose Range (µg/kg/min)**
Amrinone[a]	2–5	2–20
Dopamine	2–5	2–20
Dobutamine	2–5	2–20
Epinephrine	0.01	0.01–0.1
Isoproterenol[b]	0.05–1	0.1–1
Lidocaine	20	20–50
Milrinone	50 µg/kg (over 3 min)	0.3–0.7
Nitroglycerin	0.5	0.5–5
Nitroprusside	0.5	0.5–5
Norepinephrine	0.1	0.1–1
Phenylephrine	1	1–3
Prostaglandin E$_1$	0.05–0.1	0.05–0.2
Vasopressin		0.0004

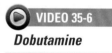

VIDEO 35-6

Dobutamine

[a]Requires initial bolus of 750 µg/kg over 3 min before start of infusion.
[b]For chronotropic effect following cardiac transplantation, doses of 0.005 to 0.010 µg/kg/min are used.
From Skubas NJ, Lichtman AD, Sharma A, et al. Anesthesia for cardiac surgery. In: Barash PG, Cullen BF, Stoelting RK, et al., eds. *Clinical Anesthesia*. 7th ed. Philadelphia: Wolters Kluwer Health/Lippincott Williams & Wilkins; 2013, with permission.

require significant inotropic support for ventricular failure may need mechanical support. Placement of an intra-aortic balloon pump should be considered when postbypass ischemia is suspected, whereas severe ventricular dysfunction may require placement of a ventricular assist device until ventricular recovery. Patients who suffer significant pulmonary failure may need oxygenation via extracorporeal membrane oxygenation as a temporary measure.

VI. Minimally Invasive Cardiac Surgery

Advances in technology have made minimally invasive cardiac surgical approaches possible in an attempt to avoid complete median sternotomy, aortic cross clamping, and cardiopulmonary bypass. Decreased time to extubation, decreased length of stay in the intensive care unit, decreased transfusion rates, and decreased incidence of postoperative atrial fibrillation are cited as benefits of minimally invasive cardiac surgery. Although reduction in neurocognitive dysfunction was a primary goal of minimally invasive cardiac surgery, randomized controlled studies have had disappointing results in this area (8). Minimally invasive cardiac surgery procedures are available for coronary artery disease as well as valvular heart disease.

However, procedures through small incisions in the chest are technically very challenging. Inexperience with minimally invasive techniques can lead to very significant complications, including inadequate valve repair, paravalvular leaks, and coronary obstruction. Catheter-based percutaneous valve repair and replacement are becoming more common in the United States. These techniques may be best suited for patients who have a history of previous sternotomy or very high perioperative risk of mortality.

VII. Postoperative Considerations

Patients in the immediate postoperative period are at high risk for developing life-threatening complications, including respiratory failure, severe hemorrhage, cardiac tamponade, acute coronary graft failure, and prosthetic valve dysfunction (Table 35-7).

A. Urgent Reoperations

The incidence of urgent chest exploration after cardiac surgery is between 3% to 5%. The most common reasons are *persistent bleeding* and cardiac *tamponade*. It is critical to distinguish whether persistent bleeding is due to a coagulopathy or inadequate surgical hemostasis. Thromboelastography or coagulation studies, including prothrombin time, activated partial thromboplastin time, fibrinogen level, and platelet count, may confirm a coagulopathy and indicate the optimal treatment. If bleeding persists and coagulopathy is excluded, the patient should return to the operating room for surgical correction of the bleeding.

If drainage from the mediastinal chest tubes is not sufficient, cardiac tamponade can result and prompt surgical treatment is imperative. Tamponade must be included in the differential diagnosis of postoperative hypotension or low cardiac output states. It results in the collapse of cardiac chambers due to elevated pressures within the pericardium exceeding the pressures within the heart (particularly the atria). The normal signs and symptoms of tamponade are hypotension, paradoxical pulse, tachycardia, dyspnea, and orthopnea. TEE is an essential tool in making the prompt diagnosis of tamponade and expediting surgical intervention.

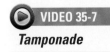

VIDEO 35-7

Tamponade

Table 35-7   Physiologic Effects of Congenital Cardiac Lesions

Volume overload of the ventricle or atrium resulting in increased pulmonary blood flow
Atrial septal defect (high flow, low pressure)
Ventricular septal defect (high flow, high pressure)
Patent ductus arteriosus (high flow, high pressure)
Endocardial cushion defect (high flow, high pressure)

Cyanosis resulting from obstruction to pulmonary blood flow
Tetralogy of Fallot
Tricuspid atresia
Pulmonary atresia

Pressure overload to the ventricle
Aortic stenosis
Coarctation of the aorta
Pulmonary stenosis

Cyanosis due to a common mixing chamber
Total anomalous venous return
Truncus arteriosus
Double outlet right ventricle
Single ventricle

Cyanosis due to separation of the systemic and pulmonary circulation
Transposition of the great vessels

From Skubas NJ, Lichtman AD, Sharma A, et al. Anesthesia for cardiac surgery. In: Barash PG, Cullen BF, Stoelting RK, et al., eds. *Clinical Anesthesia.* 7th ed. Philadelphia: Wolters Kluwer Health/Lippincott Williams & Wilkins; 2013, with permission.

B. Pain Management

The desire to rapidly awaken and extubate patients following cardiac surgery has driven changes in the pain management. The use of *shorter-acting narcotics* (fentanyl and remifentanil) has become a prominent practice along with intrathecal opioids. Studies have confirmed the safety and efficacy of intrathecal opioids to enhance postoperative pain management and facilitate earlier tracheal extubation (9). *Dexmedetomidine*, an intravenous α_2-adrenergic agonist, has both sedative and analgesic properties without significant respiratory depression. Dexmedetomidine has been shown in multiple trials to decrease the time to tracheal extubation, and, therefore, its use is increasing in postcardiac surgical patients, despite its current high cost.

VIII. Anesthesia for Children with Congenital Heart Disease

Approximately 8 children of every 1,000 live births have congenital heart disease (CHD). Ventricular septal defect is the most common CHD, and many of these defects will close spontaneously. However, others will require surgical treatment, as will the complex defects such as tetralogy of Fallot, transposition of the great vessels, hypoplastic left heart syndrome, and atrioventricular septal defects. Progress in corrective and palliative surgical techniques for CHD has been enormous in the past 2 decades. Many children with these complex

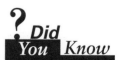

? Did You Know

In the United States, there are more adults than children with congenital heart disease.

lesions can undergo cardiac surgical procedures and live full and productive lives. In fact, there are more adults alive today with CHD than children with CHD. Full coverage of anesthesia for CHD is beyond the scope of this chapter and can be found elsewhere (10).

References

1. Nishimura RA, Otto CM, Bonow RO, et al. 2014 AHA/ACC guideline for the management of patients with valvular heart disease. *Circulation.* 2014;e521–e643.
2. Hiratzka LF, Bakris GL, Beckman JA, et al. 2010 ACCF/AHA/AATS/ACR/ASA/SCA/SCAI/SIR/STS/SVM guidelines for the diagnosis and management of patients with thoracic aortic disease: executive summary. *Anesth Analg.* 2010;111:279–315.
3. Patel HJ, Deeb GM. Ascending and arch aorta: Pathology, natural history and treatment. *Circulation.* 2008;118:188–195.
4. Augoustides JGT, Andritsos M. Innovations in aortic disease: The ascending aorta and aortic arch. *J Cardiothorac Vasc Anesth.* 2010;24:198–207.
5. Dobbs HA, Bennett-Guerrero E, White W, et al. Multinational institutional survey on patterns of intraoperative transesophageal echocardiography use in adult cardiac surgery. *J Cardiothorac Vasc Anesth.* 2014;28:54–63.
6. Hillis LD, Smith PK, Anderson JL, et al. 2011 ACCF/AHA guideline for coronary artery bypass graft surgery. *Circulation.* 2011;124:e652–e735.
7. Denault AY, Deschamps A, Couture P. Intraoperative hemodynamic instability during and after separation from cardiopulmonary bypass. *Semin Cardiothorac Vasc Anesth.* 2010;14:165–182.
8. Cheng DC, Bainbridge D, Martin JE, et al. Does off-pump coronary artery bypass reduce mortality, morbidity, and resource utilization when compared with conventional coronary artery bypass? A meta-analysis of randomized trials. *Anesthesiology.* 2005;102:188.
9. Chaney MA. Intrathecal and epidural anesthesia and analgesia for cardiac surgery. *Anesth Analg.* 2006;102:45–64.
10. Skubas NJ, Lichtman AD, Sharma A, et al. Anesthesia for cardiac surgery. In: Barash PG, Cullen BF, Stoelting RK, et al., eds. *Clinical Anesthesia.* 7th ed. Philadelphia: Wolters Kluwer Health/Lippincott Williams & Wilkins; 2013:1076.

Questions

1. The three primary determinants of myocardial oxygen demand are heart rate, contractility, and:
   A. Systolic wall tension
   B. Systemic vascular resistance
   C. Preload
   D. Systolic blood pressure
   E. None of the above

2. The most common valvular heart disease is:
   A. Mitral stenosis
   B. Mitral regurgitation
   C. Aortic stenosis
   D. Aortic regurgitation
   E. None of the above

3. Which type of aortic dissection is a surgical emergency?
   A. Type A
   B. Type B
   C. Type C
   D. Type D
   E. None of the above

4. Retrograde cardioplegia is delivered by a cannula placed into the:
   A. Right atrium
   B. Left atrium
   C. Aortic root
   D. Coronary sinus
   E. None of the above

5. At what activated clotting time is anticoagulation sufficient to initiate cardiopulmonary bypass?
   A. Greater than 200 seconds
   B. Greater than 300 seconds
   C. Greater than 400 seconds
   D. Greater than 500 seconds
   E. None of the above

6. The optimal drug for maintenance of anesthesia during cardiac surgery is:
   A. Fentanyl
   B. Isoflurane
   C. Remifentanil
   D. Propofol
   E. None of the above

36 Anesthesia for Vascular Surgery

Wendy K. Bernstein
Kyle E. Johnson

I. Vascular Disease: Epidemiologic, Medical, and Surgical Aspects

The incidence of atherosclerosis and vascular disease increases with advancing age. Therefore, it can be expected that there will be higher demand for vascular procedures, especially novel techniques such as angioplasty and endovascular stent placement. In addition, vascular surgery patients are some of the most complex patients to manage in the perioperative period. This chapter will focus on the principles of that management.

A. Pathophysiology of Atherosclerosis

Atherosclerosis describes a multifactorial *inflammatory disease* of the vascular tree. Predisposing risk factors for atherosclerosis include hypertension, dyslipidemia, abdominal obesity, insulin resistance, cigarette smoking, increasing age, family history, proinflammatory states, and prothrombotic states. The development of atherosclerosis occurs in two stages: endothelial injury and inflammatory response to injury. The primary injury occurs as low-density lipoprotein and apolipoprotein-B–containing lipoproteins invade the vascular endothelium and become proinflammatory. As the inflammatory cascade ensues, the subendothelial space is filled with atherogenic lipoproteins and macrophages, which form foam cells. Foam cells form the atheromatous core of a plaque, which becomes necrotic and further enhances the inflammatory process. Disruption of the fibrous cap over a lipid deposit can lead to plaque rupture and ulceration. Vascular disease is not a localized phenomenon, but rather a systemic one affecting multiple organs including the heart with myocardial infarction (MI) and the brain with cerebrovascular accidents (CVA).

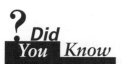

B. Natural History of Patients with Peripheral Vascular Disease

More than 25 million people in the United States have clinical manifestations of atherosclerotic vascular disease (Fig. 36-1). For example, 43% of men and 34% of women older than 65 years of age have >25% carotid stenosis, and stroke remains the leading cause of disability and the third leading cause of death in the United States. Peripheral arterial disease (PAD) can cause claudication and

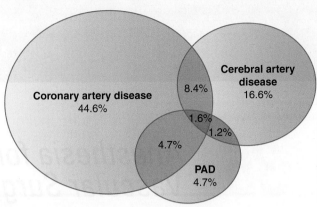

Typical overlap in vascular disease affecting different territories. Based on REACH data. PAD, peripheral arterial disease. (From Smaka TJ, Miller TE, Hutchens MP, et al. Anesthesia for vascular surgery. In: Barash PG, Cullen BF, Stoelting RK, et al. *Clinical Anesthesia*, 7th ed. Philadelphia: Lippincott Williams & Wilkins, 2013:1114.)

limb ischemia (2% prevalence in aging individuals). Aortic atherosclerotic disease can lead to abdominal aortic aneurysm (AAA), aortic dissection, peripheral atheroembolism, penetrating aortic ulcer, and intramural hematoma. Coronary atherosclerosis that leads to MI is the leading cause of death and disability worldwide.

C. Medical Therapy for Atherosclerosis

Management of contributing systemic diseases such as *hypertension* (using antihypertensives such as beta-blockers), *hyperlipidemia* (using statins or other lipid-lowering agents), *diabetes* (using oral hypoglycemic agents or insulin therapy), and obesity (through exercise, weight loss, and diet) may significantly retard the progression of atherosclerosis and may reduce perioperative morbidity and mortality after vascular surgery. Treatment with statin drugs reduces progression and may cause regression of atherosclerotic plaques, improve endothelial function, and reduce cardiovascular events. Chronic therapy with aspirin, angiotensin-converting enzyme inhibitors, and especially smoking cessation have all been shown to significantly slow or reverse the progression of atherosclerosis. Most *medical therapies*, including statins, aspirin, and beta-blockers, should be continued up to and throughout the perioperative period to reduce the risk of perioperative cardiovascular events (Table 36-1).

? **Did You Know**

As many as 25% of adults presenting for vascular surgery have severe coronary artery disease.

II. Chronic Medical Problems and Management in Vascular Surgery Patients

The patient undergoing vascular surgery likely has systemic vascular disease complicated by medical problems such as coronary artery disease, systemic hypertension, hyperlipidemia, diabetes, obesity, and tobacco abuse.

A. Coronary Artery Disease in Patients with Peripheral Vascular Disease

As many as 25% of patients presenting for vascular surgery have severe coronary artery disease (CAD). The American Heart Association and others have published guidelines for cardiac evaluation and management prior to noncardiac surgery (Fig. 36-2) (1).

Table 36-1	Medical Therapy, Side Effects, and Current Recommendations	
Medication/Drug Class	**Side Effects**	**Perioperative Recommendations**
Aspirin	Platelet inhibition may lead to increased bleeding Decreased GFR	Continue until day of surgery, especially for carotid and peripheral vascular cases. Monitor fluid and urine output.
Clopidogrel	Platelet inhibition may lead to increased bleeding Rare thrombotic thrombocytopenic purpura	Hold for 7 days before surgery except for CEA and severe CAD or DES. Cross-match blood. Avoid neuraxial anesthesia if not held at least 7 days.
HMG CoA Reductase Inhibitors (Statins)	Liver function test abnormalities Rhabdomyolysis	Assess liver function tests. Continue through morning of surgery and continue as soon as possible postoperatively. Check CPK if myalgias.
Beta-Blockers	Bronchospasm Hypotension Bradycardia, heart block Induction hypotension Cough	Continue through perioperative period.
ACE Inhibitors	Induction hypotension Cough	Continue through perioperative period. Consider one-half dose on day of surgery.
Diuretics	Hypovolemia Electrolyte abnormalities	Continue through morning of surgery. Monitor fluid and urine output.
Calcium Channel Blockers	Perioperative hypotension (especially with amlodipine)	Continue through perioperative period. Consider withholding amlodipine on day of surgery.
Oral Hypoglycemics	Hypoglycemia intraoperatively and perioperatively Lactic acidosis with metformin	When feasible, switch to insulin preoperatively. Monitor glucose status intraoperatively and perioperatively.

GFR, glomerular filtration rate; CEA, carotid endarterectomy; CAD, coronary artery disease; DES, drug-eluting stents; HMG CoA, 3-hydroxy-3-methyl-glutaryl-CoA reductase; ACE, angiotensin-converting enzyme; CPK, creatine phosphokinase.
Adopted from Morgan GE, Mikhail MS, Murray MJ, eds. *Clinical Anesthesiology.* 4th ed. New York: Lange Medical Books/McGraw-Hill, 2006.

B. Preoperative Coronary Revascularization

The Coronary Artery Revascularization Prophylaxis trial randomized patients with coronary disease before elective vascular surgery to either coronary revascularization or medical therapy and found no benefit to coronary revascularization if aggressive medical therapy (including beta-blockers, aspirin, and statins) was instituted. *Revascularization* may therefore be of minimal value in preventing coronary events after vascular surgery, except in patients in whom revascularization is indicated for acute coronary syndrome. If a *coronary stent* is placed, elective surgery should be delayed: for bare metal stents, a minimum of 6 weeks of dual antiplatelet therapy (DAPT); and for drug-eluting stents, 12 months (or longer) of DAPT (2). Aspirin is recommended indefinitely to prevent in-stent thrombosis. With the advent of new stents, the time required for DAPT and delay of surgery will likely evolve.

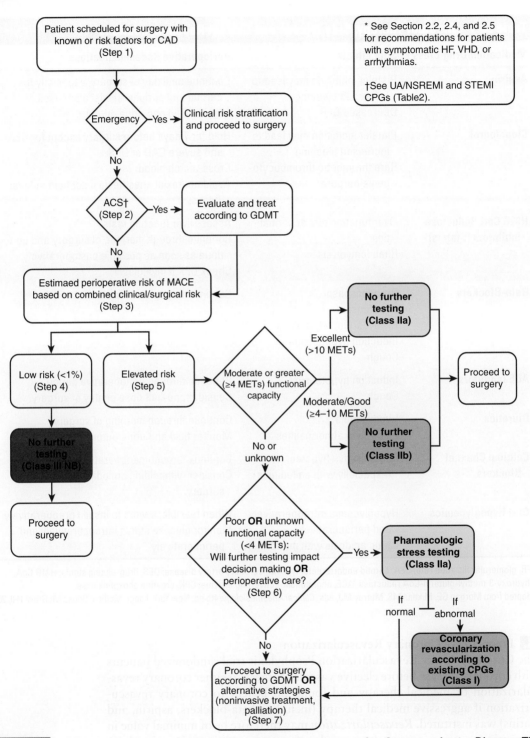

Figure 36-2 Stepwise Approach to Perioperative Cardiac Assessment for Coronary Artery Disease. The American College of Cardiology/American Heart Association (ACC /AHA) guideline calls for stepwise cardiac risk assessment involving consideration of the patient's cardiac risk factors, functional capacity, and the planned surgical procedure. See Figure 16-1 and accompanying legend for details. (From Fleisher LA, Fleischmann KE, Auerbach AD, et al. 2014 ACC/AHA Guideline on Perioperative Cardiovascular Evaluation and Management of Patients Undergoing Noncardiac Surgery: A Report of the American College of Cardiology/American Heart Association Task Force on Practice Guidelines. *J Am CollCardiol*. 2014;():. doi:10.1016/j.jacc.2014.07.944. Available at http://content.onlinejacc.org/article.aspx? articleid=1893784. Page 30 of 105)

III. Other Medical Problems in Vascular Surgery Patients

In addition to known common comorbid conditions such as CAD, systemic hypertension, hyperlipidemia, diabetes, obesity, and tobacco abuse, the vascular patient may have other undiagnosed conditions including hypercoagulable states, renal insufficiency, heart failure, chronic obstructive pulmonary disease, sleep apnea and others. If surgery is elective, preoperative management should focus on optimizing all the patient's chronic conditions, a process that cannot be accomplished if the patient presents on the morning of surgery.

IV. Organ Protection in Vascular Surgery

Many vascular procedures involve the occlusion of blood flow through the application of clamps, shunts (providing flow at a lower perfusion pressure), or bypasses (directing flow from a well perfused region to a poorly perfused region). Therefore, vital organs may suffer ischemia for varying durations.

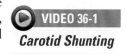

VIDEO 36-1

Carotid Shunting

A. Ischemia-Reperfusion Injury in the Vascular Surgery Patient: Fundamental Concepts

Reduction or interruption of blood flow (ischemia) compromises delivery of oxygen, glucose, and other essential nutrients for aerobic metabolism and thus slows the generation of adenosine triphosphate. When adenosine triphosphate is fully depleted, cellular processes fail and cellular integrity is lost (ischemic injury). The duration of ischemia correlates directly with the degree of cellular injury. In addition, toxic metabolites of *anaerobic metabolism* accumulate in the low or no-flow regions during the ischemic period. Upon restoration of flow and resumption of delivery of nutrients, further damage occurs via generation of toxic oxygen species, release of cytotoxic amino acids, up-regulation of nitric oxide synthase, and initiation of cellular apoptosis. In addition, toxic by-products of anaerobic metabolism are released into the systemic circulation, causing electrolyte abnormalities, labile blood pressures, alterations in systemic vascular resistance, and potentially severe acid-base disequilibrium.

B. Prevention of Myocardial Injury

Vascular surgery can result in dramatic changes in blood pressure, especially during procedures requiring *aortic clamping*. (See Chapter 35 for further discussion of myocardial oxygen supply and demand as well as techniques for monitoring and treating myocardial ischemia.)

C. Prevention of Kidney Injury

Postoperative *acute renal failure (ARF)* results in an increased length of hospital stay, as well as significant morbidity and mortality. Underlying kidney disease, cardiac disease, and especially renal ischemia contribute to its development: suprarenal aortic cross-clamping 15% and infrarenal cross-clamping 5% incidence of ARF. Additional risk factors may include advanced age, hypovolemia, and anemia. Logically, minimizing renal ischemia time and maintaining appropriate hemodynamics are important to preserving renal function. However, currently there is no clinically proven strategy to minimize the risk of postoperative renal insufficiency and ARF.

D. Prevention of Pulmonary Complications

More and more vascular procedures are done via minimally invasive or endovascular techniques for which postoperative pulmonary complications should

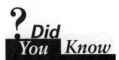

be minimal. However, for patients who require open surgical procedures, especially aortic procedures, significant pulmonary complications are a real risk due to *large fluid shifts* and *transfusion-related acute lung injury*. In addition, pain from large incisions can compromise respirations and cough. Different centers manage these challenges differently, however, minimizing transfusions and optimizing postoperative analgesia are established ways of improving outcome. After carotid endarterectomy, the carotid body on the operative side is denervated and this blunts the ventilatory response to hypoxemia and virtually eliminates this response after bilateral carotid endarterectomy. Postoperative surgical site bleeding after carotid endarterectomy can distort, compress, or occlude the trachea rapidly, necessitating emergent evacuation of the causative hematoma.

E. Protection of the Central Nervous System and Spinal Cord

In vascular surgery patients, neurologic injury is most common after carotid endarterectomy *(stroke)* and thoracic aortic procedures *(paraplegia)*. During carotid endarterectomy, emboli from the surgical site are the usual cause of stroke. However, hypoperfusion of the brain on the operative side can result during carotid clamping if the patient's perfusion via the circle of Willis or the surgical shunt around the site of carotid clamping is inadequate. In thoracic aortic procedures, compromise of the spinal cord vascular supply, especially the artery of Adamkiewicz, is a major risk. For strategies to improve neurologic outcome, please see subsequent chapters on the specific procedures (Fig. 36-3). Unfortunately, no pharmacologic intervention has proven beneficial.

V. Carotid Endarterectomy

A. Management of Asymptomatic Carotid Stenosis

Screening asymptomatic patients for carotid stenosis is not recommended, because carotid endarterectomy (CEA) is beneficial for only a very select group of asymptomatic patient and only if the expected risk of CVA is less with CEA than without it (3).

B. Management of Symptomatic Carotid Stenosis

Symptoms of carotid artery stenosis include sudden unilateral vision loss (amaurosis fugax) and unilateral changes in motor function, dysarthria, and aphasia. These symptoms require *urgent evaluation* and treatment to minimize the risk of permanent neurologic damage. If performed expertly, CEA is effective in reducing this risk in symptomatic patients with moderate and high-grade carotid stenosis.

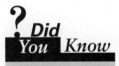

C. Preoperative Evaluation and Preparation for Carotid Endarterectomy

The preoperative evaluation of vascular surgical patient includes the essential elements required for all surgical patients (see Chapter 16). CEA is defined by the American College of Cardiology/American Heart Association (ACC/AHA) as an intermediate-risk procedure, with the possibility of cardiac death or nonfatal MI being <5% (1). The ACC/AHA algorithm defines an evidence-based approach to the preoperative evaluation (Fig. 36-2). If preoperative medical management with *anticoagulants* or *antiplatelet drugs* does not control symptoms of carotid stenosis, CEA is urgent. Preoperative reduction of hypertension is controversial especially if the carotid stenosis is severe or bilateral. Sudden reduction in blood pressure should be avoided.

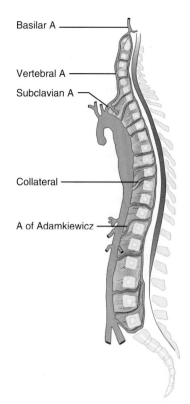

Basilar A

Vertebral A

Subclavian A

Collateral

A of Adamkiewicz

Figure 36-3 The artery of Adamkiewicz usually arises at the T11–T12 level and provides the blood supply to the lower spinal cord. Its variable location and the uncertainty of additional collateral blood supply explain, in part, the unpredictability of paraplegia following descending aortic surgery. (From: Smaka TJ, Miller TE, Hutchens MP, et al. Anesthesia for vascular surgery. In: Barash PG, Cullen BF, Stoelting RK, et al. *Clinical Anesthesia*, 7th ed. Philadelphia: Lippincott Williams & Wilkins, 2013:1122.)

D. Monitoring and Preserving Neurologic Integrity

Monitoring for cerebral ischemia during CEA is controversial. Some centers advocate providing regional anesthesia and argue that the awake patient can report neurologic changes most reliably. Others advocate general anesthesia to ensure a motionless surgical field, and they rely on continuous electroencephalogram, somatosensory-evoked potentials, transcranial Doppler, or cerebral oximetry. Each method has its limitations and challenges and neither regional nor general anesthesia has provided better *neurologic outcomes*. With either technique, if there are signs of cerebral ischemia, blood pressure should be optimized (usually to the patient's normal awake level) or a shunt placed, if not already in use.

E. Anesthetic Management for Elective Surgery

No one anesthetic approach has been proven best for patients undergoing CEA. Both regional and general anesthesia are employed safely (4). With either approach, the patient must be awake and cooperative at the end of the procedure for ongoing *neurologic assessment*. Given the very high incidence of CAD and hypertensive heart disease in this patient population, etomidate and esmolol are often used in combination for induction of general anesthesia and abatement of the stimulation of endotracheal intubation. For patients at low risk from the hypotensive effects of propofol, it may be used instead of etomidate to reduce the risk of postoperative nausea and vomiting. General anesthesia can be maintained by intravenous or inhaled anesthetics with the caveat that *blood pressure* must be maintained at or near the patient's normal resting level. Isoflurane, sevoflurane, and desflurane reduce cerebral oxygen consumption and provide ischemic preconditioning for the heart and other organs. Despite these potential advantages, they have not been proven to improve outcome, perhaps because the majority of CVAs are caused by *emboli* from the surgical site. Regional anesthesia techniques include deep and superficial cervical plexus blocks, as well as cervical epidural anesthesia and local infiltration. In addition to standard American Society of Anesthesiologists (ASA) monitors, continuous direct arterial blood pressure monitoring is highly recommended because blood pressure control is vital during CEA.

F. Carotid Angioplasty with Stenting
In the past decade, carotid angioplasty with stenting has emerged as an alternative treatment to CEA. However, compared with CEA, carotid stenting is associated with a higher risk of periprocedural stroke and death, especially in older patients. The longer-term relative outcomes remain to be defined (5).

G. Postoperative Management
The most urgent and potentially devastating complication of CEA is clot formation at the surgical site and the associated *thromboembolism* to the cerebral circulation. A new onset neurologic change after surgery requires immediate ultrasound examination of the operative site and reoperation if indicated. Other complications presenting in the early postoperative period include stroke from emboli or hypoperfusion during surgery, severe hyper- and hypotension, myocardial ischemia, cranial and recurrent nerve injuries, and wound hematoma. Control of severe hypertension is vital because if uncontrolled, it is associated with increased mortality and increased cardiac and neurologic complications. Additionally, persistent severe postoperative hypertension increases the risk of cerebral hyperperfusion syndrome, characterized by headaches, seizures, and focal neurologic signs. An *expanding wound hematoma* can obstruct the airway, necessitating emergent evacuation of the hematoma before an adequate airway can be re-established.

VI. Aortic Aneurysms
The management of patients with aortic aneurysms is evolving rapidly with innovative stenting techniques progressively replacing open surgical procedures. However, *rupture* of an aortic aneurysm is a *true surgical emergency* and one of the greatest anesthetic management challenges.

A. Epidemiology and Pathophysiology of Abdominal Aortic Aneurysms
There are approximately 200,000 AAAs diagnosed annually. Approximately 45,000 of these require surgical repair annually. Risk factors for AAA include male sex, advanced age, smoking, hypertension, low serum high-density lipoprotein cholesterol, high fibrinogen plasma levels, and low platelet count. The annual risk of aneurysmal rupture is directly related to its diameter: 1% for aneurysms measuring <4.0 cm, 2% for aneurysms 4.0 to 4.9 cm, and 20% for aneurysms >5.0 cm. All aneurysms >5.0 cm should be considered for surgical or endovascular repair. Screening is recommended by the U.S. Preventative Services Task Force for men >65 years old with a smoking history.

B. Medical Management versus Endovascular Repair versus Open Surgical Repair

Medical management of aortic aneurysms includes smoking cessation and control of hypertension, dyslipidemia, diabetes, and diet. Medical management may slow, but will not halt aneurysm progression completely. For patients with AAAs measuring 4.0 to 5.4 cm, frequent ultrasound monitoring for progression is vital. Since the 1980s, *endovascular aneurysm repair* (EVAR) has progressively become the *dominant* treatment modality. In this approach, the femoral artery is used to introduce stent graft(s) inside the aneurysm, thereby preventing further enlargement or rupture. Initially, EVAR was used on patients deemed too high risk for an open surgical repair, but now it has evolved into a first-line treatment choice. Nevertheless, EVAR is not without complications, including *graft leak* and intraoperative conversion to open repair because of aneurysm rupture, vascular injury, or inability to seal the graft against the wall of the aorta. When compared with open surgical repair, EVAR is associated with shorter recover times and lower 30-day mortality rates (1.4% vs. 4.2%) but no difference in mortality rates at intermediate and long-term follow-up. Graft costs and reoperation expenses offset other savings, so that ultimately there is no cost benefit to EVAR verses open surgical repair. EVAR is performed using local, regional, or general anesthesia depending on the preferences of the patient and the surgical team.

C. Open Surgical Repair

Open surgical repair of an abdominal aortic aneurysm is performed through either an anterior transperitoneal laparotomy incision or an anterolateral retroperitoneal approach. The surgical exposure for either approach is virtually identical, but the retroperitoneal approach is associated with less fluid shifts, faster return of bowel function, lower pulmonary complications, and shorter intensive care unit stays. After administration of intravenous heparin, the aortic cross-clamp is applied to the supraceliac, suprarenal, or infrarenal aorta, depending on the location of the aneurysm. The higher the *level of cross-clamping*, the greater the stress will be on the left ventricle and the higher the incidence of ischemic injury to the gut, kidney, and spinal cord. Intraoperative blood loss during open AAA repair can be significant, and the extensive retroperitoneal surgical dissection increases fluid requirements (up to 10 to 12 mL/kg/hr). In addition to standard ASA monitors, continuous direct arterial blood pressure monitoring is highly recommended because of the rapid and marked changes in blood pressure during the clamping and unclamping of the aorta. Central venous and pulmonary artery pressure monitoring as well as transesophageal echocardiography are often used depending on the comorbidities of the patient and preferences of the anesthesiologist. General anesthesia or combined general and epidural anesthesia are common approaches. The combined approach has the advantage of providing excellent postoperative analgesia but introduces the risk of epidural hematoma because systemic anticoagulation must be used during surgery.

 VIDEO 36-2
Aortic Cross-Clamping: Blood Volume Redistribution

D. Thoracoabdominal Aneurysm Repair

Thoracoabdominal aortic aneurysm surgery is one of the *greatest anesthetic management challenges*. Typically, thoracoabdominal aneurysms involve the descending thoracic and abdominal aorta, require an expansive incision extending into these cavities, one-lung ventilation, and the use of partial cardiopulmonary bypass. Selective ("one-lung") ventilation of the contralateral

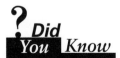
Did You Know

Spinal fluid drainage during thoracic aneurysm can be employed to enhance spinal cord perfusion pressure.

Table 36-2	Methods of Spinal Cord Protection during Descending Thoracic Aortic Surgery
Limitation of cross-clamp duration	
Distal circulatory support (partial bypass)	
Reattachment of critical intercostal arteries	
CSF drainage (lumbar drain)	
Hypothermia	Moderate systemic (32–34°C) Epidural cooling Circulatory arrest
Maintenance of proximal blood pressure	Pharmacotherapy: Corticosteroids, barbiturates, naloxone, calcium channel blockers, oxygen free radical scavengers, NMDA antagonists, mannitol, magnesium, vasodilators (adenosine, papaverine, prostacyclin), perfluorocarbons, colchicine Intrathecal: Papaverine, magnesium, tetracaine, perfluorocarbons
Avoidance of postoperative hypotension	
Sequential aortic clamping	
Enhanced monitoring for spinal cord ischemia	Somatosensory-evoked potentials Motor-evoked potentials Hydrogen-saturated saline
Avoidance of Hyperglycemia	

CSF, cerebrospinal fluid; NMDA, N-methyl-D-aspartate.
Adopted from Thomas DM, Hulten EA, Ellis ST, et al. Open versus endovascular repair of abdominal aortic aneurysm in the elective and emergent setting in a pooled population of 37,781 patients: a systematic review and meta-analysis. *ISRN Cardiol*. 2014, Apr 2;2014:149243.

lung is required for optimizing surgical exposure and to prevent the ipsilateral lung from surgical trauma. During thoracic aortic procedures, *spinal cord ischemia* may be detected through the use of somatosensory-evoked potential and motor-evoked potentials (Table 36-2). To improve spinal cord perfusion pressure, a *lumbar subarachnoid drain* can be used to remove cerebrospinal fluid. Partial cardiopulmonary bypass has been used to provide perfusion distal to the operative site. In fact, the incidence of neurologic injury in this setting has been substantially reduced when distal aortic perfusion is combined with drainage of cerebrospinal fluid. Many of the other anesthetic management considerations are the same for thoracoabdominal as noted above for AAA surgery. (See the sections in Chapter 35 on "Aortic Dissection" and "Aortic Aneurysm" and Table 35-2 for a summary of the common hemodynamic goals for all these procedures.)

E. **Management of Emergency Aortic Surgery**

Rupture or leaking of an aortic aneurysm is the most common reason for emergency aortic surgery. Aortic aneurysm rupture has a mortality rate of 85% unless surgery is performed immediately, and even then the *mortality rate is 50%*. If the patient survives emergency surgery, the incidence of renal impairment, pulmonary injury, myocardial infarction, and spinal cord injury is significantly greater than in elective aortic surgery. Ruptures most commonly occur into the retroperitoneum, and this site allows temporary tamponade of the hemorrhage. About 25% of aneurysms rupture into the peritoneal cavity, and rapid exsanguination occurs. Massive blood loss will occur during this surgery, and, therefore, preparations for blood replacement, including rapid infusion devices, are critical. For this true surgical emergency, both EVAR and open surgical repair are used in different centers depending on the resources and expertise available (6).

VII. Lower Extremity Revascularization

The incidence of PAD is increasing, especially in the aging population. Roughly 10 million people in the United States have symptomatic PAD, and another 20 to 30 million have asymptomatic PAD. The three indications for elective revascularization procedures include claudication, ischemic rest pain or ulceration, and gangrene. High-risk procedures, including ileofemoral bypass, femoral-femoral bypass, and aortofemoral bypass, re-establish blood flow to an ischemic extremity and relieve debilitating symptoms of claudication. However, advances in minimally invasive percutaneous techniques have made *endovascular procedures* the primary modality for revascularization. Regional or local anesthesia with or without sedation is often used for endovascular approaches. The majority of the procedure is not painful. However, tunneling the graft and deployment of the stent can be quite painful and trigger patient movement or hypertension and tachycardia. Heparin is given prior to deployment of grafts or stents and anticoagulation may be needed in the postoperative period to maintain graft patency.

References

1. Fleisher LA, Beckman JA, Brown KA, et al. 2009 ACCF/AHA Focused update on periopereaitve beta blockade incorporated into the ACC/AHA guidelines on perioperative cardiovascular evaluation and care for noncardiac surgery. *Circulation.* 2009;120:e169–e276.
2. Hawn MT, Graham LA, Richman JR, et al. The incidence and timing of noncardiac surgery after cardiac stent implantation. *J Am Coll Surg.* 2012;214(4):658–666.
3. Raman G, Moorthy D, Hadar N, et al. Management strategies for asymptomatic carotid stenosis: A systematic review and meta-analysis. *Ann Intern Med.* 2013;158:676–685.
4. Vaniyapong T, Chongruksut W, Rerkasem K. Local versus general anesthesia for carotid endarterectomy. *Cochrane Database Syst Rev.* 2013;12:CD000126.
5. Bonati LH, Lyrer P, Ederle J, et al. Percutaneous transluminal angioplasty and stenting for carotid artery stenosis. *Cochrane Database Syst Rev.* 2012;12:CD000515.
6. Open versus endovascular repair of abdominal aortic aneurysm in the elective and emergent setting in a pooled population of 37,781 patients: A systematic review and meta-analysis. *ISRN Cardiol.* 2014; Apr 2;2014:149243.

Questions

1. Atherosclerosis occurs in two stages, the first is endothelial injury and the second is:
   A. An inflammatory response
   B. A thrombogenic response
   C. A cytotoxic response
   D. An angiogenic response
   E. None of the above

2. What percentage of men over the age of 65 have carotid stenosis?
   A. Over 20%
   B. Over 30%
   C. Over 40%
   D. Over 50%
   E. None of the above

3. How long should elective surgery be delayed after placement of a drug-eluting coronary stent?
   A. 6 weeks
   B. 3 months
   C. 6 months
   D. 12 months
   E. None of the above

4. The risk of cardiac-related death or nonfatal myocardial infarction after carotid endarterectomy is less than:
   A. 1%
   B. 2%
   C. 5%
   D. 10%
   E. None of the above

5. Signs and symptoms of cerebral hyperperfusion syndrome after carotid endarterectomy include headache, seizures, and:
   A. Focal neurologic deficits
   B. Hypertension
   C. Bradycardia
   D. Apnea
   E. None of the above

6. At what diameter should an aortic aneurysm be considered for surgical repair?
   A. Greater than 4 cm
   B. Greater than 4.5 cm
   C. Greater than 5.0 cm
   D. Greater than 5.5 cm
   E. None of the above

37 Management of Acute and Chronic Pain

Ashley N. Agerson
Honorio T. Benzon

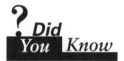

Did You Know

When chronic pain is associated with neuroplastic changes in the central and peripheral nervous systems that may manifest as hypersensitivity, windup, and allodynia, the pain itself becomes a disease state.

Pain is defined by the International Association for the Study of Pain (IASP) as "an unpleasant sensory and emotional experience associated with actual or potential tissue damage, or described in terms of such damage" (1). *Acute pain* is a normal physiologic response to injury, disease, or surgery and is usually temporally self-limited. Though unpleasant, pain is protective and serves the purpose of avoiding, stopping, or minimizing tissue damage and should be seen as a symptom of an underlying disease. *Chronic pain* is usually defined as pain lasting more than 3 months. It can be due to ongoing disease or tissue injury or can persist after resolution of or in the absence of injury. Chronic pain is associated with neuroplastic changes in the central and peripheral nervous systems that may manifest as hypersensitivity, windup, and allodynia. When these changes occur, the pain itself can be called a disease state.

Nociceptive pain results from transmission of a noxious stimulus through an intact nervous system. Nociceptive pain can be worsened by inflammation, which causes *hyperalgesia*, the phenomenon of normally painful stimuli being perceived as more painful than usual. Nociceptive pain can be somatic or visceral. *Somatic pain* originates within the skin, superficial tissue, and musculoskeletal system and is typically easy to localize and described as sharp. *Visceral pain* is typically vague, diffuse, achy, and may refer to surrounding areas.

In contrast to nociceptive pain, *neuropathic pain* results from a lesion in the central or peripheral nervous system. It is often described as electric or lancinating in character. If this is found in the distribution of a known nerve, it is termed *neuralgia*. Neuropathic pain is often associated with altered sensations. *Paresthesias* are abnormal, spontaneous, or evoked sensations. *Dysesthesia* are unpleasant abnormal sensations. *Allodynia* is the perception of pain from a normally nonpainful stimulus (such as light touch). *Hyperesthesia* is increased sensitivity to stimulation, and *hypoesthesia* is decreased sensation of stimulus.

I. Anatomy, Physiology, and Neurochemistry of Pain

A. Pain Processing

The physiology of pain processing functionally comprises four steps: transduction, transmission, modulation, and perception. These processes are clinically relevant as each provides targets for pain treatment and prevention (Fig. 37-1). *Transduction* is the generation of an action potential from a noxious chemical, mechanical, or thermal stimulus. *Transmission* is the propagation of the signal through the afferent pathway from the nociceptor to the sensory cortex. *Modulation* is the positive or negative modification of the pain signal along the afferent pathway, while *perception* is the integration of the pain signal into consciousness.

B. Transduction

Nociceptors are located in the skin, mucosa, muscle, fascia, joint capsules, dura, viscera, and adventitia of blood vessels. Most Aδ and C nociceptors are polymodal (i.e., their terminals express transducer channels that are sensitive to multiple stimuli). When they are activated by pressure, chemical, or thermal stimuli, the channels activate voltage-sensitive sodium and calcium channels, starting an action potential. Nociceptors can be activated by bradykinin, serotonin, and protons and sensitized by prostaglandins, leukotrienes, and cytokines. Glutamate, substance P, and nerve growth factor can also promote transduction of a pain signal (Table 37-1).

C. Transmission

Pain transmission occurs via a three-neuron afferent pathway, beginning in the periphery (Fig. 37-2). First-order neuronal cell bodies are located in the

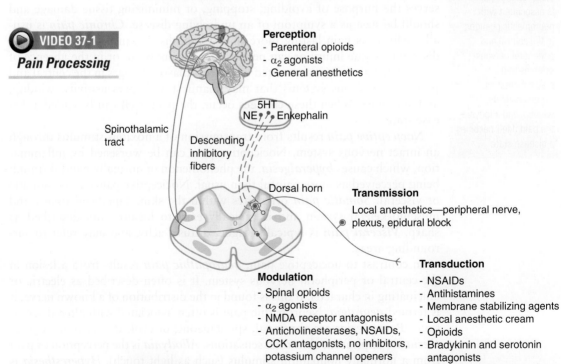

VIDEO 37-1

Pain Processing

Perception
- Parenteral opioids
- α₂ agonists
- General anesthetics

5HT
NE Enkephalin

Spinothalamic tract

Descending inhibitory fibers

Dorsal horn

Transmission
Local anesthetics—peripheral nerve, plexus, epidural block

Transduction
- NSAIDs
- Antihistamines
- Membrane stabilizing agents
- Local anesthetic cream
- Opioids
- Bradykinin and serotonin antagonists

Modulation
- Spinal opioids
- α₂ agonists
- NMDA receptor antagonists
- Anticholinesterases, NSAIDs, CCK antagonists, no inhibitors, potassium channel openers

Figure 37-1 The four elements of pain processing: transduction, transmission, modulation, and perception. (From Macres SM, Moore PG, Fishman SM. Acute pain management. In: Barash PG, Cullen BF, Stoelting RK, et al., eds. *Clinical Anesthesia*. 7th ed. Philadelphia: Lippincott Williams & Wilkins; 2013:1611–1642, with permission.)

Table 37-1	Classification of Neural Fibers			
Fiber Type	**Modality**	**Function**	**Receptor**	**Diameter**
Aα	Proprioceptive	Muscle tension, length, velocity	Golgi and Ruffini endings, muscle spindle afferents	15–20 μm
Aβ	Mechanosensitive	Touch, motion, pressure, vibration	Meissner, Ruffini, Pacinian corpuscles; Merkel disk	5–15 μm
Aδ	Thermoreceptive Nociceptive	Cold Sharp pain	Free nerve endings	1–5 μm
C	Thermoreceptive Nociceptive	Warmth Burning pain	Free nerve endings	<1 μm

Adapted from Table 57.1 in Barash PG, Cullen BF, Stoelting RK, et al., eds. *Clinical Anesthesia*. 7th ed. Philadelphia: Lippincott Williams & Wilkins; 2013.

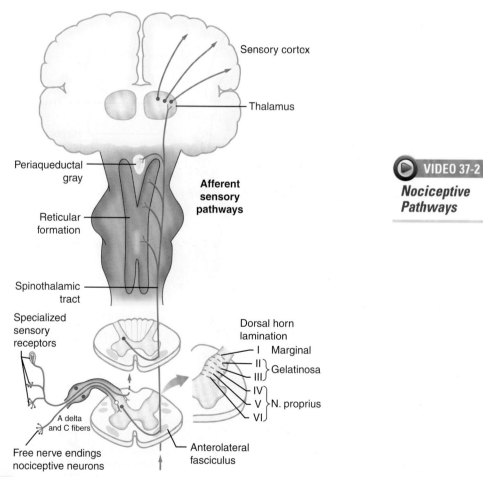

VIDEO 37-2

Nociceptive Pathways

Figure 37-2 The afferent nociceptive pathway. (From Macres SM, Moore PG, Fishman SM. Acute pain management. In: Barash PG, Cullen BF, Stoelting RK, et al., eds. *Clinical Anesthesia*. 7th ed. Philadelphia: Lippincott Williams & Wilkins; 2013:1611–1642, with permission.)

dorsal root ganglia with fibers projecting to peripheral tissue where the receptors are located. Fibers enter the spinal cord and travel up or down through the posterolateral tract before entering the dorsal horn to synapse on second-order neurons. Second-order neuron cell bodies are located in the dorsal horn and are either nociceptive specific or wide dynamic range. Axons transmitting somatic nociception decussate and ascend via the contralateral spinothalamic tract, while axons transmitting visceral nociception ascend via the ipsilateral dorsal column medial lemniscus. Both synapse on the third-order neurons in the thalamus, the axons of which terminate in the sensory cortex. In the face, the primary afferent neuron has its cell body in the trigeminal ganglion and synapses on the second-order neuron in the medulla in the spinal trigeminal nucleus. From here the signal is transmitted to the thalamus, as are pain signals from the rest of the body.

D. Modulation

Modulation of the pain response occurs at many levels and can be positive or negative (Fig. 37-3). Activity between first- and second-order neurons is decreased by feedback from interneurons and descending inhibition from

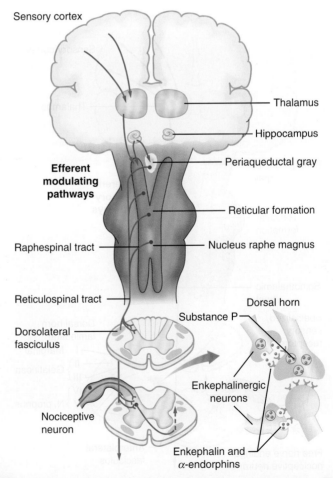

Figure 37-3 The efferent pathway for modulation of nociception. (From Macres SM, Moore PG, Fishman SM. Acute pain management. In: Barash PG, Cullen BF, Stoelting RK, et al., eds. *Clinical Anesthesia.* 7th ed. Philadelphia: Lippincott Williams & Wilkins; 2013:1611–1642, with permission.)

the periaqueductal gray matter, rostral ventromedial medulla, and the dorsolateral pontine tegmentum. Augmentation of pain may occur as part of the transition from acute to chronic pain. Repetitive activation of wide dynamic range neurons by C fibers causes windup. Axonal sprouting causes crosstalk between different fibers, causing nonnoxious stimuli to become painful. In addition, neuromas and axonal sprouting may be associated with upregulation of sodium and downregulation of potassium channels, which cause destabilized cell membranes to become more prone to forming an action potential. Normal Aβ fibers do not produce substance P, but in the presence of tumor necrosis factor-α from injury, Aβ fibers can secrete it. This transition is termed *phenotypic switch*.

E. Perception

Perception of pain is mediated by multiple structures. The primary and secondary somatosensory cortices are involved with sensory discrimination of pain. The frontal cortex and insula may facilitate learning and memory of pain. The anterior cingulate gyrus is related to emotional significance of pain, while the lentiform nucleus and cerebellum are involved in self-protective reflexes related to pain.

II. Assessment of Pain

Pain is a highly subjective experience and affects many aspects of life. As such, the evaluation of the patient in pain relies primarily on patient-reported information and should include assessment of multiple domains. Because pain is dynamic, it should be reassessed regularly and adjustments to therapy made as appropriate. The location of the pain and where it radiates, if at all, are important. In the postoperative setting, it is still necessary to ask where the pain is located rather than presume the pain is incisional. Patients may have additional pain related to pre-existing conditions, positioning or retraction during surgery, and immobility. The onset and temporal pattern as well as exacerbating and ameliorating factors are established. The quality of the pain can help indicate its origin and possible treatment options—sharp incisional pain may respond well to nonsteroidal anti-inflammatory drugs (NSAIDs), opioids, and nerve blocks, but shooting neuropathic pain may respond to an N-methyl-D-aspartate (NMDA) antagonist, clonidine, or antiepileptic agent.

The intensity of pain should be assessed in multiple contexts. The baseline level of pain is the pain that exists at all times, while breakthrough pain escalates beyond the background. Multiple tools exist to aid in the assessment of pain intensity, all of which are arbitrary, subjective, and have a high degree of variability between patients. Despite these flaws, they are useful to determine trends in pain control. The numerical rating scale is most commonly used, which asks patients to rate their pain from 0, no pain, to 10, worst pain imaginable. For young children or patients with cognitive impairments, the facial grimace scale allows for a more descriptive approach (Fig. 37-4).

Because pain impacts many activities, it is important to investigate the patient's functional status including the ability to eat, sleep, ambulate, work, and perform one's activities of daily living. Any side effects from pain therapy should be thoroughly discussed as well. Physical examination is focused on possible etiologies of pain and should include a thorough neurologic and musculoskeletal examination.

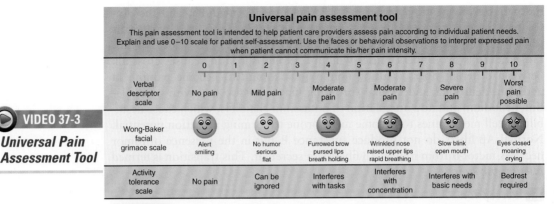

Universal pain assessment tool

This pain assessment tool is intended to help patient care providers assess pain according to individual patient needs. Explain and use 0–10 scale for patient self-assessment. Use the faces or behavioral observations to interpret expressed pain when patient cannot communicate his/her pain intensity.

	0	1	2	3	4	5	6	7	8	9	10
Verbal descriptor scale	No pain		Mild pain		Moderate pain		Moderate pain		Severe pain		Worst pain possible
Wong-Baker facial grimace scale	Alert smiling		No humor serious flat		Furrowed brow pursed lips breath holding		Wrinkled nose raised upper lips rapid breathing		Slow blink open mouth		Eyes closed moaning crying
Activity tolerance scale	No pain		Can be ignored		Interferes with tasks		Interferes with concentration		Interferes with basic needs		Bedrest required

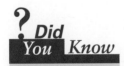

VIDEO 37-3
Universal Pain Assessment Tool

Figure 37-4 Universal pain assessment tool. Different scales can be used depending on the patient's age and other medical conditions. (From Macres SM, Moore PG, Fishman SM. Acute pain management. In: Barash PG, Cullen BF, Stoelting RK, et al., eds. *Clinical Anesthesia*. 7th ed. Philadelphia: Lippincott Williams & Wilkins; 2013:1611–1642, with permission.)

III. Pharmacologic Management of Pain

A. Opioids

Opioids are useful for acute pain and cancer-related pain and can be a component of a chronic pain regimen. In acute pain, short-acting agents are typically used alone. In chronic pain, 80% of the daily dose is given in a basal long-acting medication with the remainder given as a short acting opioid as needed for breakthrough. When assessing patients for opioid management, it is important to inquire about the level of analgesia provided, whether the patient's functional status is improved, whether there are side effects of therapy, and whether the patient displays aberrant behaviors (i.e., early refills, lost pills).

Opioids bind to the μ, κ, and δ receptors to cause analgesia and side effects, such as pruritus, nausea, constipation, and respiratory depression. Various opioids have different potencies, bioavailabilities, and dosages (Table 37-2). For ease of comparison and conversion from one medication to another, they are all compared to the prototypical opioid, morphine. When converting from one opioid to another, it is important to reduce the expected dosage by 25% to 50% to account for incomplete cross-tolerance to the new agent. When treating patients with opioids, precision of vocabulary is important. *Tolerance* is the phenomenon of decreased effect of a given amount of medication. It usually occurs after prolonged administration of the drug. *Dependence* is the physiologic condition of withdrawal symptoms when an opioid is discontinued. *Addiction* is a disease marked by altered behavior to seek the desired substance despite negative consequences. *Pseudo-addiction* is aberrant drug-seeking behavior due to undertreatment of pain.

Morphine is metabolized by the liver to morphine-6-glucuronide (M6G) and morphine-3-glucuronide (M3G), which are renally excreted. M6G is analgesic due to μ-binding activity and is responsible for respiratory depression, sedation, and nausea. M3G has no μ effect and is associated with hyperalgesia, seizures, and tolerance. Morphine's half-life is 2 hours, but its duration of action is 4 to 5 hours due to its slow elimination from the brain compartment.

Hydromorphone is five times more potent than morphine and is associated with fewer side effects. It is metabolized in the liver to dihydromorphine and dihydroisomorphine, which are active, and hydromorphone-3-glucuronide,

? Did You Know

It is important to know the differences between drug tolerance, dependence, addiction, and pseudo-addiction.

Table 37-2	Opioid Pharmacokinetics and Equianalgesic Dosing				
Drug	**Onset**	**Duration**	**Active Metabolite**	**Oral Equianalgesic Dose**	**IV Equianalgesic Dose**
Fentanyl	IV: immed IM: 7–8 min	IV: 30–60 min IM 1–2 hr Transdermal: 72 hr	—	—	100 μg
Hydromorphone	IM: 15 min PO: 30 min	4–5 hr	—	6–8 mg	1.5–2 mg
Meperidine	PO: 15 min IM/SQ: 10–15 min IV: immed	2–4 hr	Normeperidine	300 mg	100 mg
Methadone	IV: 10–20 min PO: 30–60 min	4 hr (t½ is 8–59 hr)	—	Variable	Variable
Morphine	IM: 10–30 min	4–5 hr	Morphine-6- glucuronide	30 mg	10 mg
Oxymorphone	5–10 min	3–6 hr	—	10 mg	1 mg
Oxycodone	<60 min	3–4 hr	—	20 mg	10–15 mg
Remifentanil	Rapid	5–10 min	—	—	50 μg
Sufentanil	IV: immed Epidural: 10 min	Epidural: 1.7 hr	—	—	10–40 μg

IV, intravenous; IM, intramuscular; SQ, subcutaneous; immed, immediately; PO, oral; t½, half-life.
Adapted from Benzon HT, Hurley RW, Deer T, et al. Chronic pain management. In: Barash PG, Cullen BF, Stoelting RK, et al., eds. *Clinical Anesthesia.* 7th ed. Philadelphia: Lippincott Williams & Wilkins; 2013: 1645–1669.

which does not cause analgesia but is similar in side effects to M3G. Its onset is 15 minutes when administered intravenously and its duration of action is similar to that of morphine.

Fentanyl is 80 times more potent than morphine and is associated with less histamine release and pruritus. It is more lipophilic than morphine. It is metabolized by the liver and is appropriate for patients with renal failure. It is available as a transdermal patch. Due to gradual absorption of the drug, the patch requires 6 to 8 hours to reach maximum plasma concentrations. The patch provides steady-state analgesia without periods of side effects related to high serum concentrations and periods of pain due to low serum concentrations. After removal of the patch, significant serum levels remain, hence, intramuscular opioid should not be given immediately.

Sufentanil is 1,000 times as potent as morphine and is typically used in intraoperative infusions or neuraxially. It has a slightly shorter elimination half-life than fentanyl. Alfentanil is 10 times the potency of morphine and has its peak effect within 2 minutes. It has a very short duration of action, <10 minutes, and is ideal for brief periods of intraoperative stimulation. Remifentanil is approximately 100 times the potency of morphine. Like alfentanil, it is also rapid acting. It is eliminated by plasma cholinesterases, so its terminal half-life is 10 to 20 minutes. Its termination of analgesia is so rapid that it may result in rebound hyperalgesia.

Methadone is a unique opioid because it enhances analgesia by antagonizing the NMDA receptor and inhibiting serotonin reuptake in addition to its μ effect. It is metabolized in the liver by cytochrome P450 and has many drug interactions. It has a variably long elimination half-life between 8 and 80 hours, requiring slow titration to avoid accidental overdose. After a single dose, it provides analgesia for 3 to 6 hours, but with prolonged around-the-clock dosing, the duration of analgesia can be 8 to 12 hours. Methadone can cause prolonged QT and torsades de pointes, requiring periodic electrocardiograms.

Meperidine is a short-acting opioid that is metabolized in the liver to normeperidine, which can be neurotoxic and result in seizures, especially in the setting of renal failure or prolonged dosing. It is indicated for short-term use only. Its most common usage is in low doses to treat postoperative rigors.

Oxycodone is activated by conversion to oxymorphone. Both drugs are associated with less pruritus than morphine. Tramadol, hydrocodone, and codeine are considered weak opioids. Tramadol is a μ agonist with monoaminergic properties. It carries low rates of constipation, respiratory failure, and abuse. Codeine is a prodrug that is metabolized to morphine by cytochrome P450 2D6. Reductions in enzymatic activity, as seen in children and certain ethnic groups (whites and Asians), cause decreased analgesia and increased respiratory depression.

B. Nonsteroidal Anti-inflammatory Drugs (NSAIDs)

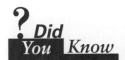

Did You Know

Acetaminophen is a centrally acting COX inhibitor with minimal peripheral action that causes analgesia and antipyrexia but has no anti-inflammatory effect.

NSAIDs work by inhibiting cyclooxygenase (COX) enzymes, exerting anti-inflammatory, antipyretic, and analgesic effects. COX-1 is present in healthy tissue and serves gastroprotective and hemostatic functions. COX-2 is induced in injury and produces prostaglandins that sensitize peripheral nociceptors to pain and promote hyperalgesia. NSAIDs are effective at reducing postoperative pain and opioid consumption and are commonly used in both acute and chronic pain. Side effects include platelet dysfunction, nephrotoxicity, and gastric ulcers. Acetaminophen is a centrally acting COX inhibitor with minimal peripheral action. It causes analgesia and antipyrexia, but has no anti-inflammatory effect.

C. Anticonvulsants

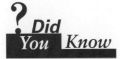

Did You Know

Chronic nerve damage is associated with spontaneous ectopic firing of neurons and anticonvulsants reduce ectopic signals by blocking sodium or calcium channels. Thus, anticonvulsants may be useful in treating neuropathic pain.

Chronic nerve damage is associated with spontaneous ectopic firing of neurons and changes in sodium and calcium channel expression. Anticonvulsants reduce ectopic signals by blocking sodium or calcium channels. Gabapentin and pregabalin both block α₂-δ subunit of calcium channels. Both have been shown to be helpful in multiple neuropathic pain syndromes, including postherpetic neuralgia (PHN), diabetic painful neuropathy (DPN), trigeminal neuralgia, human immunodeficiency virus (HIV) neuropathy, spinal cord injury pain, phantom limb pain, and poststroke pain. In acute pain, preoperative gabapentin has been shown to decrease narcotic requirements, improve pain control, and reduce opioid-related side effects. Neither gabapentin nor pregabalin have significant drug–drug interactions. Side effects of both drugs include dizziness, fatigue, peripheral edema, and cognitive slowing.

D. Antidepressants

Tricyclic antidepressants (TCAs) and serotonin-norepinephrine reuptake inhibitors (SNRIs) exert an independent analgesic effect distinct from their mood stabilizing properties. TCAs affect many pathways, including inhibition of the reuptake of serotonin and adenosine, interaction with α receptors, opioid receptor binding, and blockade of sodium channels, calcium channels, and

NMDA receptors. They are effective at treating neuropathic pain, especially postherpetic neuralgia (PHN) and diabetic peripheral neuropathy (DPN), but frequent side effects limit their use. These include sedation, xerostomia, urinary retention, and blurred vision and tend to be more pronounced in the elderly. Nortriptyline and desipramine are better tolerated than amitriptyline.

SNRIs cause pain relief by inhibiting the reuptake of norepinephrine more than serotonin. SNRIs (duloxetine and milnacipran) are effective in DPN and fibromyalgia and are commonly prescribed in other neuropathic pain syndromes because of their minimal side-effect profile compared with TCAs. Selective serotonin reuptake inhibitors (SSRIs) have not been proven to have analgesic properties outside of their beneficial effect on depressive symptoms.

E. N-methyl-d-aspartate Antagonists

NMDA receptors provide a nonopioid strategy for pain management and can be helpful in the opioid-dependent patient. NMDA stimulation is thought to play a role in development of chronic pain, opioid-induced hyperalgesia, and windup. Ketamine is the prototypical NMDA antagonist. It has poor oral bioavailability, so it is used in intravenous infusions to reduce opioid requirements. Dosage is limited by side effects, including tachycardia, salivation, and dysphoria. Dextromethorphan also antagonizes the NMDA receptor and is orally bioavailable. When given for acute or chronic pain, it is thought to reduce secondary hyperagesia and modestly reduce opioid requirements.

F. Alpha Adrenergics

Clonidine and dexmedetomidine are both central α_2 agonists. Binding causes reduced norepinephrine output, which causes sedation and analgesia in addition to reduced heart rate and blood pressure without affecting respiratory drive. The half-life of clonidine is 9 to 10 hours. It can be given orally, intravenously, or intrathecally. When given as a transdermal patch, it can be helpful to mitigate adrenergic symptoms of opioid withdrawal. The half-life of dexmedetomidine is 2 hours. Because it is much more selective for α_2 than α_1, as compared with clonidine, intravenous infusion is used for profound sedation with analgesia, with a lower incidence of bradycardia and hypotension.

G. Glucocorticoids

Glucocorticoids, including dexamethasone, inhibit phospholipase A2 to block the production of prostaglandins and leukotrienes and have analgesic and anti-inflammatory effects. They are useful perioperatively to reduce pain and nausea, but may be associated with poor wound healing. Bursts of steroids (e.g., hydrocortisone, methylprednisolone) can be useful in the management of chronic pain, such as radiculitis, but side effects such as gastric ulcers, osteoporosis, water retention, hypertension, and hyperglycemia limit long-term use.

H. Local Anesthetics

Lidocaine can be delivered in patch form directly to an area of neuropathic pain. The medication is slowly absorbed and blocks sodium channel locally, rather than a systemic effect. It can be helpful in PHN, peripheral neuropathy, osteoarthritis, myofascial pain, and low back pain. It may require as long as 2 weeks of daily patch use to obtain relief. Intravenous lidocaine infusion can be given for neuropathic pain resistant to other treatments. Dosing is typically 5 mg/kg over 30 minutes. Mexiletine is an orally available local anesthetic with a similar effect to intravenous lidocaine.

I. Topical Agents

Capsaicin's mechanism of action is to stimulate TRPV1 receptors, which then causes reduced nerve fiber density. Substance P may also be depleted. It is available in a low concentration cream, which must be applied three to four times daily for weeks to experience relief. A patch form (8%) is effective in PHN, DPN, and HIV neuropathy when applied. Local anesthetic ointment must be applied for an hour before the patch to mitigate the burning sensation of the patch; relief from one application can last 12 weeks.

IV. Acute Pain

A. Surgical Stress Response and Preventive Analgesia

Postoperative pain occurs by the mechanisms described above. The surgical stress response is the systemic response to the operation, in which cytokines are released with various negative responses. Chemical mediators of the surgical stress response include interleukin-1, interleukin-6, and tumor necrosis factor-α, which promote inflammation. Poorly controlled pain results in increased levels of catecholamine release, which in turn disrupts the neuroendocrine balance. Hormonal changes include increased secretion of cortisol and glucagon paired with decreased secretion of insulin and testosterone. Together these result in a catabolic state with a negative nitrogen balance, hyperglycemia, poor wound healing, muscle wasting, fatigue, and immune compromise. Other negative effects of the surgical stress response are tachycardia, hypertension, increased cardiac work, bronchospasm, splinting, pneumonia, ileus, oliguria, urinary retention, thromboembolism, impaired immunity, weakness, and anxiety. Preventive analgesia is the concept of perioperative strategies for reducing pain-mediated sensitization of the nervous system with the goal of reducing long-term pain. To be effective, preventive analgesia must cover the entire surgical field and be adequate enough to prevent nociception during surgery as well as the entire perioperative period (2).

B. Strategies for Acute Pain Management

Patient-controlled Analgesia

Patient-controlled analgesia (PCA) has been shown to be a safe alternative to intermittent intravenous boluses of opioids for acute pain, with improved patient satisfaction, decreased nursing requirements, and lower opioid requirements. The general principle is that the patient self-administers incremental boluses of medication at safe intervals, building up the dose until adequate analgesia is achieved. The most common agents for PCA use are morphine, hydromorphone, and fentanyl (Table 37-3). Programmable variables include starting bolus, demand dose and interval, basal infusion rate, and 1- or 4-hour

Table 37-3 Common Dosing Parameters for Patient-Controlled Analgesia in Opiate-Naïve Patients

Opioid	Demand Dose	Lockout (min)	Basal Infusion
Fentanyl	20–50 µg	5–10	0–60 µg/hr
Hydromorphone	0.2–0.4 mg	6–10	0–0.4 mg/hr
Morphine	1–2 mg	6–10	0–2 mg/hr

Adapted from Macres SM, Moore PG, Fishman SM. Acute pain management. In: Barash PG, Cullen BF, Stoelting RK, et al., eds. *Clinical Anesthesia.* 7th ed. Philadelphia: Lippincott Williams & Wilkins; 2013: 1611–1642.

limit. The demand dose should be a fraction of the usual therapeutic dose. The dosing interval should be after the medication effect begins and before it starts to wane to allow for cumulative effect. A basal infusion may be employed in a patient on long-term opioid therapy, but should not be used in the opioid naïve. The 1- and 4-hour limits may be used to limit overall dosage, but care must be taken not to limit it so severely that the patient uses all the allowable boluses in the first portion of the time interval and is without analgesia for the remainder. PCA may result in overdose and respiratory depression. Side effects include nausea, pruritus, and altered mental status. Risk factors include obstructive sleep apnea, congestive heart failure, pulmonary disease, renal or hepatic failure, head injury, and altered mental status.

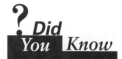

Did You Know

The programmable variables when administering intravenous patient-controlled analgesia include starting bolus, demand dose and interval, basal infusion rate, and 1- or 4-hour limit.

Neuraxial and Regional Analgesia

Epidural infusion provides improved pain control with activity, decreased respiratory complications, and decreased postoperative ileus compared with systemic opioids. The placement of the catheter should correspond to the dermatome level of the surgical incision. Epidural local anesthetic provides somatic analgesia but may cause hypotension and weakness. Epidural opioids provide analgesia with good coverage of visceral pain but can cause pruritus and respiratory depression. The combination of opioids and local anesthetics is synergistic and allows for reduced dosage compared with single-agent infusions, minimizing side effects. Clonidine may be a useful adjuvant, but could cause hypotension and sedation. Hypotension usually responds to fluid administration. Pruritus is due to spinal μ binding and is independent of histamine. Therefore, treatment is best accomplished with a low dose of mixed opioid agonist-antagonist, such as nalbuphine. Epidural infusions are usually continuous and may have a patient-administered bolus programmed as well.

Peripheral nerve blocks and continuous catheters are an important component of multimodal pain therapy as well. The discussion of this branch of anesthesia is beyond the scope of this chapter but is well discussed in Chapter 21.

C. Special Cases in Acute Pain

Pediatrics

Acute pain management in children must be tailored to the individual child and family. Assessment of pain is sometimes difficult in younger children, but family and other caregivers can aid in this evaluation. The same techniques can be employed in children as in adults. PCA in older children is safe, as long as no one other than the patient delivers a bolus dose. Epidural infusions and ultrasound-guided peripheral nerve blocks are useful and are commonly placed after induction of anesthesia, rather than awake, as in adults. Caudal injection of local anesthetic is an excellent treatment for postoperative pain for perineal, lower extremity, and lower abdominal cases. Local anesthetic must be dosed appropriately for weight.

The Opioid-dependent Patient

Controlling the pain of the opioid-dependent patient can be challenging in the perioperative setting and usually requires a multimodal approach. Successful treatment relies on identification of these patients and appropriate goal setting, so attention to pain medications is important in the preoperative assessment.

As a general rule, the perioperative period is not a time to wean opioid usage. Clinical observations show that opioid requirements are approximately doubled from baseline in the postoperative period. The patient's long-acting opioid should be continued unchanged. If fasting status prohibits dosing of oral medication, the equianalgesic amount should be administered as the baseline infusion in a PCA. The bolus dose should be set 25% to 50% higher than for an opioid-naïve individual. Regional and epidural analgesia is helpful in reducing overall opioid dosage, though care should be taken not to administer opioids in more than one route. To avoid cumulative effect, epidural infusions often consist of local anesthetic only, paired with intravenous opioid PCA. Ketamine, NSAIDs, antiepileptics, acetaminophen, and antidepressants can assist with pain control and limit opioids as well. Medications should be weaned to baseline postoperatively.

V. Chronic Pain

A. Management of Common Pain Syndromes

Low back pain is a very common complaint worldwide, accounting for many visits to emergency departments, primary care providers and specialists, as well as billions of dollars in health care costs and lost productivity. Low back and buttock pain can have a number of possible etiologies, including disk herniation or internal disruption, facet joint syndrome, piriformis syndrome, sacroiliac joint syndrome, myofascial pain, and fibromyalgia, as well as vertebral body compression fractures, spinal metastatic lesions, and spinal infections (3).

Low Back Pain: Radicular Pain Syndromes

When pain radiates in a dermatomal distribution, it is considered *radicular* and can be accompanied by weakness, depressed reflexes, numbness, and tingling in the same dermatomal distribution (Fig. 37-5, Table 37-4). Pain is typically sharp and lancinating. Physical examination often reveals antalgic gait, a positive straight leg raise test, diminished or absent reflexes, reduced strength, and decreased sensation in the affected spinal level. Radicular pain is typically the result of irritation or dysfunction of the spinal nerve root in the epidural space, which can be due to neuroforaminal stenosis or disk herniation, causing compression and initiation of the inflammatory cascade. Spinal imaging may be helpful in diagnosis, but herniated disks are commonly asymptomatic.

Treatment of radicular pain syndromes is best managed in a multimodal fashion. NSAID medications, oral steroids, physical therapy, short periods of bed

Table 37-4	Muscle Innervation and Deep Tendon Reflexes by Spinal Level	
Spinal Level	**Muscle Action**	**Reflexes**
C5	Shoulder abduction	Biceps
C6	Elbow flexion	Brachioradialis
C7	Elbow extension	Triceps
C8	Thumb extension	—
L2	Hip flexion	—
L3	Knee extension	—
L4	Ankle dorsiflexion	Patella
L5	Great toe extension	Medial hamstring
S1	Ankle plantar flexion	Achilles

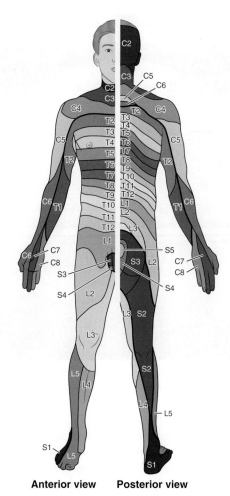

Anterior view   Posterior view

Figure 37-5 Dermatome map for localization of affected level, planning appropriate epidural placement. (From Moore KL, Agur AMR, Dalley II AF. *Clinically Oriented Anatomy,* 7th ed. Philadelphia: Lippincott Williams & Wilkins, 2013, with permission.)

rest, and neuropathic pain medications such as gabapentin or pregabalin can be helpful. If symptoms do not respond to these measures, *epidural steroid injection (ESI)* of corticosteroid can reduce inflammation in the epidural space by reducing the activity of phospholipase A2. Corticosteroids also block C-fibers, causing antinociception directly. ESIs have been shown to provide short-term (<3 months) relief of radicular pain. ESIs are most effective in patients with acute radiculitis and less effective for management of chronic symptoms and nonradicular pain. Surgery does not appear to produce better long-term outcomes for radiculitis than a more conservative approach. The natural history of low back and radicular pain due to a herniated disk is one of gradual improvement with conservative measures. Thus, the use of epidural steroids can minimize the use of other systemic medications and their attendant side effects.

ESI are performed for low back pain with or without radiculitis. Once the intended level is localized by fluoroscopy, the skin is anesthetized. In the interlaminar approach, an epidural needle is advanced through the skin, subcutaneous tissue, supraspinous ligament, interspinous ligament, and finally the ligamentum flavum. A loss of resistance technique is employed to detect penetration of the ligamentum flavum and presence in the posterior epidural space. Alternatively, the transforaminal approach may be used, which directs the

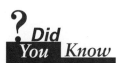

Epidural steroid injections are most effective in patients with acute radiculitis and less effective for management of chronic symptoms and nonradicular pain. Surgery does not appear to produce better long-term outcomes for radiculitis than a more conservative approach.

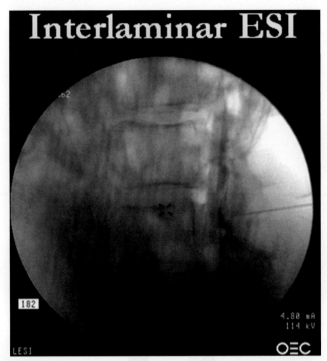

Figure 37-6 Lateral view of an interlaminar approach showing predominant spread of the contrast in the posterior epidural space with minimal spread into the anterior epidural space.

steroid more anteriorly, closer to the disk–nerve interface. In this technique, the entry point is off midline to the affected side and the needle is directed through skin and paraspinal musculature, traveling medially to the intervertebral foramen. In both techniques, a small amount of radiopaque contrast is injected to confirm epidural placement without vascular uptake, followed by corticosteroid diluted in local anesthetic or saline (Fig. 37-6).

There are multiple randomized controlled trials investigating the efficacy of ESI with varying results (4). Most show short-term relief of lumbar radiculopathy symptoms. There are fewer studies of epidural steroid injections in cervical radiculopathy, but those also generally show short-term relief of symptoms (5). There have been comparisons between the transforaminal and interlaminar approaches, which generally favor the transforaminal technique. Comparison of transforaminal to far-lateral interlaminar (parasagittal) showed better contrast spread in parasagittal injections but overall similar efficacy. The short-term relief achieved from ESI can be helpful in returning a patient to function and reducing the toxicity from systemic medications, but it should be used as an adjuvant to multimodal therapy, not a sole treatment.

ESI is safe when performed by a trained practitioner in an appropriate patient. Complications include epidural hematoma and infection, both of which can cause irreversible neurologic deficit. The incidence of hematoma is reduced by the timely discontinuation of antiplatelet and anticoagulant agents (6). Penetration of the radicular artery during lumbar transforaminal ESI or the vertebral artery during cervical transforaminal ESI can result in traumatic shearing, vasospasm, or embolism of particulate steroid, which, in turn, can cause infarction to the brain or spinal cord.

In addition, systemic corticosteroid absorption can cause side effects. Blood pressure and serum glucose levels can be elevated for a week after ESI.

Exogenous corticosteroids can suppress the hypothalamic–pituitary–adrenal axis, with even a single dose reducing plasma cortisol and corticotropin levels for weeks. Blood pressure can be elevated as well.

The patient should be re-evaluated 2 to 3 weeks after the ESI. If there is no response to a single injection, it can be repeated once, because some patients who did not have relief after one injection have relief after the second. A third injection can be performed if partial relief occurs, but a series of three regardless of relief is not advised.

Low Back Pain: Facet Syndrome

Another common diagnosis causing low back pain is *lumbar facet syndrome*. There are two columns of facet joints in the spine located posterior and lateral to the intervertebral disks bilaterally. They normally transmit 10% to 15% of the body's weight and are subject to arthritis and increased forces in the presence of spondylolisthesis and disk degeneration. Pain is axial and can radiate to the buttock and posterior thigh on the affected side. Physical examination is positive for paraspinal muscle tenderness and pain with ipsilateral rotation during extension. Facet joints are innervated by the medial branches of the dorsal rami, so pain relief from medial branch blocks or facet joint injections can confirm diagnosis. Intra-articular facet joint injections can produce long-lasting analgesia. If pain relief is transient and there is relief from medial branch blocks, radiofrequency ablation of the medial branches can be performed (7).

Buttock Pain: Sacroiliac Joint Syndrome

Sacroiliac (SI) joint pain is commonly described near the posterior superior iliac spine (PSIS) and the buttock. It may radiate to the posterior thigh and calf as well as the groin. Physical examination is significant for pain with palpation of the PSIS and stressing of the joint, such as by the FABER, Gaenslen, or Yeoman maneuvers. Treatment of SI joint syndrome may include physical therapy, NSAIDs, intra-articular steroid injections, radiofrequency denervation of the L5 medial branch and sacral (S1 to S3) lateral branches, and surgical fusion.

Buttock Pain: Piriformis Syndrome

Piriformis syndrome is another etiology of buttock and leg pain. The piriformis muscle originates in the ventral sacrum, exits the pelvis through the greater sciatic foramen, and inserts in the greater trochanter. It internally rotates the extended hip and externally rotates the flexed hip. Buttock pain occurs from muscular irritation, such as from trauma, infection, or surgery. Pain may radiate to the posterior thigh and calf, indicating irritation of the sciatic nerve by the piriformis muscle. The pain is typically worse with prolonged sitting or moving from sitting to standing. Physical examination reveals pain with *f*lexion, *a*dduction, and *i*nternal *r*otation (FAIR, Laseque), pain or weakness with resisted abduction with hip flexed (Pace), and pain with passive internal rotation of an extended thigh (Freiberg sign). Computed tomography (CT) or magnetic resonance imaging may show enlarged piriformis; electromyogram may show signs of neuropathy or myopathy, but the diagnosis is clinical. Treatment includes physical therapy, NSAIDs, and muscle relaxants. Injections of local anesthetic and steroid into the muscle belly can also be helpful.

Myofascial Pain Syndrome

Trigger points are focal, palpable areas of pain in muscle or fascia. Palpation of these nodules may provoke a twitch response or reproduce radiating pain in a distribution characteristic of the muscle involved. *Myofascial pain syndrome* is local, regional, and referred pain that originates from these trigger points. Treatment of myofascial pain syndrome includes massage and stretching, postural training, physical therapy, trigger point injections with local anesthetic or botulinum toxin, and dry needling.

Fibromyalgia

Fibromyalgia is a chronic pain disorder associated with widespread pain and abnormally sensitive soft tissue. The diagnosis is made when there is a history of at least 3 months of diffuse pain and allodynia to palpation at 11 of 18 tender points. Associated symptoms are sleep disturbance, fatigue, and cognitive dysfunction. Other regional pain syndromes (headaches, irritable bowel syndrome, temporomandibular joint dysfunction, interstitial cystitis) may also be present. Treatment of fibromyalgia is multimodal and should include an exercise program, cognitive behavioral therapy, and medications. Opiates are typically not effective, but SNRIs (e.g., milnacipran, duloxetine), pregabalin, and amitriptyline can be helpful.

Neuropathic Pain Syndromes

Herpes Zoster and Postherpetic Neuralgia

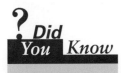

Did You Know

The likelihood of developing PHN is reduced by prompt administration of antiviral drugs.

Pain associated with herpes zoster accompanies and occasionally precedes the rash. It is typically well managed with analgesics and resolves as the rash heals, but can persist for over 3 months and become postherpetic neuralgia (PHN). The overall incidence of developing PHN is between 10% and 15%, but the rate rises steeply after age 65, such that 30% to 50% of elderly patients with zoster develop PHN. Besides older age, other risk factors include high intensity of pain during zoster, severity of zoster rash, and painful prodrome. The likelihood of developing PHN is reduced by prompt administration of antiviral drugs such as acyclovir, famciclovir, and valacyclovir. There are conflicting data regarding the use of epidural steroid injections as prophylaxis against PHN, but they may be considered among high-risk individuals within 2 to 4 weeks of the onset of the rash.

Treatment of PHN is primarily medical, relying on the use of anticonvulsants such as gabapentin and pregabalin, opioids, and antidepressants such as nortriptyline. Topical medications such as lidocaine patch and capsaicin can also be helpful. If medications are ineffective, a procedural approach may be helpful. Spinal cord stimulation and intrathecal alcohol can be considered (8).

Diabetic Painful Neuropathy

Peripheral neuropathy is a common consequence of chronic neural ischemia in patients with long-term diabetes. Incidence increases with age, duration of diabetes, and severity of hyperglycemia. The most common subtypes are distal symmetric polyneuropathy, median neuropathy, and visceral autonomic neuropathy. It is unknown why some patients experience painful neuropathy and others do not.

The serotonin-norepinephrine reuptake inhibitors (e.g., duloxetine, milnacipran) are considered first-line therapy due to their efficacy and favorable side-effect profile. Other useful medications include gabapentin, pregabalin, and nortriptyline. If these are ineffective, opioids can provide additional analgesia. SSRIs are not thought to be effective. In addition to these medications, tight glucose control is necessary.

Did You Know

Complex regional pain syndrome is diagnosed clinically by meeting specified historical and physical criteria.

Complex Regional Pain Syndrome

Complex regional pain syndrome (CRPS) is a chronic pain syndrome that can develop after a known nerve injury (type II, formerly causalgia) or in the absence of previous nerve injury (type I, formerly reflex sympathetic dystrophy). It is characterized by symptoms and signs in multiple categories: sensory, sudomotor, vasomotor, and motor/trophic (9). Sensory changes include allodynia, hyperalgesia, hyperesthesia, or spontaneous pain. Sudomotor changes are sweating

Table 37-5	Budapest Criteria for Complex Regional Pain Syndrome

1. Continuing pain, which is disproportionate to any inciting event
2. Must display at least one sign at time of evaluation in two or more of the following categories:
   a. Sensory
   b. Vasomotor
   c. Sudomotor/edema
   d. Motor/trophic
3. Must report at least one symptom in three of the four following categories:
   a. Sensory
   b. Vasomotor
   c. Sudomotor/edema
   d. Motor/trophic
4. There is no other diagnosis that better explains the signs and symptoms

From Harden RN, Bruehl S, Stanton-Hicks M, et al. Proposed new diagnostic criteria for complex regional pain syndrome. *Pain Med.* 2007;8:326–331, with permission.

abnormalities or edema. Vasomotor symptoms are temperature abnormalities or skin color changes. Motor deficiencies include decreased range of motion, weakness, tremor, or neglect. Trophic changes are changes in hair or nail growth (Table 37-5). Risk factors include female sex, work-related injury, and previous surgery. The diagnosis is made clinically but can be supported by osteopenia on radiographs and metabolic alterations on three-phase bone scan.

Treatment should be multimodal and focus on functional restoration, pain management, and psychological treatment. Physical therapy is useful for desensitization and strengthening. Medications can include gabapentin, pregabalin, duloxetine, nortriptyline, memantine, opioids, calcitonin, and bisphosphonates. Sympathetic blocks and spinal cord stimulation are procedural approaches to analgesia.

Human Immunodeficiency Virus Neuropathy
Neuropathy in HIV can be viral related or due to nucleoside reverse transcriptase inhibitors used for treatment of the infection. Allodynia and hyperalgesia are most commonly located in the lower extremities and may respond to lamotrigine or gabapentin (Table 37-6).

Table 37-6	Recommended Medications for Chronic Pain Conditions			
Postherpetic Neuralgia	**Diabetic Painful Neuropathy**	**Spinal Cord Injury**	**Fibromyalgia**	**Human Immunodeficiency Virus**
Pregabalin	Duloxetine	Pregabalin	Duloxetine	Lamotrigine
Gabapentin	Pregabalin	Gabapentin	Pregabalin	Gabapentin
Opioid	Gabapentin	Lamotrigine	Milnacipran	
Antidepressants	Antidepressants	IV lidocaine	Tramadol	
Tramadol		Mexiletine		
Lidoderm patch				

IV, intravenous.
Adapted from Macres SM, Moore PG, Fishman SM. Acute pain management. In: Barash PG, Cullen BF, Stoelting RK, et al., eds. *Clinical Anesthesia.* 7th ed. Philadelphia: Lippincott Williams & Wilkins; 2013: 1611–1642.

Phantom Pain

Phantom limb sensation may be experienced by up to 80% of patients with amputated extremities, but phantom pain is significantly less common. The incidence may be reduced by adequate preoperative pain control prior to the amputation. Methods have included epidural infusion and continuous plexus blocks. Treatment includes opioids, gabapentin, NMDA antagonists like ketamine and memantine, and antidepressants. Nonpharmacologic techniques include biofeedback, mirror therapy, transcutaneous electrical nerve stimulation, and spinal cord stimulation.

Cancer Pain

Cancer pain is common in up to 90% of patients with advanced disease. It can be somatic pain, which responds well to opioids, NSAIDs, and neural blockade; visceral pain, which responds well to sympathetic blocks; or neuropathic pain, which is best treated with opioids, SNRIs, antiepileptics, and TCAs. Although opioids are the mainstay of treatment for cancer-related pain, management should include a combination of pharmacologic agents, antineoplastic treatment (chemotherapy, radiation), interventional procedures as necessary, and psychological care (10).

Neurolytic Blocks for Visceral Pain from Cancer

The abdominal organs, with the exception of the descending colon, are innervated by the *celiac plexus*, which lies on the anterior surface of the aorta at L1. The celiac plexus is made up of sympathetic fibers from the greater, lesser, and least splanchnic nerves, as well as parasympathetic fibers from the vagus nerve. Reduction of pain from the abdominal organs, such as that associated with pancreatic cancer, can be accomplished by the blockade of the splanchnic nerves at the anterior margin of T12 or the retrocrural or anterocrural blockade of the plexus anterior to the L1 vertebral body. Fluoroscopic or CT guidance is mandatory. Alcohol (50% to 100%) or phenol (6% aqueous) is used to coagulate the target nerves, allowing for weeks to months of pain relief before the nerves regenerate. Complications can include orthostatic hypotension, transient diarrhea, aortic dissection, back pain, retroperitoneal hematoma, hematuria, pleurisy, hiccups, and paraplegia.

The pelvic organs are innervated via the superior hypogastric plexus, the continuation of the sympathetic chain. It is located anterior to the L5-S1 disk space and can be blocked bilaterally or with a single needle transdiscally.

The perineal area, including the distal rectum, anus, vulva, distal vagina, and distal urethra, are innervated via the ganglion impar, the termination of the sympathetic chain. It is a midline structure located anterior to the sacrococcygeal junction. The transcoccygeal approach is most commonly employed, wherein a needle is placed through the sacrococcygeal ligament until its tip is just anterior to the distal sacrum.

Interventional Procedures

Intradiscal Procedures

Discography is a diagnostic procedure used to determine the presence of internal disk disruption and to correlate this finding with symptoms. It is useful when the symptomatic disk is not known or to confirm a symptomatic disk is included within a planned fusion. During the procedure, contrast is injected into the disks under pressure using a manometer. Fluoroscopy is used to visualize the distribution of contrast within the disk and the patient reports whether the pain produced with pressurization is concordant with their usual pain.

Complications of discography include worsened pain, disk injury, and discitis. Prophylactic antibiotics are routinely given.

Intradiscal electrothermal therapy (IDET) is a therapeutic procedure for discogenic pain wherein a thermal resistance catheter is percutaneously positioned in the posterior disk between the annulus fibrosis and nucleus pulposus. The catheter is then heated, causing the contraction of the cartilage in the posterior disk wall and disruption of nerve fibers. Despite evidence for the efficacy of the procedure, IDET is seldom performed due to lack of insurance coverage. Nucleoplasty, or percutaneous disk decompression, is a therapeutic procedure to remove or coagulate part of the nucleus pulposus in a herniated disk. An introducer needle is placed, through which an electrode enters the disk and vaporizes or removes sections of disk. The intradiscal pressure is lowered, alleviating symptoms. The evidence for nucleoplasty is limited and it is rarely performed. The complications of IDET and nucleoplasty are similar and include nerve root injury, leg pain, infection, hematoma, dural puncture, catheter breakage, and damage to the spinal cord or cauda equina.

Minimally Invasive Lumbar Decompression Procedure

The minimally invasive lumbar decompression procedure is indicated to treat spinal stenosis related to ligamentum flavum hypertrophy. An epidural needle is placed and an epidurogram is performed, followed by contouring of the lamina and partial debulking of the hypertrophic ligamentum flavum. This partially decompresses the central canal and alleviates symptoms of back pain and neurogenic claudication.

Vertebroplasty and Kyphoplasty

Vertebroplasty and *kyphoplasty* are procedures to treat painful vertebral body compression fractures, usually due to osteoporosis. In both procedures, trocars are inserted percutaneously into the fractured vertebral body, either through the pedicle or extrapedicularly. A biopsy of the bone may be taken. In kyphoplasty, a balloon is inflated within the vertebral body fracture to restore height and correct the kyphotic defect. The balloon cavity is then filled with cement. In vertebroplasty the cement is injected directly into the fractured trabeculae. In both procedures, the patient remains supine for several hours during observation of neurologic status. Complications can include hematoma, cement leakage into vasculature resulting in pulmonary embolism, and retropulsion of bone fragments or cement into the spinal canal causing neurologic deficit. Long-term sequelae can include return of pain and fracture at another vertebral level.

Neuromodulation

Spinal cord stimulation is a modality that is used to treat chronic pain in which electrodes are placed in the epidural space along the dorsal columns. Stimulation of these tracts causes a sensation of vibration or tingling, which replaces the sensation of pain. The stimulator increases the output of larger Aβ fibers responsible for the sensation of touch. These Aβ fibers cause excitation of interneurons in the substantia gelatinosa, which inhibit transmission of signals from smaller pain-mediating C fibers. Spinal cord stimulation may be helpful to control symptoms and reduce opioid usage in patients with failed back surgery syndrome, neuropathic pain, CRPS, angina, and chronic limb ischemia. Patients should first undergo a psychological screening process to determine appropriateness for therapy and have excellent pain relief from temporary trial leads prior to permanent implantation. Trial leads may be implanted percutaneously in an outpatient clinic and are typically left in 5 to 7 days. Permanent leads may be implanted percutaneously or via laminectomy. The leads exit the epidural space and are tunneled to a battery implanted subcutaneously.

Peripheral nerve stimulation is indicated to treat pain originating from a single peripheral nerve, such as occipital or supraorbital neuralgia. Leads are implanted using ultrasound guidance to lie adjacent to the painful nerve. Similar to spinal cord stimulation, the mechanism of peripheral nerve stimulation is thought to involve gate control.

Intrathecal Drug Delivery

Intrathecal drug delivery systems, or intrathecal pumps, consist of an intrathecal catheter tunneled under the skin to an internalized pump and drug reservoir. Infused medications may include opioids, bupivacaine, and clonidine. Ziconotide is used for neuropathic pain and baclofen is indicated for spasticity. The most common opioids used are morphine, hydromorphone, and fentanyl. Intrathecal opioids are indicated in malignant pain when oral and transdermal opioids have failed to provide adequate relief despite appropriate dosing or when side effects limit upward titration of opioids. Medications are placed in the spinal fluid, bypassing the blood–brain barrier and allowing for much lower effective doses and an improved side-effect profile. Side effects can include respiratory depression, headache, pruritus, peripheral edema, granuloma formation, and hormone disruption.

References

1. Merksey H, Boguk N. A current list with definitions and notes on usage. In *Classification of Chronic Pain,* 2nd ed. Seattle: IASP Press; 1994. Available at: www.iasp-pain.org/Education/Content.aspx?ItemNumber=1698.
2. Macres SM, Moore PG, Fishman SM. Acute pain management. In: Barash PG, Cullen BF, Stoelting RK, et al., eds. *Clinical Anesthesia.* 7th ed. Philadelphia: Lippincott Williams & Wilkins; 2013:1611–1644.
3. Benzon HT, Hurley RW, Deer T, et al. Chronic pain management. In: Barash PG, Cullen BF, Stoelting RK, et al., eds. *Clinical Anesthesia.* 7th ed. Philadelphia: Lippincott Williams & Wilkins; 2013:1645–1671.
4. Benyamin RM, Manchikanti L, Parr AT, et al. The effectiveness of lumbar interlaminar epidural injections in managing chronic low back and lower extremity pain. *Pain Phys.* 2012;15:E363–E404.
5. Diwan S, Manchikanti L, Benyamin RM, et al. Effectiveness of cervical epidural injections in the management of chronic neck and upper extremity pain. *Pain Phys.* 2012; 15:E405–E434.
6. Horlocker TT, Wedel DJ, Rowlingson JC, et al. Regional anesthesia in the patient receiving antithrombotic or thrombolytic therapy: American Society of Regional Anesthesia and Pain Medicine Evidence-Based Guidelines (third edition). *Reg Anesth Pain Med.* 2010;35:64–101.
7. Lord SM, Barnsley L, Wallis BJ, et al. Percutaneous radio-frequency neurotomy for chronic cervical zygapophyseal-joint pain. *N Engl J Med.* 1996;23:1721–1726.
8. Hurley RW, Henriquez OH, Wu CL. Neuropathic pain syndromes. In: Benzon HT, ed. *Raj's Practical Management of Pain.* 5th ed. Philadelphia: Mosby Elsevier; 2014:346–361.
9. Harden RN, Bruehl S, Stanton-Hicks M, et al. Proposed new diagnostic criteria for complex regional pain syndrome. *Pain Med.* 2007;8:326–331.
10. Swarm R, Abernethy AP, Anghelescu DL, et al. Adult cancer pain. *J Natl Comp Canc Netw.* 2010;9:1046–1086.

Questions

1. Drug dependence is best described as:
   A. The phenomenon of decreased effect of a given amount of medication
   B. The physiologic condition of withdrawal symptoms when an opioid is discontinued
   C. A disease marked by altered behavior to seek the desired substance despite negative consequences
   D. Aberrant drug-seeking behavior due to undertreatment of pain

2. Which of the following drugs provides analgesia but no anti-inflammatory effects?
   A. Ibuprofen
   B. Naproxen
   C. Acetaminophen
   D. Ketorolac

3. Why are anticonvulsants useful in treating neuropathic pain?
   A. Anticonvulsants reduce ectopic signals from neurons
   B. Neuropathic pain is caused by seizures
   C. Chronic peripheral nerve damage causes seizures
   D. They enhance transmission through sodium channels

4. For which patient is an opioid basal infusion rate indicated for intravenous patient-controlled analgesia?
   A. Patients whose pain is not controlled with bolus doses
   B. Patients who are at risk for ventilatory depression
   C. Patients who are opioid tolerant
   D. Elderly patients

5. The best strategy for providing perioperative analgesia for NPO opioid dependent patients is:
   A. Wean the patient from chronic opioid usage
   B. Use continuous IV infusion of opioid to replace oral long-acting opioid and increased demand dose of opioid PCA
   C. Add opioid epidural analgesia to opioid intravenous PCA that provides opioid dose equianalgesic to chronic oral consumption
   D. Avoid the use of ketamine

6. Epidural steroid injections are most effective in patients:
   A. With chronic pain
   B. With nonradicular pain
   C. With acute radiculitis
   D. Where surgery fails to alleviate pain

7. The likelihood of developing postherpetic neuralgia is best reduced by:
   A. Prompt administration of antiviral drugs
   B. Use of anticonvulsant drugs during the acute herpetic eruption
   C. Administration of oral steroids
   D. Use of lidocaine patch in the affected dermatome

8. The diagnosis of complex regional pain syndrome:
   A. Requires positive findings on magnetic resonance imaging
   B. Cannot be made without a plain x-ray of the affected area
   C. Requires assessment by a psychiatrist
   D. Is a diagnosis of exclusion

38 Nonoperating Room Anesthesia and Special Procedures

Karen J. Souter
Isuta Nishio

Nonoperating room anesthesia (NORA) refers to anesthesia services that are provided outside of traditional surgical operating rooms. These locations include, but are not limited to, radiology departments, endoscopy suites, magnetic resonance imaging (MRI) and computerized tomography (CT) scanners, and cardiac catheterization (*cardiac cath*) and electrophysiology (EP) laboratories. NOR cases account for a significant proportion of the procedural work of hospitals, and, increasingly, patients or the proceduralists require or request anesthesia or sedation to facilitate these procedures. This chapter will discuss the care of patients requiring anesthesia or sedation for procedures in NOR locations. Anesthesia for surgical procedures performed in offices and ambulatory surgery centers is addressed Chapter 25, and anesthesia and analgesia provided for labor and delivery is discussed in Chapter 31.

I. The Three-Step Approach to Nonoperating Room Anesthesia

NORA covers a diverse spectrum of patients, procedures and locations and a systematic approach is recommended. The simple *three-step paradigm*—the *patient*, the *procedure*, and the *environment*—may be a useful mnemonic for NORA (Fig. 38-1).

A. The Patient

Patients may require sedation or anesthesia to tolerate NOR procedures for a number of reasons (Table 38-1). Children often require sedation or anesthesia for diagnostic and therapeutic procedures. Patients with significant comorbidities or surgical disease may be too ill to tolerate a major operative procedure, whereas a palliative, less-invasive NOR procedure may be possible. All patients presenting for NORA require a thorough *preanesthesia assessment* and the development of a sound anesthetic plan with appropriate levels of monitoring.

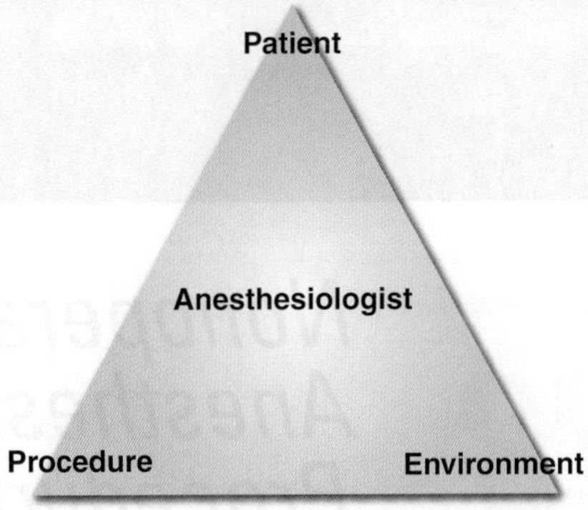

Figure 38-1 A simple three-step paradigm for nonoperating room anesthesia.

B. The Procedure

Common NOR procedures for which the patient may require anesthesia or sedation are listed in (Table 38-2). The anesthesiologist must understand all the details of the NOR procedure, specifically the position the patient will be in, how painful the procedure will be, how long it will take, and any special requirements (such as use of contrast media or the need to wake the patient up halfway through). ***Preoperative communication*** with the proceduralist is essential and must include discussion of contingency plans for emergencies and complications.

VIDEO 38-1
Anesthesia in Remote Locations

C. The Environment

Unlike in operating rooms, the conditions under which NORA services are delivered may vary greatly in terms of the space, equipment, and staff available. A number of factors contribute to NORA sites being unfamiliar and less optimal environments for anesthesia providers (Fig. 38-2):

1. These locations were often designed before or without considering whether anesthesia would be needed for patients undergoing care. Access to the patient by the anesthesia provider is often limited by diagnostic and therapeutic equipment such as CT and MRI scanners, fluoroscopes, or endoscopy towers.
2. Hazards unique to specific locations exist such as radiation in fluoroscopy and CT and the magnetic field in MRI.

Table 38-1 Patient Factors Requiring Sedation or Anesthesia for Nonoperating Room Procedures
• Claustrophobia, anxiety, and panic disorders
• Cerebral palsy, developmental delay, and learning difficulties
• Seizure disorders, movement disorders, and muscular contractures
• Pain, related to the procedure or the positioning, or unrelated pain
• Acute trauma with unstable cardiovascular, respiratory, or neurologic function
• Increased intracranial pressure
• Significant comorbidity and patient frailty (American Society of Anesthesiologists grades III and IV)
• Child's age, especially children <10 years old

Table 38-2	Common Nonoperating Room Anesthesia Procedures
Radiologic imaging	Computed tomography Magnetic resonance imaging Positron emission tomography
Diagnostic and therapeutic interventional radiology	Various vascular imaging, stenting, and embolization procedures Radiofrequency ablation Transjugular intrahepatic portosystemic shunt

Diagnostic and therapeutic interventional neuroradiology	Occlusive ("closing") procedures
	    Embolization of cerebral aneurysm/arteriovenous malformations/
	        highly vascular tumors (e.g., meningiomas)
	Opening procedures
	    Angioplasty/stenting/thrombolysis in stroke or cerebral vasospasm

Radiotherapy	Radiation therapy Intraoperative radiotherapy Diagnostic and therapeutic interventional cardiology
Cardiac catheterization laboratory	Diagnostic cardiac catheterization Percutaneous coronary interventions Interventional techniques for structural heart disease Transcatheter aortic valve implantation or replacement Placement of left ventricular cardiac assist devices for hemodynamic support
Electrophysiology laboratory	Electrophysiology studies and radiofrequency ablation Implantation of biventricular pacing systems and cardioverter defibrillators
Other Procedures	Cardioversion and transesophageal echocardiography
Diagnostic and therapeutic interventional gastroenterology	Upper gastroenterology endoscopy Esophageal dilatation or stenting Percutaneous endoscopic gastrostomy tube placement Endoscopic retrograde cholangiopancreatography Colonoscopy Liver biopsy
Psychiatry	Electroconvulsive therapy
Dentistry	Dental extractions Restorative dentistry

3. Proceduralists and ancillary staff may be unfamiliar with the requirements for safe anesthesia care and how to assist anesthesia providers when a difficulty is encountered.
4. Away from the operating room, immediate help from anesthesia colleagues in case of emergency may not be readily available.

The American Society of Anesthesiologists (ASA) has developed *standards* for NORA (1). Prior to the anesthetic, the presence and proper functioning of all equipment needed for safe patient care must be established; this is described in Table 38-3.

The location of immediately available resuscitation equipment should be noted and protocols developed with the local staff for dealing with

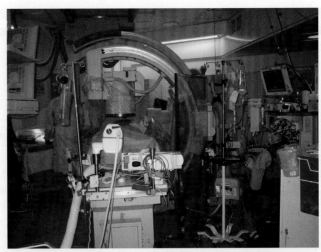

Figure 38-2 A radiology suite showing a C-arm and the high density of equipment that may separate the anesthesiologist from the patient.

emergencies, including cardiopulmonary resuscitation and the management of anaphylaxis.

II. Standards of Care for Nonoperating Room Anesthesia

Many NOR procedures are performed under *sedation* or *monitored anesthesia care*. Anesthesia care may be thought of as a continuum, with a gradual transition from the awake state, through progressively deepening sedation to general anesthesia (Table 38-4) (2).

As sedation deepens, progressive blunting of the airway reflexes, with the potential for airway obstruction, together with depression of spontaneous ventilation can ensue. The individual responsiveness of patients to different sedative agents varies, as do the levels of stimulation during the course of a procedure. Consequently, during the course of a NOR procedure under sedation, the patient may drift to a deeper level than is intended, resulting in airway and respiratory depression. It is, therefore, essential that the person providing sedation be properly trained to care for a patient who drifts to a deeper level of sedation than the level originally intended.

At the conclusion of the NOR procedure, the patient should be transported by a member of the anesthesia team to a recovery area that is equipped to the same standards as for all postoperative patients.

III. Adverse Events

Significant adverse events in NORA are rare; however, the number of deaths associated with NORA is higher than for operating room anesthesia (3). Complications related to the airway and respiratory system, such as airway obstruction and respiratory depression as a result of oversedation, are the most common complications associated with NORA. This is particularly relevant in patients with obstructive sleep apnea, who are more prone to airway and respiratory complications during and after anesthesia and sedation.

? Did You Know
The same standards for operating rooms should be applied to patients being cared for in all nonoperating room sites.

? Did You Know
More than 80% of surgical patients are unaware that they have obstructive sleep apnea prior to undergoing surgery.

Table 38-3	American Society of Anesthesiologists' Standards for Nonoperating Room Anesthesia Locations

1. Oxygen-reliable source and full backup E-cylinder

2. Suction adequate and reliable and meets operating room standards

3. Scavenging system if inhalational agents are administered

4. Anesthetic equipment
   - Backup self-inflating bag capable of delivering at least 90% oxygen by positive-pressure ventilation
   - Adequate anesthetic drugs and supplies
   - Anesthesia machine with equivalent function to those in the operating rooms and maintained to the same standards
   - Adequate monitoring equipment to allow adherence to the ASA standards for basic monitoring

5. Electrical outlets
   - Sufficient for anesthesia machine and monitors
   - Isolated electrical power or ground fault circuit interrupters if "wet location"

6. Adequate illumination of patient, anesthesia machine, and monitoring equipment
   - Battery-operated backup light source

7. Sufficient space for:
   - Personnel and equipment
   - Easy and expeditious access to patient, anesthesia machine, and monitoring equipment

8. Resuscitation equipment immediately available
   - Defibrillator/emergency drugs/cardiopulmonary resuscitation equipment

9. Adequately trained staff to support the anesthesiologist and a reliable means of two-way communication

10. All building and safety codes and facility standards should be observed

11. Postanesthesia care facilities:
    - Adequately trained staff to provide postanesthesia care
    - Appropriate equipment to allow safe transport to main postanesthesia care unit

ASA, American Society of Anesthesiologists.
From Statement on Nonoperating Room Anesthetizing Locations. Committee of Origin: Standards and Practice Parameters. Approved by the ASA House of Delegates on October 19, 1994 and last amended on October 16, 2013. Available at: www.asahq.org/For-Members/Standards-Guidelines-and-Statements.aspx.

IV. Environmental Considerations for Nonoperating Room Anesthesia

A. X-rays and Fluoroscopy

Fluoroscopy (C-arm) is widely used in many NOR locations, including interventional radiology, cardiac catheterization, electrophysiological procedures, and in the gastroenterology suite. The C-arm moves back and forth around the patient during the procedure, requiring large amounts of space, limiting access to the patient, and serving as a means of dislodging intravenous lines and endotracheal tubes (Fig. 38-2).

B. Computed Tomography

The CT procedure is painless, and most adults do not require sedation or anesthesia. For children or adults with neurologic or psychological disorders, sedation or anesthesia may be required. CT scanning may be employed to facilitate invasive and painful procedures such as abscess localization and drainage and

Table 38-4   Definition of General Anesthesia and Levels of Sedation or Analgesia

Vital Sign	Minimal Sedation (*Anxiolysis*)	Moderate Sedation (*Conscious Sedation*)	Deep Sedation	General Anesthesia
Responsiveness	Normal response to verbal stimulation	Purposeful response to verbal or tactile stimulation	Purposeful response after repeated or painful stimulation	Unarousable, even with painful stimulus
Airway	Unaffected	No intervention required	Intervention may be required	Intervention often required
Spontaneous ventilation	Unaffected	Adequate	May be inadequate	Frequently inadequate
Cardiovascular function	Unaffected	Usually maintained	Usually maintained	May be impaired

From Practice guidelines for sedation and analgesia by non-anesthesiologists. An updated report by the American Society of Anesthesiologists task force on sedation and analgesia by non-anesthesiologists. *Anesthesiology.* 2002;96:1004–1017.

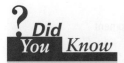

Always secure the airway and resuscitate hemodynamically unstable patients before they undergo CT or any other form of emergency diagnostic imaging!

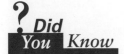

The intensity of the radiation is inversely proportional to the *square* of the distance from the source (the inverse square law).

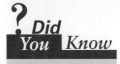

Thirty percent of adult patients experience some degree of anxiety during MRI scanning.

ablation of tumors. Patients with acute thoracic, abdominal, and cerebral trauma often require urgent imaging to facilitate diagnosis. These patients may develop hemorrhagic shock, increased intracranial pressure (ICP), depression of consciousness, and cardiac arrest while in the CT scanner.

Hazards of Ionizing Radiation

The effects of *ionizing radiation* on biologic tissues are classified as deterministic (severity of tissue damage is dose dependent, such as in cataract or infertility) and stochastic (probability of occurrence is dose related, such as in cancer or genetic effect) (4). Protective measures to reduce patient exposure to radiation should always be taken. Staff exposure to radiation can be minimized by:

1. Limiting the time of exposure to radiation
2. Increasing the distance from the source of radiation
3. Using protective shielding (lead aprons, thyroid shields, and leaded eyeglasses)
4. Using dosimeters.

C. Magnetic Resonance Imaging

MRI, like CT, is painless and does not require sedation or anesthesia (5). However, the scanning sequences are considerably longer than for CT, so a scan of ≥30 minutes for younger children as well as adults with neurologic or psychological disorders, including claustrophobia, often requires sedation or anesthesia.

Hazards of Magnetic Resonance Imaging

MRI is devoid of the risks related to ionizing radiation. However, magnetizable materials and electronic devices represent potential hazards to the patient and staff. For example, cardiac pacemakers may malfunction, intracerebral aneurysm clips may move, and transdermal medication patches may cause burns. Before entering the vicinity of the magnet, patients and staff need to complete a rigorous checklist to ensure they are not carrying any ferrometallic objects. Ferromagnetic equipment such as intravenous poles, gas cylinders, laryngoscopes, and pens become potentially lethal projectiles if brought too close to the magnetic field. Patient monitors, ventilators, and electrical infusion pumps may malfunction in proximity to the scanner, and magnet-safe technology is available for these times. In the case of an emergency, resuscitation attempts should take place outside the scanner because equipment such as laryngoscopes and cardiac defibrillators cannot be taken close to the magnet.

D. Intravenous Contrast Agents

Intravenous contrast agents are commonly used in CT and MRI scans to highlight organs, vessels, and tumors. Adverse reactions to contrast agents may occur and can be divided into renal adverse reactions and hypersensitivity reactions.

Renal Adverse Reactions

Contrast agents are eliminated via the kidneys, and patients with pre-existing chronic renal disease, diabetes mellitus, dehydration, advanced age, and concomitant use of nephrotoxic drugs (e.g., nonsteroidal anti-inflammatory drugs) are at risk of developing contrast-induced nephropathy. Preventative measures against contrast-induced nephropathy include adequate hydration, maintaining a good urine output, and using sodium bicarbonate infusions to improve elimination of the contrast agent. Gadolinium-containing contrast agents used in MRI scans may cause nephrogenic systemic fibrosis in patients with renal insufficiency.

Hypersensitivity Reactions

Hypersensitivity reactions to contrast media are divided into immediate (<1 hour) and nonimmediate (>1 hour) reactions. The clinical manifestations of various hypersensitivity reactions to contrast media are outlined in Table 38-5. Treatment of moderate and severe immediate hypersensitivity reactions is identical to that of anaphylaxis.

> **? Did You Know**
>
> MRI field strength is measured in the units Gauss (G) and Tesla (T). 1T = 10,000 G. The Earth's magnetic field is approximately 0.3 to 0.7 G, whereas the standard MRI generates a field of 1.5 to 3T!!

V. Specific Nonoperating Room Procedures

A. Diagnostic and Interventional Radiology

Angiography

Angiography causes minimal discomfort and may be performed under local anesthesia with or without light sedation (6). Lengthy procedures and patients

Table 38-5	Clinical Manifestations of Immediate and Nonimmediate Hypersensitivity Reactions to Radiocontrast Agents	
Immediate Reactions	**Nonimmediate Reactions**
Pruritus	**Pruritus**
Urticaria	**Exanthema (mostly macular or maculopapular drug eruption)**
Angioedema/facial edema	Urticaria, angioedema
Abdominal pain, nausea, diarrhea	Erythema multiforme minor
Rhinitis (sneezing, rhinorrhea)	Fixed drug eruption
Hoarseness, cough	Stevens-Johnson syndrome
Dyspnea (bronchospasm, laryngeal edema)	Toxic epidermal necrolysis
Respiratory arrest	Graft-versus-host reaction
Hypotension, cardiovascular shock	Drug-related eosinophilia with systemic symptoms
Cardiac arrest	Symmetrical drug-related intertriginous and flexural exanthema
	Vasculitis

Note: Most frequent reactions are in bold.

with recent cerebral vascular accidents, depressed levels of consciousness, or raised ICP may necessitate anesthesia with formal airway protection (tracheal intubation).

Interventional Neuroradiology
Endovascular embolization may be used to treat cerebral aneurysms, arteriovenous malformations, and certain vascular tumors such as meningiomas. General anesthesia and conscious sedation are both suitable techniques for interventional neuroradiology depending on the complexity of the procedure, the need for blood pressure manipulation, and the requirement for neurologic assessment during the procedure.

Radiofrequency Ablation
CT-guided percutaneous radiofrequency ablation (RFA) is carried out for treatment of primary and metastatic tumors in solid organs. One-lung ventilation and high-frequency jet ventilation may be used in patients for RFA of liver tumors to minimize motion associated with diaphragm excursions from standard ventilation.

Transjugular Intrahepatic Portosystemic Shunt
A transjugular intrahepatic portosystemic shunt (TIPS) procedure is carried out using fluoroscopy and is performed to help alleviate portal hypertension in patients with advanced cirrhosis. The procedure may be performed under sedation or general anesthesia. Patients presenting for a TIPS procedure, in general, have significant hepatic dysfunction and require careful preoperative assessment and intraoperative management.

B. Radiation Therapy
External beam radiation is a common treatment for children with malignancies (Table 38-6) (7). The doses of radiation used are very high, and all personnel must leave the room during the treatment. An interfaced system of closed-circuit television, telemetric microphones, and standard monitoring is used to allow close observation of the patient during the procedure. Complete absence of movement is crucial during radiation therapy and general anesthesia or deep sedation techniques, with propofol the anesthetic of choice during these procedures.

C. Interventional Cardiology
Diagnostic and therapeutic interventional procedures are carried out in the cardiac catheterization laboratory (*cath lab*) and the electrophysiology laboratory (*EP lab*) (8). These procedures are outlined in Table 38-2. Light or

Table 38-6   Common Radiosensitive Tumors in Children
Primary CNS tumor: neuroblastoma, medulloblastoma
Acute leukemia: CNS leukemia
Ocular tumors: retinoblastoma
Intra-abdominal tumors: Wilms' tumor
Rhabdomyosarcoma
Other tumors: Langerhans cell histiocytosis

CNS, central nervous system.

moderate sedation is commonly used under supervision of the cardiologist. However, general anesthesia is increasingly required for more lengthy and complex procedures. The ability to move the patient rapidly to the operating room and the availability of cardiopulmonary bypass are essential backups for cath lab and EP lab procedures.

Electrophysiologic studies (EPS) and ablation of abnormal conduction pathways are performed for the treatment of dysrhythmias caused by aberrant conduction pathways. EPS are lengthy and can cause discomfort, especially when intraoperative dysrhythmias are provoked by the procedure and then terminated using overdrive pacing, or if unsuccessful, by external cardioversion. Despite the fact that volatile anesthetic agents may interfere with cardiac conduction, these agents can be successfully used during EPS and cardiac ablation procedures.

D. Cardioversion

Transthoracic cardioversion is commonly used electively to treat dysrhythmias, especially atrial fibrillation and atrial flutter. Cardioversion takes a few seconds; however, it is distressing, and deep sedation is preferable except in life-threatening situations. A small bolus of intravenous induction agent such as propofol or etomidate is usually sufficient for the procedure.

E. Nonoperating Room Pediatric Cardiac Procedures

Cardiac catheterization is performed in children with congenital heart disease for both hemodynamic assessment and interventional procedures. These children are often very sick and may present with cyanosis, dyspnea, congestive heart failure, and intracardiac shunts. In patients with a patent ductus arteriosus, high oxygen tension can lead to premature closure, and prostaglandin infusions are often used to maintain duct patency.

F. Gastroenterology

Procedures commonly performed in the gastrointestinal endoscopy suite are outlined in Table 38-2. The majority of these procedures may be performed with light sedation (commonly fentanyl and midazolam or propofol infusion) without the involvement of an anesthesiologist.

Gastroenterologists, however, universally agree that patients in ASA classes III and IV who are undergoing complex procedures or have histories of adverse or inadequate responses to sedation require the care of an anesthesiologist.

The patient's condition and the specific procedure determine the anesthetic technique to be used. Local anesthetic is sprayed into the oropharynx to facilitate passage of the endoscope. This can abolish the gag reflex and increase the risk of aspiration. Under general anesthesia, patients usually require tracheal intubation to protect the proximal airway, which is shared with the endoscope during the procedure.

G. Electroconvulsive Therapy

Electroconvulsive therapy (ECT) has been used in the management of severe depression, mania, and affective disorders (9). Patients typically undergo a series of regular treatments (three times a week for 6 to 12 treatments, followed by weekly or monthly maintenance). The procedures are usually performed in the postanesthesia care unit, where there is close access to anesthesia support service. Alternately, they may be performed in the psychiatric unit where these services may not be so readily available. ECT is distressing and possibly dangerous because generalized convulsions may result in limb injuries and significant cardiovascular reactions may occur. Light general anesthesia

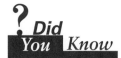

Did You Know

Transcatheter aortic valve implantation or replacement allows replacement of the aortic valve percutaneously in the cath lab. Patients in their 80s and 90s who are too sick for open heart surgery may be treated successfully!

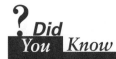

Did You Know

Pay meticulous attention to preventing air bubbles entering intravenous lines shunts in children with right-to-left shunts because they may cross to the arterial circulation, causing stroke or cardiac arrest.

with muscle relaxation, usually provided with the short-acting muscle relaxant succinylcholine, is used to mitigate the unpleasant effects of a generalized seizure. The anesthesiologist should be aware of the patient's medication regimes because drug interactions between anesthetic agents and psychotropic medications, particularly monoamine oxidase inhibitors, may be occur. Skillful airway management using bag and mask ventilation is usually sufficient to maintain oxygenation during anesthesia for ECT.

References

1. Statement on Nonoperating Room Anesthetizing Locations. Committee of Origin: Standards and Practice Parameters. Approved by the ASA House of Delegates on October 19, 1994 and last amended on October 16, 2013. Available at: www.asahq.org/For-Members/Standards-Guidelines-and-Statements.aspx.
2. Practice guidelines for sedation and analgesia by non-anesthesiologists. An updated report by the American Society of Anesthesiologists task force on sedation and analgesia by non-anesthesiologists. *Anesthesiology*. 2002;96:1004–1017.
3. Metzner J, Posner KL, Domino KB. The risk and safety of anesthesia at remote locations: The US closed claims analysis. *Curr Opin Anaesthesiol*. 2009;22:502–508.
4. Miller DL, Vañó E, Bartal G, et al. Occupational radiation protection in interventional radiology: A joint guideline of the Cardiovascular and Interventional Radiology Society of Europe and the Society of Interventional Radiology. *Cardiovasc Intervent Radiol*. 2010;33:230–239.
5. Veenith T, Coles JP. Anesthesia for magnetic resonance imaging and positron emission tomography. *Curr Opin Anaesthesiol*. 2011;24:451–458.
6. Varma MK, Price K, Jayakrishnan V, et al. Anaesthetic considerations for interventional neuroradiology. *Br J Anaesth*. 2007;99:75–85.
7. McFadyen GJ, Pelly N, Orr RJ. Sedation and anesthesia for the pediatric patient undergoing radiotherapy. *Curr Opin Anaesthesiol*. 2011;24:433–438.
8. Faillace, RT, Kaddaha R, Bikkina R, et al. The role of the out-of-operating room anesthesiologist in the care of the cardiac patient. *Anesthesiol Clin*. 2009;27:29–46.
9. Ding Z, White PF. Anesthesia for electroconvulsive therapy. *Anesth Analg*. 2002;94:1351.

Questions

1. What are the most common complications associated with NORA?
   A. Airway obstruction and respiratory depression
   B. Tachycardia and hypertension
   C. Pain and agitation
   D. Nausea and vomiting

2. When a patient inside the MRI machine requires resuscitation, the following procedure should be followed:
   A. Turn off the magnet before entering the MRI scanner room to resuscitate the patient
   B. Immediately bring an external defibrillator into the MRI scanner room
   C. Remove the patient from the MRI scanner room prior to resuscitation
   D. Those responding to the emergency should don protective lead aprons prior to entering the MRI scanner room

3. Anesthesia for electroconvulsive therapy requires the administration of a muscle relaxant because:
   A. It is imperative to intubate the trachea
   B. Patients having seizures should receive muscle relaxants to stop movement caused by the seizure
   C. Use of muscle relaxants creates a more hemodynamically stable treatment
   D. Electrical stimulation of the motor cortex causes violent muscle contraction

4. Adult patients undergoing MRI scans may need monitored anesthesia care because:
   A. They experience anxiety in the MRI scanner
   B. MRI scanning can be painful for some patients
   C. 30% of patients undergoing MRI scans have psychiatric diagnoses
   D. Patients frequently experience airway obstruction in the MRI scanner

39 *Postoperative Recovery*

Roger S. Mecca

I. Selecting Appropriate Postoperative Care

The appropriate level of postoperative care should be determined by the patient's underlying illness, the complexity of anesthesia and surgery, and the potential associated complications. Matching the level of care with need improves patient satisfaction and optimizes postanesthesia care unit (PACU) use without affecting quality or safety. Patients should be individualized regardless of whether they are inpatients or outpatients. If patients meet PACU discharge criteria after surgery, regardless of whether they have had deep sedation, regional anesthesia, or general anesthesia, they could possibly go directly to lower intensity recovery settings, although pain or postoperative nausea and vomiting (PONV) often precludes PACU bypass. If any doubt exists about safety, patients should be admitted to a full-service PACU.

II. Admission to the Postanesthesia Care Unit

Upon arrival in the PACU, the anesthesiologist should provide a thorough, yet concise, report on the patient (Table 39-1). As a minimum of care upon a patient's arrival in the PACU, vital signs, airway patency, ventilation, oxygen saturation, and level of pain should be documented initially, then three times every 5 minutes and every 15 minutes thereafter. Temperature, level of consciousness, mental status, neuromuscular function, hydration status, and degree of nausea should be assessed at least on admission and again at discharge. The patient should be continuously monitored with a pulse oximeter and a single-lead electrocardiogram. Capnography should be used when appropriate, and diagnostic tests should be ordered when indicated.

III. Postoperative Pain Management

Effective control of surgical pain with minimal side effects during and beyond the PACU interval should be a high priority, even if large doses of analgesics are necessary (see Chapter 37). The correlation between the patient's

733

Table 39-1	Items to Consider upon Postanesthesia Care Unit Admission
Underlying medical illness, chronic medications, pertinent previous surgery	
Medication allergies or reactions, nothing by mouth status, premedications	
Surgical procedure, type of anesthetic, ancillary nerve blocks	
Time and amount of opioids, relaxants, reversal agents, local anesthetics	
Estimated blood loss, urine output, crystalloid or blood component replacement	
Intraoperative vital sign ranges, laboratory findings, unexpected events	
Other drugs (e.g., steroids, diuretics, antibiotics, vasoactive medications)	
Airway patency, ventilatory adequacy, level of consciousness, level of pain	
Acceptable ranges for vital signs and monitored parameters, therapeutic endpoints	
Anticipated cardiovascular, respiratory, or renal problems	
Indwelling devices (intravenous, intraarterial, or epidural catheters)	
If intubated, endotracheal tube position, plans for ventilation and extubation	
Orders for therapeutic interventions, diagnostic tests, how to contact the responsible physician	

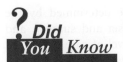

Did You Know

Opioids are relatively ineffective sedatives, and benzodiazepines are ineffective analgesics. It is important to choose the correct class of drug when treating postoperative pain and/or anxiety.

Did You Know

Some PACU discharge criteria, such as ability to void or recovery from a peripheral nerve block, can be bypassed following a few procedures in selected patients, but the patients must be given explicit instructions and capable of following them.

perception of pain and observed sympathetic nervous system (SNS) response varies widely due to cardiovascular, psychological, and cultural factors. Assessment of discomfort is difficult and imprecise. Use of a *quantitative pain scale* yields more reliable results. PACU staff should ensure that the nature and intensity of the patient's pain are appropriate so as to avoid masking an evolving complication. For example, tachycardia or hypertension can reflect pain, but they can also be caused by hypoxemia, cerebral hypoperfusion, or hypovolemia. Administration of analgesia may accentuate these phenomena. Fear and anxiety accentuate pain, so titration of an intravenous sedative such as midazolam may be a useful adjunct to analgesics.

IV. Discharge Criteria

Prior to PACU discharge, patients should be assessed using consistent criteria that ensure that the patient will have *sufficient reserve* to tolerate minor deterioration after discharge (Table 39-2). Simple scoring systems exist, such as the Aldrete scale, which quantifies physical status and vital sign thresholds, but they lack sensitivity and specificity for identifying subtle problems. Oxygen saturation as measured by pulse oximetry (SpO$_2$) should be satisfactory while the patient breathes room air prior to discharge. Inpatients and selected ambulatory patients can be discharged before they void if urination is carefully tracked after discharge.

V. Postoperative Hypotension

There are multiple causes for hypotension in the PACU. Hypotension causes hypoperfusion of vital organs, anaerobic metabolism, and lactic acidemia. Symptoms referable to the brain or heart (e.g., disorientation, nausea, unconsciousness,

Table 39-2   Guidelines for Postanesthesia Care Unit Discharge

Oriented, adequate muscular strength, and mobility for minimal self-care

Control of nausea, emesis, agitation, and pain: temperature >97 °F, shivering resolved

Vital signs 20% or more of preoperative value, stable for 30 minutes

Urine output >30 mL/hr

Ventilatory rate >10, <30 breaths/min, SpO_2 >93%

Airway patency acceptable, protective reflexes (swallow, gag) intact

Control of surgical complications (e.g., bleeding, edema, pulses)

Exacerbation of pre-existing conditions (e.g., bronchospasm, myocardial ischemia, hyperglycemia)

Test results (e.g., hematocrit, blood glucose, electrolytes, chest radiograph, electrocardiogram)

Destination unit appropriate for patient's status and likely clinical course

SpO_2, oxygen saturation as measured by pulse oximetry.
Note: Not all criteria will be satisfied by every patient. Clinical judgment supersedes guidelines.

angina) indicate that the patient's ability to compensate for hypotension is exhausted. Morbidity is higher in patients with chronic hypertension, arteriosclerotic disease, increased intracranial pressure (ICP), and renal insufficiency.

Low intravascular volume (absolute hypovolemia) caused by inadequate replacement of fluid deficits and blood loss decreases cardiac output. SNS-mediated tachycardia, vasoconstriction, and venoconstriction compensate for a 15% to 20% deficit before hypotension occurs. In hypothermic patients, rewarming often unmasks hypovolemia. A "normal" intravascular volume can be inadequate to maintain blood pressure (relative hypovolemia) if increased venous capacity (histamine release, sympathectomy), thoracic vein compression (positive pressure ventilation, tension pneumothorax), or pericardial tamponade impair venous return. Using urine output to assess intravascular volume can be misleading. Impaired renal tubular concentrating ability or glycosuria can maintain output despite hypovolemia.

Hypotension caused by ventricular dysfunction often indicates acute myocardial ischemia precipitated by either tachycardia or inadequate diastolic pressure. Hypoxemia or anemia will exacerbate ischemia. Chest pain might be masked by analgesia or confused with surgical pain or gastric distention. Ischemia is sometimes silent in patients with diabetic neuropathy. The ST segment and T-wave morphology on electrocardiogram should be evaluated, as well as pulmonary artery pressures and echocardiography if available. Some patients with nonischemic cardiomyopathy require high left ventricular end diastolic pressure and elevated SNS activity to maintain blood pressure. Right ventricle dysfunction caused by pulmonary thromboembolism often presents with hypotension.

Heart rate below 40 to 45 beats per minute (sinus or nodal bradycardia, complete heart block) decreases both cardiac output and blood pressure. A tachydysrhythmia above 140 to 150 beats per minute (bpm) can compromise ventricular filling, especially if atrial kick is absent. Changes in heart rate place patients with aortic or mitral stenosis at particular risk of hypotension.

Decreased systemic vascular resistance from regional anesthesia, α-adrenergic blockade, warming, or sepsis may also generate hypotension. Rarely, hypotension reflects acute steroid deficiency.

Indications to treat hypotension include symptoms of vital organ hypoperfusion or a 20% to 30% reduction of blood pressure (BP) below preoperative levels. *Tighter control* of BP is indicated in high-risk patients. Always ensure that hypotension is real before treating. A BP cuff that is too large or a transducer that is improperly calibrated may yield false values. Before administering potent drugs to treat BP, consider using simple maneuvers (e.g., repositioning, reducing airway pressure) when appropriate. A 500-mL crystalloid infusion often improves hypotension in the PACU because hypovolemia is by far the most common etiology. Plasma expanders or blood products may be required in some circumstances. Administration of an α-adrenergic pressor (e.g., phenylephrine) may provide temporary support of BP until sufficient volume is infused. Treat myocardial ischemia with control of precipitating factors, support of diastolic pressure, β-adrenergic blocking agents, and nitrates. Bradycardia usually responds to atropine, glycopyrrolate, or ephedrine. Refractory bradycardia should be managed with epinephrine or with cardiac pacing.

VI. Postoperative Hypertension

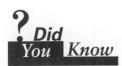
? Did You Know

Non-invasive measurement of BP requires a properly fitting cuff. A cuff that is too wide will yield falsely low values, and one that is too narrow will yield falsely high values.

Moderate hypertension in response to noxious stimuli (pain, surgical stress) is common in the PACU. High BP can increase blood loss, ventricular wall tension, and intraocular or ICP. *Indications* to treat hypertension include a BP 20% to 30% above preoperative baseline, an unusual risk of morbidity (e.g., increased ICP, mitral regurgitation, open eye injury), or evidence of complications (e.g., bleeding, headache, visual changes, ischemia). As in the case of hypotension, a BP cuff that is too small or an improperly calibrated transducer can yield erroneously high BP values. The treatment of hypertension in the PACU should be aimed at addressing causes of increased SNS activity. Common causes include pain, anxiety, or a full bladder. If hypertension persists, intravenous antihypertensive medications such as labetalol, esmolol, hydralazine, or nicardipine can achieve temporary control. Potent vasodilators such as nitroprusside or nitroglycerin should be reserved for refractory or profound hypertension.

VII. Inadequate Ventilation

Unfortunately, hypoventilation is *common* in the PACU. Frequent causes include residual effects of inhaled anesthetics or opioids, residual neuromuscular relaxation, pain, respiratory secretions, airway edema, hypothermia, and physical limitations to breathing associated with the surgical procedure (e.g., increased abdominal pressure).

Elevated exhaled carbon dioxide (CO_2) or arterial partial pressure of CO_2 ($PaCO_2$) usually reflects hypoventilation (see "Acid–Base Disorders" below). Ventilation is likely to be inadequate if (a) hypercarbia occurs coincident with tachypnea, anxiety, dyspnea, or increased SNS activity; (b) if the arterial pH falls below 7.30; or (c) if there is a progressive decrease in arterial pH.

Hypoventilation can also result from airway obstruction, increased airway resistance, or decreased lung compliance. High resistance to gas flow increases the work of breathing and CO_2 production. If inspiratory muscles cannot maintain sufficient ventilation, respiratory acidemia and hypoxemia occur. Increased upper airway resistance or obstruction can occur in the pharynx (posterior tongue displacement, edema, soft tissue collapse, secretions), the larynx (laryngospasm, edema), or the large airways (extrinsic compression, tracheal stenosis). Initial assessment and treatment of these problems should include arousal of the patient, lateral head positioning, chin lift, mandibular advancement, airway suctioning, or placement of an oropharyngeal or nasopharyngeal airway. Soft tissue edema may respond to nebulized racemic epinephrine. During emergence, pharyngeal or vocal cord stimulation can generate laryngospasm, especially in patients who smoke, have had recent upper respiratory infections, or have undergone upper airway surgery. Laryngospasm can usually be effectively treated with mandibular advancement and positive pressure ventilation with oxygen and a tight-fitting mask. Rarely, a small dose of succinylcholine (0.1 mg/kg) may be required. Pathologic upper airway obstruction, such as an impingement from an expanding hematoma, might require emergency decompression of the hematoma, tracheal intubation, or cricothyroidotomy. Pharyngeal or tracheal stimulation can trigger reflex bronchospasm in patients with reactive airways, as can histamine release. Flow might be so impeded that no wheezing is appreciated. To treat, administer albuterol via an inhaler. Some patients may require an anticholinergic medication such as ipratropium. If bronchospasm is life-threatening, administer an intravenous epinephrine infusion.

Low pulmonary compliance causes respiratory muscle fatigue, hypoventilation, and respiratory acidemia. Collapsed airspaces are difficult to re-expand. Excess lung water increases the lung's inertia and elevates surface tension. Extrathoracic factors such as adipose tissue, tight dressings, intragastric gas, or high intra-abdominal pressure impair thoracic expansion. Placement of the patient in a semisitting position may be useful to improve compliance. Note that signs of increased airway resistance mimic those of decreased compliance. Spontaneously breathing patients exhibit labored ventilation, while mechanically ventilated patients exhibit high peak inspiratory pressures.

VIII. Neuromuscular Problems

Residual paralysis compromises ventilation, airway patency, and airway protection. Partial paralysis is also dangerous because a somnolent patient with mild stridor and shallow ventilation might be overlooked, promoting insidious hypoventilation or aspiration. Overdosing patients with nondepolarizing relaxants or incomplete reversal after surgery can lead to residual weakness in the PACU. Neuromuscular abnormalities (myasthenia gravis) or medications (antibiotics, furosemide, phenytoin) can prolong the action of relaxants. In addition to the use of a nerve stimulator, recovery from muscle relaxants in the PACU can be assessed by observing sustained supine head elevation, a vital capacity of 10 to 12 mL/kg, or an inspiratory pressure more negative than –25 cm H_2O. Occasionally, painful chest expansion, thoracic restriction, low compliance, or hyperventilation will generate dyspnea, labored breathing, or rapid, shallow breathing that can mimic ventilatory insufficiency due to residual paralysis.

IX. Postoperative Hypoxemia

Arterial partial pressure of oxygen (PaO_2) is the best indicator of pulmonary oxygen transfer. Pulse oximetry, although easy to measure, yields less information on the alveolar–arterial gradient. A PaO_2 above 80 mm Hg (93% saturation) with an acceptable hemoglobin level ensures adequate oxygen content, but the lowest acceptable PaO_2 varies among individuals. Elevating PaO_2 above 110 mm Hg (100% saturation) offers little benefit because the additional oxygen dissolved in plasma is negligible. Elevating PaO_2 to above normal levels can also *mask dangerous hypoventilation*. That is, $PaCO_2$ may be quite high yet the patient will appear to be ventilating well because of a high arterial oxygen saturation. During mechanical ventilation, a PaO_2 above 80 mm Hg with 0.4 fraction of inspired oxygen and 5 cm H_2O continuous positive airway pressure usually predicts sustained oxygenation after extubation. Adequate PaO_2 does not guarantee that cardiac output, arterial pressure, or distribution of blood flow will maintain oxygen delivery. Lactic acidemia best reflects inadequate tissue oxygenation.

There are many causes for hypoxemia in the PACU. Loss of dependent lung volume causes maldistribution of ventilation, ventilation perfusion ($\dot{V}/\dot{Q}$) ratio mismatching, and hypoxemia. During surgery, obesity, abdominal retraction, peritoneal insufflation, or unusual positions reduce functional residual capacity (FRC), causing small airways to collapse and distal atelectasis. Older patients and those with obstructive airway disease often exhibit airway closure at end expiration. Right upper lobe atelectasis is frequent after inadvertent partial right endobronchial intubation. During one-lung anesthesia, parenchymal compression and lymphatic obstruction reduce dependent lung volume. Acute pulmonary edema from ventricular dysfunction or inspiratory efforts against an obstruction seriously compromises ($\dot{V}/\dot{Q}$) matching. Conservative measures to restore lung volume (semisitting position, analgesia) often improve oxygenation. Cough, incentive spirometry, chest physiotherapy, or face-mask continuous positive airway pressure (5 to 7 cm H_2O) help expand FRC.

Hypoxemia sometimes reflects a global reduction of alveolar partial pressure of oxygen (PAO_2) from severe hypoventilation. Complete upper airway obstruction or apnea will cause rapid reduction of PAO_2 at a rate that varies with age, body habitus, underlying illness, and initial PAO_2 (Fig. 39-1).

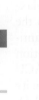

VIDEO 39-1

Apneic Oxygen Saturation

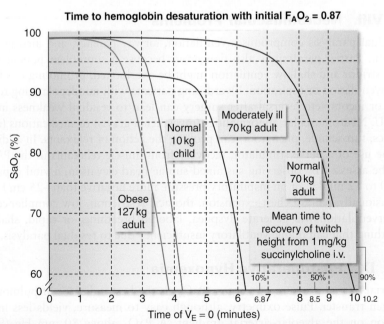

Figure 39-1 Rate of oxygen saturation as measure by pulse oximetry declines after onset of apnea. IV, intravenous; SaO_2, arterial oxygen saturation; FAO_2, alveolar fraction of oxygen; $\dot{V}_E$, expired volume per unit of time. (From Benumof JL, Dagg R, Benumof R: Critical hemoglobin desaturation will occur before return to an unparalyzed state following 1 mg/kg intravenous succinylcholine. *Anesthesiology.* 1997;87:979, with permission.)

Low venous oxygen content from decreased cardiac output, anemia, shivering, or hypermetabolism magnifies the impact of shunted blood on PaO_2 and increases oxygen extraction from poorly ventilated alveoli.

One cannot predict which patients will become hypoxemic during a stay in the PACU, so monitoring with oximetry is essential following most surgical procedures, particularly those where general anesthesia or deep sedation was employed. Patients arriving in the PACU should receive supplemental oxygen until such time they have been stabilized, they are able to maintain an airway, and ventilation is adequate. Cost, inconvenience, and risk of temporary oxygen administration is negligible. However, as mentioned above, oxygen may delay recognition of hypoventilation and does not address underlying causes of hypoxemia.

X. Postoperative Nausea and Vomiting

PONV is a *common and significant problem* in the PACU. In addition to the misery experienced by the patient, there may be a concomitant elevated heart rate, BP, and central venous pressure, which can increase morbidity, especially in patients with coronary artery disease or after ocular, tympanic, or intracranial procedures. Gagging and retching might also elicit parasympathetic nervous system responses with bradycardia and hypotension. Serious causes for PONV must be excluded, such as hypotension, hypoxemia, hypoglycemia, or increased ICP.

When treating PONV, it is often effective to *combine agents* with different sites of action such as serotonin blocking agents (ondansetron 4 mg) and dexamethasone (4 to 8 mg). Droperidol (1 to 2 µg/kg; 0.625 to 1.25 mg in adults) can be useful to treat breakthrough nausea, although mild sedation, transient restlessness, and hypotension can occur. Isolated cases of Q-T interval prolongation and cardiac dysrhythmia have decreased the use of this agent. Propofol's short-term antiemetic properties do not compare with the first-line antiemetics. Supplemental oxygen and hydration might reduce the incidence or severity of PONV, however, drinking beverages in the immediate postoperative period can be a triggering event.

XI. Perioperative Aspiration

The risk of pulmonary aspiration is elevated in the PACU due to PONV coupled with impaired airway reflexes from sedation or residual weakness. If patients have had their mandible wired following orofacial surgery, a wire cutter must be immediately available in the event the patient vomits or the airway obstructs. Aspiration of clear oral secretions is usually insignificant, but cough, tracheal irritation, or transient laryngospasm can occur. Aspirated sterile blood is cleared by mucociliary transport and phagocytosis, but clots can obstruct airways. Aspiration of acidic gastric contents is rare, but it can cause diffuse bronchospasm, atelectasis, and chemical pneumonitis. Morbidity increases directly with volume and inversely with the pH of the aspirate. Food particles obstruct airways and promote bacterial infection. After serious aspiration, epithelial degeneration with interstitial and alveolar edema rapidly progresses to acute respiratory distress syndrome with high-permeability pulmonary edema. Prevention is critical because effective therapy is limited. If gastric secretions are observed in the patient's pharynx, this should be immediately suctioned and the patient's head turned laterally. Tracheal intubation should be considered if airway reflexes are compromised. After intubation, suction the trachea before applying positive-pressure ventilation to avoid disseminating aspirate distally.

XII. Ability to Void, Oliguria, and Polyuria

Oliguria (≤0.5 mL/kg/hr) in the PACU usually reflects a normal renal response to hypovolemia but might indicate abnormal renal function, especially following intraoperative events such as severe hypotension or aortic cross-clamping, which can jeopardize renal function. Urinary retention is common after opioid administration, neuraxial regional anesthesia, and urologic, inguinal, or genital surgery. Measurement of bladder volume with a portable ultrasonic bladder scanning device can help to differentiate between the inability to void and oliguria. If indicated, urine can be checked for sodium and osmolarity, because a urine osmolarity >450 mOsm/L or a urine sodium concentration <50 meq/L indicates intact tubular concentrating ability. The initial treatment for suspected hypovolemia should be to administer 5 to 7 mL/kg intravenous crystalloid. If oliguria persists, consider a second fluid bolus or furosemide 5 mg intravenously. Persistence of oliguria despite adequate perfusion pressure, rehydration, and a furosemide challenge might indicate acute tubular necrosis. Profuse urine output in the PACU usually reflects generous intraoperative fluid administration, but osmotic diuresis caused by glycosuria is also seen. Sustained polyuria (4 to 5 mL/kg/hr) might reflect diabetes insipidus or high output renal failure, especially if diuresis compromises intravascular volume.

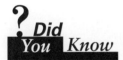

XIII. Acid–Base Disorders

Moderate respiratory acidemia (PaCO$_2$ 45 to 50 mm Hg, pH 7.36 to 7.32) is common due to the respiratory depressant effects of residual anesthetics, opioids, and sedatives. Central nervous system depression also blunts agitation, tachypnea, and SNS responses, which are usually seen with acidemia or hypoxemia. Patients with abnormal CO$_2$ or pH responses (e.g., morbid obesity, sleep apnea) are more sensitive to the respiratory depressant effects of drugs. Impaired mechanics of ventilation can also lead to hypercapnia, especially if shivering increases CO$_2$ production. Respiratory acidemia increases cerebral blood flow and ICP. The obvious treatment for respiratory acidemia is to improve ventilation. If dangerous hypoventilation from opioids is suspected, arouse the patient or carefully titrate intravenous naloxone (0.04 mg every 2 minutes, up to 0.12 mg).

Metabolic acidemia almost always reflects lactic acidemia from *insufficient tissue oxygenation.* Assess the patient for hypotension, hypoxemia, low cardiac output, hypothermia, severe anemia, or carbon monoxide poisoning. Occasionally, ketoacidosis occurs in type 1 diabetics, presenting with ketones in blood and urine. A spontaneously breathing patient should hyperventilate to compensate, but ventilatory depression from inhaled anesthetics and opioids blunts this response. To treat metabolic acidemia, the etiology must be resolved. Improving cardiac output, blood pressure, hypothermia, PaO$_2$, or hemoglobin concentration will reduce lactic acid production. Ketoacidosis is treated with intravenous crystalloids, insulin, glucose, and potassium. Renal excretion of hydrogen ions will then restore normal pH. For severe or progressive acidemia, intravenous bicarbonate or calcium gluconate might be necessary.

Transient respiratory alkalemia from hyperventilation is rare in the PACU but can be caused by pain, anxiety, stormy emergence reactions, or excessive mechanical ventilation. Respiratory alkalemia can cause confusion and dizziness. Treatment typically requires the administration of analgesics and sedatives for pain and anxiety. Metabolic alkalemia is rare unless alkalosis existed before surgery.

XIV. Glucose and Electrolyte Disorders

Moderate *hyperglycemia* (150 to 200 mg/dL) usually resolves spontaneously, but higher glucose levels cause glycosuria and osmotic diuresis. In type 1 diabetics, severe hyperglycemia causes ketoacidosis, increased serum osmolality, cerebral disequilibrium, and even hyperosmolar coma. Treatment consists of carefully titrated administration of insulin. *Hypoglycemia* can be a complication of overly aggressive treatment of hyperglycemia, but can be treated with intravenous 50% dextrose and a glucose infusion. Importantly, the signs of hypoglycemia are masked by both sedation and excessive SNS activity.

Hyponatremia occurs with respiratory uptake of nebulized water, inappropriate antidiuretic hormone secretion, or uptake of sodium-free irrigating solution during transurethral surgical procedures. Rarely, excessive infusion of isotonic saline leads to excretion of hypertonic urine and iatrogenic hyponatremia. Moderate hyponatremia causes agitation, disorientation, visual disturbances, and nausea, whereas severe hyponatremia causes unconsciousness, impaired airway reflexes, and grand mal seizures. Therapy includes intravenous normal saline and intravenous furosemide to promote free water excretion. Infusion of hypertonic saline should be used sparingly as it can cause central pontine myelinosis.

Hypokalemia is usually inconsequential but can cause serious dysrhythmias if exacerbated by acute respiratory alkalemia, insulin therapy, or beta-mimetic medications. Adding potassium to peripheral intravenous fluids or slowly infusing a concentrated solution through a central catheter may be necessary. *Hyperkalemia* often reflects a hemolyzed specimen or sampling near an intravenous containing potassium or banked blood. Severe hyperkalemia occurs in patients with rhabdomyolysis or malignant hyperthermia. Acute acidemia exacerbates hyperkalemia. Hyperventilation, hydration, beta-mimetic medications and intravenous insulin with glucose acutely lowers potassium, while intravenous calcium counters myocardial effects.

Symptomatic *hypocalcemia* seldom occurs in the PACU, although massive blood and fluid replacement reduces total-body and ionized calcium. Anesthesiologists should be alert for laryngospasm from hypocalcemia after parathyroid excision. Decreased ionized calcium during acute respiratory alkalemia, as during mechanical ventilation, may cause myocardial conduction and contractility abnormalities, decreased vascular tone, or tetany. Administration of calcium chloride or calcium gluconate to hypocalcemic patients improves cardiovascular dynamics.

XV. Incidental Trauma and Adverse Side Effects from Surgery

Corneal abrasion caused by drying or inadvertent eye contact is a common eye injury in the elderly, following lateral or prone positioning, and during head or neck surgery. Corneal injury can occur in the PACU if the eye is accidently scraped by a piece of apparatus. Abrasion causes tearing, decreased visual acuity, pain, and photophobia, but usually heals without scarring within 72 hours if the eye is taped shut. Regardless, it is prudent to obtain an ophthalmology consultation to evaluate the extent of injury. Autonomic side effects of medications administered in the perioperative period can impair visual acuity and accommodation, while residual ocular lubricants can cloud vision. It is important to be alert for visual impairment in patients who have had prolonged surgical procedures in the prone position. Ocular compression can impair retinal perfusion and cause blindness. Ischemic optic atrophy also occurs without compression.

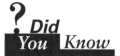
? Did You Know

While significant hyperglycemia is undesirable, overzealous treatment can potentially be worse. Sedation from residual anesthesia and SNS stimulation from pain or hypothermia can mask the signs of hypoglycemia. Frequent measurement of blood glucose is recommended.

Oral trauma can be caused by laryngoscope blades, surgical instruments, rigid airways, and dentition. Treat lip, tongue, or gum abrasions with icing and analgesia. Penetrating injury of soft tissue caught between teeth and rigid devices may require topical antibiotics. If dentition is damaged by airway manipulation or jaw clenching, obtain a dental consultation and observe for foreign body aspiration. Sore throat, unquenchable dryness, and hoarseness occur in up to 50% of patients after laryngoscopy and intubation, varying with degree of trauma, duration of intubation, and use of local anesthetic lubricants. This problem is also caused by suctioning, drying from inhalation of unhumidified gases, and placement of oral or laryngeal mask airways. Treat with cool mist therapy, analgesia, nebulized racemic epinephrine, or dexamethasone. Intubation can also cause temporomandibular joint dysfunction, hypoglossal, lingual, or recurrent laryngeal nerve damage, vocal cord evulsion, or tracheoesophageal perforation.

Intraoperative **nerve injuries** often manifest in the PACU. Spinal cord injury caused by neck positioning or by a hematoma after neuraxial regional block placement can cause acute motor deficits. Immediate radiologic evaluation and surgical consultation is indicated. Peripheral nerve compression or plexus stretch from hyperextension can lead to permanent sensory and motor impairment. Evaluate the patient for nerve damage with any complaint of nonsurgical discomfort, numbness, or weakness and with any bruising or skin breakdown. Many neuropathies have no identifiable cause (see Chapter 22).

Postdural puncture headache can occur after subarachnoid anesthesia, dural puncture during epidural placement, myelography, or following any procedure accompanied by a loss of cerebrospinal fluid. Treat with aggressive hydration, analgesia, and positioning. In severe cases, consider an early epidural blood patch. After spinal anesthesia, some patients experience transient neurologic symptoms with leg discomfort and buttock pain, especially with 5% lidocaine and lithotomy positioning. This should be treated supportively. Nerve injury from needle contact or intraneuronal injection during regional anesthesia is unusual but can result in pain, focal numbness, residual paresthesia, or dysesthesia.

Muscle pain, aching, or stiffness may reflect lack of motion or muscle stretch associated with positioning during surgery, particularly if the procedure is prolonged. Fasciculation associated with succinylcholine has been implicated, but myalgia also occurs after nondepolarizing relaxation and in patients receiving no relaxant. Excessive joint extension can lead to backache, joint pain, and even joint instability. Soft tissue ischemia and necrosis can occur if pressure points are improperly padded, especially during lateral or prone positioning. Prolonged scalp pressure may cause localized alopecia, whereas entrapment of ears, genitalia, or skin folds can cause inflammation or necrosis. Extravasation of intravenous medications might result in sloughing, localized chemical neuropathy, or compartment syndromes. Thermal, electrical, or chemical burns from cautery equipment, preparatory solutions, or adhesives may also happen. In the event of significant tissue injury or a suspected compartment syndrome, urgent surgical consultation is indicated.

? **Did You Know**

Postoperative peripheral neuropathy may be caused by compression or stretching of the nerve. However, many postoperative neuropathies can occur in the absence of any obvious cause.

XVI. Hypothermia and Hyperthermia

Hypothermia in the PACU is common, despite the widespread use of thermal blankets intraoperatively. *Hypothermia* elevates vascular resistance and heart rate, increases risk of myocardial ischemia, and promotes tissue hypoperfusion.

Platelet sequestration, impaired platelet function, and reduced clotting factors contribute to coagulopathy. Moderately hyperglycemia, increased residual sedation, prolonged weakness from relaxants, and compromised immune responses might occur. Shivering can double oxygen consumption and CO_2 production, risking ventilatory failure in patients with limited reserve or myocardial ischemia in those with coronary artery disease. Shivering also promotes incidental trauma and interferes with monitoring. Movement is accentuated by tonic-clonic tremors related to emergence from inhalation anesthesia. Shivering usually requires only rewarming with forced air devices. Several medications might suppress shivering, but meperidine seems most effective.

Rarely, transient hyperthermia appears after overly aggressive measures are taken to prevent intraoperative heat loss. Fever sometimes reflects bacteremia from a pre-existing infection or the surgical procedure. Elevated temperature from atelectasis usually appears after PACU discharge. Fever might indicate a drug or transfusion reaction or a hypermetabolic state. Ambient cooling, chest physiotherapy, incentive spirometry, and antipyretics are usually sufficient for treatment.

XVII. Altered Mental Status

For any patient who exhibits an unusual mental status in the PACU, immediately rule out life-threatening conditions such as hypotension, hypoxemia, hypoglycemia, severe hyponatremia, or CO_2 narcosis ($PaCO_2$ >150 mm Hg).

Failure to awaken from anesthesia that lasts 15 minutes beyond admission to the PACU is prolonged and *requires explanation.* The most common cause is residual effects of drugs administered during anesthesia. Assess for pre-existing mental dysfunction, intoxication with alcohol or drugs, or use of long-acting sedatives and review unusual intraoperative events. The spontaneous ventilatory rate reflects residual anesthesia depth, while BP reflects adequacy of cerebral perfusion. Include a tactile stimulus to elicit arousal. The diagnostic value of pupillary size and response is low. Low solubility inhalation anesthetics such as sevoflurane or desflurane seldom cause prolonged unconsciousness. If the level of consciousness is depressed by opioids, low-dose intravenous naloxone can be beneficial. Flumazenil (0.2 mg/min intravenously up to 1.0 mg) reverses sedation from benzodiazepines. Physostigmine (1.25 mg intravenously) counteracts but does not reverse sedation caused by other medications. If naloxone, flumazenil, and physostigmine do not elicit a response, unconsciousness is likely not caused by medications. Profound neuromuscular paralysis might rarely mimic unconsciousness, but spontaneous ventilation or reflex activity eliminates this possibility. Patients awaken slowly after long intracranial procedures. Exhausted children are often difficult to awaken, especially after emergency surgery at night. If a diagnosis remains elusive, consult a neurologist. Consider subclinical seizures, cerebral anoxia, increased ICP, cerebral thromboembolism, paradoxical air embolism, or fat embolism syndrome. Risk of stroke is high after cardiac, major vascular, or invasive neck surgery.

During emergence, some patients exhibit somnolence, disorientation (emergence delirium), and sluggish mental reactions that usually clear spontaneously. Others manifest wide emotional swings, weeping, or combativeness. The emotional significance of the surgical procedure (e.g., therapeutic abortion, amputation) can play a role. A stormy emergence reaction causes tachycardia and hypertension, risks incidental trauma, and jeopardizes suture lines, grafts, and indwelling devices. Risk of injury to PACU staff is real. *Emergence*

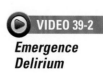

VIDEO 39-2

Emergence Delirium

reactions are prevalent in children, especially after ear, nose, or throat procedures. Patients with pre-existing intoxication, mental disorders, or organic brain dysfunction often act out in the PACU. Pain amplifies agitation, as do urinary urgency, gastric distention, residual paralysis, nausea, pruritus, or dyspnea. Emerging patients often exhibit escalating resistance to unpleasant positioning, restraint, or limitation of inspiratory volume. Most emergence reactions resolve quickly. Disorientation, paranoia, dysphoria, and combativeness might occur after use of scopolamine, ketamine, or droperidol. Treat emergence reactions by eliminating obvious causes and checking for entrapment of body parts, infiltrated vascular catheters, or small devices left beneath the patient. In selected cases, parenteral sedation smooths emergence. It is important to identify whether a patient is reacting to pain or to anxiety. Benzodiazepines are ineffective analgesics, while opioids are poor sedatives. Use physical restraint only as a last resort.

Suggested Readings

Aldrete JA. The post-anesthesia recovery score revisited. *J Clin Anesth*. 1995;7:89.

American Society of PeriAnesthesia Nurses. *2012–2014 Perianesthesia Nursing Standards, Practice Recommendations and Interpretive Statements*. Cherry Hill, NJ: American Society of Post Anesthesia Nursing; 2012.

A report by the American Society of Anesthesiologists Task Force on Postanesthetic Care: Practice guidelines for postanesthetic care. *Anesthesiology*. 2002;96:742.

A report by the American Society of Anesthesiologists Task Force on Prevention of Perioperative Peripheral Neuropathies: Practice advisory for the prevention of perioperative peripheral neuropathies. *Anesthesiology*. 2000;92:1168.

An updated report by the American Society of Anesthesiologists Task Force on Acute Pain Management. *Anesthesiology*. 2004;100:1573.

Benumof JL, Dagg R, Benumof R. Critical hemoglobin desaturation will occur before return to an unparalyzed state following 1 mg/kg intravenous succinylcholine. *Anesthesiology*. 1997;87:979.

Gan TJ, Meyers T, Apfel CC, et al. Consensus guidelines for managing postoperative nausea and vomiting. *Anesth Analg*. 2003;97:67.

Hines R, Barash PG, Watrous G, et al. Complications occurring in the postanesthesia care unit: A survey. *Anesth Analg*. 1992;74:503.

Sessler DI. Complications and treatment of mild hypothermia. *Anesthesiology*. 2001;95:531.

Questions

1. A 40-year-old patient underwent surgical repair of a calcaneus fracture. A sciatic nerve block was administered at the completion of surgery but before the patient was awakened from general anesthesia. Ten minutes after arrival in the PACU, she complained of severe pain in the operative foot. The most appropriate next step would be to:
   A. Obtain an x-ray of the foot
   B. Administer 5 mg of midazolam intravenously
   C. Administer 25 μg of fentanyl intravenously
   D. Repeat the sciatic nerve block

2. A 72-year-old man underwent total hip replacement. His preoperative BP and heart rate averaged 140/90 mm Hg and 82 beats per minute, respectively. His hematocrit was 34% shortly before emergence from anesthesia. Thirty minutes after arrival in the PACU, his BP was 100/75 mm Hg and heart rate was 105 beats per minute. He was awake and coherent. The next best step would be:
   A. Phenylephrine 10 mg intravenously
   B. Ephedrine 15 mg intravenously
   C. Lactated Ringer's solution 500 mL intravenously
   D. Repeat the hematocrit

3. Which of the following will cause an erroneously high BP measurement?
   A. A BP cuff that is too small for the arm
   B. Overinflation of the BP cuff
   C. An arterial line transducer that is above the patient's heart
   D. Hypothermia

4. A patient's endotracheal tube is electively removed in the PACU. Immediately after removal, the patient exhibits inspiratory stridor and sternal retraction. All of the following are appropriate next steps EXCEPT:
   A. Anterior displacement of the mandible
   B. Administration of oxygen
   C. Gentle positive pressure ventilation with a bag and mask
   D. Administration of inhaled albuterol

5. In the PACU, after which of the following surgical procedures is atelectasis most likely to be present?
   A. Tonsillectomy
   B. Simple mastectomy
   C. Laparoscopic cholecystectomy
   D. Inguinal hernia repair

6. Atelectasis is effectively treated with all of the following EXCEPT:
   A. Oxygen administered via nasal prongs
   B. Continuous positive airway pressure with a mask
   C. Incentive spirometry
   D. Chest physiotherapy

7. Effective remedies for PONV include all of the following EXCEPT:
   A. Droperidol
   B. Fentanyl
   C. Ondansetron
   D. Dexamethasone

8. Tracheal and pulmonary aspiration of which of the following is most likely to cause acute respiratory disease?
   A. Nonclotted blood
   B. Ringer's lactate used for oral irrigation
   C. Gastric acid
   D. Pus from a ruptured tonsillar abscess

9. The LEAST likely explanation for oliguria in the PACU is:
   A. Acute tubular necrosis
   B. Inadequate intravascular volume
   C. Residual effects of spinal anesthesia
   D. Inguinal hernia repair

10. Effective strategies for treatment of postdural puncture headache include all of the following EXCEPT:
    A. Bedrest
    B. Oral analgesics
    C. Hydration
    D. Epidural blood patch

Complications, Risk Management, Patient Safety, and Liability

40

James E. Szalados

William Osler once commented "errors in judgment must occur in the practice of an art which consists largely of balancing probabilities." The practice of medicine applies as much art as science to the treatment of diverse and unique individuals. The 20th century witnessed a transformation of medicine from a largely humanistic art into a technologically driven enterprise accounting for one-eighth of the US gross domestic product. Nonetheless, many critical clinical decisions are made in the context of rapidly deteriorating physiology, relatively sparse data, and subjective clinical judgment. Given enormous human variability and its consequent potential for both unforeseen biologic variations and idiosyncratic physiologic and psychological reactions, the risk of anesthesia-related complications cannot be completely eliminated at the present time.

VIDEO 40-1

Rates of Selected Anesthetic Complications

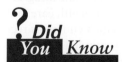

The estimated anesthesia-specific mortality risk has steadily declined from approximately 1 in 1,000 in the 1940s to 1 in 10,000 in the 1970s to 1 in 100,000 in the 2000s.

I. Risks and Complications

A. Mortality and Major Morbidity Related to Anesthesia

With the advent of specialty training and certification, advances in pharmacology and monitoring technology, and improved perioperative medical care, the *anesthesia mortality risk* has declined from about 1 in 1,000 anesthesia procedures in the 1940s to 1 in 10,000 in the 1970s and to 1 in 100,000 in the early 2000s, and it was most recently reported to be 8.2 in 1 million hospital surgical discharges (11.7 for men and 6.5 for women) (1). Although the reliability of these statistics is undermined by the lack of a centralized data repository, the indirect sources of the data (typically incident reports and *International Classification of Diseases*–based codes), the multifactorial and interdisciplinary management of such cases, and the undefined postoperative time period, available data generally show that anesthesia-related mortality is directly related to the age (higher at both extremes of age) and the physical status of the patient.

The risk of *anesthesia-related morbidity* is also difficult to quantify because such data are similarly subject to limitations in reporting and disclosure. It is estimated that more than 1 in 10 patients will have an intraoperative

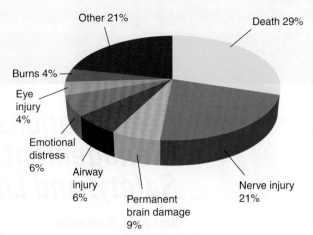

Figure 40-1 Most common injuries leading to anesthesia malpractice claims 2000 to 2009. Other category includes aspiration (4%), pneumothorax (3%), back pain (3%), myocardial infarction (3%), newborn injury (2%), headache (2%), and awareness/recall during general anesthesia (2%). Damage to teeth and dentures excluded. American Society of Anesthesiologists' Closed Claims Project (*n*–9,214). (From: Posner KL, Adeogba S, Domino K. Anesthesia risk, quality improvement, and liability. In: Barash PG, Cullen BF, Stoelting RK, et al. *Clinical Anesthesia*, 7th ed. Philadelphia: Lippincott Williams & Wilkins, 2013:100.)

incident and 1 in 1,000 will suffer an actual injury such as a dental damage, an inadvertent dural puncture, peripheral nerve injury, or significant pain (2). Some morbidity, such as venous thromboembolism, myocardial infarction, or catheter-related bloodstream infections, can be predicted and managed. Some morbidity, such as aspiration, previously unknown allergies, nerve injuries, or retained awareness, might be mitigated. However, some morbidity such as stroke can neither be well predicted nor consistently mitigated (Fig. 40-1).

II. Risk Management and Patient Safety

A. Ethics

The term *ethics* is derived from the Greek *ethos*, translated as "custom" or "habit," and is a branch of philosophy dedicated to the study of values and customs of groups. In its contemporary applications, ethics relates to the analysis and application of precepts such as right and wrong, good and evil, and norms for interactions between people. Because it is inevitable that disagreements will arise when individual preferences form the basis for health care and end-of-life decisions, ethics provides a framework within which clinicians reconcile differing beliefs and values. Thus, ethics is an open-minded structural framework that facilitates *discourse* and *problem solving* in highly complex clinical dilemmas for which there are no clear-cut answers and for which decisions are frequently subject to retrospective scrutiny.

Medical ethics refers to the systematic study of ethical or moral values as they apply to the practice of medicine. Medical ethics addresses issues such as do-not-resuscitate (DNR) orders, medical futility, withdrawal of life support, terminal sedation, research subject protections, placebo therapy, access to health care, and the meaning of brain death. However, because ethics is a branch of philosophy, it is as important to understand that it is as much about discourse—structured argumentation representing disparate points of view—as it is about a study of values and customs. Ethics provides the theoretical foundation, structure, and context with which health care providers can have meaningful discussions with patients, families, and among one another regarding deeply personal topics.

Although ethics is widely believed to represent a branch of legal doctrine, it applies equally to all professions. Nonetheless, laws apply to interactions between individuals and between individuals and society. Lawyers are trained to manage opposing points of view and are trained to develop arguments on behalf of their clients. In the United States, laws are derived from the shared ethical and moral principles inherent in the US Constitution. Laws, much like ethical concepts, form the structure and context within which lawyers argue the merits of their clients' cases. The important relationship of professions with society suggests that *professional values* must be congruent with the societal values in which the professionals practice. Ethical decisions made in the medical context are subject to public review and must be as unbiased, carefully reasoned, well documented, and as transparent as possible.

The goal of communication in medicine is the formation of a *therapeutic alliance* that facilitates *shared decision making*. Many so-called ethical conflicts in clinical practice can be traced to a lack of effective communication. Medical malpractice litigation is very closely linked to the perceptions of patients and families regarding honest communication, team cohesiveness, disclosure of adverse events, and, therefore, their subjective impressions regarding the quality of care. *Litigation* is more likely to result when there is a significant discrepancy between a patient's or family's expectations and perceptions regarding the care that was rendered. In the absence of true medical negligence, patients and families are most likely to remember the respect, caring, and attentiveness (ethical behavior) they encountered during the time of the patient's health care encounter.

Ethical codes or *codes of conduct* are largely a set of aspirational values, which are the ethical guiding principles for professions, and apply equally to each and every member of the health care team. The Oath of Hippocrates, the Nightingale Pledge, Thomas Percival's Code of Medical Ethics, the Oath of Maimonides, the Declaration of Geneva, and the American Medical Association's Principles of Medical Ethics represent such foundational professional documents. The four formal principles of medical ethics—beneficence, nonmaleficence, autonomy, and justice—represent a set of precepts that must be considered in any discussion of medical ethics, and commonly apply to medical ethics decision making.

The principle of *beneficence* represents that each health care practitioner should knowingly strive to always act in the best interests of each individual patient (*salus aegroti suprema lex*). Thus, health care decisions should reflect the highest level of care for each patient, without regard to personal gain, societal interests, or the interests of family.

The principle of *nonmaleficence* is embodied in the concept of *primum non nocere*—"first, do no harm." Harm may be variably interpreted and includes either willful omission or commission of an act that inflicts emotional or psychologic distress, pain and suffering, or physical injury. Nonmaleficence is also inherent in the fiduciary duty (i.e., acting in the patient's best interests) that physicians owe to their patients. Nonmaleficence can become legally operative with medical interventions that have risks that cannot be eliminated no matter how much care and attention is rendered. Where a therapeutic intervention is prescribed with the intent of "doing good" and an unavoidable but recognized harm may ensue, this is known as the *double effect.* For example, respiratory depression caused by the administration of opiates for palliative sedation is well recognized, but its intended desired effect is not respiratory depression, but rather relief from suffering. Thus, palliative sedation is ethically acceptable, whereas euthanasia and assisted suicide are not. The process is similar but the intent is dichotomous.

The principle of *autonomy* addresses the patient's right to choose (*voluntas aegroti suprema lex*) and to make informed, uncoerced, voluntary decisions. Autonomy refers to each individual's right to *self-determination.* Historically, US culture has placed great importance on and has had great respect for the principle of individual autonomy, a notion embodied in the Declaration of Independence, the US Constitution, and the Bill of Rights. The principle of autonomy is exemplified in the obligations to obtain informed consent, the adoption of living wills and advance directives, and health care proxy designations. The principle of autonomy requires health care *surrogates* (proxies) to use *substituted judgment* in decision making, whereby the surrogate decides for the patient as he or she believes the patient would have done.

The principle of *justice* is bifurcated into distribution and retribution. *Distributive justice* is an ideal that concerns the hope that all are treated equally and with clear transparency with respect to access to and distribution of limited health care resources. *Retributive justice* addresses retrospective retaliation as punishment or prospective warnings of imminent punishment as a deterrent to certain actions. In some ways, justice represents the antithesis of the principle of autonomy. Whereas autonomy dictates that a patient's interests are determinative, the principle of distributive justice dictates that the physician must consider the fair allocation of resources without discrimination. *Triage* in emergencies and in critical care settings represents application of the principle of distributive justice. Retributive justice is largely reserved for disciplinary and legal review.

The principle of *paternalism* refers to the instinct for professionals to unilaterally make decisions on behalf of others, regardless of their capability to do so themselves. In its extreme form, the paternalistic provider ignores the wishes and needs of the patient and is not reconcilable with the precept of autonomy. Less obtrusively, paternalism is also manifested when the physician subconsciously withholds crucial information in the belief that bad news, such as a terminal diagnoses or a poor prognosis, might inflict undue emotional distress. Paternalistic decision making is no longer acceptable in modern medicine.

B. Medical Errors and Patient Safety

The topics of medical error and patient safety attained national prominence in 2000 when the Institute of Medicine (IOM) published *To Err Is Human: Building a Safer Health System.* In it the IOM purported that medical errors accounted for at least 98,000 inpatient deaths annually, or, at least 270 deaths daily (3). Medical error can be defined as a mistake, *inadvertent occurrence*, or *unintended event* in health care delivery that may or may not result in patient injury. The Institute of Medicine defines patient safety as "freedom from accidental injury" and has suggested 10 recommendations for improving both quality of care and patient safety (4):

1. Care based on continuous healing relationships
2. Customization based on patient needs and values
3. Establishment of the patient as the source of control

4. Shared knowledge and the free flow of information
5. Evidence-based decision making
6. Safety as a priority
7. Transparency
8. Anticipation of needs
9. Continuous reduction of waste
10. Cooperation among clinicians

Anesthesiology has a long history of leadership in quality and safety and was the first specialty to adopt a national standard for safety improvements and the first national foundation dedicated to patient safety (Anesthesia Patient Safety Foundation). In 1978, Cooper et al. (5) retrospectively examined the role of human factors in anesthesia incidents and determined that 82% of the incidents deemed to be preventable involved human error and 14% involved equipment failures. Less commonly, errors were deemed due to faulty equipment design, experience, insufficient familiarity with equipment or with the surgical procedure, poor communication among personnel, haste or lack of precaution, and distraction. Critical cognitive processes that predispose to errors include unintentional actions in the performance of routine tasks, mistakes in judgment, and inadequate plans of action. In addition, errors are classified as either *active failures* (e.g., violations of rules) or latent failures (e.g., faulty organizational or systemic processes). *Latent failures* are often unrecognized and have high potential for future repetition. *Error-prone systems* are exemplified by the concept of the *Swiss-cheese model* of error, whereby each layer of activity within a system contains embedded latent failures (holes) that allow errors to pass undetected through the system resulting in an adverse event. When the error penetrates all but a final barrier, the result is a near miss. In general, the more complex the system is, the greater the potential for error. Lastly, anesthesia practice shares common characteristics of many complex systems: high-level technical requirements, the need for quick reaction times, 24-hour-a-day operations, fatigue related to long hours, production pressure that frequently involves tradeoffs between service and safety, and multidisciplinary team coordination.

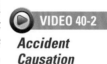

VIDEO 40-2

Accident Causation

The medical model for team coordination for error prevention has its origins in the aviation industry, which developed the *crew resource management* (CRM) paradigm in 1978 (Table 40-1). CRM fosters an organizational culture that encourages each team member to respectfully question authority,

Table 40-1   The Structure of Crew Resource Management
Communication: Leadership and team management
Workload management: Mission planning, stress management, and workload distribution
Decision making: Integration and proceduralization (standard operating procedure)
Conflict resolution
Leadership
Team management
Stress management

while preserving authority and chain of command. CRM encompasses knowledge, skills, and attitudes including communications, situational awareness, problem solving, decision making, and teamwork. CRM is a team management system that makes optimum use of all available resources. These include equipment, procedures, and people in order to promote safety, enhance operational efficiency, and foster teamwork, as well as allowing patient involvement, transparency, and accountability. CRM has become an integral part of both anesthesiology simulator training and interdisciplinary trauma care (see Chapter 32).

C. Informed Consent

A separate and distinct documentation of informed consent for anesthesia and for anesthesia-related procedures is widely held to be the standard. In addition, a patient's ability to refuse a proposed intervention; to place limits, restrictions, or conditions on treatment; or disregard the advice of a physician altogether are all corollaries of the informed consent doctrine. Providers must understand and respect the fact that what may be consented to may also be refused. Documentation of refusal to consent is equally as important as the documentation of informed consent to treatment.

The doctrine of informed consent is premised on the ethical principle of autonomy that obliges physicians to respect patients' right to bodily self-determination and therefore share medical decision-making authority with patients. The cornerstone of valid informed consent is effective communication—a *two-way dialogue*. There are two distinct legal standards that are applied to the informed consent process: the reasonable physician standard or the reasonable patient standard.

The *reasonable patient standard* is more commonly applied and is consistent with a respect for patient autonomy. It requires disclosure of the relevant information that a typical and reasonable patient would want to know in order to make an informed decision. The process of informed consent requires disclosure and discussion of all material risks, benefits, and alternatives to proposed therapeutic or investigational interventions.

All disclosure standards require that information and choices be presented comprehensively and in clear terms. This should include a concomitant explanation of the meaning of the terms, potential short-term and long-term implications of each option, discussions regarding the option to change the plan of care at a later time and the implications of such withdrawal, and reassurance that such decisions will be respected. The dialogue, including an opportunity for patients to ask questions and receive honest answers regarding the proposed treatment, should occur in an atmosphere devoid of any sense of duress or coercion in order for the consent to be truly valid.

Finally, after all disclosures have been made, the options considered, and the accord reached, then the signed form within the record will represent the formal documentation of the process. Consent is therefore somewhat analogous to a contract that not only requires truthful disclosure, consideration, and acceptance, but also imposes duties and obligations on the parties.

Similar to *contracts*, there are potential legal challenges regarding to the validity of the consent or contract. Such challenges include fraudulent facts or pretenses, duress, lack of capacity, or impaired judgment. A legally competent patient is one who is legally able to make decisions on his or her own behalf. Unemancipated minors, the mentally challenged, or the permanently disabled are possible examples of patients who may lack competency for autonomous decision making and therefore family or court-appointed guardians will make decisions on their behalf. The term *capacity* refers to an impairment in decision making that is more situational in context, for example, medications that impair judgment and reasoning; metabolic disturbances; or mental states such as depression, mania, psychosis, and delirium or confusion.

The majority of states have **statutory requirements** regarding informed consent, where failure to comply with statutory requirements for informed consent can put the provider at risk for a charge of professional misconduct. Medicare's conditions of participation and the Joint Commission also separately mandate informed consent. If a course of medical care is litigated for any reason, the lack of documented informed consent can compromise the legal defensibility of that case.

The doctrine of *implied consent* can sometimes address the relatively common clinical situation where the provider could reasonably infer that a patient would have consented to the treatment. Implied consent is essentially a matter of the provider's reasonable interpretation of the overall patient's conduct to be consistent with an intention to authorize a procedure, even though express consent to treatment is lacking. Implied consent should be reserved for emergency care and situations where informed consent from a patient or surrogate is either very impracticable or impossible.

In the instance where a previously competent patient, or a patient with capacity, has clearly expressed their directives, these directives remain binding even after the patient loses competence or capacity. For example, in the case of an adult Jehovah's Witness patient who expressly refuses blood transfusion and this directive is documented clearly in the record, most courts have held the family cannot overrule the patient's decision after he or she loses capacity.

D. Importance of the Medical Record
The medical record serves medical, legal, and business purposes. It is an ongoing **record of treatment** that is used to record and communicate the circumstances of patient care to other providers, to substantiate and justify the medical reasoning involved in reaching a diagnosis and determining a plan of care, and to support a claim for reimbursement. The medical record is legally the **work product** of the health care team (Table 40-2). There are two aspects of medical records: the physical chart and the information contained on it. The patient has both the right of possession and the right of confidentiality to his

Table 40-2 Purposes of the Medical Record
Written documentation of the health care encounter
Basis for longitudinal comparisons of a patient's clinical course over time
Communication and continuity of care among the health care team
Basis for coding and billing claims in support of reimbursement for services
Utilization review
Peer review and quality-of-care evaluations
Collection of research data

or her medical information. The physical chart is the property of the medical provider who is the *legal custodian* of the chart and assumes responsibility for its integrity, whereas the information contained within the medical record is legally the property of the patient.

With widespread adoption of the electronic medical record (EMR), there are new risks for providers and institutions. The risk for breach of confidentiality is enhanced with EMRs mainly because unprotected (lost or unencrypted) portable devices can store and access data remotely. The potential for unauthorized access to repositories of records through hacking is great, and electronic data transmission can disseminate confidential data faster and farther than was possible with photocopy or fax technologies in the past.

Many doctrines, laws, regulations, and policies address the confidentiality of medical information, including the *Health Insurance Portability and Accountability Act* of 1996 (HIPAA) and the *Health Information Technology for Economic and Clinical Health Act* of 2009. These laws address the privacy of personally identifiable health information and security concerns associated with the electronic transmission of health information and penalties for violations for unauthorized disclosures, respectively. Breaches of medical record privacy are enforced by the *Office of Civil Rights*.

The *metadata* embedded within EMRs provide details regarding the records and images accessed for review, the time and duration of document review and record entry, and any changes made. Thus, a detailed log of the exact data and documentation reviewed by a clinician during a patient's evaluation can be retrospectively reconstructed in the event of a lawsuit. Maintaining timely and accurate documentation in the EMR can be a challenge, however, given the possibilities for delayed or late entries, typographical and word-recognition transcription errors that can be perpetuated through cut-and-paste charting, and the rigidity of templates, checkboxes, and pull-down menus. Thus, a clear, organized, timely, and carefully proofread narrative will best reflect the clinician's thought process, differential diagnosis, and clinical judgment as well as provide the most defensible clinical work product.

E. Responding to an Adverse Event

A serious adverse perioperative event, especially one that results in severe disability or death to an otherwise healthy patient during elective surgery, can have tremendous psychological impact on the anesthesia care team. Because such events are likely to be rare occurrences during a single practice career, the Anesthesia Patient Safety Foundation has developed an *adverse event protocol* to facilitate an effective, efficient, and coordinated response to a perioperative incident (6). The verbal, written, and behavioral responses of involved providers after a perioperative incident have potentially enormous legal ramifications. Therefore, a well-designed adverse event protocol is communicated to all members of the anesthesia care team before any incident occurs. It has been sanctioned by providers, administrators, and legal counsel and is both protocolized and automatically triggered.

The formal discussion of the circumstances surrounding an adverse event has come to be known as *disclosure*. The term *disclosure* is most frequently used in the context of a disclosure of a medical error. However, disclosure of the circumstances relating to an adverse event that results in patient harm frequently occurs before it is clear that a medical error did in fact occur. Truthfulness is widely recognized as an ethical tenet and therefore a professional responsibility of physicians. Whereas it is widely recognized that identification and scrutiny of error with implementation of corrective feedback loop (*root cause analysis [RCA]*) is a critical mechanism to enhance patient safety, the dissemination of specific data regarding an adverse event or medical error has administrative and legal implications to both providers and institutions.

Numerous but not well-controlled studies have suggested that patients are more likely to seek legal counsel to explore their legal rights and to bring suit in the absence of a formal explanation or apology, presumably because of an innate sense of suspicion and a need to reach closure. The legal quandary with respect to disclosure meetings is that potentially self-implicating statements made during such meetings can be later discovered by plaintiff attorneys and admitted into evidence. With the intent of facilitating truthful communication between providers and patients, all but 14 states have enacted *Apology Statutes*, which are safe harbors designed to protect physicians who apologize to patients for medical errors. Under an Apology Statute, expressions of apology are excluded from discoverable evidence in the event of a malpractice claim. Apology Statutes allow "offers of expressions of grief" and are primarily intended to encourage open communication through informal conversations between the patient or family and the health care provider. In general, although it is sound practice for medical staff to adhere to regulatory and administrative policies and procedures mandating disclosure of medical errors, it is equally important that the circumstances surrounding the discussion are carefully controlled to the extent possible. Legal advice should be sought before a disclosure policy is implemented, and legal opinion should be obtained prior to a formal disclosure meeting.

? *Did* *You* *Know*

Apology statutes vary by state and are of two types: sympathy statutes, which protect physicians' expressions of sympathy, regret, and condolences, and admission of fault statutes, which protect physicians' admissions of fault or error.

F. National Practitioner Data Bank

The National Practitioner Data Bank (NPDB) was created in 1990 through the Medicare and Medicaid Patient and Program Protection Act of 1987 and represents a federal data repository to collect and maintain quality-related information about health care providers (Table 40-3). The HIPAA law of 1996 created the Healthcare Integrity and Protection Data Bank (HIPDB) in response to fraud and abuse in health insurance and health care delivery. In 2013, the NPDB merged with the HIPDB and now serves as the central data

Table 40-3 Examples of Events Reportable to the National Practitioner Data Bank
Medical malpractice payments
Health care–related civil or criminal actions
Adverse licensure actions
Adverse clinical privileging actions
Adverse professional society membership actions
Drug Enforcement Agency actions
Exclusions from federal- or state-funded health care programs
Private accreditation organization actions
Other due-process adjudications pertinent to health care

clearinghouse that collects and releases information related to the professional conduct and competence of physicians, nurses, dentists, and other health care practitioners. The intent of the NPDB is to support professional peer review by requiring hospitals, state licensing boards, professional societies, and other health care entities to report adverse actions against providers and also to query the databank as part of the credentialing and privileging process. The NPDB contains information about health care practitioners' malpractice history, adverse licensure actions, restrictions on professional membership, and negative privileging actions by hospitals. It is important to realize that uncontested adverse actions such as *settlements before judgment* in malpractice litigation, uncontested denials for medical staff credentialing, and resignations from medical staff while a peer review investigation is ongoing are all reportable to the NPDB.

G. Advance Directives

An *advance directive* is a statement of instruction that is anticipated to potentially take effect at some point in the future. The purpose of an advance directive is to make one's wishes known to others in the event that one later loses the ability to communicate, so that one's wishes can be known and respected. Advance directives represent a practical application of the ethical principle respecting autonomous decision making. Examples of advance directives include *living wills* and health care proxies, *durable powers of attorney*, general DNR requests, or the specific documentation of preferences for interventions such as prolonged mechanical ventilation, artificial nutrition and hydration, or dialysis in the event of severe incapacitating injury.

A *living will* is a common form of advance directive that defines a patient's expectations from providers and the health care system. It almost always delineates specific or general parameters for the initiation, continuation, or termination of various levels of life-sustaining medical treatment. Living wills can be prepared by the patient alone or more often in consultation a physician or attorney. One limitation of living wills is insufficient specificity so as to unequivocally define a patient's wishes for all contingencies. As a result, most living wills are practically little more than a general guide to patients' wishes. Thus, even when a living will is available, the patient's surrogate decision makers are still tasked with interpreting the patient's wishes in that specific circumstance.

A *health care proxy* is a surrogate decision maker who is specifically and legally appointed by the patient, by way of a written designation, for the purpose of making health care decisions on the patient's behalf. The health care proxy need not be a relative, and this person supersedes statutorily defined *surrogacy hierarchies*. The proxy or surrogate is merely conveying indirectly the wishes and directions of the patient and should not engage in unilateral decision making. In the absence of a previously designated health care proxy, providers should consult their state laws regarding statutes of surrogacy that define the hierarchy of decision makers who can speak on a patient's behalf.

A *power of attorney* is a legal document empowering another person with authority of agency—the authority to act in one's place. Powers of attorney can be specific to financial, administrative, or health care matters or may be more general and even unrestricted. Simple powers of attorney are in effect only as long as the patient also has the capacity to make decisions and become void when a patient loses decision-making capacity. On the other hand, a *durable power of attorney* is a more powerful document that retains its effect even after a patient loses decision-making capacity. Again, even durable powers of attorney may be restricted in scope and may not necessarily extend to health care decisions.

Advance directives also include orders regarding preferences for resuscitation. DNR or do-not-attempt-resuscitation (DNAR) orders represent provider orders that are based on the completion of a standardized form that outlines a patient's resuscitation preferences. The DNR form is similar to the living will but it is more specific and is frequently a legal form designed and regulated by individual state statutes. DNR forms closely resemble a refusal to consent to treatment because they specify a limitation of medical care. The general legal and ethical considerations that apply to the informed consent process also apply to end-of-life discussions and the DNR order. For a DNR to be legally valid, it must be obtained after full disclosure in a competent patient with capacity and without duress or coercion.

III. Quality Improvement and Patient Safety

A. Structure, Process, and Outcome: The Building Blocks of Safety

The *Donabedian model* (7) is a conceptual framework for evaluating quality and designing and quality-of-care improvements using three categories of analysis: structure, process, and outcome. *Structure* describes factors that impact the context in which care occurs (e.g., hospital physical plant, staff, training, equipment, and administration). *Process* relates to the normative behaviors, relationships, and interactions (e.g., preventive care, patient education) throughout health care delivery. *Outcome* refers to the results obtained and the effect of health care encounters on patients or populations (e.g., mortality, health status, patient satisfaction, or health-related quality of life). The Donabedian model can be used to modify a health care delivery unit and to evaluate the effects of changes on specified external indicators of quality. However, the model itself does not contain an implicit definition of quality or value.

The Donabedian model is relevant to discussions of patient safety and quality of care for two reasons: (a) patient safety is related to structure and process, and quality describes outcomes and the manner in which they are achieved; (b) legislators, regulators, health care administrators, and payors uniformly require and rely on this framework. The model describes how regulators, policymakers, and stakeholders analyze the health care system. Therefore, every health care system's licensure, regulatory compliance, condition of participation requirement, and accreditation standard is in some way a structure, process, or outcome measure.

Several other quality improvement models also apply to anesthesiology, including Total Quality Management model, the Continuous Quality Improvement model, the PDSA (plan, do, study, act) cycle, the Six Sigma model, and RCA. The RCA model differs from the other models in that it represents a retrospective rather than prospective model of quality improvement. It is a two-step quality improvement process that examines adverse outcomes and develops plans to strengthen or develop safety systems through data collection and analysis.

B. Difficulty of Outcome Measurement in Anesthesia

Quality of care is obviously challenging to define and measure clinically. The first clinical quality indicators relied on the identification of specific adverse outcomes and subsequent analysis through individual case review to identify potential quality of care issues. Subsequently, the Joint Commission developed a series of anesthesia-related *quality indicators* by which organizational performance could be continuously monitored and evaluated. This national Indicator Measurement System evaluated two categories of performance: (a) sentinel event indicators (unexpected occurrences involving death or serious physical injury), and (b) rate-based indicators (trends in a particular type of process or outcome of care).

Unfortunately, the validation of anesthetic clinical indicators is largely limited to expert opinion because at this time there is insufficient evidence to demonstrate that compliance with evidence-based best practice will systematically and universally result in better patient outcome. For example, compliance with perioperative beta-blockade was initially instituted as a national quality indicator after data suggested that perioperative beta-blockade reduced the incidence of myocardial infarction in high-risk patients undergoing noncardiac surgery. However, subsequent data also demonstrated that the risk of death and blindness were increased in noncardiac surgery patients receiving perioperative beta-blockade.

Outcome measurement in anesthesiology is also complicated by the lack of standardized and consensus definitions across systems and countries. For example, the American Society of Anesthesiologists' Physical Status Classification System is related to perioperative risk but is largely subjective and results in inconsistent categorization. The complexity of clinical care systems is such that multiple variables are involved in every outcome. Thus, anesthesia-specific outcomes remain elusive because it is difficult to attribute causality for the outcome to either a specific surgical, anesthetic, or medical intervention as opposed to the totality of the medical care. With respect to the Donabedian model, practical quality improvements based on connections between process and outcomes require large sample populations, adjustments by case mix, and long-term follow-up. As a result, the meaningful impact of specific interventions on relatively low-frequency adverse outcomes is largely lost in the complexity of the individual patient and multiple health care interventions.

C. Regulatory Requirements for Quality Improvement

The Flexner Report established standards for modern medical education and provided an impetus for the development of state departments of public health that were later charged with the supervision of health care institutions. In 1917, the American College of Surgeons established minimum quality standards for hospitals and introduced a voluntary compliance system. In 1946, the US Congress enacted the Hill-Burton Act to provide funds for states to build hospitals and conditioned the funds on minimum standards regarding the maintenance and operation of health care facilities. In the 1950s, the Joint Commission on Accreditation of Hospitals, later known as the Joint Commission on Accreditation of Healthcare Organizations and now referred to simply as the Joint Commission, established an accreditation process for hospitals that became a compulsory standard for facilities seeking state licensure and Medicare participation.

State licensure is a statutory *condition of participation* for hospitals, while accreditation is a voluntary means of meeting the conditions for participation. Regulatory oversight for health care quality occurs at many levels, including professional licensure, conditions of participation, training, certification or accreditation, mandatory reporting, and pay-for-performance plans. *Compliance* with such regulatory mandates has made health care the most regulated of all industries in the United States.

? Did You Know

Participation in Medicare and Medicaid Electronic Health Record (EHR) Incentive programs requires that physicians and hospitals demonstrate "meaningful use" of the EHR by collecting and submitting data on specified clinical quality measures using certified EHR technology.

IV. Professional Liability

A. Professionalism and Licensure

A professional is one who practices within a profession. Professionals have met standards of education and training through which specialized knowledge and skills are acquired. Professional standards of practice and ethics are codified in professional codes of conduct specific to the profession. By virtue of this imbalance in their education, training, and knowledge, professionals owe a *fiduciary duty* to their clients.

Professionalism is challenging to define in more practical terms. Epstein and Hundert (8) define professionalism as a "habitual and judicious use of communication, knowledge, technical skills, clinical reasoning, emotions, values, and reflection in daily practice for the benefit of the individual and community being served." The ***Medical Professionalism Project*** (9) represents a collaboration of the American Board of Internal Medicine Foundation, the American College of Physicians Foundation, and the European Federation of Internal Medicine, and it defined three fundamental principles of professionalism: (a) the primacy of patient welfare, which addresses altruism, trust, and patient interest; (b) patient autonomy addressing the importance of honesty with patients and the need to empower patients in medical decision making; and (c) social justice addressing physicians' societal contract and distributive justice in consideration of the finite nature of health care resources (Table 40-4).

Tetzlaff (10) has defined the essentials of professionalism to include (a) accountability, (b) humanism, (c) personal well-being, and (d) ethics. Lastly and more practically, the three pillars of clinical excellence that impact professionalism can been defined as availability, affability, and ability.

B. The Adversarial System

The adversarial system refers to a common law legal system whereby advocates represent their parties' positions before an impartial person or group of people, usually a judge or jury, who attempt to determine the truth of the matters alleged. The aggrieved patient who initiates a medical malpractice lawsuit is the plaintiff who seeks a legal remedy from the court. If the plaintiff is successful, the court will enter judgment for the plaintiff and issue a court order

Table 40-4　Commitments Inherent to Professionalism
Professional competence
Honesty
Patient confidentiality
Appropriate relations with patients
Improving quality of care
Improving access to care
Just distribution of finite resources
Scientific knowledge
Maintaining trust by managing conflicts of interest
Professional responsibilities

for damages with the intention of making the plaintiff whole in compensation for having been wronged. The party against whom the complaint is directed is the defendant. In litigation, cases are identified by citing the plaintiff name first. Thus, a lawsuit is cited as "Plaintiff vs. Defendant." In a *civil lawsuit*, the burden of proof rests with the plaintiff who must establish the requisite elements of his or her case by a *"preponderance of evidence"* that all the alleged facts have been presented and are more likely than not to be true.

The party who initiates the lawsuit (plaintiff) must file the claim within a specified period of time, a statutorily defined and state-specific time period known as the *statute of limitations*. A lawsuit is formally commenced when the plaintiff's attorney files a complaint with the court and the clerk of the court issues a summons. A civil lawsuit in the United States is initiated by filing a summons, claim form, or complaint, documents that are collectively referred to as the *pleadings*. **Pleadings** describe in detail the alleged wrongs committed by the defendant and include a demand for relief. The legal action is initiated by physical delivery of the pleadings to the defendant. The pleadings are then filed with the court that has jurisdiction over the parties, together with an affidavit verifying that they have served on the defendant.

Typically, service of the **summons** is made on the defendant physician, not on the insurer, and it is important that the physician notify the insurance carrier immediately because the defendant has only a limited period of time during which to answer the complaint. If the answer is not filed by the physician's defense counsel within the statutory time limits, the plaintiff can obtain a default judgment against the defendant physician, forfeiting the right to contest the matter in court.

If the action is not dismissed, then both parties will begin a process of *discovery*. **Discovery** relates to the opportunity of each party to obtain relevant information and documents from the parties to the lawsuit. Discovery may include interrogatories, **depositions** of key parties, support staff, families, chart reviews, expert reviews, and determination of relevant supporting materials. Interrogatories refer to written questions served on parties, whereas depositions represent formal oral sworn testimony obtained under oath and transcribed by a court reporter.

All states have trial courts where civil disputes are filed and litigated, and there is usually a system of appeals courts, with final judicial authority resting in the state court of final appeal. If the malpractice claim involves the federal government acting through a federally funded clinic or a Veterans Administration facility, then the action is filed in a federal district court. Federal courts will also hear malpractice claims when there is diversity of state citizenship, such as when the parties are domiciled in different states or if a federal question is at issue, such as a violation of a fundamental constitutional right during the alleged negligent conduct. The place where the case is filed is usually guided by where the incident occurred, or the residence of the parties involved, and is known as the *venue*.

At various times during the litigation process, the parties might choose to settle, attempt alternative dispute resolution such as mediation or arbitration, proffer motions for either summary judgment or dismissal, or voluntarily discontinue the action. **Settlement** prior to trial is generally encouraged by the courts in the interests of judicial efficiency. Medical malpractice cases frequently settle out of court because there are many potential advantages of doing so: (a) juries are unpredictable; (b) the negative consequences and publicity of a guilty verdict are lessened; (c) defense attorney, expert witness, and court costs are potentially lessened; and (d) the precedential impact of the verdict to future similar cases is eliminated. If the matter proceeds to trial, the court will set a trial date on the *docket* (trial calendar). A party generally has the right to appeal a judgment to at least one higher court, which has the power to affirm, reverse, or modify the judgment of the trial court.

C. Elements of Medical Malpractice

Because medicine involves decision making of high complexity, it is an area of professional practice wherein the risk of adverse outcomes and litigation is high. Nonetheless, physicians must understand that a bad outcome does not equate with medical malpractice. A physician is generally not liable for negligence for errors in judgment. Rather, liability can only legitimately be inferred where the treatment rendered clearly falls outside recognized standards of good medical practice. In order to prove medical malpractice, the plaintiff must show that the physician or provider deviated from the standard of care relevant to the specific treatment setting in question. The *standard of care* is further defined as that care which a reasonably competent and skilled health care professional, with a similar training, would have provided under similar circumstances.

Medical malpractice is a specific type of *negligence* within a group of legal causes of action known as *civil torts,* and it is governed by the laws of state-specific civil statutes. To be found liable under any specific cause of action, the trial court will require that the plaintiff demonstrates each legal element of that particular cause of action. The legal elements of the civil tort of medical negligence are (a) the existence of a duty, (b) a breach of that duty, (c) proof that the breach of duty was the actual and proximate cause of the adverse outcome, and (d) demonstration that ascertainable damages resulted as a cause of that breach. Medical malpractice usually involves issues that are beyond the usual understanding of laypersons. Therefore, the courts require that the elements of malpractice, including standard of care, breach, and proximate cause, must be proved through expert testimony.

Duty is created by the physician–patient relationship and requires that the physician adhere to that degree of skill and learning ordinarily possessed and employed by other members of the same profession, who are in good standing, and are engaged in the same type of practice or specialty. In practice, however, the norms of generally accepted medical practice, which form the basis for a definition of a relevant standard of care, can be difficult to define because the medical literature is replete with controversy and new advances, and there can be great variation between patients. Therefore, both plaintiff and defendant will each introduce *expert opinion* testimony regarding the applicable standard of care. In order to prove that the defendant physician committed a breach of duty, the plaintiff must demonstrate that the defendant did not act in accordance with the applicable standard of care.

The plaintiff must prove *causation* by showing of a reasonably close causal connection between the alleged negligent act (or omission) and the resulting injury. The malpractice must be shown to be a cause in fact (i.e., actual cause) of the plaintiff's injury. However, in addition, the alleged act of malpractice must be shown to also be the *proximate cause* (i.e., legal cause) of the plaintiff's injury. The concept of legal causation can be difficult for physicians to comprehend because it does not refer to a strict scientific causation. Legal causation considers both causation in fact and foreseeability. *Causation in fact* is defined using the *"but for" test,* which requires a showing that "but for" the act or failure to act, the complication or injury would not have occurred.

> **? Did You Know**
>
> In medical malpractice cases, physicians are generally not liable for negligence for errors in judgment, but can be liable for care that falls outside recognized standards of good medical practice, defined as care that a reasonably competent and skilled health care professional, with similar training, would provide under similar circumstances.

Foreseeability requires that the patient's injuries be a ***reasonably foreseeable*** result of the defendant physician's actions.

The term *damages* attempts to quantify the actual ascertainable injuries suffered by the plaintiff. The term damages is broad and encompasses a range of financial, physical, and emotional injuries. The intent of awarding compensatory damages in a tort action is to "make the plaintiff whole again," which, in most medically related injuries, is an obvious legal fiction but nonetheless the best attempt at compensation. There are two types of compensatory damages: special and general. ***Special damages*** include economic injuries such as subsequent hospitalization or rehabilitation costs, costs of assistance or custodial care, lost wages, or lost earning capacity. ***General or noneconomic damages*** address emotional injuries such as loss of companionship (consortium), mental anguish, grief and pain, and suffering. ***Punitive, or exemplary damages***, may also be sought if the alleged conduct can be shown to be wanton and willful, reckless, fraudulent, intentional, grossly negligent, or malicious.

In the event that the elements of medical negligence cannot be proven or the case is relatively straightforward, a theory of medical liability can also be premised in the doctrine of *res ipsa loquitur,* which literally translates as "the facts speak for themselves." The specific elements of a ***res ipsa loquitur*** claim vary by state. However, in general, a case can be submitted to the jury on the theory of *res ipsa loquitur* only when the plaintiff can establish that (a) the event is one that ordinarily does not occur in the absence of negligence; (b) the event was caused by an agency or instrumentality within the exclusive control of the defendant; and (c) the event cannot have been due to any voluntary action or contribution on the part of the plaintiff. Examples of *res ipsa loquitur* claims include retained instruments, positioning injuries, and intraoperative burns and do not usually require expert testimony.

Medical malpractice insurance indemnity policies provide insurance coverage for claims arising from alleged malpractice. The malpractice carrier has two principal obligations to the insured: the ***duty to defend*** and the ***duty to indemnify***. In order to provide a legal defense, an insurance carrier will typically retain knowledgeable and experienced defense counsel and pay the legal fees on behalf of the defendant physician. The duty to indemnify requires the carrier to pay the amount of a settlement or judgment on a covered claim within the set policy limits. There are two general types of medical malpractice insurance policies. ***Occurrence policies*** cover incidents that occur during the policy period, even if it is reported in the future following expiration or discontinuance of that policy. ***Claims-made policies*** will only cover occurrences where both the event and the claim occur during the life of the policy. Because the average malpractice claim is made 1 to 2 years following an incident, claims-made policies usually require that the physician purchase either "nose" or "tail" coverage in order to maintain coverage during job or insurer-to-insurer transitions.

References

1. Li G, Warner M, Lang BH, et al. Epidemiology of anesthesia-related mortality in the United States, 1999–2005. *Anesthesiology.* 2009;110(4):759–765.
2. Haller G, Laroche T, Clergue F. Morbidity in anaesthesia: Today and tomorrow. *Best Pract Res Clin Anaesthesiol.* 2011;25(2):123–132.
3. Institute of Medicine. *To Err Is Human: Building a Safer Health System.* Washington, DC: National Academy Press; 1999.
4. Institute of Medicine. *Crossing the Quality Chasm: A New Health System for the 21st Century.* Washington, DC: National Academy Press; 2001.

5. Cooper JB, Newbower RS, Long CD, et al. Preventable anesthesia mishaps: A study of human factors. *Anesthesiology.* 1978;49(6):399–406.
6. Cooper JB, Cullen DJ, Eichhorn JH, et al. Administrative guidelines for response to an adverse anesthesia event. The Risk Management Committee of the Harvard Medical School's Department of Anaesthesia. *J Clin Anesth.* 1993;5(1):79–84.
7. Donabedian A. The role of outcomes in quality assessment and assurance. *Qual Rev Bull.* 1992;18:356–360.
8. Epstein RM, Hundert EM. Defining and assessing professional competence. *JAMA.* 2002;287(2):226–235.
9. American Board of Internal Medicine Foundation. American College of Physicians– American Society of Internal Medicine Foundation. European Federation of Internal Medicine Medical professionalism in the new millennium: A physician charter. *Ann Intern Med.* 2002;136(3):243–246.
10. Tetzlaff JE. Anesthesiology. Professionalism in anesthesiology: "What is it?" or "I know it when I see it." *Anesthesiology.* 2009;110(4):700–702.

Questions

1. Which of the following is a formal principle of medical ethics?
   A. Patient autonomy
   B. Beneficence
   C. Nonmaleficence
   D. All of the above

2. Which of the following is an example of the medical ethical principle of "justice"?
   A. An anesthesiologist decides on a perioperative care plan based on careful review of the patient's medical history, without discussion with the otherwise mentally competent and communicative patient.
   B. An anesthesiologist working in a mass casualty incident triages patients to settings of emergent care, delayed care, or expectant care.
   C. An anesthesiologist provides the highest level of care, without regard to personal gain or societal interests.
   D. The concept of *primum non nocere* (first, do no harm).

3. A healthy 2-month-old, former preterm boy is undergoing an elective inguinal hernia repair under general anesthesia. The "crew resource management" paradigm for perioperative care team coordination includes all of the following examples EXCEPT:
   A. A preoperative "timeout" takes place for all members of the team to review the surgical safety checklist.
   B. Prior to administering a local anesthetic field block, the surgeon, nursing staff, and anesthesiologist review and agree on the correct drug and dose for the child.
   C. When the surgeon and anesthesiologist disagree on the maximum local anesthetic dose for the child, the procedure is briefly halted to consult with the hospital pharmacy.
   D. On her first day in her anesthesiology clerkship, the medical student assisting the anesthesiologist notices a large volume of air in the intravenous tubing, but refrains from telling the anesthesiologist due to her insecurity.

4. A healthy, mentally competent, 55-year-old married father of three teenage children is about to undergo an elective open repair of an iliac artery pseudoaneurysm. The patient is a Jehovah's Witness who has noted in writing on both his hospital admission form and his surgical consent form that he will not accept any type of blood product under any condition. The anesthesiologist should:
   A. Contact hospital risk management to obtain a court order to transfuse blood products, should unexpected life-threatening bleeding occur intraoperatively.
   B. Discuss the issue with the patient to confirm his wishes (even if doing so might put his life in danger) and to discuss potential alternative treatments (e.g., intraoperative blood salvage and return).
   C. Arrange for intraoperative blood salvage (e.g., cell-saver) to be used without informing the patient.
   D. Refuse to participate in the procedure.

5. The National Practitioner Data Bank collects and releases information related to the professional conduct and competence of physicians and other health care providers, including which of the following?
   A. Negative privileging actions by a hospital
   B. Previous malpractice claims, irrespective of settlement
   C. Adverse licensure actions by state authorities
   D. All of the above

6. Which of the following is an example of an advance directive?
   A. Living will
   B. Do-not-resuscitate (DNR) order
   C. Durable power of attorney
   D. All of the above

7. Medical malpractice is a type of negligence that is argued in civil court, as opposed to criminal court. Related to the initiation, location, and appeals process for such proceedings, all of the following are true EXCEPT:
   A. Civil lawsuits are initiated by postal mailing of a summons, claim form, or complaint document to the defendant physician's malpractice insurer.
   B. Civil malpractice disputes are generally filed in state trial courts and final judicial authority generally rests in the state court of appeals.
   C. Civil malpractice disputes can be filed in federal courts only in specific instances where federal issues are involved.
   D. Once a defendant physician receives a proper summons, the defendant has only a limited time to respond to the complaint (i.e., statutory time limit).

8. Regarding medical malpractice insurance indemnity policies, which of the following is TRUE?
   A. Defendant physicians generally must retain their own defense counsel.
   B. Occurrence policies only cover occurrences where both the event and the claim occur during the life of the policy.
   C. Claims-made policies usually require the physician to purchase a "tail" policy to maintain malpractice coverage for incidents that occurred during the life of the policy but the malpractice claim was filed after the policy ended.
   D. Insurance carriers are not required to pay the amount of a settlement or judgment, even if the amount is within set policy limits.

9. A 75-year-old mentally competent woman with no living relatives is scheduled to undergo hip replacement surgery and has granted legal and documented "simple power of attorney" to her otherwise unrelated and mentally competent housemate. Is the following statement true or false? "While under general anesthesia, the housemate may make health care decisions on behalf of the patient."
   A. True
   B. False

10. The Donabedian model, root cause analysis, the PDSA cycle, and the Six Sigma model are all examples of which of the following:
    A. Adverse event reporting systems
    B. Strategies to document "meaningful use" of electronic health records
    C. Paradigms for decision making in medical ethics
    D. Quality improvement models

41 Critical Care Medicine

Matthew R. Hallman

The practice of critical care medicine (CCM) and development of intensive care units (ICUs) date to at least the 1940s and perhaps earlier. Advances in surgical interventions along with increased incidences of respiratory failure due to polio epidemics led to an increased demand for physicians specializing in the care of critically ill patients, especially patients with respiratory failure. To meet this demand, the first CCM training program was established by Peter Safar, an anesthesiologist at the University of Pittsburgh, in the 1960s, but it was not until 1986 that the first CCM board certification examination was administered by the American Board of Anesthesiology. As of 2010, approximately 1,300 anesthesiologists had completed the CCM certification process. However, <10% of practicing intensivists are anesthesiologists, and the majority of intensivists in the United States continue to be pulmonary physicians. Fortunately for those interested in this specialty, the future need for intensivists is expected to be much greater than the supply.

The scope of CCM is vast, covering nearly every aspect of illness and injury and drawing upon knowledge from nearly every medical and surgical specialty. It is also a specialty that continues to undergo tremendous change. New technologies, equipment, and medications along with increased understanding of diseases and pathophysiology allow for the treatment of increasingly ill patients. More recently, as the economics of health care delivery have received increased attention, the focus on delivering evidence-based, cost-effective care has also increased. Because the ICU is one of the most resource-intensive areas of modern hospitals, care of patients in the ICU has been identified as an obvious target for increased efficiency.

Although the entire spectrum of critical care is beyond the scope of this chapter, widely applicable aspects of contemporary critical care are reviewed here. The first part of the chapter addresses processes of care that are applicable to most ICU settings, including both medical and surgical ICUs. The second part of the chapter provides an overview of the management for some commonly encountered diagnoses. The entire chapter focuses on evidence-based practices that may improve both patient outcomes and health care system performance in the perioperative setting.

I. Processes of Care

A. Staffing

Advances in medical and surgical therapeutics have increased the complexity of care for an aging and increasingly ill population. It has become clear that providing the best care for such a population requires a knowledge base and skill set that are highly specialized and that involving intensivists in the care of critically ill patients is desirable. Compared with low-intensity staffing models, *high-intensity staffing* models (i.e., an intensivist-led team or mandatory consultation of an intensivist) are associated with lower hospital and ICU mortality as well as shorter hospital and ICU lengths of stay (1).

Patient outcomes appear to be further improved by the addition of *multidisciplinary* providers to intensivist led teams. Examples include pharmacist participation in daily rounds, as well as the inclusion of nurses, dieticians, and respiratory therapists. These practices significantly reduce costs and medication-related adverse events and are also associated with decreased patient mortality (2).

B. Checklists

Despite the improvement in communication and information transfer that occurs with multidisciplinary teams, high stress and a massive volume of information in the ICU environment can lead to errors. Checklists have been widely implemented on ICU rounds as cognitive aids that serve as daily reminders to evaluate a limited number of interventions, preventative measures, bundles, and processes of care that can improve outcomes. Their implementation is associated with decreased mortality and ICU length of stay, and their cost is negligible (3). Considering the potential benefits and the minimal economic investment required for checklist implementation, their use is strongly recommended. In fact, many of the care processes discussed in this chapter commonly appear on checklists and should be considered for every patient, every day. Suggested content for consideration and inclusion in a daily ICU checklist is listed in Table 41-1. Content might be added or removed based on local ICU considerations.

C. Resource Management

In 2014, the Critical Care Societies Collaborative released a list of "Five Things Physicians and Patients Should Question" in critical care as part of the Choosing Wisely campaign. The campaign is designed to reduce unnecessary interventions that lack cost-effectiveness and has been supported by many medical specialties. At the top of the list is a recommendation to not order diagnostic studies (chest x-rays, blood gases, blood chemistries and counts, and electrocardiograms) at regular intervals (e.g., daily) unless there is a clear indication. Compared with the practice of ordering tests only to answer clinical questions or when doing so will directly affect management, the routine ordering of tests increases costs, does not benefit patients, and may in fact harm them. This and other efforts to minimize unnecessary interventions recognize both the

Table 41-1 Suggested Daily Intensive Care Unit Checklist	
• Spontaneous awakening trial	• Unnecessary labs and imaging discontinued
• Spontaneous breathing trial	
• Nutrition/diet ordered	• Antibiotics discontinued
• Glucose control adequate	• Foley catheter removed
• Deep vein thrombosis prophylaxis initiated	• Central venous catheter and arterial line removed

financial impact medical practice decisions have on individual patients and the health care system overall. These efforts also emphasize the physician's role in providing not just effective care, but efficient care.

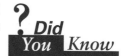

D. Analgesia and Sedation

Pain

Pain, agitation, and delirium (PAD) are closely linked and are often experienced by critically ill patients. There are many causes of PAD related to the underlying medical conditions and also to the assessments and interventions that occur as part of care. ***An effective PAD management program should be tailored to each individual patient and involve steps to prevent, detect, quantify, treat, and reassess PAD.*** Current guideline recommendations are summarized in Figure 41-1 (4).

Opioids are the primary modality of treating moderate to severe pain in critically ill adults. However, they have undesirable side effects including nausea, constipation, respiratory depression, and alteration of mental status. When titrated to similar endpoints, there is not one opioid medication that has been shown to be superior to others. In order to reduce opioid-related side effects, nonopioid analgesics such as acetaminophen, nonsteroidal anti-inflammatory drugs, local anesthetics, ketamine, and γ-aminobutyric acid analogues may be used in conjunction with opioids. In the case of mild pain, acetaminophen or nonsteroidal anti-inflammatory drugs may replace opioids altogether. Regional anesthesia techniques may also be helpful in managing a variety of types of pain including extremity injuries, incisional pain on the torso, and rib fractures. Neuropathic pain, commonly related to diabetes and vascular disease, can be just as debilitating as nonneuropathic pain and therefore deserves equal attention. Although all these medications can play a role in the management of neuropathic pain, the γ-aminobutyric acid analogues, such as gabapentin, pregabalin, and carbamazepine, are recommended as first-line agents. In all instances, before and after assessments of pain severity should be made to guide further analgesic administration. A number of validated assessment instruments exist including the Numeric Rating Scale, Behavioral Pain Scale, and the Critical care Pain Observation Tool. It is important to note that vital signs alone should not be used to assess pain but may be a clue (i.e., pain-induced sympathetic nervous system activation) to further investigate whether pain is present.

Agitation and Delirium

A variety of factors may contribute to the development of agitation and delirium including pain, hypotension, hypoxemia, hypoglycemia, alcohol and other drug intoxication or withdrawal, sleep cycle alteration, light, noise, and mechanical ventilation. These contributing factors should be sought out and aggressively corrected. Similar to pain treatment, treating agitation and delirium effectively requires patient assessment followed by an intervention, with a subsequent reassessment to determine the effectiveness of the intervention. There are multiple validated agitation and delirium assessment tools, including the Richmond Agitation Sedation Score and the Sedation Agitation Scale for agitation and the Confusion Assessment Method for the ICU and ICU Delirium Screening Checklist for delirium. All patients should have daily screening with one of these tools. When agitation and delirium are detected, it is especially important to differentiate pain from other etiologies as appropriate treatment of pain may eliminate the need for additional sedatives. Efforts should also be made in all patients to minimize sleep interruption and to maintain a normal sleep–wake cycle. Opening the window shades, turning on

	PAIN	AGITATION	DELIRIUM
ASSESS	Assess pain ≥4x/shift & prn Preferred pain assessment tools: • Patient able to self-report → NRS (0–10) • Unable to self-report → BPS (3–12) or CPOT (0–8) Patient is in significant pain if NRS ≥ 4, BPS > 5, or CPOT ≥ 3	Assess agitation, sedation ≥4x/shift & prn Preferred sedation assessment tools: • RASS (−5 to +4) or SAS (1 to 7) • NMB → consider using brain function monitoring Depth of agitation, sedation defined as: • *agitated* if RASS = +1 to +4, or SAS = 5 to 7 • *awake and calm* if RASS = 0, or SAS = 4 • *lightly sedated* if RASS = −1 to −2, or SAS = 3 • *deeply sedated* if RASS = −3 to −5, or SAS = 1 to 2	Assess delirium Q shift & prn Preferred delirium assessment tools: • CAM-ICU (+ or −) • ICDSC (0 to 8) Delirium present if: • CAM-ICU is positive • ICDSC ≥ 4

TREAT	Treat pain within 30' then reassess:
	• Non-pharmacologic treatment–relaxation therapy
	• Pharmacologic treatment:
	  – Non-neuropathic pain → non-opioid analgesics, +/− opioids
	  – Neuropathic pain → gabapentin or carbamazepine, + opioids
	  – S/p abdominal or thoracic incision, rib fractures → thoracic epidural
		Targeted sedation or DSI (*Goal: patient purposely follows commands without agitation*):
		RASS = −2 – 0, SAS = 3 – 4
		• If *under sedated* (RASS > 0, SAS >4) assess/treat pain → treat w/sedatives prn (non-benzodiazepines preferred, unless ETOH or benzodiazepine withdrawal is suspected)
		• If *over sedated* (RASS < −2, SAS <3) hold sedatives until at target, then restart at 50% of previous dose
			• Treat pain as needed
			• Reorient patients; familiarize surroundings; use patient's eyeglasses, hearing aids if needed
			• Pharmacologic treatment of delirium:
			  – Avoid benzodiazepines unless ETOH or benzodiazepine withdrawal is suspected
			  – Avoid rivastigmine
			  – Avoid antipsychotics if ↑ risk of Torsades de pointes

PREVENT	• Administer pre-procedural analgesia and/or non-pharmacologic interventions (e.g., relaxation therapy)
	• Treat pain first, then sedate
		• Consider daily SBT, early mobility and exercise when patients are at goal sedation level, unless contraindicated
		• EEG monitoring if:
		  – at risk for seizures
		  – burst suppression therapy is indicated for ↑ ICP
			• Identify delirium risk factors: dementia, HTN, ETOH abuse, high severity of illness, coma, benzodiazepine administration
			• Avoid benzodiazepine use in those at ↑ risk for delirium
			• Mobilize and exercise patients early
			• Promote sleep (control light, noise; cluster patient care activities; decrease nocturnal stimuli)
			• Restart baseline psychiatric meds, if indicated

Figure 41-1 Pain, Agitation and Delirium Guideline Implementation. NRS, Numeric Rating Scale; BPS, Behavioral Pain Scale; CPOT, Critical care Pain Observation Tool; RASS, Richmond Agitation Sedation Score; SAS, Sedation Agitation Scale; CAM-ICU, Confusion Assessment Method for the intensive care unit; ICDSC, Delirium Screening Checklist; DSI, Daily Sedation Interruption; SBT, spontaneous breathing trial; IV, intravenous; NMB, neuromuscular blockade; ETOH, ethanol; nonbenzodiazepines, propofol (use in intubated/mechanically ventilated patients), dexmedetomidine (use in either intubated or nonintubated patients); EEG, electroencephalography; ICP, intracranial pressure; HTN, hypertension. (Reproduced from Barr J, Fraser GL, Puntillo K, et al. Clinical practice guidelines for the management of pain, agitation, and delirium in adult patients in the intensive care unit. *Crit Care Med.* 2013;41:263–306, with permission.)

lights, engaging the patient with conversation, television, and radio during the day, while turning off lights, minimizing noise, and minimizing procedures at night all help to achieve this goal.

When pharmacologic intervention is necessary, the goal is to use the smallest amount of sedative possible. Although deeper states of sedation may make patient care easier, minimal sedation is associated with improved outcomes including reduced duration of mechanical ventilation and shorter ICU stays. Pharmacologic treatment of agitation commonly involves benzodiazepines, propofol, and dexmedetomidine. Although all three agents are potentially useful for agitation treatment, benzodiazepines are associated with increased delirium and should be minimized unless alcohol withdrawal is suspected. Regardless of the agent used, unless there is a specific contraindication to stopping sedation, all patients should have a daily *spontaneous awakening trial (SAT)*.

II. Ventilator Liberation and Spontaneous Breathing Trials

Liberation (sometimes called weaning) from mechanical ventilation is a process that requires, at a minimum, adequate oxygenation and ventilation without mechanical assistance. However, safe removal of the endotracheal tube requires patients to meet additional criteria including the ability to manage secretions and protect their airway from aspiration and obstruction.

Both objective and subjective parameters should be examined in order to determine a patient's suitability for liberation from mechanical ventilation. Table 41-2 lists commonly used criteria for extubation. The objective criteria require the patient to undergo a *spontaneous breathing trial (SBT)*. The SBT is a 30- to 120-minute trial of breathing with little or no assistance from the ventilator. It may be performed with a variety of techniques including T-piece trials, pressure support ventilation trials, and continuous positive airway pressure trials, although no single technique is superior to another. An SBT should be performed daily on all patients who qualify. Typically this includes mechanically ventilated patients requiring <60% fraction of inspired oxygen

? Did You Know

For mechanically ventilated patients in the intensive care unit who are recovering respiratory function, a spontaneous breathing trial (reduced ventilator support while the trachea is still intubated) is often coupled with a spontaneous awakening trial (reduced administration of sedative medications) to determine the likelihood of successful tracheal extubation.

Table 41-2   Criteria for Extubation

Subjective Criteria
- Indication for intubation is resolved
- Adequate airway reflexes to handle secretions and avoid upper airway obstruction
- No signs of increased work of breathing (e.g., nasal flairing, accessory muscle use, sternal retractions, diaphoresis)

Objective Criteria (based on spontaneous breathing trial performance)
- Hemodynamic stability: Heart rate and blood pressure change <20% from baseline
- Adequate oxygenation: SaO_2 >90%, PaO_2 >60 mm Hg, PaO_2/FiO_2 >150
- PEEP <8 cm H_2O and FiO_2 <0.5
- Adequate ventilation: $PaCO_2$ <60 mm Hg, pH >7.25
- Rapid shallow breathing index (RR/Vt) <105
- Negative inspiratory force >30 cm H_2O
- Vital capacity >10 cc/kg

SaO_2, arterial oxygen saturation; PaO_2, arterial partial pressure of oxygen; FiO_2, fraction of inspired oxygen; PEEP, positive end-expiratory pressure; $PaCO_2$, arterial partial pressure of carbon dioxide; RR/Vt, respiratory rate/tidal volume.
Note: These criteria are only guidelines. Decisions regarding extubation should be made on an individual basis.

(FiO_2) and positive end-expiratory pressure (PEEP) <8 cm H_2O. When combined with a protocolized daily SAT, the daily SBT has been shown to shorten the duration of mechanical ventilation and may improve mortality.

A. Venous Thromboembolism

Deep venous thrombosis (DVT) and venous thromboembolism (VTE) are common problems in critically ill patients. The incidence may be as high as 30% for DVTs and 5% for pulmonary embolism (PE) depending on the population. The pathologist Rudolph Virchow was the first to describe the combination of three factors that predispose patients to venous thrombosis. The triad of hypercoagulability, venous stasis, and vascular endothelial damage bare his name, and almost all ICU patients have at least one of these risk factors. A simple scoring system for VTE risk stratification is shown in Table 41-3. Determining VTE risk is important in that it helps in choosing

Table 41-3　Caprini Risk Assessment Model for Venous Thromboembolism

1 Point	2 Points	3 Points	5 Points
Age 41–60 years	Age 61–74 years	Age >75 yr	Stroke <1 month
Minor surgery	Arthroscopic surgery	Personal history of VTE	Elective lower extremity arthroplasty
Body mass index >25 kg/m²	Major open surgery >45 min	Family history of VTE	Hip, pelvis, or leg fracture
Swollen legs	Laparoscopic surgery >45 min	Any thrombophilia	Acute spinal cord injury <1 month
Varicose veins	Bed rest >72 hr	Elevated serum homocysteine	Multiple trauma <1 month
Pregnant or postpartum <1 month	Immobilizing plaster cast	Heparin-induced thrombocytopenia	
History of miscarriage	Central venous access		
Oral contraceptives or hormone replacement therapy		High Risk: ≥5 points	
Sepsis <1 month		Intermediate Risk: 3–4 points Low Risk: 1–2 points Very Low Risk: 0 points	
Serious lung disease <1 month			
Abnormal pulmonary function			
Acute myocardial infarction			
Congestive heart failure <1 month			
History of inflammatory bowel disease			
Medical patient on bed rest			

VTE, venous thromboembolism.
Adapted from Pollak AW, McBane RD 2nd. Succinct review of the new VTE prevention and management guidelines. *Mayo Clin Proc.* 2014;89:394–408.

prophylactic therapy and in determining the level of suspicion for VTE in individual patients (5). *The clinical decision of which patients to treat prophylactically and how to treat them always balances the risk of VTE with the risks of VTE prophylaxis*, including heparin-induced thrombocytopenia and bleeding. It is generally agreed that high-risk patients without contraindications should receive prophylaxis with low molecular-weight heparin (LMWH). Patients with low to moderate risk should receive either low-dose unfractionated heparin (UFH) or LMWH. Patients with contraindications to LMWH or UFH may receive prophylaxis with mechanical devices (serial compression devices), and in some cases inferior vena cava (IVC) filters. But IVC filters should be reserved for the setting of high VTE risk and ongoing contraindications to anticoagulation. There is no evidence to support the routine preventive placement of IVC filters in the critically ill, including those with traumatic injuries. UFH and LMWH do not need to be routinely held prior to most surgical procedures (unless regional anesthesia is under consideration), but decisions regarding perioperative anticoagulation should be made in conjunction with the surgical team.

Although routine DVT screening studies are not recommended, asymptomatic DVTs are common. Thus, VTE should be considered in patients with nonspecific findings such as tachycardia, tachypnea, fever, asymmetric extremity edema, and gas exchange abnormalities. *Compression Doppler ultrasonography* is the most commonly used test for diagnosis of DVT. It has a good positive and negative predictive value. However, regularly scheduled screening compression Doppler ultrasonography is not generally recommended. The Well's criteria and D-dimer levels, tests commonly used in the outpatient setting, have little role in critically ill patients due to their lack of specificity.

The mainstay of treatment for VTE is heparin, which should be started prior to confirmatory studies if clinical suspicion is high. The advantage of UFH over LMWH in the ICU population is its titratability and rapid reversibility, which may be desirable in patients at high risk for bleeding and in those with renal insufficiency. In patients with PE and hemodynamic instability, chemical thrombolytic therapy or mechanical thrombectomy should be considered (if not contraindicated). Although the data supporting thrombolytic therapy for treatment of PE are limited, patients with massive PE or shock are likely to benefit.

B. Nutrition

Critical illness can lead to hypermetabolic states and an early risk of malnutrition. Poor nutritional status is associated with increased mortality and morbidity among critically ill patients. Therefore, appropriate nutrition is an important aspect of critical care, and adequate nutritional support should be considered a standard of care. The American Society for Parenteral and Enteral Nutrition regularly publishes and updates evidence-based guidelines for best nutritional practices (6). The most recent guidelines recommend the following practices in the ICU setting:

- Caloric needs for most patients can be predicted with a simple formula based on ideal body weight (25 to 30 kcal/kg/day). Proteins should represent 15% to 20% of this (1.2 to 2 g/kg/day). In the obese patient (body mass index >30), permissive underfeeding at a level 60% to 70% of ideal body weight–predicted needs is acceptable.
- Nutrition should be initiated in the first 24 to 48 hours after ICU admission. In patients unable to take a volitional oral diet, a feeding tube should be placed.

- Postpyloric positioning of the feeding tube (vs. gastric positioning) is not necessary prior to the start of tube feedings.
- Enteral feeds should not be held for residual volumes >500 mL unless there is other evidence of feeding intolerance. In the event of gastric feeding intolerance, postpyloric positioning of the feeding tube and prokinetic agents (e.g., metoclopramide, erythromycin) may be considered.
- Total parenteral nutrition should not be used unless enteral nutrition is anticipated to be inadequate for at least 7 days, as parenteral nutrition is associated with increased infectious complications.

? Did You Know

Vigilant glucose control is required in the intensive care unit to minimize morbidity associated with both hyperglycemia and hypoglycemia, although the most appropriate serum glucose range in this setting remains controversial.

C. Glucose Control

Hyperglycemia is common in critically ill patients. It can occur in both diabetics and nondiabetics. It results from both a primary increase in glucose production as well as insulin resistance due to inflammatory and hormonal mediators that are released in response to injury. It can be exacerbated by therapeutic interventions, including corticosteroids and total parenteral nutrition. Hyperglycemia is associated with increased risks of infection as well as poorer outcomes in patients with stroke, traumatic brain injury, and myocardial infarction.

Considering the association of hyperglycemia with negative outcomes, it is not surprising that efforts to improve outcomes by treating hyperglycemia have been made. Although targeting serum glucose levels of 80 to 110 mg/dL (commonly called tight control) was advocated in the past, more recent evidence suggests that this level of control is associated with significant *hypoglycemia* and possibly increased mortality (7). Current serum glucose targets are somewhat variable, but 140 to 180 mg/dL is acceptable in most patients. As insulin delivery and glucose monitoring systems improve, it may become possible to safely target levels less than 140 mg/dL.

D. Stress Ulcer Prophylaxis

Gastric mucosal breakdown with resulting gastritis and ulceration (stress ulceration) is common in critically ill patients, but significant bleeding from the ulcerations is uncommon. Significant bleeding occurs in <4% of high-risk patients (those with a coagulopathy or more than 48 hours of mechanical ventilation) and in <1% of patients without these risk factors. Despite this being a relatively uncommon event, the mortality from significant bleeding (requiring blood transfusion or resulting in hemodynamic instability) is >45% and has resulted in the common use of pharmacologic agents including H_2 receptor antagonists, proton pump inhibitors, and cytoprotective agents such as sucralfate for stress ulcer prophylaxis (SUP). These medications are not benign and are associated with increased costs, drug interactions, and adverse drug reactions. In addition, due to changes in the pH of gastric contents, H_2 receptor antagonists and proton pump inhibitors may be associated with increased rates of pneumonia and *Clostridium difficile* infection. Considering this, routine SUP in critically ill patients is not recommended. Further, enteral feeding may be a safe and more effective strategy for SUP than pharmacologic agents. Among high-risk patients, pharmacologic SUP may be considered, but no agent has been shown to be clearly superior to the others.

E. Transfusion Therapy

Anemia is common in critical illness. Most patients admitted to the ICU are anemic at some point during their hospital stay, and many will receive a blood transfusion. Although both anemia and blood transfusions are associated with mortality, it is important to note this does not imply cause and effect and may simply reflect the severity of illness. Anemia in critical illness has many causes, including blood loss from the primary injury or illness, iatrogenic blood loss due to daily blood sampling, nutritional deficiencies, and marrow suppression.

Transfusion thresholds are a source of ongoing debate. Historically, a hemoglobin (Hb) concentration of 10 g/dL was advocated. This was based on the assumption that critically ill patients have reduced physiologic reserve and require this level for adequate tissue oxygen delivery. However, red blood cell transfusion carries a risk of infection, transfusion-related acute lung injury, transfusion-associated circulatory overload, transfusion-related immunomodulation, microchimarism, and more (see Chapter 24). The undesired effects of transfusion may explain why a large, randomized, prospective trial of transfusion requirements in critical illness failed to show a mortality difference when a restrictive transfusion threshold (Hb <7 g/dL) was compared with a more conventional threshold of <10 g/dL (8). These data strongly suggest that routine transfusion of critically ill patients is not necessary and may be harmful unless the Hb concentration is below 7 g/dL. Based largely on the results of this trial, most critical care guidelines now suggest a transfusion threshold of 7 g/dL unless there is evidence of ongoing blood loss, acute myocardial infarction, unstable angina, or possibly acute neurologic injury.

III. Common Diagnoses in the Intensive Care Unit

A. Nosocomial Infections

Nosocomial infections are a major source of morbidity and mortality in the critically ill, but many of them are preventable with relatively simple interventions. There are four types of infection that are relatively unique to inpatient and ICU care that should be considered when signs suggestive of infection arise. They are ventilator-associated pneumonia (VAP), central line-associated blood stream infection (CLABSI), catheter-associated urinary tract infection (UTI), and *C. difficile* infection (CDI).

Ventilator-associated Pneumonia
The risk of developing VAP increases with the duration of mechanical ventilation. This underscores the importance of any intervention that can reduce the duration of mechanical ventilation such as SATs, SBTs, and sedation minimization. The exact definition and diagnostic criteria for VAP are controversial, but most agree that radiologic evidence of pneumonia, fever, leukocytosis, increasing sputum production, and quantitative culture results all may support the diagnosis. VAP is typically classified as early-onset (occurring within the first 48 to 72 hours of intubation or ventilation) or late-onset (occurring thereafter). Antibiotic-sensitive bacteria including *Hemophilus influenza,* *Streptococcus pneumonia,* and methicillin-sensitive *Staphylococcus aureus* are often the causal organisms. In contrast, late-onset VAP is associated with more antibiotic-resistant organisms, including methicillin-resistant *Staphylococcus aureus* (MRSA), *Pseudomonas aeruginosa,* and *Acinetobacter.*

A number of simple and low-cost interventions may reduce the incidence of VAP, including strict handwashing between patients, positioning the patient with at least 30 degrees of head elevation, avoiding inappropriate use of gastric stress ulcer prophylaxis, using closed tracheal suction systems, and the use of chlorhexidine for daily oral decontamination. These practices should be rigorously applied in all ICUs.

Once VAP has developed, early detection and appropriate treatment are essential to reducing morbidity and mortality. As noted previously, the diagnostic criteria for VAP are controversial. However, an invasive diagnostic strategy is likely more accurate than traditional clinical criteria to diagnose VAP and is recommended whenever possible. Invasive strategies typically involve collection of bronchial-alveolar specimens using lavage or protected brushes and then quantitating bacterial growth in the laboratory.

Because delayed treatment of VAP is associated with increased mortality, treatment should not be delayed pending diagnostic evaluation. Treatment should be started after culture specimens are sent if the clinical suspicion of VAP is high. Antibiotics can then be narrowed in spectrum or discontinued depending on the results from quantitative cultures after 48 to 72 hours. This approach of de-escalating therapy is designed to both ensure adequate initial antibiotic treatment and also to avoid development of antibiotic resistance. In general, antibiotic treatment for early-onset VAP can be relatively narrow in spectrum and limited to a single agent. Late-onset VAP requires broader spectrum antibiotics covering resistant gram-negative organisms and MRSA. Table 41-4 lists common antibiotic selections for a variety of common infections. However, antibiotic selection should always consider local patterns of

Table 41-4   Suggested Empiric Antibiotic Regimens for Common Intensive Care Unit Infections

Ventilator-associated Pneumonia	
• Early (<72 hr of intubation and hospital admission)	Ceftriaxone PLUS azithromycin Consider adding vancomycin or linezolid if known history of MRSA
• Late (>72 hr of intubation or hospital admission)	Vancomycin OR linezolid AND cefepime Consider adding ciprofloxacin if high incidence of MDR GNRs
Bloodstream	Vancomycin OR linezolid AND cefepime
Urinary Tract	
• Noncatheter-associated	Ceftriaxone
• Catheter-associated	Ceftazidime ADD vancomycin if GPCs on Gram stain CONSIDER meropenem instead of ceftazidime if concerned for MDR GNRs or ESBLs
***Clostridium difficile* diarrhea**	Vancomycin (oral dosing) IF shock, megacolon or ileus, then ADD intravenous metronidazole
Meningitis	
• Nonsurgical	Dexamethasone AND ceftriaxone AND vancomycin AND ampicillin AND acyclovir
• Postsurgical	Cefepime AND metronidazole AND vancomycin
Intra-abdominal	
• Community acquired	Ceftriaxone AND metronidazole
• Hospital acquired	Vancomycin AND either piperacillin-tazobactam OR meropenem
Sepsis, site unknown	Vancomycin AND meropenem Consider adding ciprofloxacin if concern for MDR GNRs or ESBLs

MRSA, methicillin-resistant *Staphylococcus aureus;* MDR, multidrug resistant; GNR, gram-negative rods; GPC, gram-positive cocci; ESBL, extended spectrum beta-lactamase.
Note: Antibiotic regimens should be narrowed once culture results are available.

Table 41-5 Best Practices for Central Venous Catheter Placement

Subclavian and internal jugular veins are preferred over femoral veins

Prep skin with chlorhexidine (if chlorhexidine allergy, 70% alcohol or tincture of iodine are acceptable alternatives)

Full barrier precautions (full body sterile drape)

Strict aseptic technique (handwashing, sterile gloves and gown, mask, and surgical cap)

Use ultrasound guidance to minimize number of needle passes

Choose a catheter with the minimum number of lumens possible for the clinical situation

Use a chlorhexidine impregnated sponge and sterile, transparent semipermeable dressing

Inspect the catheter site daily for signs of infection

Do not routinely replace catheters unless medically indicated[a]

Remove catheters as soon as possible

[a]When adherence to aseptic technique cannot be maintained (e.g., catheters placed emergently), the catheter should be replaced with aseptic technique as soon as possible.

infection and hospital specific antibiograms. Optimal therapy duration is not clear, but 8 days is typically sufficient unless multidrug resistant organisms are present. In that case, 14 days or longer may be appropriate.

Central Line–associated Bloodstream Infections

The Centers for Disease Control and Prevention has a complex but strict definition for central line–associated bloodstream infection (CLABSI). The specific criteria have changed over time and are important for epidemiologic and payment reasons but are less important clinically. Conceptually, CLABSIs are infections arising from the placement or use of a central venous catheter. They have received a great deal of attention due to their common occurrence, high financial costs associated with treating these infections, significant mortality, and, most important, preventable nature. The Centers for Disease Control and Prevention's recommendations for practices that minimize such catheter-associated infectious risk are summarized in Table 41-5.

CLABSIs are commonly caused by a number of bacteria including *Staphylococcus epidermidis* and *S. aureus*, enteric gram-negative bacteria, *P. aeruginosa* and *Acinetobacter*, and occasionally *Enterococcal* species. Although coagulase-negative staphylococci are commonly isolated from blood cultures, they are in most cases contaminants. When catheter-related bacteremia is suspected, blood cultures should be tested from the catheter and peripheral sites, and consideration should be given to catheter removal. If infection is confirmed, the catheter should be removed promptly and replaced if necessary. As with other infections, prompt initiation of antibiotics may be lifesaving. High clinical suspicion of infection should trigger the initiation of broad-spectrum antibiotic coverage. Table 41-4 lists the common antibiotic regimens for CLABSI treatment.

Catheter-associated Urinary Tract Infection

UTIs are the second most common source of ICU infection. Because the incidence of catheter-associated UTI (CAUTI) increases with the duration of bladder catheterization, the necessity of an indwelling catheter should be reviewed daily and it should be removed as soon as possible. Other strategies to minimize the risk of CAUTIs include adherence to aseptic technique during placement, using bladder scans to minimize unnecessary catheter insertion, and maintaining the drainage bag below the level of the bladder. The responsible organisms are similar to those causing other nosocomial infections, including *Staphylococcal* species, *Enterococcus*, enteric gram-negative bacteria, and nonlactose fermenting gram-negative bacteria such as *Pseudomonas*. Once the diagnosis of a CAUTI has been made, it is reasonable to remove and replace the catheter (if still indicated) in an effort to reduce the microbiologic burden while also starting antibiotics. Recommended antibiotic treatment for UTIs is presented in Table 41-4.

Clostridium difficile *Diarrhea*

CDI has surpassed MRSA as the most common hospital-acquired infection. Pharmacologic risk factors for CDI include the use of antibiotics, antineoplastic agents, corticosteroids, and proton pump inhibitors. Although clindamycin, third-generation cephalosporins, and ampicillin are the most commonly implicated antibiotics, nearly all antibiotics, including metronidazole and vancomycin, may increase the risk. Other significant risk factors include prior CDI, chronic dialysis, gastrointestinal surgery, recent hospitalization, and postpyloric feeding. Diarrhea is the most common symptom, but it is not always present. Fever, abdominal pain, constipation, and leukocytosis (commonly with white blood cell counts >20,000/mm^3) should prompt consideration of the diagnosis, which can be further confirmed by a number of laboratory methods. It should be noted, however, that all currently available laboratory tests are imperfect and considerable debate exists as to which is the best. Once the diagnosis is confirmed, the treatments outlined in Table 41-4 can be initiated.

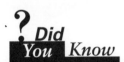

? *Did* *You* *Know*

With adoption in 2012 of the Berlin definition of acute respiratory distress syndrome (ARDS), the previous distinction between acute lung injury and ARDS has been replaced by the classification of ARDS into mild, moderate, or severe based on the degree of hypoxemia.

IV. Acute Lung Injury and Acute Respiratory Distress Syndrome

Acute respiratory distress syndrome (ARDS) occurs commonly in the ICU. It is characterized by the acute onset of hypoxemic respiratory failure, diffuse alveolar damage, noncardiogenic edema, reduced thoracic compliance, and both increased dead space and shunt. ARDS can occur as a result of direct injury to the lung (e.g., aspiration or pneumonia) or in association with extrapulmonary infection (e.g., sepsis) or injury (e.g., multiple trauma).

The definition of ARDS has changed over time. In 2012, a new consensus conference proposed the Berlin definition, which eliminates the distinction between acute lung injury and ARDS, and instead categorizes ARDS as mild, moderate, or severe based on the degree of hypoxemia (9). The classification system is summarized in Table 41-6.

Although ARDS appears to be a diffuse process by chest x-ray, computerized tomography imaging and histopathologic specimens demonstrate heterogeneity with severely damaged areas of lung existing next to normal appearing areas. Treatment of ARDS is largely supportive and consists mainly of attempting to preserve the uninjured lung.

A. Lung Protective Ventilation

Lung protective ventilation (LPV) describes a mechanical ventilation strategy that restricts tidal volumes (Vt) to ≤6 mL/kg and targets a static (plateau) airway pressure of ≤30 cm H_2O. Because minute ventilation can be maintained by increasing the respiratory rate only so far, it is commonly inadequate to eliminate all carbon dioxide that is produced. This results in a state of hypercapnea and respiratory acidosis called *permissive hypercapnea*. LPV is

Table 41-6	The Berlin Definition of the Acute Respiratory Distress Syndrome
Timing	Within 1 week of a known clinical insult or new or worsening respiratory symptoms
Chest imaging[a]	Bilateral opacities not fully explained by effusions, lobar/lung collapse, or nodules
Origin of edema	Not fully explained by cardiac failure or fluid overload. Need objective assessment (e.g., echocardiography) if no risk factor present
Oxygenation	
Mild:	200 mm Hg < PaO_2/FiO_2 ≤300 mm Hg; PEEP or CPAP ≥5 cm H_2O
Moderate:	100 mm Hg < PaO_2/FiO_2 ≤200 mm Hg; PEEP ≥5 cm H_2O
Severe:	PaO_2/FiO_2 ≤100 mm Hg with PEEP ≥5 cm H_2O

PaO_2, arterial partial pressure of oxygen; FiO_2, fraction of inspired oxygen; PEEP, positive end-expiratory pressure; CPAP, continuous positive airway pressure.
[a]Chest radiography or computed tomography scan.
Adapted from Force ADT, Ranieri VM, Rubenfeld GD, et al. Acute respiratory distress syndrome: The Berlin definition. *JAMA.* 2012;307:2526–2533.

the only intervention that has been shown to significantly reduce mortality in patients with ARDS compared with conventional ventilator strategies that rely on Vt >6 mL/kg.

LPV strategies would result in substantial atelectasis and increased shunt if a reduction in Vt were the only intervention. In order to maintain a nonatelectatic and open lung, low Vt is typically bundled with higher levels of PEEP. The optimal balance between PEEP and FiO_2 continues to be debated. Alternative approaches to *open lung ventilation* include the use of intermittent high-level end expiratory pressure or sigh breaths, pressure controlled ventilation, inverse ratio ventilation (prolonged inspiratory time), prone positioning, and high-frequency ventilation, which have all been used successfully.

B. Rescue Techniques
In instances when oxygenation is severely impaired, prone positioning, inhaled vasodilators, and extracorporeal life support (also known as extracorporeal membrane oxygenation) may be used. Of these techniques, only prone positioning has shown a mortality benefit in severe ARDS. Inhaled nitric oxide and inhaled prostacyclins variably and transiently improve oxygenation in ARDS by improving blood flow to ventilated alveoli, but they do not have a proven mortality benefit. Similarly, extracorporeal life support may improve oxygenation, but it has not been shown to reliably improve outcomes. Other therapies for ARDS that do not have strong evidence in support of their efficacy include inhaled beta-agonists, albumin infusions, and systemic steroids.

C. Sepsis and Septic Shock
Septic shock is a form of distributive shock associated with the activation of the systemic inflammatory response and is usually characterized by low systemic vascular resistance, hypotension, and regional blood flow redistribution, resulting in tissue hypoperfusion. In patients with systemic infections, the physiologic response can be staged on a continuum from a systemic inflammatory response syndrome (SIRS), to sepsis, to severe sepsis, to septic shock. SIRS has traditionally been defined as the presence of any two of the following: temperature >38°C or <36°C, white blood cell count >11 k/cc^3 or <4 k/cc^3 or

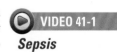
VIDEO 41-1
Sepsis

Table 41-7   Expanded Indications of Sepsis and Hypoperfusion

SIRS	Hypoperfusion
• Significant edema or positive fluid balance (>20 mL/kg over 24 hr)	• Sepsis-induced hypotension
• Hyperglycemia (plasma glucose > 140 mg/dL or 7.7 mmol/L) in the absence of diabetes	• Lactate above the upper limits of normal
• Plasma C-reactive protein more than two standard deviations above the normal value	• Urine output <0.5 mL/kg/hr for more than 2 hr despite adequate fluid resuscitation
• Plasma procalcitonin more than two standard deviations above the normal value	• Acute lung injury with PaO_2/FiO_2 <250 in the *absence* of pneumonia as the infection source
• Arterial hypotension (SBP <90 mm Hg, MAP <70 mm Hg, or an SBP decrease >40 mm Hg in adults or less than two standard deviations below normal for age)	• Acute lung injury with PaO_2/FiO_2 <200 in the *presence* of pneumonia as the infection source
• Arterial hypoxemia (PaO_2/FiO_2 <300)	• Creatinine >2.0 mg/dL (176.8 µmol/L)
• Acute oliguria (urine output <0.5 mL/kg/hr for at least 2 hr despite adequate fluid resuscitation)	• Bilirubin >2 mg/dL (34.2 µmol/L)
• Creatinine increase >0.5 mg/dL	• Platelet count <100,000 µL
• Coagulopathy (INR >1.5 or aPTT >60 s)	• Coagulopathy (INR >1.5)
• Ileus (absent bowel sounds)	• Altered mental status
• Thrombocytopenia (<100,000 μL^{-1})	• Cardiac dysfunction
• Hyperbilirubinemia (total bilirubin >4 mg/dL)	
• Hyperlactemia (>1 mmol/L)	
• Decreased capillary refill or mottling	

PaO_2, arterial partial pressure of oxygen; FiO_2, fraction of inspired oxygen; SBP, systolic blood pressure; MAP, mean arterial pressure; INR, international normalized ratio; aPTT, activated partial thromboplastin time.

>10% band forms, heart rate >90 beats per minute, or respiratory rate >20 per minute, or arterial carbon dioxide partial pressure <30 mm Hg. Although there are many noninfectious causes of SIRS, the presence of SIRS in the setting of suspected infection defines sepsis. Sepsis with evidence of organ hypoperfusion is considered severe sepsis, and the persistence of organ hypoperfusion despite adequate fluid resuscitation is considered septic shock. Unfortunately, these simple criteria lack sensitivity. Because the effective treatment of sepsis depends heavily on early recognition, the most recent guidelines for the treatment of sepsis list an expanded set of criteria that should alert clinicians to both sepsis and hypoperfusion (Table 41-7) (10).

Clinical management of sepsis is summarized in Table 41-8. The mainstay of early treatment is prompt and appropriate antibiotic administration, intravascular fluid resuscitation using crystalloids, vasopressors if hypotension persists after adequate fluid resuscitation, and inotropes if low cardiac output is suspected.

Fluid Resuscitation

Sepsis commonly causes a state of systemic vasodilation that results in a low effective circulating volume. Restoration of an effective circulating volume

Table 41-8   Management of Severe Sepsis and Septic Shock

- Early recognition of systemic inflammatory response syndrome or sepsis
- Obtain cultures prior to starting antibiotics, but do not delay antibiotics
- Administer empiric, broad-spectrum antibiotics within 1 hr of diagnosis
- Control the source of infection if appropriate (i.e., surgical intervention if appropriate)
- Administer crystalloids for fluid resuscitation
- Fluid challenge to achieve adequate filling pressures, and reduction of rate of fluids with rising filling pressure and no improvement in tissue perfusion
- Use norepinephrine as the first-line vasopressor for a target mean arterial pressure of ≥65 mm Hg
- Consider adding vasopressin at a fixed rate as an adjunct to catecholamines
- Consider dobutamine if low cardiac output persists despite fluid resuscitation
- Consider stress-dose steroid therapy if blood pressure is poorly responsive to fluid and vasopressors
- Targeting a hemoglobin of 7 to 9 g/dL in the absence of tissue hypoperfusion, coronary artery disease, or acute hemorrhage

Adapted from Dellinger RP, Levy MM, Rhodes A, et al. Surviving sepsis campaign: International guidelines for management of severe sepsis and septic shock: 2012. *Crit Care Med.* 2013;41:580–637.

may be achieved by increasing absolute intravascular volume with fluid resuscitation or by increasing vascular tone with vasopressors. A wide variety of fluids including blood products, albumin, synthetic colloid solutions, and many different crystalloid solutions have been extensively studied (see Chapter 23). Albumin has generally proven no more effective than crystalloid solutions, and synthetic colloids are associated with increased harm. Older guidelines have advocated that red blood cell transfusion be used as a way to increase oxygen delivery, but newer data suggest that targeting a Hb of 7 g/dL, the same as in most critically ill patients, is appropriate. *Crystalloids remain the preferred resuscitation fluid in most septic patients.*

Vasopressors

A number of vasopressors, including phenylephrine, norepinephrine, epinephrine, dopamine, and vasopressin, have been evaluated for systemic vascular resistance augmentation in sepsis. Norepinephrine is the recommended first-line agent owing to evidence of improved outcomes and reduced side effects. Epinephrine may be considered an alternative agent, but it is associated with increased arrhythmias. There is evidence that endogenous vasopressin production is suppressed in sepsis, and this provides the theoretical basis for considering the addition of vasopressin to norepinephrine. However, this has not been shown to improve outcomes. Dopamine and phenylephrine are generally not recommended.

Inotropes

Myocardial depression is a common phenomenon in patients with septic shock and may result in inadequate cardiac output and oxygen delivery. Once adequate intravascular volume and systemic vascular resistance have been achieved by the administration of fluid therapy and vasopressors, dobutamine or epinephrine may be used to augment cardiac output. Because pulmonary artery catheters are no longer recommended for the routine management of septic patients, central venous oxyhemoglobin saturation of ≥70% is a commonly used surrogate marker for adequate cardiac output and oxygen

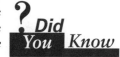
? *Did* **You Know**

Of the various vasopressors used to augment systemic vascular resistance in the setting of septic shock, norepinephrine is the first-line agent owing to evidence of improved outcomes and reduced side effects.

delivery. This may help guide decisions about the addition of inotropes. Both agents may precipitate arrhythmias.

Antibiotics

Identifying the source of the infection, attaining source control, and initiating appropriate antibiotic therapy early are at least as important as providing hemodynamic support in sepsis. Appropriate cultures should always be obtained before antimicrobial therapy is initiated and may include blood, sputum, urine, cerebrospinal fluid, and wounds and other fluid cultures (e.g., pleural fluid or ascites). Empiric antibiotic therapy should be started within 1 hour of recognition of sepsis (see Table 41-4 for antibiotic recommendations). After antibiotic susceptibility testing is available, narrowing the spectrum of antimicrobial treatment is appropriate.

Corticosteroids

The use of stress dose steroids (e.g., hydrocortisone 200 to 300 mg/day) in sepsis is controversial. Current guidelines recommend they be considered as an adjunct in patients with septic shock who remain hypotensive despite adequate volume resuscitation and vasopressor therapy. Cosyntropin stimulation testing prior to steroid initiation is not recommended. Steroids may also be considered in patients with recent steroid use.

References

1. Wilcox ME, Chong CA, Niven DJ, et al. Do intensivist staffing patterns influence hospital mortality following ICU admission? A systematic review and meta-analyses. *Crit Care Med.* 2013;41:2253–2274.
2. Lane D, Ferri M, Lemaire J, et al. A systematic review of evidence-informed practices for patient care rounds in the ICU. *Crit Care Med.* 2013;41:2015–2029.
3. Hales BM, Pronovost PJ. The checklist—a tool for error management and performance improvement. *J Crit Care.* 2006;21:231–235.
4. Barr J, Fraser GL, Puntillo K, et al. Clinical practice guidelines for the management of pain, agitation, and delirium in adult patients in the intensive care unit. *Crit Care Med.* 2013;41:263–306.
5. Guyatt GH, Akl EA, Crowther M, et al. Executive summary: Antithrombotic Therapy and Prevention of Thrombosis, 9th ed: American College of Chest Physicians Evidence-Based Clinical Practice Guidelines. *Chest.* 2012;141:7S–47S.
6. McClave SA, Martindale RG, Vanek VW, et al. Guidelines for the provision and assessment of nutrition support therapy in the adult critically ill patient: Society of Critical Care Medicine (SCCM) and American Society for Parenteral and Enteral Nutrition (A.S.P.E.N.). *JPEN.* 2009;33:277–316.
7. Kansagara D, Fu R, Freeman M, et al. Intensive insulin therapy in hospitalized patients: A systematic review. *Ann Intern Med.* 2011;154:268–282.
8. Hebert PC, Wells G, Blajchman MA, et al. A multicenter, randomized, controlled clinical trial of transfusion requirements in critical care. Transfusion Requirements in Critical Care Investigators, Canadian Critical Care Trials Group. *N Engl J Med.* 1999; 340:409–417.
9. Force ADT, Ranieri VM, Rubenfeld GD, et al. Acute respiratory distress syndrome: The Berlin definition. *JAMA.* 2012;307:2526–2533.
10. Dellinger RP, Levy MM, Rhodes A, et al. Surviving sepsis campaign: International guidelines for management of severe sepsis and septic shock: 2012. *Crit Care Med.* 2013;41:580–637.

Questions

1. The implementation of checklists for various ICU activities is associated with decreased mortality and decreased length of ICU stay at negligible cost. Examples of clinical activities frequently incorporated into such checklists include which of the following?
   A. Deep venous thrombosis prophylaxis
   B. Urinary catheter indications and removal
   C. Central venous catheter placement
   D. All of the above

2. Because before and after assessments are necessary to determine the effectiveness of a given clinical intervention, which of the following assessment instruments is validated and useful for the assessment of agitation and delirium?
   A. Richmond Agitation Sedation Score (RASS)
   B. Behavioral Pain Scale (BPS)
   C. Critical care Pain Observation Tool (CPOT)
   D. Spontaneous Awakening Trial (SAT)

3. A 45-year-old female recovering from severe aspiration pneumonia has been mechanically ventilated for 7 days and is now being considered for tracheal extubation. Each of the following techniques may be considered part of a spontaneous breathing trial (SBT) EXCEPT:
   A. Spontaneous ventilation with pressure support assistance
   B. Lung protective ventilation
   C. Spontaneous ventilation on a T-piece
   D. Spontaneous ventilation with continuous positive airway pressure

4. A 66-year-old morbidly obese male with a history of a previous myocardial infarction is scheduled for arthroscopic meniscus repair on his right knee. Using the Caprini Risk Assessment Model, his risk for postoperative venous thromboembolism is:
   A. Very low (<0.5%)
   B. Low (~1.5%)
   C. Intermediate (~3%)
   D. High (~6%)

5. For the patient described in question 4, the most appropriate venous thromboembolism prophylaxis technique would be mechanical, serial compression devices placed on both lower extremities. TRUE or FALSE?
   A. True
   B. False

6. Evidence-based guidelines of the American Society for Parenteral and Enteral Nutrition support each of the following nutritional practices in the ICU setting EXCEPT:
   A. Nutrition should be initiated in the first 24 to 48 hours after ICU admission.
   B. Total parenteral nutrition is associated with increased infectious complications compared with enteral nutrition; therefore, enteral feeding is preferred.
   C. Postpyloric feeding tube positioning is required prior to starting tube feeds.
   D. Protein should generally comprise 15% to 20% of the calculated daily caloric needs.

7. A 27-year-old female with insulin-dependent, type 1 diabetes is cared for in the ICU due to extensive necrotizing soft tissue infection of her left arm and septic shock. The generally accepted target serum glucose level in her case would be 140 to 180 mg/dL. TRUE or FALSE?
   A. True
   B. False

8. A recent, large, multicenter, randomized, controlled clinical trial of transfusion requirements in critical care reported which of the following conclusions regarding red blood cell transfusions?
   A. Transfusion threshold of Hb <7 g/dL was superior to Hb <10 g/dL
   B. Transfusion threshold of Hb <7 g/dL was no different from Hb <10 g/dL
   C. Transfusion threshold of Hb <7 g/dL was inferior to Hb <10 g/dL
   D. Transfusion threshold of Hb <7 g/dL was inferior to Hb >10 g/dL

9. Best practice recommendations of the Centers for Disease Control and Prevention to minimize catheter-related infections for central venous catheters include all of the following EXCEPT:
   A. Remove catheters as soon as possible
   B. Use chlorhexidine sponge for skin preparation prior to catheter placement
   C. Use ultrasound guidance to minimize the number of needle passes during placement
   D. Routinely replace catheters every 7 days

10. A previously healthy 57-year-old man is admitted to the ICU postoperatively following an open appendectomy with intraoperative findings of appendical rupture and fecal contamination of the peritoneum. In the ICU, he has a blood pressure of 82/46 mm Hg, heart rate of 114 beats per minute, a core temperature of 39.1°C, a blood Hb of 7.9 g/kL, and is mechanically ventilated. The presumptive diagnosis is septic shock. Which of the following would be the most appropriate initial treatment?
    A. Transfuse packed red blood cells to restore circulating volume
    B. Administer dopamine to augment systemic vascular resistance
    C. Administer norepinephrine to augment systemic vascular resistance
    D. Administer hydrocortisone 100 mg

Anesthesia for Urologic Surgery

Aymen A. Alian

Urologic procedures are some of the most common procedures done in the general operating rooms of many hospitals. Advances in noninvasive techniques have transformed urologic surgery to provide greater effectiveness, less cost, and improved outcomes for patients. This chapter provides an overview of those procedures and reviews the core anesthetic concerns associated with them.

I. Transurethral Procedures

A. Cystoscopy and Ureteroscopy

Cystoscopy and ureteroscopy are endoscopic procedures that provide visualization and treatment of lower and upper urinary tract disease, respectively. Depending on the extent and duration of the planned surgery, cystoscopy can be performed under local anesthesia, conscious sedation, or regional or general anesthesia. Ureteroscopy provides access to the upper urinary tract and kidney for diagnostic endoscopy and biopsy, removal of ureteral and renal calculi (Fig. 42.1), passage of ureteral stents, dilatation and incision of strictures, fulguration of tumors, and laser treatments. Ureteroscopy usually requires regional or general anesthesia.

B. Resection of Bladder Tumors

Bladder cancer is the second most common urologic malignancy, with superficial transitional cell carcinoma accounting for ~90% of bladder cancers. In diagnosing and treating this cancer, most patients undergo endoscopic transurethral resection. This procedure can be performed with either regional or general anesthesia. For laterally located bladder tumor, general anesthesia with muscle relaxant is the preferred technique to avoid obturator nerve stimulation and inadvertent bladder perforation. Bladder perforation with extravasation of the irrigating fluid is a well-known risk of transurethral bladder resection. During regional anesthesia in a conscious patient, bladder perforation results in sudden severe abdominal pain. This is often accompanied by referred pain from the diaphragm to the shoulder, as well as pallor, sweating, abdominal

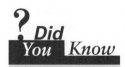

? Did You Know

Bladder perforation with extravasation of the irrigating fluid is a well-known risk of transurethral bladder resection.

785

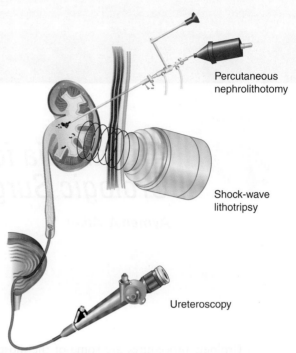

Figure 42-1 Urinary tract stones: Intervention choices. (From Stafford-Smith M, Shaw A, Sandler A, et al. The renal system and anesthesia for urologic surgery. In: Barash PG, Cullen BF, Stoelting RK, et al. *Clinical Anesthesia*, 7th ed. Philadelphia: Lippincott Williams & Wilkins, 2013:1114.)

rigidity, nausea, and vomiting. If extravasation is suspected, the operation should be terminated as quickly as possible. Small perforations with minimal intraperitoneal leakage rarely cause hemodynamic changes and can usually be managed with catheter drainage and diuretics. The consequences of a large intraperitoneal accumulation of irrigating fluid (especially sterile water) can be life-threatening. Open laparotomy for drainage and bladder perforation repair is recommended in these cases.

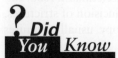

VIDEO 42-1

Transurethral Resection of the Prostate

? *Did* *You* *Know*

Most of the irrigating solutions are hypoosmolar and acidic. Transient blindness is associated with glycine irrigation, hyperglycemia is associated with sorbitol and volume overload is associated with the use of mannitol.

C. Resection of the Prostate

Benign prostatic hyperplasia (BPH), the most common benign tumor in men, is responsible for the majority of urinary symptoms in men older than 50 and results in a need for prostatectomy in approximately one-third of all men who live to age 80. *Transurethral resection of the prostate (TURP)* is the primary treatment for symptomatic BPH. In this procedure, a resectoscope is used to remove prostatic tissue that is protruding into the urethra with preservation of the prostatic capsule. Continuous irrigation of the bladder and prostatic urethra is required to maintain visibility, distend the operative site, and remove dissected tissue and blood. During TURP, violation of the prostatic capsule results in absorption of large amounts of irrigation solution into the circulation and the periprostatic and retroperitoneal spaces.

Irrigating Solutions for Transurethral Resection of the Prostate

The ideal irrigating fluid should be isotonic, nonhemolytic, nontoxic, electrically inert (if a monopolar electrical resecting electrode is used), transparent, rapidly excreted, and inexpensive. Most of the irrigating solutions are hypo-osmolar and acidic, as shown in Table 42-1. Isotonic irrigation solutions

Table 42-1	Properties of Commonly Used Irrigating Solution during Transurethral Resection of Prostate Procedure		
Solution	**Osmolality (mOsm/L)**	**Advantage**	**Disadvantage**
Distilled water	0	Improved visibility	Hemolysis Hemoglobinemia Hemoglobinuria Renal failure Hyponatremia
Glycine (1.5%)	200	Less likelihood of TURP syndrome	Transient blindness Hyperammonemia Hyperoxaluria
Sorbitol (3.3%)	165	Same as glycine	Hyperglycemia, Lactic acidosis (possible) Osmotic diuresis
Mannitol (5%)	275	Isomolar Not metabolized	Osmotic dieresis Acute volume overload

TURP, transurethral resection of prostate.

(normal saline and lactated Ringer's solution) are available, but these electrolyte solutions are ionized and conduct electrical currents.

Transurethral Resection Syndrome
Absorption of large volumes of irrigating solution leads to respiratory distress secondary to intravascular volume overload, hyponatremia, and hypoosmolality (1). The average amount of irrigating fluid absorbed during TURP is ~20 mL/min of resection time. The volume of fluid absorbed during the procedure can be estimated with the following formula:

$$\text{Volume Absorbed} = \frac{\text{Preoperative Serum Na}^+}{\text{Postoperative Serum Na}^+} \times \text{ECF} - \text{ECF}$$

where ECF is extracellular fluid volume and Na$^+$ is the sodium ion.

Absorption of the irrigating fluid during TURP is directly related to the number and size of venous sinuses opened, the duration of resection, and the height of the bag of irrigating solution above the surgical table, which determines the hydrostatic pressure driving fluid into prostatic veins and sinuses. Resection time should be limited to <1 hour and the bag of irrigating solution should be suspended no more than 30 cm above the operating table at the beginning of the resection and 15 cm in the final stages of resection. Irritability, restlessness, nausea, shortness of breath, dizziness, hypertension, and headache are early manifestations of *TURP syndrome*. They provide an early warning of developing *hyponatremia* and *serum hypo-osmolality*. The acute decrease in serum sodium concentration is responsible for many of the signs and symptoms of TURP syndrome, as shown in Table 42-2.

Symptoms related to absorption of a specific irrigating solution during the procedure may further complicate TURP syndrome, as shown in Table 42-1. Prompt treatment is necessary when neurologic or cardiovascular complications of TURP are recognized. Table 42-3 summarizes those treatments.

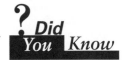

Absorption of large volumes of irrigating solution leads to intravascular volume overload, hyponatremia and hypoosmolality.

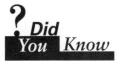

Absorption of the irrigating fluid during TURP is directly related to the number and size of opened venous sinuses, duration of resection, and the height of the bag of irrigating solution above the surgical table.

Table 42-2	Signs and Symptoms Associated with Acute Changes in Serum Na⁺ Levels	
Serum Na⁺ (mEq/L)	Central Nervous System Changes	Electrocardiogram Changes
120	Confusion, restlessness	Possible widening of QRS complex
115	Somnolence, nausea	Widened QRS complex, Elevated ST segment
110	Seizure, coma	Ventricular tachycardia or fibrillation

Bleeding and Coagulopathy

Several factors influence blood loss during TURP, such as the vascularity and size of the gland, duration of surgery, the number of sinuses opened during resection, and the presence of infection (2). Blood loss is difficult to assess because of its mixing with the irrigating fluid. Therefore, both intravascular volume assessment and serial hematocrit values may be necessary to estimate blood loss and the need for red cell transfusion. Excessive bleeding after TURP occurs in <1% of cases. In theory, primary fibrinolysis may result from prostatic release of tissue plasminogen activator, which converts plasminogen to plasmin. However, there is little evidence to support this factor as clinically significant or to support the practice of administering an antifibrinolytic such as aminocaproic acid. Disseminated intravascular coagulopathy is the likely etiology of abnormal bleeding after TURP.

Bladder Perforation

The incidence of bladder perforation is ~1%, and most perforations are extraperitoneal, resulting in periumbilical, inguinal, or suprapubic pain in a conscious patient. The urologist may suspect perforation by noting the irregular return of irrigating fluid. Intraperitoneal bladder perforation occurs less

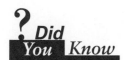

Did You Know?

Disseminated intravascular coagulopathy is the likely etiology of abnormal bleeding after TURP.

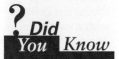

Did You Know?

The urologist may suspect perforation by noting the irregular return of irrigating fluid.

Table 42-3   Treatment of Transurethral Resection of Prostate Syndrome
Ensure oxygenation, ventilation, and circulatory support
Notify surgeon to terminate procedure as soon as possible
Consider insertion of invasive monitors if cardiovascular instability occurs
Send blood to laboratory for electrolytes, creatinine, glucose, and arterial blood gases
Obtain 12-lead electrocardiogram
Treat mild symptoms (serum Na⁺ concentration >120 mEq/L) with fluid restriction and loop diuretic (furosemide)
Treat severe symptoms (if serum Na⁺ <120 mEq/L) with 3% sodium chloride intravenously at a rate <100 mL/hr
The rate at which serum sodium is increased should not exceed 12 mEq/L in a 24-hr period to a void *pontine myelinolysis*
Discontinue 3% sodium chloride when serum Na⁺ >120 mEq/L

frequently, and pain is more generalized in the upper part of the abdomen or referred to the precordial or shoulder. Pallor, restlessness, sweating, abdominal rigidity, nausea, vomiting, and hypotension usually accompanied this generalized pain.

Transient Bacteremia and Septicemia

Bacteremia is usually asymptomatic and easily treated with commonly used antibiotic combinations that are effective against gram-positive and gram-negative bacteria. In 7% of patients, septicemia may occur. Common manifestations include chills, fever, and tachycardia. In severe cases, bradycardia, hypotension, and cardiovascular collapse may occur, with mortality rates of 25% to 75%. Aggressive treatment with antibiotics and critical care support employing a sepsis protocol should be instituted.

Hypothermia

Heat loss results from irrigation, and absorption of room temperature irrigating fluid may lead to a significant decrease in the patient's body temperature and shivering. The use of warmed irrigating solutions has been shown to minimize or prevent this problem.

Positioning Complications

TURP is performed in the lithotomy position with slight Trendelenburg. Without proper positioning and padding, the common peroneal, sciatic, and femoral nerves may be injured.

Anesthetic Techniques

Regional anesthesia (spinal or epidural) has been the technique of choice for TURP because the conscious patient can alert the clinicians to the early signs of TURP syndrome or bladder perforation. A sensory level to T10 is required to eliminate the discomfort caused by bladder distention. Spinal anesthesia is usually preferred over lumbar epidural anesthesia because sacral segments are sometimes inadequately blocked with lumbar epidural techniques. However, general anesthesia can be used safely as well, and the anesthetic technique should be tailored to the individual patient and surgical requirements.

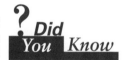

? Did You Know

Regional anesthesia has been the anesthetic technique of choice for TURP as the conscious patient can alert the clinicians to the early signs of TURP syndrome or bladder perforation.

Morbidity and Mortality After Transurethral Resection of the Prostate

In a recent retrospective review of 722 who underwent TURP, the authors found 244 complications in 145 patients (3). Most of the complications were relatively minor, but 16 patients required blood transfusions, 5 had capsule perforation, 2 had pulmonary thromboembolism, 7 had myocardial infarction, 4 had urosepsis, 7 had TURP syndrome, and 3 died. Patient age, comorbidities, and duration of surgery were independent predictors of the complications.

The Future of Transurethral Resection of the Prostate

Less invasive surgical treatments include balloon dilatation, prostate stents, transurethral incision of the prostate, and laser prostatectomy. These less invasive procedures usually can be done on an outpatient basis, as they are associated with minimal blood loss and less risk of TURP syndrome. These techniques may be preferred for elderly patients with significant medical comorbidities (4).

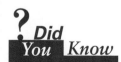

? Did You Know

ESWL has become the treatment of choice for disintegration of urinary stones in the kidney and upper part of the ureters.

II. Extracorporeal Shock Wave Lithotripsy

In the United States, 12% of the population will experience calculus disease in their lifetimes. The optimal therapy is based on the size of the stone (<4.0 mm usually pass spontaneously), location in the urinary tract, and stone

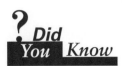

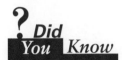

composition. With the introduction of extracorporeal shock wave lithotripsy (ESWL), only 5% of all urinary calculi require open surgical procedures. ESWL has become the treatment of choice for disintegration of urinary stones in the kidney and upper part of the ureters. It has the advantages of being minimally invasive, performed on an outpatient basis, and associated with minimal perioperative morbidity and significant cost reduction.

The original, first-generation lithotripter required the patient to be placed in a hydraulically supported gantry chair and immersed in a water bath. Modern lithotripters do not require water immersion and thus greatly simplify the procedure and eliminate the many adverse effects and difficulties of water immersion. As a result, most *ESWL* can be done on an outpatient basis and rarely require deep sedation or general anesthesia (Fig. 42.1).

Pregnancy, untreated bleeding disorders, or anticoagulation and obstruction distal to the renal calculi are contraindications to lithotripsy. Patients with a pacemaker or internal cardiac defibrillator are acceptable candidates for lithotripsy provided the pacemaker is set to the asynchronous mode (if the patient's normal heart rate is pacemaker dependent) and the defibrillator is turn off during the procedure. Renal parenchymal damage is believed to be responsible for the hematuria that occurs in nearly all patients, whereas subcapsular hematoma is seen in only 0.5% of patients after lithotripsy. A decrease in postoperative hematocrit should arouse suspicion of a large perinephric hematoma. Up to 10% of patients have significant urinary tract colic, occasionally requiring hospitalization and opioid analgesics. Shock waves lithotripsy can cause damage to adjacent tissues such as the lungs and pancreas. Despite the wide array of potential complications, mortality after ESWL is very rare.

III. Percutaneous Renal Procedures

Percutaneous nephrostomy (PCN) is a commonly performed procedure that entails using ultrasound guidance to percutaneously puncture the renal pelvis, creating a nephrostomy tract. PCN is used to diagnose and treat a wide variety of urologic problems, including relief of renal obstruction, stone removal, biopsy of tumors, and ureteral stent placement (Fig. 42.1).

Nephroscopy involves passing an endoscope through the nephrostomy tract to examine the kidney. For this procedure, the patient is placed in the oblique prone position and provided local anesthesia and intravenous sedation. Percutaneous nephrolithotomy, a procedure to remove renal calculi too large to be treated with lithotripsy, is one of the most common urologic endosurgical procedures. Anesthesia (general or regional) is required for dilatation of the nephrostomy tract.

Although percutaneous surgical techniques are considerably less invasive than open surgical procedures, a variety of complications can occur. During insertion of the nephrostomy tube, trauma to adjacent structures such as spleen, liver, and colon can result in acute blood loss necessitating an emergency open surgical procedure. Lung and pleural injury may occur during nephrostomy tract placement when access is created above the 12th rib or the kidney lays in a more cephalad position than normal. In order to improve the surgical field for the surgeon during nephroscopy, continuous irrigation of fluid through the endoscope is necessary. Extravasation of irrigation fluid into the retroperitoneal, intraperitoneal, intravascular, or pleural spaces is possible and can result in electrolyte abnormalities, fluid overload, and other complications.

Table 42-4	Lasers Used for Urologic Surgery	
Type of Laser	**Characteristics**	**Uses**
Carbon dioxide (CO_2)	Intense heat with vaporization, minimal tissue penetration	Cutaneous lesions of the external genitalia
Argon	Selectively absorbed by hemoglobin and melanin	Coagulation of bleeding sites in the bladder
Pulsed dye	Generates a pulsed output	Destruction of ureteral calculi
Nd-YAG laser (most versatile and widely used)	Can be used in water or urine without loss of effectiveness, deep tissue penetration	Lesions of the penis, urethra, bladder, ureters, and kidneys
KTP-532 laser (double the frequency of Nd-YAG laser)	Better cutting effect, less deep tissue penetration	Urethral strictures and bladder neck contractures

Nd-YAG, neodymium-yttrium aluminum garnet.

IV. Laser Surgery in Urology

Numerous urologic problems have been treated effectively by laser therapy, such as condyloma acuminatum of the external genitalia, ureteral stricture or bladder neck contracture, interstitial cystitis, BPH, ureteral calculi, and superficial carcinoma of the penis, bladder, ureter, and renal pelvis. Minimal blood loss, decreased postoperative pain, and tissue denaturation are major advantages of laser surgery over traditional surgical approaches. Laser lithotripsy is used for ureteral stones that are low in the ureter and not amenable to ESWL. The stones absorb the laser beam, resulting in their disintegration. Ideally, general anesthesia with paralysis should be maintained to avoid patient movement together with generous intravenous hydration. If regional anesthesia is chosen, a spinal level of T8 to T10 is required. Because lasers are an integral part of urologic surgery, understanding the indications and limitations of each type of laser is essential (Table 42-4).

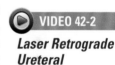

VIDEO 42-2

Laser Retrograde Ureteral Lithotripsy

Protective goggles with appropriate filtering lenses are available for each type of laser to minimize eye damage. The laser equipment should not be activated until all operating room personnel and the patient are wearing the appropriate goggles. All operating room personnel involved in carbon dioxide (CO_2) laser procedures for condyloma acuminatum should wear protective laser masks that prevent inhalation of the plume (smoke) from the vaporization of tissue. This smoke may contain active human papilloma virus. In addition, the laser plume should be removed from the operating room with a smoke evacuation system.

V. Urologic Laparoscopy

Urologic laparoscopy procedures have gained wide acceptance because they are minimally invasive and more surgically precise, with better preservation of periprostatic vascular, muscular, and neurovascular structures, less painful postoperatively, and less costly than open surgical procedures. Laparoscopic procedures performed in urology include diagnostic procedures for evaluating undescended testis, orchiopexy, varicocelectomy, bladder suspension, pelvic lymphadenectomy, nephrectomy, partial nephrectomy, nephroureterectomy, adrenalectomy, prostatectomy, and cystectomy. Many structures in the genito-urinary system are extraperitoneal (i.e., pelvic lymph nodes, bladder, ureters, adrenal glands, kidneys), and urologists use extraperitoneal insufflation during laparoscopic surgery on these organs. CO_2 absorption is greater with extra-peritoneal compared with intraperitoneal insufflation. General anesthesia with controlled ventilation is the method of choice to maintain normocarbia. Extra-peritoneal insufflation results in subcutaneous emphysema that may extend all the way up to the head and neck. Please refer to Chapter 27 for a detailed dis-cussion of the physiologic impact and potential complications of laparoscopy.

VI. Radical Cancer Surgery

?Did You Know

Radical surgical procedures are associated with extensive blood loss, complications related to positioning and venous air embolism.

Radical surgical procedures are performed to treat prostate, bladder, or kidney cancer. They are often lengthy procedures, requiring a steep Trendelenburg position to facilitate surgical access to the pelvis. As a result of this position-ing, the lower extremities have decreased perfusion while the brain experiences increased mean arterial pressure and decreased venous drainage. Lung com-pliance and functional residual capacity are decreased, resulting in increased ventilation-perfusion mismatching. Pulmonary congestion and edema have been reported as have increased intracranial pressure and intraocular pres-sure. Other complications that result from the positioning include ischemic muscle damage in the lower extremities and pelvis and lower-extremity and upper-extremity nerve injuries. When the operative site in the pelvis is above the heart, the patient is at risk for venous air embolism. In addition to all of these concerns, radical cancer surgery poses a substantial risk for extensive blood loss and the need for transfusion.

A. Radical Prostatectomy

Prostate cancer is the one of the most commonly diagnosed cancer in men. In the United States, men with clinically localized prostate cancer whose life expec-tancy is 10 years or longer tend to undergo radical prostatectomy. Radical prostatectomy can be performed by a perineal, retropubic, or laparoscopic surgi-cal approach. During radical perineal or retropubic prostatectomy, general or regional (epidural or spinal) anesthesia may be used. If regional anesthesia is used, a sensory block of T6-8 is adequate. During the laparoscopic surgical approach, general anesthesia is the technique of choice for the reasons noted above (dura-tion of surgery and steep Trendelenburg positioning). Robotic-assisted radical prostatectomy is associated with better visualization and better surgical dissec-tion, decreased blood loss, less scaring and postoperative pain, shorter hospital stay, and faster return to daily activity. However, considerable debate remains regarding the associated cost and long-term outcome of the robotic technique.

?Did You Know

During radical procedures, the anesthesiologist should identify the chemotherapeutic agents used, be aware of the side effects of these drugs, and should be prepare for significant intraoperative hemorrhage.

B. Radical Cystectomy

Radical cystectomy involves en bloc removal of the bladder, prostate, semi-nal vesicles, and proximal urethra in men, while in women, it is necessary to remove the bladder, urethra, and anterior vaginal wall, as well as to perform a total hysterectomy and bilateral salpingo-oophorectomy. At completion of the procedure, a urinary diversion is performed, most commonly as an ileal or colon conduit. Significant intraoperative hemorrhage can occur during radical cystectomy. The extent and duration of this surgery mandate general anesthe-sia. Patients with bladder cancer may have been treated with chemotherapy before their procedure. The anesthesiologist should be aware of prior use of any chemotherapeutic agent so any possible drug toxicity can be elucidated. In particular, doxorubicin has cardiotoxic effects, methotrexate may cause hepatic toxicity, and both cisplatin and methotrexate are associated with neurotoxicity and renal injury.

C. Radical Nephrectomy

Radical or partial nephrectomy is the treatment of choice for renal cell carcinoma (5). It involves en bloc removal of the kidney and surrounding fascia, the ipsilateral adrenal gland, and the upper ureter. In 5% to 10% of right-sided renal cell carcinomas, the tumor extends into the renal vein, the inferior vena cava, and the right atrium. To operate on these patients safely, the extent of the lesion must be defined preoperatively. If there is tumor extension into the vena cava or right atrium, cardiopulmonary bypass is often required to safely resect it.

Transesophageal echocardiography may be of value in confirming complete removal of the tumor or identifying intraoperative embolization of the tumor and the need to emergently institute cardiopulmonary bypass. Nephrectomy may be performed through a lumbar, transabdominal, or thoracoabdominal incision. If a lumbar approach is used, the patient is placed in the flexed lateral decubitus position with the operative side up and the mechanical kidney support elevated beneath the 12th rib. This mechanical kidney support has been associated with hypotension due to decreased venous return, nerve damage, decreased thoracic compliance, and pulmonary atelectasis. General anesthesia is used for patients placed in this position because it is so uncomfortable. Pneumothorax can occur during surgery if the chest is inadvertently entered. Venous air embolisms are also possible during nephrectomy procedures if the positioning places the operative site above the heart.

D. Radical Surgery for Testicular Cancer

All intratesticular masses are considered cancerous until proven otherwise. Radical orchiectomy is performed for both definitive diagnosis and as the initial step of most treatment regimens, and regional or general anesthesia can be used for this procedure.

The anesthesiologist should identify the chemotherapeutic agents used and be aware of the side effects of these drugs. One commonly used chemotherapeutic agent, bleomycin, is an antitumor antibiotic used against germ cell tumors of the testis. Bleomycin use is associated with pulmonary toxicity, and postoperative respiratory failure usually occurs 3 to 10 days after surgery. Risk factors for postoperative respiratory distress include preoperative evidence of pulmonary injury, recent exposure to bleomycin (within 1 to 2 months), a total dose of bleomycin >450 mg, or a creatinine clearance of <35 mL/min. A retrospective study found that intravenous fluid management, including blood transfusion, was the most significant factor affecting postoperative pulmonary morbidity and clinical outcomes. The authors recommend that intravenous fluid administration consist primarily of colloid and be limited to the minimum volume necessary to maintain hemodynamic stability and adequate renal output.

> **? Did You Know**
>
> In 5% to 10% of right-sided renal cell carcinomas, the tumor extends into the renal vein, inferior vena cava, and the right atrium, and thus TEE is of crucial value.

> **? Did You Know**
>
> Hypotension during radical nephrectomy can be multifactorial; mechanical effect, pneumothorax, air embolism and bleeding.

References

1. Hawary A, Mukhtar K, Sinclair A, et al. Transurethral resection of the prostate syndrome: Almost gone but not forgotten. *J Endourol.* 2009;23(12):2013–2020.
2. Kavanagh LE, Jack GS, Lawrentschuk N. Prevention and management of TURP-related hemorrhage. *Nat Rev Urol.* 2011;8(9):504–514.

3. Mandal S, Sankhwar SN, Kathpalia R, et al. Grading complications after transurethral resection of prostate using modified Clavien classification system and predicting complications using the Charlson comorbidity index. *Int Urol Nephrol.* 2013;45(2):347–354.

4. Strope SA, Yang L, Nepple KG, et al. Population based comparative effectiveness of transurethral resection of the prostate and laser therapy for benign prostatic hyperplasia. *J Urol.* 2012;187(4):1341–1345.

5. Cohen HT, McGovern FJ. Renal-cell carcinoma. *N Engl J Med.* 2005;353(23):2477–2490.

Questions

1. Under what condition would general anesthesia with muscle paralysis be preferred over regional anesthesia for a patient undergoing transurethral resection of a bladder tumor?
   A. The tumor involves the lateral wall of the bladder
   B. The tumor involves the posterior wall of the bladder
   C. The tumor involves the anterior wall of the bladder
   D. The tumor involves either ureteral insertion site in the bladder
   E. None of the above.

2. Following transurethral resection of the prostate in an 80 kg patient, the serum Na^+ is 120. The preoperative value was 140. Assuming the patient's extracellular volume is 25% of his weight, what approximate volume of irrigating fluid did he absorb during this surgery?
   A. 2.5 liters
   B. 3.5 liters
   C. 4.5 liters
   D. 5.5 liters
   E. None of the above

3. Correction of severe hyponatremia following transurethral resection of the prostate should not exceed:
   A. 8 mEq/liter in a 24 hour period
   B. 10 mEq/liter liter in a 24 hour period
   C. 12 mEq/liter liter in a 24 hour period
   D. 14 mEq/liter liter in a 24 hour period
   E. None of the above

4. Regional anesthesia is preferred to general anesthesia for transurethral resection of the prostate because:
   A. mortality rate is lower
   B. postoperative myocardial infarction rate is lower
   C. TURP syndrome can be detected earlier
   D. transfusion rates are less
   E. None of the above

5. Five to ten percent of right sided renal cell carcinomas extend into:
   A. the bowel
   B. the adrenal gland
   C. the aorta
   D. the vena cava
   E. None of the above

Electrical Safety and Fire

Christopher W. Connor
Wissam Mustafa

The physics and engineering principles involved in electrical supply and electrical safety are very well established, although they may not be immediately or intuitively obvious. Many clinicians, as well as most citizens of developed countries, presume that the electrical supply will be present and equipment will be working safely every day. Little thought is given as to how this is achieved until a power system failure unexpectedly occurs. Furthermore, the terminology of electrical engineering is commonly misused by laypeople so that the meaning becomes imprecise or incorrect. For instance, during the course of a surgical procedure, many overlapping meanings for the word "ground" or "grounded" might be encountered, such as:

1. The physical surface of the Earth.
2. The voltage ascribed, by convention, to the Earth: 0 V.
3. Describing an electrical plug or socket that has three pins.
4. The green electrical wire, the ground lead, found within electrical power cables.
5. The adhesive pad that forms the dispersive return electrode for an electrosurgical unit.
6. The act of connecting a patient to some form of electrical apparatus such as the electrosurgical unit ("Is the patient grounded?").
7. A state of failure of the operating room's isolated electrical power system, in which the system "becomes grounded."

Imagine the scenario of an anesthesiologist performing anesthesia for a shoulder arthroscopy in an ambulatory surgery center in which arthroscopic video cameras, instruments, and an electrosurgical unit are being used. A large puddle of joint irrigation solution has begun to accumulate on the floor and is spreading among cables on the floor and toward the anesthesiologist's feet. Is the anesthesiologist safe? Now, imagine an anesthesiologist performing cardiac anesthesia emergently at night. While the patient is on bypass, the electrical safety monitors in the room begin to alarm. What should the anesthesiologist do? In order to respond appropriately in these and similar situations, it is necessary for the anesthesiologist to understand the electrical principles involved.

I. Principles of Electricity

A. Introduction

Electrical *current* (*I*, measured in amperes) will flow through an electrically conductive substance (a conductor) when there is a difference in electrical *potential* (*E*, measured in volts) across that conductor.

Therefore, if a person (being a potential conductor of electricity) touches a live domestic electrical wire (at, for example, 120 V) while in good contact with the ground (the person's feet are at 0 V), electrical current will flow through the person and he or she will receive a shock. However, in the unlikely situation of a person standing on a metal plate that is at a voltage of 120 V while simultaneously touching a wire at a voltage of 120 V, no shock would be received because there would be no difference in voltage and no current would flow.

It is the difference in electrical potential (called the *potential difference*) that generates the current and the delivery of energy, not the absolute voltage. As an analogy, imagine two patients who accidentally fall from their beds. One patient is on the sixth floor of the hospital so his bed is 20 m above ground level; the other patient is on the third floor so his bed is 10 m above ground level. Of course, it is not the patients' absolute height in the building (i.e., absolute voltage) that matters, but instead the height of the fall from their beds to the floor of their rooms (i.e., potential difference).

Conductors have a property called *resistance* (*R*, measured in ohms), which is their tendency to resist the flow of a current for a given potential difference. Potential difference, current, and resistance are related by *Ohm's law*, represented with the following equation:

$$E = I \times R \quad \text{or equivalently} \quad I = E/R.$$

The electrical resistance of the human body is not constant; it depends strongly on the wetness of the skin, ranging from approximately 1,000 Ω with wet skin, to approximately 100,000 Ω with dry skin.

B. Direct and Alternating Current

The current flow in a circuit may be either *direct current (DC)* or *alternating current* (AC) depending on whether the direction of current flow in that circuit remains constant or oscillates. Batteries produce DC; the positive terminal of the battery remains at a constant higher electrical potential relative to the negative terminal of the battery until the battery is exhausted. The current always flows from the positive to the negative terminal. Conversely, as with common household electricity, the electrical current obtained from the "mains" power supply is AC; the potential difference of the live conductor oscillates around the neutral conductor. It is possible to convert AC to DC using a simple circuit called a *rectifier,* where AC voltages are specified in terms of the equivalent DC voltage that would make the same amount of electrical power available. The main power supply in the United States, which is nominally 120 V, actually has a live conductor whose potential difference oscillates sinusoidally between ±170 V relative to the neutral conductor 60 times each second. The frequency of AC oscillation is expressed in terms of Hertz (Hz); thus, common household current is 60 Hz.

C. Capacitors and Inductors, Reactance, and Impedance

Capacitors and inductors are both devices capable of storing electrical energy (1). A *capacitor* consists of two electrical plates, separated by an insulating material called the *dielectric.* As a DC voltage is applied to the capacitor, positive charge begins to accumulate on one plate of the capacitor, while negative charge begins to build up on the opposite plate. Eventually, a sufficient charge accumulates such that an equilibrium state is produced in which no further current can flow. The capacitor can be rapidly discharged from this state, producing a pulse of current through the desired part of the circuit. This is similar to how a camera flash operates. Once the capacitor is fully charged, however, no additional electrical current can flow onto it and its resistance to DC becomes effectively infinite. An *inductor* consists of a coil of wire wrapped in a spiral fashion around a ferromagnetic core. As electrical current passes through the coil of wire, an equal and opposing magnetic field is created in the core. An opposing electrical voltage occurs in the coil. In this regard, an inductor is similar to a simple electromagnet. However, once the current to the inductor is interrupted, the magnetic field in the core collapses, inducing a strong, opposing voltage spike in the electrical coil. From these simple analogies in DC, it can be seen that these devices can store charge and also cause electrical and magnetic fields that can exist beyond the physical boundaries of the device itself.

When alternating current is applied to a capacitor, the voltage on the plates of the capacitor switches polarity as the AC voltage cycles. This causes electrical charge, in the form of electrical current, to flow on and off the plates of the capacitor. Therefore, even though there is no direct electrical connection between the two plates of the capacitor and the effective electrical resistance to DC is infinite, the act of repeatedly charging and discharging the capacitor allows alternating current to be able to flow through it. This "resistance" to alternating current is called *reactance*. It is a property of both capacitors and inductors and is dependent on the frequency of the alternating current. The simple and familiar expression of Ohm's law, in which resistance is expressed as *R*, is only true for direct current. In order to model alternating current at different frequencies, a quantity called *impedance* is used. Impedance represents a combination of both resistance and reactance.

More precisely, impedance is a complex number whose real component is the electrical resistance and whose imaginary component is the reactance. From a practical standpoint, the existence of reactance makes it possible to design circuits that only allow electrical signals at certain frequencies to pass through them. This is the basis of, for example, graphic equalizers for music and medical signal filters for electrocardiograms (ECGs) that filter and amplify only those frequencies associated with cardiac conduction.

By carefully arranging capacitors and inductors, it is possible to design circuits that can receive and respond to external electromagnetic signals as well as to circuits that optimally radiate electromagnetic energy into the environment. Such circuits form the basis of radio reception and broadcasting. However, these properties can also exist in an unwanted form in electrical devices. For example, the proximity of electrical conductors within the power cord of a device or between the windings of an electric motor and its metal case, cause *stray capacitance* or *parasitic capacitance*. In turn, these produce the phenomena of *electrical interference* and *leakage current*.

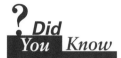

? *Did* **You** *Know*

It is possible for electricity to be transmitted from one circuit to another without direct contact. This is an important part of the isolation transformer in use in most operating rooms.

II. Electrical Shock Hazards

A. Alternating and Direct Currents

Electrical current can stimulate nerves and muscle contraction. This leads to the possibility of its therapeutic uses; however, it also leads to the risk of

Table 43-1	Physical Effects of Exposure to a 60 Hz Electrical Current, Measured in Amperes for 1 Second	
Electrical Current		**Physical Effect**
Macroshock (to body via skin contact)		
1 mA	(0.001 A)	Threshold of perception
5 mA	(0.005 A)	Maximum harmless current
10–20 mA	(0.01–0.02 A)	Maximum current before sustained muscle contraction prevents voluntary release of the conductor ("let-go threshold")
50 mA	(0.05 A)	Pain, risk of mechanical injury from muscle contractions
100–300 mA	(0.1–0.3 A)	Threshold for ventricular fibrillation, respiration drive is preserved
6000 mA	(6 A)	Sustained myocardial contraction, followed by resumption of heart rhythm; temporary respiratory paralysis; burns at areas of high current density
Microshock (to heart via wire or conducting cannula)		
10 µA	(0.01 mA)	Maximum recommended 60 Hz leakage current
100 µA	(0.1 mA)	Ventricular fibrillation

A, ampere; mA, milliampere; µA, microampere.

injury or death. Direct current is generally considered to be safer than alternating current. The amount of direct current necessary to induce ventricular fibrillation is around three times higher than the amount of alternating current required to produce the same effect. Table 43-1 summarizes the physical effects that are experienced from exposure to different thresholds of 60 Hz alternating current, as would be encountered in the standard US "mains" electricity supply.

The perception of the safety of direct current is reinforced by daily experience of "mains" alternating current being more powerful and dangerous than the relatively small amounts of direct current that are produced from standard batteries. However, a large direct current source such as an automobile battery or marine battery should not be considered harmless. The direct current discharge that can be produced between the terminals can cause significant burns and musculoskeletal injury.

B. Source of Shocks

Whenever a difference in electrical potential exists, current will flow through a suitable conductor placed between those electrical potentials. Consequently, there is always a risk of electrical shock whenever an external source of electricity is touched. The severity of the physical effect of the shock depends on both the magnitude of the electrical current and the duration of time for which that current is applied. At lower current levels, the electrical shock is first felt as a sensory tingling sensation, rising to pain with increased levels of current. Greater levels of current are able to stimulate contraction of muscles directly; furthermore, beyond a certain current level, it becomes impossible to release the contraction of these muscles voluntarily. Beyond this "let-go" threshold, it may no longer be possible for a victim to break contact with the source of electrical shock, further sustaining the electrical exposure (2). Further escalations in current can cause the onset of ventricular fibrillation as the electrical shock interferes with cardiac conduction and causes direct paralysis of the respiratory muscles. The flow of electrical current through the body also generates heat and can destroy tissue through direct thermal injury. The risk of burn injury is greatest at the points where the electrical current is entering or leaving the body, as the concentration of electrical current (the *current density*) is greatest there.

C. Grounding

When electrical current flows through a person, causing a shock, the current is usually flowing from some other electrical potential to ground. The body of the person is usually either in direct contact with the ground or electrically connected to the ground via a conductor such as an item of metal furniture. Because an electrical shock can only occur when there is a difference in electrical potential, the aim of electrical safety is to minimize that potential difference so that the magnitude of that electrical shock is made as small as possible. One approach, as seen in small battery-powered devices, is to minimize the total electrical voltage used by the device to such an extent that even the maximum possible shock current that could be generated by it is harmless. However, for devices that require significant electrical power, electrical safety must be achieved by more active means. In this case, "grounding" refers to the various steps that can be taken to reduce the magnitude of the possible electrical shock.

The simplest of these is illustrated in Figure 43-1. On the right, a malfunctioning device is shown. It has developed a fault in which a conductor connected to the "hot" or "live" wire of the electrical supply has broken and is now in contact with the casing of the device. Touching the case poses an immediate risk of electric shock because it is possible for this live voltage to flow through a person's body to ground. However, as a safety precaution, the device also contains a "ground" or "earth" wire that is connected to ground voltage, which is also connected to the casing of the device. The electrical current from the case fault is therefore able to flow to ground either through the body of the person touching the device or through the ground wire. Because the electrical resistance of the ground wire is much lower than the resistance

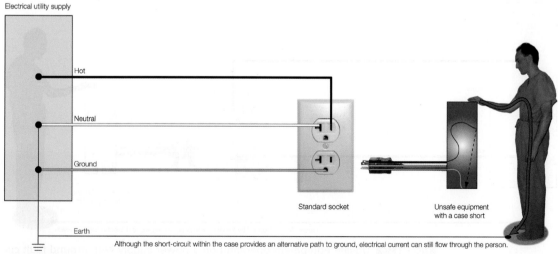

Electrical utility supply

Hot

Neutral

Ground

Earth

Standard socket

Unsafe equipment with a case short

Although the short-circuit within the case provides an alternative path to ground, electrical current can still flow through the person.

Figure 43-1 Unsafe equipment operating on a standard power supply.

of the body, most of the electrical current will preferentially travel to ground through the ground wire, reducing but not eliminating the magnitude of the electrical shock current passing through the person. However, if the ground wire were to break or if the device was instead connected to a two-pin electrical socket without a ground pin, then the protection afforded by the ground wire would be entirely lost and the person touching the case would be exposed to the full magnitude of the electrical shock current.

III. Electrical Power and Isolation

A. Grounded Power Systems and the Ground Fault Circuit Interrupter

The electrical power supply illustrated in both Figures 43-1 and 43-2 is referred to as a *grounded power system.* It is given this name because the potential of the neutral wire is fixed at the same potential as the ground wire, which in turn is fixed at the same potential as the actual ground (i.e., the physical surface of the Earth).

Although a ground wire within a malfunctioning device can reduce the amount of electric shock current flowing through a person touching that device, it cannot eliminate that shock current entirely. In the scenario shown in Figure 43-1, the device will continue to pose an ongoing risk of electrical shock. Furthermore, this risk of shock will not likely be discovered until someone touches the device and experiences a shock from it. The grounded power system shown in Figure 43-1 represents the standard for domestic electrical wiring, but it is inadequately safe for the operating room (3).

Figure 43-2 demonstrates a refinement of this electrical system, making use of a device called a *ground fault circuit interrupter* (GFCI). A GFCI is an electrical device, common in hazardous locations, such as in a bathroom or outdoors, that monitors the ground wire to detect whether any current is flowing in that wire. GFCIs are available as individual units that can be plugged into normal electrical sockets. Alternatively, electrical sockets can be purchased and installed so that the GFCI circuitry is contained within the socket itself. Figure 43-2 shows this latter type of installation.

Under normal operating conditions, no electrical current should be flowing in the ground wire. However, if a piece of equipment with an electrical fault,

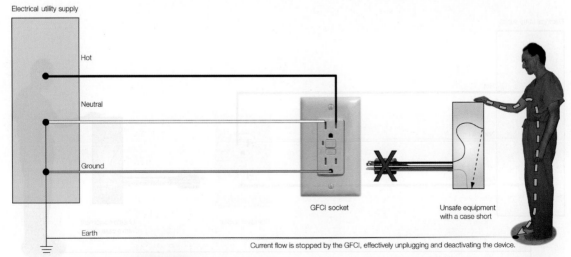

Current flow is stopped by the GFCI, effectively unplugging and deactivating the device.

Figure 43-2 Unsafe equipment operating on a power supply with ground fault circuit interrupter protection.

that makes the casing of the device electrically live, is plugged into a GFCI, then some of that fault current will be carried away in the ground wire. The GFCI detects that anomalous current flow. In response, the GFCI automatically interrupts the electrical supply to the device, deactivating the electrical socket and producing the same effect as if the malfunctioning device were suddenly unplugged. The GFCI also displays a warning light on the socket (shown red in Fig. 43-2), indicating that the safety provisions of the GFCI have been triggered and that power output from the socket has been disabled. The malfunctioning device (and anyone who may touch it) is rendered electrically safe, in that the device no longer has any electrical power flowing to it; however, it is also rendered inactive.

In many regards, this is a significant improvement over the preceding scenario in Figure 43-1 where there is no GFCI. However, there are some notable drawbacks. First, once the GFCI is triggered, electrical power to all equipment plugged into that circuit is immediately interrupted. This may be dangerous if any of the equipment items are necessary for life support, such as a cardiac bypass machine or a ventilator. Second, the GFCI can only work if the ground wire is intact. If the ground wire is broken or is not connected to the GFCI because an intervening two-pin plug has been used, then the GFCI can never detect current flow in the ground wire and its safety features are ineffective. Third, the GFCI relies on an active mechanical circuit breaker to interrupt electrical power to the device. If this mechanical circuit breaker itself were to fail or jam, then theoretically the GFCI might be unable to interrupt the electrical power to the device. For these reasons, GFCIs are not approved for electrical safety in all operating rooms. GFCIs may be installed for electrical safety only if the operating room is certified as a dry location (4).

B. Isolated Power Systems, Isolation Transformers, and the Line Isolation Monitor

The limitations of the GFCI can be overcome by creating what is known as an *isolated power system.* The purpose of the design of an isolated power system is to create an electrical power supply that can tolerate an electrical fault to the casing of a device while simultaneously:

- Raising an alarm that an electrical fault has occurred
- Allowing the malfunctioning device to continue to operate
- Preventing a risk of shock from the malfunctioning device to a person touching it.

Figure 43-3 illustrates an electrical fault occurring in an isolated power system. The two important new components in this diagram are the *isolation transformer* and the *line isolation monitor (LIM).*

An isolation transformer allows electrical power to be transmitted from one circuit to another without the existence of a direct electrical connection between them. In Figure 43-3, the standard, grounded electrical power supply is connected to the primary coil of the isolation transformer. The primary coil consists of a single wire, wrapped in a spiral fashion around a ferromagnetic core. The current flowing in this wire causes a magnetic field to be created in the core, in the manner described earlier for an inductor. However, in this case, the ferromagnetic core is shaped like a loop (here, a square), and the magnetic field is trapped within the body of this loop. A secondary coil is wrapped around the opposite side of the core. The magnetic field generated by the current in the primary coil circulates around within this ferromagnetic loop. As

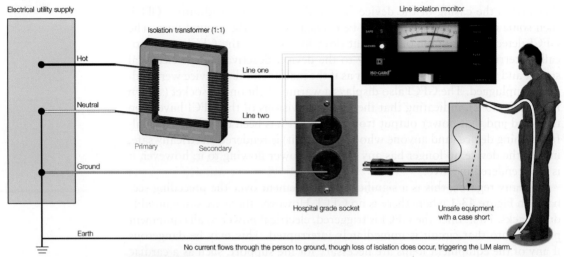

No current flows through the person to ground, though loss of isolation does occur, triggering the LIM alarm.

Figure 43-3 Unsafe equipment operating on an isolated power supply.

the magnetic field passes through the windings of the secondary coil, it induces an electrical potential difference, allowing power to be transmitted from the primary to the secondary. In an isolation transformer, the number of windings in the primary and secondary coils is the same, so that the current flowing in the primary and secondary coils is the same. The purpose of an isolation transformer, therefore, is to convert electrical power into a magnetic field and then convert it immediately back into electrical power. Although this may initially appear redundant, it produces two important effects:

1. An electrical fault on one side of the transformer cannot spread to the other side because the two coils of the transformer are physically separated and linked only by a magnetic field.
2. The isolation transformer transmits only the potential difference across the primary coil, not the absolute voltage. A potential difference of 120 V AC exists between the hot and neutral wires attached to the primary coil. It is the hot wire that is at 120 V AC and the neutral wire that is fixed at ground (0 V). The outputs from the secondary coil are called line 1 and line 2, and there is a potential difference of 120 V AC between them. The absolute voltages of line 1 and line 2 are not known; they are now isolated. Yet, any equipment plugged into the isolated circuit will still operate normally.

Suppose now an electrical device with an internal fault is connected to this isolated power supply, as shown in Figure 43-3. The electrical paths through the ground wire and through the person touching the device now provide an electrical connection from the isolated line 1 to ground. The effect of this is that line 1 has now become grounded, and its voltage has become fixed at 0 V. Line 1 is said to have lost isolation. Line 2 will continue to have a potential difference of 120 V AC relative to line 1, so the device will continue to operate. However, because line 1 has taken on the same absolute voltage as ground, no current can flow through the person to the ground and no electrical shock is produced.

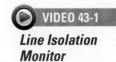

VIDEO 43-1

Line Isolation Monitor

The LIM monitors the electrical potentials and leakage currents that exist between line 1 and line 2 and ground. The LIM is designed to alarm when the isolation of the electrical power system has degraded to the extent that an electrical shock of greater than 5 mA could be produced with the next electrical fault. As shown in Table 43-1, a shock current of 5 mA applied to the body is the threshold below which no physical harm can result. Figure 43-3 shows that the LIM has detected a loss of isolation and has triggered a hazard alarm.

In summary, in an isolated power system, neither line 1 nor line 2 are the hot or neutral wires. However, if a fault occurs such that, for example, line 1 is brought into contact with a grounded object or person, then line 1 will immediately become the neutral wire (having lost isolation and becoming grounded) and line 2 will in turn become the equivalent of the hot wire. However, no shock will occur and all equipment will continue to receive electrical power. An isolated power system can therefore accommodate a single electrical fault without producing a shock and without having to shut down potentially life-sustaining medical devices. Of course, once a fault has occurred and the isolated power system has become grounded, then it is only as safe as the standard, grounded power system, as shown in Figures 43-1 and 43-2.

If a LIM alarms during a surgical case, the anesthesiologist and operating room (OR) personnel should try to identify which device in the OR is faulty. Each electrical device should sequentially be unplugged until the alarm stops, thus identifying the piece of equipment that contains the electrical fault. Once the offending device has been disconnected and quarantined, the other devices can progressively be reconnected. If the source of the fault cannot be identified or if the fault lies within an essential piece of equipment that cannot be disconnected or replaced, then it is acceptable to continue and complete the surgical procedure while remaining aware that the margin of safety provided by the isolated power system has been lost and that particular attention must be paid to the arrangement of electrical devices around the patient. It is, however, contraindicated to begin a subsequent surgical case in an operating room in which an electrical fault is known to exist.

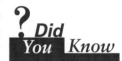

? Did You Know

If the line isolation monitor alarms all equipment plugged into that circuit will remain operative. However, if the faulty device causing the alarm is not identified and removed, the LIM will no longer provide protection against shock if a second defective piece of equipment is plugged into the circuit.

IV. Microshock

Table 43-1 shows that a current threshold of between 100 to 300 mA is required to induce ventricular fibrillation with a 60 Hz AC electrical shock. However, these results are calibrated for electrical current applied to the body surface. Electrical current that bypasses the skin and is applied directly to the heart can induce ventricular fibrillation with currents as low as 100 µA (0.1 mA) and is known as *microshock*. The patient can be placed at risk for microshock by any conductive medium that is in contact with the myocardium and that also extends outside the body. Examples would be temporary pacemaker wires or a pulmonary artery (PA) catheter containing a conductive electrolyte solution such as normal saline. Because the LIM does not usually alarm until there is a possible shock current of at least 5 mA, the use of an isolated power system and a LIM does not necessarily protect against the risk of microshock. The anesthesiologist must remember that a risk of microshock to the myocardium exists whenever devices such as pacemaker wires or PA catheters are manipulated. These devices should not be handled while the anesthesiologist is simultaneously in physical contact with any other piece of electrical apparatus (5).

V. Electrosurgery

The use of electrosurgery in clinical practice was pioneered in 1926 through a collaboration between the neurosurgeon Harvey Cushing and physicist William Bovie (6). Electrosurgery is different from electrocautery. *Electrocautery* is the process of using electricity (commonly DC current) to generate heat, and then applying that heat to tissue to cauterize it. In electrocautery, the electricity is simply a convenient form of energy to convert to heat at the surgical site. *Electrosurgery* instead makes use of alternating current at very high frequencies, of the order of 300 to 500 kHz, generated by an electrosurgical unit (ESU). These frequencies are sufficiently high that they are close to the radio frequencies (RF) used to transmit medium-wave AM radio. Electrosurgery is therefore sometimes referred to as RF electrosurgery in order to further distinguish it from simple cautery. The power output from an ESU operating in "cut" mode exceeds the power required to simply burn or desiccate tissue; it is sufficient to convert the water within the tissue into vapor, effectively exploding or vaporizing the tissue itself. The use of a fine-pointed surgical electrode produces a region of very high current density around the tip and permits precisely controllable surgical tissue dissection.

However, once this electrical current has been introduced into the body, it is important to consider how this current will travel through the body and return to the ESU in such a way that no destructive effects occur outside the desired region. Many electrosurgical tools have two electrodes, referred to as *bipolar instruments.* The current is introduced to tissue through one electrode at the tip of the instrument and a second electrode nearby receives the return current. This design is appropriate for instruments such as laparoscopic scissors, in which the two blades of the scissors act as the two electrodes. The current transmitted to or through neighboring anatomical structures is very small. Therefore, bipolar units are also commonly employed in neurosurgery. Alternatively, an electrosurgical device may consist of only one electrode—described as *monopolar.* These devices require a separate electrical return path from the patient to the ESU (7). This return path is created by sticking a large electrically conductive pad to a substantial part of the body such as the patient's thigh. This pad is often referred to as a *grounding pad,* but that description is unfortunately misleading. The pad does not ground the patient to earth potential because the patient and the electrosurgical device are electrically isolated by an isolated power system. The purpose of the pad is to act as an electrode to receive the electrosurgical current. The current is retrieved over a large tissue surface area so that the tissue current density is low; otherwise, the tissue under the pad might be accidently burned or cauterized. The grounding pad should therefore, more correctly, be called a *dispersive electrode.* If the dispersive electrode is improperly applied so that it only contacts the patient's skin in a few small locations, the return current will be concentrated at these points, the current density will be high, and accidental burns may result. Current might also be inappropriately directed to ECG electrodes. Additionally, patients should be strongly encouraged to remove metal jewelry because of the risk that, for example, a metal wedding ring may come to rest against a metal part of the OR table and form an electrically conductive path back to the dispersive electrode. The wedding ring would then effectively act as an unintended return electrode and potentially cause a circumferential burn to the finger. Metal jewelry that cannot be removed can be covered with tape to provide a layer of electrical insulation.

The frequency of the electrosurgical current is so high that it does not cause depolarization of nerves or muscle fibers. Nerves and muscles possess a property called *chronaxy,* which is the shortest duration of electrical impulse to which they can respond. Because the frequency of the AC current produced by an ESU is at several hundred kilohertz, the duration of one oscillation of

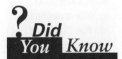

Did You Know

A large dispersive electrode ("grounding pad") is not required for bipolar electrosurgical instruments. The current in one electrode is returned to the adjacent electrode and does not pass elsewhere in the body.

the electrosurgical current is far shorter than the chronaxy of these tissues. The electrosurgical current can therefore pass through the body without triggering ventricular fibrillation, unlike an electrical shock from equivalent mains power supply current at 60 Hz. However, special care must be taken with patients who have an automatic implantable cardioverter defibrillator (AICD). The AICD continuously monitors the electrical activity of the patient's heart. It may misinterpret the high-frequency electrical interference from the electrosurgical current as being an episode of ventricular fibrillation requiring a defibrillatory shock. Therefore, the AICD must be inhibited from administering this shock during surgery. The AICD can either be reprogrammed (pre- and postsurgery), or it can be temporarily inhibited by placing a large magnet on the patient's chest over the AICD insertion site. The AICD detects the presence of this magnetic field; it responds by emitting an audible warning tone, and then the defibrillatory action of the AICD is inhibited while the magnet remains in place.

VI. Fire Safety

Starting a fire requires the presence of each element of the "fire triad"—a source of ignition, a fuel to burn, and an oxidizer (i.e., a source of oxygen) (8). The most common sources of ignition in the operating room are electrosurgical units or laser light sources, which are usually under the control of the surgical team. The most common sources of fuel are drapes, dressings, or gauzes, which may have additionally become soaked in alcohol-based preparation solutions or petroleum jelly. These materials are usually under the control of nursing personnel. The most common oxidizers are oxygen itself, spreading into the operating room environment from a face mask or nasal cannulae, or nitrous oxide, which is also capable of supporting combustion. These factors are usually under the control of the anesthesiologist. The operating room environment therefore contains ample equipment and materials to fulfill the three parts of the required triad for the outbreak of an operating room fire. Worse, each part of the triad is usually under the control of a different part of the overall operating room team. Therefore, it is possible for all three parts of the fire triad to come together in the same location without any one person being immediately aware that this has occurred.

Although the anesthesiologist must always be aware of the potential risk of an intraoperative fire, some procedures present a clearly foreseeable risk (9).

- During a tracheostomy, the opening of the trachea can potentially release a high concentration of oxygen into the surgical field. This can combine with the presence of gauze and electrosurgical instruments to produce an imminent risk of fire.
- The surgical site preparation solution for procedures on the upper chest or neck (e.g., portacatheter placement) may tend to pool or accumulate within the material of the surgical drapes, producing a potent fuel source. These procedures are commonly performed under sedation and oxygen from a face mask or nasal cannulae can accumulate underneath the drapes and residual preparation solution. The use of an electrocautery device on the surgical side of the drape can then be sufficient to ignite the drapes over the patient's head. This sudden flash fire, combined with melting of the plastic of the face mask or nasal cannulae, can produce disfiguring head and facial burn injuries within only a few seconds (10).
- Laser laryngoscopic surgery typically involves the use of laser surgical tools in close proximity to an airway that has been secured with an endotracheal

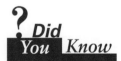
? Did You Know

Although modern inhaled anesthetics are considered non-explosive or non-flammable, disastrous fires can still occur because both oxygen and nitrous oxide support combustion. Caution must be exercised when these gases come in contact with a source of ignition (e.g. laser, ESU) and fuel (e.g. paper drapes, prep solution, endotracheal tube).

tube. Appropriate "laser-safe" endotracheal tubes should be used during this type of surgery, but a risk of igniting the endotracheal tube itself is always present. In the event of the endotracheal tube catching fire, the patient must be immediately extubated at the same time that the endotracheal tube is disconnected from the anesthesia circuit. The surgical field should be drenched with sterile water or saline, and any remaining burning material should be removed from the airway. The primary goal is to terminate the injury from the fire in the shortest possible time. Once the airway fire is extinguished, the patient can be mask ventilated, the airway can be examined by laryngoscopy or bronchoscopy, and the airway can be re-established with a new endotracheal tube.

When an ignition source (e.g. laser, electrocautery) is used in close proximity to the airway, regardless of the type of anesthesia employed (local with sedation, regional, or general), it is incumbent on the anesthesiologist to administer supplemental oxygen only in an amount that is sufficient to keep the patient's blood oxygen saturation at a safe level. Delivered oxygen should be diluted with nitrogen or air, but not nitrous oxide.

References

1. Horowitz P, Hill W. *The Art of Electronics*. 2nd ed. Cambridge, Engl.: Cambridge University Press; 1989;1125.
2. Cadick J, Capelli-Schellpfeffer M, Neitzel D, et al. *Electrical Safety Handbook*. 4th ed. New York: McGraw-Hill, 2012.
3. Chambers JJ, Saha AK. Electrocution during anaesthesia. *Anaesthesia*. 1979;34(2): 173–175.
4. Wills JH, Ehrenwerth J, Rogers D. Electrical injury to a nurse due to conductive fluid in an operating room designated as a dry location. *Anesth Analg*. 2010;110(6):1647–1649.
5. Baas LS, Beery TA, Hickey CS. Care and safety of pacemaker electrodes in intensive care and telemetry nursing units. *Am J Crit Care*. 1997;6(4):302–311.
6. O'Connor JL, Bloom DA. William T. Bovie and electrosurgery. *Surgery*. 1996;119(4): 390–396.
7. Brill AI, Feste JR, Hamilton TL, et al. Patient safety during laparoscopic monopolar electrosurgery—principles and guidelines. Consortium on Electrosurgical Safety During Laparoscopy. *JSLS*. 1998;2(3):221–225.
8. Culp WC Jr, Kimbrough BA, Luna S, et al. Mitigating operating room fires: Development of a carbon dioxide fire prevention device. *Anesth Analg*. 2014;118(4):772–775.
9. Kaye AD, Kolinsky D, Urman RD. Management of a fire in the operating room. *J Anesth*. 2014;28(2):279–287.
10. Culp WC Jr, Kimbrough BA, Luna S. Flammability of surgical drapes and materials in varying concentrations of oxygen. *Anesthesiology*. 2013;119(4):770–776.

Questions

1. All of the following are characteristics of common "household" electricity EXCEPT:
   A. The electrical potential is nominally 120 V
   B. The current oscillates at 60 Hz
   C. Current always flows from the positive (black) wire to the neutral (white) wire
   D. The potential difference between the "hot" and neutral conductor oscillates sinusoidally between ±170 V

2. In a hospital operating room, the MOST efficacious way to reduce the possibility of harmful shock to personnel is to:
   A. Use a system that transmits power from one circuit to another without a direct electrical connection between them
   B. Install GFCI devices at all electrical outlets
   C. Use only equipment that has a three-pin (conductor) plug
   D. Only use items of equipment that have been serviced and checked for the absence of leakage current

3. All of the following statements regarding a GFCI device are true, EXCEPT:
   A. It senses current flow in the ground wire of any device plugged into it
   B. If triggered, it will disconnect ("unplug") all devices plugged into it
   C. If triggered, a red light will come on, but it will not sound an alarm
   D. It will remain operative if a two-pin adapter is inserted between a three-pin plug and the outlet

4. All of the following statements regarding electrical power supplied to an OR by an isolation transformer, in conjunction with a line isolation monitor (LIM) are true EXCEPT:
   A. Electrical power is delivered by induction of a magnetic field across two separated wire coils.
   B. Under normal operation, the output of the isolation transformer is through two wire leads, one at 120 V and the other at 0 V (ground).
   C. Electrical power will continue to be provided at the outlet if a malfunctioning piece of equipment is plugged in.
   D. If a person touches a malfunctioning piece of equipment plugged into a properly functioning isolation circuit, some current will flow through the person but no shock will be perceived.

5. If the LIM alarms, the most appropriate next action for the anesthesiologist is to:
   A. Convert to manual ventilation and prepare to administer intravenous anesthesia
   B. Have the LIM alarm reset, but be prepared to have all electrical equipment checked at the end of the case
   C. Recommend the surgical procedure be rapidly aborted and have someone unplug all nonessential pieces of equipment
   D. Have someone sequentially unplug single pieces of equipment until the LIM alarm stops and the offending device is discovered

6. Which of the following statements is TRUE?
   A. A dispersive pad applied to the patient is required for both mono- and bipolar electrosurgical instruments.
   B. Use of electrosurgical devices is contraindicated when patients have an implanted cardioverter defibrillator (AICD).
   C. The current frequency of the electrosurgical unit is so high that if passed through the heart, ventricular fibrillation is unlikely.
   D. The dispersive plate is grounded so that the patient does not receive a shock.

7. All of the following scenarios represent a significant risk for fire associated with use of an electrosurgical device EXCEPT:
   A. Tracheostomy during anesthesia with isoflurane, 70% nitrous oxide and 30% oxygen.
   B. Laparoscopy during which the pneumoperitoneum is achieved with carbon dioxide.
   C. Laser surgery for laryngeal papilloma with general anesthesia achieved via a standard endotracheal tube.
   D. Facial plastic surgery performed during conscious sedation with 100% oxygen administered via plastic face mask under the drapes.

44 Wellness Principles and Resources for Anesthesiologists

Amy E. Vinson
Robert S. Holzman

In dealing with those who are undergoing great suffering, if you feel "burnout" setting in, if you feel demoralized and exhausted, it is best, for the sake of everyone, to withdraw and restore yourself. The point is to have a long-term perspective.

—Dalai Lama

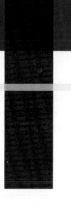

VIDEO 44-1

Wellness Principles

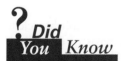

? Did You Know

Wellness is a complex and personal endeavor, defined by the collective thought processes, values, and attitudes that lead to increased resilience, decreased burnout, and an enhanced sense of well-being, including job and life satisfaction.

I. Wellness and the Anesthesiologist

Wellness is personal; therefore, a single definition is elusive. Of diverse cultural and spiritual backgrounds, anesthesiologists operate in a high-stress environment physically, mentally, and emotionally. They work alongside one another while experiencing vastly different life stages, thereby "wellness" means something entirely different to each member of the team. Compare the 29-year-old residency graduate in her second year of marriage, starting a family, and paying down medical school debt while learning how to become an autonomous physician and teacher, with the 63-year-old seasoned practitioner celebrating her first grandchild while contemplating retirement, her own health, and the illness or death of a parent. Here the commonality of wellness is defined as the collective thought processes, behaviors, values, and attitudes that lead to increased resilience, decreased burnout, an enhanced sense of well-being, and improved job and life satisfaction. Given that wellness is a multivariate, complex, and personal endeavor, it is not the purpose of this chapter to provide a personal guide to wellness. Rather, this chapter will provide a summary of wellness issues specific to the anesthesiologist, the practice of anesthesiology, and to leaders within anesthesiology-related organizations.

Several organizations have incorporated wellness as a group of competencies to be achieved during training. For example, the Royal College of Physicians and Surgeons of Canada lists: "Demonstrate a commitment to physician health and sustainable practice" as the third competency of professionalism in their 2005 framework (1). More recently, as part of the Milestones project, well-being has been addressed as a training requirement: "Professionalism: Responsibility to maintain personal emotional, physical, and mental health."

Although the concept of wellness remains somewhat nebulous, the concept of burnout is well established. The "burnout syndrome" gained attention in the 1970s and 1980s, when Maslach et al. (2) developed and marketed the "Maslach Burnout Inventory" (MBI). They defined *burnout* as "a syndrome of emotional exhaustion and cynicism that occurs frequently among individuals who do 'people work' of some kind." The MBI characterizes burnout based on three major psychological characteristics: *emotional exhaustion, depersonalization,* and a *low sense of personal accomplishment.* The MBI has since become the gold standard in quantifying burnout.

In 1999, in response to a growing body of literature concerning higher rates of suicide, substance abuse, and depression among anesthesiologists, Jackson (3) contemplated the role of stress, closely examining aspects such as personality type, physical implications of stress, life-cycle changes, sex stress differences, self-esteem, and workplace stress abatement. He defined stress as the "nonspecific adaptive response of the body to any change, demand, pressure, challenge, threat or trauma" and related this to the particular stressors encountered within the practice of anesthesiology. Jackson offered that a humanistic approach to medical education, coupled with the teaching of stress management techniques, could improve the overall professional and personal lives of anesthesiologists. Following this, a body of literature has amassed exploring the epidemiology and impact of burnout in the larger community of physicians (Table 44-1).

Shanafelt et al. (4) surveyed over 27,000 US physicians, with 46% of them reporting at least one burnout symptom (emotional exhaustion, depersonalization, or low sense of personal accomplishment). Physicians and osteopaths reported higher rates of burnout than the average high school graduate. However, a comparison group holding nonmedical graduate degrees had lower rates of burnout than the average high school graduate. Anesthesiologists ranked 7 of 23 medical specialties in burnout among physicians. Of all respondents, 38% screened positive for depression and 6% reported suicidal ideations within the past 12 months.

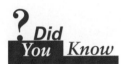

? Did You Know

In one large national study, physicians reported higher burnout rates than the average high school graduate, whereas those with nonmedical graduate degrees reported lower burnout rates than the average high school graduate.

II. Special Circumstances

Some stressors are so vital they require intervention to continue practice. This has resulted in various legislative efforts, as described in the sections that follow.

A. Americans with Disabilities Act

The *Americans with Disabilities Act (ADA)* is "An Act to establish a clear and comprehensive prohibition of discrimination on the basis of disability" that was signed into law by George H. W. Bush in 1990. This was followed in 2008 by the *ADA Amendments Act (ADAAA)*, which broadened the protections offered in the original bill. In order to be protected by the ADA, a person must demonstrate a disability to qualify for protection and then request reasonable accommodation. A major focus of the ADAAA was to clarify the meaning of disability and broaden its definition to include any impairment that "substantially limits" a "major life activity." Although patients' safety must take primary focus, there will occasionally be physicians who have physical or mental limitations, including visual and auditory impairments. Often, reasonable accommodations can be made to enable the anesthesiologist to perform in an acceptable manner. When this is possible, the patient is protected by the ADA. Controversy is introduced, however, when there is a question of whether the proposed accommodations are reasonable or when patient safety

Table 44-1   Physician Burnout: Causes, Consequences, and Epidemiology

Study	Methods and Focus	Findings
Shanafelt TD, Bradley KA, Wipf JE, et al. Burnout and self-reported patient care in an internal medicine residency program. *Ann Intern Med.* 2002;136:358–367	Survey of 115 internal medicine residents. Maslach Burnout Inventory (MBI)	• 76% response rate. • 76% fulfilled criteria for burnout (either emotional exhaustion or depersonalization). • Those with burnout more likely to espouse "suboptimal patient care practices."
Nyssen AS, Hansez I, Baele P, et al. Occupational stress and burnout in anaesthesia. *Br J Anaesth.* 2003;90:333–337	Survey of 318 anesthetists in Belgium University Network. Psychological state of stress measure, working conditions, and control questionnaire	• Stress level 50.6 (same as general population). • Stress sources: lack of control over time, risk, and work planning. • 40.4% with high emotional exhaustion (e.g., burnout), worse in younger cohort.
Kluger MT, Townend K, Laidlaw T. Job satisfaction, stress and burnout in Australian specialist anaesthetists. *Anaesthesia.* 2003;58:339–345	Survey of 700 Australian anesthetists. MBI	• 60% response rate. • Anesthesia stressors: interference with home life, time constraints. • Stress reduced with assistants and organization. • Burnout symptoms reported by 20% (emotional exhaustion), 20% (depersonalization), and 36% (low sense of accomplishment).
Thomas NK. Resident burnout. *JAMA.* 2004;292:2880–2889	Review of 15 studies of resident burnout	• 15 articles identified—heterogeneous composition. • Data suggesting high levels of resident burnout impacting patient care. • Data insufficient to assign causal relationship or identify risk factors.
Kuerer HM, Eberlein TJ, Pollock RE, et al. Career satisfaction, practice patterns and burnout among surgical oncologists: Report on the quality of life of members of the Society of Surgical Oncology. *Ann Surg Oncol.* 2007;14:3043–3053	Survey of 1,519 Society of Surgical Oncology members. Queried burnout (MBI) and quality of life (QOL)	• 36% response rate, 72% academic, 26% at least one-fourth research. • 79% would pursue the same career again. • 28% with symptoms of burnout, more common in those <50 years old, and in women. • Associated factors with burnout: lower physical QOL, <25% of time in research.
Shanafelt TD, Balch CM, Bechamps GJ, et al. Burnout and career satisfaction among American surgeons. *Ann Surg.* 2009;250:463–471	Survey of 24,922 American College of Surgeons (ACS) members. MBI and QOL data	• 32% response rate. • 40% with symptoms of burnout, 30% with symptoms of depression. • 36% felt their schedule allowed sufficient personal time. • Independent factors associated with burnout: younger age, having children, number of on-call nights weekly, and billing-based compensation.

Table 44-1   Physician Burnout: Causes, Consequences, and Epidemiology (*Continued*)

Study	Methods and Focus	Findings
West CP, Tan AD, Habermann TM, et al. Association of resident fatigue and distress with perceived medical errors. *JAMA*. 2009;302:1294–1300	Prospective longitudinal cohort study of 430 internal medicine residents. Survey: MBI, QOL, PRIME-MD depression screen, and self-reported medical errors	• 67.5% response rate to individual surveys (average). • 39% self-reported at least one major medical error. • Errors positively associated with increased sleepiness scale score, fatigue score and burnout. • Self-reported medical errors associated with fatigue and markers of distress.
Shanafelt TD, Balch CM, Bechamps G, et al. Burnout and medical errors among American surgeons. *Ann Surg*. 2010;251:995–1000	Survey of 7,905 ACS members. MBI, QOL and depression screens	• 32% response rate. • 8.9% reporting a major medical error in past 3 months, with 70% citing individual, not systems, errors. • Recent error associated with all three components of burnout, lower mental QOL, and depression.
Dyrbye LN, Massie FS, Eacker A, et al. Relationship between burnout and professional conduct and attitudes among US medical students. *JAMA*. 2010;304:1173–1180	Survey of medical students at 7 US medical schools. MBI, PRIME-MD depression screen, QOL survey	• 61% response rate. • 52.8% incidence of burnout. • Reporting unprofessional behavior more common among students with burnout. • Burnout associated with lower rates of altruistic views.
Balch CM, Shanafelt TD, Sloan JA, et al. Distress and career satisfaction among 14 surgical specialties, comparing academic and private practice settings. *Ann Surg*. 2011; 254:558–568	14 surgical specialties from ACS data— demographics, career satisfaction, distress parameters	• Academic surgeons less likely to experience burnout, depression, or suicidal ideation and more likely to have career satisfaction. • Academic burnout associations: Negative (older children, pediatric surgery, cardiothoracic surgery, male); Positive (trauma surgery, nights on call, hours worked). • Private practice burnout associations: Negative (older children, physician spouse, older age); Positive (urologic surgery, 31–50% nonclinical time, incentive-based pay, nights on call, hours worked).
Shanafelt TD, Boone S, Tan L, et al. Burnout and satisfaction with work-life balance among US physicians relative to the general US population. *Arch Intern Med*. 2012;172:1377–1385	Survey of 27,276 US physicians from American Medical Association Physician Masterfile, compared with probability-based sample of the general US population. MBI	• 26.7% response rate. • 45.8% of physicians with at least one symptom of burnout. • Burnout more common in MD and DO cohorts than in the average high school graduate. • Burnout less common in those with nonphysician graduate degrees than the average high school graduate. • Burnout most common in emergency medicine and general internal medicine (anesthesiology was 7th of 23 specialties listed).

PRIME-MD, Primary Care Evaluation of Mental Disorders.

appears to be compromised. Further questions—and controversies—arise at the local level with regard to credentialing and privileges and at the indemnification level with liability insurance underwriting. These cases are rare and are generally dealt with on a case-by-case basis.

B. Family and Medical Leave Act

The *Family and Medical Leave Act* of 1993 was signed into law by President Bill Clinton and was a federal attempt at protecting work–life balance by ensuring covered employees job-protected, albeit unpaid, leave during times of family need, such as an illness in the family, military leave, personal illness or recovery, pregnancy, or adoption. Certain stipulations (e.g., who is considered a covered employee, including employment of 12 months prior to leave) are made, but most employed physicians and trainees fall within this category. Many employers also provide paid leave for various periods of time and circumstances. Controversies persist regarding the relatively higher use by women for maternity leave, although the use of paternity leave does appear to be increasing.

III. Considerations for the Physician

A. The Impaired Physician

The current body of literature relating to physician impairment, with few exceptions, focuses on impairment from substance use disorders. However, it must be noted that factors other than substance use may impair professional performance. These include other forms of addiction (e.g., gambling, sex, food), psychiatric conditions (e.g., anxiety, depression, obsessive–compulsive disorder), and medical conditions or treatments leading to fatigue or altered mental status (e.g., obstructive sleep apnea, seizure disorder, prescribed narcotics).

Anesthesiologists have, for years, been considered at high risk for *substance use disorder (SUD)*. However, until recently, strong data did not exist to support this assertion or its consequences. In 2013, Warner et al. (5) reported on the prevalence of SUD in those entering Accreditation Council for Graduate Medical Education–accredited anesthesiology residencies between 1975 and 2009. Although their primary objective was to define the *incidence* of SUD during training, they also reported on the types of substances abused, episodes of relapse, and consequences, including death attributed to SUD. The most commonly abused substances were opioids, with intravenous fentanyl being the most common. Other commonly abused substances were alcohol, anesthetics or hypnotics, marijuana, and cocaine, with many abusing multiple substances. Despite the varied treatment and support programs offered to physicians with SUDs, the incidence of relapse does not appear to have declined since 1975. Additionally, the risk of death was high: 11% of trainees identified as having SUD during training died from a SUD-related cause during the study period. From an occupational health perspective, the rates of SUD-related death make anesthesiology relatively more dangerous than being a firefighter and only slightly less dangerous than being a police officer.

In response to the growing requirements by the Joint Commission, most states now offer specialized support programs for physicians struggling with SUD. These programs vary in their relation with their respective state medical boards. Anesthesiologists can easily find a local program by doing an online search for "physician health program" in their state. Alternatively, one can simply visit the Federation of State Physician Health Programs (http://www.fsphp.org) and select the appropriate state or access aggregated information

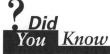

? Did You Know

For anesthesiologists who developed a substance use disorder (SUD) during their training, the subsequent risk of death from relapse and SUD-related causes is reported to be 11%—an occupational hazard rate higher than being a firefighter and only slightly lower than being a police officer.

links via the American Society of Anesthesiologists Wellness website (http://www.asahq.org/resources/resources-from-asa-committees/work-life-balance-asa-wellness-resources).

B. The Aging Physician

With time, physicians gain experience, attain knowledge, advance within the field, pass skills on to trainees, and shape the practice environment. Unfortunately, aging physicians are increasingly distant from their initial education and training and may eventually experience cognitive decline and changes in sensory perception, despite garnering the respect and admiration of their colleagues. How should the competency of the aging physician population be assessed, and at what point should clinical practice be limited or ceased? There is no set retirement age for physicians, and this question is arising more frequently as many physicians choose to delay retirement following the most recent recession. In 2013, Haddad (6) published a review of the literature relating to the aging physician. It was noted in this study that the airline industry requires routine neurocognitive testing after age 40 and has mandated a retirement age for commercial airline pilots.

The requirements for continuing medical education and maintenance of certification in anesthesiology have been promulgated, in part, to address the aging workforce. However, participation is not clearly linked to improved knowledge retention or patient care. Several studies have also demonstrated a disconnect between self-assessment and cognitive performance in an aging physician population, while others demonstrate an increase in certain adverse outcomes as physician age increases. Many institutions have mandated neuro-cognitive testing to begin at a certain threshold age (often 70 years), but this testing has fallen under scrutiny due to the low positive predictive value and high potential for psychological stress from false positive results. More frequent ongoing professional performance evaluations have been recommended by the Joint Commission to address competency more frequently. As institutions implement such evaluations, they will hopefully become more valid and sensitive to instances of true cognitive decline.

IV. Providing Support

At some point in the anesthesiologist's career, an extraordinarily stressful event will be encountered that will require additional assistance with either processing or navigating the situation. It is unfortunate that not everyone faced with these situations seeks or accepts such assistance. Two specific situations arise during the careers of many anesthesiologists: adverse clinical events and malpractice litigation (see Chapter 40).

A. After an Adverse Event

"War stories" of perioperative catastrophes are occasionally shared in the anesthesia lounge, but until recently, the prevalence and impact of these events was not fully described. In 2012, a survey study was sent to 1,200 members of the American Society of Anesthesiologists. Gazoni et al. (7) reported on this survey and found that, with a 56% response rate, 84% of respondents had experienced at least one unexpected perioperative catastrophe. Of these, 19% reported never having fully recovered from the event, nearly all (88%) required some time to recover emotionally, and 67% felt the care they were delivering over the subsequent 4 hours was compromised. Despite this, only 7% were given any time off to recover. The most common emotional reactions included reliving the event, anxiety, guilt, fear of litigation, depression, and sleeplessness. The respondents felt that if they had experienced a subsequent catastrophic event, they would most likely have found the following interventions helpful: "talking with anesthesia personnel," "debriefing with entire operating room team," "talking with the patient's family," "talking with one's own spouse/family," and "talking with a professional counselor."

Many hospitals, universities, malpractice providers, and other organizations offer support following adverse events. These come in the form of peer support, formal counseling, debriefing, and even mandatory time away from clinical practice. Some have advocated for an organized and stepwise response in the wake of an adverse event in order to better support the providers as "second victims" (8). It is wise to become familiar with the support resources available in one's practice environment in the event that such assistance is someday required following an adverse clinical event.

B. During or After a Malpractice Claim

Despite the historical role of anesthesiologists in improving patient safety, anesthesiologists can still find themselves named in a malpractice claim. A recent study of malpractice claims for a national carrier demonstrated anesthesiologists to have an annual risk of malpractice claims and payment similar to that of other medical specialists (9). This can be one of the most stressful events in a physician's life, with distress arising from the uncertainty of outcomes, the prolonged nature of many lawsuits, and the sense of isolation that can occur when advised to not discuss the case with others. Although physicians' ego, financial security, and career are seemingly at risk during the litigation process, they also must repeatedly relive a potentially traumatizing adverse clinical event, adding to the psychological impact of the experience. Many malpractice carriers offer support and assistance during the difficult process of a medical malpractice lawsuit.

V. Promoting Wellness

Although many suggest that personal well-being is an individual responsibility, recent data highlighting rates of burnout, SUD, and SUD-related death underscore the obligation of the profession in promoting well-being for its members. Moreover, as wellness principles become integrated into training and practice, there will likely be an inevitable extension into the concept of personal well-being as a "duty owed" to patients.

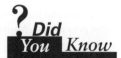

The components of wellness are varied, but certain approaches to decrease stress or increase resilience have been well validated and studied. Although fitness, nutrition, proper rest, fiscal responsibility, and work–life balance are all important components of wellness, none have been as solidly linked to improved physician well-being as *mindfulness-based stress reduction (MBSR)*. Mindfulness carries many different definitions, all of which express the concept of an intentional, enhanced, and nonjudgmental awareness of one's environment and an inclination for living in the present moment. Rooted in Buddhist philosophy, the incorporation of mindfulness in contemporary medical practice has been led by the work of Jon Kabat-Zinn. Decreases in chronic pain and anxiety and improved wound healing have been reported, with some recent studies demonstrating changes in brain architecture and gene expression. The practice of MBSR is starting to be studied in health care professionals, with results showing clear improvements in perceived levels of stress (Table 44-2).

Did You Know

Although fitness, nutrition, proper rest, fiscal responsibility, and work–life balance are all important components of wellness, mindfulness-based stress reduction—an intentional, enhanced, and nonjudgmental awareness of one's environment and an inclination for living in the present moment—is most strongly linked to physician well-being.

Table 44-2   Effect of Meditation Practices[a] on Brain Function and Architecture and Gene Expression

Study	Methods and Focus	Findings
Davidson RJ, Kabat-Zinn J, Schumacher J, et al. Alterations in brain and immune function produced by mindfulness meditation. *Psychosom Med.* 2003;65:564–570	MBSR intervention (25 in study group, 16 control). Measured brain electrical activity and immune response to influenza vaccination	• Increased left anterior activation (associated with positive affect) in meditator group. • Increase in antibody titers to vaccination in meditator group (degree of increase correlating with degree of left anterior activation).
Dusek JA, Otu HH, Wohlhueter AL, et al. Genomic counter-stress changes induced by the relaxation response. *PLoS ONE.* 2008;3:e2576	Whole blood transcription profiles 19 LTMs, 19 controls, 20 in RR intervention group	• 2,209 differentially expressed genes in LTM vs. controls. • 1,561 differentially expressed genes in RR group vs. controls. • 433 genes shared between 2,209 and 1,561 groups (suggesting short-term inducible expression). • Genes involved in cellular response to stress response, oxidative stress, and cellular damage.
Sharma H, Datta P, Singh A, et al. Gene expression profiling in practitioners of Sudarshan Kriya. *J Psychosom Res.* 2008;64:213–218	42 LTMs eliciting RR via Sudarshan Kriya (SK, breathing exercise) and 42 controls	• SK group: higher levels of glutathione, glutathione peroxidase, and super oxide dismutase. • SK group: higher expression of antioxidant enzymes. • Authors suggest SK group has higher resistance to oxidative stress and a protective advantage to cancer and cardiovascular disease.
Luders E, Toga AW, Lepore N, et al. The underlying anatomical correlates of long-term meditation: Larger hippocampal and frontal volumes of gray matter. *Neuroimage.* 2009;45:672–678	22 LTMs and 22 controls High resolution MRI and voxel-based morphometry	• LTMs: significantly larger gray matter volumes, particularly in right orbitofrontal cortex and right hippocampus, both thought to be involved in emotional regulation and response control. • Authors postulate this change may be responsible for the emotional stability, mindfulness, and positivity typical of the LTM cohort.
Hölzel BK, Carmody J, Vangel M, et al. Mindfulness practice leads to increases in regional brain gray matter density. *Psychiatry Res.* 2011;191:36–43	Pre-post gray matter density (voxel-based morphometry, MRI) in 16 MBSR class participants, compared with 17 controls	• MBSR group: increased gray matter density in left hippocampus, posterior cingulate cortex, temporoparietal junction, and cerebellum. • These regions involved in emotional regulation, self-referential processing, perspective taking, and learning and memory.
Kilpatrick LA, Suyenobu BY, Smith SR, et al. Impact of mindfulness-based stress reduction training on intrinsic brain connectivity. *Neuroimage.* 2011;56:290–298	Functional connectivity MRI (fcMRI) in 17 MBSR participants, compared with 15 controls. All healthy women	• MBSR group: increased functional connectivity in auditory and visual networks, between auditory cortex and attentional and self-referential process areas, as well as greater anticorrelation between auditory and visual cortices and visual cortex and attentional and self-referential process areas. • Authors suggest MBSR improves sensory processing, attentional focus, and reflective awareness.

Table 44-2 Effect of Meditation Practices[a] on Brain Function and Architecture and Gene Expression (*Continued*)

Study	Methods and Focus	Findings
Ives-Deliperi VL, Solms M, Meintjes EM. The neural substrates of mindfulness: An fMRI investigation. *Soc Neurosci.* 2011;6:231–242	Functional MRI (fMRI) during meditation of 10 LTM subjects (following MBSR course and at least 4 years of daily meditation)	• Meditation decreased signal in midline cortical structures (implicated in interoception). • Meditation increased signal in right posterior cingulate cortex. • Consistent signal change among participants. • Authors postulate a disidentification mechanism for mindfulness meditation state.
Bhasin MK, Dusek JA, Chang B-H, et al. Relaxation response induces temporal transcriptome changes in energy metabolism, insulin secretion and inflammatory pathways. *PLoS ONE.* 2013;8:e62817	Measured rapid time-dependant genomic changes before and after meditation in 26 LTMs and 26 controls (before and after an 8-week RR training in novice controls)	• RR-enhanced expression of genes implicated in metabolism, mitochondrial function, telomere maintenance, and insulin secretion (especially mitochondrial ATP synthase), but decreased expression of genes involved in inflammatory and stress responses (especially NF-κB). • Response was more pronounced in LTMs. • Authors stipulate enhanced mitochondrial resilience induced by RR.
Luders E, Kurth F, Toga AW, et al. Meditation effects within the hippocampal complex revealed by voxel-based morphometry and cytoarchitectonic probabilistic mapping. *Front Psychol.* 2013;4:398	Focused and detailed MRI examination of hippocampus in 50 LTMs and 50 controls using voxel-based morphometry	• Significant changes noted in the hippocampal subiculum in LTMs. • This region is responsible in part for stress regulation. • Authors suggest that meditation may lead to neuronal preservation, attenuated stress response, and decreased neurotoxicity.
Black DS, Cole SW, Irwin MR, et al. Yogic meditation reverses NF-κB and IRF-related transcriptome dynamics in leukocytes of family dementia caregivers in a randomized controlled trial. *Psychoneuroendocrinology.* 2013;38:348–355	Immune cell gene expression during yogic meditation in caregivers (presumed stressful life event) of dementia patients (23 in meditation group, 16 controls)	• In meditation group, increased expression of 19 genes (including immunoglobulin-related genes) and decrease in pro-inflammatory cytokines. • Promotor-based bioinformatics suggest a NK-κB pathway reduction and IRF1 activity increase. • Results suggest that meditation may attenuate the typical immunologic stress response
Kaliman P, Alvarez-López MJ, Cosín-Tomás M, et al. Rapid changes in histone deacetylases and inflammatory gene expression in expert meditators. *Psychoneuroendocrinology.* 2014;40:96–107	Gene expression in peripheral blood mononuclear cells in 19 LTMs compared with 21 controls. Intervention was a Trier Social Stress Test (TSST)	• Groups had similar levels of baseline regulatory and inflammatory genes. • TSST led to a reduced expression of histone deacetylase genes and pro-inflammatory genes in the LTM group compared with the control group. • Two of these genes (*HDAC2* and *RIPK2*) correlated with a faster return to cortisol baseline.

LTM, long-term meditator; MBSR, mindfulness-based stress reduction; RR, relaxation response; MRI, magnetic resonance imaging; ATP, adenosine triphosphate; NF-κB, nuclear factor kappa-B.
[a]Meditation practices include focused and intentional mental practices, such as meditation, mindfulness meditation, yogic meditation, and the relaxation response, among others.

Many medical schools are also starting to integrate MBSR into their curricula as a concept of mindful practice. These curricula vary, yet they generally seek to prevent compassion fatigue (characterized by a lessening of compassion over time) and burnout, increase physician engagement and self-awareness, and decrease stress. Many consider engagement to be the psychological opposite of burnout. A recent review of mindfulness curricula provides summaries of existing mindfulness curricula and raises critical questions of if, when, and how mindfulness should be introduced during medical training (10).

VI. Conclusions

In order to provide sustained care, a person must have a degree of well-being. Given the data accumulating on anesthesiologist burnout, depression, suicidality, SUD, and SUD-related death, there should be substantial concern that common, as well as unique, problems exist within the specialty of anesthesiology. Fortunately, research and a body of literature are emerging on recognition and interventions focused on decreasing burnout and improving physician well-being.

References

1. Frank JR, ed. *The CanMEDS 2005 Physician Competency Framework. Better Standards. Better Physicians. Better Care.* Ottawa: Royal College of Physicians and Surgeons of Canada; 2005.
2. Maslach C, Jackson SE, Leiter MP. *The Maslach Burnout Inventory.* 3rd ed. Palo Alto, CA: Consulting Psychologists Press; 1996.
3. Jackson SH. The role of stress in anaesthetists' health and well-being. *Acta Anaesthesiol Scand.* 1999;43:583–602.
4. Shanafelt TD, Boone S, Tan L, et al. Burnout and satisfaction with work-life balance among US physicians relative to the general US population. *Arch Intern Med.* 2012;172:1377–1385.
5. Warner DO, Berge K, Sun H, et al. Substance use disorder among anesthesiology residents, 1975–2009. *JAMA.* 2013;310:2289–2296.
6. Haddad T. Cognitive assessment in the practice of medicine—dealing with the aging physician. *Phys Exec.* 2013;39:14–20.
7. Gazoni FM, Amato PE, Malik ZM, et al. The impact of perioperative catastrophes on anesthesiologists. *Anesth Analg.* 2012;114:596–603.
8. Cooper JB, Cullen DJ, Eichhorn JH, et al. Administrative guidelines for response to an adverse anesthesia event. The Risk Management Committee of the Harvard Medical School's Department of Anaesthesia. *J Clin Anesth.* 1993;5:79–84.
9. Jena AB, Seabury S, Lakdawalla D, et al. Malpractice risk according to physician specialty. *N Engl J Med.* 2011;365:629–636.
10. Dobkin PL, Hutchinson TA. Teaching mindfulness in medical school: Where are we now and where are we going? *Med Educ.* 2013;47:768–779.

Questions

1. The Maslach Burnout Inventory is a tool that quantifies physician burnout by assessing all of the following characteristics EXCEPT:
   A. Low sense of personal accomplishment
   B. Presence of substance abuse
   C. Emotional exhaustion
   D. Depersonalization

2. Which of the following federal legislation is designed to address life stressors associated with adoption of a teenage child?
   A. Americans with Disabilities Act (ADA)
   B. Americans with Disabilities Amendments Act (ADAAA)
   C. Family and Medical Leave Act (FMLA)
   D. Health Insurance Portability and Accountability Act (HIPAA)

3. According to a recent study, the thoughtful expansion of treatment and support programs for anesthesiology trainees with substance use disorders between 1975 and 2009 has resulted in an almost 50% reduction in the relapse rate for such substance use. TRUE or FALSE?
   A. True
   B. False

4. Which of the following programs has a high positive predictive value for detecting clinical impairments associated with aging?
   A. Continuing Medical Education (CME) performance
   B. Neurocognitive testing
   C. Maintenance of Certification in Anesthesiology (MOCA) programs
   D. None of the above

5. All of the following statements regarding mindfulness-based stress reduction (MBSR) techniques are true EXCEPT:
   A. Medical school curricula are increasingly incorporating MBSR techniques
   B. Nonjudgmental awareness of one's environment is a key concept of MBSR
   C. Nutrition, fitness, and proper rest are key components of MBSR
   D. MBSR is rooted in Buddhist philosophy of living in the moment

Formulas

Hemodynamic Formulas
Respiratory Formulas
Lung Volumes and Capacities

Hemodynamic Formulas

Hemodynamic Variables: Calculations and Normal Values

Variable	Calculation	Normal Values
Cardiac index (CI)	CO/BSA	2.5–4.0 L/min/m^2
Stroke volume (SV)	CO × 1000/HR	60–90 mL/beat
Stroke index (SI)	SV/BSA	40–60 mL/beat/m^2
Mean arterial pressure (MAP)	Diastolic pressure + $\frac{1}{3}$ pulse pressure	80–120 mm Hg
Systemic vascular resistance (SVR)	$\dfrac{\text{MAP} - \overline{\text{CVP}}}{\text{CO}} \times 79.9$	1,200–1,500 dyne-cm-sec^{-5}
Pulmonary vascular resistance (PVR)	$\dfrac{\overline{\text{PAP}} - \overline{\text{PCWP}}}{\text{CO}} \times 79.9$	100–300 dyne-cm-sec^{-5}
Right ventricular stroke work index (RVSWI)	0.0136 (PAP − CVP) × SI	5–9 g-m/beat/m^2
Left ventricular stroke work index (LWSWI)	0.0136 (MAP − PCWP) × SI	45–60 g-m/beat/m^2

HR = heart rate; $\overline{\text{CVP}}$ = mean central venous pressure; BSA = body surface area; CO = cardiac output; PAP = mean pulmonary artery pressure; PCWP = pulmonary capillary wedge pressure; MAP = mean arterial blood pressure.

Respiratory Formulas

	Normal Values (70 kg)
Alveolar oxygen tension $P_{AO_2} = (P_B - 47)\, F_{IO_2} - P_{ACO_2}$	110 mm Hg ($F_{IO_2} = 0.21$)
Alveolar-arterial oxygen gradient $Aa_{O_2} = P_{AO_2} - P_{aO_2}$	<10 mm Hg ($F_{IO_2} = 0.21$)
Arterial-to-alveolar oxygen ratio, a/A ratio	>0.75
Arterial oxygen content $Ca_{O_2} = (Sa_{O_2})(Hb \times 1.34) + Pa_{O_2}\,(0.0031)$	21 mL/100 mL
Mixed venous oxygen content $C\bar{v}_{O_2} = (S\bar{v}_{O_2})(Hb \times 1.34) + P\bar{v}_{O_2}\,(0.0031)$	15 mL/100 mL
Arterial-venous oxygen content difference $av_{O_2} = Ca_{O_2} - C\bar{v}_{O_2}$	4–6 mL/100 mL
Intrapulmonary shunt $\dot{Q}_S/\dot{Q}_T = (Cc_{O_2} - Ca_{O_2})/(Cc_{O_2} - C\bar{v}_{O_2})$ $Cc_{O_2} = (Hb \times 1.34) + (P_{AO_2} \times 0.0031)$	<5%
Physiologic dead space $\dot{V}_D/\dot{V}_T = (P_{aCO_2} - P_{ECO_2})/P_{aCO_2}$	0.33
Oxygen consumption $\dot{V}_{O_2} = CO(Ca_{O_2} - C\bar{v}_{O_2})$	240 mL/min
Oxygen transport $O_2T = CO\,(Ca_{O_2})$	1,000 mL/min

Ca_{O_2} = arterial oxygen content; $C\bar{v}_{O_2}$ = mixed venous oxygen content; Cc_{O_2} = pulmonary capillary oxygen content; CO = cardiac output; F_{IO_2} = fraction inspired oxygen; O_2T = oxygen transport; P_B = barometric pressure; $\dot{Q}_S/\dot{Q}_T$ = intrapulmonary shunt; P_{ACO_2} = alveolar carbon dioxide tension; P_{aCO_2} = arterial carbon dioxide tension; P_{AO_2} = alveolar oxygen tension; P_{aO_2} = arterial oxygen tension; P_{ECO_2} = expired carbon dioxide tension; V_D = dead space gas volume; V_T = tidal volume; $\dot{V}_{O_2}$ = oxygen consumption (minute).

Lung Volumes and Capacities

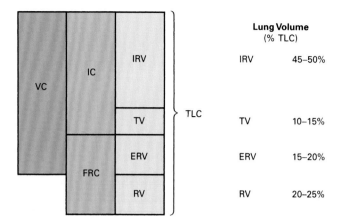

	Lung Volume (% TLC)
IRV	45–50%
TV	10–15%
ERV	15–20%
RV	20–25%

		Normal Values (70 kg)
Vital capacity	VC	4,800 mL
Inspiratory capacity	IC	3,800 mL
Functional residual capacity	FRC	2,400 mL
Inspiratory reserve volume	IRV	3,500 mL
Tidal volume	TV	1,500 mL
Expiratory reserve volume	ERV	1,200 mL
Residual volume	RV	1,200 mL
Total lung capacity	TLC	6,000 mL

Atlas of Electrocardiography

Gina C. Badescu
Benjamin M. Sherman
James R. Zaidan
Paul G. Barash

Lead Placement

	Electrode	
	Positive	**Negative**
Bipolar Leads		
I	LA	RA
II	LL	RA
III	LL	LA
Augmented Unipolar		
aVR	RA	LA, LL
aVL	LA	RA, LL
aVF	LL	RA, LA
Precordial		
V_1	4 ICS–RSB	
V_2	4 ICS–LSB	
V_3	Midway between V_2 and V_4	
V_4	5 ICS–MCL	
V_5	5 ICS–AAL	
V_6	5 ICS–MAL	

Sections and images of this Appendix were developed, in part, for both Barash PG, Cullen BF, Stoelting RK, et al., eds. *Clinical Anesthesia*, 7th ed. Philadelphia: Wolters Kluwer Health/Lippincott Williams & Wilkins; 2013, and Kaplan JA, Reich DL, Savino JS, eds. *Kaplan's Cardiac Anesthesia: The Echo Era*. Philadelphia: Elsevier; 2011 with permission of the editors and publishers.

Abbrev.	Meaning
LA	Left arm
RA	Right arm
LL	Left leg
ICS	Intercostal space
RSB	Right sternal border
LSB	Left sternal border
MCL	Midclavicular line
AAL	Interaxillary line
MAL	Midaxillary line

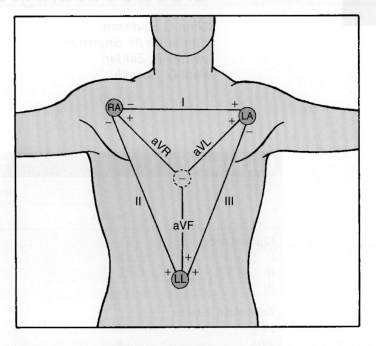

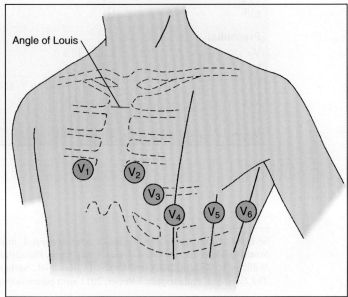

THE NORMAL ELECTROCARDIOGRAM—CARDIAC CYCLE

The normal electrocardiogram is composed of waves (P, QRS, T, and U) and intervals (PR, QRS, ST, and QT).

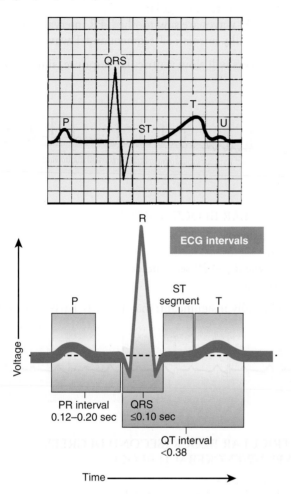

ATRIAL FIBRILLATION

Rate: Variable (~150–200 beats/min)
Rhythm: Irregular
PR interval: No P wave; PR interval not discernible
QT interval: QRS normal

Note: Must be differentiated from atrial flutter: (1) absence of flutter waves and presence of fibrillatory line; (2) flutter usually associated with higher ventricular rates (>150 beats/min). Loss of atrial contraction reduces cardiac output (10–20%). Mural atrial thrombi may develop. Considered controlled if ventricular rate is <100 beats/min.

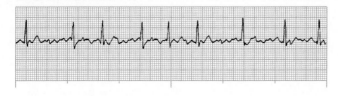

ATRIAL FLUTTER

Rate: Rapid, atrial usually regular (250–350 beats/min); ventricular usually regular (<100 beats/min)
Rhythm: Atrial and ventricular regular
PR interval: Flutter (F) waves are saw-toothed. PR interval cannot be measured.
QT interval: QRS usually normal; ST segment and T waves are not identifiable.

Note: Vagal maneuvers will slow ventricular response, simplifying recognition of the F waves.

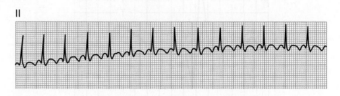

ATRIOVENTRICULAR BLOCK (FIRST DEGREE)

Rate: 60–100 beats/min
Rhythm: Regular
PR interval: Prolonged (>0.20 sec) and constant
QT interval: Normal

Note: Usually clinically insignificant; may be early harbinger of drug toxicity.

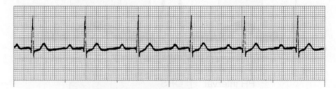

ATRIOVENTRICULAR BLOCK (SECOND DEGREE), MOBITZ TYPE I/WENCKEBACH BLOCK

Rate: 60–100 beats/min
Rhythm: Atrial regular; ventricular irregular
PR interval: P wave normal; PR interval progressively lengthens with each cycle until QRS complex is dropped (dropped beat). PR interval following dropped beat is shorter than normal.
QT interval: QRS complex normal but dropped periodically.

Note: Commonly seen in trained athletes and with drug toxicity.

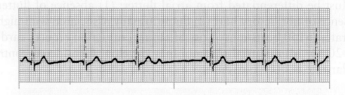

ATRIOVENTRICULAR BLOCK (SECOND DEGREE), MOBITZ TYPE II

Rate: <100 beats/min

Rhythm: Atrial regular; ventricular regular or irregular

PR interval: P waves normal, but some are not followed by QRS complex.

QT interval: Normal but may have widened QRS complex if block is at level of bundle branch. ST segment and T wave may be abnormal, depending on location of block.

Note: In contrast to Mobitz type I block, the PR and RR intervals are constant and the dropped QRS occurs without warning. The wider the QRS complex (block lower in the conduction system), the greater the amount of myocardial damage.

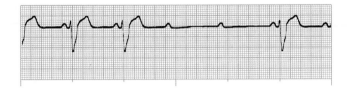

ATRIOVENTRICULAR BLOCK (THIRD DEGREE), COMPLETE HEART BLOCK

Rate: <45 beats/min

Rhythm: Atrial regular; ventricular regular; no relationship between P wave and QRS complex

PR interval: Variable because atria and ventricles beat independently.

QT interval: QRS morphology variable, depending on the origin of the ventricular beat in the intrinsic pacemaker system (atrioventricular junctional vs. ventricular pacemaker). ST segment and T wave normal.

Note: AV block represents complete failure of conduction from atria to ventricles (no P wave is conducted to the ventricle). The atrial rate is faster than ventricular rate. P waves have no relationship to QRS complexes (e.g., they are electrically disconnected). In contrast, with AV dissociation, the P wave is conducted through the AV node and the atrial and ventricular rate are similar. Immediate treatment with atropine or isoproterenol is required if cardiac output is reduced. Consideration should be given to insertion of a pacemaker. Seen as a complication of mitral valve replacement.

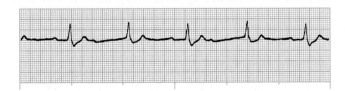

BUNDLE-BRANCH BLOCK—LEFT (LBBB)

Rate: <100 beats/min

Rhythm: Regular

PR interval: Normal

QT interval: Complete LBBB (QRS >0.12 sec); incomplete LBBB (QRS = 0.10–0.12 sec); lead V_1 negative RS complex; I, aVL, V_6 wide R wave without Q or S component. ST segment and T-wave direction opposite direction of the R wave.

Note: LBBB does not occur in healthy patients and usually indicates serious heart disease with a poor prognosis. In patients with LBBB, insertion of a pulmonary artery catheter may lead to complete heart block.

Left Bundle Branch Block

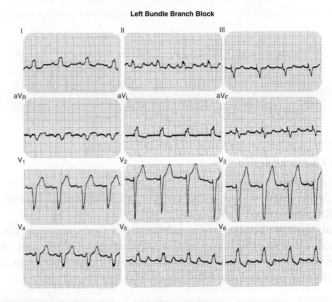

BUNDLE BRANCH BLOCK—RIGHT (RBBB)

Rate: <100 beats/min

Rhythm: Regular

PR interval: Normal

QT interval: Complete RBBB (QRS >0.12 sec); incomplete RBBB (QRS = 0.10–0.12 sec). Varying patterns of QRS complex; rSR (V_1); RS, wide R with M pattern. ST segment and T wave opposite direction of the R wave.

Note: In the presence of RBBB, Q waves may be seen with a myocardial infarction.

Right Bundle Branch Block

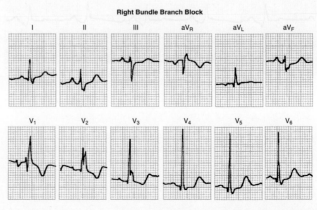

Coronary Artery Disease

TRANSMURAL MYOCARDIAL INFARCTION (TMI)

Q waves seen on ECG, useful in confirming diagnosis, are associated with poorer prognosis and more significant hemodynamic impairment. Arrhythmias frequently complicate course. Small Q waves may be normal variant. For myocardial infarction (MI), Q waves >0.04 seconds or depth exceeds one-third of R wave. For inferior wall MI, differentiate from RVH by axis deviation.

Myocardial Infarction			
Anatomic Site	**Leads**	**ECG Changes**	**Coronary Artery**
Inferior	II, III, AVF	Q, ↑ST, ↑T	Right

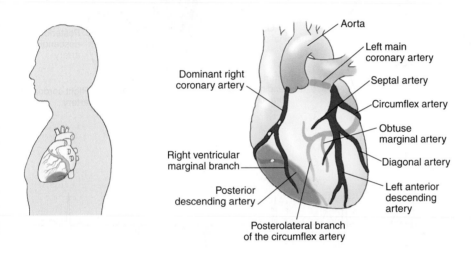

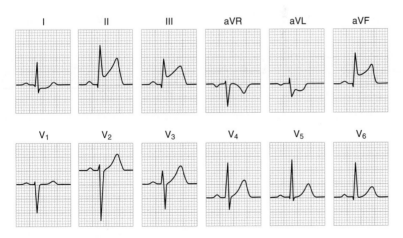

Myocardial Infarction			
Anatomic Site	**Leads**	**ECG Changes**	**Coronary Artery**
Posterior	V_1–V_2	↑R, ↓ST, ↓T	Left circumflex

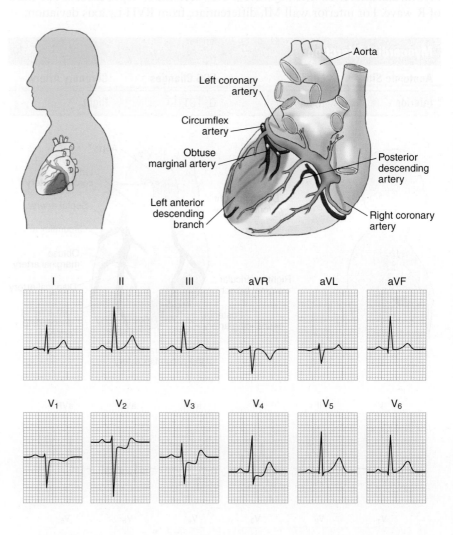

Myocardial Infarction

Anatomic Site	Leads	ECG Changes	Coronary Artery
Lateral	I, aVL, V$_5$–V$_6$	Q, ↑ST, ↑T	Left circumflex

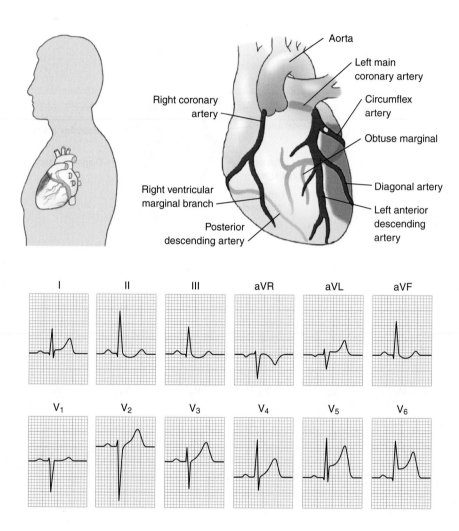

Myocardial Infarction			
Anatomic Site	Leads	ECG Changes	Coronary Artery
Anterior	I, aVL, V_1–V_4	Q, ↑ST, ↑T	Left anterior descending

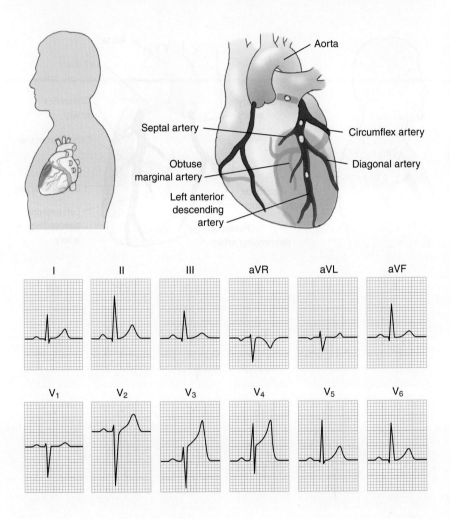

Myocardial Infarction

Anatomic Site	Leads	ECG Changes	Coronary Artery
Anteroseptal	V_1–V_4	Q, ↑ST, ↑T	Left anterior descending

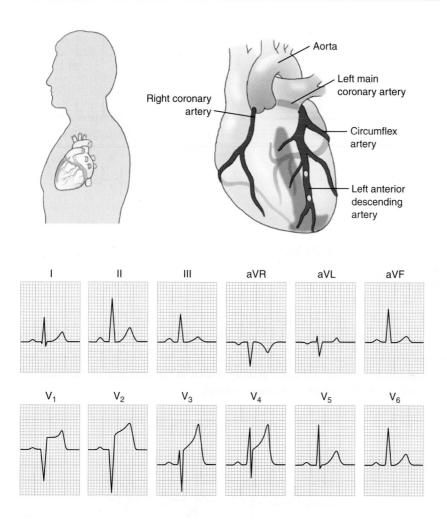

SUBENDOCARDIAL MYOCARDIAL INFARCTION (SEMI)

Persistent ST-segment depression and/or T-wave inversion in the absence of Q wave. Usually requires additional laboratory data (e.g., isoenzymes) to confirm diagnosis. Anatomic site of coronary lesion is similar to that of TMI electrocardiographically.

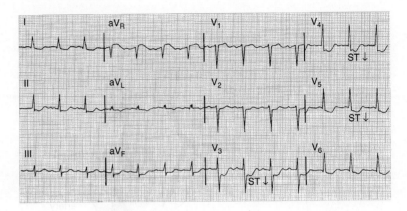

MYOCARDIAL ISCHEMIA

Rate: Variable
Rhythm: Usually regular but may show atrial and/or ventricular arrhythmias.
PR interval: Normal
QT interval: ST segment depressed; J-point depression; T-wave inversion; conduction disturbances. **(A)** TP and PR intervals are baseline for ST-segment deviation. **(B)** ST-segment elevation. **(C)** ST-segment depression.

Note: Intraoperative ischemia usually is seen in the presence of "normal" vital signs (e.g., ± 20% of preinduction values).

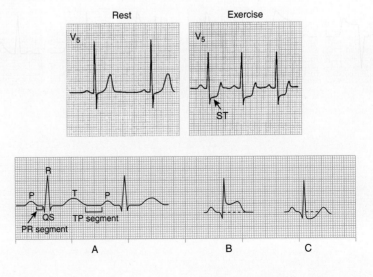

DIGITALIS EFFECT

Rate: <100 beats/min
Rhythm: Regular
PR interval: Normal or prolonged
QT interval: ST-segment sloping ("digitalis effect")

Note: Digitalis toxicity can be the cause of many common arrhythmias (e.g., premature ventricular contractions, second-degree heart block). Verapamil, quinidine, and amiodarone cause an increase in serum digitalis concentration.

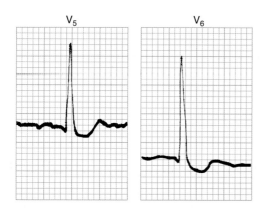

Electrolyte Disturbances				
	↓Ca^{2+}	↑Ca^{2+}	↓K^+	↑K^+
Rate	<100 beats/min	<100 beats/min	<100 beats/min	<100 beats/min
Rhythm	Regular	Regular	Regular	Regular
PR interval	Normal	Normal/increased	Normal	Normal
QT interval	Increased	Decreased	Normal	Increased
Other			T wave flat U wave	T wave peaked

Note: ECG changes usually do not correlate with serum calcium. Hypocalcemia rarely causes arrhythmias in the absence of hypokalemia. In contrast, abnormalities in serum potassium concentration can be diagnosed by ECG. Similarly, in the clinical range, magnesium concentrations are rarely associated with unique ECG patterns. The presence of a U wave (>1.5 mm in height) can also be seen in left main coronary artery disease, with certain medications and long QT syndrome.

CALCIUM

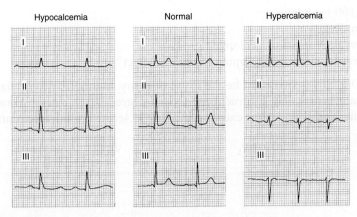

POTASSIUM

Hypokalemia (K^+ = 1.9 mEq/L)

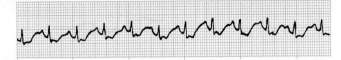

Hyperkalemia (K^+ = 7.9 mEq/L)

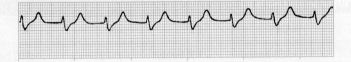

HYPOTHERMIA

Rate: <60 beats/min
Rhythm: Sinus
PR interval: Prolonged
QT interval: Prolonged

Note: Seen at temperatures below 33°C with ST-segment elevation (J point or Osborn wave). Tremor due to shivering or Parkinson's disease may interfere with ECG interpretation and may be confused with atrial flutter. May represent normal variant of early ventricular repolarization. (*Arrow* indicates J point or Osborn waves.)

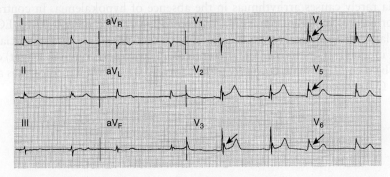

MULTIFOCAL ATRIAL TACHYCARDIA

Rate: 100–200 beats/min
Rhythm: Irregular
PR interval: Consecutive P waves are of varying shape.
QT interval: Normal

Note: Seen in patients with severe lung disease. Vagal maneuvers have no effect. At heart rates <100 beats/min, it may appear as wandering atrial pacemaker. May be mistaken for atrial fibrillation. Treatment is of the causative disease process.

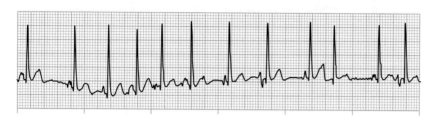

PAROXYSMAL ATRIAL TACHYCARDIA (PAT)

Rate: 150–250 beats/min
Rhythm: Regular
PR interval: Difficult to distinguish because of tachycardia obscuring P wave. P wave may precede, be included in, or follow QRS complex.
QT interval: Normal, but ST segment and T wave may be difficult to distinguish.

Note: Therapy depends on the degree of hemodynamic compromise. Carotid sinus massage, or other vagal maneuvers, may terminate rhythm or decrease heart rate. In contrast to management of PAT in awake patients, synchronized cardioversion, rather than pharmacologic treatment, is preferred in hemodynamically unstable anesthetized patients.

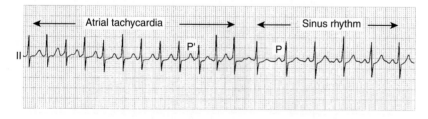

PERICARDITIS

Rate: Variable

Rhythm: Variable

PR interval: Normal

QT interval: Diffuse ST and T-wave changes with no Q wave and seen in more leads than a myocardial infarction.

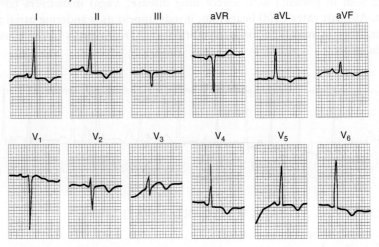

PERICARDIAL TAMPONADE

Rate: Variable

Rhythm: Variable

PR interval: Low-voltage P wave

QT interval: Seen as electrical alternans with low-voltage complexes and varying amplitude of P, QRS, and T waves with each heart beat.

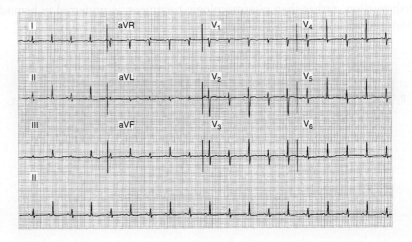

PNEUMOTHORAX

Rate: Variable
Rhythm: Variable
PR interval: Normal
QT interval: Normal

Note: Common ECG abnormalities include right-axis deviation, decreased QRS amplitude, and inverted T waves V_1–V_6. Differentiate from pulmonary embolus. May present as electrical alternans; thus, pericardial effusion should be ruled out.

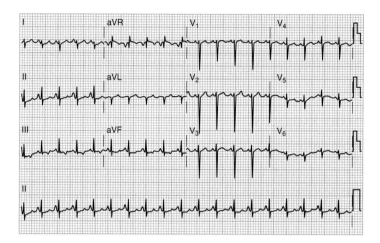

PREMATURE ATRIAL CONTRACTION (PAC)

Rate: <100 beats/min
Rhythm: Irregular
PR interval: P waves may be lost in preceding T waves. PR interval is variable.
QT interval: QRS normal configuration; ST segment and T wave normal.

Note: Nonconducted PAC appearance similar to that of sinus arrest; T waves with PAC may be distorted by inclusion of P wave in the T wave.

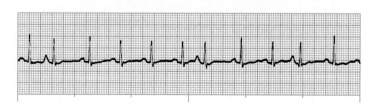

PREMATURE VENTRICULAR CONTRACTION (PVC)

Rate: Usually <100 beats/min

Rhythm: Irregular

PR interval: P wave and PR interval absent; retrograde conduction of P wave can be seen.

QT interval: Wide QRS (>0.12 sec); ST segment cannot be evaluated (e.g., ischemia); T wave opposite direction of QRS with compensatory pause. Fourth and eighth beats are PVCs.

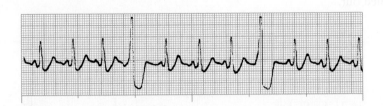

PULMONARY EMBOLUS

Rate: >100 beats/min

Rhythm: Sinus

PR interval: P-pulmonale waveform

QT interval: Q waves in leads III and aVF

Note: Classic ECG signs S1Q3T3 with T-wave inversion also seen in V_1–V_4 and RV strain (ST depression V_1–V_4). May present with atrial fibrillation or flutter.

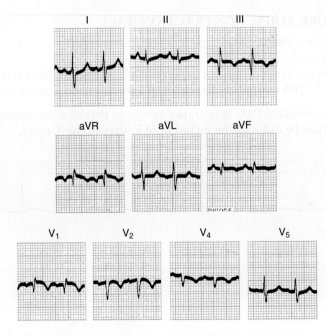

SINUS BRADYCARDIA

Rate: <60 beats/min
Rhythm: Sinus
PR interval: Normal
QT interval: Normal

Note: Seen in trained athletes as normal variant.

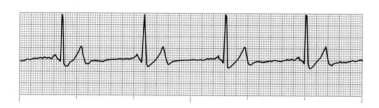

SINUS ARRHYTHMIA

Rate: 60–100 beats/min
Rhythm: Sinus
PR interval: Normal
QT interval: R-R interval variable

Note: Heart rate increases with inhalation and decreases with exhalation + 10–20% (respiratory). Nonrespiratory sinus arrhythmia seen in elderly with heart disease. Also seen with increased intracranial pressure.

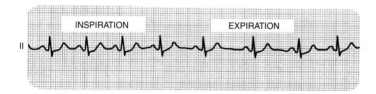

SINUS ARREST

Rate: <60 beats/min
Rhythm: Varies
PR interval: Variable
QT interval: Variable

Note: Rhythm depends on the cardiac pacemaker firing in the absence of sino-atrial stimulus (atrial pacemaker 60–75 beats/min; junctional 40–60 beats/min; ventricular 30–45 beats/min). Junctional rhythm most common. Occasional P waves may be seen (retrograde P wave).

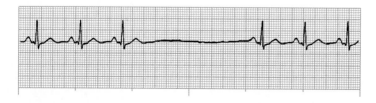

SINUS TACHYCARDIA

Rate: 100–160 beats/min
Rhythm: Regular
PR interval: Normal; P wave may be difficult to see.
QT interval: Normal

Note: Should be differentiated from paroxysmal atrial tachycardia (PAT). With PAT, carotid massage terminates arrhythmia. Sinus tachycardia may respond to vagal maneuvers but reappears as soon as vagal stimulus is removed.

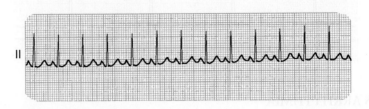

SUBARACHNOID HEMORRHAGE

Rate: <60 beats/min
Rhythm: Sinus
PR interval: Normal
QT interval: T-wave inversion is deep and wide. Prominent U waves are seen. Sinus arrythmias are observed. Q waves may be seen and may mimick acute coronary syndrome.

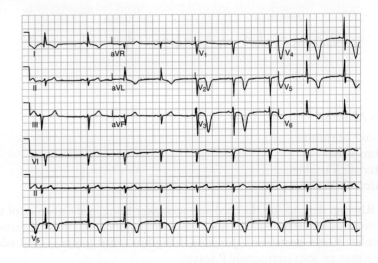

TORSADES DE POINTES

Rate: 150–250 beats/min
Rhythm: No atrial component seen; ventricular rhythm regular or irregular.
PR interval: P wave buried in QRS complex
QT interval: QRS complexes usually wide and with phasic variation twisting around a central axis (a few complexes point upward, then a few point downward). ST segments and T waves difficult to discern.

Note: Type of ventricular tachycardia associated with prolonged QT interval. Seen with electrolyte disturbances (e.g., hypokalemia, hypocalcemia, and hypomagnesemia) and bradycardia. Administering standard antiarrhythmics (lidocaine, procainamide, etc.) may worsen torsades de pointes. Prevention includes treatment of the electrolyte disturbance. Treatment includes shortening of the QT interval, pharmacologically or by pacing; unstable polymorphic VT is treated with immediate defibrillation.

Torsades de Pointes: Sustained

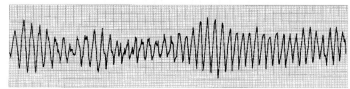

VENTRICULAR FIBRILLATION

Rate: Absent
Rhythm: None
PR interval: Absent
QT interval: Absent

Note: "Pseudoventricular fibrillation" may be the result of a monitor malfunction (e.g., ECG lead disconnect). Always check for carotid pulse before instituting therapy.

Coarse Ventricular Fibrillation

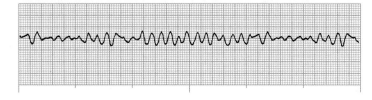

Fine Ventricular Fibrillation

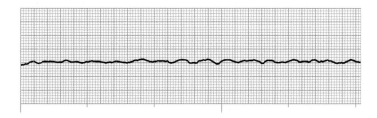

VENTRICULAR TACHYCARDIA

Rate: 100–250 beats/min
Rhythm: No atrial component seen; ventricular rhythm irregular or regular.
PR interval: Absent; retrograde P wave may be seen in QRS complex.
QT interval: Wide, bizarre QRS complex. ST segment and T wave difficult to
determine.

Note: In the presence of hemodynamic compromise, VT with a pulse is treated
with immediate synchronized cardioversion, whereas VT without a pulse is
treated with immediate defibrillation. If the patient is stable, with short bursts
of ventricular tachycardia, pharmacologic management is preferred. Should
be differentiated from supraventricular tachycardia with aberrancy (SVT-A).
Compensatory pause and atrioventricular dissociation suggest a PVC. P waves
and SR′ (V_1) and slowing to vagal stimulus also suggest SVT-A.

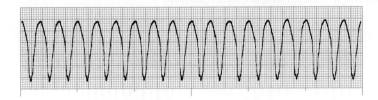

WOLFF-PARKINSON-WHITE SYNDROME (WPW)

Rate: <100 beats/min
Rhythm: Regular
PR interval: P wave normal; PR interval short (<0.12 sec)
QT interval: Duration (>0.10 sec) with slurred QRS complex (delta wave). Type A
has delta wave, RBBB, with upright QRS complex V_1. Type B has delta wave
and downward QRS-V_1. ST segment and T wave usually normal.

Note: Digoxin should be avoided in the presence of WPW because it increases
conduction through the accessory bypass tract (bundle of Kent) and decreases
AV node conduction; consequently, ventricular fibrillation can occur.

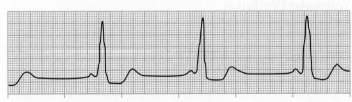

ATRIAL PACING

Pacemaker Tracings

Atrial pacing as demonstrated in this figure is used when the atrial impulse can proceed through the AV node. Examples are sinus bradycardia and junctional rhythms associated with clinically significant decreases in blood pressure. (*Arrows* are pacemaker spikes.)

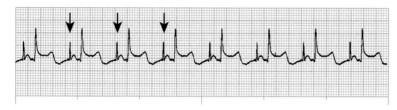

VENTRICULAR PACING

In this tracing, ventricular pacing is evident by absence of atrial wave (P wave) and pacemaker spike preceding QRS complex. Ventricular pacing is employed in the presence of bradycardia secondary to AV block or atrial fibrillation. (*Arrows* are pacemaker spikes.)

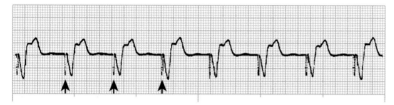

DDD PACING

DDD pacing, one of the most commonly used pacing modes, paces and senses both the right atrium and right ventricle (A-V sequential pacing). Each atrial and the right ventricular complex are preceded by a pacemaker spike.

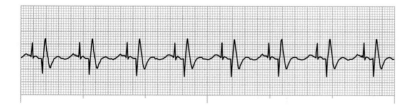

ACKNOWLEDGMENTS

Illustrations in the atlas are reprinted from Aehlert B. *ECGs made easy*, 4th ed. St. Louis: Mosby/Elsevier; 2011; Goldberger AL. *Clinical electrocardiography: a simplified approach*, 7th ed. Philadelphia: Mosby/Elsevier; 2006; Groh WJ, Zipes DP. Neurological disorders and cardiovascular disease. In Bonow RO, Mann DL, Zipes DP, et al., eds. *Braunwald's heart disease: a textbook of cardiovascular medicine*, 9th ed. Philadelphia: Saunders/Elsevier; 2012; Huszar RJ. *Basic dysrhythmias: interpretation and management*, 2nd ed. St. Louis: Mosby Lifeline; 1994; and Soltani P, Malozzi CM, Saleh BA, et al. Electrocardiogram manifestation of spontaneous pneumothorax. *Am J Emerg Med* 2009;27:750.e1–e5.

Pacemaker and Implantable Cardiac Defibrillator Protocols

Gina C. Badescu
Benjamin M. Sherman
James R. Zaidan
Paul G. Barash

Cardiac Implantable Electronic Devices (CIED)—Pacemakers
Cardiac Implantable Electronic Devices (CIEDs)—Implantable Cardiac Defibrillators (ICDs)
Potential Intraoperative Problems with Cardiac Electronic Implantable Devices
General Principles of Perioperative Management of Patients with CIED
Risk Mitigation Strategies
Recommendations for Postoperative Follow-up of the Patient with CIED
Optimization of Pacing after Cardiopulmonary Bypass (CPB)

Table 1   Abbreviation Table

Abbrev.	Meaning
3D	Three dimensional
ASA	American Society of Anesthesiologists
ATP	Antitachycardia pacing
AV	Atrioventricular
AVB	Atrioventricular block
BPEG	British Pacing and Electrophysiology Group
bpm	Beats per minute
CAD	Coronary artery disease
CIED	Cardiac implantable electronic devices
CPB	Cardiopulmonary bypass
CRP	Current return pad
CRT	Cardiac resynchronization therapy
CRT-D	Cardiac resynchronization therapy-defibrillation
CT	Cautery tool
DCM	Dilated cardiomyopathy
ECG	Electrocardiogram
ECT	Electroconvulsive therapy
EF	Ejection fraction
EMI	Electromagnetic interference
HCM	Hypertrophic cardiomyopathy
HR	Heart rate
HRS	Heart Rhythm Society
HV	HV interval
ICD	Implantable cardiac defibrillators
LV	Left ventricle
LVOT	Left ventricular outflow tract
MRI	Magnetic resonance imaging
NASPE	North American Society of Pacing and Electrophysiology
NBG	N (NASPE), B (BPEG), G (GENERIC)
PG	Pulse generator
PP	External cardioversion-defibrillation pads or paddles
RA	Right atrium
RF	Radio frequency
R&R	Rate and rhythm
RT	Radiation therapy
RV	Right ventricle
SCD	Sudden cardiac death
SND	Sinus node dysfunction
STEMI	ST-segment elevation myocardial infarction
TUNA	Transurethral needle ablation
TURP	Transurethral resection of prostate
VT	Ventricular tachycardia
VF	Ventricular fibrillation

Cardiac Implantable Electronic Devices (CIED)—Pacemakers

Pacemakers are devices that deliver electrical energy and control the patient's conduction system when necessary.

Common indications for permanent pacemaker implantation: (For a complete list of indications, please refer to the ACC/AHA/HRS 2008 Guidelines for Device-Based Therapy of Cardiac Rhythm Abnormalities.)

1. Sinus node dysfunction:
   - Documented symptomatic bradycardia
   - Documented symptomatic chronotropic incompetence
   - Documented symptomatic bradycardia induced by essential medical therapy
   - Syncope of unexplained origin with inducible sinus bradycardia or pauses on electrophysiologic studies
   - Symptomatic patients with assumed sinus bradycardia and no other possible etiologies
2. Atrioventricular (AV) node dysfunction:
   - Third-degree AV block
   - Type II second-degree AV block
   - Symptomatic type I second-degree AV block
   - Symptomatic first-degree AV block
   - Asymptomatic first-degree AV block with coexisting disease that can impair the conduction system (i.e., sarcoidosis, amyloidosis, neuromuscular diseases)
   - Drug- or medication-induced AV block that is thought to recur despite discontinuation of the drug or medication.
3. Bifascicular block and:
   - Alternating bundle branch block
   - Electrophysiologic evidence of a markedly prolonged HV interval ≥100 ms. (His bundle [H] potential and the onset of ventricular activity, also known as the HV interval, is normally 35–45 ms)
   - Concomitant neuromuscular disease (i.e., myotonic muscular dystrophy, Erb dystrophy)
4. ST-segment elevation myocardial infarction (STEMI) with second- or third-degree AV block
5. Hypersensitive carotid sinus syndrome and neurocardiogenic syncope
6. Cardiac transplantation patients who develop persistent inappropriate bradycardia.
7. Prevention and termination of certain arrhythmias such as:
   - Sustained pause-dependant VT
   - High-risk patients with congenital long-QT syndrome
   - Recurrent refractory symptomatic atrial fibrillation and SND
   - Symptomatic recurrent SVT that is reliably terminated by pacing and catheter ablation and medication management has failed
8. Hemodynamic indications:
   - Cardiac resynchronization therapy (CRT) in patients with NYHA class III or ambulatory class IV heart failure with optimal medical management and an ejection fraction (EF) ≤35% and QRS ≥120 ms
   - Hypertrophic cardiomyopathy with sinus node dysfunction (SND) or AV node dysfunction
9. Congenital heart diseases with associated bradyarrhythmias or AV block.

Cardiac Implantable Electronic Devices (CIEDs)— Implantable Cardiac Defibrillators (ICDs)

Implantable cardiac defibrillators (ICDs) are rhythm management devices that consist of a generator and a lead system. One lead is usually placed in the right atrium and the second lead in the right ventricular apex. A specific type of ICD is the biventricular pacemaker, used for cardiac resynchronization therapy (CRT). This device will have a third lead placed in the coronary sinus to pace the left ventricular (LV) lateral wall in synchrony with the right ventricle (RV), in the patient with EF ≤35% and a QRS duration ≥120 msec.

Common indications for ICD implantation: (For a complete list of indications, please refer to the ACC/AHA/HRS 2008 Guidelines for Device-Based Therapy of Cardiac Rhythm Abnormalities.)

1. Prevention of sudden cardiac death (SCD) in survivors of prior cardiac arrest due to VF or unstable VT without a reversible cause.
2. Structural heart disease with spontaneous sustained VT or syncope not otherwise specified.
3. Sustained VT with normal or near normal LV function.
4. Syncope of undetermined origin with clinically relevant, hemodynamically significant, sustained VT or VF induced by an electrophysiologic study.
5. Unexplained syncope with significant LV dysfunction and nonischemic DCM.
6. Prior myocardial infarction (not within 40 days) and an EF ≤35%.
7. Nonischemic dialated cardiomyopathy (DCM) and an EF ≤35%.
8. Nonsustained VT due to prior MI with an EF ≤–40% and inducible VF or sustained VT on electrophysiologic study.
9. HCM with one or more risk factors for SCD.
10. Arrhythmogenic right ventricular dysplasia/cardiomyopathy with one or more risk factors for SCD.

Table 2　Generic Pacemaker Code: NASPE/BPEG Revised (2002)

Position I, Pacing Chamber(s)	Position II, Sensing Chamber(s)	Position III, Response(s) to Sensing	Position IV, Programmability	Position V, Multisite Pacing
0 = none	0 = none	0 = none	0 = none	0 = none
A = atrium	A = atrium	I = inhibited	R = rate modulation	A = atrium
V = ventricle	V = ventricle	T = triggered		V = ventricle
D = dual (A + V)	D = dual (A + V)	D = dual (T + I)		D = dual (A + V)

NASPE, North American Society of Pacing and Electrophysiology, now called the Heart Rhythm Society; BPEG, British Pacing and Electrophysiology Group.
Reproduced with permission from: Practice advisory for perioperative management of patients with cardiac rhythm management devices: Pacemakers and implantable cardioverter-defibrillators. A report by the American Society of Anesthesiologists Task Force on Perioperative Management of Patients with Cardiac Rhythm Management Devices. *Anesthesiology* 2011;114:247–261.

11. Long QT syndrome with syncope and/or VT due to beta-blocker therapy or other risk factors for SCD.
12. Brugada syndrome with syncope or VT.
13. Catecholaminergic polymorphic VT with syncope while receiving beta-blocker therapy.
14. Diseases associated with cardiac involvement (i.e., Chagas disease, giant cell myocarditis, sarcoidosis).
15. Familial cardiomyopathy associated with SCD.
16. LV noncompaction.

Potential Intraoperative Problems with Cardiac Electronic Implantable Devices

Electromagnetic interference (EMI) with a CIED is more likely when electrocautery is used above the umbilicus in a patient with the CIED implanted in the subclavicular region. Current expert opinion further states that the region 15 cm around the generator and cardiac leads is with the highest risk of EMI interference. For generators placed elsewhere (e.g., abdominal site), this 15-cm rule still applies.

EMI interference leads to:

1. Inhibition of pacemaker by EMI
2. Inappropriate delivery of antitachycardia therapy by ICD
3. Changes in lead parameters:
   a. Atrial mode switching
   b. Inappropriate ventricular sensing
   c. Electrical reset
   d. Increase in ventricular thresholds
4. "Runaway" pacemaker
5. Conversion from VOO back to backup mode (reprogramming)
6. Transient or permanent loss of capture

Table 3 Generic Defibrillator Code (NBG): NASPE/BPEG			
Position I, **Shock** **Chamber(s)**	**Position II,** **Antitachycardia** **Pacing Chamber(s)**	**Position III,** **Tachycardia** **Detection**	**Position IV,**[a] **Antibradycardia** **Pacing Chamber(s)**
0 = none	0 = none	E = electrogram	0 = none
A = atrium	A = atrium	H = hemodynamic	A = atrium
V = ventricle	V = ventricle		V = ventricle
D = dual (A + V)	D = dual (A + V)		D = dual (A + V)

NBG: N refers to North American Society of Pacing and Electrophysiology (NASPE), now called the Heart Rhythm Society (HRS); B refers to British Pacing and Electrophysiology Group (BPEG); and G refers to generic.
[a]For robust identification, position IV is expanded into its complete NBG code. For example, a biventricular pacing defibrillator with ventricular shock and antitachycardia pacing functionality would be identified as VVE-DDDRV, assuming that the pacing section was programmed DDDRV. Currently, no hemodynamic sensors have been approved for tachycardia detection (position III).
Reproduced with permission from: Practice advisory for perioperative management of patients with cardiac rhythm management devices: Pacemakers and implantable cardioverter-defibrillators. A report by the American Society of Anesthesiologists Task Force on Perioperative Management of Patients with Cardiac Rhythm Management Devices. *Anesthesiology* 2011;114:247–261.

7. Noise reversal mode
8. Pacemaker failure after direct contact with electrocautery and cardioversion
9. Myocardial burns with increased pacing thresholds if electrocautery travels through leads into the myocardium
10. Rate-adaptive pacing (interaction of minute ventilation sensor with ECG/plethysmography)
11. Oversensing and inhibition with use of lithotripsy
12. Radiofrequency ablation has a high risk of interference due to long episodes of exposure to current.
13. Therapeutic ionizing radiation is especially damaging to CIEDs by damaging internal components.

General Principles of Perioperative Management of Patients with CIED

- The perioperative management of the patient with a CIED is via an individualized recommendation, made by the CIED team (electrophysiologist cardiologist), in collaboration with members of the surgical/anesthesia team (perioperative team). The recommendations should not be made by the industry representative without supervision by a physician who is qualified to manage these devices.
- The perioperative team should provide information to the CIED team regarding the upcoming procedure (see Table 4).
- The CIED team should in turn provide information about the device and a recommendation for perioperative management of the device (see Table 5).
- The patient with a pacemaker should have had an interrogation of the device in the 12 months prior to the surgical procedure, whereas the patient with an ICD should have had the device interrogated within 6 months prior to the scheduled procedure.

Table 4   Essential Elements of the Information Given to the CIED Physician

- Type of procedure
- Anatomic location of surgical procedure
- Patient position during the procedure
- Will monopolar electrosurgery be used? (If so, anatomic location of EMI delivery.)
- Will other sources of EMI likely be present?
- Will cardioversion or defibrillation be used?
- Surgical venue (operating room, procedure suite, etc.)
- Anticipated postprocedural arrangements (anticipated discharge to home <23 hours, inpatient admission to critical care bed, telemetry bed)
- Unusual circumstances: Cardiothoracic or chest wall surgical procedure that could impair/damage or encroach upon the CIED leads, anticipated large blood loss, operation in close proximity to CIED

Reproduced with permission from Crossley GH, Poole JE, Rozner MA, et al. The Heart Rhythm Society (HRS)/American Society of Anesthesiologists (ASA) Expert Consensus Statement on the Perioperative Management of Patients with Implantable Defibrillators, Pacemakers, and Arrhythmia Monitors: Facilities and Patient Management: This document was developed as a joint project with the American Society of Anesthesiologists (ASA), and in collaboration with the American Heart Association (AHA), and the Society of Thoracic Surgeons (STS). Heart Rhythm 2011;8(7):1114–1154.

Table 5   Essential Elements of the Preoperative CIED Evaluation to be Provided to the Operative Team

- Date of last device interrogation
- Type of device: Pacemaker ICD, CRT-D, CRT-P, ILR, implantable hemodynamic monitor
- Manufacturer and model
- Indication for device
  - Pacemaker: Sick sinus syndrome, AV block, syncope
  - ICD: Primary or secondary prevention
  - Cardiac resynchronization therapy
- Battery longevity documented as >3 months
- Are any of the leads <3 months old?
- Programming
  - Pacing mode and programmed lower rate
  - ICD therapy
    - Lowest heart rate for shock delivery
    - Lowest heart rate for ATP delivery
  - Rate-responsive sensor type, if programmed on
- Is the patient pacemaker dependent, and what is the underlying rhythm and heart rate if it can be determined?
- What is the response of this device to magnet placement?
  - Magnet pacing rate for a pacemaker
  - Pacing amplitude response to magnet function
  - Will ICD detections resume automatically with removal of the magnet? Does this device allow for magnet application function to be disabled? If so, document programming of patient's device for this feature.
- Any alert status on CIED generator or lead
- Last pacing threshold: Document adequate safety margin with the date of that threshold

Reproduced with permission from Crossley GH, Poole JE, Rozner MA, et al. The Heart Rhythm Society (HRS)/American Society of Anesthesiologists (ASA) Expert Consensus Statement on the Perioperative Management of Patients with Implantable Defibrillators, Pacemakers, and Arrhythmia Monitors: Facilities and Patient Management: This document was developed as a joint project with the American Society of Anesthesiologists (ASA), and in collaboration with the American Heart Association (AHA), and the Society of Thoracic Surgeons (STS). *Heart Rhythm* 2011;8(7):1114–1154.

- The inactivation of the ICD or programming of a pacemaker to asynchronous mode is recommended when electromagnetic interference (EMI) is likely to occur.
- In patients in whom the ICD antiarrhythmia detection is turned off, an external defibrillator should be immediately available and ready to deliver therapy.
- In cases where EMI is likely, the function of the CIED can be altered either by a ferrous magnet or by reprogramming. (See below for magnet response for ICD.)
- Magnet response: Placing a magnet over a pacemaker generator will turn the pacemaker to asynchronous mode in most models. Placing a magnet over an ICD will suspend the arrhythmia detection. It will not switch the pacemaker function to asynchronous mode; therefore, in patients who are pacemaker dependent, the team must be aware of the risk of inhibition of the pacemaker by EMI. If EMI is likely to occur, the recommendation is

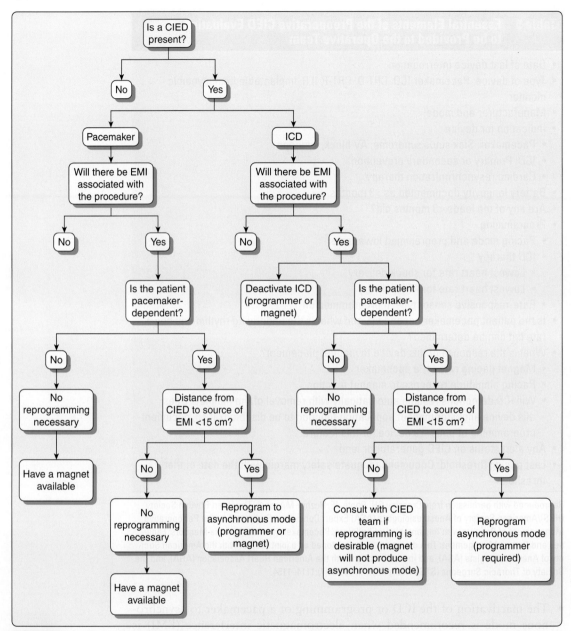

Figure 1 Example of an algorithm for perioperative management of patients with CIED. From Stone ME, Salter B, Fischer A. Perioperative management of patients with cardiac implantable electronic devices. *Br J Anaesth* 2011;107(Suppl 1):i16–26, with permission.

Table 6 Example of a Stepwise Approach to the Perioperative Management of the Patient with a Cardiac Implantable Electronic Device

Perioperative Period	Patient/CIED Condition	Intervention
Preoperative evaluation	Patient has CIED	Focused history
		Focused physical examination
	Determine CIED type (PM, ICD, CRT)	Manufacturer's CIED identification card
		Chest x-ray (no data available) Supplemental resources[a]
	Determine if patient is CIED-dependent for pacing function	Verbal history
		Bradyarrhythmia symptoms
		Atrioventricular node ablation
		No spontaneous ventricular activity[b]
	Determine CIED function	Comprehensive CIED evaluation[c]
		Determine if pacing pulses are present and create paced beats
Preoperative preparation	EMI unlikely during procedure	If EMI is unlikely, then special precautions are not needed
	EMI likely; CIED is PM	Reprogram to asynchronous mode when indicated
		Suspend rate adaptive functions[d]
	EMI likely; CIED is ICD	Suspend antitachyarrhythmia functions. If patient is dependent on pacing function, then alter pacing function as above
	EMI likely; All CIED	Use bipolar cautery; ultrasonic scalpel
		Temporary pacing and cardioversion-defibrillation available
	Intraoperative physiologic changes likely (e.g., bradycardia, ischemia)	Plan for possible adverse CIED-patient interaction
Intraoperative management	Monitoring	Electrocardiographic monitoring per ASA standard
		Peripheral pulse monitoring
	Electrocautery interference	CT/CRP no current through PG/leads
		Avoid proximity of CT to PG/leads
		Short bursts at lowest possible energy
		Use bipolar cautery; ultrasonic scalpel
	RF catheter ablation	Avoid contact of RF catheter with PG/leads
		RF current path far away from PG/leads
		Discuss these concerns with operator
	Lithotripsy	Do not focus lithotripsy beam near PG
		R wave triggers lithotripsy? Disable atrial pacing
	MRI	Generally contraindicated
		If required, consult ordering physician, cardiologist, radiologist, and manufacturer
	Radiation therapy	PG/leads must be outside of RT field
		Possible surgical relocation of PG
		Verify PG function during/after RT course
	ECT	Consult with ordering physician, patient's cardiologist, a CIED service, or CIED manufacturer

(*continued*)

Table 6   Example of a Stepwise Approach to the Perioperative Management of the Patient with a Cardiac Implantable Electronic Device (*Continued*)

Perioperative Period	Patient/CIED Condition	Intervention
Emergency defibrillation-cardioversion	ICD: magnet-disabled	Terminate all EMI sources Remove magnet to re-enable therapies Observe for appropriate therapies
	ICD: programming disabled	Programming to re-enable therapies or proceed directly with external cardioversion/defibrillation
	ICD: either of above	Minimize current flow through PG/leads PP as far as possible from PG PP perpendicular to major axis PG/leads To extent possible, PP in anterior–posterior location
	Regardless of CIED type	Use clinically appropriate cardioversion/defibrillation energy
Postoperative management	Immediate postoperative period Postoperative interrogation and restoration of CIED function	Monitor cardiac R&R continuously Back-up pacing and cardioversion/defibrillation capability Interrogation to assess function Settings appropriate?[e] Is CIED an ICD?[f] Use cardiology/PM-ICD service if needed

[a]Manufacturer's databases, pacemaker clinic records, cardiology consultation.
[b]With cardiac rhythm management device (CRMD) programmed VVI at lowest programmable rate.
[c]Ideally, CIED function assessed by interrogation, with function altered by reprogramming if required.
[d]Most times this will be necessary; when in doubt, assume so.
[e]If necessary, reprogram appropriate setting.
[f]Restore all antitachycardia therapies.
Reproduced with permission from: Practice advisory for perioperative management of patients with cardiac rhythm management devices: Pacemakers and implantable cardioverter-defibrillators. A report by the American Society of Anesthesiologists Task Force on Perioperative Management of Patients with Cardiac Rhythm Management Devices. *Anesthesiology* 2011;114:247–261.

to reprogram the CIED prior to the operation, by turning off the arrhythmia detection function and programming the pacemaker to asynchronous mode. Due to the fact that a minority of models do not respond to magnet application in the fashion described above, it is always recommended to contact the manufacturer and confirm the response to a magnet for the specific model one is dealing with.

Risk Mitigation Strategies

- Have a magnet available.
- Use bipolar cautery where possible.
- Use short bursts of monopolar cautery (5 seconds or less).
- Place the return current pad in such a way to avoid current crossing the generator.
- Have rescue equipment, including external pacemaker/defibrillator, immediately available for all patients with a CIED.
- Be aware of other potential sources of EMI in addition to electrocautery.
- Be aware of dislodgement of leads during atrial fibrillation ablations, central intravenous catheter insertions, or other catheter-based procedures.

Recommendations for Postoperative Follow-up of the Patient with CIED (see Tables 7 and 8)

- Note the *Practice Advisory for the Perioperative Management of Patients with Cardiac Implantable Electronic Devices: Pacemakers and Implantable Cardioverter-Defibrillators* states that "postoperative patient management should include interrogating and restoring CIED function in the post anesthesia care unit or intensive care unit."

Table 7	Specific Procedures and Writing Committee Recommendations on Postoperative CIED Evaluation
Procedure	**Recommendation**
Monopolar electrosurgery	CIED evaluated[a] within 1 month from procedure unless Table 8 criteria are fulfilled
External cardioversion	CIED evaluated[a] prior to discharge or transfer from cardiac telemetry
Radiofrequency ablation	CIED evaluated[a] prior to discharge or transfer from cardiac telemetry
Electroconvulsive therapy	CIED evaluated[a] within 1 month from procedure unless fulfilling Table 8 criteria
Nerve conduction studies (electroneurography [ENG])	No additional CIED evaluation beyond routine
Ocular procedures	No additional CIED evaluation beyond routine
Therapeutic radiation	CIED evaluated prior to discharge or transfer from cardiac telemetry; remote monitoring optimal; some instances may indicate interrogation after each treatment (see text)
TUNA/TURP	No additional CIED evaluation beyond routine
Hysteroscopic ablation	No additional CIED evaluation beyond routine
Lithotripsy	CIED evaluated[a] within 1 month from procedure unless fulfilling Table 8 criteria
Endoscopy	No additional CIED evaluation beyond routine
Iontophoresis	No additional CIED evaluation beyond routine
Photodynamic therapy	No additional CIED evaluation beyond routine
X-ray/CT scans/mammography	No additional CIED evaluation beyond routine

CIED, cardiac implantable electronic device; CT, computed tomography; TUNA, transurethral needle ablation; TURP, transurethral resection of prostate.

[a]This evaluation is intended to reveal electrical reset. Therefore, an interrogation alone is needed. This can be accomplished in person or by remote telemetry.

Reproduced with permission from: Crossley GH, Poole JE, Rozner MA, et al. The Heart Rhythm Society (HRS)/American Society of Anesthesiologists (ASA) Expert Consensus Statement on the Perioperative Management of Patients with Implantable Defibrillators, Pacemakers, and Arrhythmia Monitors: Facilities and Patient Management: This document was developed as a joint project with the American Society of Anesthesiologists (ASA), and in collaboration with the American Heart Association (AHA), and the Society of Thoracic Surgeons (STS). *Heart Rhythm* 2011;8(7):1114–1154.

Table 8	Indications for the Interrogation of CIEDs Prior to Patient Discharge or Transfer from a Cardiac Telemetry Environment

- Patients with CIEDs reprogrammed prior to the procedure that left the device non-functional such as disabling tachycardia detection in an ICD.
- Patients with CIEDs who underwent hemodynamically challenging surgeries such as cardiac surgery or significant vascular surgery (e.g., abdominal aortic aneurysmal repair).[a]
- Patients with CIEDs who experienced significant intraoperative events including cardiac arrest requiring temporary pacing or cardiopulmonary resuscitation and those who required external electrical cardioversion.
- Emergent surgery where the site of EMI exposure was above the umbilicus.
- Cardiothoracic surgery.
- Patients with CIEDs who underwent certain types of procedures (Table 7) that emit EMI with a greater probability of affecting device function.
- Patients with CIEDs who have logistical limitations that would prevent reliable device evaluation within 1 month from their procedure.

CIED, cardiac implantable electrical device; EMI, electromagnetic interference; ICD, implantable cardiac defibrillator.
[a]The general purpose of this interrogation is to ensure that reset did not occur. In these cases, a full evaluation including threshold evaluations is suggested.
Reproduced with permission from Crossley GH, Poole JE, Rozner MA, et al. The Heart Rhythm Society (HRS)/American Society of Anesthesiologists (ASA) Expert Consensus Statement on the Perioperative Management of Patients with Implantable Defibrillators, Pacemakers, and Arrhythmia Monitors: Facilities and Patient Management: This document was developed as a joint project with the American Society of Anesthesiologists (ASA), and in collaboration with the American Heart Association (AHA), and the Society of Thoracic Surgeons (STS). *Heart Rhythm* 2011;8(7):1114–1154.

Optimization of Pacing after Cardiopulmonary Bypass (CPB)

During separation from CPB, it is not uncommon for a patient to develop a conduction abnormality, ranging from the more benign first-degree AV block or sinus bradycardia to the more severe interventricular delays or third-degree AV block.

Optimizing pacing:

1. **Lead placement:** Right atrial (RA) lead—place at the cephalic atrial wall, between the atrial appendages. Right ventricular lead—place at the level of the right ventricle outflow tract (RVOT). For the patient with obstructive cardiomyopathy, the RV lead is better placed in the RV apex, for less dynamic obstruction of the LVOT. Biventricular pacing can be initiated for patients with intraventricular conduction lesions and dyssynchrony of contraction. The LV lead should be placed at the basal posterolateral wall and the two ventricular leads can be connected through a Y piece to the ventricular output of the temporary pacemaker box.
2. **Rate:** Program to obtain the best improvement in cardiac output and improvement in mixed venous saturation and arterial blood pressure.
3. **AV delay:** In patients with LV dysfunction, we can maximize the contribution of the atria to the preload. Use pulse wave Doppler through the mitral valve inflow, and modify the AV delay to obtain clear E and A waveforms and to ensure that the A wave ends before the onset of the QRS. The closure of the mitral valve should happen at the end of the A

Table 9 Treatment of Pacemaker Failure

Rate	Possible Response
Adequate to maintain blood pressure	1. Oxygen, airway control 2. Place magnet over pacemaker 3. Atropine if sinus bradycardia
Severe bradycardia and hypotension	1. Oxygen, airway control 2. Place magnet over pacemaker 3. Other types of pacing if magnet does not activate the pacemaker (transcutaneous, esophageal, or transvenous) 4. Atropine if sinus bradycardia 5. Isoproterenol to increase ventricular rate
No escape rhythm	1. Cardiopulmonary resuscitation 2. Place magnet over pacemaker 3. Other types of pacing if magnet does not activate the pacemaker (transcutaneous, esophageal, or transvenous) 4. Isoproterenol to increase ventricular rate

From Zaidan JR, Youngberg JA, Lake CL, et al., eds. *Pacemakers, Cardiac, Vascular and Thoracic Anesthesia.* New York: Churchill Livingstone; 2000, with permission.

wave but before any diastolic mitral regurgitation. If echocardiography is not available, adjust the AV interval to achieve highest cardiac output.

4. **Pacing mode:** Three modes are explained here. In the patient with normal AV conduction, AAI mode allows for an increase in HR and a physiologic depolarization of the ventricles. If inhibition by electrocautery is a concern, use asynchronous pacing in AOO mode. For the patient with AV conduction delay, DOO or DDI should be used. DDI mode also avoids tracking of rapid atrial rates in cases of postbypass atrial fibrillation.

5. **Biventricular pacing:** In patients with EF ≤35% and QRS ≥120 ms, acute biventricular pacing improves torsion and mechanics of contraction, particularly in patients with mitral regurgitation due to papillary muscle dyssynchrony. Speckle-tracking, 3D echocardiography, M-mode definition of septal to wall motion delay, color Doppler tissue imaging, and analysis of segmental velocity are used to characterize ventricular dyssynchrony. Currently available temporary pacemakers only allow biventricular pacing through a Y connection of the two ventricular epicardial wires to the ventricular output of the box. Acute CRT leads to an increase in myocardial performance with a slight decrease in myocardial oxygen consumption.

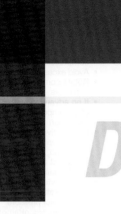

American Heart Association (AHA) Resuscitation Protocols

Adult
  Advanced Cardiac Life Support (ACLS) Cardiac Arrest Algorithm
  ACLS Bradycardia Algorithm
  ACLS Tachycardia Algorithm
  Maternal Cardiac Arrest Algorithm

Pediatric
  Pediatric Health Care Provider Basic Life Support (BLS) Algorithm
  Pediatric Advanced Life Support (PALS) Medications for Cardiac Arrest
    and Symptomatic Arrhythmias
  PALS Pulseless Arrest Algorithm
  PALS Bradycardia Algorithm
  PALS Tachycardia Algorithm
  PALS Newborn Resuscitation Algorithm

For more detailed information, the reader is referred to the American Heart Association: 2010 American Heart Association Guidelines for cardiopulmonary resuscitation and emergency cardiovascular care. *Circulation* 2010;122(Suppl 3).

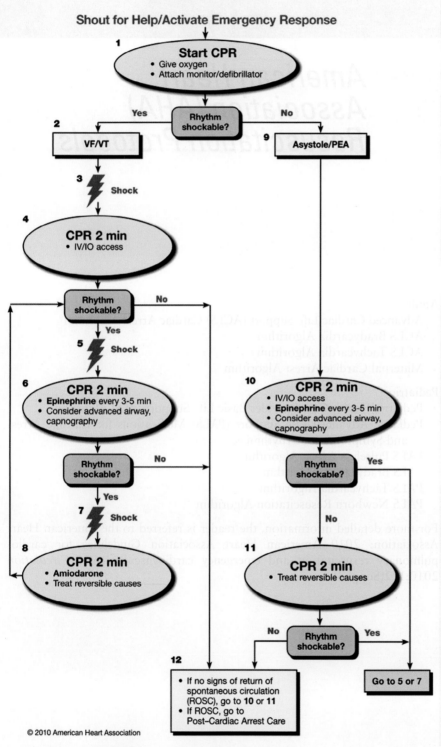

Adult Cardiac Arrest

Shout for Help/Activate Emergency Response

1 Start CPR
- Give oxygen
- Attach monitor/defibrillator

Rhythm shockable?
Yes / No

2 VF/VT

9 Asystole/PEA

3 Shock

4 CPR 2 min
- IV/IO access

Rhythm shockable?
No / Yes

5 Shock

6 CPR 2 min
- Epinephrine every 3-5 min
- Consider advanced airway, capnography

Rhythm shockable?
No / Yes

7 Shock

8 CPR 2 min
- Amiodarone
- Treat reversible causes

10 CPR 2 min
- IV/IO access
- Epinephrine every 3-5 min
- Consider advanced airway, capnography

Rhythm shockable?
Yes / No

11 CPR 2 min
- Treat reversible causes

Rhythm shockable?
No / Yes

Go to 5 or 7

12
- If no signs of return of spontaneous circulation (ROSC), go to **10** or **11**
- If ROSC, go to Post–Cardiac Arrest Care

© 2010 American Heart Association

CPR Quality
- Push hard (≥2 inches [5 cm]) and fast (≥100/min) and allow complete chest recoil
- Minimize interruptions in compressions
- Avoid excessive ventilation
- Rotate compressor every 2 minutes
- If no advanced airway, 30:2 compression-ventilation ratio
- Quantitative waveform capnography
  – If P_{ETCO_2} <10 mm Hg, attempt to improve CPR quality
- Intra-arterial pressure
  – If relaxation phase (diastolic) pressure <20 mm Hg, attempt to improve CPR quality

Return of Spontaneous Circulation (ROSC)
- Pulse and blood pressure
- Abrupt sustained increase in P_{ETCO_2} (typically ≥40 mm Hg)
- Spontaneous arterial pressure waves with intra-arterial monitoring

Shock Energy
- **Biphasic:** Manufacturer recommendation (eg, initial dose of 120-200 J); if unknown, use maximum available. Second and subsequent doses should be equivalent, and higher doses may be considered.
- **Monophasic:** 360 J

Drug Therapy
- **Epinephrine IV/IO Dose:** 1 mg every 3-5 minutes
- **Vasopressin IV/IO Dose:** 40 units can replace first or second dose of epinephrine
- **Amiodarone IV/IO Dose:** First dose: 300 mg bolus. Second dose: 150 mg.

Advanced Airway
- Supraglottic advanced airway or endotracheal intubation
- Waveform capnography to confirm and monitor ET tube placement
- 8-10 breaths per minute with continuous chest compressions

Reversible Causes
- Hypovolemia
- Hypoxia
- Hydrogen ion (acidosis)
- Hypo-/hyperkalemia
- Hypothermia
- Tension pneumothorax
- Tamponade, cardiac
- Toxins
- Thrombosis, pulmonary
- Thrombosis, coronary

Figure 1 Adult advanced cardiac life support pulseless arrest algorithm.

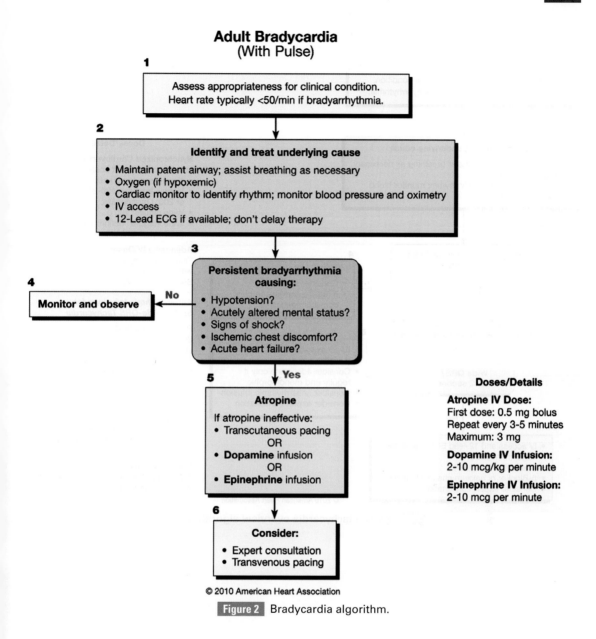

Figure 2 Bradycardia algorithm.

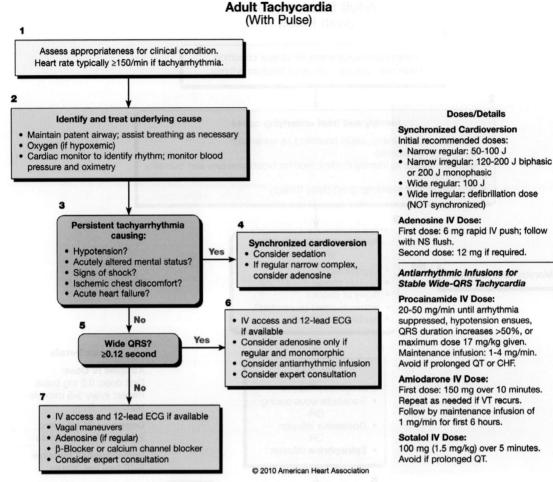

Figure 3 The tachycardia overview algorithm.

Maternal Cardiac Arrest

First Responder

- Activate maternal cardiac arrest team
- Document time of onset of maternal cardiac arrest
- Place the patient supine
- Start chest compressions as per BLS algorithm; place hands slightly higher on sternum than usual

---

Subsequent Responders

Maternal Interventions

Treat per BLS and ACLS Algorithms

- Do not delay defibrillation
- Give typical ACLS drugs and doses
- Ventilate with 100% oxygen
- Monitor waveform capnography and CPR quality
- Provide post–cardiac arrest care as appropriate

Maternal Modifications

- Start IV above the diaphragm
- Assess for hypovolemia and give fluid bolus when required
- Anticipate difficult airway; experienced provider preferred for advanced airway placement
- If patient receiving IV/IO magnesium prearrest, stop magnesium and give IV/IO calcium chloride 10 mL in 10% solution, or calcium gluconate 30 mL in 10% solution
- Continue all maternal resuscitative interventions (CPR, positioning, defibrillation, drugs, and fluids) during and after cesarean section

Obstetric Interventions for Patient With an Obviously Gravid Uterus*

- Perform manual left uterine displacement (LUD)— displace uterus to the patient's left to relieve aortocaval compression
- Remove both internal and external fetal monitors if present

Obstetric and neonatal teams should immediately prepare for possible emergency cesarean section

- If no ROSC by 4 minutes of resuscitative efforts, consider performing immediate emergency cesarean section
- Aim for delivery within 5 minutes of onset of resuscitative efforts

*An obviously gravid uterus is a uterus that is deemed clinically to be sufficiently large to cause aortocaval compression

---

Search for and Treat Possible Contributing Factors (BEAU-CHOPS)

Bleeding/DIC
Embolism: coronary/pulmonary/amniotic fluid embolism
Anesthetic complications
Uterine atony
Cardiac disease (MI/ischemia/aortic dissection/cardiomyopathy)
Hypertension/preeclampsia/eclampsia
Other: differential diagnosis of standard ACLS guidelines
Placenta abruptio/previa
Sepsis

© 2010 American Heart Association

Figure 4 Maternal cardiac arrest algorithm.

Pediatric BLS Healthcare Providers

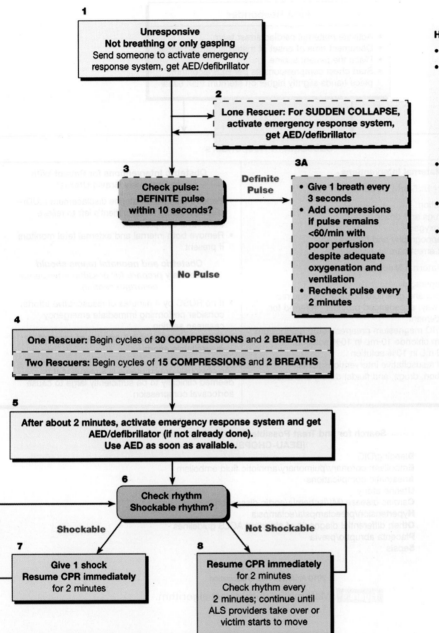

1
Unresponsive
Not breathing or only gasping
Send someone to activate emergency
response system, get AED/defibrillator

2
Lone Rescuer: For SUDDEN COLLAPSE,
activate emergency response system,
get AED/defibrillator

3
Check pulse:
DEFINITE pulse
within 10 seconds?

Definite Pulse →

3A
• Give 1 breath every
  3 seconds
• Add compressions
  if pulse remains
  <60/min with
  poor perfusion
  despite adequate
  oxygenation and
  ventilation
• Recheck pulse every
  2 minutes

No Pulse

4
One Rescuer: Begin cycles of 30 COMPRESSIONS and 2 BREATHS
Two Rescuers: Begin cycles of 15 COMPRESSIONS and 2 BREATHS

5
After about 2 minutes, activate emergency response system and get
AED/defibrillator (if not already done).
Use AED as soon as available.

6
Check rhythm
Shockable rhythm?

Shockable   Not Shockable

7
Give 1 shock
Resume CPR immediately
for 2 minutes

8
Resume CPR immediately
for 2 minutes
Check rhythm every
2 minutes; continue until
ALS providers take over or
victim starts to move

High-Quality CPR

• Rate at least 100/min
• Compression
  depth to at least
  ⅓ anterior-posterior
  diameter of chest,
  about 1½ inches
  (4 cm) in infants
  and 2 inches (5 cm)
  in children
• Allow complete
  chest recoil after each
  compression
• Minimize interruptions
  in chest compressions
• Avoid excessive
  ventilation

Note: The boxes bordered with dashed lines are performed
by healthcare providers and not by lay rescuers

© 2010 American Heart Association

Figure 5 Pediatric health care provider basic life support algorithm.

Table 1 Pediatric Advanced Life Support Medications for Cardiac Arrest and Symptomatic Arrhythmias

Drug	Dosage (Pediatric)	Remarks
Adenosine	0.1 mg/kg (maximum, 6 mg) Repeat: 0.2 mg/kg (maximum, 12 mg)	Monitor ECG during dose Rapid IV/IO bolus
Amiodarone	5 mg/kg IV/IO Repeat up to 15 mg/kg Maximum: 300 mg	Monitor ECG and blood pressure Adjust administration rate to urgency Use caution when administering with other drugs that prolong QT

Atropine	0.02 mg/kg IV/IO
	0.03 mg/kg ET[a]
	Repeat once if needed
	Minimum dose: 0.1 mg
	Maximum single dose:
	  Child, 0.5 mg
	  Adolescent, 1.0 mg
		Higher doses may be given with organophosphate poisoning

Calcium chloride (10%)	20 mg/kg IV/IO (0.2 mL/kg)	Give slow IV push for hypocalcemia, hypermagnesemia, calcium channel blocker toxicity
Epinephrine	0.01 mg/kg (0.1 mL/kg 1 : 10,000) IV/IO 0.1 mg/kg (0.1 mL/kg 1 : 1,000) ET[a] Maximum dose: 1 mg IV/IO; 10 mg ET	May repeat every 3–5 min
Glucose	0.5–1.0 g/kg IV/IO	$D_{10}W$: 5–10 mL/kg $D_{25}W$: 2–4 mL/kg $D_{50}W$: 1–2 mL/kg
Lidocaine	Bolus: 1 mg/kg IV/IO Maximum dose: 100 mg Infusion: 20–50 /g/kg/min ET[a]: 2–3 mg/kg	—
Magnesium sulfate	25–50 mg/kg IV/IO over 10–20 min; faster in torsades Maximum dose: 2 g	—
Naloxone	≤5 years or <20 kg: 0.1 mg/kg IV/IO/ET[a] ≥5 y or >20 kg: 2 mg IV/IO/ET[a]	Use lower doses to reverse respiratory depression associated with therapeutic opioid use (1–15 /µg/kg)
Procainamide	15 mg/kg IV/IO over 30 to 60 min Adult dose: 20 mg/min IV infusion up to total maximum dose of 17 mg/kg	Monitor ECG and blood pressure Use caution when administering with other drugs that prolong QT
Sodium bicarbonate	1 mEq/kg IV/IO slowly	After adequate ventilation

ECG, electrocardiogram; IV, intravenous; IO, intraosseous; ET, endotracheal.
[a]Flush with 5 mL of normal saline and follow with five ventilations.
Adapted from: 2005 American Heart Association Guidelines for cardiopulmonary resuscitation and emergency cardiovascular care. *Circulation* 2005;112(Suppl IV):IV.

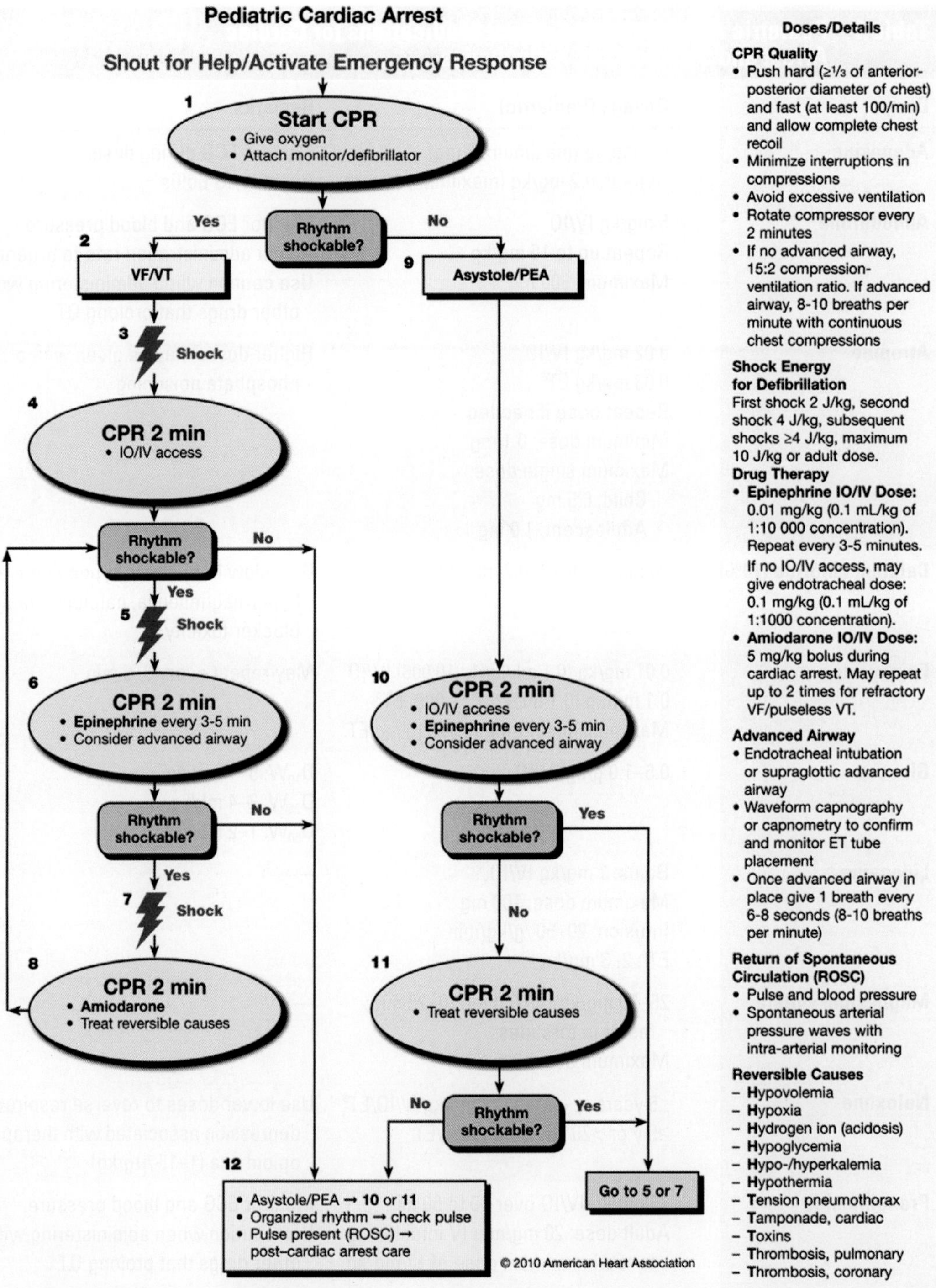

Pediatric Cardiac Arrest

Shout for Help/Activate Emergency Response

1
Start CPR
- Give oxygen
- Attach monitor/defibrillator

Rhythm shockable?

Yes → **2** VF/VT
No → **9** Asystole/PEA

3 Shock

4
CPR 2 min
- IO/IV access

Rhythm shockable?
No →

Yes ↓
5 Shock

6
CPR 2 min
- Epinephrine every 3-5 min
- Consider advanced airway

Rhythm shockable?
No →

Yes ↓
7 Shock

8
CPR 2 min
- Amiodarone
- Treat reversible causes

10
CPR 2 min
- IO/IV access
- Epinephrine every 3-5 min
- Consider advanced airway

Rhythm shockable?
Yes →

No ↓
11
CPR 2 min
- Treat reversible causes

Rhythm shockable?
Yes → Go to 5 or 7

No ↓

12
- Asystole/PEA → 10 or 11
- Organized rhythm → check pulse
- Pulse present (ROSC) → post–cardiac arrest care

© 2010 American Heart Association

Doses/Details

CPR Quality
- Push hard (≥1/3 of anterior-posterior diameter of chest) and fast (at least 100/min) and allow complete chest recoil
- Minimize interruptions in compressions
- Avoid excessive ventilation
- Rotate compressor every 2 minutes
- If no advanced airway, 15:2 compression-ventilation ratio. If advanced airway, 8-10 breaths per minute with continuous chest compressions

Shock Energy for Defibrillation
First shock 2 J/kg, second shock 4 J/kg, subsequent shocks ≥4 J/kg, maximum 10 J/kg or adult dose.

Drug Therapy
- **Epinephrine IO/IV Dose:** 0.01 mg/kg (0.1 mL/kg of 1:10 000 concentration). Repeat every 3-5 minutes. If no IO/IV access, may give endotracheal dose: 0.1 mg/kg (0.1 mL/kg of 1:1000 concentration).
- **Amiodarone IO/IV Dose:** 5 mg/kg bolus during cardiac arrest. May repeat up to 2 times for refractory VF/pulseless VT.

Advanced Airway
- Endotracheal intubation or supraglottic advanced airway
- Waveform capnography or capnometry to confirm and monitor ET tube placement
- Once advanced airway in place give 1 breath every 6-8 seconds (8-10 breaths per minute)

Return of Spontaneous Circulation (ROSC)
- Pulse and blood pressure
- Spontaneous arterial pressure waves with intra-arterial monitoring

Reversible Causes
– Hypovolemia
– Hypoxia
– Hydrogen ion (acidosis)
– Hypoglycemia
– Hypo-/hyperkalemia
– Hypothermia
– Tension pneumothorax
– Tamponade, cardiac
– Toxins
– Thrombosis, pulmonary
– Thrombosis, coronary

Figure 6 PALS pulseless arrest algorithm.

Pediatric Bradycardia
With a Pulse and Poor Perfusion

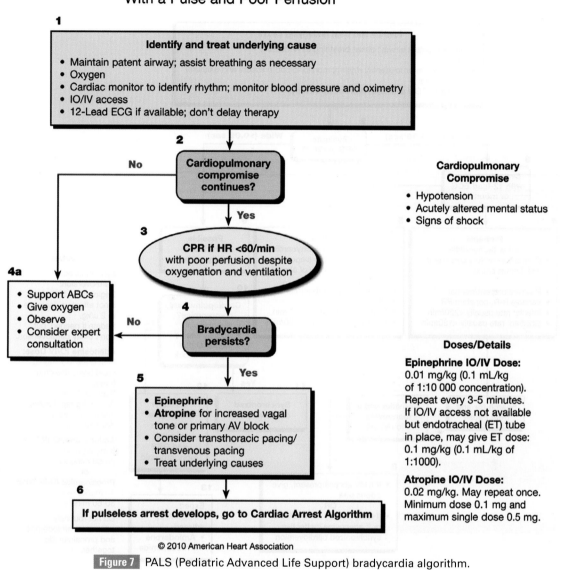

1

Identify and treat underlying cause
- Maintain patent airway; assist breathing as necessary
- Oxygen
- Cardiac monitor to identify rhythm; monitor blood pressure and oximetry
- IO/IV access
- 12-Lead ECG if available; don't delay therapy

2

No

Cardiopulmonary compromise continues?

Yes

3

CPR if HR <60/min
with poor perfusion despite oxygenation and ventilation

4a
- Support ABCs
- Give oxygen
- Observe
- Consider expert consultation

4

No

Bradycardia persists?

Yes

5
- **Epinephrine**
- **Atropine** for increased vagal tone or primary AV block
- Consider transthoracic pacing/transvenous pacing
- Treat underlying causes

6

If pulseless arrest develops, go to Cardiac Arrest Algorithm

Cardiopulmonary Compromise
- Hypotension
- Acutely altered mental status
- Signs of shock

Doses/Details

Epinephrine IO/IV Dose:
0.01 mg/kg (0.1 mL/kg of 1:10 000 concentration). Repeat every 3-5 minutes. If IO/IV access not available but endotracheal (ET) tube in place, may give ET dose: 0.1 mg/kg (0.1 mL/kg of 1:1000).

Atropine IO/IV Dose:
0.02 mg/kg. May repeat once. Minimum dose 0.1 mg and maximum single dose 0.5 mg.

© 2010 American Heart Association

Figure 7   PALS (Pediatric Advanced Life Support) bradycardia algorithm.

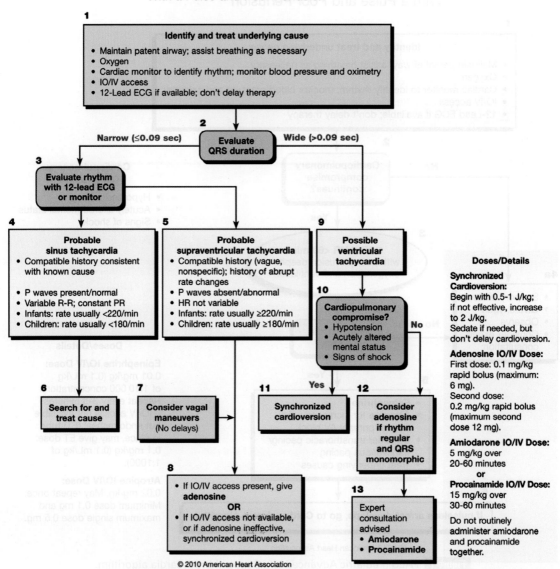

Figure 8 PALS tachycardia algorithm for infants and children with rapid rhythm and evidence of poor perfusion.

Newborn Resuscitation

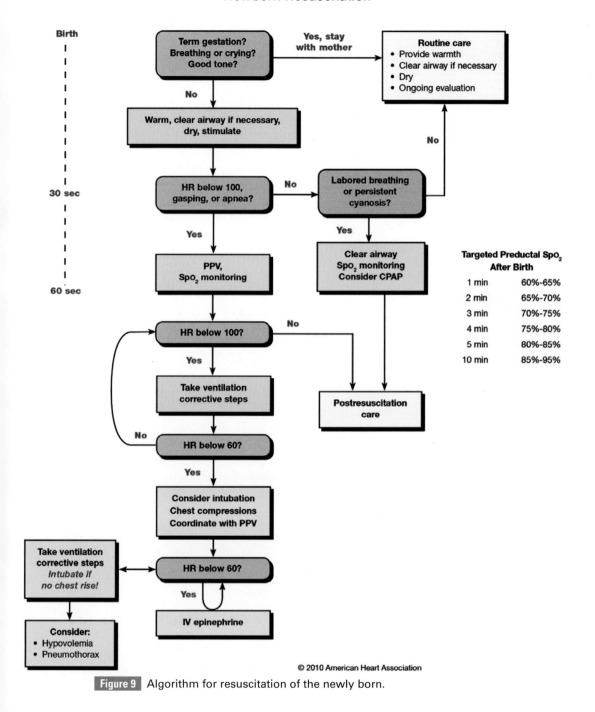

© 2010 American Heart Association

Figure 9 Algorithm for resuscitation of the newly born.

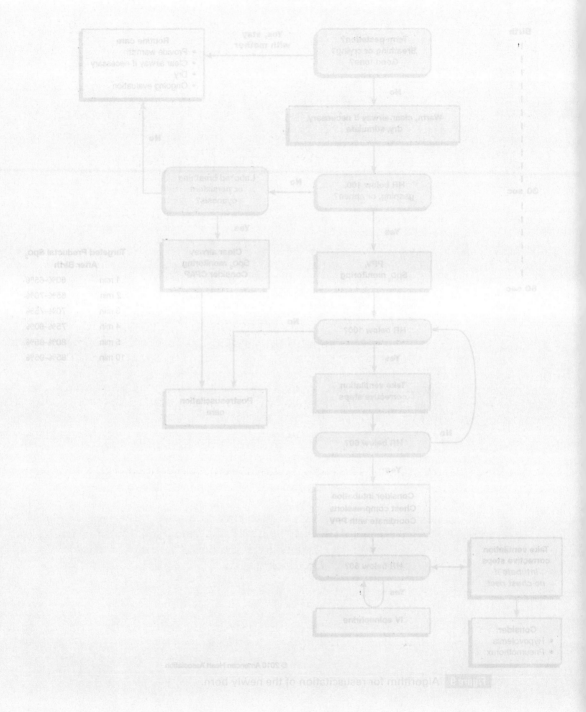

American Society of Anesthesiologists Standards, Guidelines, and Statements

E

*This is not an ASA document but is included because of its relevance to fire safety. (*APSF Newsletter* 2012;26:43, www.apsf.org)

Standards for Basic Anesthetic Monitoring

Committee of Origin: Standards and Practice Parameters

(Approved by the ASA House of Delegates on October 21, 1986, and last amended on October 20, 2010, with an effective date of July 1, 2011)

These standards apply to all anesthesia care although, in emergency circumstances, appropriate life support measures take precedence. These standards may be exceeded at any time based on the judgment of the responsible anesthesiologist. They are intended to encourage quality patient care, but observing them cannot guarantee any specific patient outcome. They are subject to revision from time to time, as warranted by the evolution of technology and practice. They apply to all general anesthetics, regional anesthetics and monitored anesthesia care. This set of standards addresses only the issue of basic anesthetic monitoring, which is one component of anesthesia care. In certain rare or unusual circumstances, 1) some of these methods of monitoring may be clinically impractical, and 2) appropriate use of the described monitoring methods may fail to detect untoward clinical developments. Brief interruptions of continual* monitoring may be unavoidable. These standards are not intended for application to the care of the obstetrical patient in labor or in the conduct of pain management.

Standard I

Qualified anesthesia personnel shall be present in the room throughout the conduct of all general anesthetics, regional anesthetics and monitored anesthesia care.

Objective

Because of the rapid changes in patient status during anesthesia, qualified anesthesia personnel shall be continuously present to monitor the patient and provide anesthesia care. In the event there is a direct known hazard, e.g., radiation, to the anesthesia personnel which might require intermittent remote observation of the patient, some provision for monitoring the patient must be made. In the event that an emergency requires the temporary absence of the person primarily responsible for the anesthetic, the best judgment of the anesthesiologist will be exercised in comparing the emergency with the anesthetized patient's condition and in the selection of the person left responsible for the anesthetic during the temporary absence.

Standard II

During all anesthetics, the patient's oxygenation, ventilation, circulation and temperature shall be continually evaluated.

Oxygenation
Objective

To ensure adequate oxygen concentration in the inspired gas and the blood during all anesthetics.

Methods

1. Inspired gas: During every administration of general anesthesia using an anesthesia machine, the concentration of oxygen in the patient breathing

---

*Note that "continual" is defined as "repeated regularly and frequently in steady rapid succession" whereas "continuous" means "prolonged without any interruption at any time."

system shall be measured by an oxygen analyzer with a low oxygen concentration limit alarm in use.[†]

2. Blood oxygenation: During all anesthetics, a quantitative method of assessing oxygenation such as pulse oximetry shall be employed.[†] When the pulse oximeter is utilized, the variable pitch pulse tone and the low threshold alarm shall be audible to the anesthesiologist or the anesthesia care team personnel.[†] Adequate illumination and exposure of the patient are necessary to assess color.[†]

Ventilation
Objective
To ensure adequate ventilation of the patient during all anesthetics.

Methods
1. Every patient receiving general anesthesia shall have the adequacy of ventilation continually evaluated. Qualitative clinical signs such as chest excursion, observation of the reservoir breathing bag and auscultation of breath sounds are useful. Continual monitoring for the presence of expired carbon dioxide shall be performed unless invalidated by the nature of the patient, procedure or equipment. Quantitative monitoring of the volume of expired gas is strongly encouraged.[†]
2. When an endotracheal tube or laryngeal mask is inserted, its correct positioning must be verified by clinical assessment and by identification of carbon dioxide in the expired gas. Continual end-tidal carbon dioxide analysis, in use from the time of endotracheal tube/laryngeal mask placement, until extubation/removal or initiating transfer to a postoperative care location, shall be performed using a quantitative method such as capnography, capnometry or mass spectroscopy.[†] When capnography or capnometry is utilized, the end tidal CO_2 alarm shall be audible to the anesthesiologist or the anesthesia care team personnel.[†]
3. When ventilation is controlled by a mechanical ventilator, there shall be in continuous use a device that is capable of detecting disconnection of components of the breathing system. The device must give an audible signal when its alarm threshold is exceeded.
4. During regional anesthesia (with no sedation) or local anesthesia (with no sedation), the adequacy of ventilation shall be evaluated by continual observation of qualitative clinical signs. During moderate or deep sedation the adequacy of ventilation shall be evaluated by continual observation of qualitative clinical signs and monitoring for the presence of exhaled carbon dioxide unless precluded or invalidated by the nature of the patient, procedure, or equipment.

Circulation
Objective
To ensure the adequacy of the patient's circulatory function during all anesthetics.

Methods
1. Every patient receiving anesthesia shall have the electrocardiogram continuously displayed from the beginning of anesthesia until preparing to leave the anesthetizing location.[†]

[†]Under extenuating circumstances, the responsible anesthesiologist may waive the requirements marked with an dagger (†); it is recommended that when this is done, it should be so stated (including the reasons) in a note in the patient's medical record.

2. Every patient receiving anesthesia shall have arterial blood pressure and heart rate determined and evaluated at least every five minutes.[†]
3. Every patient receiving general anesthesia shall have, in addition to the above, circulatory function continually evaluated by at least one of the following: palpation of a pulse, auscultation of heart sounds, monitoring of a tracing of intra-arterial pressure, ultrasound peripheral pulse monitoring, or pulse plethysmography or oximetry.

Body Temperature
Objective
To aid in the maintenance of appropriate body temperature during all anesthetics.

Methods
Every patient receiving anesthesia shall have temperature monitored when clinically significant changes in body temperature are intended, anticipated or suspected.

Continuum of Depth of Sedation: Definition of General Anesthesia and Levels of Sedation/Analgesia*

Committee of Origin: Quality Management and Departmental Administration

(Approved by the ASA House of Delegates on October 13, 1999, and last amended on October 15, 2014)

	Minimal Sedation (Anxiolysis)	Moderate Sedation/ Analgesia ("Conscious Sedation")	Deep Sedation/ Analgesia	General Anesthesia
Responsiveness	Normal response to verbal stimulation	Purposeful[†] response to verbal or tactile stimulation	Purposeful[†] response following repeated or painful stimulation	Unarousable even with painful stimulus
Airway	Unaffected	No intervention required	Intervention may be required	Intervention often required
Spontaneous Ventilation	Unaffected	Adequate	May be inadequate	Frequently inadequate
Cardiovascular Function	Unaffected	Usually maintained	Usually maintained	May be impaired

---

*Monitored Anesthesia Care ("MAC") does not describe the continuum of depth of sedation, rather it describes "a specific anesthesia service in which an anesthesiologist has been requested to participate in the care of a patient undergoing a diagnostic or therapeutic procedure."
[†]Reflex withdrawal from a painful stimulus is NOT considered a purposeful response.

Minimal Sedation (Anxiolysis) is a drug-induced state during which patients respond normally to verbal commands. Although cognitive function and physical coordination may be impaired, airway reflexes, and ventilatory and cardiovascular functions are unaffected.

Moderate Sedation/Analgesia ("Conscious Sedation") is a drug-induced depression of consciousness during which patients respond purposefully[†] to verbal commands, either alone or accompanied by light tactile stimulation. No interventions are required to maintain a patent airway, and spontaneous ventilation is adequate. Cardiovascular function is usually maintained.

Deep Sedation/Analgesia is a drug-induced depression of consciousness during which patients cannot be easily aroused but respond purposefully[†] following repeated or painful stimulation. The ability to independently maintain ventilatory function may be impaired. Patients may require assistance in maintaining a patent airway, and spontaneous ventilation may be inadequate. Cardiovascular function is usually maintained.

General Anesthesia is a drug-induced loss of consciousness during which patients are not arousable, even by painful stimulation. The ability to independently maintain ventilatory function is often impaired. Patients often require assistance in maintaining a patent airway, and positive pressure ventilation may be required because of depressed spontaneous ventilation or drug-induced depression of neuromuscular function. Cardiovascular function may be impaired.

Because sedation is a continuum, it is not always possible to predict how an individual patient will respond. Hence, practitioners intending to produce a given level of sedation should be able to rescue[‡] patients whose level of sedation becomes deeper than initially intended. Individuals administering Moderate Sedation/Analgesia ("Conscious Sedation") should be able to rescue[‡] patients who enter a state of Deep Sedation/Analgesia, while those administering Deep Sedation/Analgesia should be able to rescue[‡] patients who enter a state of General Anesthesia.

[†]Reflex withdrawal from a painful stimulus is NOT considered a purposeful response.
[‡]Rescue of a patient from a deeper level of sedation than intended is an intervention by a practitioner proficient in airway management and advanced life support. The qualified practitioner corrects adverse physiologic consequences of the deeper-than-intended level of sedation (such as hypoventilation, hypoxia and hypotension) and returns the patient to the originally intended level of sedation. It is not appropriate to continue the procedure at an unintended level of sedation.

Basic Standards for Preanesthesia Care

Committee of Origin: Standards and Practice Parameters

(Approved by the ASA House of Delegates on October 14, 1987, and last affirmed on October 20, 2010)

These standards apply to all patients who receive anesthesia care. Under exceptional circumstances, these standards may be modified. When this is the case, the circumstances shall be documented in the patient's record.

An anesthesiologist shall be responsible for determining the medical status of the patient and developing a plan of anesthesia care.

The anesthesiologist, before the delivery of anesthesia care, is responsible for:

1. Reviewing the available medical record.
2. Interviewing and performing a focused examination of the patient to:
   a. Discuss the medical history, including previous anesthetic experiences and medical therapy.
   b. Assess those aspects of the patient's physical condition that might affect decisions regarding perioperative risk and management.
3. Ordering and reviewing pertinent available tests and consultations as necessary for the delivery of anesthesia care.
4. Ordering appropriate preoperative medications.
5. Ensuring that consent has been obtained for the anesthesia care.
6. Documenting in the chart that the above has been performed.

Standards for Postanesthesia Care

Committee of Origin: Standards and Practice Parameters

(Approved by the ASA House of Delegates on October 27, 2004, and last amended on October 15, 2014)

These standards apply to postanesthesia care in all locations. These standards may be exceeded based on the judgment of the responsible anesthesiologist. They are intended to encourage quality patient care, but cannot guarantee any specific patient outcome. They are subject to revision from time to time as warranted by the evolution of technology and practice.

Standard I

All patients who have received general anesthesia, regional anesthesia or monitored anesthesia care shall receive appropriate postanesthesia management.[1]

1. A Postanesthesia Care Unit (PACU) or an area which provides equivalent postanesthesia care (for example, a Surgical Intensive Care Unit) shall be available to receive patients after anesthesia care. All patients who receive anesthesia care shall be admitted to the PACU or its equivalent **except** by specific order of the anesthesiologist responsible for the patient's care.
2. The medical aspects of care in the PACU (or equivalent area) shall be governed by policies and procedures which have been reviewed and approved by the Department of Anesthesiology.
3. The design, equipment and staffing of the PACU shall meet requirements of the facility's accrediting and licensing bodies.

Standard II

A patient transported to the PACU shall be accompanied by a member of the anesthesia care team who is knowledgeable about the patient's condition. The patient shall be continually evaluated and treated during transport with monitoring and support appropriate to the patient's condition.

Standard III

Upon arrival in the PACU, the patient shall be re-evaluated and a verbal report provided to the responsible PACU nurse by the member of the anesthesia care team who accompanies the patient.

1. The patient's status on arrival in the PACU shall be documented.
2. Information concerning the preoperative condition and the surgical/anesthetic course shall be transmitted to the PACU nurse.
3. The member of the Anesthesia Care Team shall remain in the PACU until the PACU nurse accepts responsibility for the nursing care of the patient.

Standard IV

The patient's condition shall be evaluated continually in the PACU.

1. The patient shall be observed and monitored by methods appropriate to the patient's medical condition. Particular attention should be given to monitoring oxygenation, ventilation, circulation, level of consciousness and temperature. During recovery from all anesthetics, a quantitative method of assessing oxygenation such as pulse oximetry shall be employed

---

[1]Refer to *Perianesthesia Nursing Standards, Practice Recommendations and Interpretive Statements,* published by ASPAN, for issues of nursing care.

in the initial phase of recovery.* This is not intended for application during the recovery of the obstetrical patient in whom regional anesthesia was used for labor and vaginal delivery.

2. An accurate written report of the PACU period shall be maintained. Use of an appropriate PACU scoring system is encouraged for each patient on admission, at appropriate intervals prior to discharge and at the time of discharge.

3. General medical supervision and coordination of patient care in the PACU should be the responsibility of an anesthesiologist.

4. There shall be a policy to assure the availability in the facility of a physician capable of managing complications and providing cardiopulmonary resuscitation for patients in the PACU.

Standard V
A physician is responsible for the discharge of the patient from the postanesthesia care unit.

1. When discharge criteria are used, they must be approved by the Department of Anesthesiology and the medical staff. They may vary depending upon whether the patient is discharged to a hospital room, to the Intensive Care Unit, to a short stay unit or home.

2. In the absence of the physician responsible for the discharge, the PACU nurse shall determine that the patient meets the discharge criteria. The name of the physician accepting responsibility for discharge shall be noted on the record.

---

*Under extenuating circumstances, the responsible anesthesiologist may waive the requirements marked with an asterisk (*); it is recommended that when this is done, it should be so stated (including the reasons) in a note in the patient's medical record.

Practice Advisory for the Prevention and Management of Operating Room Fires

American Society of
Anesthesiologists®

OPERATING ROOM FIRES ALGORITHM

Fire Prevention:
- Avoid using ignition sources[1] in proximity to an oxidizer-enriched atmosphere[2]
- Configure surgical drapes to minimize the accumulation of oxidizers
- Allow sufficient drying time for flammable skin prepping solutions
- Moisten sponges and gauze when used in proximity to ignition sources

Is this a High-Risk Procedure?
An ignition source will be used in proximity to an oxidizer-enriched atmosphere

YES / No

- Agree upon a team plan and team roles for preventing and managing a fire
- Notify the surgeon of the presence of, or an increase in, an oxidizer-enriched atmosphere
- Use cuffed tracheal tubes for surgery in the airway; appropriately prepare laser-resistant tracheal tubes
- Consider a tracheal tube or laryngeal mask for monitored anesthesia care (MAC) with moderate to deep sedation and/or oxygen-dependent patients who undergo surgery of the head, neck, or face.
- *Before* an ignition source is activated:
  - o *Announce* the intent to use an ignition source
  - o *Reduce* the oxygen concentration to the minimum required to avoid hypoxia[3]
  - o *Stop* the use of nitrous oxide[4]

Fire Management:

Early Warning Signs of Fire[5]

Fire is not present; Continue procedure

HALT PROCEDURE Call for Evaluation

FIRE IS PRESENT

AIRWAY[6] FIRE:

IMMEDIATELY, without waiting
- Remove tracheal tube
- Stop the flow of all airway gases
- Remove sponges and any other flammable material from airway
- Pour saline into airway

NON-AIRWAY FIRE:

IMMEDIATELY, without waiting
- Stop the flow of all airway gases
- Remove drapes and all burning and flammable materials
- Extinguish burning materials by pouring saline or other means

If Fire is Not Extinguished on First Attempt
Use a CO_2 fire extinguisher[7]
If FIRE PERSISTS: activate fire alarm, evacuate patient, close OR door, and turn off gas supply to room

Fire out / Fire out

- Re-establish ventilation
- Avoid oxidizer-enriched atmosphere if clinically appropriate
- Examine tracheal tube to see if fragments may be left behind in airway
- Consider bronchoscopy

- Maintain ventilation
- Assess for inhalation injury if the patient is not intubated

Assess patient status and devise plan for management

[1] Ignition sources include but are not limited to electrosurgery or electrocautery units and lasers.
[2] An oxidizer-enriched atmosphere occurs when there is any increase in oxygen concentration above room air level, and/or the presence of any concentration of nitrous oxide.
[3] After minimizing delivered oxygen, wait a period of time (*e.g.*, 1-3 min) before using an ignition source. For oxygen dependent patients, *reduce* supplemental oxygen delivery to the minimum required to avoid hypoxia. Monitor oxygenation with pulse oximetry, and if feasible, inspired, exhaled, and/or delivered oxygen concentration.
[4] After stopping the delivery of nitrous oxide, wait a period of time (*e.g.*, 1-3 min) before using an ignition source.
[5] Unexpected flash, flame, smoke or heat, unusual sounds (*e.g.*, a "pop," snap or "foomp") or odors, unexpected movement of drapes, discoloration of drapes or breathing circuit, unexpected patient movement or complaint.
[6] In this algorithm, airway fire refers to a fire in the airway or breathing circuit.
[7] A CO_2 fire extinguisher may be used on the patient if necessary.

Figure 1 Operating room fires algorithm. CO_2, carbon dioxide; OR, operating room. (From Caplan RA, Barker SJ, Connis RT, et al; American Society of Anesthesiologists Task Force on Operating Room Fires. Practice advisory for the Prevention and Management of Operating Room Fires: a report by the American Society of Anesthesiologists Task Force on Operating Room Fires. *Anesthesiology.* 2008 108:786–801, with permission.)

OR Fire Prevention Algorithm*

Start Here

Is patient at risk for surgical fire?

Procedures involving the head, neck and upper chest (above T5) *and* use of an ignition source in proximity to an oxidizer.

NO → **Proceed, but frequently reassess for changes in fire risk.**

Nurses and surgeons avoid pooling of alcohol-based skin preparations and allow adequate drying time. Prior to initial use of electrocautery, communication occurs between surgeon and anesthesia professional.

YES ↓

Does patient require oxygen supplementation?

NO → **Use room air sedation.**

YES ↓

Is >30% oxygen concentration required to maintain oxygen saturation?

NO → **Use delivery device such as a blender or common gas outlet to maintain oxygen below 30%.**

YES ↓

Secure airway with endotracheal tube or supraglottic device.

Although securing the airway is preferred, for cases where using an airway device is undesirable or not feasible, oxygen accumulation may be minimized by air insufflation over the face and open draping to provide wide exposure of the surgical site to the atmosphere.

Provided as an educational resource by the
Anesthesia Patient Safety Foundation

www.apsf.org

Copyright ©2014 Anesthesia Patient Safety Foundation   **www.apsf.org**

The following organizations have indicated their support for APSF's efforts to increase awareness of the potential for surgical fires in at-risk patients: American Society of Anesthesiologists, American Association of Nurse Anesthetists, American Academy of Anesthesiologist Assistants, American College of Surgeons, American Society of Anesthesia Technologists and Technicians, American Society of PeriAnesthesia Nurses, Association of periOperative Registered Nurses, ECRI Institute, Food and Drug Administration Safe Use Initiative, National Patient Safety Foundation, The Joint Commission

*This is not an ASA document but is included because of its relevance to fire safety. (http://www.apsf.org/newsletters/html/Handouts/ORFireAlgorithmPoster8.5x11.pdf)

Position on Monitored Anesthesia Care

Committee of Origin: Economics

(Approved by the House of Delegates on October 25, 2005, and last amended on October 16, 2013)

Monitored anesthesia care is a specific anesthesia service for a diagnostic or therapeutic procedure. Indications for monitored anesthesia care include the nature of the procedure, the patient's clinical condition and/or the potential need to convert to a general or regional anesthetic.

Monitored anesthesia care includes all aspects of anesthesia care—a preprocedure visit, intraprocedure care and postprocedure anesthesia management. During monitored anesthesia care, the anesthesiologist provides or medically directs a number of specific services, including but not limited to:

- Diagnosis and treatment of clinical problems that occur during the procedure
- Support of vital functions
- Administration of sedatives, analgesics, hypnotics, anesthetic agents or other medications as necessary for patient safety
- Psychological support and physical comfort
- Provision of other medical services as needed to complete the procedure safely.

Monitored anesthesia care may include varying levels of sedation, analgesia and anxiolysis as necessary. The provider of monitored anesthesia care must be prepared and qualified to convert to general anesthesia when necessary. If the patient loses consciousness and the ability to respond purposefully, the anesthesia care is a general anesthetic, irrespective of whether airway instrumentation is required.

Monitored anesthesia care is a physician service provided to an individual patient. It should be subject to the same level of payment as general or regional anesthesia. Accordingly, the ASA Relative Value Guide® provides for the use of proper base units, time and any appropriate modifier units as the basis for determining payment.

Distinguishing Monitored Anesthesia Care ("MAC") from Moderate Sedation/Analgesia (Conscious Sedation)

Committee of Origin: Economics

(Approved by the ASA House of Delegates on October 27, 2004, last amended on October 21, 2009, and reaffirmed on October 16, 2013)

Moderate Sedation/Analgesia (Conscious Sedation; hereinafter known as Moderate Sedation) is a physician service recognized in the CPT procedural coding system. During Moderate Sedation, a physician supervises or personally administers sedative and/or analgesic medications that can allay patient anxiety and control pain during a diagnostic or therapeutic procedure. Such drug-induced depression of a patient's level of consciousness to a "moderate" level of sedation, as defined in the Joint Commission (TJC) standards, is intended to facilitate the successful performance of the diagnostic or therapeutic procedure while providing patient comfort and cooperation. Physicians providing moderate sedation must be qualified to recognize "deep" sedation, manage its consequences and adjust the level of sedation to a "moderate" or lesser level. The continual assessment of the effects of sedative or analgesic medications on the level of consciousness and on cardiac and respiratory function is an integral element of this service.

The American Society of Anesthesiologists has defined Monitored Anesthesia Care *(see Position on Monitored Anesthesia Care, updated on October 16, 2013).* This physician service can be distinguished from Moderate Sedation in several ways. An essential component of MAC is the anesthesia assessment and management of a patient's actual or anticipated physiological derangements or medical problems that may occur during a diagnostic or therapeutic procedure. While Monitored Anesthesia Care may include the administration of sedatives and/or analgesics often used for Moderate Sedation, the provider of MAC must be prepared and qualified to convert to general anesthesia when necessary. Additionally, a provider's ability to intervene to rescue a patient's airway from any sedation-induced compromise is a prerequisite to the qualifications to provide Monitored Anesthesia Care. By contrast, Moderate Sedation is not expected to induce depths of sedation that would impair the patient's own ability to maintain the integrity of his or her airway. These components of Monitored Anesthesia Care are unique aspects of an anesthesia service that are not part of Moderate Sedation.

The administration of sedatives, hypnotics, analgesics, as well as anesthetic drugs commonly used for the induction and maintenance of general anesthesia is often, but not always, a part of Monitored Anesthesia Care. In some patients who may require only minimal sedation, MAC is often indicated because even small doses of these medications could precipitate adverse physiologic responses that would necessitate acute clinical interventions and resuscitation. If a patient's condition and/or a procedural requirement is likely to require sedation to a "deep" level or even to a transient period of general anesthesia, only a practitioner privileged to provide anesthesia services should be allowed to manage the sedation. Due to the strong likelihood that "deep" sedation may, with or without intention, transition to general anesthesia, the skills of an anesthesia provider are necessary to manage the effects of general anesthesia on the patient as well as to return the patient quickly to a state of "deep" or lesser sedation.

Like all anesthesia services, Monitored Anesthesia Care includes an array of post-procedure responsibilities beyond the expectations of practitioners providing Moderate Sedation, including assuring a return to full consciousness, relief of pain, management of adverse physiological responses or side effects from medications administered during the procedure, as well as the diagnosis and treatment of co-existing medical problems.

Monitored Anesthesia Care allows for the safe administration of a maximal depth of sedation in excess of that provided during Moderate Sedation. The ability to adjust the sedation level from full consciousness to general anesthesia during the course of a procedure provides maximal flexibility in matching sedation level to patient needs and procedural requirements. In situations where the procedure is more invasive or when the patient is especially fragile, optimizing sedation level is necessary to achieve ideal procedural conditions.

In summary, Monitored Anesthesia Care is a physician service that is clearly distinct from Moderate Sedation due to the expectations and qualifications of the provider who must be able to utilize all anesthesia resources to support life and to provide patient comfort and safety during a diagnostic or therapeutic procedure.

Ethical Guidelines for the Anesthesia Care of Patients With Do-Not-Resuscitate Orders or Other Directives that Limit Treatment

Committee of Origin: Ethics

(Approved by the ASA House of Delegates on October 17, 2001, and last amended on October 16, 2013)

These guidelines apply both to patients with decision-making capacity and also to patients without decision-making capacity who have previously expressed their preferences.

I. Given the diversity of published opinions and cultures within our society, an essential element of preoperative preparation and perioperative care for patients with Do-Not-Resuscitate (DNR) orders or other directives that limit treatment is communication among involved parties. It is necessary to document relevant aspects of this communication.

II. Policies automatically suspending DNR orders or other directives that limit treatment prior to procedures involving anesthetic care may not sufficiently address a patient's rights to self-determination in a responsible and ethical manner. Such policies, if they exist, should be reviewed and revised, as necessary, to reflect the content of these guidelines.

III. The administration of anesthesia necessarily involves some practices and procedures that might be viewed as "resuscitation" in other settings. Prior to procedures requiring anesthetic care, any existing directives to limit the use of resuscitation procedures (that is, do-not-resuscitate orders and/or advance directives) should, when possible, be reviewed with the patient or designated surrogate. As a result of this review, the status of these directives should be clarified or modified based on the preferences of the patient. One of the three following alternatives may provide for a satisfactory outcome in many cases.

A. Full Attempt at Resuscitation: The patient or designated surrogate may request the full suspension of existing directives during the anesthetic and immediate postoperative period, thereby consenting to the use of any resuscitation procedures that may be appropriate to treat clinical events that occur during this time.

B. Limited Attempt at Resuscitation Defined With Regard to Specific Procedures: The patient or designated surrogate may elect to continue to refuse certain specific resuscitation procedures (for example, chest compressions, defibrillation or tracheal intubation). The anesthesiologist should inform the patient or designated surrogate about which procedures are 1) essential to the success of the anesthesia and the proposed procedure, and 2) which procedures are not essential and may be refused.

C. Limited Attempt at Resuscitation Defined With Regard to the Patient's Goals and Values: The patient or designated surrogate may allow the anesthesiologist and surgical/procedural team to use clinical judgment in determining which resuscitation procedures are appropriate in the context of the situation and the patient's stated goals and values. For example, some patients may want full resuscitation procedures to be used to manage adverse clinical events that are believed to be quickly and easily reversible, but to refrain from treatment for conditions that are likely to result in permanent sequelae, such as neurologic impairment or unwanted dependence upon life-sustaining technology.

IV. Any clarifications or modifications made to the patient's directive should be documented in the medical record. In cases where the patient or designated surrogate requests that the anesthesiologist use clinical judgment in determining which resuscitation procedures are appropriate, the anesthesiologist should document the discussion with particular attention to the stated goals and values of the patient.

V. Plans for postoperative/postprocedural care should indicate if or when the original, pre-existent directive to limit the use of resuscitation procedures will be reinstated. This occurs when the patient leaves the postanesthesia care unit or when the patient has recovered from the acute effects of anesthesia and surgery/procedure. Consideration should be given to whether continuing to provide the patient with a time-limited or event-limited postoperative/postprocedure trial of therapy would help the patient or surrogate better evaluate whether continued therapy would be consistent with the patient's goals.

VI. It is important to discuss and document whether there are to be any exceptions to the injunction(s) against intervention should there occur a specific recognized complication of the surgery/procedure or anesthesia.

VII. Concurrence on these issues by the primary physician (if not the surgeon/proceduralist of record), the surgeon/proceduralist and the anesthesiologist is desirable. If possible, these physicians should meet together with the patient (or the patient's legal representative) when these issues are discussed. This duty of the patient's physicians is deemed to be of such importance that it should not be delegated. Other members of the health care team who are (or will be) directly involved with the patient's care during the planned procedure should, if feasible, be included in this process.

VIII. Should conflicts arise, the following resolution processes are recommended:
   A. When an anesthesiologist finds the patient's or surgeon's/proceduralist's limitations of intervention decisions to be irreconcilable with one's own moral views, then the anesthesiologist should withdraw in a nonjudgmental fashion, providing an alternative for care in a timely fashion.
   B. When an anesthesiologist finds the patient's or surgeon's/proceduralist's limitation of intervention decisions to be in conflict with generally accepted standards of care, ethical practice or institutional policies, then the anesthesiologist should voice such concerns and present the situation to the appropriate institutional body.
   C. If these alternatives are not feasible within the time frame necessary to prevent further morbidity or suffering, then in accordance with the American Medical Association's Principles of Medical Ethics, care should proceed with reasonable adherence to the patient's directives, being mindful of the patient's goals and values.

IX. A representative from the hospital's anesthesiology service should establish a liaison with surgical, procedural, and nursing services for presentation, discussion and procedural application of these guidelines. Hospital staff should be made aware of the proceedings of these discussions and the motivations for them.

X. Modification of these guidelines may be appropriate when they conflict with local standards or policies, and in those emergency situations involving patients lacking decision-making capacity whose intentions have not been previously expressed.

Practice Guidelines for Preoperative Fasting and Use of Pharmacologic Agents to Reduce Risk of Pulmonary Aspiration: Application to Healthy Patients Undergoing Elective Procedures

Summary of Fasting Recommendations

Ingested Material	Minimum Fasting Period
Clear liquids	2 h
Breast milk	4 h
Infant formula	6 h
Nonhuman milk	6 h
Light meal	6 h

These recommendations apply to healthy patients who are undergoing elective procedures. They are not intended for women in labor. Following the Guidelines does not guarantee complete gastric emptying. The fasting periods noted above apply to patients of all ages.

Examples of clear liquids include water, fruit juices without pulp, carbonated beverages, clear tea, and black coffee. Because nonhuman milk is similar to solids in gastric emptying time, the amount ingested must be considered when determining an appropriate fasting period.

A light meal typically consists of toast and clear liquids. Meals that include fried or fatty foods or meat may prolong gastric emptying time. Additional fasting time (e.g., 8 h or more) may be needed in these cases. Both the amount and type of food ingested must be considered when determining an appropriate fasting period.

Summary of Pharmacologic Recommendations
For each medication type and common drug example listed below, the medications are not recommended for routine use.

Gastrointestinal Stimulants
Metoclopramide

Gastric Acid Secretion Blockers
Cimetidine
Famotidine
Ranitidine
Omeprazole
Lansoprazole

Antacids
Sodium citrate
Sodium bicarbonate
Magnesium trisilicate

Antiemetics
Droperidol
Ondansetron

Anticholinergics
Atropine
Scopolamine
Glycopyrrolate

Multiple Agents
No routine use

The Airway Approach Algorithm and Difficult Airway Algorithm

F

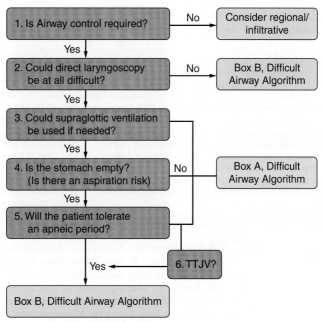

Airway Approach Algorithm

Figure 1 The airway approach algorithm: A decision tree approach to entry into the American Society of Anesthesiologists difficult airway algorithm.TTJV, transtracheal jet ventilation. (From Rosenblatt WH, Sukhupragarn W. Airway management. In: Barash PG, Cullen BF, Stoelting RK, et al., eds. *Clinical Anesthesia.* 7th ed. Philadelphia: Lippincott Williams & Wilkins; 2013:788, with permission.)

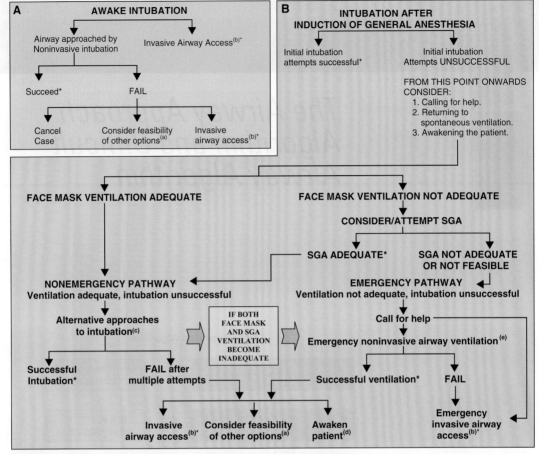

A   AWAKE INTUBATION

Airway approached by   Invasive Airway Access[(b)*]
Noninvasive intubation

Succeed*   FAIL

Cancel   Consider feasibility   Invasive
Case   of other options[(a)]   airway access[(b)*]

**B   INTUBATION AFTER
     INDUCTION OF GENERAL ANESTHESIA**

Initial intubation   Initial intubation
attempts successful*   Attempts UNSUCCESSFUL

FROM THIS POINT ONWARDS
CONSIDER:
1. Calling for help.
2. Returning to
   spontaneous ventilation.
3. Awakening the patient.

FACE MASK VENTILATION ADEQUATE

FACE MASK VENTILATION NOT ADEQUATE

CONSIDER/ATTEMPT SGA

SGA ADEQUATE*   SGA NOT ADEQUATE
                       OR NOT FEASIBLE

NONEMERGENCY PATHWAY
Ventilation adequate, intubation unsuccessful

EMERGENCY PATHWAY
Ventilation not adequate, intubation unsuccessful

Alternative approaches
to intubation[(c)]

IF BOTH
FACE MASK
AND SGA
VENTILATION
BECOME
INADEQUATE

Call for help

Emergency noninvasive airway ventilation [(e)]

Successful   FAIL after
Intubation*   multiple attempts

Successful ventilation*   FAIL

Invasive   Consider feasibility   Awaken
airway access[(b)*] of other options[(a)]   patient[(d)]

Emergency
invasive airway
access[(b)*]

*Confirm ventilation, tracheal intubation, or SGA placement with exhaled CO$_2$.

a. Other options include (but are not limited to): surgery utilizing face mask or supraglottic airway (SGA) anesthesia (e.g., LMA, ILMA, laryngeal tube), local anesthesia infiltration or regional nerve blockade. Pursuit of these options usually implies that mask ventilation will not be problematic. Therefore, these options may be of limited value if this step in the algorithm has been reached via the Emergency Pathway.

b. Invasive airway access includes surgical or percutaneous airway, jet ventilation, and retrograde intubation.

c. Alternative difficult intubation approaches include (but are not limited to): video-assisted laryngoscopy, alternative laryngoscope blades, SGA (e.g., LMA or ILMA) as an intubation conduit (with or without fiberoptic guidance), fiberoptic intubation, intubating stylet or tube changer, light wand, and blind oral or nasal intubation.

d. Consider re-preparation of the patient for awake intubation or canceling surgery.

e. Emergency non-invasive airway ventilation consists of a SGA.

Figure 2 The American Society of Anesthesiologists difficult airway algorithm. **A:** Awake intubation. **B:** Intubation after induction of general anesthesia. (From Apfelbaum JL, Hagberg CA, Caplan RA, et al; American Society of Anesthesiologists Task Force on Management of the Difficult Airway. Practice guidelines for management of the difficult airway: an updated report by the American Society of Anesthesiologists Task Force on Management of the Difficult Airway. *Anesthesiology*. 2013 Feb;118(2):251-70, with permission.)

G

Malignant Hyperthermia Protocol

Reproduced with permission Malignant Hyperthermia Association of the United States (MHAUS)

MH Hotline
1-800-644-9737
Outside the US:
1-315-464-7079

Effective Sept 2011

EMERGENCY THERAPY FOR

MALIGNANT HYPERTHERMIA

DIAGNOSIS vs. ASSOCIATED PROBLEMS

Signs of MH:
- Increasing $ETCO_2$
- Trunk or total body rigidity
- Masseter spasm or trismus
- Tachycardia/tachypnea
- Respiratory Acidosis, Metabolic Acidosis may be present
- Increased temperature (may be late sign)
- Myoglobinuria

Sudden/Unexpected Cardiac Arrest in Young Patients:
- Presume hyperkalemia and initiate treatment (see #6)
- Measure CK, myoglobin, ABGs, until normalized
- Consider dantrolene
- Usually secondary to occult myopathy (e.g., muscular dystrophy)
- Resuscitation may be difficult and prolonged

Trismus or Masseter Spasm with Succinylcholine
- Early sign of MH in many patients
- If limb muscle rigidity, begin treatment with dantrolene
- For emergent procedures, continue with non-triggering agents, evaluate and monitor the patient, and consider dantrolene treatment
- Follow CK and urine myoglobin for 36 hours.
- Check CK immediately and at 6 hour intervals until returning to normal. Observe for dark or cola colored urine. If present, liberalize fluid intake and test for myoglobin
- Observe in PACU or ICU for at least 12 hours

ACUTE PHASE TREATMENT

❶ GET HELP. GET DANTROLENE – Notify Surgeon
- Discontinue volatile agents and succinylcholine.
- Hyperventilate with 100% oxygen at flows of 10 L/min. or more.
- Halt the procedure as soon as possible; if emergent, continue with non-triggering anesthetic technique.
- Don't waste time changing the circle system and CO_2 absorbent.
- If available, place charcoal filter in anesthesia circuit

❷ Dantrolene 2.5 mg/kg rapidly IV through large-bore IV, if possible

> To convert kg to lbs for amount of dantrolene, give patients 1 mg/lb (2.5 mg/kg approximates 1 mg/lb).

- Repeat until signs of MH are reversed.
- Sometimes more than 10 mg/kg (up to 30 mg/kg) is necessary.

❸ Bicarbonate for metabolic acidosis
- 1-2 mEq/kg if blood gas values are not yet available.

❹ Cool the patient with core temperature >39ºC, Lavage open body cavities, stomach, bladder, or rectum. Apply ice to surface. Infuse cold saline intravenously. Stop cooling if temp. <38ºC and falling to prevent drift < 36ºC.

❺ Dysrhythmias usually respond to treatment of acidosis and hyperkalemia.
- Use standard drug therapy.

❻ Hyperkalemia – Treat with hyperventilation, bicarbonate, glucose/insulin, calcium.
- Bicarbonate 1-2 mEq/kg IV.
- For **pediatric,** 0.1 units insulin/kg and 1 ml/kg 50% glucose or for **adult,** 10 units regular insulin IV and 50 ml 50% glucose.
- Calcium chloride 10 mg/kg or calcium gluconate 10-50 mg/kg for life-threatening hyperkalemia.
- Check glucose levels hourly.

❼ Follow $ETCO_2$, electrolytes, blood gases, CK, core temperature, urine output and color, coagulation studies. If CK and/or K+ rise more than transiently or urine output falls to less than 0.5 ml/kg/hr, induce diuresis to >1 ml/kg/hr and give bicarbonate to alkalanize urine to prevent myoglobinuria-induced renal failure. (See D below)
- Venous blood gas (e.g., femoral vein) values may document hypermetabolism better than arterial values.
- Central venous or PA monitoring as needed and record minute ventilation.
- Place Foley catheter and monitor urine output.

POST ACUTE PHASE

Ⓐ Observe the patient in an ICU for at least 24 hours, due to the risk of recrudescence.
Ⓑ Dantrolene 1 mg/kg q 4-6 hours or 0.25 mg/kg/hr by infusion for at least 24 hours. Further doses may be indicated.
Ⓒ Follow vitals and labs as above (see #7)
- Frequent ABG as per clinical signs
- CK every 8-12 hours; less often as the values trend downward

Ⓓ Follow urine myoglobin and institute therapy to prevent myoglobin precipitation in renal tubules and the subsequent development of Acute Renal Failure. CK levels above 10,000 IU/L is a presumptive sign of rhabdomyolysis and myoglobinuria. Follow standard intensive care therapy for acute rhabdomyolysis and myoglobinuria (urine output >2 ml/kg/hr by hydration and diuretics along with alkalinization of urine with Na-bicarbonate infusion with careful attention to both urine and serum pH values).
Ⓔ Counsel the patient and family regarding MH and further precautions; refer them to MHAUS. Fill out and send in the Adverse Metabolic Reaction to Anesthesia (AMRA) form (www.mhreg.org) and send a letter to the patient and her/his physician. Refer patient to the nearest Biopsy Center for follow-up.

Non-Emergency Information
MHAUS
PO Box 1069 (11 East State Street)
Sherburne, NY 13460-1069
Phone
1-800-986-4287
(607-674-7901)
Fax
607-674-7910
Email
info@mhaus.org
Website
www.mhaus.org

Since 1981
Dedicated to Patient Safety

CAUTION: This protocol may not apply to all patients; alter for specific needs.

CAPO 5/00/5K   Produced by the Malignant Hyperthermia Association of the United States (MHAUS). MHAUS is a non-profit organization under IRS-Code 501(c)3. It operates solely on contributed funds. All contributions are tax deductible. For more information, go to www.mhaus.org.

H

Herbal Medications

The authors and publisher have exerted every effort to ensure that the herbal medication selection in this appendix is in accord with current recommendations and practice at the time of publication.

The editors wish to acknowledge the contribution of Stella A. Haddadin, BSc, PharmD, Yale–New Haven Hospital, Department of Pharmacy Services, in the preparation of this appendix.

ALFALFA

Uses: Diuretic, kidney, bladder and prostate conditions, hyperglycemia, asthma, arthritis, indigestion

Interaction/toxicity: Excessive use may interfere with anticoagulant therapy, potentiate drug-induced photosensitivity, and interfere with hormone therapy.

ANGELICA ROOT

Uses: Gastrointestinal spasm, loss of appetite, feeling of fullness, and flatulence

Interaction/toxicity: Can cause photodermatitis, claims to increase stomach acid, therefore, interferes with antacids, sucralfate, H2 antagonists, and proton pump inhibitors. Potentiates the effects and adverse effects of anticoagulants and antiplatelet drugs.

ANISE

Uses: Dyspepsia and as a pediatric antiflatulent and expectorant

Interaction/toxicity: Excessive doses can prolong coagulation, increasing PT/INR because of coumarin contained in anise. An interaction exists with anticoagulant therapy, MAOIs, and hormone therapy. Catecholamine activity might increase blood pressure readings and increase heart rate.

ARNICA FLOWER

Uses: Antiphlogistic, antiseptic, anti-inflammatory, analgesic
Interaction/toxicity: Potentiates anticoagulant and antiplatelet effect of drugs and possibly increases risk of bleeding.

ASAFOETIDA

Uses: Chronic bronchitis, asthma, pertussis, hoarseness, hysteria, flatulent colic, chronic gastric, dyspepsia, irritable colon, and convulsions
Interaction/toxicity: Might increase the risk of bleeding, and excessive doses might interfere with blood pressure control. Can irritate GI tract and is contraindicated in patients with infectious or inflammatory GI conditions.

BILBERRY

Uses: Peripheral vascular disease, diabetes, ophthalmologic diseases, peptic ulcer disease and scleroderma.
Interaction/toxicity: Excessive use may interfere with coagulation and inhibit platelet aggregation; alters glucose regulation.

BOGBEAN

Uses: Rheumatism, loss of appetite, dyspepsia
Interaction/toxicity: Potentiates anticoagulant and antiplatelet drugs and possibly increases risk of bleeding.

BROMELAIN

Uses: Acute postoperative and posttraumatic conditions of swelling, especially of the nasal and paranasal sinuses, osteoarthritis
Interaction/toxicity: Potentiates anticoagulant and antiplatelet drugs and possibly increases risk of bleeding. Increases plasma and urine tetracycline level.

CAYENNE

Uses: Muscle spasms, chronic pain
Interaction/toxicity: Overdose may cause hypothermia. May cause skin blisters.

CELERY

Uses: Rheumatism, gout, hysteria, nervousness, weight loss as a result of malnutrition, loss of appetite, exhaustion, sedative, mild diuretic, urinary antiseptic, digestive aid, antiflatulent, blood purification
Interaction/toxicity: Potentiates anticoagulant and antiplatelet drugs and possibly increases risk of bleeding. There is an additive effect with drugs with sedative properties and may cause increase in phototoxic response to psoralen plus ultraviolet light A (PUVA) therapy because of its psoralen content.

CHAMOMILE

Uses: Flatulence, nervous diarrhea, restlessness, insomnia, antispasmodic
Interaction/toxicity: Concomitant use with benzodiazepines might cause additive effects and side effects. Potentiates anticoagulant and antiplatelet drugs and possibly increases risk of bleeding. Is an inhibitor of the cytochrome P450 3A4 enzyme system.

CLOVE

Uses: Flatulence, nausea, and vomiting
Interaction/toxicity: Potentiates anticoagulant and antiplatelet drugs and possibly increases risk of bleeding.

DANDELION

Uses: Diuretic, GI disorders and anti-inflammatory effect
Interaction/toxicity: Excessive use may interfere with coagulation and inhibit platelet aggregation; alters glucose regulation. Do not use in the presence of biliary obstruction. Interactions with digoxin, lithium, insulin, oral hypoglycemics, cytochrome P450, ciprofloxacin, disulfram and metronidazole.

DANSHEN

Uses: Circulation problems, cardiovascular diseases, chronic hepatitis, abdominal masses, insomnia because of palpitations and tight chest, acne, psoriasis, eczema, aids in wound healing
Interaction/toxicity: Potentiates anticoagulant and antiplatelet drugs and possibly increases risk of bleeding. Increases the cardiovascular effects and side effects of digoxin.

DEVIL'S CLAW

Uses: Osteoarthritis, rheumatoid arthritis, gout, myalgia, fibrositis
Interaction/toxicity: Can affect heart rate, contractility of heart, and blood pressure. Might decrease blood glucose levels and have additive effects with medications used for diabetes. May cause an increase in gastric acid secretions.

DONG QUAI

Uses: Gynecologic ailments, menopausal symptoms
Interaction/toxicity: Potentiates anticoagulant and antiplatelet drugs and possibly increases risk of bleeding.

ECHINACEA

Uses: Common colds, urinary tract infections
Interaction/toxicity: May cause hepatotoxicity especially with other concomitant hepatotoxins. Antagonizes steroids and immunosuppressants. May possess immunosuppressive activity after long-term use.

EPHEDRA

Uses: Diet aid, bacteriostatic, antitussive
Interaction/toxicity: May cause arrhythmias with inhalation anesthetics and cardiac glycosides. Life-threatening reaction with MAOIs. May cause depletion of catecholamines and lead to perioperative hemodynamic instability. Can cause death.

FENUGREEK

Uses: Lower blood sugar in diabetics
Interaction/toxicity: Potentiates anticoagulant and antiplatelet drugs and possibly increases risk of bleeding. Inhibits corticosteroid drug activity, interferes with hormone therapy, can alter blood glucose control, and potentiate effect of MAOIs.

FEVERFEW

Uses: Migraine prophylaxis, antipyretic

Interaction/toxicity: Inhibit platelet activity. Potentiates anticoagulants. Abrupt withdrawal may cause rebound headaches. Uterine stimulant. Associated with serotonin syndrome.

FISH OIL

Uses: Cardiovascular disease, colon cancer, psychiatric disorders, diabetes, inflammatory disease, inflammatory bowel diseases, premenstrual syndrome and scleroderma

Interaction/toxicity: Excessive use may interfere with coagulation and inhibit platelet aggregation; alters glucose regulation; potentiates anti-hypertensive drugs.

FLAXSEED OIL

Uses: Cardiovascular disease, colon cancer, psychiatric disorders, diabetes, inflammatory disease, inflammatory bowel diseases, breast cancer and depression

Interaction/toxicity: Excessive use may interfere with coagulation and inhibit platelet aggregation; alters glucose regulation.

GARLIC (PERTAINS TO SUPPLEMENT PRODUCT)

Uses: Lower lipids, antihypertensive, antiplatelet, antioxidant, antithrombolytic

Interaction/toxicity: Potentiates anticoagulants, especially in the presence of drugs that inhibit platelet function. Potentiates vasodilator drugs and antihypertensives. May decrease blood glucose levels as a result of increased serum insulin levels.

GINGER (PERTAINS TO SUPPLEMENT PRODUCT)

Uses: Antinauseant, antispasmodic

Interaction/toxicity: Inhibits thromboxane synthetase. Potentiates anticoagulants. May alter effects of calcium channel blockers.

GINKGO

Uses: Circulatory stimulant, inhibit platelets

Interaction/toxicity: Potentiates anticoagulants, especially in the presence of aspirin, NSAIDs, heparin, and warfarin.

GINSENG

Uses: Antioxidant

Interaction/toxicity: Antagonize anticoagulants. Avoid use of sympathetic stimulants, which may result in tachycardia or hypertension. Possesses hypoglycemic effects. Potentiates digoxin and MAOIs.

GOLDENSEAL

Uses: Diuretic, anti-inflammatory, hemostatic

Interaction/toxicity: May worsen edema and hypertension. Oxytocic possesses activity.

GRAPE SEED

Uses: Anti-oxidant, cardiovascular disorders, peripheral circulatory disorders, multiple sclerosis, Parkinson's disease

Interaction/toxicity: Excessive use may interfere with coagulation and inhibit platelet aggregation; may inhibit xanthine oxidase.

GREEN TEA

Uses: Improves cognitive performance, lowers cholesterol and triglycerides, aids in the prevention of breast, bladder, esophageal, and pancreatic cancers. Decreased risk of Parkinson's disease, gingivitis, obesity

Interaction/toxicity: Concomitant use might inhibit effect of adenosine and antagonize effect of warfarin. Because of the caffeine content, there is an increase in cardiac inotropic effects of beta-adrenergic agonist drugs, an increase in the effects and toxicity of clozapine, and an increased risk of agitation, tremors, and insomnia in combination with ephedrine. It might precipitate hypertensive crisis with MAOIs as well. Might reduce sedative effects of benzodiazepines.

HORSE CHESTNUT

Uses: Scleroderma, peripheral vascular disorders, varicose veins and relieving pain, tiredness, tension, swelling in legs, itching, and edema

Interaction/toxicity: Excessive use may interfere with coagulation and inhibit platelet aggregation; phosphodiesterase inhibitor and alters glucose regulation. Potentiates anticoagulant and antiplatelet drugs and possibly increases risk of bleeding, hypoglycemic effects, might interfere with binding of protein binding drugs.

KAVA-KAVA

Uses: Anxiolytic, analgesic

Interaction/toxicity: Potentiates barbiturates, opioids, and benzodiazepines.

LICORICE

Uses: Heal gastric and duodenal ulcers

Interaction/toxicity: May cause hypertension, hypokalemia, and edema.

LOVAGE ROOT

Uses: Used for inflammation of the lower urinary tract and prevention of kidney gravel; in "irrigation therapy," it is used as a mild diuretic

Interaction/toxicity: Might increase sodium retention and interfere with diuretic therapy.

MEADOWSWEET

Uses: Supportive therapy for colds

Interaction/toxicity: Can potentiate narcotic effects. Contains a salicylate constituent.

ONIONS

Uses: Loss of appetite, preventing atherosclerosis, dyspepsia, fever, colds, cough, tendency toward infection, and inflammation of the mouth and pharynx

Interaction/toxicity: May enhance antidiabetic drug effects and alter blood sugar control. Might enhance antiplatelet drug activity and increase bleeding risk.

PAPAIN
Uses: Inflammation and swelling in patient with pharyngitis
Interaction/toxicity: Concomitant use with anticoagulant and antiplatelet drugs may increase risk of bleeding.

PARSLEY
Uses: Breath freshener, urinary tract infections, and kidney or bladder stones
Interaction/toxicity: Might interfere with oral anticoagulant therapy because of the Vitamin K contained in parsley. May interfere with diuretic therapy by enhancing sodium retention. Might potentiate MAOI drug therapy.

PASSION FLOWER
Uses: Generalized anxiety disorder
Interaction/toxicity: Concomitant use with barbiturates can increase drug-induced sleep time; can potentiate the effects of sedatives and tranquilizers, including sedative effects of antihistamines.

QUASSIA
Uses: Anorexia, indigestion, fever, mouthwash, as an anthelmintic for thread worms, nematodes, and ascaris
Interaction/toxicity: Stimulates gastric acid and might oppose effect of antacids and H2 antagonists. Excessive doses might have additive effects with anticoagulant therapy with Coumadin. Concomitant use of potassium-depleting diuretics or stimulant laxative abuse might increase risk of cardiac glycoside toxicity as a result of potassium loss.

RED CLOVER
Uses: Hot flashes
Interaction/toxicity: Can increase the anticoagulant effects and bleeding risk because of its coumarin content. May interfere with hormone replacement therapy or oral contraceptives, and may interfere with tamoxifen because of its potential estrogenic effects. Can inhibit cytochrome P450 (cyp450) 3A4.

SAW PALMETTO
Uses: Benign prostatic hypertrophy, antiandrogenic
Interaction/toxicity: Potentiates birth control pills and estrogens. May cause hypertension.

ST. JOHN'S WORT
Uses: Depression, anxiety
Interaction/toxicity: Possible interaction/toxicity with MAOIs and meperidine. May prolong anesthetic effects. Potentiates digoxin. May decrease effects of warfarin, steroids, and possibly benzodiazepines and calcium channel blockers.

SWEET CLOVER

Uses: Chronic venous insufficiency, including leg pain and heaviness, night-time leg cramps, itching and swelling, for supportive treatment of thrombo-phlebitis, lymphatic congestion, postthrombotic syndromes, and hemorrhoids
Interaction/toxicity: Use with hepatotoxic drugs might increase risk of hepa-totoxicity. Concomitant use with anticoagulant and antiplatelet drugs may increase risk of bleeding.

TURMERIC

Uses: Dyspepsia, jaundice, hepatitis, flatulence, abdominal bloating
Interaction/toxicity: Concomitant use with anticoagulant and antiplatelet drugs may increase risk of bleeding.

VALERIAN

Uses: Sedative, anxiolytic
Interaction/toxicity: Potentiates barbiturates and anesthetics. May blunt symptoms of benzodiazepine withdrawal.

VITAMIN E

Uses: Vitamin E deficiency, heart disease
Interaction/toxicity: Concomitant use with anticoagulant and antiplatelet drugs may increase risk of bleeding. Might prevent tolerance to nitrates.

WILLOW BARK

Uses: Lower back pain, fever, rheumatic ailments, headache
Interaction/toxicity: Enough salicylate is present in willow bark to cause drug interactions common to salicylates or aspirin. Can impair effectiveness of beta-adrenergic blockers, probenecid, and sulfinpyrazone. Can increase effects, side effects, or toxicity of alcohol, anticoagulants, carbonic anhydrase inhibitors, heparin, methotrexate, NSAIDs, sulfonylureas, and valproic acid.

Answer Section

1. B

On October 16, 1846, William T. G. Morton induced general anesthesia with ether, which allowed surgeon John Collins Warren to remove a vascular tumor from Edward Gilbert Abbott. This demonstration is considered the first successful public administration of anesthesia for a surgical procedure. Charles Jackson, a notable Boston physician, chemist, and Morton's preceptor, stated that he counseled Morton on the use of inhaled ether for insensibility to pain, but was not the first to publicly demonstrate its use as a surgical anesthetic. Priestley lived in the 1700s and was known for his isolation of oxygen in its gaseous form and his isolation of nitrous oxide. Bigelow observed Morton's demonstration and wrote about it in the *Boston Medical and Surgical Journal*.

2. C

Various anesthetics such as ethyl chloride, ethylene, and cyclopropane, had a variety of drawbacks such as their pungent nature, weak potency, and flammability. The discovery that fluorination contributed to making anesthetics more stable, less toxic, and less combustible led to the introduction of halothane in the 1950s. The 1960s and 1970s would bring about various fluorinated anesthetics such as isoflurane, which is still widely used today.

3. D

The first medically used NMBA, Intocostrin, was based on the drug curare. Applied to arrows and darts, its paralyzing effects were originally employed for hunting and warfare. Pancuronium and vecuronium belong to the class of NMBA's known as nondepolarizing and were introduced into clinical practice much later. Succinylcholine was developed in 1949 by Nobel Laureate Daniel Bovet and is depolarizing NBMA.

4. A

In 1926, Lundy introduced the term balanced anesthesia to describe a combination of several anesthetic agents and strategies to produce unconsciousness, neuromuscular block, and analgesia, which included an opioid and an inhalant anesthetic.

5. C

Cocaine, originally described by Austrian ophthalmologist Carl Koller in 1884 as a local anesthetic, became a mainstay for regional anesthesia through the early 1900s. However, adverse effects, including postdural puncture headache, vomiting, and its addictive quality, necessitated the development of local anesthetics such as procaine in 1905 and lidocaine in 1943, which were much safer. Bupivacaine was synthesized in 1957.

1. D

There are no signals from the peripheral chemoreceptors to the respiratory centers when $PaO_2 > 100$ mm Hg. Signaling to the respiratory centers is initiated at arterial partial pressure of oxygen (PaO_2) 100 mm Hg, but minute ventilation does not begin to increase until oxygen partial pressure falls below 65 mm Hg, at which point tidal volume and ventilation rate are increased.

2. A

During spontaneous ventilation, both ventilation and perfusion are greater in gravity-dependent areas.

3. D
Arterial hypoxemia does not occur instantaneously during apnea because the capillary blood that continues to perfuse the alveoli extracts oxygen from within the functional residual capacity (FRC), the volume of gas left in the lung after passive end-expiration. The extraction of oxygen is influenced minimally by the decrease in oxygen consumption caused by zero work of breathing and has nothing to do with total lung capacity. Lung perfusion does not decrease because of apnea; it is primarily determined by the cardiac output, which does not change because of apnea alone.

4. B
During nonstrenuous (resting) breathing, the diaphragm does the vast majority of work of inspiration (active) and exhalation is mainly due to the relaxation of inspiratory muscles (passive).

5. B
Body chemoreceptors respond primarily to lack of oxygen, whereas central chemoreceptors react to elevations in carbon dioxide.

Answers Chapter 3

1. A
The subendocardium is exposed to higher pressures than the subepicardium throughout the cardiac cycle, particularly during systole: thus, the former requires a greater perfusion pressure that may not be possible in the presence of coronary stenosis. With a coronary circulation oxygen extraction ratio of ~70%, oxygen content normally decreases from 20 to 6 mL O_2/100 mL blood. Resting coronary blood flow is normally ~5% of total cardiac output. Coronary perfusion of the LV is dependent on the difference between diastolic aortic pressure and LV diastolic pressure.

2. C
As shown in Figure 3-10, cardiac output is determined by SV and heart rate. SV is the difference between EDV and ESV in the LV and is determined by the ejection fraction. Ejection fraction is a function of preload (EDV), afterload (SVR), and contractility. Although the atrial kick may enhance LV EDV, end-diastolic LA pressure does not determine cardiac output.

3. D
Diastolic dysfunction occurs when the ventricle cannot adequately collect blood due to insufficient LV filling time (tachycardia), obstruction to LV filling (mitral stenosis), or resistance to filling by reduced LV wall compliance (compression by external mediastinal mass). A mixed venous pO_2 of 45 mm Hg is normal and does not affect diastolic function.

4. B
The normal mixed venous pO_2 in the pulmonary artery is 40 mm Hg. Because the P50 of normal hemoglobin A is 27 mm Hg, a blood sample pO_2 of 23 mm Hg corresponds to an oxygen saturation of 30% to 40%, which can only be found near the coronary sinus due to the high oxygen extraction ratio (~70%) in the coronary circulation.

5. C
With spontaneous inspiration, venous return to the RV is increased, resulting in prolonged RV ejection time compared with the LV. This causes the pulmonic valve to close later than the aortic valve, producing respiration-induced variation in splitting of S_2 (physiologic splitting).

6. D
Myocardial oxygen supply increases to match oxygen demand under normal conditions. When supply cannot increase to meet demand (coronary artery disease), myocardial ischemia is first manifest by decreased LV compliance and increased LV EDV. If demand further exceeds supply, wall motion abnormalities (TEE) appear next, followed by reduced LV ejection fraction, and eventual ST segment changes, CHF, and cardiogenic shock.

7. C
As shown in Figure 3-8, the area within the LV pressure-volume diagram corresponds to stroke work (SW). If the MAP is known, SV can be

calculated (SV = SW/MAP). If the heart rate (HR) is also known, then cardiac output (CO) can be calculated (CO = SV * HR). Myocardial oxygenation consumption requires measurement of oxygen content in the aorta and the coronary sinus and cannot be determined from the pressure-volume diagram.

8. B
Frank-Starling ventricular function plots require information for LV end-diastolic pressure (x-axis) and SV (y-axis). The former can be estimated from the pulmonary artery wedge pressure, while the latter can be calculated either from the cardiac output (CO) and heart rate (HR) (SV = CO/HR) or from the LV stroke work (SW) and the MAP (SV = SW/MAP). SVR is not needed to construct such a curve.

9. C
Venous return to the RA is enhanced by the combination of extremity muscle contractions and passive one-way valves in extremity veins (muscle pump), as well as by spontaneous ventilation (thoracoabdominal pump). Skeletal muscle paralysis impairs venous return by impairing both the muscle pump and the thoracoabdominal pump. Trendelenburg position enhances venous return by increasing the hydrostatic pressure gradient to the RA. Passive one-way valves in extremity veins are not affected by general anesthesia. Positive pressure ventilation impairs venous return by reducing the hydrostatic pressure gradient to the RA.

10. D
Plasma oncotic pressure is primarily determined by circulating albumin; thus, hypoalbuminemia will reduce oncotic pressure, but will not affect either hydrostatic pressure or capillary membrane permeability. If all other variables in the Starling equation are held constant, the lower oncotic pressure gradient across the capillary membrane in the setting of hypoalbuminemia will favor increased fluid movement from the intravascular compartment to the extravascular space.

Answers | Chapter 4

1. C
Physostigmine crosses the blood–brain barrier to exert its central effect. Pyridostigmine does not cross the blood–brain barrier and therefore it is the reason the drug is used to reverse nondepolarizing muscle relaxants.

2. A
A known complication of interscalene nerve block is development of Horner syndrome due to blockade, hematoma, or injury to the stellate ganglion. Hoarseness is the result of similar mechanisms to the recurrent laryngeal nerve.

3. D
In many cases of cerebral spinal fluid leakage, ocular and auditory signs can appear. In this case the patient is manifesting neurologic signs of an abducens nerve (cranial nerve) injury (external rectus muscle). This occurs with spinal fluid loss because the abducens nerve has the longest pathway in the skull and is thus prone to injury when the cushioning effect of spinal fluid is lost.

Cranial nerve III controls the internal rectus, which is not consistent with the findings of the image (unopposed pull of medial rectus muscle).

4. C
The only two hormones synthesized in the hypothalamus are antidiuretic hormone and oxytocin. Other than these two compounds, the hypothalamus synthesizes releasing factors (e.g., corticotropin releasing factor, thyrotropin releasing hormone, etc.), which are discharged from the hypothalamus to the pituitary gland.

5. B
In the somatic nervous system, the motor cell bodies are located within the CNS. In the autonomic nervous system, the analogous structures are located in ganglia, outside the CNS. Further, the parasympathetic nervous system ganglia are peripherally located near the target organ. Somatic efferent nerves transverse the anterior root of the spinal cord. The somatic efferent nerve interneuron is in the spinal cord.

6. C
The nerves with the fastest neural transmission are myelinated, α-motor neurons (at ~100 m/sec). In contrast, slow pain neuron transmit impulses at ~1 m/sec.

7. C
A transient decrease in cardiac output is observed. This is associated with a more sustained increase in heart rate as seen in patients with autonomic dysfunction tested with a Valsalva maneuver. The systolic arterial pressure decrease is significant, averaging 20–30 mm Hg.

Answers   Chapter 5

1. D
No compound or ion is actively transported across the thin descending loop of Henle.

2. D
Autoregulation of renal blood pressure occurs between mean arterial pressure of 70 to 125 mm Hg and results in the maintenance of renal blood flow and glomerular filtration rate within relatively tight levels.

3. C
Arterial oxygen saturation has little to do with renal autoregulation of renal blood flow.

4. B
Nitric oxide is the predominant intrinsic renal vasodilator. Both prostaglandins and endothelial-derived hyperpolarizing factor contribute a smaller vascular action. Aldosterone is part of a chain of events that leads to increased blood pressure, including the renal artery.

5. A
This graph shows that as GFR is reduced and serum creatinine rises asymptotically.

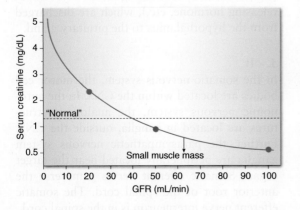

6. A
GFR is employed in the RIFLE classification but not for AKIN. The other choices are used in both classification systems.

7. A
This patient has respiratory acidosis. The renal compensation for this acid-base abnormality is excretion H^+ and generating new HCO_3^- to restore normal acid base balance.

8. A
The predominant renal diuretic action of dopamine is to reduce Na^+ reabsorption in the proximal tubule, thus producing natriuresis. Its cardiac effects contribute little to the diuretic effect. Dopamine is not protective against renal injury. Fenoldopam, although a diuretic and used by some clinicians for renal protection, is approved by the U.S. Food and Drug Administration only for treatment of hypertension.

9. A
The tubule is very sensitive to hypoxemia. In this situation, the efferent arteriole constricts to maintain glomerular pressure and filtration. Thus, there is a reduction in blood flow to the capillaries and tubular apparatus. Due to its high metabolic demands for filtration, the tubule is highly vulnerable to ischemia.

10. A
As a nonsteroidal anti-inflammatory drug, ibuprofen will constrict the renal afferent arteriole, reducing renal plasma flow, which decreases glomerular pressure. This results in a decrease GFR, with less creatinine filtered, leading to an increase in serum creatinine.

Answers Chapter 6

1. C
The liver receives 25% of total cardiac output, with 25% of the blood supply coming from the hepatic artery (oxygenated blood) and 75% from the portal vein (deoxygenated blood). Because of the differences in blood flow and oxygenation, each blood supply delivers a similar amount of oxygen content to the liver.

2. C
Because hepatic Kupffer cells and dendritic cells comprise part of the mononuclear phagocyte system, liver failure increases the frequency and severity of systemic infections. Because impaired hepatic protein synthesis reduces both plasma oncotic pressure and the production of various coagulation factors, liver failure results in increased extravascular fluid accumulation (edema, ascites) and impaired coagulation, respectively. However, impaired glycogen storage in patients with liver failure is more likely to result in hypoglycemia, rather than hyperglycemia.

3. B
Dynamic laboratory tests of liver function include measure of substrate half-life, elimination capacity, and metabolite formation (Fig. 6-5); thus, they are likely more indicative of liver function than static tests (e.g., blood AST, ALT). However, dynamic tests require specialized facilities and procedures and are not widely available.

4. B
An elevated AST/ALT ratio (>2) is most likely associated with alcoholic hepatitis or cirrhosis. Biliary obstruction due to gallstones or pancreatic masses is unlikely to result in an elevated AST/ALT ratio, although the AP and GGT would likely be elevated. Acute viral hepatitis may result in elevated AST and ALT, but the AST/ALT ratio is unlikely to be elevated.

5. C
Drugs with a high extraction ratio are cleared quickly, with significant first-pass liver metabolism. However, elimination of such drugs is highly dependent on hepatic blood flow. Therefore, in the case of hypovolemic shock, drug X will be cleared rapidly by Patient NL, but more slowly by Patient HS.

Answers Chapter 7

1. D
Oral administration results in first-pass metabolism by the liver and reduces bioavailability. Further, lower perfusion of the gastrointestinal system also decreases bioavailability.

2. C
Oral administration results in first-pass metabolism via the liver. Oral administration results in both lower peak plasma concentrations and time to peak plasma concentration. Plasma concentrations are affected by gastrointestinal perfusion.

3. A
Anesthetic drug transport to or from the tissue is usually not saturable. Drug uptake by the tissue is limited by blood flow to the tissue (flow limited drug uptake). The other choices will not have a major effect on equilibration.

4. C
Fentanyl is lipophilic. To be excreted, it must be transformed to a hydrophilic compound or a glucuronide, which is excreted by both kidney and liver.

5. B
Clearance of these drugs is affected by blood flow (e.g., decrease in blood flow decreases clearance). Midazolam clearance is predominantly determined by an enzymatic reaction.

6. B
Half-life is useful in estimating the rise in drug concentration to a steady state. Half-life combines the concepts of volume of distribution and elimination clearance.

7. C

Most opioids and hypnotics are lipophilic (required to pass the blood–brain barrier). Dosing to actual body weight overshoots dose; targeting to ideal body weight underestimates dose. Many clinicians use a combination of both, the pharmacologic body weight (ideal body weight + 0.33 [actual body weight – ideal body weight]).

8. C

The dose–response relation is unable to correctly identify whether pharmacodynamics, pharmacokinetics, or both are responsible for interpatient variability. The curvilinear dose–response curve is a more appropriate manner in describing this relation.

9. C

The addition of an opioid to a volatile anesthetic produces a supra-additive (synergistic) effect.

Therefore, even a small dose of remifentanil (i.e., a 0.05 μg/kg/min infusion) decreases the amount of sevoflurane required to prevent nociception induced movement or hemodynamic responses by 30–40%. Isoproterenol decreases the level of plasma propofol. SSRI's decrease the clinical effectiveness of codeine. Methylene blue can result in serotonin syndrome given to patients taking selective serotonin reuptake inhibitors (SSRI's).

10. D

The graphic displays the context sensitive half-time (CSt₁/₂) of four commonly used opioids (fentanyl [F], alfentanil [A], sufentanil [S], and remifentanil [R]). Of these compounds, remifentanil has the most unique CSt₁/₂, which accounts for shorter offset. CSt₁/₂ is not a pharmacokinetic parameter, but is derived from computer simulation. As the duration of infusion increases, the CSt₁/₂ increases, but the least with remifentanil.

Answers   Chapter 8

1. A

Xenon is a gas that is stored in a tank and does not require vaporization.

2. C

Inhaled anesthetics that have low solubility in blood can induce anesthesia most rapidly, as well as allow rapid awakening from anesthesia.

3. C

Induction of anesthesia with inhaled anesthetics (rate of rise of F_A relative to F_I) is increased by an increase in alveolar ventilation. It is slower when cardiac output is high. It is relatively unaffected by blood pressure or obesity.

4. A

Because blood flow to fat is a small fraction of total cardiac output, it does not play a significant role in determining the rate of induction with inhaled anesthetics.

5. D

MAC is a tool for comparison of potency of inhaled anesthetics. It is determined in patients

by measuring the alveolar concentration of anesthetic required to prevent movement in response to a skin incision in 50% of patients. Patients are unconscious at 1 MAC but not adequately anesthetized for surgery.

6. C

All of the volatile inhaled anesthetics increase cerebral blood flow despite a modest reduction in blood pressure and cardiac output.

7. B

Sevoflurane causes minimal irritation of the upper respiratory tract. Nitrous oxide is not a complete anesthetic. Induction with desflurane and isoflurane is commonly associated with coughing and laryngospasm.

8. D

Abrupt discontinuation of nitrous oxide and inhalation of air can cause diffusion hypoxia. Alveolar oxygen is diluted by an effusion of nitrous oxide into the alveoli from the blood and inhalation of a high concentration of nitrogen.

9. A
All of the volatile anesthetics produce relaxation of uterine muscle. Contraction of the uterus is necessary to control bleeding following delivery of an infant.

10. D
Xenon has many properties of the ideal anesthetic (such as high potency, rapid onset of action, few side effects, no metabolites). However, because it must be extracted from the atmosphere, it is extremely expensive.

Answers | Chapter 9

1. B
Barbiturates depress the reticular activating system in the brainstem and are believed to potentiate the action of $GABA_A$ receptors, increasing the duration of an associated chloride ion channel opening. Barbiturates also decrease cerebral metabolic rate of oxygen, cerebral blood flow, and intracranial pressure.

2. D
Benzodiazepines can be pharmacologically reversed with flumazenil, a specific competitive antagonist with a high affinity for the benzodiazepine receptor site. Flumazenil is cleared more rapidly than the benzodiazepines, so patients must be monitored as resedation may occur and additional doses of flumazenil may be required.

3. B
Similar to propofol, etomidate can cause pain upon injection. Etomidate transiently inhibits 11-β-hydroxlase (not methionine synthetase).

Etomidate is frequently used because it causes minimal hemodynamic depression. Lastly, it is capable of producing convulsion-like EEG potentials in epileptic patients.

4. A
Unlike propofol and etomidate, ketamine's major effects are mediated through its potent antagonism of the NMDA receptor, rather than action at the $GABA_A$ receptor. Dexmedetomidine acts only on α_2 receptors.

5. C
Dexmedetomidine produces sedation and analgesia by acting only on α_2 receptors. These receptors are not involved with respiration, thus minimal respiratory depression is observed. It is metabolized in the liver and the by-products are excreted via bile and urine. Compared to benzodiazepines in the intensive care unit, dexmedetomidine is associated with a lower incidence of delirium.

Answers | Chapter 10

1. A
NSAIDs inhibit the synthesis of prostanoids including thromboxane A2 as well as prostacycline. Thus, NSAIDs decrease the concentration of these two prostanoids but not their inflammatory and other effects. Arachidonic acid is released from cell membranes during tissue injury and is not directly affected by NSAIDs.

2. C
Celecoxib is relatively selective in its inhibition of cyclooxygenase COX-2 and not COX-1, which is the enzyme responsible for the platelet

effects of the nonselective COX inhibitors including ketorolac. Rofecoxib and valdecoxib are selective COX-2 inhibitors but they have been removed from the market because of increased cardiac-related morbidity and mortality.

3. D
Clonidine and dexmedetomidine are α_2 adrenergic receptor agonists. These receptors are found throughout the brain and the posterior horn of the spinal cord, which is the most significant site of their analgesic effects. The other mechanisms listed are not applicable.

4. A

The context-sensitive half-time of a drug is a key parameter when the duration of a drug infusion is significant. For all opioids except remifentanil, the context-sensitive half-time increases substantially as the duration of the infusion increases. Thus, the duration of their action increases as well. Remifentanil is the exception because it is so rapidly metabolized by plasma esterases.

5. B

Sufentanil is approximately 10 times more potent than fentanyl, 40 times more than hydromorphone, and 200 times more than methadone.

6. B

The formula for the calculation is: modified fat free mass = fat free mass + 0.4 (total body mass – fat free mass), so 70 – 0.4 (140 – 70) = 98 kg.

Answers   Chapter 11

1. B

Both hypermagnesemia and hypocalcemia antagonize release of acetylcholine from the nerve terminal. The potassium channels limit calcium entry into the terminal.

2. B

Potency, as described by degree of depression of normal muscle contraction, is best expressed as the ED_{95}. The RI_{25-75} and TOF >0.9 are not appropriate descriptors of potency.

3. C

A phase II block exhibits all the muscle contraction characteristics of a nondepolarizing block EXCEPT it cannot be reversed by an anticholinesterase drug.

4. A

The most consistent manner to reduce postsuccinylcholine myalgias is by use of nonsteroidal anti-inflammatory drugs. Although defasciculating doses of nondepolarizing neuromuscular blockers are commonly used, their effect is inconsistent.

5. B

Use of ideal body weight will result in underdosing of succinylcholine and will fail to rapidly secure an airway.

6. C

The plasma/biophase concentration effect explains the rapidity of onset for rocuronium, for example. The greater concentration difference

between plasma and biophase helps explains rocuronium's rapid onset because it is much less potent.

7. B

Inhalation agents potentiate the effect of neuromuscular blockers. Desflurane potentiates to the greatest degree. Higher concentration of inhalation agents and prolonged exposure to the agent will further potentiate the neuromuscular block.

8. A

Muscle failure (myopathy) is commonly seen in mechanically ventilated intensive care patients. All nondepolarizing neuromuscular blockers share this characteristic. Administration of steroids, particularly of long duration, can increase the incidence of myopathy in patients who are also receiving neuromuscular blockers.

9. D

Use of TOF (TOF ≥0.9) to guide therapy for reversal of neuromuscular blockade suggests that since baseline has almost been reached, no additional anticholinergic is required. This is not unique to the neuromuscular blocker, but rather to the detection of residual blockade.

10. C

The pharmacokinetic profile (onset) of glycopyrrolate (2 to 3 minutes) most closely matches that of neostigmine (~5 minutes).

Answers Chapter 12

1. C
In myelinated nerve fibers, local anesthetics bind voltage-gated Na^+ channels at the nodes of Ranvier (such channels do not exist under the myelin sheath) and do not bind to voltage-gated K^+ channels. Local anesthetics have no effect on either the cell's resting membrane potential or its threshold potential.

2. A
Only 1% to 2% of accurately administered local anesthetic reaches the neural membrane due to (a) the very small fraction of local anesthetic present in lipid-soluble form at physiologic pH and (b) the need for anesthetic molecules to penetrate nearby cell walls and multiple layers of perineural connective tissue, including the epineurium, perineurium, and endoneurium.

3. B
Maneuvers that increase the pH of the injected solution (e.g., adding sodium bicarbonate) will increase the lipid-soluble fraction of the solution. In contrast, maneuvers that decrease the pH (adding epinephrine) or clinical conditions that lower tissue pH (infection) will reduce the lipid-soluble fraction of the solution. Injection rate does not affect the lipid-soluble fraction.

4. A
Systemic absorption of local anesthetics depends on total local anesthetic dose, site of administration, physiochemical properties of individual local anesthetics, and addition of vasoconstrictors (epinephrine). Injecting 15 mL of 0.25% bupivacaine results in a lower total dose than 10 mL of 0.5% bupivacaine. Because perineural tissue perfusion is less in the epidural space than in the intercostal spaces, injections into this region result in lower systemic drug uptake.

5. B
Within a typical peripheral nerve, nerve fibers in the outer mantle of the nerve are typically distributed to more proximal anatomic structures, while those in the inner core innervate more distal structures. Therefore, following a successful sciatic nerve block, the skin on the proximal calf would typically lose sensation before

the skin on the sole of the foot because local anesthetic diffusion progresses from the outer surface toward the center of the nerve.

6. C
Plasma cholinesterase metabolizes aminoester local anesthetics and plays no role in aminoamide elimination.

7. C
Cirrhotic liver disease impairs both protein-binding and metabolism of local anesthetics, thereby increasing the risk of local anesthetic systemic toxicity. Epinephrine has minimal effect on extending the duration of blockade when using bupivacaine or ropivacaine. In contrast, because of its piperidine ring substitution and formulation as an S-enantiomer, ropivacaine is less cardiotoxic than bupivacaine.

8. B
Ensuring adequate oxygenation and ventilation is the first step in resuscitation from central nervous system manifestations of local anesthetic systemic toxicity. If this is not successful due to ongoing seizure activity, then antiseizure medication (e.g., benzodiazepines, propofol) should be given and tracheal intubation performed if necessary. Intralipid emulsion may be given for those who do not respond to such initial therapy and may prevent cardiovascular collapse.

9. B
Transient (24 to 48 hours) impairment of adrenocorticoid release is associated with etomidate, not local anesthetics.

10. D
Cardiopulmonary bypass may be considered in patients with refractory ventricular dysrhythmias unresponsive to standard advanced cardiac life support resuscitation protocols, including intravenous epinephrine (reduced dose) and amiodarone. Lidocaine is contraindicated in treating ventricular dysrhythmias caused by bupivacaine systemic toxicity because its similar mechanism of blocking cardiac voltage-gated Na^+ channels may exacerbate the dysrhythmias.

Answers Chapter 13

1. B

Choice "A" is the mechanism responsible for β_1-mediated stimulation including increased heart rate and ventricular contractility. Choices "C" and "D" are erroneous distractors.

2. C

The nonspecific blockade of β receptors by propranolol blunts epinephrine's vasodilatory effects in the peripheral circulation and its inotropic and chronotropic effects on the heart. As a result, the heart rate and contractility response are decreased and the blood pressure and systemic vascular resistance response are increased.

3. C

Norepinephrine stimulates α and β_1 receptors but, unlike epinephrine, not β_2 receptors. Thus, it lacks the peripheral dilating effects due to β_2 stimulation. As a result, the systemic vasoconstriction effects of α stimulation predominate, causing a marked increase in systemic vascular resistance and less increase in cardiac output and heart rate than seen with epinephrine. Although norepinephrine increases inotropy and venous return, these are not the primary causes of its greater effect on blood pressure.

4. A

Ephedrine acts by releasing norepinephrine from the presynaptic terminals of sympathetic neurons. Repeated administration of ephedrine depletes the presynaptic stores of norepinephrine and accounts for the diminishing response.

5. D

By blocking the vasoconstricting effects of the α receptors on the arteriolar vessels, labetalol decreases systemic vascular resistance. In addition, labetalol has direct agonist effects on β_2 receptors and, in stimulating these receptors, further lowers systemic vascular resistance.

6. C

Nitroprusside produces a redistribution of blood flow away from ischemic myocardium (coronary steal) by causing a greater increase in coronary vasodilation in vessels that perfuse normal myocardium than those that perfuse ischemic myocardium. Answers "A", "B," and "D" are correct statements about nitroprusside, but they are not the reason that nitroprusside is relatively contraindicated in patients with myocardial ischemia.

Answers Chapter 14

1. C

The modern anesthesia workstation combines all of the features of older devices into a compact, sophisticated piece of equipment that oversees many of the tasks formerly performed by the anesthesiologist. However, the convenience provided comes at the expense of complexity. When a malfunction occurs, rapid troubleshooting of that problem by the user is not always quickly possible.

2. B

A full E cylinder of oxygen contains roughly 625 L of gas at a pressure of 2,200 psi. As oxygen is used, the pressure in the tank falls linearly in proportion to the amount remaining. A tank approximately half full will have a pressure of 1,100 psi.

3. A

When the flush actuator is activated, oxygen is delivered from the inline source in the anesthetic machine at a pressure of 50 psi directly to the common gas outlet. Vaporizers are bypassed and no anesthetic is delivered to the patient.

4. C

The wall pressure for oxygen and air are similar so the fail-safe, low pressure alarm, and flowmeter proportioning system would not be activated. Unexpectedly low readings on the oxygen analyzer would be the only way to make the diagnosis.

5. A

Desflurane has a boiling point near room temperature, which prevents it from being safely used in a conventional variable bypass vaporizer. Active heating of the vaporizer is required.

6. D

A common cause for an increase in airway pressure during spontaneous ventilation is overexpansion of the rebreathing bag. To relieve the pressure, the APL valve must be opened to vent the excess gas in the system.

7. D

The pressure-limiting relief valve of a ventilator is closed during the inspiratory phase of ventilation. The high fresh gas inflow will add significantly to the preset inspiratory volume and place the patient at risk for barotrauma to the lung.

8. D

Extraction of carbon dioxide by absorbent creates heat as a by-product. A warm canister indicates normal function. Exhaustion of carbon dioxide absorbent is shown by color change of a dye to violet, but the canister will still function if only half exhausted. Compound A is not sensed by capnography. Rebreathing of exhaled carbon dioxide will occur if a unidirectional valve is malfunctioning.

9. C

If a hole existed in the bellows, the "drive gas" (air) would enter the bellows and circle system. This would dilute the oxygen, lower the oxygen analyzer reading, increase the tidal volume delivered to the patient, and allow the bellows to partially collapse between breaths.

10. B

A failure of piped oxygen is rare and should be recognized by a functioning pressure alarm.

Answers | Chapter 15

1. A

These two wavelengths are absorbed differently by oxygenated and deoxygenated blood.

2. D

All of the above can increase alveolar dead space and thus decrease end-tidal carbon dioxide concentration, but a pulmonary embolism would be the most likely to produce a sudden large decrease.

3. B

Cardiac ischemia is best detected by monitoring a five-lead ECG and displaying both leads II and V_5, a technique that can have a sensitivity of up to 80%. V_3 and V_4 may provide sensitivity as good or better than V_5, but their placement may interfere with the surgical field.

4. B

The transducer is zeroed by opening it to atmospheric pressure. Thus, the pressures it measures subsequently are relative to ambient atmospheric pressure.

5. C

The x descent occurs during early ventricular systole as the base of the heart descends, pulling the tricuspid and mitral valves with it and thereby expanding the potential volume of the atria and lowering their pressure.

Answers | Chapter 16

1. B

The patient has no functional limitation. Age alone is not a factor in assigning ASA physical status.

2. D

Although these and other drugs may have significant potentially harmful side effects due to interactions with other drugs used in anesthesia, there is no absolute contraindication to their use during an anesthetic. The decision whether to discontinue treatment should be based on the individual patient, surgical procedure, and drug.

3. B

Excessive bleeding is most problematic when surgery is performed in a closed space, such as following intracranial, middle ear, or intraocular procedures.

4. D

Patients who are addicted to opioids should not have their drugs discontinued preoperatively. To do so will place them at risk for withdrawal. These patients may require immense doses of opioid to control pain. Regional anesthetic techniques are particularly beneficial if continued into the postoperative period.

5. B

Body weight alone does not reliably signify a potentially difficult intubation. The vocal cords can be easily visualized during laryngoscopy in many morbidly obese patients.

6. B

Evidence of unstable coronary artery disease, such as angina at rest, is a major risk factor for cardiovascular complications and a thorough workup is warranted.

7. C

Malfunction of a cardiac implantable electronic device, such as a pacemaker, is most likely when monopolar cautery is used and the surgical site is within 6 inches of the device.

8. B

Due to the risk of undiagnosed hypoglycemia during general anesthesia, blood glucose levels should be maintained slightly above normal.

9. A

Malignant hyperthermia is an inherited disease not linked to rheumatoid arthritis.

10. A

There is general agreement that prophylactic administration of antibiotics reduces the incidence of surgical site infections even when patients are healthy and the surgical procedure does not involve a high risk for contamination.

Answers Chapter 17

1. C

Duchenne muscular dystrophy is characterized by proximal muscle weakness and painless muscle atrophy. Cardiac dysfunction and delayed gastric emptying are common findings. Succinylcholine is contraindicated due to risk of rhabdomyolysis and acute hyperkalemia.

2. A

Myasthenia gravis (MG) is an autoimmune disease that targets postsynaptic, acetylcholine receptors in the neuromuscular junction available for acetylcholine binding. Tensilon testing is the gold standard for MG diagnosis and produces a transient improvement in strength in affected patients. Acute decompensation of MG, or *myasthenic crisis,* is unpredictable and can occur in pregnancy, progressing to profound weakness and acute respiratory failure. Anticholinesterase inhibitors (AChEIs) are typically used as first-line therapy for symptom alleviation. However, in excess, AChEI can induce a *cholinergic crisis,* characterized by hypersalivation, weakness, and bradycardia.

3. C

Malignant hyperthermia (MH) is an autosomal dominant, hypermetabolic disease that can be provoked by potent volatile anesthetics and succinylcholine. Diagnosis can be made clinically, that is, if the signs of a hypermetabolic state—hyperthermia, rigidity, and hypercapnia—occur in the setting of triggering agents, or by the *in vitro contracture test,* also known as the caffeine-halothane contraction test.

4. D

Pseudo-cholinesterase (PChE) deficiency is a disorder that results inefficient ester substrate metabolism. Prolonged muscle relaxation after succinylcholine usually reveals this deficiency. Specific esters agents, such as mivacurium, cocaine, chloroprocaine, procaine, and tetracaine, undergo delayed metabolism in PChE.

5. B

Acute chest syndrome is a life-threatening manifestation of sickle cell disease that presents with acute dyspnea, chest pain, cough, and hypoxia. Aggressive fluid therapy, intravenous opioids, and exchange transfusion should be started immediately to avoid progression to respiratory failure and death. Pulmonary embolism and myocardial infarction may have similar presentations, but are less likely in a young adult.

Answers Chapter 18

1. B

Hypoglycemia in the anesthetized patient can be difficult to recognize. The typical changes of mental status, blood pressure, and heart changes may be obscured by the anesthetic or adjuvants but patients may develop hypertension and tachycardia. Therefore, in many cases the patient is thought to be "light anesthetized." Hypoglycemia is defined as a blood sugar <60 mg/dL and severe hypoglycemia is <40 mg/dL. An increased incidence of hypoglycemia is seen in renal failure patients.

2. C

Acute hypomagnesemia causes increases in parathyroid hormone and thus ionized Ca^{++}. Increases in serum albumin, hyperphosphatemia, and respiratory alkalosis decrease Ca^{++}.

3. C

Dexamethasone is the most clinically used anti-inflammatory corticosteroid. Cortisone is the least potent, and prednisone and triamcinolone occupy a midposition in potency.

4. B

Of the commonly used corticosteroids, prednisone and methylprednisone are the most potent mineralocorticoids. Triamcinolone and dexamethasone do not possess mineralocorticoid actions.

5. D

Of the drugs affecting thyroid function, amiodarone is the most deleterious. Propanolol does not raise thyroid-stimulating hormone. The remaining choices do not affect thyroid function.

6. A

See table below. The patient has the classic features of a hyperthyroid patient (Graves' disease). The other profiles represent different subsets of patients and their thyroid biochemical profile.

	Free Thyroxine (T₄)	Free Triiodothyronine (T₃)	Thyroid-Stimulating Hormone
Hyperthyroid	↑	↑	↓
Hypothyroid	↓	↓	↓
Sick euthyroid	→	↓	→
Pregnancy	↑	→	→

7. A

Studies have shown that mild to moderate hypothyroid patients do not require preoperative thyroid supplementation. Only patients with severe hypothyroidism are sensitive to the sedative effects of anesthetics. The coronary artery disease patient may have an attack of angina with increased preoperative thyroid supplementation. Low levels of thyroid disease are not associated with an increased need for ventilatory support postoperatively.

8. C

At 10 minutes, the radionuclide is seen in both the thyroid and parathyroid tissue. However, at 2 hours, it is confined to the right parathyroid gland. Thus, the appropriate operation is a right parathyroidectomy.

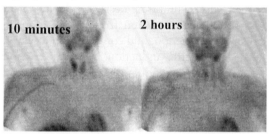

9. C

Adrenal insufficiency is the only choice that can result in *both* hypoglycemia and elevated blood ketones. The other choices can result in nonketotic hypoglycemia.

10. A

Adequate preoperative preparation for a patient with Graves' disease requires *both* potassium iodide and a beta-blocker. T₄ is contraindicated in Graves' disease, because T₄ levels are already elevated. Propylthiouracil requires a longer duration of treatment (~6 to 8 weeks). Iodine-131 treatment has poorer results compared with medical therapy. Medical treatment carries a high risk of relapse in 5 years (~30% to 40%).

Answers   Chapter 19

1. D

To minimize the risk of aspiration, American Society of Anesthesiologists' guidelines recommend patients to be NPO for 6 hours after a light meal and 8 hours after a fatty or fried meal before general anesthesia can be safely induced. Here, the patient is undergoing emergent surgery and the risks of delaying surgery outweigh the risks of possible aspiration. Therefore, the patient should be taken to surgery; however, rapid sequence induction should be performed to minimize the risk of aspiration.

2. D

The operating room is often kept cold for the comfort of surgeons and ancillary surgical staff, who perform operations in sterile gowns and under intense lights. As a result, patients' core temperature will often decrease due to heat loss through evaporation from exposed surgical sites, conduction, and convection. However, immediately after induction, the main reason for heat loss is vasodilation and redistribution of the blood supply to the periphery.

3. B

The endotracheal tube can be very uncomfortable and on emergence may cause the patient to gag and cough. This may interfere with the surgical closure and even lead to development of hematomas in the surgical field. To circumvent such an emergence, the trachea can be extubated while still under general anesthesia. However, deep extubation may lead to hypoventilation and airway obstruction; candidates for this procedure have to be selected carefully. The mask ventilation and intubation of the patient has to be easy before deep extubation can be considered. In addition, the patient cannot have any risk factors for aspiration or airway swelling.

4. B

Induction of general anesthesia can be challenging when the patient is hemodynamically unstable or has baseline cardiovascular dysfunction. Therefore, it is crucial for the anesthesiologist to be aware of the effects of different induction agents. In this case, the patient is hypotensive and may be actively bleeding. Taking time to normalize the blood pressure is not an option as that would delay the surgery and may worsen the hemodynamic state. Avoiding the use of an induction agent would result in suboptimal intubation conditions and possible injury to the patient's airway. Of the two suggested induction agents, etomidate results in fewer hemodynamic changes and may be tolerated by patients in shock.

5. C

The process of informed consent requires that the patient fully understands the risks and benefits of the anesthetic plan. For patients who do not have the mental capacity to do so, a health care proxy, or in an emergent setting, the next of kin, can make this decision. However, in order to determine if a patient has the mental capacity to consent, a formal psychiatric evaluation has to be completed. Here, the acuity of the patient's mental status change is unclear. The first step would be to obtain more information on whether this is the patient's baseline or if this is a new pathologic process. If this is a chronic condition, the assigned health care proxy should be contacted. Immediately canceling the case would not be the first step.

Answers   Chapter 20

1. A

Although the Mallampati score has a good negative predictive value, it has a very poor positive predictive value. There is no one scoring system or collection of risk variables that will *consistently* predict a difficult laryngoscopy.

2. D

According to the ASA fasting guidelines, the chart lists the relevant time intervals between food/liquid ingestion and an elective general anesthetic in normal patients.

Ingested Material	Minimum Fasting Period
Clear liquids	2 hours
Breast milk	4 hours
Infant formula	6 hours
Nonhuman milk	6 hours
Light meal	6 hours

From Practice guidelines for preoperative fasting and the use of pharmacologic agents to reduce the risk of pulmonary aspiration. Application to healthy patients undergoing elective procedures. *Anesthesiology.* 2011;114:495–511.

3. B
Injury to the recurrent laryngeal nerve results in paralysis of the abductor muscle of the vocal cords (posterior cricoarytenoid muscle). On laryngoscopy, the vocal cord is seen to remain in the median or paramedian position throughout the respiratory cycle. Sensory innervation above the vocal cords is via the internal laryngeal nerve. The cricothyroid muscle receives innervation from the external laryngeal nerve.

4. D
An uncooperative patient is a contraindication to awake fiber-optic intubation. Secretions if cleared by an antisialagogues or suction does not represent a contraindication.

5. A
A call for help is the highest priority in the "cannot ventilate, cannot intubate" clinical scenario. The remainder of the choices for this question follow the ASA difficult airway recommendations (Fig. 20-7 Box B).

6. B
The correct placement of the Macintosh 3 blade may stimulate the glossopharyngeal cranial nerve (the internal laryngeal nerve), which does not have major hemodynamic consequences. However, correct placement of the Miller 3 blade may stimulate the vagus nerve and will reflexively intensify the degree of bradycardia.

7. C
Of the choices given, the presence of a beard has the highest odds ratio for difficult mask ventilation (odds ratio [OR] >3), other than the history of snoring (OR >1), the others have an OR >2.

8. B
To have adequate denitrogenation, plus a safety factor for prolonged satisfactory oxyhemoglobin saturation, *both* a tight mask fit and FiO$_2$ are required. With room air, desaturation occurs within 2 minutes. In contrast, use of 100% oxygen increases the time to desaturation to approximately 8 minutes.

9. D
In an airway compromised by the presence of blood, key anatomic landmark structures may be hidden from view. The other choices may give rapid access to the airway without the necessity for direct visualization of anatomic structures.

10. C
Although lower intracuff pressures are preferred, up to 60 cm H$_2$O is acceptable. Adequate cuff inflation is not governed by volume.

Answers   *Chapter 21*

1. B
Unilateral phrenic nerve blockade is the side effect seen in highest frequency following interscalene block, although its incidence may be lowered further with lower concentrations or volumes. The other complications/side effects occur in much lower frequency.

2. D
Either supraclavicular, infraclavicular, or axillary blocks may be utilized. Bier block is not ideal it will require a tourniquet to be inflated

for the entire surgery duration, which may place the patient at risk for limb ischemia. Bupivacaine should NEVER be injected intravascularly. Interscalene block, typically utilized for upper arm/shoulder surgery, will likely miss the inferior brachial plexus blockade (ulnar sparing) needed for this operation.

3. A
The tibial and common peroneal nerves make up the sciatic nerve, which is the largest component of the sacral plexus. The other listed nerves

(femoral, obturator, lateral femoral cutaneous) are derived from the lumbar plexus.

4. C
The inversion response indicates that both the tibial and common peroneal nerve components

of the sciatic nerve are being stimulated. A dorsiflexion or eversion response indicates common peroneal stimulation, while plantar flexion indicates tibial stimulation.

Answers | Chapter 22

1. C
Due to gravity and a hydrostatic pressure gradient, the blood pressure will be less in structures above the site of blood pressure measurement.

2. B
Postoperative ulnar nerve neuropathy can result from pressure on the nerve (blood pressure cuff, inadequate padding) and from unknown factors such as inflammation. The ulnar nerve innervates the fourth and fifth fingers and does not run through the antecubital fossa.

3. D
The motor fibers in the ulnar nerve are primarily located in its middle. Injury to those fibers usually follows a significant ischemic or pressure insult, which also affects sensory nerve fibers. Recovery is prolonged and the nerve deficit may be permanent.

4. A
Brachial plexus injury is most commonly associated with sternotomy, shoulder surgery, and procedures performed in the prone or lateral position with one or both arms abducted.

5. B
Median nerve injury is common in men with well-developed biceps muscle and primarily results from stretching of the nerve when the

arm is fully extended. Median nerve injuries are less likely to rapidly resolve than injuries to the radial or ulnar nerves.

6. C
The lateral femoral cutaneous nerve innervates the lateral thigh and contains sensory fibers only.

7. A
If a patient develops a postoperative peripheral neuropathy with a sensory-only deficit, it is reasonable to watch the patient daily for 5 days. Many sensory deficits resolve within that time. If the deficit is prolonged, referral to the patient's primary physician or a neurologist is indicated.

8. D
When patients with thoracic outlet syndrome raise their arms above their heads, there is compression of vessels supplying the extremity and they report ischemic pain.

9. B
Male genitalia, ostomy stomas, and breast tissue can easily be compressed and damaged when patients are prone, despite the use of padded "rolls" that run from the chest to the pelvis. The femoral vessels are relatively well protected and are not easily injured.

Answers | Chapter 23

1. D
Respiratory compensation can normalize pH within minutes due to rapid changes in minute ventilation that swiftly alter the $PaCO_2$. In contrast,

metabolic compensation requires adjustment of plasma HCO_3^- levels that result from changes in renal tubular excretion and reabsorption, and occur over a much slower time frame.

2. B

The ABG indicates an uncompensated, acute respiratory acidosis. Elevated $PaCO_2$ levels can result from insufficient CO_2 removal (e.g., low tidal volume due to elevated intra-abdominal pressure associated with laparoscopy), excessive CO_2 production (e.g., hypermetabolism associated with hyperthyroidism), or rebreathing of CO_2 in a circle system (e.g., exhausted soda lime). In contrast, prolonged gastric suctioning removes gastric acid and can result in metabolic alkalosis.

3. B

Isotonic fluids are defined as those whose osmolarity is similar to serum (285 to 295 mOsm/L). As shown in Table 23-7, Ringer's lactate, Plasmalyte, and 0.9% normal saline have osmolarities in this approximate range, whereas the osmolarity of 25% albumin is 1,500 mOsm/L (hypertonic).

4. B

Crystalloids are inexpensive, nonallergenic, and do not inhibit coagulation. However, their administration results in tissue edema, leading to gut flora translocation, poor wound healing, impairment of alveolar gas exchange, limited intravascular volume expansion, and metabolic derangements. Conversely, colloids are expensive, allergenic, and linked to renal failure and coagulopathy.

5. A

Due to limited liver glycogen stores, young infants are at risk of hypoglycemia when oral intake is restricted and therefore should generally receive glucose (in the form of intravenous dextrose solutions) in the perioperative period until oral intake resumes.

6. D

The patient's maximal pulse pressure is 36 mm Hg and his minimal pulse pressure is 30 mm Hg. Using Equation 23-6, his PPV = $([36 - 30]/34) \times 100 = 18\%$. Based on this PPV (>12%), the patient is hypovolemic and would likely benefit from additional fluid or blood product resuscitation.

7. A

See Figure 23-5. Hyponatremia most commonly presents with concomitant hypotonic serum osmolarity, possible etiologies of which include syndrome of inappropriate antidiuretic hormone, primary polydipsia, and heart failure (depending on urine osmolarity, intravascular volume status, and extracellular volume status). However, in this case of isotonic hyponatremia, one possible etiology is hyperglycemia.

8. B

See Figure 23-6.

9. A

Because calcium in serum is largely bound to circulating albumin, low total calcium levels can reflect either hypocalcemia or hypoalbuminemia. Thus, in the presence of hypoalbuminemia, the ionized calcium level is a more accurate measure of body calcium homeostasis.

10. D

See step-wise approach to ABG interpretation in Table 23-6:

1. pH >7.45 → alkalemia is present
2. $PaCO_2$ <40 mm Hg → primary respiratory alkalosis is present
3. Not applicable
4. HCO_3^- is normal → no compensation is present, thus process is acute
5. ABG indicates an acute respiratory alkalosis, with the most likely cause being iatrogenic hyperventilation

Answers   Chapter 24

1. D
Whole blood is only indicated in rare circumstances (such as a war zone) where there is no ability to separate whole blood into components or to store those components. Hemorrhage from trauma can be effectively treated with PRBC and crystalloid fluids, with plasma given if there is evidence of a coagulopathy or factor deficiency.

2. A
In an otherwise healthy patient who is hemodynamically stable, there is no need to treat moderate anemia with a hemoglobin >7 g/dL. It is important to determine the cause of the anemia, but surgery need not be delayed to perform the evaluation.

3. C
Indications for FFP are treatment of dilutional coagulopathy, factor deficiency, and as a second-line agent for warfarin reversal. FFP should not be administered solely for volume replacement.

4. B
Bleeding during craniotomy or intraocular procedures is a serious complication. The threshold for platelet transfusion is more liberal at <100,000 per microliter. For patients having other major surgical procedures the threshold for platelet transfusion is <50,000 per microliter. Patients who are not bleeding will usually not incur spontaneous hemorrhage until the platelet count is <10,000 per microliter.

5. A
In an emergency, uncross-matched type O blood is best as a "universal donor" for patients of unknown blood type. While Rh-negative blood is preferred, particularly for women of childbearing age, administration of Rh-positive to men (particularly those who have never been transfused before) is associated with a low risk of a severe hemolytic reaction.

6. D
Unfortunately, there is no precise sign for diagnosis of AHTR in the anesthetized patient. Tachycardia and hypotension could be secondary to AHTR or hypovolemia from surgical hemorrhage. Bleeding could be due to surgery or due to AHTR-induced DIC.

7. B
Although transmission of hepatitis C and HIV are commonly discussed in the media, the incidence of transmitted hepatitis B is most prevalent due to a higher prevalence of the disease in the population and a longer window of time between infection and the ability to test blood for the virus. Bacterial contamination of banked blood is rare.

8. A
Although there are several alternatives to RBC transfusion, and each method has peculiar risks and benefits, overall blood salvage techniques have the lowest risk, lowest cost, and are most effective for general use.

9. C
TF and factor VIII are involved early in the coagulation pathway. Thrombin converts fibrinogen to fibrin. Factor XIII crosslinks and stabilizes the fibrin clot.

10. D
Aspirin is an irreversible inhibitor of cyclo-oxygenase, thereby preventing the synthesis of thromboxane, a major stimulant for platelet activation.

Answers   Chapter 25

1. B
According to the ASA position statement, MAC is a specific anesthesia service for a diagnostic or therapeutic procedure and does not describe the continuum of depth of sedation (2).

2. D
MAC includes all aspects of anesthetic care, including a preprocedure visit, intraprocedure care, and postprocedure recovery management (2). Patients scheduled for MAC should receive

a preoperative assessment similar to any other preoperative patient.

3. D
ASA standard monitoring, which includes continuous electrocardiography, pulse oximetry, noninvasive blood pressure and end-tidal carbon dioxide monitoring must be used for every anesthetic including MAC.

4. D
Context-sensitive half-time refers to the time it takes for the plasma concentration to decline by 50% after discontinuing an infusion. Option B describes the concept of effect-site equilibration.

5. C
Dexmedetomidine is a selective alpha2 agonist that can be used to provide sedation. It has no intrinsic amnestic properties.

6. C
Ketamine is a phencyclidine derivative that produces intense analgesia and amnesia. Its primary mechanism of action is as an NMDA receptor antagonist. It has minimal effect on respiration in contrast to other sedatives and opioids.

7. A
Opioids alone do not provide amnesia.

8. B
According to the ASA fasting guidelines for elective surgery, the fasting time for breast milk is 4 hours. The fasting time for clear liquid is 2 hours, and infant formula is 6 hours.

9. B
The Postanesthetic Discharge Scoring System (PADSS) has established parameters for evaluation for home readiness after ambulatory surgery (17). It includes assessment of vital signs relative to baseline, ability to ambulate, as well as level of nausea, pain and surgical bleeding. A score of 9 to 10 indicates patient is fit for discharge. A patient with uncontrolled nausea would not qualify for discharge using this scoring system.

10. D
All of the items listed are goals of an ambulatory anesthetic.

Answers | Chapter 26

1. D
Primary injury to neuronal structures occurs immediately at the time of traumatic injury, whereas secondary injury can occur in the immediate minutes to days following the injury. Secondary neuronal injury is largely caused by spinal cord ischemia and neuronal hypoxia that can result from systemic hypotension, inadequate local tissue perfusion, arterial hypoxemia, or local postinjury inflammatory responses including neuronal and interstitial edema.

2. C
Neurogenic shock results from the loss of sympathetic vascular tone (i.e., reduced systemic vascular resistance) to large portions of the arterial vascular system. Generally, spinal cord injuries at the level of T6 and higher that result in complete motor and sensory deficits below the level of injury will functionally denervate enough of the arterial vasculature to result in hypotension and neurogenic shock, whereas injuries below this level will not. Bradycardia may or may not be present depending on whether sympathetic innervation of the sinoatrial node of the heart is also affected.

3. B
Acute intraoperative changes in neurophysiologic monitoring of the spinal cord must be immediately communicated to the surgeon in the event that reversible surgical manipulations of the cord have occurred. Other steps should include repositioning the patient to maintain neutral spinal column alignment, correcting hypotension, metabolic abnormalities, anemia, and hypo- or hyperthermia, and minimizing volatile anesthetic agents (due to their dose-dependent negative impact on evoked potential signals).

4. D
The etiologies and risk factors for POVL are described in Table 26-6. Due to the significant morbidity of this complication and its incidence of up to 2% following spine surgery, explicit discussion of POVL should occur with the patient during the preanesthetic visit as well as with the surgeon prior to the procedure. Careful blood pressure monitoring and judicious use of crystalloid fluids should take place during the intraoperative period.

5. A
The presentation and management of VAE are described in Table 26-7. Due to accumulation of air in the right heart, VAE impedes venous return and pulmonary blood flow, leading to an abrupt decrease in expired carbon dioxide. VAE can be immediately treated by flooding the surgical field with irrigation fluid and lowering the surgical site to a level below the right heart (to prevent further entry of air into the venous circulation). Air can potentially be removed from the right heart by placing the patient in the left lateral decubitus position and by aspirating a central venous catheter placed at the junction of the superior vena cava and the right atrium.

6. C
In addition to the general benefits of regional anesthesia or analgesia, orthopedic surgery patients have a high incidence of perioperative deep venous thrombosis and are frequently required to begin extremity movement and rehabilitation therapy as soon as possible. Regional anesthesia may be advantageous in both instances. Sympathectomy due to regional blockade causes peripheral vasodilation.

7. B
Proximal upper extremity (shoulder and upper arm) surgery requires proximal brachial plexus blockade, most commonly achieved by the interscalene approach. The other blocks listed may insufficiently anesthetize branches of the C5 and C6 nerve roots supplying sensory innervation to the superior or lateral shoulder. Conversely, the interscalene block may spare sensory branches of C8 and T1 nerve roots and, therefore, is inadequate for some types of hand surgery.

8. B
Tourniquet inflation pressures must exceed systolic pressure to prevent blood flow to the surgical field. This is generally accomplished in the upper extremity with inflation pressure 100 mm Hg over systolic pressure and in the lower extremity with inflation pressure 150 mm Hg over systolic pressure. Because of additional soft tissue in the extremities of the morbidly obese, higher inflation pressures may be needed to effectively prevent arterial inflow. The maximal tourniquet inflation duration is not well defined. It should generally be limited to 2 hours, but may be used longer depending on the tourniquet location and surgical procedure.

9. A
Major criteria for fat embolism syndrome diagnosis include acute changes coincident with increases in intramedullary pressure at the surgical site, such as respiratory distress (hypoxia, pulmonary edema), neurologic impairment ranging from confusion or lethargy to seizures and coma, and petechia on the conjunctiva and upper trunk. Minor diagnostic criteria include fever, tachycardia, fat globules in sputum and urine, and decreased platelets and hematocrit. Initial treatment focuses on aggressive cardiovascular and pulmonary supportive therapy.

10. D
Anesthetic options for forefoot surgery are described in Table 26-10.

Answers | Chapter 27

1. B
The initial pressure is limited to this level to minimize the adverse hemodynamic and respiratory consequences.

2. C
Pneumoperitoneum induces a modest splanchnic hyperemia due to the vasodilating effects of the absorbed CO_2. In contrast, pneumoperitoneum

decreases renal blood flow, glomerular filtration rate and urine output by up to 50%. Cerebral blood flow increases during pneumoperitoneum due to an increase in $PaCO_2$.

3. D
A large intravascular CO_2 embolism should be suspected when sudden, severe hypotension is accompanied by a marked decrease in end-tidal CO_2 occurring during insufflation. A capnothorax can present with hypotension but end-tidal CO_2 should be elevated. A pneumothorax can present with both decrease blood pressure and decreased end-tidal CO_2, but is less likely than a CO_2 during insufflation.

4. C
Shoulder pain referred from the diaphragm is common after laparoscopy. Complete clearance of intra-abdominal CO_2 may require over one hour and during that time patients may experience severe shoulder pain referred from diaphragmatic irritation. The other answers are plausible but much less likely.

5. B
Severe hypothermia is a significant risk during laparoscopy because in addition to the usual mechanisms of heat loss during anesthesia (convection, conduction, radiation and evaporation), insufflation of cold CO_2 (at 23 degrees C) causes additional heat loss.

Answers | Chapter 28

1. C
Morbid obesity is defined as ≥ 40 kg/m^2. Patient C's height is 4 ft 8 in = 56 in = 56×0.0254, or 1.42 m. Weight is 180 lb = 180/2.2, or 81.82 kg. The BMI is $81.81/(1.42)^2$, or 40.44 kg/m^2.

2. A
Lower doses of succinylcholine, using LBW instead of TBW, will result in poor intubating conditions due to increased extracellular volume and increased activity of pseudo-cholinesterase activity in obese patients.

3. D
The head-down (Trendelenburg) position causes the highest degree of respiratory compromise, with a decrease in FRC and lung compliance, due in large part to the weight of the abdominal contents and elevation of the diaphragm.

4. B
Whereas a longer cuff may be necessary to encircle a large arm, in an obese patient the cuff should be wider, not more narrow, than normal to be accurate.

5. D
Placing the obese patient in a semisitting position with a ramp, achieved with towels, folded blankets under the patient's shoulders, or with a commercially available device, elevates the head and shoulders above the chest, with the goal of elevating the external auditory meatus to the level of the anterior chest wall.

6. B
In the absence of surgical complications or significant presurgical comorbidities, the goal should be to avoid tracheal intubation and mechanical ventilation. It is preferred to extubate the patient and institute measures to improve ventilation such as CPAP, opioid-sparing analgetic techniques, and use of the semisitting position.

7. A
Single induction doses of intravenous induction agents are short acting despite liver disease, because cardiac output is elevated and drug effect is terminated primarily by redistribution. The duration of action of continuous infusions may be prolonged due to deposition of drug in fat and delayed metabolism.

8. C
With reanastomosis of the hepatic vein and reperfusion of the new liver, rapid blood loss, academia, and embolism can cause severe cardiopulmonary instability. Vasopressors, inotropes, and pulmonary vasodilators are often necessary. Patients are also at risk of hypocalcemia due

to high-volume infusion of citrated blood and hyperkalemia because of underlying renal function, blood transfusion, splanchnic ischemia, and acidosis.

9. A
Nitrous oxide will diffuse into distended bowel, which can result in increased intraluminal pressure

and difficulty with abdominal closure or, in extreme situations, bowel ischemia.

10. D
Clear fluids (water, fat-free and protein-free liquids, pulp-free fruit juice, carbonated drinks, black tea, and black coffee) are emptied from the stomach within 2 hours of ingestion.

Answers | Chapter 29

1. B
Otitis media has a peak incidence at 1 year of age. This is due to a variety of factors in this age group, including that the eustachian tube drains poorly due to its small cross-sectional area and its floppy cartilaginous walls. Additionally, its short length increases exposure of the middle ear to the mucous and bacteria of the nasopharynx.

2. D
The short length of performing myringotomy and ear tube placement and its noninvasive nature allow use of inhaled anesthetics alone. Inhalation induction and maintenance using a face mask is frequently sufficient. Myringotomy and ear tube placement requires general anesthesia to provide the surgeon with the absolute immobility required for working under a microscope. These procedures are most frequently performed without intravenous access or endotracheal intubation.

3. D
Epiglottitis is a life-threatening condition typically caused by a bacterial infection. It often affects the epiglottis, aryepiglottic folds, arytenoids, and uvula. Clinical signs include stridor, drooling, odynophagia, outright avoidance of food and drink, and high fever.

4. B
A sudden decrease in heart rate during ophthalmologic procedures is usually caused by the oculocardiac reflex. Treatment begins with cessation of any stimuli. Atropine may be required and, in rare situations, epinephrine, if the bradycardia progresses to cardiac arrest.

5. B
Sulfur hexafluoride is used in retinal detachment repair to replace the volume of vitreous humor lost during surgery. Because nitrous oxide is much more soluble than nitrogen, it can enter the bubble quicker than nitrogen can exit, causing expansion of the gas bubble, increasing the IOP, and potentially causing retinal ischemia.

Answers | Chapter 30

1. C
The cervical spinal cord is supplied by the posterior Circle of Willis (vertebral arteries). The aortic arch, via the internal carotid arteries, supplies the anterior Circle of Willis. The artery of Adamkiewicz supplies the thoracolumbar spinal cord anteriorly, while the external carotid arteries supply the face.

2. B
Cerebral perfusion pressure is the difference between mean arterial pressure and intracranial

pressure or central venous pressure, whichever is higher. Cerebral blood flow equals cerebral perfusion pressure divided by cerebrovascular resistance.

3. D
Autoregulation in the brain generally refers to the control of cerebral blood flow. Cerebral blood flow remains constant between a range of cerebral perfusion pressures (or mean arterial pressures).

4. A
Cerebral blood flow is controlled by $PaCO_2$, PaO_2, MAP, and $CMRO_2$. pH in the CNS does not directly influence cerebral blood flow, except as it relates to changes in $PaCO_2$.

5. D
The administration of mannitol, hyperventilation, a total intravenous anesthetic technique, and elevation of the head of the bed will all affect intracranial pressure by lowering it. The administration of opioids *in a ventilated patient* will have no appreciable effect on intracranial pressure.

6. E
Muscle relaxants may improve SSEPs and EEG (by removing EMG artifact), will have no appreciable effect on BAEPs and VEPs, and may ablate EMG activity at moderate-to-high doses.

7. E
Focal cerebral ischemia may be ameliorated by barbiturates. In humans, global cerebral ischemia has not been definitively shown to be improved by any modality of treatment or prophylaxis.

8. B
In order to avoid secondary injury to the brain, acute traumatic brain injury should be treated very carefully. Hypotension and hypoxia should be avoided at all costs, GCS < 8 warrants intubation, and mannitol should be given to lessen intracranial pressure. There is a role for hyperventilation in the first 6 hours, but hyperventilation should be avoided after this period as its effect will wane after this time and it may actually contribute to cerebral ischemia.

9. A
Acute cervical spine injury may lead to bradycardia, respiratory impairment, hypotension, and flaccid paralysis (because of effects on the cardioaccelerator fibers, which originate from the high thoracic spinal cord, and the phrenic nerve, which originates from C3-C5). *Hypothermia* may result from such an injury, due to dysregulation of temperature control mechanisms.

Answers | Chapter 31

1. B
During pregnancy, blood volume increases by 40% to approximately 100 mL/kg; plasma volume increases by 30% to 50% and red blood cell volume by 20% to 30%, causing a physiologic anemia of pregnancy. Red blood cell production and circulating half-life are normal during pregnancy. Pregnant women may be iron deficient, but this condition accentuates the physiologic anemia of pregnancy (which includes red blood cells of normal size).

2. D
Pregnant women develop mucosal edema and capillary engorgement, creating mechanical obstruction to the instruments used for mask ventilation and tracheal intubation. Pregnancy does not alter neck range of motion. Whether pregnant women have dyspnea in the supine position is immaterial as they would be paralyzed at the time of the attempts to mask ventilate or intubate. Finally, although pregnant women's Mallampati scores tend to increase over the course of gestation, the score is a measure designed to predict difficult intubation, and it does not cause difficult intubation.

3. A
All the listed transport mechanisms are active in the placental–fetal circulatory interface. Oxygen and carbon dioxide exchange occurs via simple diffusion; higher maternal PaO_2 favors diffusion to the fetus, and fetal carbon dioxide is higher than maternal carbon dioxide, favoring diffusion back to the mother.

4. C
Most anesthetic drugs cross the placenta, with the exception of paralyzing agents (such as succinyl choline) and glycopyrrolate. Heparin and insulin also do not cross the placenta. Transient fetal or neonatal depression can be seen after administration of induction agents (such as propofol), anesthetic gases (such as

sevoflurane), opioids (such as fentanyl), and benzodiazepines.

5. B
Pain during the first stage of labor, which commences with the beginning of regular contractions and cervical dilation and ends at complete cervical dilation, is transmitted via visceral afferent fibers entering the spinal cord from T10-L1. Therefore, these are the only afferent fibers that are targeted to provide analgesia during the first stage of labor.

6. A
Avoiding excessive motor blockade, while still providing adequate analgesia, is ideal in labor. This goal is commonly accomplished by administering low-concentration (0.0625% to 0.125% bupivacaine), high-volume, patient-controlled epidural anesthesia, with small amounts of opioid in the solutions. Adding epinephrine does not influence motor blockade.

The administration of epidural local anesthetics may cause sufficient motor blockade so as to prevent ambulation. However, ambulation does not prevent this effect of epidural local anesthetic administration. Finally, patient-controlled epidural anesthesia causes less motor blockade than intermittent boluses delivered by anesthesia providers.

7. C
Fetal heart rate (FHR) tracing interpretation is very sensitive but not very specific. Therefore, a normal FHR and variability without decelerations almost always indicate a nonacidotic fetus, but a healthy fetus may have FHR abnormalities not due to acidosis or distress. Fetal tachycardia may be due to hypoxemia but may also result from maternal fever or infection or maternally administered drugs (β agonists in particular). Many maternally administered drugs, including magnesium and opioids, may decrease FHR variability.

Answers   Chapter 32

1. B
Because properly applied MILS limits both flexion and extension of the cervical spine and atlanto-occipital joint, laryngoscopic view of the vocal cords may be restricted and increase the difficulty of tracheal intubation.

2. B
The neurologic examination translates into a Glasgow coma scale motor score of 4, a verbal score of 2, and an eye score of 2, for a total Glasgow coma scale score of 8 (see Fig. 32-2).

3. D
The "Emergency and Trauma Anesthesia Checklist" can be of particular value in preparing to anesthetize a critically ill patient on short notice or in the middle of the night by providing a specific list of trauma-specific equipment and procedures that should be available (see Fig. 32-1).

4. A
Hypotensive resuscitation temporarily targets a lower-than-normal blood pressure until major hemorrhage is controlled and is more likely to

benefit patients with penetrating trauma due to the presence of anatomically distinct and reparable injuries. It should not be attempted in patients with TBI due to the risk of secondary neurologic injury and neuronal ischemia.

5. A
The goal of 1:1:1 volume resuscitation is to maintain proper oxygen carrying capacity (i.e., red cell mass) and normal coagulation function and to avoid the anemia and dilutional coagulopathy that can occur with high-volume isotonic crystalloid resuscitation. Studies in both military and civilian populations suggest that this resuscitation strategy improves survival compared with high-volume crystalloid resuscitation.

6. B
Hyperkalemia can occur when potassium is released from lysed red blood cells, such as following transfusion in small children of old units of packed red blood cells (that may have undergone lysis during prolonged storage) or acute, immune-mediated hemolysis. Succinylcholine can precipitate hyperkalemia in patients with large

burn injuries >48 hours old because of quantitative and qualitative changes in neuromuscular acetylcholine receptors that accompany burn injuries.

7. C
Pelvic fractures are accompanied by significant internal hemorrhage—2 to 3 L (see Table 32-5)—due to bleeding from the large bone fragments, as well as injury to nearby retroperitoneal veins. Because approximately half the patient's blood volume could be lost into the pelvis, crystalloid resuscitation to euvolemia would be expected to dilute his remaining red cell mass to a hematocrit approximately 50% below his baseline.

8. C
The Parkland formula (Table 32-6) calculates isotonic fluid resuscitation for the first 24 hours after injury as 4.0 mL × body weight (kg) × %TBSA burn. Thus, the total 24-hour resuscitation volume would be (4 × 21 × 29) = 2,436 mL. Since half of this volume is to be administered in the first 8 hours, her 8-hour fluid volume would be (2,436/2) = 1,218 mL.

9. C
With a history of smoke inhalation in an enclosed space and carbonaceous sputum, significant inhalation injury is likely, including carbon monoxide poisoning. Carbon monoxide poisoning would be reflected in an elevated carboxyhemoglobin and a low oxyhemoglobin saturation, both measured by arterial blood co-oximetry in the laboratory. Peripheral pulse oximetry is typically normal because this device only measures the relative values of oxyhemoglobin and deoxyhemoglobin, and does not measure carboxyhemoglobin. Arterial PO_2 would be normal because carboxyhemoglobin does not affect the partial pressure of oxygen dissolved in the plasma.

10. B
Because emergency medical care resources are limited and insufficient to treat all victims of mass casualty incidents, those with the most severe injuries and near death (e.g., cardiac arrest) are managed expectantly. Instead, the highest priority for care is given to those who are in need of emergent surgery to save life, limb, or eyesight.

Answers | Chapter 33

1. C
According to the American Society of Anesthesiologists' fasting guidelines, clear liquids can be given up to 2 hours prior to surgery, breast milk up to 4 hours, formula up to 6 hours, and solid food up to 8 hours.

2. C
The only pediatric indication for succinylcholine, according to the package insert is: "It is recommended that succinylcholine chloride use in children be restricted to emergency intubation or instances where immediate securing of the airway is necessary." Many clinicians administer rocuronium in this situation but modify the dose. Preceding the administration of succinylcholine with a neuromuscular blocker may add complications.

3. B
Use of the 4-2-1 fluid administration formula yields the following answer: fasting requirements (2 hr NPO) = (2)(4 mL/kg × 10 kg) = 80 mL + maintenance fluids for hour 1 (4 mL/kg × 10 kg) = 40 mL. Of the total 120 mL, 50% of the fasting deficit is replaced in first hour, followed by 25% of the deficit replaced in hour 2, and hour 3 to complete the entire deficit.

4. B
The greatest risk for postoperative apnea is prematurity. The other choices do not present as high a risk.

5. D
In comparison to the adult, the vocal cords of the neonate slant caudally for their attachment to the arytenoids.

6. C
Oxygen consumption (mL/kg/min) is three times greater in the neonate (9 cc mL/kg/min) versus the adult (3 mL/kg/min).

7. A
The classic electrolyte picture in the setting of pyloric stenosis is hyponatremic, hypokalemic, hypochloremic metabolic alkalosis with compensatory respiratory acidosis.

8. B
Line A represents the fetal arterial blood gases (ABG) at the end of labor; line C is the ABG term newborn at 1 hour, and line D is the ABG at 1 week.

9. D
Facemask fit is not a primary design goal of the pediatric (Mapleson) circuits. Decreased

resistance to gas flow, maintenance of body temperature, and minimal dead space volume are the major aims.

10. D
The infant has a much higher oxygen consumption than the adult. The variables are within a similar range for infants and adults. See Table 33-2.

Answers   Chapter 34

1. A
The calculation is made by the formula: postoperative FEV_1 = preoperative FEV_1 × (1 − resected segments/total lung segments). The right upper lobe contains 6 of the 42 total lung segments and thus 60% × (1 − 6/42) = 51%.

2. B
Chronic obstructive pulmonary disease is the comorbidity most commonly established preoperatively. Many patients have the other comorbidities listed, especially occult coronary artery disease, but they are not established diagnoses.

3. D
By increasing ventilation to the dependent lung, one-lung ventilation matches ventilation with the majority of perfusion, which goes to the dependent lung due to the effects of gravity.

4. D
Although all the maneuvers listed may help resolve hypoxia, positioning problems with double-lumen endobronchial tubes and bronchial

blockers are so common that their positioning should be rechecked whenever unexplained changes in saturation or ventilation occur.

5. C
Endobronchial blockers are much less stable than double-lumen endobronchial tubes, making protection from the spread of infection less reliable. Both right- and left-sided endobronchial tubes would be better choices, but the left-sided tube is the best choice because the left main stem bronchus is longer than the right main stem, making obstruction of the upper lobe bronchus less likely.

6. D
Profuse bleeding during mediastinoscopy results from injury to the great vessels of the upper thorax, including the innominate vein and superior vena cava. Fluids administered through the upper extremities or internal jugular vein may not reach the heart and could impede the efforts to repair the site of injury.

Answers   Chapter 35

1. A
In its calculation, systolic wall stress incorporates the size of the ventricle (preload) and the systolic blood pressure. Systemic vascular resistance may or may not correlate with myocardial oxygen consumption, but it does not take into account the size of the ventricle or blood pressure.

2. C
Approximately 1% to 2% of the population in the United States have bicuspid aortic valves, a

special risk factor for early development of aortic stenosis.

3. A
A type A dissection involves the ascending aorta. It may cause disruption of blood flow to the coronaries or the arch vessels, or it can rupture into the pericardium, causing cardiac tamponade. The mortality without surgical correction increases exponentially by the hour. Type B dissections can be managed medically

in most patients. There are no type C or D dissections.

4. D
The cannula for delivery of retrograde cardioplegia is placed through the right atrium and into the coronary sinus. Cardioplegia solution is infused via this cannula and travels retrograde through the coronary circulation. Antegrade cardioplegia is administered through the aortic root.

5. C
A level >400 seconds prevents activation of the clotting cascade and clot formation in the CPB machine due to the exposure of blood to CPB circuitry.

6. E
Outcome studies have not demonstrated the optimal anesthetic agent for patients undergoing cardiac surgery.

Answers Chapter 36

1. A
In response to the injury, an inflammatory cascade ensues, causing the subendothelial space to be filled with atherogenic lipoproteins and macrophages, which form foam cells.

2. C
Forty-three percent of men and 34% of women older than 65 years of age have >25% carotid stenosis due to atherosclerosis, and stroke remains the leading cause of disability and the third leading cause of death in the United States.

3. D
If a coronary stent is placed, elective surgery should be delayed: for bare metal stents, a minimum of 6 weeks of DAPT; and for drug-eluting stents, 12 months (or longer) of DAPT.

4. C
The American Heart Association defines carotid endarterectomy as an intermediate-risk procedure, with the possibility of cardiac death or nonfatal MI <5%.

5. A
Persistent severe postoperative hypertension increases the risk of cerebral hyperperfusion syndrome, characterized by headaches, seizures, and focal neurologic signs. Although hypertension is very common after carotid endarterectomy, it is not a sign of hyperperfusion syndrome.

6. C
The annual risk of aneurysmal rupture is directly related to its diameter: 1% for aneurysms measuring <4.0 cm, 2% for aneurysms 4.0 to 4.9 cm, and 20% for aneurysms >5.0 cm.

Answers Chapter 37

1. B
Tolerance is the phenomenon of decreased effect of a given amount of medication. It usually occurs after prolonged administration of the drug. *Dependence* is the physiologic condition of withdrawal symptoms when an opioid is discontinued. *Addiction* is a disease marked by altered behavior to seek the desired substance despite negative consequences. *Pseudo-addiction* is aberrant drug-seeking behavior due to undertreatment of pain.

2. C
Acetaminophen is a centrally acting COX inhibitor with minimal peripheral action. It causes analgesia and antipyrexia but has no anti-inflammatory effect. Ibuprofen, naproxen, and ketorolac are all NSAIDs, which work by inhibiting cyclooxygenase enzymes, exerting anti-inflammatory, antipyretic, and analgesic effects. NSAIDs are effective at reducing postoperative pain and opioid consumption and are commonly used in both acute and chronic pain. Side effects

include platelet dysfunction, nephrotoxicity, and gastric ulcers.

3. A

Chronic nerve damage is associated with spontaneous ectopic firing of neurons and changes in sodium and calcium channel expression. Anticonvulsants reduce ectopic signals by blocking sodium or calcium channels. Thus, anticonvulsants may be useful in treating neuropathic pain. Neuropathic pain is not caused by seizures, nor does chronic peripheral nerve damage cause seizures.

4. C

Programmable variables include starting bolus, demand dose and interval, basal infusion rate, and 1- or 4-hour limit. The demand dose should be a fraction of a usual therapeutic dose. The dosing interval should be after the medication effect begins and before it starts to wane to allow for cumulative effect. A basal infusion may be employed in a patient on long-term opioid therapy but should not be used in the opioid naïve. The 1- and 4-hour limits may be used to limit overall dosage, but care must be taken not to limit so severely that the patient uses all the allowable boluses in the first portion of the time interval and is without analgesia for the remainder.

5. B

As a general rule, the perioperative period is not a time to wean opioid usage. Clinical observations show that opioid requirements are approximately doubled from baseline in the postoperative period. The patient's long-acting opioid should be continued unchanged. If fasting status prohibits dosing of oral medication, the equianalgesic amount should be

administered as the baseline infusion in a PCA. The bolus dose should be set 25% to 50% higher than for an opioid-naïve individual. Regional and epidural analgesia is helpful in reducing overall opioid dosage, although care should be taken not to administer opioids in more than one route. To avoid cumulative effect, epidural infusions often consist of local anesthetic only, paired with intravenous opioid PCA. Ketamine, NSAIDs, antiepileptics, acetaminophen, and antidepressants can assist with pain control and limit opioids as well. Medications should be weaned to baseline postoperatively.

6. C

Epidural steroid injections are most effective in patients with acute radiculitis and less effective for management of chronic symptoms and nonradicular pain. Surgery does not appear to produce better long-term outcomes for radiculitis than a more conservative approach.

7. A

The likelihood of developing postherpetic neuralgia is reduced by prompt administration of antiviral drugs such as acyclovir, famciclovir, and valacyclovir. There are conflicting data regarding the use of epidural steroid injections as prophylaxis against PHN, but they may be considered among high-risk individuals within 2 to 4 weeks of the onset of the rash.

8. D

Table 37-5 gives the Budapest criteria for diagnosis of CRPS. The fourth criteria is that there is no other diagnosis that better explains the signs and symptoms. Imaging studies are not usually helpful in the diagnosis of CRPS. Psychiatrists may help with therapy but are not required for diagnosis.

Answers | Chapter 38

1. A

Significant adverse events in NORA are rare, however, the number of deaths associated with NORA is higher than with operating room anesthesia. Complications related to the airway and respiratory system, such as airway obstruction and respiratory depression as a result of

oversedation, are the most common complications associated with NORA. This complication is particularly relevant in patients with obstructive sleep apnea who are more prone to airway and respiratory complications during and after anesthesia and sedation.

2. C

Before entering the vicinity of the magnet, patients and staff need to complete a rigorous checklist to ensure that they are carrying no ferrometallic objects. Ferromagnetic equipment such as intravenous poles, gas cylinders, laryngoscopes, and pens become potentially lethal projectiles if brought too close to the magnetic field. Patient monitors, ventilators, and electrical infusion pumps may malfunction in proximity to the scanner, and magnet-safe technology is available. In the case of an emergency, resuscitation attempts should take place outside the scanner because equipment such as laryngoscopes and cardiac defibrillators cannot be taken close to the magnet.

3. D

Light general anesthesia with muscle relaxation, usually provided with the short-acting muscle relaxant succinylcholine, is used to mitigate the unpleasant effects of a generalized seizure. The anesthesiologist should be aware of the patient's medication regimes because drug interactions between anesthetic agents and psychotropic medications, particularly monoamine oxidase inhibitors, may occur. Skillful airway management using bag and mask ventilation is usually sufficient to maintain oxygenation during anesthesia for ECT.

4. A

MRI, like CT, is painless and does not require sedation or anesthesia. However, the scanning sequences are considerably longer than for CT, ≥ 30 minutes, and younger children as well as adults with neurologic or psychological disorders, including claustrophobia, often require sedation or anesthesia. Approximately 30% of adults report experiencing anxiety during MRI scans.

Answers Chapter 39

1. C

Treatment of severe pain with an opioid should be an immediate priority, followed by an assessment to determine the cause of the pain.

2. C

The patient's BP was only 20% lower than his preoperative value. He was awake and alert. Vasopressors would have short action. The most likely cause for moderate hypotension is hypovolemia. Laboratory studies can be drawn after initiation of fluid therapy.

3. A

Overinflation of a BP cuff has no effect. An elevated transducer will yield erroneous low BP. Hypothermia does not cause an artifact in the absence of shivering.

4. D

The most likely cause of stridor in this circumstance is laryngospasm. Administration of an inhaled bronchodilator at this point would be inappropriate.

5. D

Collapse of small airways is most likely following procedures in the abdomen associated with organ retraction or pneumoperitoneum.

6. A

Administration of oxygen may slightly elevate PaO_2 but will not help to expand collapsed airways and increase functional residual capacity.

7. B

Fentanyl is an opioid. Opioids are known to cause nausea and vomiting.

8. C

Blood is cleared by mucociliary transport. Balanced salt solution is harmless if aspirated. Infected drainage may contribute to pneumonia, but it is the bronchospasm, atelectasis, and chemical pneumonitis associated with material of low pH that is most damaging.

9. A

Renal dysfunction after common anesthetic and surgical procedures is rare.

10. A

Studies have shown that keeping a patient at bedrest does not reduce the incidence or severity of postdural puncture headache.

Answers   Chapter 40

1. D

The four formal principles of medical ethics are patient autonomy, beneficence, nonmaleficence, and justice, and they provide a structure for case discussions and application to medical ethics decision making.

2. B

The medical ethical principle of justice has components of distribution and retribution. Distributive justice addresses aspects of providing access to equitable and transparent care within the confines of limited health care resources (e.g., triage). Retributive justice addresses retaliation or punishment for certain actions and is largely applicable to disciplinary and legal reviews. Making unilateral decisions on behalf of patients without their input is a form of paternalism. Providing the highest level of care typifies the ethical principle of beneficence, whereas *primum non nocere* typifies that of nonmaleficence.

3. D

As shown in Table 40-1, the general structure of the crew resource management paradigm in the operating room is focused on team communication and leadership, workload management, structured decision making, and stress management. One key tenet is that any team member—regardless of their position in the chain of command—is free and encouraged to respectfully question issues related to patient safety.

4. B

When clearly documented in the medical record, the directive of a mentally competent, adult Jehovah's Witness to not receive intraoperative blood products is binding, even after the patient loses competence or capacity under general anesthesia. The anesthesiologist should explicitly confirm these directives prior to surgery and then agree to follow the directives. If the anesthesiologist has personal or religious objections to carrying out such directives, he or she should arrange for a colleague to provide such care.

5. D

The purpose of the National Practitioner Data Bank is to support professional peer review by requiring hospitals (patient care privileges), state licensing boards (licensure actions), professional societies (restrictions on membership), and other health care entities (malpractice claims) to report such adverse actions. Such data can then be released (under strict control) for future physician credentialing and privileging purposes.

6. D

Examples of advance directives include living wills and health care proxies, durable powers of attorney, general do-not-resuscitate requests, or the specific documentation of preferences for interventions such as prolonged mechanical ventilation, artificial nutrition and hydration, or dialysis in the event of severe incapacitating injury.

7. A

All states have trial courts where civil disputes such as medical malpractice are filed and litigated, up to and including the appeals process. However, when there is diversity of state citizenship among parties, if a federal question (e.g., violation of a constitutional right) is at stake, or if care occurred in a federally funded health care facility, the disputes (and possible appeals) will be litigated in federal court. Medical malpractice lawsuits are initiated by physical delivery of the summons, claim form, or complaint to the defendant physician, who must them immediately inform his or her insurance carrier due to the limited time to respond to the complaint (i.e., statutory time limit).

8. C

To meet their dual obligations to defend and to indemnify, insurance carriers (not the defendant physician) will typically retain experienced defense council and also pay the amount of a settlement or judgment on a covered claim (within set policy limits). Occurrence policies cover events even if the claim is filed after discontinuation or expiration of the policy. In contrast, claims-made policies only cover events that both occur and are claimed during the life of the policy; thus, a "tail" policy is generally required for such policies.

9. B

Simple power of attorney is in effect only as long as the patient also has the capacity to make decisions but becomes void when a patient loses that capacity. In contrast, a durable power of attorney retains its effect after the patient loses decision-making capacity. Thus, only someone with legal and documented durable power of attorney specifically for health care decisions can make such decisions on behalf of the patient while the patient is under general anesthesia.

10. D

The models and strategies noted above can all be used for quality improvement purposes by providing structures to link clinical outcomes with quality-of-care improvements. Key factors in each approach can include data collection, error identification, clinical outcomes, patient satisfaction, process measures, and analysis.

Answers | Chapter 41

1. D

See Table 41-1.

2. A

The RASS specifically assesses agitation and delirium, in contrast to the BPS and CPOT that assess pain. The SAT is not an assessment tool, but rather a technique used to intermittently assess baseline neurologic function in patients receiving pharmacologic sedatives.

3. B

Spontaneous ventilation with pressure support ventilation, on a T-piece, or with continuous positive airway pressure can all be used during an SBT, with no technique yet proven to be superior. Lung protective ventilation (i.e., low tidal volume, high respiratory rate) is performed in settings of ARDS and is associated with reduced mortality compared with ventilation strategies using high tidal volumes.

4. D

Using Table 41-3, the patient receives the following points: age 66 (2 points), morbidly obese (1 point), previous MI (1 point), arthroscopic surgery (2 points). This total of 6 points puts him in the high-risk category.

5. B

It is generally agreed that high-risk patients without contraindications should receive prophylaxis with low molecular-weight heparin. Mechanical devices are generally used in patients with contraindications to pharmacologic anticoagulation.

6. C

Gastric (prepyloric) feeding tube positioning is acceptable in most cases unless there is evidence of gastric feeding intolerance.

7. A

Although tight control of serum glucose (80 to 110 mg/dL) has been proposed to minimize morbidity associated with hyperglycemia, evidence suggests that such tight control carries a significant risk of hypoglycemia and possible increased mortality.

8. B

In the absence of ongoing blood loss, acute myocardial infarction, unstable angina, or possibly acute neurologic injury, routine red blood cell transfusion of critically ill patients is not necessary—and may be harmful—unless the Hb concentration is <7 g/dL.

9. D
See Table 41-5.

10. C
Initial treatment of septic shock generally involves administering isotonic crystalloid solutions to restore circulating volume and increasing systemic vascular resistance, preferably with norepinephrine. Red blood cell transfusion is only indicated if the Hb is <7 g/dL. Alternative vasopressors to norepinephrine include epinephrine or vasopressin, but generally not phenylephrine or dopamine. Exogenous steroids are controversial and generally indicated only for refractory hypotension, despite adequate volume resuscitation and vasopressor therapy.

Answers | Chapter 42

1. A
When the tumor involves the lateral wall, it is near the obturator nerve where electrocautery can stimulate the nerve and induce the thigh muscles to contract violently, potentially resulting in bladder rupture.

2. B
The formula for this calculation is:

$$\text{Volume Absorbed} = \frac{\text{Preoperative Serum Na}^+}{\text{Postoperative Serum Na}^+} \times \text{ECF} - \text{ECF}$$

Thus, $(80 \times 0.25) = 20$ liters $= \text{ECF}$, and $(140/120) \times 20 = 23.33 - 20 = 3.33$ liters absorbed.

3. C
The maximum rate should not exceed 12 mEq/liter in a 25 hour period. Faster correction has been associated with pontine myelinolysis.

4. C
The earliest signs of the transurethral resection of the prostate (TURP) syndrome include irritability, restlessness, nausea, shortness of breath, dizziness, and headache. These signs and symptoms can be reported to the anesthesiologist by a conscious patient under regional anesthesia. They are concealed by general anesthesia. Postoperative mortality, myocardial infraction, and transfusion rates are not different between regional and general anesthesia.

5. D
In 5% to 10% of right-sided renal cell carcinomas, the tumor extends into the renal vein, the inferior vena cava, and right atrium.

Answers | Chapter 43

1. C
Typical "household" electrical supply is AC. The potential difference of the live conductor oscillates in a sinusoidal manner at ±170 V around the neutral conductor, but is nominally 120 V. The current therefore changes direction at a rate of 60 Hz (cycles per second).

2. A
No system is absolutely foolproof; but, the best system is one that employs an isolation transformer that allows power to be supplied to the OR, without the need for a direct wire connection. The system is even more foolproof when combined with a line isolation monitor.

3. D
A GFCI senses current flow in the ground wire of equipment plugged into it. Eliminating the ground connection by use of a two-pin adapter renders the GFCI inoperative. If the equipment malfunctions (e.g., metal casing becomes "live"), the GFCI will cut off power to the outlet and a red light will appear. All items of equipment plugged into outlets controlled by the GFCI will also be turned off. No alarm will sound.

4. B
The isolation transformer "isolates" the electrical power in the OR by inducing a magnetic field across two physically separated wire coils. The

output from the secondary coil has a potential difference of 120 V but neither lead is grounded (at 0 V). If a person touches a malfunctioning piece of equipment, one wire from the outlet becomes grounded, the LIM will alarm, power will continue to the equipment, and the person will not receive a shock.

5. D

If the LIM alarms, it is not an emergency. Electrical power will continue to be supplied, but the safety feature of the isolation circuit has been bypassed. Each electrical device should sequentially be unplugged until the alarm stops. The faulty piece of equipment must then be removed or replaced. If it is an essential piece of equipment, it is acceptable to continue and complete the surgical procedure.

6. C

A dispersive electrode is only required for monopolar electrosurgical instruments. The current frequency of an ESU is very high and can safely pass through the heart without risk of fibrillation. The dispersive plate, although commonly referred to as a "ground" plate, is not connected to ground. It is safe to use an ESU when patients have an AICD, but a magnet must be placed over it or the AICD must be reprogrammed prior to surgery to prevent the AICD from misinterpreting the ESU as ventricular fibrillation.

7. B

Carbon dioxide does not support combustion so that use of an ESU intraperitoneally is safe. Nitrous oxide supports combustion so it should not be administered if the ESU is to be used at the time of tracheal incision. Oxygen should be diluted with air or nitrogen. Only "laser safe" endotracheal tubes may be used during laser surgery in proximity to the airway. Oxygen administered via a plastic face mask can contribute to a devastating fire in the event that it is exposed to an ESU or ignited drapes. Administer only enough oxygen to keep the oxygen saturation as measured by pulse oximetry at a safe level.

Answers | Chapter 44

1. B

The MBI is considering the gold standard for assessing burnout and assesses three psychological characteristics. Substance use is not a component of the tool.

2. C

FMLA attempts to protect work–life balance by ensuring covered employees protected leave during times of family need, such as family illness, military leave, personal illness, pregnancy, and adoption. ADA and ADAAA clarify the meaning of disability and prohibit discrimination on the basis of disability. HIPAA protects health insurance coverage for workers and their families when they lose or change jobs and also provides national standards for electronic health care transactions and protection of personal identifiers.

3. B

Despite expanded treatment and support programs for anesthesiology trainees during this time period, the incidence of relapse does not appear to have declined in this particular population. There does seem to be some improvements made for established anesthesiologists.

4. D

Neither CME or MOCA performance have been clearly linked to improved knowledge retention or patient care, and neurocognitive testing can have both low positive predictive value and high potential for psychological stress from false positive results.

5. C

MBSR is distinct from other common approaches to stress reduction, including proper nutrition, physical fitness, proper rest, and fiscal responsibility.

...put from the secondary coil has a potential difference of 120 V but neither lead is grounded (Fig. 11A-7). If a person touches a malfunctioning piece of equipment, one wire from the outlet becomes grounded, the LIM will alarm, power will continue to the equipment, and the person will not receive a shock.

5. D
If the LIM alarms, it is not an emergency. Electrical power will continue to be supplied, but the safety feature of the isolation circuit has been bypassed. Each electrical device should sequentially be unplugged until the alarm stops. The faulty piece of equipment must then be removed or replaced. If it is an essential piece of equipment, it is acceptable to continue and complete the surgical procedure.

6. C
A dispersive electrode is only required for monopolar electrosurgical instrument. The current frequency of an ESU is very high and can safely pass through the heart without...

1. B
The MBI is considering the gold standard for assessing burnout and assesses three psychological characteristics. Substance use is not a component of the tool.

2. C
FMLA attempts to protect work–life balance by ensuring covered employees protected leave during times of family need, such as family illness, military leave, personal illness, pregnancy, and adoption. ADA and ADAAA clarify the meaning of disability and prohibit discrimination on the basis of disability. HIPAA protects health insurance coverage for workers and their families when they lose or change jobs and also provides national standards for electronic health care transactions and protection of personal identifiers.

3. B
Despite expanded treatment and support programs for anesthesiology trainees during this...

Index

Note: Page number followed by f and t indicates figure and table respectively.